CW00693113

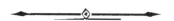

ISBN 978-0-265-96945-8
PIBN 10917218

MINNESOTA MEDICINE

Journal of the Minnesota State Medical Association, Southern Minnesota Medical Association, Northern Minnesota Medical Association, Minnesota Academy of Medicine, and Minneapolis Surgical Society

Owned and Published by
The Minnesota State Medical Association
Under the Direction of Its

EDITING AND PUBLISHING COMMITTEE

T. A. Peppard, M.D., Minneapolis   J. T. Christison, M.D., St. Paul

C. B. Wright, Minneapolis   E. M. Hammes, M.D., St. Paul

Waltman Walters, M.D., Rochester

EDITOR

Carl B. Drake, M.D., St. Paul

ASSOCIATE EDITORS

W. F. Braasch, M.D., Rochester

Gilbert Cottam, M.D., Minneapolis

VOLUME 21

JANUARY TO DECEMBER, 1938

EDITORIAL AND BUSINESS OFFICES

2642 University Avenue - - - - - - - - - Saint Paul, Minn.

BUSINESS MANAGER

J. R. Bruce

MINNESOTA MEDICINE

Journal of the Minnesota State Medical Association, Southern Minnesota Medical Association, Northern Minnesota Medical Association, Minnesota Academy of Medicine and Minneapolis Surgical Society.

| Volume 21 | JANUARY, 1938 | Number 1 |

UNILATERAL AND BILATERAL CARCINOMA OF THE BREAST*
(Including Paget's Disease)

Results Three, Five, Ten, Fifteen And Twenty Years After Operation

STUART W. HARRINGTON, M.D.

Rochester, Minnesota

CANCER of the breast is one of the most easily diagnosable forms of malignant tumor and it is probable that no form of cancer receives more surgical attention with such excellent results when treated by early primary radical operation. In spite of the fact, however, that countless patients, who otherwise would have died, have been operated on for cancer of the breast with excellent results, the general mortality from the disease has constantly increased, which indicates that there is an actual and not an apparent increase in the incidence of the disease.

The most important consideration in the treatment of cancer of the breast is early recognition of the disease and its immediate radical surgical treatment. There are no pathognomonic signs or symptoms by which all mammary malignant growths can be recognized. This, unfortunately, is particularly true of early lesions, and it emphasizes the importance of considering every lesion of the breast as being potentially malignant because delay in treatment may result in death from metastasis.

The educational program which members of the medical profession have for many years participated in, has been of great benefit in that a greater number of patients are seeking medical advice for lesions of the breast earlier in the course of the disease. This increases the responsibility of the physician, for lesions of the

breast are seen before the characteristic signs of malignancy are present and it is often difficult to distinguish benign from malignant lesions on the basis of clinical signs and symptoms. In those cases in which carcinoma is suspected and in which the diagnosis is definite, the subsequent course and planning of treatment should be carried out by one who is thoroughly familiar with the management of such lesions of the breast. The initial treatment is by far the most important procedure and the possibility of cure often depends on its effectiveness.

I have recently made another complete study of the cases of all patients with carcinoma of the breast who have been operated on at The Mayo Clinic from 1910 to 1933, inclusive. In an effort to make this study as accurate as possible, I have again reviewed the cases from a pathologic standpoint, and in a few cases in which the pathologic classification was not definite, additional microscopic studies were made which in some instances have changed the classification. There were relatively few of these cases; however, the figures which I have previously published have not been materially changed.

This present study comprises 4,628 cases in which patients were operated on in the period from 1910 to 1933 inclusive. The results have been tabulated in terms of "percentage survival rates" after operation, that is, the percentage of patients who were living, three, five, ten, fifteen and twenty years after operation. The five-year "percentage survival rate" is what is

*From the Division of Surgery, The Mayo Clinic, Rochester, Minnesota. Read before the annual meeting of the Minnesota State Medical Association, Saint Paul, Minnesota, May 4, 1937.

sometimes referred to in surgical parlance as a "five-year cure." A word about the way in which the calculations were made is in order: Patients who were treated for the requisite number of years prior to the time of inquiry, which was as of January 1, 1937, were first selected for the three-year survival rate, patients treated in 1933 or earlier for the five-year rate, patients treated in 1928 or earlier, for the ten-year rate, and so forth. Obviously, therefore, the three-year rate was calculated on the basis of a larger number of patients than the five-year rate, and the five-year rate was calculated on a larger number of patients than the ten-year rate, and so forth. Of the patients who were operated on, any patient who was traced for an insufficient number of years was considered to be "untraced" and was therefore excluded from the calculation. For instance in calculating the five-year survival rate, a patient who had been operated on five years prior to the time of the inquiry but who was traced only for four years after operation and who was living at that time was considered as "untraced," for one cannot know whether that patient did or did not survive until the fifth year after the operation. For the purposes of calculating the three-year survival rate that patient is traced, however, for we do know that the patient survived more than three years after operation.

An exhaustive effort was made to trace all patients. When patients were delinquent in answering routine follow-up letters, local health departments, vital statistics bureaus, and so forth, were consulted to learn whether there was any record of death. In the end, only a small number of the patients remained untraced, 97 per cent of the patients who were operated on five or more years before the investigation having been traced for a period of five years or more. It is to be noted that hospital deaths are not subtracted from the traced group, so that hospital deaths are counted as are other deaths in the first year after operation. In the 4,628 cases in which patients were operated on, which constitutes the total group dealt with in this paper, there were thirty-eight hospital deaths, or a rate of 0.8 per cent. In this paper, therefore, I shall report the three, five, ten, fifteen and twenty-year results in cases in which patients were operated on for unilateral carcinoma

of the breast and bilateral carcinoma of the breast, as well as the three, five, ten, fifteen and twenty-year results according to the grade of the malignancy in cases of unilateral carcinoma of the breast and the results of radical amputation for Paget's disease:

That malignant disease is not confined to any definite period of life is evidenced by the age incidence in this series. The youngest patient was seventeen, the oldest eighty-six years of age. In Table I is shown the age distribution of the patients for the entire series and also for those with and those without glandular involvement.

The results of operation depend on four important factors: (1) the extent of the disease at the time of operation, (2) the thoroughness with which the operation is performed, (3) the degree of the malignancy as measured by its list of pathologic grade at the time of operation, and (4) the age of the patient. Statistical studies are often misleading and may fail to give the true conception of the results obtained if proper attention is not paid to the specific character of the material dealt with. In studying carcinoma of the breast the first important consideration is the extent of the disease at the time of operation, and therefore the results will depend considerably on where the line is drawn between operable and inoperable conditions. I believe that this is one of the most important factors to be kept in mind in evaluating the results of statistical studies because, if only the small lesions without demonstrable axillary metastasis are considered surgical, the results would be unrepresentatively favorable. This method, however, would include only a relatively small number of patients, for the majority of patients present fairly well advanced lesions at the time of the initial examination. But even in this larger group of cases, in which there are more extensive lesions with ulceration and axillary metastasis, comfort and additional life can be given by proper surgical treatment and the patients deserve the benefit of this treatment.

There are varied opinions as to what constitutes operability. I will state briefly the criteria of operability which have been followed in this series of cases: Any lesion of the breast was considered to be operable if it was freely movable from the thoracic wall regardless of ulceration. In some cases even if there were cutane-

2

TABLE I. CARCINOMA OF BREAST (1910-1933)
Cases in Which Operation was Performed
Age Distribution

Age, Years	Total		With Glandular Involvement		Without Glandular Involvement	
	Number	Per Cent	Number	Per Cent	Number	Per Cent
10-19	2	0.0	1	0.0	1	0.1
20-29	70	1.5	38	1.3	32	1.9
30-39	664	14.3	434	14.7	230	13.7
40-44	707	15.3	453	15.3	254	15.2
45-49	862	18.6	566	19.2	296	17.7
50-54	719	15.5	462	15.7	257	15.3
55-59	646	14.0	414	14.0	232	13.8
60-64	464	10.0	308	10.4	156	9.3
65-69	286	6.2	172	5.8	114	6.8
70-74	149	3.2	80	2.7	69	4.1
75+	59	1.3	24	0.8	35	2.1
Total	4628	100	2952	100	1676	100
Per Cent of Total	100		63.8		36.2	
Mean Age	49.7 yrs.		49.4 yrs.		50.2 yrs.	
Youngest	17 yrs.		17 yrs.		18 yrs.	
Oldest	86 yrs.		82 yrs.		86 yrs.	

ous nodules proximal to the tumor, regardless of the presence or absence of palpable axillary lymph nodes, the lesion was considered operable. The same view of operability was held in most cases in which supraclavicular nodes were palpable but were confined to one side. In addition, patients were accepted for operation if they had a diffuse type of malignant growth, if malignancy was associated with lactation and, in most cases, if malignancy was associated with pregnancy. Those conditions were considered to be inoperable in which a large growth was fixed to the thoracic wall and there was very extensive metastasis to the regional lymph nodes or distant metastasis to other parts of the body. A few patients with distant metastasis were accepted for operation because of exceptional circumstances.

As those indicated, it is difficult to draw any sharp line between operable and inoperable lesions, and in each case treatment must be according to the findings. I have accepted for operation all patients to whom, I felt, there

was a reasonable chance of offering comfort or greater length of life as well as those whose disease, I felt, there was a reasonable chance of curing. It may seem that these rules of operability have not been drawn strictly enough and that I am accepting for operation cases in which the growth is too extensive. This is a matter of opinion, however, and justification has been found in many cases in which the condition was thought to be absolutely hopeless before operation, but in which the patients have lived and enjoyed many years of comfort afterward.

I have ascertained for each year from 1910 through 1933 the percentage of cases in which there was lymphatic involvement at the time of operation. This percentage for the entire series was 64.0 and it has shown little variation in the last ten years of this period. In 1933, however, the percentage was 55.7. This relatively low percentage is very encouraging as it is the next to the lowest for cases presenting glandular involvement that have been seen since 1910, the lowest being 54.3 in that year. However, it is

TABLE II. CARCINOMA OF BREAST
(1910-1933)
Per Cent Survivals for Various Years after Operation*
Comparison of cases with and without glandular involvement

Axillary Metastasis	Patients Operated on	Patients Traced	LIVED		
			Years After Operation	Number	Percentage of those Traced
Present	2952	2882	3 or more	1208	41.9
Absent	1676	1624		1334	82.1
Present	2736	2666	5 or more	746	28.0
Absent	1520	1460		1052	72.1
Present	1963	1901	10 or more	297	15.6
Absent	1066	1011		544	53.8
Present	1219	1173	15 or more	117	10.0
Absent	696	649		275	42.4
Present	545	529	20 or more	39	7.4
Absent	329	307		100	32.6

*Investigation as of January 1, 1937. The three-year group comprises patients who were operated on three years or more prior to the investigation, the five-year group patients who were operated on five years or more prior to investigation, and so forth.

TABLE III. UNILATERAL CARCINOMA OF BREAST
(1910-1933)
Percentage Survival Rates for Various Years after Operation*
Comparison of primary and secondary operations

GROUP	Patients Operated on	Patients Traced	LIVED		
			Years After Operation	Number	Per Cent of those Traced
Primary operation	3883	3777	3 or more	2122	56.2
Secondary operation	488	475		255	53.7
Primary operation	3591	3482	5 or more	1500	43.1
Secondary operation	426	408		173	42.4
Primary operation	2572	2476	10 or more	703	28.4
Secondary operation	285	269		73	27.1
Primary operation	1624	1546	15 or more	332	21.5
Secondary operation	169	157		24	15.3
Primary operation	733	700	20 or more	118	16.9
Secondary operation	79	75		9	12.0

*Investigation as of January 1, 1937. The three-year group comprises patients operated on three years or more prior to investigation, the five-year group five years or more prior to investigation, and so forth.

TABLE IV.   UNILATERAL CARCINOMA OF BREAST
(1910-1933)
Distribution by Grade of Malignancy

Grade of Malignancy	Total Cases		With Glandular Involvement		Without Glandular Involvement	
	Number	Per Cent of those Graded	Number	Per Cent	Number	Per Cent
1	129	3.8	10	7.8	119	92.2
2	427	12.7	183	42.9	244	57.1
3	1091	32.4	782	71.7	309	28.3
4	1721	51.1	1520	88.3	201	11.7
Total Graded	3368	100	2495		873	
Not Graded	1003		298		705	
Total	4371		2793		1578	

only the sixth time that the percentage has been in the fifties. Our experience at the clinic during this period indicates that the medical profession's educational program is hopeful of bearing results, although this percentage of 55.7 is still too high and indicates that we are seeing patients too late in the course of the disease to expect the best results from surgical treatment. Table II shows how much better the results are in cases in which patients are operated on before glandular invasion has occurred and again strongly emphasizes the importance of early operation. As has been pointed out in Table I, more than half the cases (64 per cent) presented evidence of glandular metastasis at the time of operation. It will be noted in Table II that the percentage of patients who were traced, and who were living three or more years after operation, is nearly twice as great for the group without axillary metastasis at the time of operation as for the group with axillary metastasis; for patients who were living five years after operation the percentage was about two and a half times greater; for patients who were living ten years after operation, three and a half times greater; for patients who were living fifteen years after operation, four times greater, and for patients who were living twenty years after operation four and a half times greater for those who did not have axillary metastasis at the time of operation than for those who did.

A comparison was made of the results of primary as opposed to secondary operations, and

the results for unilateral carcinoma are given in Table III. Those operations were considered secondary in which there had previously been a primary minor operation, elsewhere, for the same condition, and they comprised 11.2 per cent of all the operations for unilateral carcinoma. As Table III shows, the results for primary operations as indicated by the percentage survivals for the different years are better for the primary group than they are for the secondary group.

A study was also made to determine the results of amputation for unilateral carcinoma of the breast according to the grade of malignancy (Broders). This grading is based on the presence of cell differentiation, the greater the tendency of the cells to differentiate or to approach the normal, the lower being the grade of the malignancy. Lesions are graded on a basis of 1 to 4, grade 1 being the least and grade 4 the most malignant. A study was first made as to the relative frequency of each of the four grades of malignancy in cases of unilateral carcinoma. Not all the lesions in these cases were graded; 3,368, which comprised 77.1 per cent of the lesions, were graded, and 1,003, or 22.9 per cent, were not graded. Table IV shows the distribution of the various grades of malignancy for the entire group and compares the percentages in cases with and without glandular involvement for the various grades of malignancy. It is to be noted in this table that the high grades of malignancy comprise the largest percentage of all

TABLE V. UNILATERAL CARCINOMA OF BREAST
(1910-1933)

Percentage Survival Rates According to Glandular Involvement
and Grade of Malignancy*

Grade	Axillary Metastasis	Lived 3 or More Years After Operation				Lived 5 or More Years After Operation				Lived 10 or More Years After Operation			
		Patients Operated on	Patients traced	Number	Per Cent of those Traced	Patients Operated on	Patients traced	Number	Per Cent of Those Traced	Patients Operated on	Patients traced	Number	Per Cent of Those Traced
1	Present	10	10	10	100.0	10	10	10	100.0	8	7	5	71.4
	Absent	119	111	107	96.4	97	91	87	95.6	49	48	41	85.4
2	Present	183	178	121	68.0	177	172	89	51.7	149	142	43	30.3
	Absent	244	236	210	89.0	211	202	163	80.7	93	87	48	55.2
3	Present	782	770	385	50.0	743	724	221	30.5	533	519	74	14.3
	Absent	309	303	241	79.5	252	247	154	62.3	127	122	55	45.1
4	Present	1520	1484	483	32.5	1362	1334	281	21.1	945	921	110	11.9
	Absent	201	197	134	68.0	173	168	96	57.1	115	112	44	39.3

*Investigation as of January 1, 1937. The three-year group comprises patients operated on three years or more prior to investigation, the five-year group five years or more prior to investigation, and so forth.

TABLE VI. BILATERAL CARCINOMA OF BREAST
(1910-1933)

Percentage Survival Rates According to Whether Carcinoma Developed Simultaneously
in Both Breasts or Not*

Group	Patients Operated on	Patients Traced	LIVED		
			Years After Operation	Number	Per Cent of Those Traced
Simultaneous	47	47	3 or more	15	31.9
Not simultaneous	210	206		150	72.8
Simultaneous	42	42	5 or more	8	19.0
Not Simultaneous	195	189		115	60.8
Simultaneous	31	30	10 or more	2	6.7
Not simultaneous	141	135		63	46.7
Simultaneous	19	19	15 or more	0	0.0
Not simultaneous	103	99		36	36.4
Simultaneous	14	14	20 or more	0	0.0
Not simultaneous	48	47		12	25.5

*Investigation as of January 1, 1937. The three-year group comprises patients operated on three years or more prior to investigation, the five-year group five years or more prior to investigation, and so forth.

TABLE VII. PAGET'S DISEASE OF BREAST
(1910-1933)
Percentage Survival Rates*

				LIVED	
Axillary Metastasis	Patients Operated on	Patients Traced	Years After Operation	Number	Per Cent of Those Traced
Present	11	11	3 or more	5	45.5
Absent	23	23		20	87.0
Present	7	7	5 or more	3	42.9
Absent	20	20		16	75.0
Present	2	2	10 or more	1	50.0
Absent	13	13		6	46.2
Present	0	–	15 or more	–	–
Absent	6	6		2	33.3
Present	0	–	20 or more	–	–
Absent	2	2		0	0

*Investigation as of January 1, 1937. The three-year group comprises patients operated on three years or more prior to investigation, the five-year group five years or more prior to investigation, and so forth.

cases, and that glandular involvement is present relatively less frequently when the lesion is of the lower grades of malignancy than when it is of the high grades. Thus for lesions of grade 1, only 7.8 per cent showed glandular involvement, whereas for lesions of grade 4, 88.3 per cent showed glandular involvement.

The grade of the malignancy is probably the most important indication as to the prognosis. This is again made more significant when considered in connection with glandular invasion. As has been previously shown, the higher the degree of malignancy the greater the percentage of cases with glandular involvement. The fact that the lesions in most of the cases I am dealing with were of a high grade of malignancy accounts for the high percentage of cases with glandular involvement, as these high grade lesions metastasize early to the regional lymph nodes. This again emphasizes the importance of early operation. The best results are therefore obtained in the case of lesions of lower degrees of malignancy without glandular involvement. The least satisfactory results are obtained in cases of grade 4 lesions with glandular involvement, and this holds true for the various years of survival after operation (Table V).

The results of the surgical treatment of bilateral carcinoma of the breast are shown for two groups: (1) those cases in which the carcinoma occurred in both breasts at the same time, designated as "simultaneous" carcinoma of the breast, and (2) those in which the carcinoma occurred in the second breast at a later time. The results for bilateral simultaneous carcinoma, which comprise forty-seven cases or 1.0 per cent of all cases of carcinoma of the breast, are, as would be expected, much less satisfactory than for those cases in which the carcinoma occurred in the breasts at different times. There were 210 of these latter cases, or 4.5 per cent of the total cases of carcinoma of the breast. The results in this latter group are better than would be expected, although it must be taken into consideration that these are the most favorable cases in the group, as many patients who later had carcinoma in the remaining breast had distant metastasis, which contraindicates any radical procedure on the remaining breast (Table VI).

Of all the cases of carcinoma of the breast in this series, only thirty-four patients, or 0.7 per cent, were classified as having Paget's disease. Like other forms of carcinoma, Paget's disease comes into existence by differentiation of epithelial cells which appear to be practically limited in origin to protective or closely allied epithelium. It seems reasonable to classify Paget's disease with the squamous cell or epidermoid type of carcinoma. These cases are often associated with a ductal type of adenocarcinoma in the underlying mammary tissue. There is some difference of opinion pathologically as to whether malignancy originates in the epithelial structures or in the glandular structures in these cases; from a surgical standpoint, however, I believe that these patients should receive the same surgical treatment as those with adenocarcinomas. As will be shown in Table VII a relatively high percentage of these cases show glandular invasion, the percentage being 32.4. This is only half as great as that for all cases of carcinoma of the breast with glandular invasion, which was shown in a previous table to be 64.0 per cent. This proves very definitely that the lesions in these cases metastasize to the regional lymph nodes, necessitating a thorough radical procedure. As shown in Table VII, the results of radical amputation in cases of Paget's disease presenting glandular invasion are less satisfactory than in similar cases of the entire group of adenocarcinomas of the breast (Table II). In cases without glandular metastasis the results are more satisfactory for the three, and five-year periods and not as satisfactory for the ten and fifteen-year periods.

Summary and Conclusions

A review has been made of all cases of carcinoma of the breast encountered at the clinic from 1910 to 1933, inclusive. Of the total of 4,628 patients, 97.4 per cent have been traced three years or more and the results of operation have been determined for three, five, ten, fifteen and twenty-year periods in cases of unilateral carcinoma of the breast, bilateral carcinoma of the breast, and Paget's disease (Tables I to VII inclusive).

The best surgical results were obtained in cases in which metastasis to the lymph nodes had not taken place. In this series of 4,628 cases, 1,676 cases (36.2 per cent) did not present axillary metastasis at the time of operation. It was found that 82.1 per cent of these patients were living three years, 72.1 per cent were living five years, 53.8 per cent were living ten years, 42.4 per cent were living fifteen years and 32.6 per cent were living twenty years or more after operation. In cases in which there had been lymphatic involvement, the results were less satisfactory. There were 2,952 cases in this group, or 63.8 per cent of the total; 41.9 per cent of these patients were living three years, 28.0 per cent were living five years, 15.6 per cent were living ten years, 10.0 per cent were living fifteen years and 7.4 per cent were living twenty years after operation.

As is shown by this study, the important indications as to prognosis following surgical treatment are the extent of the malignancy at the time of operation, particularly as to the presence or absence of axillary metastasis, and the degree of the malignancy, as shown by the miscropic examination of the primary malignant lesion.

NEW AUTOMOBILES AND NEW FRACTURES*

HARRY B. MACEY, M.D.

Rochester, Minnesota

TURRET tops, all steel bodies and shatter-proof glass have not compensated for fast driving, reckless driving and driving while drunk. This is attested by the 36,000 deaths from automobile accidents in 1936 and by the recent enactment in Minnesota of a law prohibiting speeds in excess of sixty miles an hour in the daytime or in excess of fifty miles an hour after dark.

By the title of this paper, I do not mean to suggest that the fractures now incurred in automobile accidents are unheard of. It is true, however, that, in comparison with former days, physicians are seeing more uncommon and more multiple fractures.

TABLE I.   PATIENTS, FRACTURES AND TYPES OF
ACCIDENTS

Patients	100
Fractures	164
Patients in overturn accidents	42
Patients in impact accidents	43
Patients in impact and overturn accidents	3
Type of accident unknown	12
Patients who had multiple fractures, 33 per cent	

The frame of the older type of automobile was chiefly of wood. There was very little steel support and the outcome of severe accidents was practically demolition of the car. Its parts were scattered, its doors were unhinged and, not infrequently, motors were driven into the front seat. As for the passengers, frequently they suffered compound fractures, together with laceration of soft tissue.

Today soft tissue is better preserved, but the feature of present day accidents which makes their human products more difficult to handle is the fact that the multiplicity of fractures, which previously has been mentioned, leaves the

patient in a state of more or less profound shock. The energy concealed in increased velocity has got to be absorbed somewhere.

Statistical Study

A statistical study of 100 consecutive cases, exclusive of those in which the skull was fractured, was made in an effort to give a cross section of the bones fractured and of the types of fractures sustained. The study is best re-

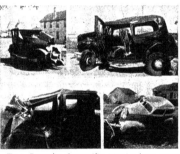

Fig. 1. Destruction of automobiles *(above)* in impact type of accident, and *(below)* in overturn type of accident.

viewed from the point of view of the types of accidents (Table I). Automobile accidents in general entail either impact, defined as striking together, or overturning. Impact accidents (Fig. 1, *above*) result from head-on collisions or from striking bridge abutments, trees or any object which stops or impedes progress. Overturn accidents (Fig. 1, *below*) commonly occur secondary to cars being sideswiped or forced off the road by inconsiderate drivers. Blowouts and falling asleep while driving are less frequent causes.

Thirty-three per cent of the individuals sustained multiple fractures; 100 patients sustained 164 fractures. Impact and overturn accidents occurred in about the same frequency. In our geographical district, with its long distances and high speed highways, a preponderance of over-

*From the Section on Orthopedic Surgery, The Mayo Clinic, Rochester, Minnesota. Read before the annual meeting of the Minnesota State Medical Association, St. Paul, Minnesota, May 5, 1937.

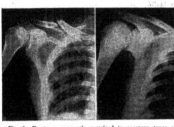

Fig. 2. Fractures commonly sustained in overturn types of accidents. *a*, Fracture of clavicle and scapula; *b*, fracture of scapula (the line across the surgical neck of the humerus is the epiphysis).

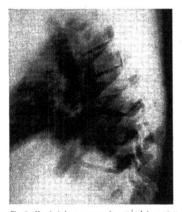

Fig. 3. Vertebral fracture commonly sustained in overturn type of accident.

turn accidents would be expected, whereas in large cities and more densely populated areas the impact type of accident would be expected to prevail.

As to bones injured, fractures of the ribs occurred in the highest proportion, 28.9 per cent (Table II). However, this high percentage is misleading in that only 17 per cent of the patients had fractures of the ribs: The high percentage is accounted for by the fact that usually several ribs were fractured. Twenty-four per cent of the individuals had vertebral fractures. These represented 20.2 per cent of the total number of fractures. The fact that a high per-

TABLE II. STRUCTURES FRACTURED

Structure	Per Cent
Vertebrae and processes	20.2
Ribs	28.9
Upper extremity and shoulder girdle	26.8
Lower extremity and pelvic girdle	22.3
Sternum	1.8
Total	100

centage of fractures occurred about the upper extremity and shoulder girdle, was attributable chiefly to the large number of clavicular and scapular fractures. Clavicular fractures were sustained commonly whether the accident was of the impact or of the overturn type. As compared with the upper extremity and shoulder girdle, the lower extremity and pelvic girdle suffered less. The sternum usually is thought of as an unusual situation for fracture to occur; yet the sternums of 3 per cent of the individuals were fractured.

Carrying the statistical study further, and reviewing the fractures in relation to the type of accident, several definite facts were brought out.

Overturn Accidents

Following overturn accidents, the frequency of fractures of the shoulder girdle (Fig. 2, *a* and *b*) and vertebral column (Fig. 3) was outstanding; 48.5 per cent of the fractures (representing 54.8 per cent of the patients) were of one of these structures (Table III). There was a tendency for these fractures to occur in combination, indicating that in this type of accident there is a common mechanism in their production. In the production of vertebral fractures of the compression type, and this is the type found after automobile fractures, force must be applied to the spinal column while it is in a flexed or jack-knife position; therefore, it would be logical to assume that, as the occupants are seated in a flexed posture, force is applied back and forth from the top of the car to the seat, as the car rolls over and over. This may further explain the situation of the fracture. Cervical fractures are produced by force applied from the top of the car to the skull, with the cervical portion of the spinal column flexed. In the pro-

TABLE III.   FRACTURES FROM OVERTURN
ACCIDENTS

Structures fractured		Per Cent
Upper extremity and shoulder girdle		34.6
	Clavicle 18 per cent	
	Scapula 8.3 per cent	
Ribs		29.2
Vertebrae and processes		22.2
Lower extremity		7
Pelvis		4.2
Sternum		2.8
Total		100
42 patients sustained 72 fractures		

TABLE IV.   FRACTURES FROM IMPACT ACCIDENTS

Structures fractured		Per Cent
Lower extremity and pelvic girdle		43.0
	Femur 12.7 per cent	
	Patella 9.5 per cent	
Ribs		27.0
Vertebrae		11.1
Upper extremity and shoulder girdle		18.9
	Upper extremity 11.0 per cent	
Total		100
43 patients sustained 63 fractures		

duction of fractures of the thoracic and lumbar portions of the spinal column, direct force probably is applied to the shoulders, with the spinal column in a flexed, sitting position, or possibly the force is applied to the head, with the cervical portion of the spinal column in a neutral position. As the car continues to roll, the spinal column may assume different flexed positions and, with the reapplication of force, fractures may be produced at different levels.

In the production of clavicular fractures, indirect force is the most likely factor; probably, as the occupants are tossed from side to side, force is transmitted to the clavicle through the shoulder. These fractures are chiefly of the middle and outer third of the clavicle. Frac-

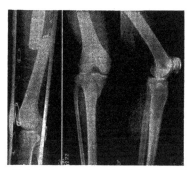

Fig. 4. Fractures commonly sustained in impact types of accidents. *a,* Fracture of shaft of femur; *b,* intra-articular fracture of knee; *c,* fracture of patella.

tures of the outer third probably occur as a result of force applied to the shoulder in a slightly downward plane; fractures of the middle third probably result from force transmitted through the shoulder in a horizontal, or in a slightly upward, plane.

The mechanism of the scapular fractures that occur in this type of accident is difficult to explain; however, I assume that force is applied directly to the body of the scapula rather than indirectly to the glenoid. This assumption seems reasonable because scapular fractures in this series involved chiefly the body of the scapula rather than the processes or glenoid.

Impact Accidents

In the impact accident, in contradistinction to the overturn accident, there was an outstanding occurence of fractures of the lower extremities (Fig. 4, *a, b* and *c*). Forty-three per cent of the fractures (representing 46.5 per cent of the patients) were of the lower extremity and pelvic girdle. In Table IV, certain fractures of the lower extremity are mentioned; other fractures were of the leg, tarsus, hip, and ankle.

In many instances the position of the individual in the car could be learned. All of the patellar fractures, and 75 per cent of the fractures of the femoral shaft, affected occupants of the front seat. The patellar fractures probably result from striking the dashboard and the fractures of the femur result either from direct force transmitted from the dashboard to the shaft of the femur or from indirect force exerted on the patella, with or without associated muscular action. An individual riding in the front seat probably would be aware of an impending accident and there would result a pro-

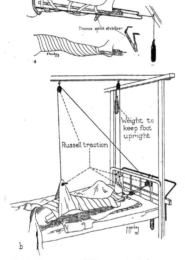

Fig. 5. Skin traction applied by means of adhesive tape and *a*, the Thomas splint; *b*, Russell method.

tective muscular reaction in which the feet would be pressed against the floor board and the muscles of the leg and thigh would be rendered tense. With the impact, the individual is thrown forward in accordance with the force of the impact. Thus it is conceivable that if the occupant is thrown forward, in a semi-crouching position, direct force on the knee, plus the powerful muscular action, could snap the femur. If the individual is thrown forward with the legs outstretched, direct force exerted by the lower margin of the dash may produce a fracture of the femur. The driver may sustain fractures of the femoral shaft from force exerted directly against the steering wheel.

The percentage of vertebral fractures sustained in impact accidents was about half that

sustained in overturn accidents. A large majority of fractures of the vertebræ in impact accidents probably result from the spine being snapped forward into flexion at the time of the impact. The percentage of fractures of the shoulder girdle and vertebræ sustained in overturn accidents also was only about half that sustained in impact accidents. Fractures of the shoulder girdle and upper extremities in the impact type of accident probably result from instinctive thrusting forward of the hand as a protective mechanism in bracing for the impact, with consequent direct or indirect exertion of force.

Treatment

In discussing the treatment of automobile fractures my remarks will be confined chiefly to the immediate care of these fractures. Not infrequently the patients are in poor general condition and treatment cannot be elective. Therefore, means of treatment or of protection of the fracture must be limited to those which will not make worse the general condition of the patient.

The Thomas splint, simple of construction and easy of application, is one of the most useful devices. It is made for use on the lower extremity but occasionally it can be successfully used in the immediate care of fractures of the upper extremity. The fixation and supporting functions of the Thomas splint often are employed in conjunction with skeletal or skin traction.

Skeletal traction can be facilitated by employment of the Kirschner wire. The wire can be inserted at the bedside, under local anesthesia. The sites of election for introduction of the wire are through the femoral condyles or tibial tubercle. By means of this wire, adequate traction can be instituted early, commonly as an emergency measure and, frequently, as an elective measure in cases of fracture of the femur. In the same manner, fractures of the leg can be treated by applying the traction to the calcaneus or to the lower third of the tibia just proximal to the ankle joint. Should the general condition of the patient permit an elective course of management, traction by Kirschner wire offers an excellent method of treatment of fractures that are compounded or associated with badly traumatized surrounding soft tissue.

Skin traction can be applied by use of adhesive

tape or moleskin, and is efficient for short periods with heavy traction, or for longer periods with light traction. It is well used in certain instances. The Thomas splint also can be used in the immediate care of fractures about the hip (Fig. 5, a).

A third method of skin traction, reported by Russell, can be applied without detriment to the patient's general condition (Fig. 5, b). This has been found to be effective in treating fractures about the tibial tuberosities of adults and fractures of the femoral shaft of children. It is most effectively used on children if applied bilaterally for unilateral fractures of the femoral shaft.

Fractures of the patella usually require open operation. This is particularly true of fractures of the patella acquired in automobile accidents, because of their comminuted nature. Emergency measures consist of splinting, and possibly of aspiration of the hemarthrosis. Surgical treatment, as employed today for fracture of the patella, consists of internal fixation. In one method of fixation that is widely used, fascia lata is passed through the fragments, or encircles the fragments, and is sutured in position; in another, a rustless steel wire is introduced anteriorly and encircles the fragments of the patella. In its insertion the wire loop is passed through the quadriceps, patellar tendon and lateral capsular expanse, or if preferred, may be passed through the bony fragments, thereby insuring stability. Should fascia lata be employed as a means of fixation it is advisable to repair the usually associated lateral tear in the expanse of the capsule, using either chromic catgut or strips of fascia lata.

Hyperextension, the treatment for compression fractures of the vertebral bodies, is best maintained by well fitting plaster-of-paris casts. The danger of injuring the spinal cord by hyperextension should be kept in mind, and the method should not be applied until roentgenograms have made it evident that this danger does not exist. Frequently the condition of the patient necessitates delaying the application of plaster-of-paris casts, in which case hyperextension should be instituted in some simple and convenient manner. In cases of fracture of the lower thoracic and lumbar portions of the spinal column, hyperextension can be attained by means

of rolled blankets, suspension slings (Fig. 6, a and b) or ingeniously devised frames. In cases of cervical fracture and in cases of fracture of the upper part of the thoracic portion of the column, traction by some type of head sling,

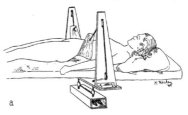

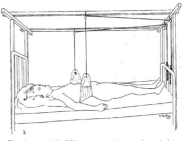

Fig. 6. a, and b, Different types of suspension sling for use in vertebral and pelvic fractures.

with or without hyperextension, can be instituted easily.

In considering vertebral fractures, I would urge that all complaints referable to the back, particularly a complaint of persistent soreness, be thoroughly investigated roentgenologically. Soreness, often mistaken for that of muscular contusion, may be the result of a fracture which can be revealed only by roentgenologic examination. I would urge that lateral roentgenograms always be included in the examination, for frequently a vertebra which appears normal in the anteroposterior roentgenogram will be found to be the site of a compression fracture when viewed laterally.

Fractures of the ribs, although painful, rarely are difficult to treat and simple immobilization for several weeks usually suffices.

Fractures of the shoulder girdle, so common in the overturn type of accident, usually can be treated by elective measures from the beginning. In a rare case, surgical measures may be resorted to from the beginning. The clavicle most commonly is fractured in its middle third; less frequently in its outer third. In this series of

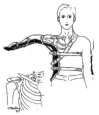

Fig. 7. Abduction humerus splint in treatment of clavicular fracture.

cases, none of the fractures were of the inner third. Treatment of fracture of the outer, or of the middle, third is directed toward correction of the deformity. This deformity usually consists in separation of the fragments, with the outer fragment carried downward by the weight of the upper extremity and the proximal fragment pulled upward by the sternocleidomastoid muscle. Correction is attained by elevation and extension of the shoulder. If manipulative reduction is employed for the simpler type of fracture, fixation is best afforded by a combined Sayre and Velpeau dressing. If delayed reduction is employed, and the fracture is simple, treatment can be carried out by the clavicular T splint, by clavicular rings, or by some type of special splint or some form of traction. If the fracture is comminuted, delayed reduction is in-

dicated. Manipulative procedures are rarely employed. A device which we, at the clinic, have found particularly effective for treatment of both simple and comminuted fractures of the clavicle is the abduction humerus splint, made in such a manner that the arm is held abducted about 110° and in slight extension (Fig. 7).

In scapular fractures, it is the body of the bone which usually is broken. Fortunately, the scapula is so placed that it is well protected posteriorly by muscles and anteriorly by the thoracic wall. Because of this, simple immobilization of the associated upper extremity for a period of two to three weeks usually suffices.

In this series, none of the sternal fractures required other than simple strapping by means of adhesive tape applied across the anterior thoracic wall. However, should gross displacement take place, open operation and reduction often will be required.

Comment

In closing, I would like to emphasize that in this review of 100 cases there occurred three sternal fractures and ten scapular fractures, fractures heretofore considered rare. Several textbooks either omit discussion of these fractures or give them slight mention. Furthermore, I would like to call attention to the fact that multiple fractures now are common results of automobile accidents. The overturn type of accident commonly produced fractures of the vertebra and shoulder girdle, whereas the impact type of accident commonly produced fractures of the lower extremities. Skull fractures, most commonly the cause of death in automobile accidents, have purposely been omitted in this discussion.

PERIPHERAL NERVE INJURIES*

ARTHUR A. ZIEROLD, M.D.

Minneapolis, Minnesota

INJURIES to the peripheral nerves, while not of frequent occurrence, are of importance by reason of the prolonged and many times permanent disability which accompanies them. The end-results following treatment are probably not

*Presented before the annual meeting of the Minnesota State Medical Association, Saint Paul, Minnesota, May 5, 1937.

the best possible. This is true not because nerve injuries pass unrecognized or because the possibilities of treatment are not known but because most of us have no definite plan of procedure. Only too often we are confronted with permanent disabilities that might have been avoided had the patient been aware of what he might reasonably expect from treatment and, what is of prime importance, when that treatment should be undertaken. This paper will discuss briefly the development of a reasonable plan of treatment that will best conserve the factors necessary for success.

Nerve injuries in themselves are relatively simple in their nature but are often complicated by association with other injuries to tendons, muscles, vessels, and bones. A primary nerve injury may consist in nothing more than a concussion. This is manifested by a loss of function without structural damage. Next in order of severity is contusion of the nerve wherein there is actual cell damage and often interstitial hemorrhage. Last and most severe of the primary injuries is partial or complete section of the nerve trunk. Classed as secondary injuries are those compressions of the nerve resulting from the development of scar within the nerve trunk which frequently follows contusion or the external scar which results from lacerations of the surrounding tissue. Included in this and differing only in the character of the tissue is the compression of the nerve trunk by bone fragments or callus.

While symptoms of nerve injuries may by careful study be elaborated into a very complex syndrome, they may also be reduced to simple terms. When a nerve is injured there is a partial or complete loss of motor power or sensation or both. These are the primary signs of nerve damage and the areas affected can usually be identified with the affected nerve without a great deal of difficulty. Most prolonged study is undertaken in the attempt not to identify which nerve is injured but rather the nature and extent of the injury and its progression. If definite organic nerve injuries occur, secondary symptoms and signs will develop in the course of time. Vasomotor disturbances giving rise to changes in color and temperature develop so early as to be almost primary symptoms. The unopposed muscles give rise to deformities and finally, as atrophy and fibrosis of the muscles develop, these deformities become permanent. In the latest stages the involved joints become fixed by reason of muscle contracture or shrinkage of the capsule. Together with the muscular atrophy, atrophy of the skin frequently occurs and, with this, changes in nail structure and hair distribution. In some instances, particularly in the

lower extremities, ulceration may occur. These signs and symptoms are the gross outward evidence of nerve injury and may all or in part disappear with regeneration of the nerve. The manner of this may perhaps be best understood by a brief consideration of the histopathology.

What we class as peripheral nerves are those spinal nerve trunks consisting of sensory fibers from the posterior spinal roots and motor fibers from the anterior roots together with fibers communicating with the sympathetic ganglia. These are united in cable-like strands surrounded by a fibrous tissue sheath and subdivided by fibrous tissue septa. There are few if any purely motor or sensory nerves if we exclude the cranial nerves, although in some one element may predominate almost to the exclusion of the other. Although in our consideration of nerve injuries we are dealing with nerve trunks made up of numerous smaller fiber bundles, these fibers are all projections of cell bodies within the central nervous system or the sympathetic ganglia. Therefore, the changes which occur in peripheral nerve injuries must be considered in terms of a single cell. For example, an anterior horn cell of the spinal cord sends out its neuraxis which transverses the spinal nerve uninterruptedly to the muscle to which it is joined by specific end plates. This neuraxis is made up of numerous protoplasmic fibrils and is surrounded by myelin and the tubular sheath of Schwann. When section of the neuraxis occurs, degeneration promptly begins. This consists of fragmentation of the neuraxis fibrils and final decomposition attended by proliferation of neurilemma cells until the end-result is a tubular sheath filled with an undifferentiated, nucleated strand of protoplasm. This occurs almost simultaneously throughout the length of the distal fragments and is complete within two weeks. This state of affairs may persist unchanged for several months. As time progresses, however, the tubular sheath contracts until finally the degenerated distal fragment of nerve is represented by nothing more than a fibrous tissue strand with a few inclusions of protoplasm. As the distal fragment of nerve degenerates, the central stump also degenerates for a distance of two or three millimeters. Following this, however, regeneration of the nerve begins. The fine fibrils of the neuraxis proliferate and grow distally with rounded bulb-like ends, into the exudate at the site of the injury. If uninterrupted by scar or undue separation of the fragments they pass into the previously mentioned neuraxis tube of degenerated nerve substance and grow in a rather regular manner toward the periphery. Because a sensory fibril may grow into a motor ending and vice versa, the mathematical chances of perfect anatomical regeneration are slight, but because of the great number of fibrils the chance of functional results is good, once the site of injury has been passed. It might be supposed that a nerve trunk with its included fibers laid down in a regular arrangement would not regenerate successfully after section unless each fiber tract had opportunity to grow into its proper and corresponding tube in the distal fragment. Because of the many intra-neural communications and plexuses this is found not to be necessary. It is, of course, obvious that the more nearly a nerve approaches an unmixed type the more satisfactory will be the end-result and the less will be the misfit of nerves and nerve endings.

If, however, a nerve be sectioned and the fragments separated, allowing scar tissue to intervene, the outgrowing fibrils in the central stump will turn upon themselves and form a loose network together with the newly formed scar, giving rise to a bulb-like stump which is the neuroma commonly found at operation. If this condition is allowed to persist for many months the distal degenerated portion of the nerve gradually contracts until the pathway for regenerating fibrils is lost. If instead of section the nerve has sustained a contusion with injury to nerve tissue the distal part may degenerate and regeneration from the proximal stump may take place uninterruptedly and successfully. On the other hand, if the contusion is severe, sufficient scar tissue may develop within the nerve to cause pressure enough to kill the newly growing fibrils and regeneration not only stops but what has previously grown following the initial injury is often lost. This process is duplicated in cases in which the nerve is compressed by bone or callus or other extraneous scar. Although the continuity of the nerve may be intact, function is lost by the injury of compression.

From this brief pathology, I believe, may be gathered the manner in which peripheral nerves

16

early to afford the best opportunity for complete nerve regeneration. If, on exploration, the continuity of the nerve is found to be intact, no damage is done by the exploration and conservative measures can be employed. On the other hand, if exploration is delayed several months awaiting regeneration (and, to be logical, this period should be at least six months) many operable cases will be unnecessarily handicapped, regeneration will be less prompt and sure, and many secondary complications will be developed which otherwise might have been avoided. Furthermore, the status of the nerve which does not require immediate suture will not be improved.

If confronted with a fresh wound and exploration reveals section of a nerve, the nerve should be united by suture even in the face of possible infection. There is everything to gain and nothing to lose. If the wound heals without pus formation, regeneration is well on its way with a minimum of scar and the best possible chance of success. If, on the contrary, the wound suppurates, the nerve ends are in better position than if allowed to separate and become imbedded in the resultant scar tissue. When sepsis subsides and the wound has healed, resuture of the nerve is usually necessary but this cannot be done immediately. An infected wound should not be reopened within a six-months period. At the end of this time successful regeneration is still quite possible and the chances of a clean field are reasonably good.

Summary

From the foregoing plan of procedure what may be reasonably expected?

1. Roughly, 50 per cent of all injuries to the peripheral nerves recover function without operation.

2. Of the uncomplicated cases which require neurolysis or nerve suture, 75 per cent may expect functional recovery.

3. Of those cases which require nerve transplant, the percentage of success is considerably less.

4. Following nerve suture, the first evidence of regeneration seldom appears before four months and may be delayed two or three months longer.

5. Improvement may be expected for twenty-four to thirty months.

6. The results from primary suture are much better than the results from secondary or delayed suture: recovery is more often complete and the time of regeneration shortened and the secondary complications are obviated.

7. Of the various nerves subject to operation it is probable that one regenerates about as rapidly and as successfully as the other although from the published figures almost anything may be proven. It is probable, however, that the nearer a nerve approaches a pure type, either sensory or motor, the better are the chances of regeneration.

THE TREATMENT OF BURNS*

ROBERT F. McGANDY, M.D.

Minneapolis, Minnesota

ANY consideration of burns, like other injuries, from an industrial viewpoint should have the following objectives:

1. Prevention.
2. Lowering of the mortality rate.
3. Returning the patient to employment in the shortest possible healing period and with a minimum of permanent disability.

As a matter of fact there is no difference between these objectives from an industrial viewpoint than from that of private practice.

Ninety per cent of all burns are due to carelessness. Industry attempts to prevent burns as well as other accidents by:

1. Rigid physical examination of all applicants for employment.
2. Reëxamination of all employees at stated intervals and following illnesses.
3. The activity of safety crews and safety appliances.

A similar campaign might be carried on for the prevention of so-called non-industrial burns. This might be done by impressing the lay people, particularly women, with the hazard of their

*Presented before the annual meeting of the Minnesota State Medical Association, St. Paul, May 5, 1937.

clothing. Special precaution should be taken in protecting children in the preschool age.

Outside of industry, women are burned more frequently then men. The mortality rate in hospital cases in the past ten to twelve years has been reduced to one-half. It is significant, however, that 45 per cent of all deaths due to burns are in children between one and five years.

Historically, there is nothing new in the treatment of burns. At the present time, and for many years past we have been employing methods which were in vogue at one time or another, over many centuries, and which have been recently reintroduced and exploited. The treatment of burns really started with man's discovery of fire. Salves, ointments and oils have been used for ages, and their value can be attributed to the fact that anything covering a burn allayed pain. Hippocrates, in 430 B. C., used a combination of oil and resin in the treatment of burns. Alum and other astringents were used in the sixth century, A. D. The use of limewater and oil, which was the forerunner of carron oil, was recorded in the third century, B. C. Tait used paraffin in 1864 but it did not become popular until 1915. Picric acid was first used in 1864. Open air treatment was recorded as early as 1867. Water baths were used in 1858. Lister used boric acid compresses for burns exclusively and it is possible that he had the present popular infection theory for the toxemia of burns in mind at that time. The Chinese, in the sixth century, B. C., used a strong infusion of tea as wet dressings. One might say that one of the earliest treatments recently has become one of the most modern treatments. In general, one might say that burns have passed through periods of fads and fancy without much real investigation, until the last twelve years.

The various agents producing burns are too numerous and familiar to everyone to enumerate here. I am going to limit this paper to consideration of superficial burns and scalds in general, rather than to those due to specific agents, as electricity, et cetera. Burns vary in extent and degree, depending primarily on the agent producing the burn. The American classification of burns into three degrees is the one most generally used, and I am sure all of you are familiar with it. I feel that Berkow's method of estimation of the extensiveness of surface burns showing the percentage ratio of parts

burned to the total body surface, is of great value. One must remember, however, that burns, regardless of their extent, are more serious in some localities than in others. This is especially true in burns about the genitals, neck and orifices. Briefly, the prognosis of burns depends on the burning agent; sex, age, and occupation of the burned patient; depth and extent of the region involved, as well as the physical condition of the patient at the time of the burn.

The general course of extensive superficial burns, and by this I mean burns involving 15 to 20 per cent of the body surface, can be divided into the following stages:

1. Initial shock.
2. Secondary shock.
3. Toxemia or sepsis.
4. Healing.

Initial shock, when present, begins immediately and is coincident with the occurrence of the burn. It is now thought that it is due to an upset of the vasomotor mechanism caused by afferent nerve impulses from the injured area. It is characterized by an anxious expression on the face and a moist grey skin. The temperature may drop slightly while the respirations become elevated and shallow. Blood pressure as a rule falls, but as the systolic and diastolic pressure usually fall together, there is little if any change in pulse pressure. This stage passes off as a rule with heat, opiates, et cetera.

Secondary shock usually follows in two to ten hours. There have been numerous theories advanced for this stage. The theory accepted now by most authorities is that of blood concentration. It is thought that the burn alters the permeability of the capillary walls. This, in turn, allows the escape of blood plasma from the body into the burned area. There is a definite measurable increase in blood viscosity. Blood concentration can be estimated by using a hemoglobinometer and this fact should be remembered, as it gives an easy method of determining the amount of fluid intake. As you know, a marked concentration of blood results in failure of circulation with an inefficient oxygen carrier. This means oxygen starvation of the tissues, resulting in falling of the temperature and finally death, if allowed to continue. One of the earliest signs of secondary shock is lowered pulse pressure with or without a fall of the systolic pressure. A drop of less than 30 mm. in an adult, especial

18

ly if the systolic is below 100, is definite evidence of early secondary shock. The pulse becomes rapid and, if at the same time it becomes feeble, it is an indication of advanced shock. The respirations become rapid as well. These in general are some of the common findings in secondary shock. As these conditions can be aggravated by exposure, coarse cleansing or scrubbing of the burned area, and the application of irritating antiseptics, et cetera, it is very obvious that one should forget the local burn and treat the patient systemically until the shock has safely passed or is under control.

In view of these facts, and others which I will take up later, I am sure you can readily see why I feel that lay people coming in contact with an extensive superficial burn should wrap the victim in a blanket or sheet, keep him warm and call a doctor or transport the patient to a hospital as soon as possible. Too often, some overwilling neighbor, employee or ambitious safety man pushes the poor victim deeper into shock by applying his or her favorite ointment, salve, paste, oil or other "household" remedy and then damages the patient further by showing the bystanders what a neat bandage he can apply. The real tragedy, however, is the fact that these applications must be removed by the doctor when the patient reaches him, so that the more necessary water-soluble escharotics can be applied. Fortunately the doctor can use nitrous oxide if the patient's condition does not permit otherwise. I cannot too strongly impress upon you my feeling that, from the standpoint of everybody concerned, the patient with extensive burns is best let alone, with the exception of course of wrapping him in a blanket or sheet and keeping him warm. A patient seen some some time after a burn has been received should be given opiates to relieve pain and prevent the further development of shock.

When the patient reaches the hospital, he should be placed in bed under a cradle where the temperature is kept at about 90 degrees. Fluids should next be started. These can be given intravenously, but, if the patient's condition warrants, any method may be used. It is generally accepted that saline and glucose be used in order to take care of the blood chlorides lost and to protect the liver. If the patient's temperature is subnormal, these fluids are best given at 105 to 110 degrees. Blood transfusion,

except for sepsis, is best reserved for shock from trauma rather than burns. Many men recommend gum acacia in this stage as an initial measure and I heartily approve of it. A severe burn usually requires intravenous fluids for three days. A good rule for quantity is 1,000 c.c. per twenty-five pounds of body weight in twenty-four hours. A good adjuvant measure in the treatment of burns in this stage is the use of extract of suprarenal cortex. This is used in one c.c. doses and repeated at intervals. This extract, as in the case of Addison's disease, increases the efficiency of the circulatory mechanism and apparently checks some of the salt loss through the kidneys. So much for the control of fluid intake in combating blood concentration.

How may we now control fluid loss? It is definitely known that blood concentration and subcutaneous edema of the tissues following burns reaches its peak in twenty-four to thirty-six hours following injury. A hemoglobin determination may reach as high as 180. It has also been demonstrated that a third degree burn involving one-sixth of the body surface results in a fluid loss of 70 per cent of the total blood volume in twenty-four hours. This means that an adult weighing 65 kilograms having a blood volume of about 5,000 c.c. would lose 3,500 c.c. of fluid from the blood stream in twenty-four hours. Two out of three deaths in burns occurring in the first twenty-four hours, excluding of course those who die of primary shock and in those cases immediately hopeless, are attributed to the rapid concentration of blood and the great loss of blood plasma. So the ideal first dressing in extensive burns is one which not only allays pain by covering the burned surfaces but also, what is more important, prevents the loss of fluids from the blood stream. Too much credit cannot be given to Davidson, who, in 1925, called attention to the use of tannic acid in precipitating broken down burned tissue and thereby sealing off the capillary bed at the outset and preventing loss of body fluid. Time does not permit me to go into the details of this technic, and it is familiar to you. In review, may I state that most men now use tannic acid in a 10 per cent freshly prepared aqueous solution rather than the more dilute solution first advocated. There are many who use a 20 per cent solution, as coagulation takes place more rapidly with the stronger solution. This, however, does more damage to the normal epithelial cells left in the burn, as I will explain later. Of the three methods of applying tannic acid, I believe the spray method far exceeds the other two. Immersion of the patient in a tub of tannic acid solution, although it can be done, requires a large amount of help and solution. Wet tannic acid dressings, like the objection to wet dressings in general, are painful to change because they adhere to the underlying structures and oftentimes reduce the patient's temperature and increase shock. The spray method is simple and can be carried out under a tent with ease or with the aid of a warm air blower or lamp in smaller areas, such as on the extremities. It is essential that the tannic acid result should be obtained as quickly as possible in order to retain body fluids. By the same token, tannic acid is of little value after fluid loss has reached its peak. For then, the reverse process takes place and fluid loss is not a factor. With the aid of heat and warm air, coagulation can be completed in six to twelve hours, and in eighteen hours at the outside. The use of silver nitrate with tannic acid is painful in extensive burns, and what is worse destroys unburned epithelial tissue which is invaluable for regeneration.

Picric acid in aqueous solution will coagulate tissue, but, due to its toxicity, I believe it should be limited, if used at all, to the ointment preparation for the emergency treatment of small burns and scalds. Alcohol, which is an excellent esclarotic, I reserve for the treatment of minor burns. Here I feel it is of considerable value.

At this point, I wish to call your attention to a new group of escharotics, namely, the dyes, but before discussing these, I am first going to briefly consider toxemia. For many years, we have heard about toxic substances originating at the site of burns, circulating through the blood stream, causing elevation of temperature and other symptoms. Robertson and Boyd, in 1923, published an article describing primary and secondary proteoses. Various articles enumerate, in all, about ten or twelve so-called toxic substances. Many feel the evidence in support of the theory of absorption of toxins from the burned area back into the body is indefinite and contradictory. There has never been a constant toxic agent described nor has there been any agreement as to the nature of the toxin or the manner in which it works. The best evidence seems to be based on clinical observation. Recently, Underhill and Kapsinow repeated the work of Robertson and Boyd, injecting an extract of burned skin into an animal and producing toxemia. By the same technic, however, they made an extract of normal skin and obtained the same results. On further analysis, they found the extract according to the original technic contained alcohol. As a control, therefore, they injected a like amount of alcohol into the experimental animal and got the same toxic results that they obtained from both the burned and normal skin. They concluded, therefore, that Robertson and Boyd's results were due to the alcohol. Underhill has injected whole blood from a burned patient into an animal and produced no toxicity. Harrison and Blalock grafted burned skin into a fresh wound on a normal dog and didn't produce toxemia. Later, Underhill, Hapsinow and Fisk injected methylene blue and another dye into burned animals and found the dyes rapidly went into the edema fluid but did not go back into the blood stream to any significant extent. They also injected five times the lethal dose of strychnine about the burned area and found no symptoms of poisoning in the animal. They concluded that, due to the change in capillary permeability, the body fluid shifted from within outward and that if methylene blue and strychnine could not get back into the body, how could some vague toxin be absorbed in sufficient quantity to account for the so-called toxemia of burns. Neither can we attribute toxemia to blood concentration. This is evidenced by the fact that fluids can be kept up to a normal level by watching the blood chlorides and hemoglobin, and yet symptoms of toxemia will appear.

It was in 1929 that Aldrich of Boston and Firor of Johns Hopkins University, because they were impressed by the fact that there was enough infection present in all large superficial burns to account for the symptoms of toxemia, began an investigation along this line. They were also impressed with the fact that practically no work had been done on the bacteriology of burns. They, therefore, took careful repeated cultures from burned areas and from the fluid under the blisters. In the first twelve hours, as a rule, they got no growth. After the first twelve hour period, it was found that in 100 per cent of patients severely burned and a large majority of those with minor burns, a growth of hemolytic streptococc was found. The concentration of these organisms paralleled the increase in the signs of sepsis from the beginning of the toxic stage of the patient. At the end of forty-eight to fifty-six hours pure cultures were obtained and the organisms had outgrown all others. It is the opinion of Aldrich and Firor that a burn is a large open surgical lesion bathed in virulent pus. Moorhead has defined a burn as, "an infected wound due to heat." It is interesting that the general condition of an untreated burned patient has a course similar to many widespread hemolytic streptococcus infections. Additional evidence was obtained from blood cultures of patients after the toxic stage had started. These showed the same strain of streptococcus as was found on the burned surface. In fatal cases, cultures from the heart blood and lungs also revealed streptococcus hemolyticus. Davidson felt that tannic acid rendered the toxic substance in a burn non-absorbable, but Aldrich feels that the power of tannic acid lies in the formation of an eschar over a practically sterile burn and sealing of the burn, which prevents fluid loss and further contamination. Davidson also pointed out that the general condition of the patient depended on the condition of the eschar. The condition of the patient was good as long as the eschar remained dry. You have probably had the experience of having most large burns treated with tannic acid eventually become infected. These facts and the theory of infection caused Aldrich and Firor to look for a new escharotic which, at the same time, would prevent an infection. Such a substance, of course, would have to be non-toxic when used in large quantities for extensive burns. After considerable search they began to use gentian violet, which would not allow Gram-positive streptococci to grow even in the presence of proteins and could be used in large quantities. You, undoubtedly, have all used gentian violet in such infections as: impetigo, indolent ulcers, and certain ear conditions. The dye is not only an antiseptic, specific for streptococcus hemolyticus but also reacts with the superficial burned skin to form a light, tough, flexible eschar. The eschar is more apt to remain dry, and, what is more important, the patient is free from sepsis. Gentian violet is used the same as tannic acid, namely by the spray method. It can be applied every fifteen minutes to one-half hour and my experience with it has been very favor-

able. Aldrich later found that it had one weakness, namely, that it was not a specific against Gram-negative organisms, which enter burns secondarily. He then tried to find some one substance that would be highly antiseptic against both Gram-negatives and Gram-positives and would have the power of escharosis as well as being non-toxic when used for extensive burns. A search through the anilin dyes, as well as the azos and chloramids failed to reveal the answer. He therefore settled upon a mixture of gentian violet, brilliant green and neutral acriflavine as the answer to his problem. He uses gentian violet, three parts by weight; brilliant green two parts by weight; neutral acriflavine, one part by weight. Two grams of this mixture, commonly known as the Aldrich dye mixture, are dissolved in 100 c.c. of water and used in the same manner as gentian violet. Briefly, the patient is placed under a cradle and when shock is under control the local treatment is begun. Aldrich does not believe soap and water preparation is necessary with the dyes. Blisters are opened and loose shreds of epidermis are trimmed away. If ointments and oils were used before admission, these are removed by patting the burns gently with an ether sponge. Personally, I still use soap and water also, but heartily believe that if extensive debridement is necessary the patient should be put to sleep with nitrous oxide. The dye is then sprayed on and after it dries another coat is applied. This process is kept up until a good eschar is obtained. Pain usually disappears after the second application. Once the eschar is formed no further dye treatment is necessary unless the burn becomes secondarily infected. This is true, particularly in children where the eschar is torn off or in burns near the orifices. The eschar should be inspected every day, soft areas excised, and the dye reapplied rather than antiseptic solutions as in the case of similar situations with tannic acid. It should be kept in mind that softening of the eschar is not always due to infection in either the tannic acid or dye treatment. Necrosis from pressure and melting of fat from heat can also cause soft areas. It is the experience of all who have used the dye method that softening under the eschar due to infection is not nearly as frequent as in the case of tannic acid. In general, the advantages of the dyes over tannic acid is that the eschar with dyes is thin and pliable and is therefore more comfortable and less liable to crack and allow secondary contamination. There is little if any antiseptic value in tannic acid, whereas the dyes are specific for the bacteria found in burns. This, in turn, lessens the number of pockets of infection so common in tannic acid treatment. It is a well established fact that tannic acid, although it will not affect normal skin with the cornified layer present, will kill the prickle cell and germinal layers if this layer is absent. This retards epithelization and increases the likelihood of the need for skin grafting. The dyes, on the other hand, do not kill any of the skin layers. For the same reason, the chance of scar formation is lessened. Both methods, however, have the common properties of saving lives by sealing off the capillary bed and thereby reducing shock, allaying pain, simplifying the care of extensive burns and reducing the number of dressings required.

For those who question the use of dyes alone, I find two methods of combining them with tannic acid being used. The burned surface is prepared as usual. In one method, the surface is first sprayed or painted with a 2 per cent aqueous solution of gentian violet. After drying, the tannic acid spray is used until an eschar is formed. The other method incorporates a 2 per cent aqueous solution of gentian violet in 10 per cent tannic acid. This solution is used as tannic acid or gentian violet alone. I have used both these methods more than the gentian violet alone or the newer so-called Aldrich mixture, which has only recently come to my attention. The only objection I find to the dyes is staining of the bed linen, but this is no worse than with mercurochrome and some of the other antiseptics we have all used.

Occasionally, an extensive burn comes to the surgeon which has been poorly treated or not treated at all and has survived the stages of shock. Infection is the paramount issue in these cases and it is best taken care of locally by clearing up the infection as rapidly as possible with saline or Dakin's compresses. In addition, it has occurred to me that if the toxic stage of burns is due to a streptococcus hemolytic infection, and I believe it is, the surgeon might treat cases with prontylin or any other brand of sulfanilamide. This is merely a suggestion as I haven't had much experience with the drug in this type of case and I can find no mention of it in the literature to date.

Concerning healing of extensive burns, there seem to be two procedures where escharotics are used. One method is to leave the eschar alone until it falls away, epithelization having been completed under it. The other method hastens this process by the early removal of the eschar and stimulation of granulation tissue and epithelization by other means. As granulation tissue is not ready for grafting for three or four weeks, I recommend the eschar be left alone until this time has passed, unless it comes away before. No harm is done in removing small areas of eschar for inspection purposes before this time, however. If one decides to go ahead, and each case is an individual one, the tannic acid eschar must be cut away, whereas the dye eschar can be easily loosened by saline compresses and then peeled off. In small areas a stimulating ointment can be used such as scarlet red alone or in combination with oxyquinolin. Epithelization can be promoted also, and I am personally impressed with thioglycerol for this purpose. In large burned areas grafting is eventually necessary, and I feel the sooner it is done, the better from the economic standpoint alone. Preparation of the area for grafting is a personal matter as a rule, but I feel Dakin's pack for twenty-four hours followed by saline packs is a very effective method. Here again, the method of grafting is a personal one with most surgeons and I will not go into it. Generally speaking, small full-thickness grafts seem to be the most popular.

The indications for skin grafting in burns are:
1. To cut down the size of the lesion.
2. To fill in areas when the burn has become indolent in its ability to spread epithelium.
3. To stimulate the spread of epithelium from the periphery of a burn.
4. To prevent contractures, especially over the flexor surfaces and where there are folds in crevices and motion.

In general, early skin grafting is indicated to cover with epithelium as much of the burned surface as possible and cut down the size of the burned area as soon as possible. Late skin grafting is used to complete epithelization where nature is slow, or to prevent disability from contractures.

There are a few general considerations in the treatment of extensively burned patients that I might mention in closing. The patient should be placed in the best position to prevent con-

22

tractures. This is especially true in burns about the neck, axilla and flexor surfaces of the extremities. Competent nursing care is very essential and the patient should be kept in the best mental attitude. Food should be adequate. Carbohydrates should be pushed where the metabolism is increased due to fever. All the vitamins are necessary and especially vitamin "C," if there is infection. Secondary anemia, which is common in extensive burns, should be watched for and taken care of by the administration of iron. Lastly, I wish to remind you that two-thirds of the body sulphur is in the skin. It is a clinical fact that patients on a high sulphur intake grow epithelium faster than those on a sulphur-deficient diet. This need is taken care of by adding two or three eggs to the daily diet.

Bibliography

Aldrich, R. H.: Personal communication.
Aldrich, R. H.: The rôle of infection in burns. New England Jour. Med., 208:299, 1933.
Bettman, Adalbert G.: The tannic acid silver nitrate treatment of burns. Northwest Med., 34:46, (Feb.) 1935. Also Surg., Gyn. and Obst., 62:458, (Feb.) 1936.
Coakley, Walter A.: Burns. Amer. Jour. Surg., 46:50, (April) 1937.
Coan, Glen L.: Ferric chloride coagulation in treatment of burns; with résumé of tannic acid treatment. Surg. Gyn. and Obst., 61:687, (Nov.) 1935.
Crile, George J.: The treatment of burns. Med. Clin. of No. Am., 19:1941, (May) 1936.
Davis, J. S., and Kitlowski, E. A.: The treatment of old un-healed burns. Ann. Surg., 97:648, 1933.
Loehr, W.: The treatment of extensive superficial first, second and third degree burns with cod liver oil. Chirurg., 6:265, 1934.
Mason, James: An evaluation of tannic acid treatment. Ann. Surg., 97:641, 1933.
Mason, Robert L.: Preoperative and postoperative treatment. Saunders, 1937.
McClure, Roy D., and Allen, Clyde L.: Davidson tannic acid treatment of burns; ten years results. Am. Jour. Surg., 28:370, (May) 1935.
Pack, George T., and Davis, A. Hobson: Burns. Philadelphia. J. B. Lippincott Co., 1930.
Penberthy, Grover C.: Treatment of burns. New England Jour. Med., 214:306, (Feb.) 1936.
Penberthy, Grover C.: Tannic acid treatment of burns. Jour. Mich. State. Med. Soc., 34:1, (Jan.) 1935.
Penberthy and Weller: Complications associated with the treatment of burns. Am. Jour. Surg., 26:124, 1934.
Ritter, H. H.: Burns. Am. Jour. Surg., 31:48, 1936.
Robe, John J.: Treatment of cellulitis, suppuration and burns. British Med. Jour., 1:466 (March) 1935.
Steel, John P.: The cod liver oil treatment of wounds. Lancet, 229:290, (Aug. 10) 1935.
Taylor, Frederic: The misuse of tannic acid. Jour. Am. Med. Assn., 106:1144, (April) 1936.
Turner, A. C.: Contribution to treatment of burns. British Med. Jour., 2:995, (Nov.) 1935.
Weaver, Don: Burns—their treatment. Cal. and Western Med. 41:222, (Oct.) 1934.
Wilson, W. C.: Modern methods in the treatment of burns. Practitioner, 136:394, (April) 1936.
Wilson, W. C., Rowley, G. D., and Gray, N. A.: Acute tox-emia of burns. Extract of suprarenal cortex. Lancet, 1:1400, 1936.

CERTAIN DERANGEMENTS OF THE KNEE JOINT*

C. C. CHATTERTON, M.D., F.A.C.S.

Saint Paul, Minnesota

IN dealing with the subject it will be quite impossible to consider more than briefly injuries that take place in and around the knee joint. We must reflect on the anatomy and physiology of the knee joint, discuss the symptoms and treatment and briefly the methods of disability rating. Personally, I like very much to consider disabilities of the knee joint in two classes, based on the clinical history: (1) disabilities that are likely to cause locking of the knee joint; (2) disabilities that do not cause locking of the knee joint.

The anatomy and physiology of the knee joint.—The knee joint is more than a hinge joint. It is a so-called gliding joint because with its power of flexion of 135° it also has a rotary power of 45° to 60° and a lateral motion usually of about 5°.

Because of the great freedom of motion controlled principally by muscular and ligamentous restriction, the knee joint is not well adapted to stand stress and strain, especially rotary strain. In fact, rotation is not well controlled until the knee is in full extension, when the bony anatomy with the power of the quadriceps extensor holds the knee joint stable. Muscle control through the quadriceps extensor is the most important mechanism in maintaining stability of the knee joint, and muscle defense is the first buffer to stress and strain. After muscle defense is overcome, the ligaments and capsule next come into play, and extreme continuous force may stretch or tear the ligaments themselves or from their bony attachments, allowing extreme motion of the joint with resulting injury to the cartilage, the menisci, synovial lining, the fat pads, and the ligamenta alaria.

The lateral ligaments and capsule control lateral motion, except when the knee is in full extension. The crucial ligaments control the extreme anterior and posterior motion.

The semilunar cartilages by their shape tend

*Presented before the annual meeting of the Minnesota State Medical Association, Saint Paul, Minnesota, May 5, 1937.

to deepen the tibial tuberosities and make compensation through their slight motion for a better fit between the condyles of the femur and tibia, and it is believed that they also act as the spreaders of synovial lubrication and help prevent friction. The semilunar cartilages are maintained in position by the coronary ligament to which they are attached.

Abnormal Conditions Which May Produce Locking in the Knee Joint

1. Injury to the cartilages (menisci), external or internal.
2. Loose bodies or joint mice.
3. Slipping patella.
4. Damage to the fat pad.
5. Fracture of the tibial spine.

1. *Injuries to the Cartilage (external or internal meniscus).*—The type of injury may be a tear or split of a portion of the cartilage with or without tags: the entire cartilage may be dislocated into the intercondyloid notch, the so-called bucket handle type of injury; or the cartilage may be torn at the attachment of the coronary ligament, which may cause extreme freedom of motion to the cartilage so it can be displaced, causing locking of the knee joint without actual fracture or damage of the cartilage itself. The meniscus has no blood supply except at the junction with the coronary ligament, and actual repair of an injury to the meniscus proper usually does not take place.

The anterior portion of the meniscus is most subject to injury and most defects are found in the anterior half of the meniscus. It has been my experience that the internal cartilage is damaged in the ratio of approximately fifteen to one compared with the external cartilage.

The mechanism producing an injury to the cartilage is usually lateral strain or rotary strain or a combination of both, and along with any severe cartilage injury we frequently expect to find injury to the lateral ligaments.

The history of injury may be of severe trauma or the condition may occur after minor stress such as assuming a squatting position. The diagnosis of damage to the cartilage after one single injury is difficult, but after recovery from swelling and inflammation, and with a history of repeated catches and localized pain along the edge of the cartilage plus the so-called positive

Jones test (pain on making pressure over the cartilage and extension of the knee), negative x-rays which exclude loose bodies, dislocated patella, surgical inspection of the knee joint is warranted. The external cartilage frequently gives, with other findings, a musical sound or click upon examination. Recently Steindler has found that auscultation of the joint may be of value in diagnosing internal derangements of the knee joint, especially those of the cartilage.

2. *Loose Bodies.*—Loose bodies found in joints are usually composed of bone and cartilage and are most frequently associated with two conditions: (1) osteochondritis dissecans, which is a separation of a small amount of bone and cartilage from the articular surface; and (2) osteochondromatosis or synovial enchondromatosa. Rarely a loose body may result from breaking off of a hypertrophic spur in osteoarthritis or after a fracture of the joint surface, or from an organization of clots of fibrin forming rice bodies in the joint.

There are several theories as to the cause of *osteochondritis dissecans.* Many feel that, because of its usual location at the site of greatest stress and strain, trauma is the sole cause. Fat or bacterial embolism is thought by some to be a causative factor. Low grade arthritis or a variant of arthritis deformans is considered by others as a predisposing cause.[1]

The symptoms of trouble in the knee joint may be noted long before the actual separation of the loose body, which may take months or years, but after the body has become separated the spasmodic locking of the joint due to the mechanical interference of free motion in the joint is quite conclusive for diagnosis. In many cases it is possible by x-ray examination to discover the punched out area before the loose body has formed, and removal of the affected area at that time may prevent the formation of a number of bodies.

Osteochondromatosis is usually easily diagnosed by the roentgen ray because of the large number of loose bodies seen. Some are bone, some are cartilage, many are pediculated, many free and they usually pack the joint and mechanically block free motion of the joint and produce locking. The real cause of osteochondromatosis is unknown, but trauma and infection seem to be the likely causative agents.

24

3. *Slipping Patella.*—While external slipping of the patella cannot be classed as a true internal derangement of the knee joint, as this condition often produces a painful twinge and occasionally definite locking, I feel that the discussion here with conditions that produce similar symptoms is proper.

This condition is seen in children and women much more frequently than in men, and because cartilage injuries are rare in children, the diagnosis after careful analysis and description is usually quite easy. Slipping patella may be unilateral or bilateral and is usually associated with a mild knock-knee and in young individuals who have unusual freedom of joints. Something occurs in the knee that temporarily restricts the motion, is usually quite painful and at the same time it is noted that the patella has assumed a position on the outer side of the knee joint. There may be an instant of restriction of motion or the knee may remain locked until manipulation releases the patella. The accident is usually followed by a period of swelling and pain about the knee.

4. *Damage to Retropatellar Fat Pad.*—This condition is quite frequently seen in middle age. My experience is that the diagnosis of injury to the cartilage has been made and upon exposure of the joint the fat pad is found to be abnormal in shape, inflamed, thickened and in such position that it could easily interfere with the mechanical motion of the knee joint. It is indeed difficult to make a positive diagnosis of locking of the joint due to the fat pad until after exposure of the joint.

5. *Fracture of the Anterior Tibial Spine* or the anterior portion of the tibia may lock the knee joint and prevent extension. X-ray studies will at once show the bone block and demonstrate the pathological condition and the diagnosis in this injury is not usually difficult.

Disabilities That Do Not Cause Locking

1. Rupture of the lateral ligaments.
2. Rupture of the crucial ligaments.
3. Fracture of the patella.

1. *Rupture of the Lateral Ligaments.*—Severe sprains with minor symptoms about the knee joint are most common, but when either of the lateral ligaments has been severely damaged,

the stability of the knee joint is greatly impaired. Rupture of the internal lateral ligament is caused by overadduction commonly seen in football accidents of line play, clipping and tackling in an open field. The external ligament is frequently injured by accidents producing overabduction.

Sprains of either ligaments are usually only partial tears, and, while there is marked limitation of motion perhaps to a small arc, absolute locking is rare and is usually produced by some internal derangement of the structures of the knee joint.

Swelling, edema, limited arc of motion, localized pain over the external or internal ligaments or their attachments with increased lateral motion are the usual signs and symptoms of ruptured lateral ligaments. It is difficult at the time of injury to evaluate the amount of injury or tear to the ligaments, but with continued abnormal lateral motion, enough to disable the patient, an attempt to repair the damaged part should be made.

2. *Rupture of the Crucial Ligaments.*—Damage to the crucial ligaments may be caused by a combination of the same force and mechanism that causes damage to the cartilages. Usually torsion is necessary along with hyperabduction and adduction, to rupture both crucial ligaments. Rupture of the anterior crucial ligament allows forward gliding of the tibia on the femur, and when the posterior ligament is ruptured the tibia can be pushed backward, and if both are backward. This condition causes a feeling of ruptured there is great instability of the tibia as it may easily be pushed well forward and insecurity or giving way of the knee joint, but true locking is absent. Tenderness is found over the spine of the tibia with injury to the anterior crucial ligament, and just below and to the inner side of the patella upon flexion when the posterior crucial is damaged. Usually in this condition the lateral ligaments also are damaged, giving the objective and subjective findings of a relaxed, unstable knee joint.

3. *Fracture of the Patella.*—Fracture of the patella, complete or partial, may cause marked instability to the knee joint. If the fracture is complete the loss of ability to extend the knee is present. True locking is not seen, but swelling and injury to the soft parts may materially

affect the range of motion. The diagnosis of fractured patella is usually easy with the roentgen ray. Usually there is pain on attempting extension of the knee joint, with the point of tenderness over the injured patella.

Treatment

The old dictum that the knee joint should be opened with caution still holds good. Infection after operation is a surgical catastrophe, usually resulting in ankylosis or perhaps an even more serious result. But we feel that the knee joint has resisting powers against infection greater than was formerly realized, and infection even after frequent opening of joints is relatively uncommon.

If, after an accident, diagnosis is not certain, it is much better to wait and treat symptomatically, giving the joint a chance to recover spontaneously. Then if symptoms return at least a tentative diagnosis can be made and operation considered.

The danger of an unstable joint which at any time may give way, causing the patient to fall, cannot in the city dweller or in any individual be lightly dismissed. Repeated injuries, with internal derangement to the joint, may also cause degenerative changes quite as damaging to the function of the joint as the original injury.

When operation is considered, I feel that the patient should present himself at the hospital at least twenty-four hours previous to the operation, and should have a normal white count, normal temperature, and be free from demonstrable infection. The leg, thigh and knee should be carefully clipped and painted with merthiolate or 3 per cent iodin, after a soap, water and ether bath, and a sterile towel bandaged over the knee. In the operating room the application of merthiolate or iodin is repeated and the leg and thigh is carefully draped in such a manner that flexion and rotary motion of the knee joint can be performed.

Nothing should enter the knee joint except the instruments, unhandled gauze or small cotton pledgets; never the gloved finger. The choice of incision depends upon the type of operation considered, and in any knee joint condition the operator may find it necessary to inspect the knee through more than one incision. The small curved incision lateral to the patella gives

wonderful exposure to the anterior knee joint compartment, and the posterior exposure of Henderson and others will expose the posterior compartment satisfactorily. Lateral incisions are very valuable, but the lateral ligaments are to be avoided as much as possible. Upon opening the knee joint one is greatly relieved if the findings exposed prove the diagnosis. Apparently normal on the first inspection, the joint must be carefully explored, the cartilages pulled and moved about and search made for tags, splits and tears, the fat pad examined, the crucial ligaments, examination for loose bodies, and the defect in the cartilage from which they came. Often the anterior portion of the internal cartilage must be removed from its insertion and pulled forward to discover injury to the posterior portion of the cartilage. Some recommend entire removal of the cartilage if damaged. It has been our experience that if the anterior two-thirds or anterior three-fifths, especially if the cartilage is damaged in this portion, be removed, the symptoms will be relieved. If the cartilages prove to be absolutely normal or are found to be freely movable, I hesitate to remove them because of this free motion alone. The fat pad, which may be enlarged, red and inflamed, should be carefully examined, especially with the absence of damage to other internal tissues of the joint. Enlarged portions of the pad are removed freely with careful control of the hemorrhage usually found after cutting this pad.

Damage to the Tibial Tubercle.—If the tibial tubercle is loose, it is sutured into place by the method of Lee.[2]

Usually the crater in osteochondritis dissecans is carefully saucerized to prevent formation of new loose bodies in the joint, that is if the knee joint proper is opened. If the loose body is removed by incision through the pouch, the area of origin is not treated. Many condemn the refraining from treatment of the crater in osteochondritis dissecans, but I personally have simply removed loose bodies in this condition without new bodies forming and without further trouble to the patient.

Treatment of Injuries to Ligaments.—Following injuries to either or both of the ligaments, full extension of the knee joint should be main-

26

tained for at least three to four weeks without motion, and the limb held in a rigid apparatus. The apparatus should be of such character, however, that it can be removed so that massage and manipulation and contraction of the quadriceps extensor tendon can be a daily procedure. After removal of the rigid apparatus, a hinge splint or cage splint may be used for two or three months, and then a heavy, soft bandage can be used for protection. If the point of rupture can be demonstrated at the time of injury, early suture of the ligament is indicated, but if after usual care stability does not return, repair of the ligament is demanded.

Repair of Ligaments.—The internal lateral ligament is usually repaired by the use of the tendons of the gracilis and the semitendinosus muscle, freeing them from their insertion, bringing them forward and cutting them at the level of the attachment of the ligament on the condyle of the femur and either suturing or holding them with a metal staple in a groove made in the condyle. The free tendons are sutured to the tendon of the sartorius so the muscle power of these tendons is not lost. The Mauck method of suture or removing the tibial attachment and suturing the flap of bone down on the tibia seems worthy of trial in cases in which there is not a complete rupture of the ligament.[3] There are many other operations for repair of the lateral ligaments.

The external lateral ligament is usually repaired by using a tube of fascia lata, attaching it to the external condyle of the femur in a small bone cavity, pulling it down along the course of the lateral ligament and suturing it to the head of the fibula under strong tension.

Rupture of the Crucial Ligaments.—Operations for repair of crucial ligaments are rare because repair or a fair degree of stability returns after conservative treatment. Like treatment for lateral ligaments, prolonged immobilization in the greater number of cases brings satisfactory results. If, in spite of the usual conservative treatment, marked instability is present due to rupture of the anterior or posterior crucial ligaments, operation may be contemplated. Most of the operations are copied after the procedure made standard by Hey Groves, that is the use of a strip of fascia lata inserted to take the place

of the ruptured ligament. Recently Cubbins and Campbell have perhaps improved the original plan to perfect treatment in this serious injury.[4]

Slipping Patella.—Habitual outward dislocation of the patella is as disabling as other derangements of the knee joint and may prevent the individual from competing in sports or doing manual labor. The old method of Goldthwaite in transferring the tibial tubercle with the attached patellar tendon to the inner side of the tibia is a tried and known procedure. In young children and in adolescents my operation of choice has been reefing of the internal capsule of the knee joint with a strip of fascia attached to the patella and the internal condyle of the femur, the so-called Mouchet operation. Recently Ober has observed an abnormal relationship between the iliotibial band and the patella and concludes that recurrent dislocation of the patella is a mild congenital displacement of the patella. He uses a flap of this band after dissecting loose from above the patella and suturing it through a small tunnel cut into the inner side of the tibia. The operation relieves the pathological anatomy and supplies a tendon which maintains the normal position of the patella.[5]

Fractured Patella—Fracture of the patella with separation requires an operation. Some suture only the capsule, others suture the bone, and a combination of the two methods may be used. Fascia, wire, Kangaroo tendon, and heavy chromic catgut may be the choice of materials used as sutures. Chip or split fractures or comminuted fractures without misplacement are often treated and successfully by apparatus.

Postoperative Treatment

After inspecting a joint for a loose body or removal of a cartilage, care should be taken in closing the wound layer by layer, synovia fascia, capsule fascia and skin. A dry dressing, covered by many layers of sheet wadding, is held in place by a bandage and supported by adhesive. Motion is not restricted and after three or four days is encouraged. Weight bearing is usually allowed after seven days, stitches are removed on the eighth day, and the patient leaves the hospital on the tenth or twelfth day. A soft supporting bandage is worn for two weeks more. Motion is encouraged, and heat and gentle massage along with active motion may be given for a week or ten days after the hospital discharge with advantage to the patient.

Treatment After Injuries to Lateral Ligaments, crucial ligaments, slipping patella, or evulsion of the tibial spine, requires absolute fixation usually with a splint or a bivalved cast. About the eighth day the stitches may be removed and the retentive apparatus removed for massage, baking and contraction of the quadriceps extensor tendon, except in the case of fracture of the patella. Absolute fixation is necessary in soft parts injuries for at least three or four weeks, followed by supportive apparatus. In bony injuries six to eight weeks or even more of fixation are necessary followed by supportive apparatus. In either case gentle massage and manipulation over the ligaments and soft parts is indicated early.

The Evaluation of Disability after an injury to a knee joint in Minnesota is enumerated in percentage of loss of function of the limb as a whole. A given percentage of loss of function after injury in any case is largely a personal opinion, as evidenced by the frequent discussions before the Industrial Commission. Percentage of disability depends upon the finder's analysis of any given case, usually upon the function of the injured member.

Bibliography

1. Campbell, Willis C.: Orthopedic Surgery. Philadelphia: W. B. Saunders Co., p. 306, 1930.
2. Lee, Harold G.: Avulsion fracture to the tibial attachments of the crucial ligaments by operative procedure. Jour. Bone and Joint Surg., 19:460-468, (April) 1937.
3. Mauck, H. P.; New operative procedure for instability of the knee. Jour. Bone and Joint Surg., 18:984-990, (Oct.) 1936.
4. Cubbins, Wm. R.: Cruciate ligament injuries. Surg., Gyn. and Obst., 64:218-225, (Feb. 1) 1937.
5. Ober, F. R.: Slipping patella or recurrent dislocation of the patella. Jour. Bone and Joint Surg., 17:774-779, (July) 1935.

AN IMPROVED TREATMENT FOR OS CALCIS FRACTURES*

O. W. YOERG, M.D.

Minneapolis, Minnesota

BY the use of a method evolved about three years ago we have been able to obtain improved anatomic as well as functional results and, in the ordinary type of os calcis fracture, have been able to return men to work within three months from the time of reduction. In the more severe injuries, particularly those in which there has been a crushing of the posterior joint surface and in which the heel has been driven up and the angle either lessened or lost, convalescence has been slightly increased. But in most of these cases the men have been returned to work within four or five months from the time of reduction.

The method that we are employing consists of manually disimpacting the fracture, bringing the heel down by pulling the sole of the foot, with a sudden thrust, against a firm vertical bar, and the use of an os calcis compression clamp to overcome the broadening of the heel and to replace the loosened bones to their normal or near normal position; this followed by the application of a well molded boot cast.

In a patient with a fracture of the os calcis, the usual lateral and plantar dorsal films are made, and, in addition, an antero-posterior view is taken to visualize the anterior portion of the os calcis. He is then put to bed with the foot elevated, and hot packs employed to aid in the reduction of the swelling and to lessen his pain. Reduction can usually be made in four or five days or a week. Occasionally ten days are necessary but never more than two weeks are allowed to elapse before reduction is attempted.

We anesthetize the patient with a general anesthetic to obtain complete relaxation of the muscles of the leg. The patient is placed on the affected side so that the foot can be brought to the edge of the table, with the heel extended over the edge.

The foot and ankle are now firmly held by the left hand, and with the right hand the heel is manipulated laterally, with repeated thrusts, until the fracture has been thoroughly disimpacted.

*Presented with motion picture and x-ray slides, before the annual meeting of the Minnesota State Medical Association, Saint Paul, Minnesota, May 5, 1937.

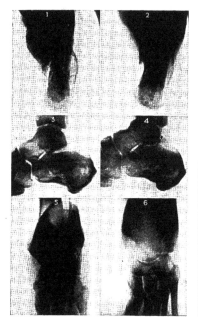

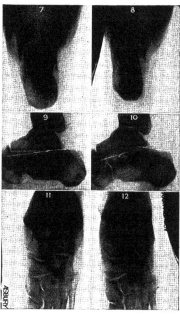

Case 1.—P.S.L., aged fifty-nine, a grain elevator foreman, fell October 13, 1936, a distance of ten feet from a ladder, sustaining a fracture of his right os calcis. Reduction was made October 18 and the cast was removed November 20. The patient began to walk on his foot December 12. He returned to light work February 18, 1937, and to regular work March 15. There is a slight limitation of motion in the sub-astragalar joint.

Fig. 1. Plantar dorsal view shows extensive fracture with lateral displacement of the tuberosity.

Fig. .2. The fracture after reduction, lateral displacement corrected.

Fig. 3. Lateral view before reduction. The posterior joint surface of the os calcis is flattened and the carrying angle negative.

Fig. 4. Lateral view after reduction. The fracture is thoroughly disimpacted and the joint surface brought up. The carrying angle is restored to normal.

Fig. 5. Antero-posterior view before reduction shows a fracture into the anterior portion of the os calcis with moderate displacement.

Fig. 6. Antero-posterior view after reduction, displacement corrected.

Case 2.—J. F. Y., aged sixty, subpostoffice superintendent, on December 2, 1936, fell six feet, fracturing his left os calcis. Reduction was made December 8, 1936, and cast was removed January 6, 1937. The patient began to walk with crutches on February 8, 1937. He returned to work on May 2, five months after the injury. He has worked regularly, on his feet at least six hours a day. Motion is excellent and there is no pain in the foot, but the patient states that calf muscles tire toward the end of the day.

Fig. 7. View of tuberosity before reduction shows a comminuted fracture with broadening and shortening.

Fig. 8. Tuberosity after reduction. The broadening has been overcome and the bone lengthened.

Fig. 9. Laterial view before reduction shows a crushing of the posterior joint surface with the carrying angle zero.

Fig. 10. The posterior joint surface of the os calcis has been brought up, and the angle restored to normal.

Fig. 11. Antero-posterior view shows the front of the os calcis and astragalus, the scaphoid and the cuboid. The anterior portion of the os calcis has been fractured into the os calcis cuboid joint with marked displacement outward under the external malleolus.

Fig. 12. Antero-posterior view after reduction. The fracture of the anterior portion of the os calcis has been reduced and the external malleolus is now clear.

Any upward displacement of the os calcis is corrected by grasping the heel with one hand, the forward portion of the foot with the other hand, and then pulling the sole of the foot with a sudden thrust against a vertical bar. The broadened but now loosened bones are squeezed into place with an os calcis clamp. All of the procedures are done with the knee flexed and the foot in plantar flexion.

A well molded boot cast is applied, with foot in full plantar flexion. Constant traction on the heel is used while the cast is molded under the malleoli, over the back of the heel and under the arch of the foot.

After reduction and the application of the cast the patient is placed in bed, with the foot elevated. He is kept in bed for three or four days, or until his pain has disappeared. Many of these patients, in spite of the fact that the fracture is forcibly manipulated, have little or no pain following reduction. When pain has subsided and we feel that there is no more likelihood of pull from the calf muscles, the patient is allowed to be up and about, using his crutches. He is discharged from the hospital, but is not allowed weight-bearing on the injured foot.

Four weeks after reduction the patient returns and the cast removed. Radiographs will show union taking place and that it is sufficiently strong so that a cast is no longer necessary. The patient is then instructed to massage and actively and passively move the boot and ankle. Particularly is he instructed to evert and invert the foot to bring about a return of motion in the subas-tragalar joint. He continues this massage and manipulation for the period of four weeks but is not allowed weight-bearing. He returns again at the end of four weeks, or two months after reduction. The radiographs then taken will show that union is firm. He is allowed to walk on the injured foot, using his crutches. In the ordinary type of fracture he does so with little or no pain, and, in a few days or a week, in most instances, will discard his crutches and walk without support.

We have now treated by this method thirty-one patients with os calcis fractures, three being bilateral. Of these, twenty-two have been restored to working capacity: five were returned to work in two and one-half months from the time of reduction, eight in three months, six in four months and three in five months.

We have one failure, in a railway mail-clerk, who fell from a ladder, a distance of twenty feet, and sustained a severe crushing fracture of the os calces of both feet. This was one of the early cases, before we pulled the heel over the vertical bar. I thought at the time we had obtained a good reduction, but I see now that we did not completely reduce the fractures. His right heel is practically well as far as pain is concerned; his left heel still causes him trouble. He has not returned to work but has been working in his yard four or five hours a day, with some pain but not enough to keep him from working.

The accompanying illustrations of two selected cases show the fracture before and after the reposition of the bones by this method.

PHYSICAL THERAPY IN RELATION TO INDUSTRIAL MEDICINE*

FRANK H. KRUSEN, M.D.

Rochester, Minnesota

PHYSICAL therapy, applied intelligently under direct medical supervision, may be of great value in hastening the rehabilitation of those injured in industry. Kessler has pointed out that the end-results of industrial accidents "should be appraised not on the basis of structural changes but on disturbed function." It is in the restoration of function that the use of physical measures is most effective. Some idea of the extensiveness of industrial injuries may be obtained from the estimate of Newquist, who said there were 16,000 accidental occupation deaths during 1935. Of course, the number who were merely maimed or injured were many times this amount.

For the most part, it becomes the duty of the medical practitioner to restore injured wor-

*From the Section on Physical Therapy, The Mayo Clinic, Rochester, Minnesota. Read before the annual meeting of the Minnesota State Medical Association, Saint Paul, Minnesota, May 5, 1937.

men to remunerative employment as soon as possible. Shinn has said of industrial medicine that: "Its purpose is to insure good health and prevent injuries, thereby promoting contentment, alleviating suffering and increasing the life span of man. It further deals with the rehabilitation of diseased and injured persons in an effort to insure them a livelihood." It cannot be stressed too strongly that there is great need for all physicians to be familiar with the best and simplest methods of treating the injured workman. As Sir John Simon has put it, "Measures, whether voluntary or compulsory, for the prevention of industrial disease and ill-health depend primarily on the knowledge, skill and coöperation of the medical profession." The objective to be attained in the treatment of all those injured in industry is the return of the involved worker to normal working status in the shortest possible time. This should be desired by the physician and the injured worker, as well as by the employer.

The chief sphere of usefulness of physical therapy in industrial injuries lies in the treatment of the large group of cases in which there has been trauma to bones, joints, muscles, nerves or skin. Hastening of restoration of articular function is one of the most important phases of this work. Another important contribution of physical therapy is in the rehabilitation of the badly maimed worker, who must be reëducated to make the best use of his limited physical capabilities. Frequently, a properly graduated routine, including surgical treatment, physical therapy, occupational therapy, the sheltered workshop, and a new type of remunerative occupation suited to the handicapped patient's limited ability, will make a happy, useful citizen and worker of a potentially permanent invalid.

Occupational therapy which plays an important part in this transition is a form of physical treatment, and properly administered under medical supervision it will aid greatly not only in restoring function but also in improving the patient's morale. Odencrantz has said: "Anything that can be done to help the handicapped build up his confidence, his morale and his ability, increases his opportunity for satisfactory adjustment."

Because of certain psychic factors which enter into the problem of the injured worker, it is essential that all phases of treatment, and particu-

ularly the details of physical therapy, be under direct supervision. No opportunity should be permitted for prolonging such treatment until it becomes a habit, and under proper medical supervision this will not occur. Physical measures should be used only when and as indicated and only when they are producing definite objective improvement. Likewise, during the application of these treatments there is an opportunity for the highly important personal contact between the physician and the patient. Eckelberry has said: "The injured workman may be just a file with a name and number in the insurance office, another case on the calendar at the hearing, and an interesting case to the doctor; but he is nevertheless a human being, influenced by his emotions, subject to hate, fear, doubt and gratitude, even as you and I. To obtain the best results in his management he should be treated as a human being."

Among the physical agents which may be applied with benefit in treating industrial injuries are heat, light, water, electricity, massage, exercise and occupational therapy. The employment of these physical measures, in their simplest form and under close supervision, frequently at the patient's home, is highly to be desired.

The physician should never write an order to some lay technician to give the patient "some physical therapy." This is just as ridiculous as if he were to write a prescription to a druggist to give the patient "some medicine," and the results are likely to be equally as unsatisfactory. The order which is frequently written for B. M. and E. (baking, massage and exercise) with no detailed instructions is likely to prove equally futile.

The Council on Physical Therapy of the American Medical Association has demonstrated that there are many physical agents which, when employed scientifically, are of great value therapeutically. Unfortunately, many physicians are little acquainted with the proper use of physical agents in treating disease because until very recently this subject was much neglected in the medical schools. At present, the intelligent employment of physical therapy in our hospitals and in private medical practice has done much to combat the charlatan who has attempted to worm his way into industrial medicine as well as other phases of medical practice.

The essentials for proper treatment of industrial injuries by means of physical therapy are: (1) devices for the production of the required physical agents (these should be as simply constructed as possible); (2) a physician skilled in the use of these devices and thoroughly familiar with the effects which they can produce; and (3) in many instances (when the physician does not wish to apply treatments himself) a trained technician who has skilled hands for massage and manipulation and who can also use various apparatus as ordered by the physician.

Light Therapy

Since the early part of the Seventeenth Century, when Isaac Newton discovered that a beam of sunlight could be split by means of a prism into the various primary colors, a series of subsequent discoveries have developed a huge electromagnetic spectrum with varying physical properties which physicians have learned to use in treating disease. Below the red end of Newton's rainbow were found invisible infra-red (heat) rays, and above the violet end were found invisible ultraviolet (chemical rays). Below the infra-red rays are hertzian waves, which physicians now utilize for short-wave diathermy. Above the ultraviolet rays lie the roentgen rays (physical rays whose therapeutic value is familiar to all physicians), and beyond these lie the gamma rays of radium (the therapeutic value of which is also well known).

Today, the injured workman may be instructed to buy a simple heat lamp which will produce either near or far infra-red rays for medical treatment. These infra-red lamps (heated by resistance coils) do not vary greatly from the ordinary household heater with the exception that the latter has a wider reflector which diffuses the heat through the room, while the therapeutic lamp has a more convex reflector which localizes the radiation of heat on the bodily surface. The so-called infra-red units (heated coils or plates) and luminous bulbs (carbon or tungsten filament lamps) may be used in the same convex reflector. The former produce less penetration of heat and more surface heat; the latter produce more hyperemia and slightly more penetration. Large lamps which have big reflectors may be used to treat extensive lesions. For use in the home, a simple home-made baker may be constructed by any tinsmith at a cost of two or three dollars. These various heat

lamps will be found extremely valuable in producing surface hyperemia to relieve the pain of sprains, contusions, fractures, and certain inflammatory lesions.

In indolent wounds and in certain types of ulcerations and lesions of the skin, the ultraviolet rays produced by a mercury quartz or by a carbon arc light may be found useful.

Time does not permit a complete consideration of all the indications for the use of light rays in industrial diseases; nevertheless, many uses are known.

Heat Therapy

One of the simplest and most effective methods of applying heat locally is by means of the paraffin bath. Extremities may be dipped in melted paraffin, a coating of which is left on the part for twenty to thirty minutes. A glove or boot of paraffin is formed, which may be stripped off with ease at the end of treatment. This leaves a marked hyperemia of the skin. The paraffin may be painted on a shoulder, arm or back and later removed, leaving a warm reddened skin which is ideally prepared for massage.

Hydrotherapy

One of the easiest ways of stimulating peripheral circulation is to apply the time-honored contrast baths. These are applied to the extremities, by using buckets or pans as containers for the hot and cold water. If a shoulder or some portion of the trunk is to be treated, an ordinary bath spray may be used to apply hot and cold water alternately to the affected region. This will produce effects comparable to those achieved by immersion contrast baths.

Whirlpool baths (baths of whirling, aerated water at a temperature of 110° F.) are excellent for the auxiliary treatment of fractures, preliminary to massage and therapeutic exercise. These baths may be constructed for a few dollars by any plumber (specifications may be obtained from the Secretary of the Council on Physical Therapy of the American Medical Association).

Recently, underwater exercises have been used not only for the treatment of poliomyelitis but also for the treatment of extensive trauma. The patient is placed in hot water in a specially constructed tub known as a Hubbard tank. In this

32

ot water the muscles usually relax, and massage administered under water during the period of aximal heating. Exercises under the water re readily performed because of its buoyancy nd it is possible to secure activity in all planes.

Electrotherapy

The use of short wave diathermy, although uch exploited, nevertheless must be considered avorably in the treatment of many types of eep trauma to soft tissues. The effects are exlained merely on the basis of heating of the issues, but this heating has been proved to reach o deeper levels than can be obtained by any ther means of application. In most instances, an nduction coil, cuffs, or air-spaced electrodes hould be applied to the area to be treated.

Massage and Corrective Exercise

Stevens in discussing the use of physical therapy in industrial injuries pointed out that by far the most valuable service which such therapy renders is in "the preservation and restoration of joint function." He believed that the technician skilled in massage and manipulation was the "sine qua non of the physical therapy set-up." In this I can heartily concur. I agree also with certain of his conclusions, namely, that "joint restriction can often be prevented by early motion which stimulates rather than hinders repair"; that "the use of apparatus has definite value but only as a preliminary to skillful manipulation at the hands of the physician or welltrained technician"; and that "active use of the part, preferably under the supervision of an occupational therapist, is a necessary supplement to other physical therapy procedures."

Occupational Therapy

Occupational therapy should be administered in conjunction with other physical measures. Devices such as the shoulder loom may be used to hasten the return of articular function in a most agreeable manner. Occupational therapy plays an important part in reëducating those who have been severely maimed in industrial accidents. Stroud has said: "The majority of the

handicapped who may be rehabilitated and placed in industry are those with cardiovascular, arthritic and orthopedic disabilities." He has recommended training in occupational therapy followed by work in sheltered workshops as a means of fitting patients for suitable industrial positions. Eckelberry has said, "One of the greatest aids in rehabilitation is the opportunity for the workman to resume work of a lighter character than his usual job and . . . gradually to approach the same work and activity he enjoyed prior to the accident."

Conclusions

1. The use of physical therapy may be of considerable value in the treatment of industrial injuries.

2. This type of therapy is particularly applicable to the hastening of restoration of function following trauma and to the rehabilitation of the severely handicapped patient.

3. The application of physical measures should be under close medical supervision, and specific instruction concerning treatment should always be given.

4. Many simple physical devices may be utilized in treating industrial injuries; these devices may frequently be constructed for home use.

5. Massage and manipulation must always be performed by skilled hands.

6. Occupational therapy in conjunction with other forms of physical therapy plays an important part in the rehabilitation and return to industry of the severely handicapped worker.

References

1. Eckelberry, N. E.: The injured workman: methods of handling to get him back on the job. Industrial Med., 5:557-560, (Nov.) 1936.
2. Kessler, H. H.: Accidental injuries: their end-results and evaluation. Am. Jour. Surg., 27:155-167, (Jan.) 1935.
3. Newquist, M. M.: Report of 1935 survey of medical services in industry by the American College of Surgeons. Surg., Gynec., and Obst., 62:485-486, (Feb. 15) 1936.
4. Odencrantz, L. C.: Occupational therapy and the placement of the handicapped in industry. Occup. Therap., 14:189-195, (June) 1935.
5. Shinn, H. L.: Industrial medicine. U. S. Nav. Med. Bull., 33:84-96, (Jan.) 1935.
6. Simon, J.: Industrial medicine: introduction. Practitioner, 137:257-259, (Sept.) 1936.
7. Stevens, J. B.: Physical therapy in industrial injuries. New York State Med. Jour., 34:841-844, (Oct. 1) 1934.
8. Stroud, W. D.: The rehabilitation and placement in industry of those handicapped with cardiovascular disease. Jour. Am. Med. Assn., 105:1401-1405, (Nov. 2) 1935.

HYSTERICAL DYSPHAGIA*

HERBERT W. SCHMIDT, M.D.
Rochester, Minnesota

THE most common conditions which cause dysphagia in the superior portion of the esophagus are:

1. Intrinsic lesions of esophagus:
   a. Carcinoma
   b. Benign stricture
   c. Pharyngo-esophageal diverticulum with secondary esophageal stenosis
2. Neurologic lesions:
   a. Bulbar palsy
   b. Amyotrophic lateral sclerosis with bulbar involvement
   c. Infantile paralysis with bulbar involvement
   d. Myasthenia gravis
3. Extrinsic lesions:
   a. Laryngeal lesions
      (1) Inflammatory
      (2) Neoplastic
   b. Tumors of the neck:
      (1) Goiter
      (2) Other tumors
4. Foreign bodies
5. Functional conditions:
   a. Functional dysphagia
   b. Hysterical dysphagia

Hysterical dysphagia was so named by H. S. Plummer, in 1914, because he believed it was a functional disturbance, of a hysterical nature, which involved deglutition.

This syndrome is characterized by a difficulty in swallowing and is associated with a hypochromic anemia; it occurs among women and there is no definite evidence of organic obstruction in the esophagus. The patients describe a dysphagia which begins suddenly, and usually is as pronounced at the onset as at any time in its course. The patients have the greatest difficulty in swallowing solid foods; they say that solid foods will not go past the level of the cricopharyngeus muscle. This difficulty may become extreme. In a recent case that was reported, the patient said that she would strain the juice from strawberry sauce to get rid of the seeds and would dilute and then strain buttermilk to get rid of the curds before ingestion, because she was afraid they would lodge in the upper portion of the esophagus and strangle her. Swallowing of pills and capsules, no matter how small, causes a great deal of trouble. Most of the patients have false teeth, and fissures at the angles of their mouths. There frequently is a glossitis which is associated with atrophy of the lingual papillæ, which

gives the tongue a red, glazed appearance which resembles the type seen in pernicious anemia. In about a third of the cases the spleen is palpable; most of the patients have an achlorhydria. It is felt that the changes in the mucous membrane and the splenomegaly are secondary to the rather severe prolonged dietary restrictions and resulting anemia.

These patients can be cured by passing an esophageal sound into the stomach over a previously swallowed silk thread, and subsequently given a good deal of reassurance. As Dr. Moersch has pointed out, this strengthens the theory that the condition is primarily of a functional nature, since the size of the sound passed is immaterial and the esophagus is not stretched.

Report of Case

The patient was a woman, forty-five years of age, who for about twenty-five years had had more or less difficulty in swallowing food. She said that a "hurting sensation" would develop in the region of the pyriform sinuses, on swallowing. She had deep fissures at the angles of her mouth and a sore tongue which had caused her much anxiety and concern. An anemia had been found ten years previously; the value for the hemoglobin had ranged from 46 to 53 per cent and the number of erythrocytes had varied from 3,-800,000 to 4,360,000 per cubic millimeter of blood. An achlorhydria had been discovered, and the possibility of pernicious anemia and Banti's disease had been considered. She had been placed on a high vitamin, high caloric diet and dilute hydrochloric acid had been administered. This treatment had produced improvement in her general physical condition and blood findings.

In May, 1936, she was seen at the clinic and said that for one year she had had an increase in the difficulty in swallowing, which had become so severe, that she had been unable to swallow aspirin tablets or even small pieces of meat because she had felt that the "opening in her esophagus was simply too small."

Examination disclosed a pale, white woman. She had false teeth, fissures at the angles of her mouth, and a red, smooth, beefy tongue. The value for the hemoglobin was 12.9 gm. per 100 c.c. of blood and there were 4,520,000 erythrocytes in each cubic millimeter of blood. Special blood smears showed nothing diagnostic. She had an absence of free hydrochloric acid in the gastric contents. The spleen was palpable. A rather large adenomatous goiter was present but there was no sign of hyperthyroidism. Her basal metabolic rate was found to be +3 per cent. It was felt that, in view of her age, the goiter should be removed. The possibility that the goiter might be a factor in the causation of her dysphagia also was considered. A thyroidectomy was performed and she made an uneventful convalescence. Her dysphagia however, failed to improve. It was then recognized that she had a true hysterical dysphagia. A No. 4 French sound was passed into the stomach; no obstruction was encountered. After the immediate effect of the passage of the sound she was able to swallow all types of foods without difficulty. Iron and ammonium citrate was given by mouth and three months after the passage of the sound the patient did not have any dysphagia.

Bibliography

1. Moersch, H. J., and Connor, H. M.: Hysterical dysphagia. Arch. Otolaryngol., 4:112-117, (Aug.) 1926.

*From the Section on Peroral Endoscopy, The Mayo Clinic, Rochester, Minnesota. Read before the annual meeting of the Southern Minnesota Medical Association, Winona, Minnesota, August 11, 1937.

Question Conference on Obstetrics and Gynecology

CHAIRMAN MUSSEY: It was suggested that a question conference or question panel be held in obstetrics and gynecology as a sort of trial flight this year. We have several men who are interested in obstetrics and gynecology or both, who have kindly consented to carry on this conference. The answers to these questions will be limited to two or two and one-half minutes, if possible. We aim to get through a fair number of them in the time allotted to us.

The first question will be answered by Dr. Randall:

"*Of what value is prepartum care?*"

DR. L. M. RANDALL (Rochester): I think the answer to this question probably is obvious to all of you, but those of us who are practicing obstetrics and gynecology feel that too much emphasis cannot be placed upon the prenatal care of the obstetrical patient.

To me, it has always seemed that this type of preventive medicine, which it is, is essentially an invoice of the patient's physical, mental and nervous assets and liabilities.

It has been shown, of course, in a great number of patients who have had what we consider to be adequate prenatal care, that the incidence of complications of pregnancy, labor and the postpartum have been reduced by one-half. We all realize that, if a patient is seen early in pregnancy, the blood pressure is taken routinely, the urine examined and pelvis measured, that we are in a much better position to guide that individual through a pregnancy than we are in the patient that we see when she is already in labor and have not had an opportunity to check these things.

In considering the blood pressure readings, it has been found that those patients who develop toxemia show first an elevation of blood pressure.

Some criticism has been made that the examinations of these patients with toxemia or suspected toxemia are too complicated.

I think, on the whole, if one reviews the situation, it will be found that the tests that will detect the presence of this condition are relatively simple: blood pressure readings, examination of the urine, and checking the patient's weight, leaving out the more complicated laboratory procedures.

I think we all need to emphasize to the patient, and I suppose to ourselves, that the chief thing to consider with these people is to see them early and do the essential, simple, routine examinations that we believe form the part of adequate prenatal care.

CHAIRMAN MUSSEY: This question is for Dr. Litzenberg:

"*Is radical treatment, that is, therapeutic abortion or cesarean section, often necessary in heart lesions during pregnancy?*"

DR. J. C. LITZENBERG (Minneapolis): Therapeutic abortion and cesarean section in heart disease are almost never necessary. The attitude towards this subject has been very rapidly changing, ever since the internists have crystallized their ideas about the treatment of the heart.

The treatment of the heart in pregnancy is the treatment of the heart, and not therapeutic abortion or cesarean section. At the University Hospital we rarely do a cesarean section for heart disease, and we almost never do early therapeutic abortions.

It can all be summed up very briefly: If every woman is examined when she comes in as to her heart condition, and then every woman with a damaged heart is treated as to the heart, a therapeutic abortion will almost never be necessary. As a matter of fact, the internists have greatly advanced in the treatment of the heart during the last decade or fifteen years.

With this modern heart treatment, if a woman does not improve under the best medical supervision, then a therapeutic abortion may be considered. Even if a woman comes in during later pregnancy and has not been properly treated before, she almost always responds to the modern treatment of the damaged heart, and cesarean section will almost never be necessary. The only operative procedure that is necessary in most of these cases is that the labor be shortened as much as possible after complete dilatation, of the cervix. Then forceps may be applied, but I have been surprised at the rapidity of the labors in these heart cases, and in most of them we don't even use forceps.

The whole question may be summed up in one sentence: The damaged heart in pregnancy should be handled by treatment of the heart and not by obstetrical interference, except to shorten labor.

CHAIRMAN MUSSEY: The next question is for Dr. Rothrock:

"*What are the indications for forceps delivery?*"

DR. J. L. ROTHROCK (Saint Paul): The indications for forceps delivery are several. Uusually, having watched the progress of labor, if we come to a time when there is no further progress, then it becomes necessary to consider the possibility of the necessity of delivering the patient with instruments.

Before this is done, it is very desirable to have, in your prenatal care, thoroughly examined the patient and to have made an exhaustive examination to know whether it is possible to deliver her with instruments. Prolonged labor is often the result of inertia of the uterus. The patients become exhausted. To allow them to go longer, perhaps, would be to their detriment. It is necessary to watch these patients, particularly, and to observe the time when it becomes desirable to interfere.

In cases of prolonged labor, it is particularly desirable, also, to handle your patients with extreme care, to prevent the possibility of infection, to eliminate, as far as possible, unnecessary examinations, and to look forward to the possibility that the patient, even though you successfully deliver her, if she becomes infected, will be in danger.

Another indication is the watching of the fetal heart sound to know whether the infant, the unborn child, is in danger. Sometimes it becomes necessary to suddenly terminate a labor with instruments, because of distress of the infant in prolonged labor.

The question is one which requires the greatest judgment, inasmuch as a certain number of borderline cases require reliance upon the so-called test of labor. How long should we permit a woman to go before we think of interfering? That depends on the condition of the patient. I would say that it may be summed up in this procedure: to carefully watch the patient, and, after there has ceased to be any progress in labor for a certain length of time, then to increase our vigilance, and, before the patient becomes exhausted, or before the fetal distress manifests itself, to prepare to interfere with the instruments.

CHAIRMAN MUSSEY: The next question is for Dr. Manley:

"If you were called to see a woman in shock in whom you suspected tubal pregnancy, how would you handle the situation?"

DR. J. R. MANLEY (Duluth): In handling tubal pregnancies, there has been, in the past, two classes of men, one who believed in waiting, and one who believed in operating. My practice has been to take care of these cases as soon as the diagnosis is made.

With one or two exceptions, the first thing to do in a case of ruptured tubal pregnancy is to transport the patient to the hospital, if possible, and give a little morphin. While waiting for the operating room to get ready, a blood transfusion or glucose intravenously should be given.

I believe the shock in tubal pregnancy is due to hemorrhage, and the logical thing to do is to stop the hemorrhage as soon as possible. A blood transfusion should always be available and may be given before, during, or after the operation. The first object during the operation is to deliver the ruptured tube and stop the bleeding. Then you may remove organized clots and complete the operation. It is not necessary or advisable to spend time removing all the blood.

CHAIRMAN MUSSEY: Dr. Hartley will answer this question:

"What are the indications for version?"

DR. E. C. HARTLEY (Saint Paul): Version is one of the oldest obstetrical operations. There are two kinds, depending on which end of the fetus you intend to cause to engage. If the head is brought down, then it becomes cephalic version. If you want to make the breech present, it becomes a podalic version.

Cephalic version is attempted when the breech presents. This may be done by external manipulation and, if it can be done, it is very desirable. If it is too difficult, it probably isn't worth doing. Often if done, unless the head can be made to engage at once, it will not stay in place.

The commonest type is podalic version. This means inserting the hand into the uterus, grasping one or two feet and bringing them down to the outlet. By means of this maneuver it is possible to convert such presentations as face, brow or shoulder into one relatively easy to deliver. For other reasons, such as hemorrhage, it may be desirable to get something down in the cervix so that delivery may be done almost at the discretion of the obstetrician.

There is a type of uterine inertia which several men have described, in which long labor finally results in the complete dilation of the cervix and yet the patient doesn't deliver. If this condition can be accurately determined in advance, and we know for certain that there is no bony obstruction, a podalic version may often be done with surprising ease.

CHAIRMAN MUSSEY: Dr. Rothrock:

"What are the outstanding indications for cesarean section?"

DR. J. L. ROTHROCK (Saint Paul): The outstanding

indication for cesarean section is a disproportion between the size of the baby and the pelvis. In other words, the most important indication is found in those patients with contraction of the pelvis. It used to be said that there were absolute indications, and indications which were under the title of emergencies. The absolute indication was a pelvis where the inlet was 7 centimeters or less. Today we recognize the fact that with inlet contraction there are a number of cases where the inlet is much more than 7 centimeters, yet the size of the head of the infant will not pass.

Then, too, we have to take into consideration contractions at the pelvic outlet, which are quite frequent. There have been added many indications for cesarean section. For example, the question of central placenta prævia in a primipara with a rigid cervix, in my opinion, becomes a perfectly justifiable indication for cesarean section. There are certain indications which arise, where it is desirable to deliver the patient, as, for example, in cases of toxemia. They are very few, however.

The premature separation of the placenta, especially the more severe form, also forms an indication where hemorrhage is going on and where, if the patient's condition is at all suitable for an operation, then sometimes the only method of rescuing that patient is to deliver as quickly as possible, and that can be done in case the patient is not in labor, by a cesarean section. These form some of the indications.

It is true that in recent years the application of cesarean section has been much extended, and some of the indications which have been alleged, have, in my opinion, brought about a situation in which far too many cesarean sections are made where the patient might be more safely delivered by other methods.

CHAIRMAN MUSSEY: Dr. McKaig is next:

"How would you manage asepsis in a farm home delivery?"

DR. C. B. McKAIG (Pine Island): My practice being mostly among the farmers makes quite a lot of difference in the handling of asepsis. The first thing I see to is that my instruments and gloves are sterilized at home in a pan contained in my grip with a good tight lid on it. The main reason for the lid is to keep the dust and flies out after you arrive at the patient's home.

The patient is scrubbed up with a combination of liquid soap and 1:2500 metaphen, half and half, which gives you a good lather. She is washed up, the legs and all sterilized but not shaved. Then after drying, the legs and vulva and parts are thoroughly sprayed with tincture of metaphen by means of an atomizer. Incidentally, at that time I strap a flashlight on the leg with adhesive plaster, so as to give me plenty of light. Usually the light isn't very much good in farm homes.

One of the main things is to impress the people that they should leave everything alone, not to handle any of the instruments, which they are very apt to do, picking one up and asking the doctor, "What is this for?" Then you have to do your sterilizing all over again.

One of the chief managements for asepsis is to do as little vaginal examination as possible. Do most all of your examination by way of rectum, keeping track of progress in that way. I carry impenetrable pads and waterproof dressings for the bed.

CHAIRMAN MUSSEY: After the program was printed, Dr. Wahlberg kindly consented to take part in this conference. The question has come in:

36

"What is the most acceptable treatment for pre-eclamptic toxemia and eclampsia?"

DR. E. W. WAHLBERG (Morgan): The treatment of preeclamptic toxemia, as you know, may be divided into prophylactic and active treatment, both of pre-eclamptic toxemia and the eclampsia.

Dr. Randall mentioned some of the indications in prenatal care. The outstanding features of the value of prenatal care in the prophylaxis of preeclamptic toxemia are the routine examination of the blood pressure, urinalysis and the recording of weight, and the recording of these so that one may detect early the development of preeclamptic toxemia and take proper steps.

How should preeclamptic toxemia be treated? In the first place, it must be considered as a medical condition to be treated by medical measures primarily. Any other measures, such as the interruption of pregnancy, are secondary to the medical measures.

In the consideration of preeclamptic toxemia, it may be considered as a disease that progresses from mild to severe forms. In other words, when we have a patient who develops a slight hypertension, with edema, and some albuminuria, even if this is very mild or slight, treatment begun then may prevent the development of a higher blood pressure and more severe symptoms.

The treatment at that time consists of bed rest, laxatives and, what is very important, sedatives, the use, if the condition progresses, of intravenous glucose and magnesium sulphate solution.

I must hurry, so I will go into the more severe form that may culminate in eclampsia: You may not have seen the patient before. Particularly in those cases where the patient is possibly far from the hospital, or where the patient has to be taken into the hospital, the very most important thing is the use of morphin sulphate in a dose of ¼ to ½ grain and used every half hour or every hour until the patient's respirations get down to 10 or 12. This will control a great many.

In the hospital, the use of intravenous glucose, the use of magnesium sulphate solutions intravenously, and other sedative measures, are carried on before any attempt is made to interrupt the pregnancy. That is the important thing. If interruption of pregnancy is determined upon, it should be done, if possible, after the patient has recovered from the acute condition, which is shown by diuresis, regaining consciousness and sweating. If cesarean section is done, it should be done on objective indications, after medical measures have been tried.

CHAIRMAN MUSSEY: Dr. Manley:

"What are the symptoms in early carcinoma of the cervix?"

DR. J. R. MANLEY (Duluth): The trouble with carcinoma of the cervix is that the symptoms do not become evident early enough. The public are pretty well trained now to see the doctor if they have postmenopausal bleeding, or if they have bleeding to any extent between their menstrual periods.

My experience is that when people come to me with that story and I look at the cervix and a carcinoma is found it is not early any more; it is almost too late to do anything. I think we have to train our patients to notice other symptoms besides bleeding. If women were trained to notice any alteration in the leukorrheal discharge which they may have had for years, just a little change in its character, a little burning, and would then come for examination, we might be able to do more.

I believe we should examine all women who come to our office, no matter what they come for. If they come for stomach ache or neuralgia, ofttimes a well directed question or two will make them willing to submit to a pelvic examination. Many women will welcome that suggestion. They do not care to ask for it because they think their symptoms are insignificant. But we can accomplish a great deal towards diagnosing early carcinoma of the cervix by educating people.

After they come, it is up to the doctor, then, to decide. The gross cases we see often enough, and it is too late, but it is the small, early ones that we do not get a chance to examine, and therefore we haven't much experience in diagnosing them. The Schiller test is one of the late methods. In my experience, it has not been of a great deal of value because it is positive in erosions and various other conditions. The Schiller test is of value only in very early lesions before there has been any breaking down of the surface epithelium, and even then a positive reaction may not always mean a carcinoma. But if our attention is called to the possibility of making an early diagnosis and we make a study of the Schiller test, we may be able to spot a few of these real early carcinomas which are evidenced by just a little, pale, thickened area in the cervix, before the mucous membrane has been eroded. That is the chance that we have to cut down the deaths from carcinoma of the cervix.

CHAIRMAN MUSSEY: We have the following hypothetical question:

"If I had a patient with occiput in the posterior position on the first labor and had only about six fingers of dilatation of the cervix after thirty hours of labor, how should I handle the situation?"

DR. J. L. ROTHROCK (Saint Paul): One of the most difficult propositions the obstetrician has to deal with is the occipitoposterior position, that is the occiput, which normally rotates anteriorly, sometimes rotates posteriorly, owing to the position of the child or to some fault in the mechanism of the labor.

The question then is what to do for this case, if it is observed early. In the first place, the first stage of labor is going to be quite normal because before any rotation possibly could take place the occiput must reach the floor of the pelvis. Almost all of these cases, if permitted to go on under careful supervision, will reach a point when the cervix is dilated.

The question of interference does not arise until the cervix is fully dilated and the head gets to the floor of the pelvis. Then the proper procedure is to conserve that patient's strength, to give her morphin to relieve the pains, and to watch her carefully, and, when the cervix is dilated, then comes the time for assistance.

It is possible sometimes in these cases, by introducing the blade of the forceps after the head has descended to the floor of the pelvis, to cause an interior rotation. In some cases the head becomes impacted, and then it is necessary to deliver with the occiput posterior.

These cases are disastrous in view of the fact that they are apt to cause deep lacerations, and, for this reason, if for no other, the patient should be permitted to go on, as far as she can with safety to the mother and the child.

I do not believe that it is necessary in these cases, as has been recommended, to resort to more radical forms of treatment, as, for example, that some of these cases should be delivered by cesarean section. I do not believe that.

OBSTETRICS AND GYNECOLOGY

CHAIRMAN MUSSEY: Dr. Randall:

"What governs the premenstrual phase of the menstrual cycle, and what happens if this is insufficient?"

DR. L. M. RANDALL (Rochester): The hormone of the corpus luteum, now known as progestin, governs the premenstrual phase of the menstrual cycle. This hormone is secreted by the corpus luteum and produces the secretory or premenstrual phase of the endometrium. It likewise not only governs the premenstrual phase of the menstrual cycle but governs the integrity of the pregnancy in the early months, before the placenta is capable of performing its own function. A lack of the corpus luetum hormone will produce sterility, a typical menstrual bleeding, and abortion.

CHAIRMAN MUSSEY: Dr. Hartley, the question has come in:

"Can you tell me something about the prenatal care, or, rather, the refresher courses in obstetrics and pediatrics that are contemplated for the state?"

DR. E. C. HARTLEY (Saint Paul): The refresher courses which have been started in Minnesota by the State Department of Health, working with the State Medical Association and the Extension Division of the State University, have been begun, on the one hand, because the physicians in the country as a whole have favored such a development, and, in the second place, because funds are now available for a purpose of this kind. These funds are made available through the Children's Bureau under the Social Security Act. Courses of this kind are being given at the present time in a number of states throughout the country.

In Minnesota we started in during the winter, after preliminary arrangements with the officers of the State Association. The general manner of presentation is as follows: We have decided that a series of six lectures, covering the most interesting or important phases of obstetrics and pediatrics, would be offered. Six obstetricians and six pediatricians were selected. These twelve men together gave the first series at the University this winter. They were given there with the idea that this would work out as sort of a demonstration as to the value of the work not only to the physicians but also as a demonstration of the technic to those who were giving it.

Having completed this series with a fair amount of success, it was decided that, in giving this series throughout the state, six more obstetricians and six more pediatricians would be added, making twelve in all. These six lectures will be repeated in six different centers throughout the state, beginning on the twenty-sixth of May and ending with the end of June. The centers chosen are, Worthington, Mankato, Fergus Falls, St. Cloud, Brainerd and Grand Rapids.

It is hoped that the course will be repeated next year.

CHAIRMAN MUSSEY: Dr. Litzenberg:

"What type of pelvic contraction is most common in Minnesota?"

DR. J. C. LITZENBERG (Minneapolis): Pelvic contractions are dependent upon early, bad nutrition. Minnesota being a rural state and a "Scandinavian province," the children of our Minnesota women, when they have grown up, haven't had to go through a childhood of poor nutrition. For that reason, we have a low percentage of rachitic pelves and general contractions of the inlet of the pelvis; we have enough, but

not as many as they do in parts of the country where they have Southern European immigrants.

In this state the contracted outlet is the most common contraction and I wish to pay particular attention to that. We are too apt to observe in our measurements only the contractions of the inlet. It is very easily detected, not only by special measuring devices but by measuring the width of the outlet by the simple device of the doubled fist. You may see that I have gained a little in weight in the last thirty-five years but that fist measurement of 8½ centimeters has never changed, because it is a bony measurement.

Every patient that I see has that outlet measurement taken with that fist. If the fist goes in between the tuberosities of the ischium with ease, I know that woman hasn't a contracted outlet. If it is tight or impossible to shove the fist in between the tuberosities of the ischium, at the level of the anterior border of the anus, I know I must give particular attention to instrumental and more careful measurements of the outlet.

There has been evolved by experience a rule, "the rule of fifteen," which is very easy to remember. If the measurements between the tuberosities of the ischium is 8 centimeters, the chances are very great that that is a normal outlet, but if it is less than 8 centimeters, then it is necessary to take the posterior sagittal measurement, which is that measurement from the tip of the sacrum (not the tip of the coccyx) to the line which runs between the tuberosities of the ischium, at the level of the anterior border of the anus.

So, if the measurement made from the tip of the sacrum to this line, added to the transverse measurement, equals 15 cm., then that outlet is capable of permitting a normal child to be born.

As to the treatment, that is a very long story. The Sims position or the exaggerated lithotomy posture may increase the outlet sufficiently to permit spontaneous delivery. If the contraction is marked, cesarean section, of course, had better be performed before a trial of labor has proven delivery impossible. When the head has reached the pelvic floor it is too late for a cesarean operation.

CHAIRMAN MUSSEY: Dr. Wahlberg, may I ask you this:

"How do you manage to get the woman in the smaller town, or in the country, to come to you for prepartum care?"

DR. E. W. WAHLBERG (Morgan): The newspapers and magazines are stressing the importance of prenatal care constantly, and most of the younger women today realize the importance of it. I think the chief drawback in country practice in getting people in to see us, is the fact that so oftentimes an extra charge is made for these individual calls.

I have gotten around that by increasing my basic charge for my confinement, and then it is up to the individual woman to either take it or leave it. Usually they will take it because they feel they are losing money if they do not come in for these visits and examinations. I think you can give just as good prenatal care in the country as you can in the city.

I usually average about six visits per patient, before delivery. The first visit includes a complete physical examination, including measurement, blood pressure, hemoglobin, and also blood Wassermanns on my new patients. In later visits I simply take the blood pressure, weight and urinalysis, except the sixth and eighth months, when I also do an external abdominal examination to determine the position of the fetus.

I don't think anyone has any difficulty in getting

their patients in. If you offer them something extra for their money the patients by word of mouth will soon spread the gospel around, and the ladies will flock to your door.

CHAIRMAN MUSSEY: Dr. Hartley:

"Puerperal sepsis is said to be the commonest cause of material mortality. What can be done about this?"

DR. E. C. HARTLEY (St. Paul): During the ten-year period ending in 1932 for the United States as a whole, about 37 per cent of all the maternal deaths were caused by sepsis. During 1936 in Minnesota, of the 198 maternal deaths, 35 per cent were caused by sepsis. Apparently the deaths from sepsis both in Minnesota and in the country as a whole run pretty close to slightly over one-third of all maternal deaths.

These are fairly evenly divided between deaths due to infected abortions and to puerperal sepsis. Regarding the deaths from abortions, probably the bulk of these are due to criminal abortions, and they are out of our hands except as to methods of treating them. The spontaneous abortions rarely end in death provided they are not neglected. Puerperal sepsis is often thought of as being something that might well be laid at the door of the medical profession; there are, however, reservations to any such a viewpoint. There is, nevertheless, much agitation and much organized effort at the reduction of maternal mortality, particularly that due to sepsis. How can such deaths be avoided? In general it may be said that these deaths may be avoided by avoiding infecting the patient or traumatizing her unnecessarily.

This can be done by having the patient go into labor with the attending physician knowing as much about her as possible. In other words, don't try to find out the size of the pelvis after the patient is in labor. Don't make numerous pelvic manipulations when the patient is in labor. Remember that in prolonged labor rest and nourishment are of vital importance to the patient.

CHAIRMAN MUSSEY: Dr. Manley:

"If the pregnant woman has a tumor of the uterus, does this tumor often seriously complicate labor?"

DR. J. R. MANLEY (Duluth): This question could almost be answered categorically, "No." The only tumors you might be afraid of would be the ones down by the cervix. As the cervix dilates, the cervix pulls up around the head, rather than the head going through the cervix. Nine times out of ten it will pull the tumor up beyond the head, so there will be no obstruction to the delivery of the head. Like everything else, there may be exceptions to this.

It is quite possible that a fibroid, perhaps on a pedicle, might get down below the head and obstruct delivery. Small fibroids in the body of the uterus may interfere with contraction pains. They may cause postpartum hemorrhage, but as a rule they do not cause any trouble with the actual delivery. They may become necrotic after delivery and produce trouble in that way.

I had a recent case of that sort in which a large fibroid was left alone during pregnancy. During the puerperium, the patient had fever and swelling of the fibroid and tenderness, but it finally subsided. Later the fibroid began to grow again and was removed, and there was definite evidence of necrosis in the fibroid. But as far as actual difficulty in delivering the baby, it does not very often happen.

CHAIRMAN MUSSEY: Dr. McKaig:

"What would you do for pain relief in a long, tedious labor in a private home?"

DR. C. B. McKAIG (Pine Island): Long, tedious labors are handled in the home by first giving some sedative. I usually use chloral, about 10 grains, let the patient alone for a couple of hours, then use nembutal. Later on I resort to the Reynolds chloroform inhaler, which the patient can take herself, and she gets a great deal of relief, without anyone in attendance watching that particular case.

CHAIRMAN MUSSEY: Dr. Randall:

"To what extent is it safe to use analgesia during labor?"

DR. L. M. RANDALL (Rochester): The lay press and the medical press has been full of articles on pain relief, in the last few years. The pendulum, I think, has definitely swung from the idea that a woman in labor was not to be given any relief from pain, to the opposite extreme, which is perhaps worse, of giving the individual at the onset of labor a sufficient amount of sedative to produce complete amnesia and lack of coöperation.

This condition definitely raises the incidence of obstetrical operations and I think in the long run will increase the maternal and infant mortality. Far be it from me to say the patient is to be denied pain relief. But in between these two extremes is the safe zone in which we can give the patient reasonable relief from pain, retain her coöperation in the second stage and reduce considerably the risk of this analgesia to the mother and to the baby.

It has been said, of course, that the ideal obstetrical analgesic should be perfectly safe for the mother and for the baby. That analgesic has not yet been discovered, so far as I know.

CHAIRMAN MUSSEY: Dr. McKaig:

"I would like to know of a satisfactory method of episiotomy in the home."

DR. C. B. McKAIG (Pine Island): Out on the farm, trying to do your work without assistants or without anesthetists, you are up against it. My method of episiotomy in that case is to put in through-and-through stitches previously, before I do any cutting. I put in a row of about four or five stitches with No. 3 forty-day chromic catgut. They go right through the mucosa, into the vagina and back out again, making a row. Then the loops inside are caught with a pair of forceps, drawn out and pulled to one side. The incision is made right in between the stitches.

After delivering the placenta, it is easy enough to pull up and tie the stitches. I have found it very satisfactory in a series of thirty-seven cases.

CHAIRMAN MUSSEY: Dr. Litzenberg:

"What is the difference, if any, between the treatment of carcinoma of the cervix and carcinoma of the body of the uterus?"

DR. J. C. LITZENBERG (Minneapolis): There is a very general consensus of opinion regarding the proper treatment of carcinoma of the cervix, and that is that it is better treated by irradiation than by operation. This irradiation does not mean treatment by radium but it means treatment by radium and deep x-ray therapy.

Very briefly, the rules of the Cancer Institute for the treatment of cancer of the cervix are these: We follow the Schmitz classification of clinical grouping, 1, 2, 3 and 4. No. 1 is a very early carcinoma of the cervix; No. 2 is an early carcinoma of the cervix, but still limited to the cervix, as far as clinical findings will reveal; and in No. 3 there is evident extension beyond the cervix into the parametrium, and No. 4 is far advanced cancer of the cervix.

In these days there is an exact measure of the amount of irradiation that may be administered to a given point, in this case the cervix. We may give a certain number of milligram-hours or millicurie-hours, with radium, and then the roentgenologist knows how much irradiation by x-ray he can give to that cervix. It is a formula which involves the measurement of the patient, the distance of the cervix from the tube, and so forth, but we may sum it up by saying that we determine in each case how much irradiation this patient must have.

Inasmuch as radium will apply the irradiation to the cervix in a better manner than the x-ray, in Group 1 we give as much irradiation as possible, 3,600 or 4,000, even more, milligram-hours. Then the roentgenologist has the amount of irradiation that we have given by radium and figures out how much more he can give and not go beyond the total amount that the normal tissues will stand.

In Group 2 we give about the same treatment.

In Group 3, when the cancer has extended into the parametrium, the surrounding tissues of the cervix, it is manifestly beyond the treatment of radium. Radium inserted into the cervix has a therapeutic limit of 3 centimeters, a little over an inch in each direction. Therefore, if we give all of the radium that we can possibly give, we have only reached, therapeutically, a distance of 3 centimeters surrounding the capsule or needle of radium. Therefore, that leaves the extension into the parametrium untreated. This must be reached by deep x-ray therapy.

In these modern days, the Coutard method of giving more x-ray treatments, a larger number with little bit smaller doses, has been a very great advance in the treatment of cancer of the cervix.

The mortality of cancer of the cervix in the better equipped clinics has been improving gradually. This later Coutard multiple, although shorter, individual treatments by the x-ray has added a very great deal to the efficacy of the treatment.

The general opinion, also, is that in cancer of the body of the uterus there should be the operative method of total hysterectomy. In cancer of the body of the uterus, operation is better than irradiation.

However, the older method of making a diagnosis, say, by a frozen section, a diagnostic curettage, and then a hysterectomy at once, has fallen into disfavor because there is a large number of patients who will die of peritonitis when it is done that way. The consensus of opinion now is that, at the time of the diagnostic curettage, if a frozen section shows that there is cancer, then radium is introduced into the uterus for 2,000-3,000 millicurie-hours, and then that will stop or retard the growth of the cancer but, of course, will not cure it. Then wait six weeks and do a hysterectomy.

CHAIRMAN MUSSEY: Dr. Wahlberg:

"In the ordinary home deliveries in town or on the farm, how would you keep the patient quiet long enough to insure proper involution of the uterus?"

DR. E. W. WAHLBERG (Morgan): Postpartum care and rest, again, involve education of the patient. The average patient is willing to coöperate if she knows why she is asked to coöperate, and usually during that quiet hour after the delivery has been performed and you are waiting for possible hemorrhage, I take the father and the attendant aside and tell them the reasons for rest, why we want involution and how it aids in allowing proper healing in episiotomy wounds, and also how it prevents cystoceles, rectoceles, prolapse and other complications.

I leave a printed list of instructions as regards the care of the child and also the care of the mother. This specifically instructs her to lie in bed until the eighth day, let her sit up on the ninth, and let her be up on the tenth. The third day postpartum, I go back for a return call. Again I check up to see whether the instructions are being followed. Then I go through the same explanation with the mother and make her understand the necessity for rest. I haven't had any trouble, provided I explained thoroughly the importance of following directions.

The Apple in the Management of Diarrhea in Children

The Council on Foods reports that the use of fresh apples in the dietary treatment of diarrhea in infants and small children has been much publicized within recent years. Lately, preparations of dried and powdered apple have been similarly acclaimed. The Council on Foods has considered the available clinical reports. These reports cover practically every kind of diarrhea that is encountered in pediatric practice. The Council concludes that the evidence which is now available indicates that the apple is useful as a thera-peutic agent in the dietary management of diarrhea. The mechanism responsible for the reported success of this diet is not clear. Apple powder when suitably prepared is considered a wholesome food and offers a convenient preparation for use in the management of diarrhea of infancy and childhood. It should be emphasized, however, that the use of the fresh or dried apple does not obviate the necessity for other measures, including parenteral administration of fluids when indicated, the careful selection of a suitable transition diet, and competent pediatric supervision. (J.A.M.A., Nov. 13, 1937, p. 1636.)

AN INTRODUCTION TO THE HISTORY OF MEDICINE IN MINNESOTA

By IOHN M. ARMSTRONG

Chairman Historical Committee
Minnesota State Medical Association

A DECADE ago a committee to collect data for a "History of Medicine in Minnesota" was appointed by our State Association. This committee has been active since its establishment and considerable data have been gathered, part of which is in a form suitable for publication. Since various members of the committee have submitted material in a finished form, of necessity there is considerable overlapping, and since it has been difficult to separate subjects which have both a general and local interest and assign them to the proper place, some duplication will occur during the narration.

Since this forms an introduction to future articles which will appear in MINNESOTA MEDICINE, a brief outline of medical history in Minnesota is here presented; later contributions will be more specific as to subject matter.

The history of Minnesota may be roughly divided into five overlapping divisions: exploration, the fur trade, military occupation, the missionary and permanent settlement. Similarly, the medical history may be so divided.

The French explorers and traders came first. Many of them were educated men, among them priests who no doubt were familiar with the medical practice of the age, but we do not find among them men with the title "doctor."

British occupation and the advent of the Northwest Company, a fur trading corporation with headquarters at Montreal, came next. Physicians were employed by this company as part of their organization. They were officially classed as clerks but received additional remuneration for their medical services. These men were stationed at times within the boundaries of our present Minnesota. With the withdrawal of the Northwest Company from American territory in 1816, the American Fur Company took over their posts and form of organization and employed physicians when available.

Military occupation by the United States government took place in 1819 when Fort St. Anthony, now Fort Snelling, was established. With the troops came our first American physician. Since that time one or more medical officers have been stationed there, with the exception of the years 1857-60 when the fort was temporarily abandoned. During the periods when Forts Ridgley and Ripley were occupied, army medical men were also stationed there. Some of these army physicians later attained some eminence both in their profession and in other lines of endeavor.

During the period of military occupancy came the first American missionaries, in 1835. All, no doubt, ministered to the physical as well as to the spiritual needs of the Indian, although but few were physicians.

Following the military occupation came various government expeditions. In those of Long, in 1820, Schoolcraft, in 1832, and David Dale Owen, 1848-50, the scientists accompanying them acted as, or were qualified as, physicians.

Some of them had previously practiced medicine and some later continued the practice of medicine.

The period of settlement began in 1838 with the beginning of lumbering on the St. Croix river, and civilian physicians followed the settlers.

One may say here that the French explorers and traders penetrated Minnesota by three routes along the north shore of Lake Superior, via the Brulé-St. Croix portage and the Green Bay-Wisconsin river route; the British entered by the north shore route; and United States exploration and settlement came in by way of the Mississippi river from the south, except that the troops which established Fort Snelling came by the Green Bay-Wisconsin river. It is logical, then, to find that our civilian physicians, as did our civilian population, followed the tributaries of the Mississippi. Stillwater, St. Paul, St. Anthony, Winona, Wabasha and Taylors Falls were our first towns. Then came Minneapolis, the towns along the Minnesota river, and those on the Mississippi above St. Anthony Falls.

Population grew rapidly during the sixth decade of the nineteenth century and numbers of physicians followed the emigrants; but since at first there was not sufficient practice to support them, many abandoned their profession and went into farming or trade, while others, after a brief sojourn, moved to other parts of the territory. With the opening of the territorial road north from Iowa, emigrants came into southern Minnesota overland, and the towns of Albert Lea, Rochester, Owatonna and Faribault came into being and attracted more medical men. Likewise southwestern Minnesota was peopled via the government road west to Fort Abercrombie. Northwestern Minnesota was not well settled till the railroads entered that region about 1870. Settlement in northeastern Minnesota lagged, as the country was not suitable for agriculture. Here the first settlers came by the lake route.

As soon as there were enough physicians they associated themselves for exchange of ideas and other mutual benefits and our first medical society was organized. This was a territorial organization formed in 1853 and local societies began to be formed soon afterward, though our present societies were not established till some years after the termination of the Civil War.

The earliest literature relating to medicine in our state is to be found in the reports of the government expeditions and reports of army surgeons, which are of considerable interest though few in number.

Medical journalism began in 1870 with the publication of the *Northwestern Medical and Surgical Journal.* Since that time nearly a dozen medical journals have been published, of which but two exist at the present time.

The teaching of medicine, other than the preceptorial system, began as early as 1870 with the establishment of preparatory medical schools in St. Paul and Winona.

Later other schools were incorporated and conferred degrees. At the present time our University and its affiliate, the Mayo Foundation, are the sole teaching institutions.

Our first private hospital opened its doors in 1854 and the first state hospital in 1866.

The State Board of Health was established in 1872, preceded only by those of Massachusetts and California.

The development and progress of legislation pertaining to the practice of medicine and the status of the physician in the community have undergone various changes since the organization of Minnesota as an entity.

All these and other aspects of medicine will receive treatment at length.

Until 1854 our white population was largely composed of native Americans and French Canadians, but at that time emigrants of foreign birth began pouring in and physicians of foreign birth and training followed, giving a cosmopolitan character to our profession which has had a considerable influence on the development of medicine in our state.

In general, the preceding is an epitome, in outline, of the progress and development of medicine in Minnesota. Much interesting material relating to the services of medical men in the Army and Navy from the War of 1812 till the present has also been gathered. Biographical data, often of more than local interest, shedding considerable light on the progress of medicine and individual achievement have also been secured and will be presented separately or with the county narratives.

The committee feels that the difficulties encountered in recording the events of the last century have been much greater than any future investigator may have in recording those of the present. Hence we have confined our efforts largely to the past century.

It is the earnest desire of the committee that medical items of interest, trivial or not, be sent to the chairman. Particularly desired are old minutes of medical meetings, physicians' diaries, addresses, account books and letters. Material of this nature forms the basis of real insight into prevailing conditions as well as the thought and activities of the individual. Historians in general are turning more and more to data of this nature as source material. May we ask your coöperation in aiding us in our attempt to compile a "History of Medicine in Minnesota"?

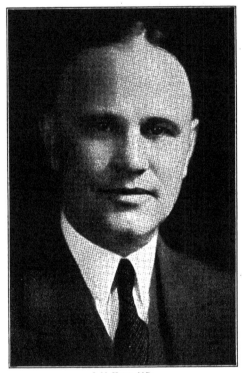

J. M. HAYES, M.D.
President, Minnesota State Medical Association

President's Message

To the Members of the Minnesota State Medical Association:

I TAKE this opportunity of wishing you all a very Happy New Year.
While I am duly grateful for the honor of being your president for the coming year, I am not unmindful of the fact that I am still only one small unit in a great organization. Whatever the administration does must be done at your bidding. You are all aware that in an organization of this magnitude, it is not the work of one individual or a small group of individuals, but the combined efforts of all members that bring about the desired results.

The problems of the medical profession have been much the same in the past as they are at present and will be in the future.

An era of depression merely magnifies the problems of those who are to be guardians of our principles, and greater efforts must be put forth to stem the tide of outside aggression. Such periods are always opportune for misguided philanthropic individuals and organizations. Improper care of the sick or the crippled child always furnished an arousing appeal to these individuals or organizations.

They all mean well, but unfortunately their information is frequently gained through improper channels. Only through the practicing physician can this information be properly obtained.

Our state and national medical organizations have the proper machinery and equipment necessary for obtaining information in regard to health problems and the care of the sick. Information obtained through other channels is frequently faulty and misleading. Such information put out to the public is bad for all concerned.

Adequate care of the sick should be the primary objective of every medical organization.

What is adequate care of the sick and how it should be administered are questions much discussed today. We know that there has never been a time when the sick were better taken care of than now. We also know that many new and fantastic schemes for improving medical care are not well founded. They are not products of the practical man.

Experience with various methods tried in other countries as well as some in our own, leads us to the conclusion that our old established Medical Guild is as good or better than any other system of medical care yet proposed.

All scientific improvement, all research or special skill of any nature may be encouraged and made use of under this system.

We do not oppose outside assistance where such assistance is necessary, but the care of the sick must always be kept in the hands of the medical profession.

> J. M. HAYES, M.D.
> President, Minnesota State
> Medical Association

EDITORIAL

MINNESOTA MEDICINE

OFFICIAL JOURNAL OF THE MINNESOTA STATE MEDICAL
ASSOCIATION

Published by the Association under the direction of its Editing
and Publishing Committee

EDITING AND PUBLISHING COMMITTEE

J. T. CHRISTISON, Saint Paul   C. B. WRIGHT, Minneapolis
E. M. HAMMES, Saint Paul   T. A. PEPPARD, Minneapolis
WALTMAN WALTERS, Rochester

EDITORIAL STAFF

CARL B. DRAKE, Saint Paul, Editor
W. F. BRAASCH, Rochester, Associate Editor
GILBERT COTTAM, Minneapolis, Associate Editor

Annual Subscription—$3.00.   Single Copies—$0.40
Foreign Subscriptions—$3.50.

The right is reserved to reject material submitted for editorial
or advertising columns. The Editing and Publishing Committee
does not hold itself responsible for views expressed either in
editorials or other articles when signed by the author.

Classified advertising—five cents a word; minimum charge,
$1.00. Remittance should accompany order.

Display advertising rates on request.

Address all communications to Minnesota Medicine, 2642 University Avenue, Saint Paul, or Suite 604, National Bldg., Minneapolis. Telephone: Nestor 2641.

BUSINESS MANAGER
J. R. BRUCE

Volume 21   JANUARY, 1938   Number 1

History of Medicine in Minnesota

BEGINNING with this issue of MINNESOTA MEDICINE, a number of pages will be devoted each month to the publication of the medical history of our state. The proposal of the Historical Committee of the Minnesota State Medical Association to publish in the journal the interesting material it has gathered on the medical activities in the state up to the year 1900, met with hearty approval. Doubtless the story of the early days will be much more widely read in piecemeal than in volume form. However, it is the present purpose of the committee eventually to publish in book form the pages appearing in MINNESOTA MEDICINE.

History, particularly medical history, has a special fascination for certain members of our profession, but it is our hope that all our readers will enjoy the published history of medicine in our state as it appears in these pages each month.

The "Elixir" of Sulfanilimide Episode

PHYSICIANS have realized for some time that the existing Food and Drugs Act does not sufficiently protect the public. Proprietaries of unknown formula are allowed to be sold directly to the public, a procedure not allowed in certain foreign countries. Opposition, however, on the part of proprietary manufacturers has been so strong that remedial legislation has been obstructed. Doubtless a certain amount of prescribing of proprietaries of unknown composition takes place although this is a drop in the bucket compared to the counter sale of these remedies. Occasionally new drugs like dinitrophenol, cinchophen and amidopyrine are offered to the profession before their dangerous qualities are realized. Rarely, fortunately, is a distinctly poisonous drug offered for general distribution.

The tragedy of seventy-three known and twenty more presumptive deaths from the dispensing of Elixir of Sulfanilimide-Massengill, serves to call attention to the inadequacy of the present laws governing the sale of drugs. The so-called elixir was not an elixir in that it contained no alcohol. Further, the elixir contained an undeclared solvent—diethylene glycol—which proved to be the fatal poison. It seems, too, that the poisonous quality of diethylene glycol should have been known to the manufacturing chemist. And finally, although this was a new preparation, no preliminary tests as to its poisonous nature were made before it was sold to the drug trade.

We are told the only law violated was the use of the term "elixir" for a preparation which was not an elixir. Had the law required revelation of the presence of the relatively unknown diethylene glycol as a solvent it is problematic how many of those physicians who prescribed the preparation would have

46

:n deterred, so great is the faith of most
rsicians in the pharmaceutical houses.
1ile these concerns are jealous of their repu-
ions and as a rule are careful not to intro-
:e drugs harmful in the recommended dos-
:, there is no law requiring such precaution.
Corrective legislation has been presented to
ngress by Senator Copeland embodying the
ommendations of the Secretary of Agricul-
·e, who investigated the tragedy. In brief
. recommendations were:

1. "License control of new drugs to insure
   that they will not be generally distributed until experimental and clinical tests
   have shown them to be safe for use."
   This is not to prevent the development of
   new drugs by experimentation in competent hands.

2. "Prohibition of drugs which are dangerous to health when administered in accordance with the manufacturers' direction for use." We presume this means
   the prohibition of direct sale to the public of such drugs.

3. "Requirement that drug labels bear appropriate directions for use and warning
   against probable misuse." Such warn-
   ings are certainly indicated in the case
   of dinitrophenol, cinchophen and amidopyrine, and their direct sale to the public
   should be prohibited.

4. "Prohibition of secret remedies by requiring that labels disclose fully the composition of drugs." Vigorous opposition
   to this proposal on the part of the proprietary manufacturers may be expected.

This proposed legislation will be lacking if
does not include the prohibition of direct
ile to the public not only of distinctly dan-
:rous drugs which should be limited to dis-
:nsation by prescription, but also of drugs
hich are habit-forming, including the bar-
:turates, the continued use of which in certain
ises results in mental changes. The proposed
1anges, along with heavier penalties for in-
ingement, will add protection to the public,
ıt too much emphasis cannot be placed on
1e importance of each physician's prescribing
nly those remedies about which he is in-
ırmed.

Health Progress

IT must be a matter of satisfaction to everyone associated with public health activities to
know that the health of our citizens as reflected
by mortality statistics has shown a marked improvement in recent years. A volume recently
published[*] by the Metropolitan Life Insurance
Company presents an analysis of the company's
mortality experience for the twenty-five years
from 1911 to 1935 inclusive, and the expert interpretation of its mortality experience over this
period supplies a confirmation of impressions and
some facts which may be new to many.

The mortality experience of this large company
corresponds very closely to that of the registration area of the United States and serves as a
check on government figures. During the twenty-
five year period reviewed the life expectancy of
the American citizen has been increased from
46.63 to 60.25 years, an increase of 30 per cent.
This has resulted in spite of a World War, a
most severe influenza epidemic and one of the
worst economic depressions this country has experienced. Most of this increase in life expectancy has been due to the marked reduction in
the diseases afflicting youth, childhood and particularly infancy.

The trend of the mortality curve for this
twenty-five year period has been downward almost constantly except during the influenza epidemic, and, strange to say, has been particularly
marked the last five years in spite of the economic depression. This does not suggest that the
people are suffering from lack of medical care.

It may not be generally realized that the mortality in the first four years of life is comparatively high, showing a marked drop in the next
four years of life until it is lowest during the
ages of ten to fourteen. The curve then rises
until at the age period of thirty-five to forty-four
it is nearly double that of the first four years of
life and, of course, is highest beyond the age of
sixty-five. For all ages combined the mortality
of males is 30 per cent higher than for females,
and for the colored population is much greater
than for the whites.

The reduction in incidence and mortality from

*Dublin, Louis I. and Lotka, Alfred J.: Twenty-five Years of
Health Progress: A Study of the Mortality Experience Among
Industrial Policyholders of the Metropolitan Life Insurance
Company, 1911 to 1935. New York: Metropolitan Life Insur-
ance Company, 1937.

the contagious diseases of childhood is particularly gratifying. Diphtheria heads the list with the most marked mortality reduction. Antitoxin and widespread immunization explains this but does not explain the marked reduction for measles, whooping cough and scarlet fever. Physicians may note that diphtheria rarely occurs in the first year of life in contrast to whooping cough and measles. The pre-school age, however, is an important period for immunization against diphtheria. The mortality for measles and its complications is greatest in the first and second years of life and the same applies to whooping cough, which in these two years of life accounts for nearly three times as many deaths as measles, scarlet fever and diphtheria combined.

Tuberculosis, though still the leading cause of death in early adult life exacts only a third the toll it did twenty-five years ago. Males die of the disease in greater numbers over the age of forty-five, while the age period of twenty to twenty-five is the worst for females. In recent years, the rate for girls ten to twenty years of age is twice that for boys, while at forty-five to fifty-five the rate for males is three and a half times that for females.

The necessary grouping of influenza and pneumonia makes deductions somewhat difficult. Some 450,000 to 600,000 deaths occurred in our population from these causes during the epidemic, and it is estimated some six to ten million throughout the world, more than from military operations throughout the World War.

We have known that lobar pneumonia is comparatively mild in Minnesota. In certain states, it is milder than in Minnesota, but is considerably more malignant in most of the Atlantic seaboard states, Missouri, Tennessee and Kentucky, and most severe in New Mexico, Arizona, and Nevada. There has been a decided decline in mortality from this disease during the past five years, for which pneumococcic serum may be partly responsible.

The increase in cancer deaths has been about 14.5 per cent. Several factors doubtless account for this. Better diagnosis and more autopsies revealing hidden cancer undoubtedly play a part. The shift of cancer mortality from seventh to second place during this period is due, however, for the most part to the reduction in other diseases.

The cardiovascular-renal group heads the and accounts for about a third of all deaths the age of forty-five almost half. Infection well as the aging process plays a part in causation of these diseases. Even in this gr there has been a slight fall in the death rate though this has been due to an improvement youth where infections such as rheumatic fe and scarlet fever are more often causative tors. While valvular heart disease has fallen half the mortality of fifteen years ago, this been for the most part in those under twenty-years of age. Heart muscle disease, howev has shown a marked increase at each age per and especially after the age of forty-five. reporting of coronary diseases has changed c siderably in recent years and the doubling reported deaths from this cause in the past years must be interpreted with caution altho most students of the question believe there been a definite increase in coronary disease, most common cause of which is hypertension.

In spite of the discovery of insulin in 1 the mortality from diabetes has increa especially in women in whom it is now alr twice that of men. The benefits of insulin seen particularly in diabetes in youth. The crease is attributed to more frequent diagnc the greater percentage of the population nov the older age groups and the increase in Jev population from one million to four million the past thirty years. Overweight and ove dulgence in food and drink along with less n ual work all play their part.

In spite of scientific advance in diagnosis treatment, the figures for the puerperal state appendicitis show no improvement during period. An appreciable percentage of such de are preventable, and concentration on lay professional education should produce resul

The story of accidental deaths in our cou is appalling. In 1934, more than 100,000 per were killed in accidents of one kind or ano In Canada the rate is 40 per cent less. We surprised to learn that the trend during twenty-five year period among policyho has been downward and in the closing five of the period was 25 per cent less than d the first five years. About a quarter of the

48

ccidents occurred at home and another quarter ere due to automobile accidents.

The rise in the number of automobile accidents :om 2,100 in 1911 to 34,000 in 1934 is disgrace- ıl and indicates the marked improvement which ust have taken place in the occurrence of other ccidents. Something will have to be done about :, but the solution is not clear.

The remarkable improvement in public health uring the past twenty-five years should be a ource of satisfaction to all these agencies de- oted to health activities. The analysis of mor- ılity statistics presented in this volume indicates here the attack should be made by medical as well as other agencies to increase life expectancy further.

MEDICAL BROADCAST FOR JANUARY

The Minnesota State Medical Association Morning Health Service.

The Minnesota State Medical Association broadcasts weekly at 9:45 o'clock every Saturday morning over Station WCCO, Minneapolis and Saint Paul (810 kilocycles or 370.2 meters).

Speaker: William A. O'Brien, M.D., Associate Professor of Pathology and Preventive Medicine, Medical School, University of Minnesota. The program for the month will be as follows:

January 1—Public Health Objectives
January 8—Pneumonia Types
January 15—Measles Prevention
January 22—Early Tuberculosis
January 29—Preventive Dentistry

Vaccines in Colds

All investigations to date have consistently shown a wide variety of bacteria present in colds. This fact necessitates the assumption either that colds are not due to any specific organism but that symptoms which we recognize by that term can be produced by a large number of different bacteria, or that the specific cause has not yet been identified. It is evident, therefore, that that any attempt made now to produce immunity by vaccines must be aimed at a combination of organisms, with the hope of chance inclusion of the right one, or that the combination also by accident contains the as yet unidentified principle which causes all colds. Neither of these possibilities seems to offer a scientifically rational approach to prophylaxis. The duration of acquired immunity is another important question. There is no real scientific evidence supporting the use of vaccines for the common cold. In those individual instances in which benefit seems to result, this apparent effect may be due either to the individual fluctuation in frequency which is generally observed or to some nonspecific stimulation of immunity created by the administered proteins. (J. A. M. A., Oct. 9, 1937, p. 1217.)

Warren Wilson
1863-1937

DR. Warren Wilson, long identified with civic and professional interests in Northfield, died September 4, 1937, from coronary thrombosis.

Dr. Wilson was born at Lyndoch, Ontario, April 24, 1863. He attended local grade schools and the high school at Simcoe and took his pre-medical course at Western University, London, Ontario. He received his medical degree at Northwestern University in 1889.

After practicing a year at Belding, Michigan, and several years at Duluth, Dr. Wilson bought the practice of Dr. S. J. Schmidt in Northfield. During the World War he headed the medical service of the S.A.T.C. at Carleton and St. Olaf with the rank of Lieutenant. In 1919 he was joined in practice by Dr. Joseph Moses and in 1924 by his son, Dr. Warren E. Wilson. In 1930, because of his health, he retired from active practice but was available for consultation.

In 1895 Dr. Wilson married Ruby Evans of Duluth. Her death occurred in 1897. In 1898 he married Bertha Schmidt who survives him. He is also survived by two sons, Dr. Warren E. Wilson of Northfield and Paul S. Wilson, who is superintendent of schools at Glencoe. A sister and three brothers reside in Ontario.

Dr. Wilson drew the plans and assisted in the management of the hospital established at Northfield by the Odd Fellows of Minnesota. Ten years later he took a leading part in the establishment of the hospital built by the Northfield Hospital Association. This hospital was eventually turned over to the city. Dr. Wilson was also a member of the Board of Education of Northfield for ten years. An active Mason, he planned the present Masonic lodge quarters at Northfield.

Dr. Wilson was an ardent golfer and became much interested in woodcraft in his later years. In his passing Northfield has lost a valuable citizen, a man of sound character and outstanding achievement.

Cobra Venom in Arthritis

For a number of years various venoms, especially those of bees and snakes, have been used in the treatment of a variety of diseases. Of commercial preparations of different venoms, those of bees have been most widely used. No extensive scientific study has been made concerning the value of cobra (or bee) toxins in chronic arthritis. Many believe that such relief as arthritis patients may obtain from bee or snake venoms is probably derived from a reaction somewhat similar to that from foreign proteins (milk, typhoid vaccine). The value of snake venom as a superior coagulant is more definitely established. (J. A. M. A., Oct. 2, 1937, p. 1143.)

MEDICAL ECONOMICS

Edited by the Committee on Medical Economics
of the
Minnesota State Medical Association

B. J. Branton, M. D.   W. F. Braasch, M. D., Chairman   J. C. Michael, M. D.
L. H. Rutledge, M. D.   A. N. Collins, M. D.

The Council Meets

THE following resolution was passed by the Council in connection with acceptance by the Council of the 1938 budget presented by Dr. H. Z. Giffin, Rochester, chairman of the Finance Committee of the Council:

"Doctor Meyerding has been on leave of absence, without salary, as to active executive duties since September 1, 1937. Mr. Rosell has been assuming responsibility under the direction of the Finance Committee for office administration and management except as to bookkeeping, receipt of mail, and custody of important documents, which have continued as under the previous regime. Bonds are required for those assuming such duties.

"The Finance Committee, in coöperation with Doctor Meyerding, has arranged for the transference of responsibility for the bookkeeping system, the custody of important documents, the opening of all mail, except that with Doctor Meyerding's name on it, and all other activities to Mr. Rosell. It has been suggested that proper bonding and other safeguards such as insurance, as well as transfer of bookkeeping, shall be completed before January 1, 1938. The books have been reviewed as of August 31, 1937, and found to be correct.

"The Council, in confirming this transfer of office management, offers the following resolution to be spread upon the minutes:

"The advantage of the past coöperation between the Minnesota Public Health Association and the Minnesota State Medical Association is fully recognized, and it is desirable that the coöperation continue as far as possible.

"The valuable services of Doctor Meyerding over a period of thirteen years in his capacity as active secretary of the Minnesota State Medical Association are appreciated by all and especially by those who best know of the struggles of the past thirteen years which have placed Minnesota medicine in its present high ranking.

"Our Association has grown and developed in many directions during Doctor Meyerding's administration. Outstanding among his services are: the growth of our membership; committee activities; development of the component society; the interesting of the county medical group in local medical relief and welfare; county contact committees; administration of finance; the public health education program; the medical economics education program; and the growth of the annual meeting with its scientific and technical exhibits. More important than all of these is our present close and friendly relationship with all large official and voluntary agencies and associations of the State.

"There never was a time when unity of thought and action on the part of all interested in public welfare and the advancement of medicine was more necessary than it is now. It is the desire and hope of the Council that Doctor Meyerding, although not responsible as to active duties, should be freely consulted regarding policies affecting the practice of medicine. We deeply appreciate the fact that he has volunteered such aid."

Thanks of the Council were extended to Doctor Giffin and members of his committee for their work.

Ready to Publish

Only a small amount of work remains to be done to complete the "History of Medicine in Minnesota" as it has been planned by the Historical Committee.

The date 1900 was chosen arbitrarily by the committee as the ending point for the history. In view of the impossibility of tracing the history of every society in the state, the committee has followed the early lines of transportation and will cover most of the settlements where pioneer medical men established themselves.

The compilation represents much devoted research on the part of members of the committee and others who have assisted them. It was close to the heart of the late Dr. H. M. Workman for many years chairman of the Council, and it has been a major interest of Dr. Arthur S Hamilton of Minneapolis, previous chairman who was forced by illness to relinquish th work, also to the present chairman, Dr. John M. Armstrong of St. Paul.

Doctor Armstrong reported upon the progress of the work, and the Council voted unanimously to publish it serially, under the editorship of Doctor Armstrong, in MINNESOTA MEDICINE.

The Council also voted an expression of appreciation for the work of Doctor Armstrong and his associates.

Care for Work Camps

The Treasury Department has asked for bids for regular sanitary inspection and medical care in the work camps of the Resettlement Administration in Northern Minnesota. Some of these camps are at some distance from resident doctors and require considerable time of the attending physician.

It is recognized that procedure for care of these camps is dictated from Washington and must be followed. The Council suggested, however, that the county societies involved make an arrangement as societies with the camp administration in St. Paul to do the work. County society members, in turn, could assign the job to the man or men nearest the camp and make mutually agreeable division or assignment of the funds.

In general, this is the scheme known as the "Iowa Plan," used first to handle care for the indigent, but well adapted, also, for special work such as care for the men in the work camps. The object, of course, is to avoid objectionable competitive bidding on contracts for medical work.

Interprofessional Meetings

Interprofessional meetings in each county and district society were approved by the Council at this meeting. These meetings are being suggested by the Interprofessional Relationship Committee of the state association, of which Dr. F. J. Savage is chairman. They are to be informal gatherings at which representatives of all the professions get together, become acquainted with mutual problems, unite for better community action on health problems. A yearly public health meeting sponsored by the entire interprofessional group is a further suggestion of the committee which met with Council approval.

These gatherings should be kept informal and without regular constitution or elected officers, in the opinion of Council and committee, since organizations thus formed are sometimes used by participating groups for purposes not contemplated by the founders.

A letter detailing the aims and purposes of these meetings has been sent to all secretaires by the Interprofessional Committee.

County Officers' Meeting

The 1938 County Officers' Conference of the State Association will be held Saturday, February 26, at the Saint Paul Hotel, Saint Paul. The date was approved by the Council and a request has subsequently been sent to all secretaries by Executive Secretary R. R. Rosell, for suggestions as to subjects that will be of most value at this meeting.

Survey in California

The California survey of sickness and sickness costs is complete at last and available to students of the subject.

This survey covers the years 1934-1935 and cost the California State Medical Association $50,000, the Federal government approximately $55,000, the California Dental Society $800, the whole making a grand total of $102,352.66.

The studies cover the medical vicissitudes of 60,033 persons out of a population of more than 5,000,000. Subject to inquiry was the general character of the population, its income, its morbidity, the medical facilities available, the extent to which they are utilized, likewise the extent to which the cost might have been instrumental in curtailing their use.

Out of the 60,003, a group of 8,260 were discovered who were in need of medical care. Of these, 4,810 were receiving care at the time of the interview, leaving 3,459, or 5.7 per cent, presumably in need of care which they were not receiving. Not a very large percentage, surely, when you consider that some of the 5.7 per cent undoubtedly did not desire medical care whether they needed it or not.

There are, in California, some 9,000 physicians licensed to practice medicine; also, 1,403 osteopaths, 2,500 chiropractors, 255 drugless therapists, 39 neuropaths and 2,000 Christian Science practitioners.

This is undoubtedly the most complete survey of its kind ever made in America. Whether it throws sufficient light on a tangled situation to repay the huge expenditure is a matter of opinion. It should be of great interest, however, to all who are concerned in the economic problems of medicine. Copies may be obtained from the office of the California State Medical Association, 450 Sutter Street, San Francisco, for $2.00.

Syphilis Campaign

The widespread campaign of publicity about venereal disease brings with it definite problems to physicians.

There is no doubt as to the worth and advisability of accurate knowledge about these diseases on the part of the public in general and the worth of routine use of the diagnostic measures.

A wave of popular enthusiasm about any health campaign carries with it possibilities of danger, however.

Lay organizers, quacks, ill-advised enthusiasts are likely to take advantage of it.

The *Journal of the American Medical Association* reports a commercial organization in Los Angeles organized to get money out of restaurants and food handling establishments in exchange for window signs to indicate that employees are free from venereal disease. Decidedly sketchy and unreliable means of vouching for the condition of employees were arranged by this company.

Doctors Must Assist

In Minnesota, the Junior Chamber of Commerce desires to make venereal disease education a major welfare project for the year. It is obvious, of course, that the Junior Chamber is incapable of carrying on any such campaign without assistance. Also it is obvious that the county medical society in every center where such a campaign is started should be the medical agency to direct and assist with the campaign. If the county medical society fails of this duty there are other agencies and individuals that will jump at the chance.

Saint Paul Project

In Saint Paul the Junior Chamber of Commerce was assisted by the Ramsey County Medical Society, with the result that every school, college, luncheon club and many other organized groups were reached by a qualified and especially trained representative of the medical society.

In Pennsylvania a state-wide educational campaign is now in progress under the auspices of the medical association committee. In the course of the campaign free Wassermann tests will be offered to all comers.

Free Tests

Free tests have been considered, also, in one of the Minnesota towns where the Junior Chamber wishes to stage a campaign. The question of whether or not free diagnostic tests should be a feature depends upon the local county medical society. If members approve and are willing to do the work in the name of the county society there can be no more objection to these tests than to other special types of public health work done by medical societies as a unit, for the period of a campaign.

Minnesota is in far better position than many other states to undertake a widespread educational campaign to bring in untreated persons for treatment as well as to extend use of the test as a routine part of every medical examination. The venereal disease program of the State Board of Health has steadily maintained laboratory service for diagnostic tests and provided drugs for those unable to pay for them for many years. There are facilities for the diagnosis and care of the disease in all parts of the state.

Handicapped

Sir Henry Brackenbury, chairman of the council of the British Medical Association, believes that a health insurance plan such as exist in England, Scotland and Wales would b enormously handicapped in the United States.

In the course of informal remarks during recent visit to this country, Sir Henry made some interesting observations on the subjec They gain significance when it is recalled tha he is an often-quoted authority on the Englis

52

system and that he has had much to do with establishment of England's rates and rules.

Sir Henry says that whatever success the English system has had is due to the homogeneity of race in England, Scotland and Wales and the likeness of the background of all their peoples. Also to the homogeneity in race-type, general professional training and outlook of their physicians. He attributes its workability, also, to the existence in Britain of a permanent civil service personnel possessed of continuous and definite authority to carry out the law, no matter what political group names the nominal heads of departments.

In the United States the difference in standards and backgrounds of the people, the differences in education and licensure of physicians from state to state and the inevitability of political control in any conceivable plan for compulsory health insurance would provide serious obstacles to success.

"1938 What"

(Monthly Editorial Prepared by the Medical Advisory Committee)

"Thank you for your interest and help in my case. I appreciate the support of the State Association more than I can say."

The above is a part of a recent letter received by your Medical Advisory Committee from one of the State Association's members following the dismissal of his case.

Only one who has gone through the ordeal of anxiously waiting for the time of trial, torn between a feeling of guilt and innocence of wrongdoing, can appreciate the sense of relief felt by the man who penned these words. His was the prayer of thanks, his evidence of applied friendship.

Could every man, each member of the Association, step into his place and feeling, we should have an Association cemented together by the common ties of mutual interest such as nothing else could do.

There can be no middle road in 1938 in dealing with the unwarranted malpractice case. If the case is one of clear responsibility on the part of physician or surgeon, the aggrieved party should be settled with. If the case is one of the usual type, purely a money-making scheme, it should be fought through all courts. Remember that, in your committee's experience,

one illegitimate case settled means at least two more will be brought in the same community within a short time.

The time is now ripe to apply that familiar phrase, "All for one and one for all." Let's make the new year a year of renewed friendships, forgotten disagreements, and forgiven quarrels. We will need patience, perseverance, endurance, and clear, concise, mutual understanding with the many problems that now beset medical practice and our Association's welfare.

Pepys in Minnesota

November 12.—More merciless days of dredging through masses of writings and what not and more than ever attracted by "Assignment in Utopia," in which Eugene Lyons tells of seven years in Russia. So now in Saint Paul, where some hundreds of doctors have feted Meyerding. At breakfast came editors of the press and then interviewers and photographers, and then to speak to the Christmas seal workers, and after that to the Junior Chamber of Commerce to speak on syphilis; and old Pepys reminded them that we must look for syphilis not only in the Junior Chamber but also in the Junior League. Next with Ben Wright to Minneapolis to speak on the radio, and after that to the annual dinner of the health association. Now here came Myers and Slater and many more, and a town crier rang out the call and an a cappella choir (no accompaniment, thank you) sang merrily. So old Pepys talked some more and a local medico came up to Mistress Pepys and said: "Your father made a swell speech"; so old Pepys decided to begin dieting again.

November 13.—At 7:30 to breakfast with the officers and council of the state medical society, talked of this and that and speaking of planning heard Chesley tell of the man in Maine where the fog was so thick that when he went up to shingle the roof and the fog cleared suddenly, he fell in the manure pile because he had shingled out ten feet from the barn onto the fog. And Adson spoke well and also Light, and then all went to see Minnesota perform against Northwestern 7 to 0; so now I get my $5.00 back. At night driving to Rochester in a blinding snow and an airplane is safer.—From Tonics and Sedatives, Pepys' Diary, *Journal of the American Medical Association,* November 27.

Illegal

Acting Comptroller-General Elliott has declared the medical plan of the Homeowners' Loan Corporation illegal. This HOLC plan provides group sickness insurance for its employees and it was financed by $40,000 of Federal funds.

In view of the special status of the HOLC the opinion of the Comptroller-General must be viewed as purely advisory. There is no specific prohibition by Congress for the action and, in any case, the money is already spent.

Minnesota State Board of Medical Examiners

Worthington Osteopath Fined $250.00 and Costs For Unlawful Practice of Medicine

State of Minnesota *vs.* Dunn.

On November 30, 1937, Donald J. Dunn, forty-five years of age, entered a plea of guilty to an information charging him with practicing medicine without a license. Dunn, who holds a license to practice osteopathy, but not medicine, and who maintains an office at Worthington, Minnesota, was sentenced by the Honorable Charles A. Flinn, Judge of the District Court, to pay a fine of $250.00 plus the court costs, or serve four months in the Nobles County Jail. Dunn paid the fine plus court costs of $6.90, or a total of $256.90.

The Minnesota State Board of Medical Examiners had received a number of complaints that the defendant was injecting medicine and furnishing medicine to be taken internally. The investigation disclosed that Dunn had written a number of prescriptions to be taken internally, but that he had neither written the name of the patient upon the prescriptions, nor had he signed them. The particular case upon which a complaint was filed concerned a young man who stated that he consulted the defendant and had been advised that he was in a run down condition and suffering from an inflammation of the kidneys and the bladder. He stated that the defendant gave him a number of hypodermic injections in the arm and some pills to be taken internally. He stated that he also received a bottle of so-called blood medicine to be taken internally and a written prescription for a second bottle of the same medicine. He stated that he received a bill from the defendant in the sum of $162.00. The patient stated that he did not get any better and, upon consulting a physician, was advised that he was suffering from a different condition from that stated by the defendant. He also stated that he has made considerable improvement since being under medical care.

The osteopathic law of Minnesota specifically provides that the practice of osteopathy

"is hereby declared distinct from that of medicine or surgery * * * Osteopathic physicians, when duly licensed, shall have the right to practice osteopathy, * * * including the use and administration in connection with the practice of obstetrics, minor surgery and toxicology only of anesthetics, narcotics, antidotes and antiseptics."

The law also provides:

"Except as hereinbefore expressly authorized as to the administration of anesthetics, narcotics, antidotes and the use of antiseptics, the license shall not authorize the holder to give or prescribe drugs for internal use."
—Section 5736-5737, Mason's Minnesota Statutes for 1927.

Itasca County Practitioner Pleads Guilty

Re: State of Minnesota *vs.* Smith

On December 10, 1937, Christopher Columbus Smith, seventy-seven years of age, entered a plea of guilty to an information charging him with practicing healing without a basic science certificate. Smith entered his plea of guilty before the Honorable Graham M. Torrance, Judge of the District Court at Aitkin, Minnesota. After hearing the facts, Judge Torrance sentenced Smith to a term of four months in the Itasca County Jail, and placed him on probation until September 13, 1938, on a number of conditions, two of which are that Smith absolutely refrain from practicing medicine in any manner, or from holding himself out to the public as a physician.

Smith moved into northern Itasca County in 1920,

and resided on a farm about a mile east of Effie. In 1930 he was given a warning by the State Board of Medical Examiners to refrain from practicing medicine, and he stated, at that time, that if given an opportunity he would return to the State of Texas. However, he did not leave and in 1933, following a fire, he moved into Effie, where he built a small place and has continued to practice medicine until the time of his arrest on December 9, 1937. Smith stated to the Court that he was born in Fannin County, Texas, and raised in Davis County, Missouri. He stated that he attended the old Medical School at Keokuk, Iowa, graduating in 1885, and being licensed by the Iowa State Board of Medical Examiners in 1886, holding license number 1050. He also stated that he had never been convicted of a crime. Judge Torrance warned the defendant that under no circumstances could he be permitted to practice medicine. It was stated to the Court that the sanitary conditions at Smith's residence, where he maintained his office, were very bad.

The State Board of Medical Examiners wishes to acknowledge the fine coöperation of John J. Benton, County Attorney, and Sheriff Elmer Madson.

List of Physicians Licensed by The Minnesota State Board of Medical Examiners, November 12, 1937

By Examination

Name	School	Address

Arkin, Archie Abraham, U. of Manitoba, M.D., 1932, Minneapolis, Minn.

Beizer, Lawrence, Harvard U., M.D., 1934, Rochester, Minn.

Bellis, Carroll Joseph, U. of Minn., M.B. and M.D., 1936, Minneapolis, Minn.

Benesh, Louis Alfred, U. of Minn., M.B., 1937, Minneapolis, Minn.

Benkwitz, Karl Burton, U. of Rochester, M.D., 1934, Minneapolis, Minn.

Bennett, Robert Leo, Jr., U. of Pittsburgh, M.D., 1936, Rochester, Minn.

Berlin, Anthony Salvatore, U. of Minn., M.B. and M.D., 1937, St. Paul, Minn.

Black, Benjamin Marden, Stanford U., M.D., 1936, Rochester, Minn.

Black, John Robert, McGill U., M.D., 1934, Rochester, Minn.

Boysen, John Edward, U. of Minn., M.B., 1936; M.D., 1937, Pelican Rapids, Minn.

Brown, Henry Allen, Med. Col. of Va., M.D., 1934, Rochester, Minn.

Browne, Harry C., Jr., U. of Ore., M.D., 1935, Rochester, Minn.

Brumm, Harold J., Rush Med. Col., M.D., 1936, Rochester, Minn.

Cabell, Charles Lorraine, U. of Va., M.D., 1934, Rochester, Minn.

Cameron, David Molloy, U. of Texas, M.D., 1935, Rochester, Minn.

Conway, John Francis, U. of Rochester, M.D., 1935, Rochester, Minn.

Cottrell, Lillian, U. of Colo., M.D., 1936, Minneapolis, Minn.

Cowan, Donald William, U. of Minn, M.B., and M.D., 1931, Minneapolis, Minn.

Craft, Charles Brigman, Tulane U., M.D., 1935, Minneapolis, Minn.

Davies, Roberts Judson, U. of Minn., M.B., 1933; M.D., 1934, Nopeming, Minn.

Dees, Myrta Susan Coons, Johns Hopkins, M.D., 1934, Minneapolis, Minn.

Delmonico, E. Joseph, Syracuse U., M.D., 1930, Rochester, Minn.

Dublin, William Brooks, U. of Cal., M.D., 1936; Rochester, Minn.

Engle, David Edwin, Indiana U., M.D., 1934, Rochester, Minn.

Foster, Furman Lamar, U. of Minn., M.B., 1936; M.D., 1937, Minneapolis, Minn.

Freedman, Harold Charles, U. of Minn., M.B., 1937, Minneapolis, Minn.

Freeman, William Neil, U. of Chicago, M.D., 1937, St. Cloud, Minn.

Goodson, William Hammack, Jr., Harvard U., M.D., 1934, Rochester, Minn.

Grindlay, John Happer, Harvard U., M.D., 1935, Rochester, Minn.

Grove, M. Stuart, U. of Minn., M.B., 1934; M.D., 1935, St. Paul, Minn.

Hammer, Howard John, Wayne U., M.B., 1934; M.D., 1935, Rochester, Minn.

Heise, William von Rohr, Northwestern, M.B., 1934; M.D., 1935, Winona, Minn.

Hildebrand, Alice Grace, U. of Neb., M.D., 1936, Rochester, Minn.

Judd, Edward Starr, Jr., Rush Med. Col., M.D., 1937, Rochester, Minn.

Kernan, Phillip Donald, U. of Wis., M.D., 1933, Minneapolis, Minn.

Kimmel, George Charles, Jr., U. of Minn., M.B., 1936; M.D., 1937, Minneapolis, Minn.

Koch, Eleanor Alice Steele, Johns Hopkins, M.D., 1934, Rochester, Minn.

Lange, Elizabeth Greason Hunter, U. of Mich., M.D., 1928, Minneapolis, Minn.

Leighton, Robert Sisson, II, U. of Minn., M.B., 1937, Minneapolis, Minn.

Madding, Gordon Francis, Northwestern, M.B., 1936; M.D., 1937, Rochester, Minn.

Mitchell, Mancel Talcott, U. of Minn., M.B., 1934; M.D., 1935, Minneapolis, Minn.

Muir, Walter Francis, U. of Minn., M.B. and M.D., 1937, Graceville, Minn.

O'Brien, Louis Timothy, U. of Minn., M.B., 1935; M.D., 1936, Wahpeton, N. Dak.

Olds, John Whitney, Rush Med. Col., M.D., 1936, Rochester, Minn.

Pearman, Robert Oliver Davidson, Harvard U., M.D., 1935, Rochester, Minn.

Peters, Stanley Bruce, U. of Rochester, M.D., 1935, Virginia, Minn.

Ralph, Robert Douglas, Queens U., M.D., 1932, Rochester, Minn.

Schiele, Burtrum Clarence, U. of Colo., M.D., 1931, Minneapolis, Minn.

Schmitz, Anthony A., U. of Minn., M.B., 1937, Minneapolis, Minn.

Schneider, Herbert Hoyt, U. of Kansas, M.D., 1936, Rochester, Minn.

Seedorf, Everett Emil, U. of Wis., M.D., 1936, Rochester, Minn.

Seldon, Thomas Harry, Queens U., M.D., 1929, Rochester, Minn.

Skinner, Ira Clifton, Jr., Tulane U., M.D., 1935, Rochester, Minn.

Smith, Baxter Allen, Jr., U. of Minn., M.B., 1936; M.D., 1937, Minneapolis, Minn.

Spink, Wesley William, Harvard U., M.D., 1932, Minneapolis, Minn.

Sturley, Rodney Francis, U. of Minn., M.B., 1937, Minneapolis, Minn.

Swartz, Frederick Charles, U. of Cincinnati, M.B., 1931; M.D., 1932, Rochester, Minn.

Templin, David Browning, U. of Chicago, M.D., 1937, Rochester, Minn.

Thomas, Margaret Jane, U. of Minn., M.B., 1936; M.D., 1937, Minneapolis, Minn.

Trach, Benedict, U. of Minn., M.B., 1937, Chicago, Ill.

Trueman, Kenneth Rankine, U. of Manitoba, M.D., 1934, Rochester, Minn.

Vickers, Paul Merton, U. of Minn., M.B., 1936; M.D., 1937, Rochester, Minn.

Waisman, Morris, U. of Ill., M.D., 1936, Rochester, Minn.

Watterson, Kenneth Ward, U. of Pittsburgh, M.D., 1929, Rochester, Minn.

Wellman, Thomas Gibbs, U. of Minn., M.B. and M.D., 1937, Lake City, Minn.

Wollaeger, Eric Edwin, Harvard U., M.D., 1934, Rochester, Minn.

By Reciprocity

Dix, Christopher Robert, U. of Wis., M.D., 1935, Rochester, Minn.

MacKay, Alexander Russell, Northwestern, M.D., 1936, Rochester, Minn.

Walsh, John Joseph, Jefferson, M.D., 1935, Rochester, Minn.

Rosenbladt, Louis Mayo, U. of Nebr., M.D., 1932, St. Paul, Minn.

Langmack, William August, Marquette U., M.D., 1936, Cloquet, Minn.

Leland, John Augustin Charles, Jr., Jefferson Med. Col., M.D., 1936, Minneapolis, Minn.

Soniat, Theodore Louis Lucian, Tulane U., M.D., 1935, Rochester, Minn.

National Board Credentials

Hartwell, Donald Clifford, Col. of Med. Evang., M.D., 1937, Wayzata, Minn.

Harris, William Elsworth Stanley, U. of Minn., M.B., 1936; M.D., 1937, St. Paul, Minn.

Pratt, Sidney Charles, U. of Minn., M.B., 1936; M.D., 1937, Minneapolis, Minn.

Sather, George Allen, Rush Med. Col., M.D., 1937, Fosston, Minn.

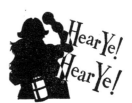

Hear Ye!
Hear Ye!

If you haven't sent in your Christmas Seal money, do so now!

Dr. Albert Goblirsch of Faribault was recently married to Miss Dorothy Fraser of Minneapolis.

* * *

Dr. M. J. Lindahl of Pipestone has moved to Sherburn, where he will practice medicine.

* * *

Dr. W. B. Beadie of Cannon Falls conducted a chest clinic early in December.

* * *

Dr. S. A. Whitson of Alden is taking postgraduate work in major surgery at the Cook County Hospital, Chicago.

* * *

Dr. Ralph E. Moyer of Minneapolis has recently been appointed to the staff at the Minnesota State School and Colony in Faribault.

* * *

Dr. Edmund V. Pellettiere of Thief River Falls was recently married in New Orleans. Dr. and Mrs. Pellettiere are now at home in Thief River Falls.

* * *

Dr. John A. Tweedy has become affiliated with his father, Dr. G. J. Tweedy, and his brother, Dr. R. B. Tweedy, of Winona, in the practice of medicine.

* * *

Dr. J. C. Masson and Dr. A. W. Adson of Rochester left early in December for a three-weeks' fishing and hunting trip in Texas and New Mexico.

* * *

A number of Willmar physicians and their wives were recently entertained by the nurses of the Rice Memorial Hospital at a housewarming for the nurses' home next to the hospital.

* * *

Dr. F. E. Harrington, Commissioner of Public Health in Minneapolis, began a new series of health talks over KSTP on December 22, at 11:15 A.M. The program is being sponsored by the Glenwood-Inglewood Pure Spring Water Company.

* * *

Dr. and Mrs. F. U. Davis of Faribault started early in December on an extended trip throughout the southern states, Mexico and California. They are traveling in their modern and well equipped house trailer. They expect to return to Faribault in the spring.

February 2, 1938, has been designated as Na Social Hygiene Day by the American Social Hy Association for the purpose of eliciting interest i various activities directed against venereal disease
The Association, with headquarters at 50 West Street, New York City, will supply interested pe or groups with suggestions for meetings and mat such as exhibits, films and literature upon reques

* * *

Dr. Wilder Penfield of Montreal, Canada, Dir of the Neurological Institute and Professor of N surgery at McGill University, will give the fift Starr Judd Lecture at the University of Minn in the Medical Science Amphitheater on Wedne February 2, at 8:15 p. m. The subject of Dr. field's lecture is "Cerebral Circulation in Epile The late E. Starr Judd, an alumnus of the M School of the University of Minnesota, establ this annual lectureship in surgery a few years b his death.

* * *

Excerpt from a recent letter from the Secreta the United States Treasury to the Attorney-Gei
(Appointment of Consulting Specialists in Psyc by the U. S. Public Health Service)
"The Department has, upon the recommendati the Surgeon-General, appointed as Consulting Spec in Psychiatry the following physicians: Dr. Jose Michael, 1945 Medical Arts Bldg., Minneapolis, Dr. Ernest Martin Hammes, 1125 Lowry Medical Bldg., Saint Paul, Minn.; Dr. William Howard H ler, 1068 Lowry Medical Arts Bldg., Saint Paul, I Dr. Gordon R. Kamman, 350 St. Peter Street, Paul, Minn., and Dr. Frank White Whitmore Lowry Medical Arts Bldg., Saint Paul, Minn. . . . specialists will, upon the request and only upon t quest of the court, examine any person held pu to a law of the United States, and will submit c ive advice and report to the court showing the status of such person or the need of further examination and observation.

"The Department desires to take this oppo of stressing the fact that the nature of the ser be furnished under the above arrangement is cor and advisory to the court, and also wishes to in tention to the importance of a realization on tl of all judicial, prosecution, and enforcement as well as defense counsel, that this service is the purpose of determining the guilt or innoce an accused; it is intended only to assist the c determine the mental state of a defendant element in the problem of the disposition to b of a case."

REPORTS and ANNOUNCEMENTS

1938 AMERICAN MEDICAL ASSOCIATION MEETING—SAN FRANCISCO

When San Francisco was selected as the host city for the 1938 Annual Session of The American Medical Association, the profession of this Golden Gate Metropolis promptly initiated plans for the comfort, pleasure and entertainment of all who come to that national meeting. A local executive committee on arrangements, composed of five members with Doctor Howard Morrow as General Chairman and Doctor Frederick C. Warnshuis as General Secretary, and eighteen sub-committees have been busy since July in developing plans and local arrangement details. Their objective is the biggest, best, and most memorable annual session in the history of the American Medical Association.

Atlantic City, Kansas City, Cleveland, Detroit, with their known facilities and attractions, have been host cities in recent years, and have justified their selection as meeting places. However, and without disparagement, none of them possess the background, the setting, the resources, the history and romance, or the facilities that are found in San Francisco and in the great state of California—the Golden Bear Empire of the Pacific Coast. To reveal these, to extend California's and San Francisco's noted hospitality, and to cause those who plan to attend the 1938 session to experience ten days of profit and pleasure midst the environs of the annual meeting city, is the goal toward which the local profession is pointing.

The Local Committee on Arrangements cordially invites the profession of the country to be San Francisco's guests this coming June. Decide now to attend the 1938 American Medical Association Meeting and plan accordingly. During the coming months an insight to some of the feature functions will be disclosed, but the final details and program of events will not be revealed until you arrive. You will long regret it if you fail to attend the coming national meeting. Talk it over tonight with the good wife and your professional associates, and join the party of your state members that is coming to San Francisco—June 12th to 17th, 1938.

THE AMERICAN BOARD OF INTERNAL MEDICINE

The American Board of Internal Medicine will hold its next written examination on Monday, February 14, 1938, in various centers of the United States and Canada.

The examination will consist of two sessions of three hours each with the morning session held at 9:00 o'clock a. m. and the afternoon session held at 2:00 o'clock p. m.

The candidates who are successful in this written examination will be eligible to take the practical examination which will be held in San Francisco the Friday and Saturday prior to the opening of the Annual Session of the American Medical Association in June, 1938.

The final date for filing applications for this written examination is January 15, 1938, and all applications should be in the office of the chairman before that date.

For further particulars and application blanks please address Dr. Walter L. Bierring, M.D., Chairman, American Board of Internal Medicine, Suite 1210, 406 Sixth Avenue, Des Moines, Iowa.

AMERICAN BOARD OF OBSTETRICS AND GYNECOLOGY

The next examination (written and review of case histories) for Group B candidates who have filed applications will be held in various cities of the United States and Canada, on Saturday, February 5, 1938.

The general oral, clinical and pathological examinations for all candidates (Groups A and B) will be conducted by the entire Board, meeting in San Francisco, California, on June 13 and 14, 1938, immediately prior to the meeting of the American Medical Association.

Applications for admission to the June, 1938, Group A examinations must be on an official application form and filed in the Secretary's Office before April 1, 1938.

For further information and application blanks address Dr. Paul Titus, Secretary, 1015 Highland Building, Pittsburgh (6), Pa.

STATE MEETING

Dr. Howard W. Haggard, of Yale, famous lecturer and writer, is one of several distinguished medical guests who will address the Minnesota State Medical Association at its 85th Annual Meeting in Duluth, June 29, 30 and July 1, at the Hotel Duluth.

Dr. Haggard will talk to the doctors at the banquet to be held on the evening of June 30. He will also address an evening health meeting to which the public is to be invited.

Dates for the meeting were set in advance of the Fourth of July holiday and at the beginning of the vacation season in the North, so that physicians and their families could combine a vacation with attendance at the meeting.

Medical men from all of the Northwest states are expected to take advantage of the opportunity.

The scientific program, now practically completed, calls for sessions on fractures, on obstetrics and pediatrics, eye, ear, nose and throat, and on use of newer drugs, also a session of clinics in the Duluth hospitals.

Exhibits and demonstrations will be a feature of the meeting.

INSTITUTE IN OPHTHALMOLOGY AND OTOLARYNGOLOGY

January 17 to 22, 1938

The next seminar for medical graduates at the Center for Continuation Study of the University of Minnesota will be on Ophthalmology and Otolaryngology, January 17 to 22, 1938. The program will occupy the full time of the physicians from Monday morning to Saturday evening. There will be no evening lectures, but a feature of the institute will be a joint meeting on Friday evening, January 21, with the Minnesota Academy of Ophthalmology and Otolaryngology.

The seminar will consist of clinics, round table discussions, and lectures illustrated by lantern slides, charts or patients. The teaching staff has been selected from the Departments of Ophthalmology and Otolaryngology of the University Medical School, Minneapolis, the Mayo Clinic, Rochester, and the General Extension Division. The meetings will be held in the Center for Continuation Study, and in the University of Minnesota Hospitals and affiliated institutions in Minneapolis and St. Paul.

It is to be noted that much of the course will be devoted to intimate clinical instruction or conferences. Those who plan to register should make their reservations as soon as possible so that proper arrangements can be made for the clinics.

Program

Monday, January 17, 1938

Morning

9:00-10:00 The Early Diagnosis and Treatment of Hearing Deficiencies, Dr. Newhart.

10:00-11:30 Operative Clinic, University Hospitals, Drs. Boies and Bryant.

11:30-12:30 Pathology of Ear, Nose and Throat Diseases, Dr. Connor.

Afternoon

2:00- 3:00 Dispensary Clinic, University Hospitals, Drs. Boies and Fjelstad.

3:00- 4:00 Malignant Tumors of the Larynx, Dr. New.

4:30- 6:00 Round Table, Surgery of Acute Mastoiditis, Dr. Boies.

Tuesday, January 18, 1938

Morning

9:00-10:00 Pitfalls in Diagnosis and Treatment of Diseases of the Eye, Dr. J. S. Macnie.

10:00-11:00 External Diseases of the Eye, Dr. Pfunder.

11:00-12:00 Pathology of Eye Diseases, Dr. Camp.

Afternoon

2:00- 3:00 Dispensary Clinic, University Hospitals, Dr. Hymes and Associates.

3:00- 4:30 Eye Operative Clinic, University Hospitals, Dr. J. S. Macnie.

5:00- 6:00 Round Table, Ophthalmological Problems, Dr. Benedict.

Wednesday, January 19, 1938

Morning

9:00-12:00 Dry and Operative Clinics, Ancker Hos tal, St. Paul, Drs. Leavenworth, Ho filzer and Associates.

Afternoon

2:00- 3:00 Endoscopic Procedures with Special Ref ence to Hoarseness and Dysphagia, Phelps.

3:00- 4:00 Management of Acute and Chronic Sii sitis, Dr. Bryant.

4:30- 6:00 Round Table, Nasal Obstruction, Hochfilzer.

Thursday, January 20, 1938

Morning

9:00-10:00 Surgery of Optical Muscles, Dr. Grant.

10:00-11:00 Fundus Findings in Blood Dyscrasias, Stanford.

11:00-12:00 Ocular Neurology, Dr. Ed. Burch.

Afternoon

2:00- 3:00 Dispensary Clinic, University Hospitals, Hanson and Associates.

3:00- 4:00 Eye Operative Clinic, University Hos tals, Dr. J. P. Macnie.

5:00- 6:00 Round Table and Pictures, Intraocular (eration, Dr. Spratt.

Friday, January 21, 1938

Morning

9:00-10:00 Demonstrations of Neurology of Eye, E Nose and Throat, Room 214, Anato Building, University, Drs. Rasmussen Newhart.

10:00-11:30 Operative Clinic, University Hospit Drs. Boies and Williams.

11:30-12:30 The Management of Chronic Otitis Me Dr. Williams.

Afternoon

2:00- 3:00 Dispensary Clinic, University Hospit Drs. Newhart, Delavan and Bryant.

3:00- 4:00 Physiology of the Nose as the Basis Treatment, Dr. Hilding.

4:30- 6:30 Round Tables (Visiting Clinicians). Section I, Ear, Nose and Throat; tion II, Eye.

6:30 Dinner meeting with Minnesota Acad of Ophthalmology and Otolaryngolog Speakers: Dr. J. P. Macnie, "Deta Retina"; and Dr. Thomas C. Gallo in the Ear, Nose and Throat field, ject to be announced later by the A emy.

Saturday, January 22, 1938

Morning

9:00-10:00 Photography of Fundus, Dr. Fellows

10:00-11:00 Ophthalmoscopy, Dr. Rucker.

11:00-12:00 Some Clinical Problems in Refraction, Prangen.

Afternoon

1:00- 3:30 Refraction Clinic, University Hospitals, Drs. Houkom, Hymes and Sandt (with a lecture by the latter on Contact Glasses).

3:30- 4:30 Allergy of Eye, Ear, Nose and Throat, Dr. Hilding.

5:00- 6:00 Round Table, Ocular Muscles and Orthoptics, Dr. Walter Fink.

Faculty

Harold S. Diehl, Professor of Preventive Medicine and Public Health, Dean of Medical Sciences, Medical School, Minneapolis.

James M. Hayes, Assistant Professor of Surgery, President, Minnesota State Medical Association, Minneapolis.

William A. O'Brien, Associate Professor of Pathology, Preventive Medicine and Public Health, Medical School. Medical Representative, Center for Continuation Study, St. Paul.

William L. Benedict, Professor of Ophthalmology, Mayo Clinic, Rochester.

Lawrence R. Boies, Assistant Professor of Otolaryngology, Medical School, Minneapolis.

Edward Burch, Special Lecturer, General Extension Division, St. Paul.

Frank L. Bryant, Instructor of Otolaryngology, Medical School, Minneapolis.

Walter E. Camp, Assistant Professor of Ophthalmology, Medical School, Minneapolis.

Charles E. Connor, Assistant Professor of Otolaryngology, Medical School, St. Paul.

Philip A. Delavan, Instructor of Otolaryngology, Medical School, St. Paul.

Manley F. Fellows, Special Lecturer, General Extension Division, Duluth.

Walter H. Fink, Instructor of Ophthalmology, Medical School, Minneapolis.

C. Alford Fjelstad, Assistant Professor of Otolaryngology, Medical School, Minneapolis.

Thomas C. Galloway, Evanston, Illinois, Guest Lecturer.

Hendrie W. Grant, Clinical Assistant Professor of Ophthalmology, Medical School, St. Paul.

Erling W. Hansen, Assistant Professor of Ophthalmology, Medical School, Minneapolis.

Anderson Hilding, Special Lecturer, General Extension Division, Duluth.

John J. Hochfilzer, Special Lecturer, General Extension Division, St. Paul.

Bjarne Houkom, Clinical Instructor of Ophthalmology, Medical School, Minneapolis.

Charles Hymes, Clinical Assistant Professor of Ophthalmology, Medical School, Minneapolis.

R. O. Leavenworth, Special Lecturer, General Extension Division, St. Paul.

John S. Macnie, Associate Professor of Ophthalmology, Medical School, Minneapolis.

John P. Macnie, Eye Institute, Medical Center, New York City, Guest Lecturer.

Gordon B. New, Professor of Laryngology, Oral and Plastic Surgery, Mayo Clinic, Rochester.

Horace Newhart, Professor of Otolaryngology, Rhinology, and Laryngology, and Director Division, Medical School, Minneapolis.

Malcolm C. Pfunder, Clinical Assistant of Ophthalmology, Medical School, Minneapolis.

Kenneth A. Phelps, Assistant Professor of Otolaryngology, Medical School, Minneapolis.

Avery D. Prangen, Associate Professor of Ophthalmology, Mayo Clinic, Rochester.

Andrew T. Rasmussen, Professor of Anatomy, Medical School, Minneapolis.

Charles W. Rucker, Assistant Professor of Ophthalmology, Mayo Clinic, Rochester.

Karl E. Sandt, Physician, Students' Health Service, Minneapolis.

Charles Spratt, Special Lecturer, General Extension Division, Minneapolis.

Charles E. Stanford, Physician, Students' Health Service, Minneapolis.

Henry L. Williams, Assistant Professor of Otolaryngology, Mayo Clinic, Rochester.

Note: Write to the Director for information, Center for Continuation Study, Minneapolis, about this and future institutes.

Medical Diagnosis and Treatment, February 7-12, 1938.

Traumatic Surgery, March 7-12, 1938.

Endocrinology, April 4-9, 1938.

Diseases of Rectum and Colon, May, 1938 (date to be announced).

Diagnostic Radiology, June 6-11, 1938.

EAST CENTRAL MINNESOTA SOCIETY

The East Central Minnesota Medical Society held its annual meeting on November 29, 1937, at the Colony for Epileptics, in Cambridge, Minnesota.

Dr. Donald Brink of Isle, Minnesota, and Dr. George Haliday of Rush City, Minnesota, were elected to membership in the society. Dr. G. L. Richey, formerly of Rochester, Minnesota, was accepted as a transfer into this society.

The following officers were elected for the coming year: Dr. George H. Schlesselman of Anoka, president; Dr. A. B. Roehlke of Elk River, vice president; Dr. Claire M. Ness of Cambridge, secretary-treasurer; Dr. H. C. Cooney of Princeton, delegate; and Dr. W. T. Nordman of Mora, alternate delegate.

Dinner was served and in the evening a scientific program was presented by guest speakers. Dr. A. W. Adson of the Mayo Clinic in Rochester, president of the Minnesota State Medical Society, spoke on the surgical treatment of hypertension. Dr. A. P. Dunnigan of the State Board of Health demonstrated the Neufield typing in pneumonia and explained the pneumonia service which is now available to physicians in this state.

KANDIYOHI-SWIFT-MEEKER COUNTY SOCIETY

The December meeting of the Kandiyohi-Swift-Meeker County Medical Society was held at the Lakeland Hotel, Willmar, on Wednesday, December 8.

Dr. J. K. Anderson of Minneapolis was the guest speaker, the subject being "The Office Treatment and Diagnosis of the Common Rectal Diseases."

The following officers were elected for 1938: Lennox Danielson, M.D., president-elect; Magnus Pederson, M.D., vice president; C. L. Scofield, M.D., secretary-treasurer; Karl Danielson, M.D., advisory committee, three years; C. L. Scofield, M.D., delegate, and J. C. Jacobs, M.D., alternate.

MOWER COUNTY SOCIETY

These officers of the Mower County Medical Society were all reëlected for 1938 at the annual meeting of the society on November 23: President, Dr. Paul C. Leck, Austin; vice president, Dr. R. S. Hegge, Austin; secretary, Dr. Paul A. Robertson, Austin; treasurer, Dr. A. E. Henslin, LeRoy.

PARK REGION MEDICAL SOCIETY

The annual meeting of the Park Region Medical Society was held on Wednesday evening, December 15, at the River Inn at Fergus Falls. About sixty physicians were present.

The principal speakers of the evening were Dr. J. A. Bargen and Dr. H. M. Weber, both of Rochester, Minnesota.

The following officers were elected for 1938: L. C. Combacker, M.D., president; Norman H. Baker, M.D., president-elect; C. J. Lund, M.D., vice president; T. S. Paulson, M.D., treasurer, and C. A. Boline, M.D., secretary.

RAMSEY COUNTY SOCIETY

Dr. R. B. J. Schoch, city health officer of Saint Paul, was elected president-elect of the Ramsey County Medical Society at the last meeting of the Society. Dr. James N. Dunn will take office as president on January 1. Other officers elected for 1938 are Dr. W. D. Brodie, vice president, and Dr. J. Allen Wilson, secretary-treasurer.

RED RIVER VALLEY MEDICAL SOCIETY

The annual meeting of the Red River Valley Medical Society was held at the Hotel Crookston in Crookston, on Tuesday, December 14.

Addresses on different phases of medical economics were given by Dr. L. J. McLeod of Grand Rapids, Dr. B. J. Branton of Willmar, and Dr. W. L. Burnap of Fergus Falls.

The following officers were elected for 1938: Baldwin Borreson, M.D., president; Eskil Erickson, M.D., vice president; C. L. Oppegaard, M.D., secretary-treasurer; J. A. Roy, M.D., and G. A. Morley, M.D., censors; J. F. Norman, M.D., and H. M. Blegen, M.D., delegates to the state convention.

ST. LOUIS COUNTY SOCIETY

Officers for 1938 for the St. Louis County Medical Society are: President, Dr. Malcolm G. Gillespie, Duluth; vice president, Dr. F. W. S. Raiter, Cloquet; president-elect, Dr. Gage Clement, Duluth; secretary-treasurer, Dr. Gordon C. MacRae, Duluth (reëlected); delegate, Dr. Harry Klein, Duluth; alternate, Dr. C. Jacobson, Chisholm.

SOUTHWESTERN MINNESOTA SOCIETY

At the annual meeting of the Southwestern Minnesota Medical Society, the following officers were elected: President, Dr. C. L. Sherman, Luverne; vice president, Dr. J. D. Waller, Wilmont; delegates, Dr. C. L. Sherman, Luverne and Dr. S. A. Slater, Worthington (reëlected); alternates, Dr. J. D. Waller, Wilmont and Dr. W. A. Piper, Mountain Lake. Dr. H. DeBoer was reëlected secretary-treasurer.

WASHINGTON COUNTY SOCIETY

The following officers were elected at the annual meeting of the Washington County Medical Society: President, Dr. Robert P. Ewald, Newport; first vice president, Dr. F. M. McCarten, Stillwater; second vice president, Dr. James H. Haines, Stillwater; secretary-treasurer, Dr. E. Sydney Boleyn, Stillwater; delegate, Dr. E. Sydney Boleyn, Stillwater (reëlected); alternate, Dr. W. R. Humphrey, Stillwater (reëlected).

WOMAN'S AUXILIARY

Mrs. J. F. Norman, Crookston, *President*
Mrs. A. A. Passer, Olivia, *Editor*

The Woman's Auxiliary again coöperated in the seventh Annual Christmas Seal High School Radio Contest which is sponsored by the Minnesota Public Health Association, and donated the awards. A total of one hundred talks were entered by the high schools of Minnesota and the judges, Dr. Kathleen Jordan of Granite Falls, Miss Melba Hurd of the University of Minnesota, and Mrs. Martin Nordland of Minneapolis, have announced the winners.

The ten best talks were broadcast over WCCO.

Mrs. F. A. Erb of Minneapolis, member of the Hennepin County Auxiliary, was in charge of the downtown Christmas Seal pay station at 612 Marquette Avenue which opened November 28 for the convenience of Christmas shoppers. A large group of volunteers, representing many organizations, assisted Mrs. Erb at the station throughout the holiday season. Proceeds from the sale of Christmas Seals go to support the tuberculosis prevention work.

Hennepin County Auxiliary

The Annual Glen Lake Sale was held at Dayton's November 18, 19 and 20, in charge of Mrs. E. S. Mariette and the Philanthropic Committee of the Hennepin County Auxiliary. The articles for sale are made by the Glen Lake Sanatorium patients and include knitted garments, toys, embroidered linens, leather goods and many novelties. Proceeds of the sale go to the patients.

The Annual Christmas party of the Hennepin County Auxiliary was held in the Hennepin County Medical Library, Friday, December 3, with the Social committee in charge of arrangements. Miss Mae Martin presented three puppet plays. Community singing of carols was led by Mrs. Herbert Jones and gifts were distributed by Mrs. H. B. Hannah, chairman of the Social Committee.

Renville County Auxiliary

Mrs. R. C. Adams, Bird Island, president of the auxiliary, entertained the members at her home Tuesday afternoon, December 7. Following the business session the auxiliary members joined their husbands at a banquet served in the Methodist Church dining hall. Music was furnished by the Bird Island High School Quartet. Dr. W. A. Brand, Redwood Falls, showed moving pictures including the national medical convention in Atlantic City and of the Renville County Society's annual picnic at Green Lake.

Mrs. H. B. Copeland of Cresco, Penn., an instructor in a school for the deaf in New York City, gave a talk on the "Care of Deafness." Very hard of hearing, she is a graduate of the Nitchie lip reading school of New York and did graduate work at Columbia.

PROCEEDINGS of the MINNESOTA ACADEMY of MEDICINE

Meeting of October 13, 1937

The regular monthly meeting of the Minnesota Academy of Medicine was held at the Town and Country Club on Wednesday evening, October 13, 1937. Dinner was served at 7 o'clock and the meeting was called to order at 8 o'clock by the president, Dr. E. M. Jones. There were forty-three members present. Minutes of the May meeting were read and approved. The scientific program followed.

BROMIDES, THEIR USE AND ABUSE

GORDON R. KAMMAN, M.D., F.A.C.P.
Saint Paul

Dr. Gordon Kamman read his Inaugural Thesis on the above subject.

Abstract

Due to the increase in functional nervous diseases, more sedatives are being prescribed than formerly. One of these sedatives is bromide, and, in susceptible individuals, bromides may produce mental symptoms even when given in therapeutic doses. The effects of bromide are confined largely to the central nervous system. The drug tends to replace chloride in the blood stream; so, with the administration of bromide, an adequate intake of chloride is necessary to prevent bromide intoxication.

The toxic effect of bromide may be described as simple bromide intoxication or depression, and bromide delirium or psychosis. Blood serum bromide in excess of 150 mgm. per 100 c.c. is said to be in the "toxic zone." The duration of symptoms of brominism following discontinuance of the drug is two to six weeks, and is roughly proportional to the length of time the symptoms existed prior to withdrawal.

The treatment of bromide intoxication consists of discontinuing the drug and all other sedatives; the administration of NaCl orally and parenterally; hydrotherapy, and, in urgent cases, quick acting and rapidly eliminated sedatives. Spinal drainage sometimes helps, and gastric aspiration has been recommended to help eliminate the bromide as the drug is reëxcreted into the stomach.

Three probable cases and three proven cases are reported.

Discussion

DR. GEORGE N. RUHBERG, St. Paul: Dr. Kamman is to be congratulated in presenting this timely and practical paper. My experience with bromide poisoning has occurred mainly among two types of cases. The first, in elderly people in whom arteriosclerosis and poor elimination tend to hasten mild symptoms of bromide poisoning. The second, are usually cases of severe functional neurosis, often seen in hospital consultation work, in whom marked symptoms of insomnia, agitation and excitement are present to a more or less marked degree. The usual amounts of sedatives have

not sufficed and, therefore, these have been repeatedly increased and continued until a toxic factor has been definitely established. Many of these cases are noisy and difficult to be taken care of properly in a general hospital. This condition also is seen occasionally in people who do not return to a doctor's office after obtaining an original prescription, but continue on their own, refilling the original until toxic symptoms have developed. In spite of all this, bromides have been, and I believe are, one of our most valuable sedatives when properly used.

DR. W. H. HENGSTLER, St. Paul: I also want to express my appreciation of Dr. Kamman's paper on this very pertinent subject, and the able presentation which he gave. I believe those of us who are interested in psychiatry are beginning to draw away from so much drug medication. We are prescribing less bromide and less of the heavy sedatives than we did ten years ago; and we are turning more to hydrotherapy than we used to. The fact that all people do not react the same way to the same drug must be taken into consideration. The use of bromides in the hospital, where the patient is under close observation, is justifiable, but the office patient should be told that the bromide prescription cannot be refilled without doctor's orders. A great many people know what bromides are and they buy them across the counter at drug stores; and the same is true of a great many other sedatives. We are not prescribing veronal as we used to and, in fact, we are eliminating, as far as possible, the use of all heavy and depressing sedatives.

DR. S. E. SWEITZER, Minneapolis: I wish to congratulate Dr. Kamman on a very fine paper. In a dermatological clinic, it has been my custom to withdraw bromides; most patients are better off without it than with it. As far as retention of bromides in the body is concerned, Wile stated that bromides would stay in the body as long as nine months. Bromide lesions on the skin stay there for a long while and Wile felt that the reason they did last so long was due to the fact that bromide stays in the body for so long; he recommended the use of chloride to eliminate the bromine. A patient who is getting bromine should be watched very carefully for some patients are more susceptible to it than others. Some patients will take only one dose of iodin and get an eruption, and often a small dose of bromine will do the same.

DR. H. Z. GIFFIN, Rochester: Does Dr. Kamman think we should prescribe salt as a routine when we prescribe bromide, and will the administration of salt prevent bromide eruption?

DR. KAMMAN (in closing): I wish to thank the gentlemen for their discussion. In answer to Dr. Giffin, it has been calculated that one should give four times as much chloride as bromide. If bromide and chloride intake are equal, intoxication is likely to occur in about three weeks. I do not know what effect an increased chloride intake would have in the prevention of skin lesions; probably the dermatologists could tell us more about that. Sir William Osler once said that a physician's skill stands in inverse proportion to the amount of opium and opium derivatives he prescribes. I think that remark might be extended to include bromide and embrace the therapeutic efforts of neuropsychiatrists.

THE ADMINISTRATION OF YELLOW BONE MARROW IN AGRANULOCYTIC ANGINA

HERBERT Z. GIFFIN, M.D., and
CHARLES H. WATKINS, M.D.

The Mayo Clinic, Rochester

Dr. H. Z. Giffin read a paper on the above subject.

Abstract

In studies made in 1928 and 1929, on the effects of the administration of bone marrow for secondary anemia, a moderate increase in the number of neutrophils and monocytes was observed in blood smears. This observation led to the administration of bone marrow in cases of granulocytopenia. The first patient with agranulocytic angina in the series was treated with bone marrow in July, 1930. Since then, twenty-four patients with agranulocytic angina have been treated with bone marrow and without other treatment than nursing care. The series includes all cases of agranulocytic angina in which an attempt was made to administer bone marrow, including those in which it was impossible, for one reason or another, to administer a sufficient amount, those in which the patients were in such serious condition that recovery could hardly be expected, and those in which patients had recovered from a former attack but could not obtain bone marrow during the fatal attack at home.

In the response during recovery, the first cells to increase in number are the monocytes, these cells not infrequently increasing to 10 or 20 per cent in the differential count. An increase up to 40 per cent has been observed. Following this, there is an increase in the number of neutrophils as the percentage of monocytes decreases. Myelocytes and even promyelocytes are seen many times during the early period of recovery. The percentage of neutrophils increases steadily to a level of 25 or 30, after which time there is a slower rise. By the end of the second week the percentage of neutrophils is approximately normal and the total leukocyte count is normal or above normal. The blood picture, however, is not regarded as entirely satisfactory until eosinophils and basophils appear.

There is apriori no reason to think that bone marrow should contain a material which produces this effect, as it consists mostly of fat, but, since even the yellow marrow contains many reticular cells and may potentially under stress be replaced by red marrow, there may be some substance retained which, when taken internally, has the power of stimulating the production or maturation of leukocytes.

Early in our experience, small doses of bone marrow were administered, with some benefit; the response was not nearly as rapid, however, as that which has been obtained with larger doses. At present we feel that the initial dose should be from 200 to 300 grains (13 to 20 gm.) daily; one patient was given as much as 800 grains (52 gm.) daily. This necessitates

the swallowing of from 75 to 100 pearls of bone-marrow extract* in twenty-four hours. This is usually not difficult except in cases in which severe ulceration or edema of the larynx is present. After recovery we have reduced the dose of bone marrow, keeping the patients on a maintenance dose of 50 to 100 grains (3.3 to 6.5 gm.) daily, for a period of three or four months longer. By this means, subsequent relapses apparently in most cases have been avoided.

As has been said, twenty-four patients with agranulocytic angina have been treated since 1930. Of this number, three were unable to obtain bone marrow during the fatal attack after having recovered from former attacks while taking bone marrow. Five were unable to take an adequate dose because of extreme illness: ulceration, edema of the larynx, nausea and vomiting. Two patients died even though an adequate dose had been given, one apparently of perforation of the bowel with peritonitis and the other of gas gangrene. The remaining fourteen patients are now living, having recovered from as many as one to four attacks. The total number of attacks in the series was twenty-nine. The number of attacks in which an inadequate dose or no bone marrow at all was given (the patients formerly having received bone marrow) was eight. The number of attacks in which adequate amounts of bone marrow were given and yet in which death resulted were two. Patients recovered from the remaining nineteen attacks. The average percentage of neutrophils on admission was 8, the average percentage ten days later, 58. The average leukocyte count on admission was 1200 per cu. mm. of blood; the average count, ten days later, 7800.

While the results of treatment of agranulocytic angina by any method are especially liable to lead to fallacious conclusions because of the frequency of spontaneous recoveries, our experience with the administration of bone marrow has, nevertheless, been sufficiently satisfactory to warrant a continuation of its administration to the exclusion, at least temporarily, of other methods of treatment such as liver extract, transfusion, and "pentnucleotide." When multiple methods of treatment are used, one cannot arrive at any sort of conclusion concerning the effectiveness of bone marrow or any other form of treatment. An accurate diagnosis is essential, and leukopenic leukemia, particularly of the monocytic type, and aplastic anemia, must especially be differentiated.

Discussion

DR. W. F. BRAASCH, Rochester: In these cases of agranulocytosis, following the use of sulfanilamide, would you use other measures than stopping the administration of the drug? Would you use bone marrow? Would it have an immediate effect?

DR. GIFFIN: I do not know whether it is advisable to use any method of treatment in cases in which the condition is apparently due to sulfanilamide. It may be that stopping administration of the drug is sufficient.

DR. C. B. WRIGHT, Minneapolis: This is a very interesting paper because of the number of cases re-

*Yellow bone-marrow extract, 3½ grain capsules, Frederick Stearns and Company, Detroit, Michigan.

ported and the length of time they have been followed. In fact, it is the largest series that I can recall seeing reported in the experience of any one man. We are recognizing more of these cases. It is true the final illness is usually very acute and tragic. We are learning more and more that these patients may have had previous attacks from which they recovered. I recently saw such a case. Her death was sudden, with high fever, normal red blood count, and a rapid disappearance of granulocytes from the blood. Transfusion did not help. Injections of blood did not help. On reviewing a previous hospitalization a year before when the patient was in for an abscess, the blood count showed that she had a marked drop in both the number of white cells and more marked still in the number of granulocytes. She promptly recovered from this attack but the last count recorded did not show a complete return to normal. In the four or five cases of this disease I have seen in practice, various procedures were tried such as pentnucleotide and transfusions. As far as could be determined, these measures had no effect on the disease. Dr. Giffin's high percentage of recoveries with the use of bone-marrow extract certainly is encouraging. As Dr. Giffin says, the cause of this condition is still undetermined. There must be something more fundamental than a mere drug reaction. Whether or not a drug reaction is an allergic reaction is not entirely agreed upon by dermatologists. Recent reports of sulfanilamide would indicate that the condition disappears rapidly with the removal of the drug. Undoubtedly, many cases recover spontaneously from attacks. With his record of recoveries from the use of yellow bone marrow, Dr. Giffin certainly should continue its use and it is hoped that some more concentrated extract may be obtained. I would like to ask Dr. Giffin if there was any way of determining in any given attack whether the outcome would or would not be fatal?

DR. MOSES BARRON, Minneapolis: Dr. Giffin was the first one to get me interested in yellow bone marrow for the treatment of agranulocytosis. It is very difficult to evaluate any kind of therapeutic measure in the treatment of this disease. The first case presented by Dr. Giffin was that of a pregnant woman who received bone marrow after the sixth day and recovered. The serious feature of this disease is that the patients may die from the second to the fifth or sixth day of this disease and if they live longer than that, many recover without any special treatment.

As Dr. Giffin emphasized, most of us do not wish to determine the efficiency of any special therapeutic agent and, for my own part, I give pentnucleotide, yellow bone marrow and liver extract all at the same time, as soon as I arrive at the diagnosis. The pathogenesis of the disease is still not understood. As Dr. Giffin pointed out, there should be no anemia along with the leukopenia for the correct diagnosis. If there is also a marked anemia present, then we must rule out other conditions such as acute leukemias and aplastic anemias.

One difficulty in the use of bone marrow is that the patients have such sore throats and find it difficult to swallow the large bulk of bone marrow necessary.

Cases in which the leukocyte count is under 300 or 400 are very serious and a large percentage die no matter what the treatment. Transfusions and x-ray treatment for stimulation of the bone marrow are practically of no value. So far, we have nothing better than the measures mentioned.

Amidopyrine may have some etiological relationship in some cases and it is not the size of the dose given but, apparently, the patient's sensitiveness to the drug which results in the leukopenia.

Prontylin has been reported to produce agranulocytosis. The nucleus in the chemical structure of pronty-

lin is similar to that of amidopyrine. Personally, I use amidopyrine a great deal and have thus far not seen a single case of agranulocytosis develop from it. At the meeting of the Central Society for Clinical Research in Chicago, three years ago, the relationship of amidopyrine to agranulocytosis was emphasized and Dr. Watkins of Rochester cited cases where the blood condition was cleared up after withholding the drug and reappeared upon administering it again. Bone marrow, along with other measures, should be used in the treatment of agranulocytosis.

DR. ALFRED HOFF, St. Paul: There are many papers about the effects of drugs, such as the barbiturates and amidopyrine, upon the bone marrow. I have had the misfortune in my own practice to have had four cases of agranulocytosis; three cases followed the use of allonal. I would like to emphasize what both Dr. Barron and Dr. Giffin said about the diagnosis. We see so much of leukopenia and we immediately begin to think what it means. Unless we have a very definite conception of what leukopenia signifies, we are in difficulty. I recall one patient at Ancker Hospital who showed various blood counts over a period of years. First she had a thyroidectomy. Her next operation was a gallbladder, and later she had backache, which was supposed to be due to some ureteral kink, and the kidney was operated upon. The patient finally came in with marked sore throat and a marked anemia and profound leukopenia. She had been given salvarsan for a Vincent's infection. Just before she died, a few immature cells were found. Autopsy revealed leukemic infiltrations in the liver and kidneys. The picture of anemia is so important in cases of agranulocytosis. We must recognize that, if the patient has anemia, we probably are not dealing with agranulocytosis.

About the treatment, I have one patient who has been well for two years. She just returned from a trip to Europe and I saw her the other day and she is perfectly well. I tried pentnucleotide. I had her husband go down to the butcher shop and get all the bone marrow he could; this was given orally, also liver extract intramuscularly. She had taken allonal for three years. She has not taken any allonal for the past two years and has remained well. I think the fundamental thing of the whole problem is, that whatever the causative action may be, there is a sensitivity in the individual. When that sensitization is recognized and the offending agent that produced the leukopenia is removed, then I think the patient will get well in the chronic recurring type of case. Bone marrow is probably an excellent thing.

DR. GIFFIN (in closing): I wish to thank the gentlemen for their discussions. In answer to Dr. Wright, I have found it almost impossible to decide beforehand whether or not a patient is likely to recover. Patients who have had edema of the larynx or incipient pneumonia at the time of admission have not survived. In the series of cases reported, patients with edema of the larynx have not been able to swallow bone-marrow capsules. The two patients who died while receiving an adequate amount of bone marrow had severe complications; one had gas gangrene and the other an abdominal abscess.

The meeting adjourned.

A. G. SCHULZE, M.D.,
Secretary.

Meeting of November 10, 1937

The regular monthly meeting of the Minnesota Academy of Medicine was held at the Town and Country Club on Wednesday evening, November 10, 1937.

Dinner was served at 7 o'clock and the meeting called to order at 8:15 by the president, Dr. E. M. Jones.

There were fifty-two members present.

Minutes of the October meeting were read and approved.

The Secretary called attention of members presenting papers and theses to the fact that abstracts should be handed in at the time, for inclusion in the published Proceedings of the Academy.

The scientific program consisted of two papers.

SYMPTOMATOLOGY OF THE VARIOUS LEUKEMIA STATES

T. A. PEPPARD, M.D.

Minneapolis

Dr. Peppard read a paper on the above subject and illustrated it with slides and charts of cases.

Abstract

Charts showing symptoms complained of and the physical signs observed in a small group of cases of leukemia were presented.

Attention was called to the great variability of the manifestations of this disease. Complete detailed records presented in four cases illustrating these variations.

Discussion

DR. H. L. ULRICH, Minneapolis: There is an immense amount of material in this study. Dr. Peppard deserves the applause and commendation of all of us for attempting such an analysis. It is difficult to discuss the rarer forms of leukemia because of our limited experience and its protean clinical manifestations. The leukemias are a paradise for the hematologist, although he gets lost in his paradise quite often. Because of the extreme difficulty in differentiating these various leukemias, I think Dr. Peppard is to be congratulated for making this clinical and hematological study.

DR. S. E. SWEITZER, Minneapolis: This is the first time I have seen a group comprising a large number of internists who were speechless after a paper. I was extremely interested in Dr. Peppard's paper and particularly interested in the fact that he did not say much about leukemia as far as the dermatologist is concerned. I am sure he must have seen some dermatological symptoms. From our standpoint, practically all our cases present dermatological symptoms. Some have exfoliative dermatitis for a long while and finally turn into leukemia, and some have minor skin symptoms at first. Some have leukemia infiltration early and no blood symptoms. I recall a patient who had been to a clinic where they had made a diagnosis of lymphosarcoma. An operation was done on the neck and six or seven years later the patient was still alive. She came in with what looked like a syphilitic serpiginous eruption on the scalp. The Wassermann reaction was negative. Biopsy showed leukemia. The blood smear was turned over to Dr. Downey who made a tentative diagnosis of leukemia. That was last summer. She came in again recently with the same type of lesion on her back. She also complained of pain in the eyeball. Dr. Peppard mentioned this, but that was the first time that I had encountered this symptom. I gave her some x-ray over that area and she was relieved. That may have been imagination but she did get relief.

I want to emphasize the point that these patients may have lesions that would lead one to suspect leukemia and yet one can't find it when examining the blood.

DR. PEPPARD (in closing): I thought I paid my respects to the dermatologists. In this group there were four who complained of skin conditions and ten who showed skin lesions on physical examination. As a rule, no biopsy is required for diagnosis for the blood examination usually suffices. However, in occasional cases, biopsy is invaluable. Whenever anyone interests himself in any one particular finding, his investigations will commonly show a higher incidence of such conditions than are found on routine examination.

THE IMPORTANCE OF IMMOBILIZATION AND POSTURE IN THE TREATMENT OF ACUTE INFECTIONS OF THE EXTREMITIES

OWEN H. WANGENSTEEN, M.D.

University Hospital

Dr. Wangensteen read a paper on the above subject, illustrated with lantern slides demonstrating methods of treatment and results.

Abstract

The rôle of the surgeon in the management of acute infections of the extremities has been reviewed. It is pointed out that his chief objective should be to assist the natural defense mechanism of the body in overcoming or localizing the infection. Other than that, his function is that of a pus evacuator—to incise an abscess when suppuration occurs.

The great virtue of rigid immobilization and elevation of the affected member in infection is described. It should be the aim of the surgeon to keep the infected extremity as quiet as physically possible; in addition, he should, through employment of elevation, strive to keep swelling at a minimum. The attainment of these objectives serves the natural defense mechanism of the body in a most helpful manner.

Discussion

DR. A. E. BENJAMIN, Minneapolis: I was very glad, indeed, to have Dr. Wangensteen bring up this method of treating wounds, injuries, or infections. It has been my practice for a number of years, in cases of infection of the extremities, to elevate the part affected about as he has demonstrated by the cases shown here tonight. I have a few cases on hand now in which this is very well illustrated. Perhaps we may be able to obviate a great many operations by following this procedure. I would further include under this method of treatment, certain leg ulcers from varicose veins. If you put the patient in bed and elevate the leg, you will note how quickly the ulcers improve. I have practiced this method in other cases, such as pelvic inflammations without any definite abscess. Cases of endometritis and non-specific salpingitis will often get well if the foot of the bed is elevated. It has been my rule always to put an inflamed part above the normal circulatory level; the swelling then disappears around the inflamed area. If there is swelling there is not the drainage of the deeper parts that otherwise obtains; and the less swelling there is the better drainage there will be of the deeper tissues. In a case of ruptured appendix, besides instituting the ordinary drainage treatment, the patient may be turned over on the abdomen. I recall one patient, a physician, who had an acute gangrenous appendix with abscess. I could not get the appendix out safely. I turned him over on his abdomen and the appendix sloughed out in three days. One should always put infection cases in a position which promotes drainage. They will recover faster that way.

I think the method of using casts, as Dr. Wangensteen has described, is a great help in treating certain cases.

Dr. L. C. Bacon, St. Paul: I listened to Dr. Wangensteen's talk with a great deal of pleasure. I am glad to hear him bring up old principles. They cannot be emphasized too much. It recalled my student days under de Nancrede. He taught that, in case of inflammation, rest and elevation of the part is the first thing to be done. It became monotonous to the students but it was repeated until it became a part of our daily lives.

Dr. J. Frank Corbett, Minneapolis: Dr. Wangensteen has given us a good deal of food for thought. I have lived long enough to see treatment of osteomyelitis progress. In the early days, wounds in the bones were opened, dressed every day, and then almost never got well. Then Orr advanced his method of treatment—complete immobilization in plaster casts, packing of the cleaned out area with vaseline and no dressing for a long time. That was a distinct advance. And now we come to another thought in regard to these cases. I recall the experience we had on the Mexican border in 1916. There were a good many gunshot wounds. That was a sterile, hot country where there was not much infection, but there were many compound fractures from gunshot wounds. Those healed very nicely without an antiseptic other than surface disinfection, but they were immobilized in plaster casts. Later on, in the World War, it was my lot to do a great number of reconstructvie operations. In wounds thought to be quiescent, infections did not occur following operation; I attributed it very largely to the fact that every one of these extremities was extensively encased in plaster, and there was absolute physiologic and complete rest to the body. However, infections vary. Every war has brought in its train a terrifically dangerous infection, and the infections of the last World War were severe in character and demanded radical treatment. We seem now to be one of the cycles of comparatively mild infection of wounds and the radical treatment of war days is no longer used.

Dr. Wangensteen's paper was very well presented.

Dr. H. P. Ritchie, St. Paul: I protest the use of Bier's hyperæmia treatment. Whatever the rationale, no cognizance is taken of the comfort of the patient. I was once subjected to this plan and testify that the method is barbarous.

I shall await, with great interest, the follow-up report on the treatment of burns by Dr. Wangensteen's plan for the fixation rest of the affected parts.

Dr. C. C. Chatterton, St. Paul: I heartily agree with Dr. Wangensteen in regard to rest and protection of parts affected with acute infection. Immobilization gives a patient comfort and prevents deformity. Until recently we were of the opinion that our treatment of osteomyelitis, so far as the end result is concerned, was perhaps superior to the treatment given years ago. In going over the records of the Gillette Hospital for Minnesota's crippled children, we find that the records of 30 or 40 years ago compare very favorably with the present records as to time in the hospital and time for the sinus to heal.

Dr. A. R. Colvin, St. Paul: The treatment of infections is perhaps the largest field of surgical endeavor and Dr. Wangensteen's paper has covered many aspects of it. His theme of "Rest in Pain" must be appreciated by all.

There is one thought concerning infections which should influence greatly our approach to the diagnosis, prognosis and treatment of infections; and that is the variability in virulence of the infecting agent and the very reliable reaction of individual tissues to infection; and, of course, our appraisal of the value of therapeutic measures—surgical or otherwise—must be influenced by an acknowledgement of these facts.

May I cite a few cases seemingly to confirm these inferences? A man of about 40 years (1908), with a suppurating tendon sheath opened on recognition, a few days later developed an abscess in the calf muscles of one leg and still a few days later developed an abscess in the other calf muscles. These were opened as soon as recognized; and very shortly there developed an acute non-suppurating infection of a shoulder and hip joint. Apparently there was no effusion, the joints were not opened, and recovery took place with saving of the tendon involved. Both joints recovered but had limited movement for some time. The closest observation was necessary to interpret the nature of the joint lesions—immediate opening saved the tendon. There, then, were different reactions of tissues at the same time in the same organism from the same infection.

The manifold nature of osteomyelitis is strikingly apparent. The infection may be fatal before there is time to do anything about it. At the other extreme is a small area of bone involvement, the size of a grain of wheat, which, as proven by radiographic study extending over a year, was entirely recovered from without any kind of treatment. There may be involvement of several bones, each bone presenting a different amount of invasion and a different grade of inflammatory reaction.

A girl of five years (1907), had five bones involved. The femur was involved in the lower third; at no time was there any operative surgery, the bone draining into the tissues of the thigh and thence through the skin. Radiographs taken at intervals showed the destruction and regeneration until at the end of a year the femur looked almost normal and remains so at the end of 30 years. The ulna showed a slow-going destruction and repair with the formation of a new shaft in the center of which were remnants of the old shaft as sequestra which had to be removed. In the humerus there was a small area about 1 cm. in length. Another child, with all the long bones of both extremities infected, presented with a very acute osteomyelitis of the femur which was opened at once. The child was very ill and, although relieved of pain, the entire femur became involved. While lying in bed, bone after bone became involved and one was conscious of this only when abscess after abscess was manifest and required opening in the various extremities. Except for the femur, first involved, the bones were not operated upon. There were no two lesions quite alike in extent of involvement. And it would seem that, as well as variability in virulence, there is a great variability also in the amount of bone involved. This, I believe to be explained by the extent of vascular territory invaded by the embolic invasion; and, too, this is, as it were, at one assault.

A boy of six years was seen six weeks after the onset of trouble, in the meantime having been treated for arthritis of the knee. His physician was insistent that the femur be opened and, although pain and fever were receding, a small opening was made in the femur. There was no pus, the spongy bone was strikingly red, the small wound in the soft parts was partially closed and finally closed completely. It was only after two months that an abscess in the soft parts was opened and in four months a sequestrum was removed.

A girl of fourteen with extreme pain and temperature of 101° to 104° lasting four months, presented herself with pain and swelling in the knee joint. The pain and elevated temperature suddenly subsided though no surgery had been done. Finally, a small abscess of the thigh opened spontaneously and ultimately a sequestrum was removed.

A boy fourteen, with multiple acute arthritis for 10 weeks and marked elevation of temperature, was reported by his physician who had at first very excusably diagnosed the case acute rheumatism. At the end of ten weeks all the joints except the hip and knee on one side were well. At that time the thigh was much swollen, there was very little pain, and the temperature was 101°. No operative measures were undertaken. He was observed for five years, during which time no abscess had as yet developed, and at this time a central sequestrum was removed.

Effusion in a joint contiguous to osteomyelitis rarely requires removal; usually it will be absorbed. The same variability as that in osteomyelitis is seen in joint infection and the treatment is just as variable. Numerous microörganisms may cause an arthritis varying from serous, fibrinous, purulent and phlegmonous. At times it is more important to know what the microörganism is doing rather than the name of it. And the treatment must be as varied as the process is variable. I am reminded of the visit of Ambroise Paré to the country to see a young man who was very ill. He said he found the young man in a most deplorable condition, lying in a filthy bed bathed in pus. He thought he could do nothing for the young man but, after taking a walk in the fields, he returned and ordered the patient bathed and supplied with clean sheets, and his thigh to be dressed with an infusion of fragrant herbs. He says that he had the pleasure of hearing that the young man recovered. I have often wondered if that case was one of neglected acute suppurative osteomyelitis. For pain, rest in bed is also valuable. Rest in a cast is of undoubted value and so is rest for the olfactories of the patient, surgeon and nurses—meaning sufficient change of dressing to accomplish this.

The treatment of chronic osteomyelitis is as variable as the result produced by the acute infection.

Just a few days ago I saw a patient on whom I operated thirty-two years ago for osteomyelitis of the lower end of the femur. He is now suffering from a very acute recrudescence of his former infection—after an interval of thirty-two years. After a few day of regrettable procrastination, a large amount of pus was evacuated from a cavity in the lower end of the bone. He will very likely never be completely cured of his trouble.

It is quite pertinent to ask when infection of bone is cured; and it is sad to say that a very large number are never cured. Microörganisms have become encapsulated in small areas of granulation tissue or in the lacunæ and canaliculi and Haversian canals of the cancellous bone which are rarely all reached by any kind of operative attack. Recurring fever and pain usually demand liberation of pus, all the more so because, in these recurring chronic cases, the pus is confined by thick-walled more or less sclerotic bone and the pain is very severe. One might say, in closing, that relief of tension by incision not only relieves pain but, in properly selected cases, leads to a subsidence of the inflammatory process.

Dr. Wangensteen (in closing) : With the development of antisepsis and asepsis the scope of the surgeon's activity broadened considerably. His ac-

tivity formerly had been concerned largely with the management of wounds. Despite his present greater field of interest, one of his major concerns is still the management of wounds. It is, therefore, very refreshing to note the manifest great interest in a subject that has perplexed surgeons ever since the humblest beginnings of their craft.

The vagaries of infection to which so many of the speakers alluded, are matters with which every one is familiar. We have all had ample opportunity to note how the mortality of pneumonia, empyema and other infections has varied from year to year independent of the mode of treatment employed. Obviously, therefore, it is an item to be reckoned with in evaluating the results of any scheme of treatment.

It is important that surgeons review critically the remedial measures which they employ in the treatment of infection. It is so easy to continue indefinitely with therapeutic agents which have not proved their worth. Surgeons generally have come to recognize their own great shortcomings in dealing with spreading infections. We no longer see surgeons making incisions in phlegmonous inflammations in the hope that they can thereby localize the infection. They have come to know that only the natural defense mechanism of the body can do that. All the surgeon can do, apart from assisting the body in its conflict with infection, is to evacuate an abscess when localization of the infection and suppuration have occurred.

I have had no experience with the conservative means of management here described in impalement types of injury which result in rapidly spreading infection and bacteremia. Instances are known to all of us in which extremities have been uselessly sacrificed in the hope of stopping the centripetal spread of the infection. The experiments of Schimmelbusch (1894) with tetanus toxin and the rat's tail are undoubtedly known to most of you. He observed that, if the denuded rat's tail was immersed in a culture of tetanus toxin, when more than 10 minutes elapsed it was futile to cut the rat's tail off at the base. The toxin had already penetrated beyond. I am inclined to believe that the interests of patients who suffer impalement types of injury giving rise to virulent infections, are better served by conservative means. Friedrich (1898) was able to show that the immediate application of antiseptics and employment of excision to tissue did exert an important influence when applied early in experimental infections in which dirt had been rubbed into wounds. After the lapse of six hours, the employment of such expedients was without value. His experiments constitute the basis of the modern débridement of soiled wounds.

The great value of immobilization and elevation in the treatment of pyogenic infections of the soft parts can be appraised now. He who will give the method a trial will observe that pain will decrease and that swelling lessens. The necessity for incision for the evacuation of exudate is less than with employment of hot fomentations with the extremity upon the bed slightly below the level of the heart. The results of treatment of acute hematogenous osteomyelitis in the manner described above must await the lapse of a sufficient interval of time. It has been intimated that the satisfactory results attending conservative treatment of acute osteomyelitis may have their explanation in rather benign forms of the disease. I value that suggestion, for an observer must always be on the alert lest he deceive himself. Yet, I would again say that many of these patients with osteomyelitis herein referred to were very ill. During the same period we have seen a few patients who had their trepanation before they came to us. The early effects, i.e., healing of the wound and subsidence of the inflammatory

(Continued on page 78)

The stated meeting of the Minneapolis Surgical Society was held Thursday, November 4, 1937, the president, Dr. O. W. Yoerg, in the chair.

The following papers were presented:

CARCINOMA OF THE GALLBLADDER WITH IMPLANTATION IN THE ABDOMINAL WALL

Case Report

JAMES A. JOHNSON, M.D.

MRS. D. W., aged seventy-three, was admitted to the Eitel Hospital October 7, 1936. Her previous history was negative except that she had a gallbladder drainage ten years ago, at which time stones were removed. She had been well until August 15, 1936, when she had an attack of vomiting which she attributed to a dietary indiscretion. On September 1, she had another attack of nausea and vomiting. There was no pain with either of these attacks. Two days after the last attack her daughter noticed that her eyes and skin were yellow. The jaundice gradually became more pronounced and she had intense itching all over the body. Her appetite had been poor and she had lost 8 pounds in weight. She consulted her family physician, Dr. S. Ericson of Le Sueur, Minnesota, who referred her for examination and also thought from his observation that there was a possibility of stone in the common duct.

Examination revealed a poorly nourished, visceroptotic, feeble old lady. The abdomen was moderately distended. The liver was smooth and extended three fingers below the right costal margin. She was deeply jaundiced. The urine was loaded with bile pigments. Exploratory operation was advised.

At operation October 9, 1936, the gallbladder and duodenum were found buried under omental adhesions. Four large stones were removed from the common duct and three stones from the right hepatic duct. The gallbladder was opened, no stones were seen, and the mucosa looked normal. The pancreas did not feel hard. The stomach and duodenum were normal. The liver was engorged with bile. A T-tube was placed in the common duct and the gallbladder was drained. Because of the extreme enlargement of the liver both drains were brought through the lower angle of the wound just inside the iliac crest.

The postoperative course was uneventful. The jaundice promptly disappeared, the liver receded to its normal size, she ate well and gained her normal weight, and continued in good health until the middle of July, 1937, when she began to have gastric distress with occasional vomiting. This increased until she was unable to retain any food. She was again admitted to the Eitel Hospital August 18, 1937. A barium meal demonstrated an obstruction at the second portion of the duodenum. At the lower angle of the scar—the site of the previous drainage—there was a hard nodule about 3 cm. in diameter.

At operation August 21, 1937, incisions were made through the old scar, and the nodule was removed separately. It was hard and on cross-section looked like a carcinoma—resembling a scirrhus carcinoma of the breast. It was confined to the tissues of the abdominal wall and did not invade the peritoneum. A microscopic examination was requested. On opening the abdomen the duodenum and omentum were firmly

fixed underneath the liver, as if there had been a perforation. When the duodenum was separated, a necrotic perforation was present which was sutured with dulox catput, and a posterior gastroenterostomy was done. The gallbladder and pancreas could not be visualized or palpated because of the large inflammatory mass which was thought to be due to the perforation. Following operation a microscopic section of the nodule by Dr. Koucky showed a fibrous tissue stroma within which were imbedded malignant carcinoma cells. Evidently the malignant cells had been carried through the drainage tube and grown by implantation in the abdominal wall.

After the operation she developed leakage from the duodenum, which resulted in peritonitis, and death occurred on the seventh day.

Postmortem.—The gallbladder was completely replaced by a white tumor mass. There was a metastatic mass on the posterior surface of the right lobe of the liver near the vena cava. The lower end of the common duct, head of pancreas, pylorus and duodenum were imbedded in a solid mass of fibrous tissue. There were small seed-like implants along the root of the mesentery and posterior abdominal wall. Microscopic examination showed primary carcinoma of the gallbladder with metastases to the liver and peritoneum. The pancreas was free.

There was a bilateral terminal bronchopneumonia.

Comment.—The extension of carcinoma from its primary focus is usually by the lymph vessels or by direct extension. A less common, but nevertheless definite, method is by direct implantation of the cancer cells at sites distant to the original tumor. In this case the cancer cells evidently were carried directly through the drainage tube into the abdominal wall, where they began to grow and formed a separate distinct tumor. There are several well-known examples in which carcinoma spreads by implantation. It is common, for instance, when a carcinoma is present in the stomach to find implant growths deep down in the pelvis. Likewise, in primary carcinoma of the ovary, it is common to find it spread uniformly throughout the abdomen in the form of miliary nodules. The cells evidently spread through the peritoneal fluid; occasionally also into the abdominal scar. It is uncommon, however, to find so striking a case as the above, where the carcinoma cell has implanted itself in entirely a different tissue at a remote distance from the original lesion. This brings us to the importance of such a clinical finding. It seems to me that it is evident that a surgeon must be careful when operating upon cancer not to invade the growth or glands in such a way that the loose implants are scattered in the healthy tissue. This is especially important for example when doing a biopsy on the breast. Here the tissue should be widely excised and gloves and instruments discarded before proceeding with the radical operation. It is also important in removing the involved glands not to macerate them and infect surrounding tissues.

My purpose in reporting this case is to stimulate an

interest in clinical evidence of cancer implants and the benefit we may derive from it. I hope members of this Society will be looking for similar cases and report them to us.

Discussion

Dr. George D. Eitel: Statistics indicate that 5 to 7 per cent of all carcinomas found at necropsy originate in the gallbladder. There is also a definite association with gallstones, and different reports indicate their presence in from 65 to 90 per cent of cases. It is more common in females and usually occurs between the ages of fifty and sixty. Walters, in 1936, reported thirteen malignant gallbladders in 808 cholecystectomies while Judd, in 1931, reported twenty-two cases in 879 cholecystectomies.

The diagnosis is usually not made except in advanced cases when the patient is very ill, usually jaundiced and presents a palpable tumor. In the earlier stages of the disease the diagnosis is usually a non-functioning gallbladder with or without stones. Because the lesion usually originates in the cystic neck of the gallbladder, there is always an obstruction to the entrance of the gallbladder and x rays fail to depict the lumen of the gallbladder.

Kirklin reports sixteen cases of carcinoma of the gallbladder in which cholecystograhpy preceded the operation, and it was found that in fourteen cases no shadow of the gallbladder appeared although gallstones were present in seven. In one case function was present but multiple stones were present and in one the shadow was normal.

The gross pathology is usually an irregular carcinomatous mass involving the wall with a stone or multiple stones in the center—probably the source of the original irritation. Perforation is rare, but when it does, secondary growths occur causing ascites or a fistulous opening between the gallbladder and a hollow viscus.

The common mode of extension is to the adjacent liver either directly or through the blood vessels or to the lymphatic glands lying in the hepatic fissure.

At operation those readily recognized as malignant are usually irremovable. Death is usually caused by hepatic insufficiency, or if removal or even biopsy is done, death may result from an associated severe hemorrhage.

The permanent cures of carcinoma of the gallbladder are usually those in which the gallbladder is removed for a chronic condition and the routine laboratory microsopic examination of the gallbladder disclosed malignancy.

The microscopic pathology is usually adenocarcinoma, although in a series of thirty-three cases careful studies revealed the presence of squamous cell carcinoma in three cases. Kaufman reports a case of sarcoma and states that only thirteen cases are on record.

Dr. Kenneth Bulkley: Might I ask the reader or his discussor as to the radio-sensitivity of these recurrences?

Dr. James A. Johnson: Dr. Bulkley asks about the sensitivity of carcinoma of the gallbladder to x-ray treatment. I am unable to answer this question directly since our experience with carcinoma of the gallbladder is rather limited. I would say in a general way, however, that it would react unfavorably because as a rule this is true of carcinoma of any of the abdominal organs.

I want again to summarize the important finding in the case just reported. At the time I first operated upon this woman, removing the stones from the common and hepatic ducts and draining the gallbladder, I was unable to find any evidence of carcinoma. She was entirely well for about one year, when she returned with an obstruction of the second part of the duodenum. The main finding, however, was a nodule which was present in the abdominal wall and was confined to the skin, fat, fascia and muscular tissues, and did not involve the peritoneum. Since it would be impossible for this to be transmitted through the blood or lymph channels, it is certain that this could only arrive through a direct transplant. The primary carcinoma was in the gallbladder and the carcinoma cells evidently drained through the drainage tube directly into the abdominal wall where they began to grow. I believe this is a significant finding.

DIVERTICULUM OF THE ESOPHAGUS

A. A. Zierold, M.D.

SOMETHING over a year ago this man was sent to me complaining of gurgling and a fullness in his neck and regurgitation of food. These symptoms had persisted over a period of ten to fifteen years, increasing to a point where he was having definite distress. The regurgitation was becoming not only embarrassing but was interfering with eating. X-ray examination revealed an esophageal diverticulum which, peculiarly enough, was in the midline. These pulsion diverticula (this discussion will be confined entirely to pulsion diverticula), are herniations of the mucosa and submucosa through the musculature at the junction of the lower portion of the pharynx and the beginning of the esophagus, forming a sac which descends usually on the left side of the neck, increasing in size, so that the esophagus is deflected to one side, making the esophagoscopy or the passage of a Bougie dangerous.

In the past, any treatment directed toward the correction of this has been attended by considerable danger because of the difficulty of removing, ligating, or suturing such a wide mouthed sac and preventing leakage into the mediastinum. The diverticulum passes downward between the prevertebral and pretracheal fascia and affords direct access to the mediastinum and any leakage is very promptly followed by a mediastinitis. In the past, attempts were made to excise the sac, exposing the sac and suturing it. The major danger was, of course, the leakage and the mediastinitis which followed. The second complication which often followed was a constricture of the esophagus. This state of affairs continued until such time as the two-stage operation was devised in which a preliminary operation for the exposure of the sac was performed. The sac was identified, dissected free and the mediastinum was walled off by adhesions between the fascial planes. At a later date an attempt was then made to tie off or suture the sac. This, while an improvement, was not entirely successful.

I am presenting this patient to you this evening to illustrate how a formidable procedure can be made easy. Dr. Lahey, I believe in 1930 or 1931, devised a method which is as near fool-proof as any and is the best example of surgical ingenuity and clear thinking that I know of. I don't know when I have seen or when I have done anything that has given me so much pleasure as Dr. Lahey's technic for the cure of esophageal diverticula. Dr. Lahey advises a longitudinal incision along the sternomastoid, retracting the sternomastoid together with the carotid sheath and the large vessels. Then, by ligating the lateral thyroid veins and the inferior thyroid vessels, direct exposure is afforded of the esophagus and of the diverticulum which, of course, begins at this point and extends downward. It is surprising what a bloodless field and what a really accessible field can be obtained with so little dissection. When this is done, the sac is carefully dissected free, remembering, of course, that it is only submucosa and mucosa. Care is taken to free the attachments at the lower angle and to reverse the angle of the sac, bringing it up to an obtuse angle and suturing the sac to the skin. That is all that is done at this operation. Care is taken, of course, to dissect well around to the right side to free any adhesions occurring on the opposite side. The fundus is sutured to the skin edge and is allowed to remain there, as in this case, eight days.

At the end of that time the end of the fundus is cut off level with the fascia and the mucosa which lines the diverticulum is separated from the submucosa as far as the esophagus. It is then cut off at a point one inch from the neck of the sac and folded upon itself. This tube of submucosa is loosely filled with some vaseline gauze. The mucosa very promptly retracts and contracts until it eventually gives a smooth lining to the esophagus. The submucosal tube becomes obliterated and at no time is there an opening or communication between the esophagus and the wound. At no time is there an opportunity for leakage into the mediastinum. In this instance, happily, there was no drainage after the second operation, no regurgitation of food and no fluid discharge through the sinus. At the end of another ten days the patient was discharged. He has had an uneventful convalescence and I present him to you this evening to show you that the residual submucosa causes no contraction deformity of the scar in the neck. It is freely movable in all directions. The patient has been symptom-free up to the present time. The only thing we haven't done is to dilate him postoperatively. Dr. Lahey advises the routine dilation of the esophagus on the assumption that the initiation of the diverticulum is due to a spasm of the beginning of the esophagus. In this instance the patient apparently successfully survived the interval and I see no reason why he should not continue.

Discussion

Dr. Orwood J. Campbell: I envy Dr. Zierold the pleasure he must have had in caring for this patient. My own experience with the surgical treatment of diverticula of the esophagus has been very limited but the few operations for diverticula which I have done have been fun and I have enjoyed doing them.

Dr. Lahey has described an ingenious operation the principal advantage of which is that it provides a

tube whereby any leakage from the esophagus is transported to the outside and not permitted to escape into the fascia layers thus to produce a mediastinitis. In some of these sacs I should anticipate considerable difficulty in shelling out the mucous membrane because of inflammation and adhesions. In such a case it would be a simple matter to do the classical two-stage resection removing the entire sac.

The principal controversy today among those who see many of these cases seems to be whether the operation shall be done in one or two stages. Dr. Jackson and his associates advocate the one stage procedure, using the esophagoscope as an aid.

The esophagoscope is passed into the diverticulum and its contents aspirated. A strong light on the end of the esophagoscope then transilluminates the sac and makes it easy for the operating surgeon to locate, free and deliver the sac into the wound. The sac is then excised and with the esophagoscope passed on down toward the stomach primary suture is done.

My limited experience does not warrant my advocating one or the other method. Personally, I like the added protection of the two-stage operation. Especially is this true if the sac is large. Smaller diverticula may be closed primarily.

Dr. Zierold mentioned narrowing of the esophagus as a complication of the usual two-stage resection. Judd, in reporting his experience with 171 operated cases, did note a small percentage of narrowing of the esophagus but stated it had not been a serious difficulty. They do not make a practice of dilating the esophagus except when indicated.

I believe the use of the esophagoscope even in the two-stage operation of resection has definite advantages. It will assist the surgeon in locating the sac and at the second stage, can be passed on down toward the stomach to prevent narrowing of the lumen when the neck of the sac is sutured. If this precaution is observed I believe a troublesome narrowing at the point of suture can be avoided.

Dr. S. R. Maxeiner: In our service at the Veterans' Hospital we have had two cases of esophageal diverticula in the last two years. Upon the first patient we performed the two-stage procedure, bringing the sac into the elevated position along the pharynx at the first stage and ten days later resected the sac. The neck of the sac was tucked beneath the muscle planes which were closed tightly. In this case healing progressed without infection and with a perfectly normal convalescence.

The second case was operated upon by Dr. Sedgely and myself by one-stage technic which I suggested and which I have not seen described any place in the literature.

Technic.—A customary incision was made along the anterior border of the left sterno-mastoid muscle. The inferior thyroid artery was ligated and the vessels retracted laterally and the thyroid retracted medially. The sac, which was of good size, was dissected free until the pedicle was well exposed, the muscle planes were separated well back from the mucosa and a small curved forceps was placed across the pedicle close to the lateral wall of the esophagus. A second forceps was placed across the pedicle of the sac parallel to and a short distance from the first pair of forceps. The pedicle was divided between the forceps with a cautery knife and the second forceps together with the diverticulum was removed. The muscle planes were then carefully sutured over the forceps which was clamped to the cut-off end of the forceps so that all of the forceps containing pedicle was completely buried by the overlapping muscle planes. The wound was then loosely closed around the forceps, which was left in situ to act as a drain. On the seventh day the forceps became spontaneously detached and fell out. There was a very small leak of a few drops of clear fluid which drained out of the sinus established by the forceps for approximately a week. The wound healed uneventfully and the patient made a splendid recovery.

The object of the two-stage operation is primarily to prevent mediastinal infection. We believe that the forceps establishes a definite sinus with the walling off of the fascial planes before the forceps separated and a leak occurs as was proven in this case. We feel that this technic in this one case proved to be entirely satisfactory and efficient and is certainly deserving of further trial.

DR. JAMES A. JOHNSON: It has been very interesting to listen to Dr. Zierold's report of removal of this esophageal diverticulum. It has been my custom to remove these diverticula in two stages, and following the second stage I have been in the habit of putting in a nasal tube for feeding purposes and to also obviate any possibility of vomiting for a few days until healing has taken place. I would like to ask Dr. Zierold what his postoperative care was in this particular case.

DR. A. A. ZIEROLD: I did not restrict him at all. He went on a general diet forty-eight hours after the resection.

ENDOMETRIOSIS

WILLIAM R. JONES, M. D.

ENDOMETRIOSIS is the presence of endometrium outside of the uterine cavity. Its cause is not definitely known. However, there are several theories as to its origin. Those most widely recognized are: (1) the implantation of Sampson, who believes that endometrial tissue finds its way through the fallopian tubes into the abdominal cavity where it implants itself and grows; (2) the embryonic rest theory advocated by Cullen and others. These men believe that the embryonic rests are activated during active menstrual life and give rise to symptoms.

Endometrial growths are found in the abdomen and pelvis from the umbilicus downward. Most frequent locations are the uterus, fallopian tubes, ovaries and the recto-genital space. Less frequently they are found in the rectum, intestines, sigmoid, appendix, vagina, uterine ligaments, umbilicus and abdominal scars following operations on the uterus.

The essential pathology is a menstruating endometrium within a closed sac and the complications of this process. The growth may vary from the size of a millet seed to a mass as large as a six months' pregnancy. As the mass enlarges it tends to infiltrate the host tissue. No definite line of cleavage is present. When the ovary is involved the cyst may rupture and a dark chocolate colored material escapes into the abdominal cavity. This material is highly irritating and stimulates dense adhesions between tissues that it contacts. These adhesions are very difficult to separate as they are infiltrative in type.

Microscopically the growth resembles endometrium very closely. Endometriosis usually occurs between thirty years of age and the menopause. According to

Sampson, it is present in from 10 to 20 per cent of women. The outstanding symptom is dysmenorrhea of the acquired type. Usually the first symptom is severe abdominal pain at the menstrual time which is most frequently lower abdominal, but may be upper abdominal or over the entire abdomen. The pain will last throughout the menstrual period, differing from that of cervical stenosis, which usually decreases after the flow has started. There may be some constant abdominal pain, but it is much more pronounced at the menstrual time. Nausea and vomiting may occur, suggesting acute appendicitis. If a chocolate cyst ruptures into the abdominal cavity, there will be signs of peritoneal irritation, nausea, vomiting and boardlike abdominal rigidity and increased leukocyte count. If the growth encroaches on the bowel, there may be symptoms of intestinal obstruction. If on the vagina or rectum, coitus may be painful or impossible and there may be pain during the act of defecation.

The treatment is surgical exploration and removal of the growth with conservation of the ovaries, if possible, in young women. In older women, both ovaries should be removed as this stops the progress of the disease and also causes a regression. For the recurrent cases and irremovable growths, sterilization by x-ray or radium is a treatment of choice.

Case 1.—The first case is that of a woman twenty-nine years of age. This patient was admitted to the Eitel hospital, January 9, 1937. She complained of severe lower right abdominal pain. There was no nausea or vomiting but the patient had lost her appetite. Her past and family histories were negative. Examination revealed an obese young woman, evidently suffering severe pain in the abdomen. There was marked tenderness and rigidity in her right lower abdomen.

Pelvic examination was negative, except tenderness on palpation. The white blood count was 16,000; polymorphonuclears 80 per cent. The urine was negative. A diagnosis of acute appendicitis was made.

Exploration of the abdomen revealed a leaking chocolate cyst of the right ovary. The entire ovary seemed to be involved and therefore was removed. The left ovary appeared to be normal. The patient had an uneventful recovery and seemed to be well for four months. Then she began having pain with each menstrual period. The past three periods have been so painful that morphine was required for relief. This patient has been advised to have x-ray treatment.

Case 2.—The second case is that of a nurse thirty years of age. The family history was negative. She had been treated for kidney stones in 1927. Her appendix was removed several years ago. She was seen by me at her home November 29, 1929, because of severe abdominal pain which began after her menstrual period started. The pain was followed by nausea and vomiting.

The patient stated that she had a similar attack in June, 1929. Severe abdominal pain was present, which appeared on the third day of her menstrual period. Her temperature at that time was 103° and leukocyte count was 16,000. She was confined to the hospital for five days. Her physician made a diagnosis of peritonitis. The July and August menses were normal. However, in September, on the third day after she began to flow, severe generalized abdominal pain again occured, which lasted until she stopped flowing. In October she experienced the same difficulty.

Examination, November 29, 1929, showed a well developed young woman evidently suffering severe pain. Her abdomen was very tender and rigid. Pelvic examination caused pain, but no abnormal pelvic masses could be palpated. The patient was taken to the Eitel hospital and a consultation was held with a gynecologist and urologist. Under ether and anesthesia, pelvic examination revealed a mass in the right adnexal region. Exploration was advised and was done.

When the abdomen was opened a cyst of the right ovary, the size of a small orange, was found, from which dark chocolate colored material was leaking. There was an unruptured cyst of the left ovary the size of a hen's egg. Because of the patients age, a conservative operation was decided upon. The cysts of both ovaries were removed and the ovaries recon structed. There was nothing unusual about her convalesence. Four years later she married and moved to another city and has not been heard from since. For these four years she was free of symptoms.

Discussion

Dr. Richard R. Cranmer: To me, endometriosis is a very unusual and peculiar condition. It has some of the earmarks of malignancy but still it is not a malignancy. The man who made a comprehensive study of endometriosis first was Sampson in 1921 and he advanced certain theories as to its etiology. He outlined, or rather, classified the different types according to the method that the endometrium reaches its ectopic positions. His first classification is that of primary endometriosis, where the endometrial cells misplaced in the uterine body develop that condition commonly known as adenomyoma and which penetrate the entire thickness of the uterine wall. Sometimes these adenomyomata, that are of mucous origin and definitely secondary to an extension process of the endometrium, are found out underneath the peritoneum, indicating that they can travel. The second classification is the implantation classification in which the endometrium is forced out of the uterine cavity through the tubes and into the peritoneal cavity and there it becomes an implant and develops and grows. Not only is it activated by the hormones just as the endometrium of the uterine cavity is, but after it has reached its location it develops and grows in size just as a malignancy does. That is the common type of endometriosis, the kind that we see most of, and it is that type that produces the so-called chocolate cyst of the ovary. The third classification is where the endometrium is transplanted into new locations due to operation. Sometimes it develops in the abdominal wound and sometimes in the perineal wound. A fourth classification, according to Sampson, is where the endometrium cells do have a metastatic action and cause metastasis into other areas in the pelvis, not in the peritoneum but in the subperitoneal areas.

Sampson also admits the possibility of endometriosis being due, in some instances, to misplaced endometrial tissue in the Wolffian body. He said he had never had any cases that he thought developed in that way but he admits the possibility of it.

As far as the treatment is concerned, Dr. Jones has covered that; the prophylactic treatment is to prevent those things which cause an expression of the endometrial cells through the tube and then into the peritoneal cavity. Sampson thinks that the inflation test of Rubin for determining the patency of the tubes should not be done soon after menstruation. He recites a case where some of the implants developed following such a procedure. Curettage soon after menstruation is also advised against.

As far as the operative treatment is concerned, he

thinks that if it is a young woman with a single ovary involved, the ovary should be removed but not the other ovary. If it is a widespread process the best thing to do is double oöphorectomy and possibly a panhysterectomy. Then, if all the implants cannot be removed, radio therapy should be used. However, there is an argument against the use of the x-ray because usually in this condition there are a lot of adhesions and the x-ray increases adhesions and might increase the symptoms resulting from them. There are very interesting cases reported. Dr. Ikeda, St. Paul, reported a case the other night. The patient was being operated on for suspected appendicitis and the patient had, implanted on the appendix, a section of endometrial tissue which evidently was the cause of the trouble. Dr. Gingold reported a case where the body of the uterus was involved and multiple implants were on the peritoneal covering of the uterus. In that case he did a panhysterectomy besides a double oöphorectomy. I think we have all seen chocolate cysts. At Asbury Hospital the pathologist told me that fifteen cases were operated upon in the last year and I would estimate probably 125 or 150 are operated upon each year in Minneapolis.

An interesting experiment was done on the eye of a monkey by Cullen. Endometrial tissue was implanted in the anterior chamber and its development was watched. It was found that blood appeared in the anterior chamber about three hours before menstruation, indicating again that this misplaced tissue does respond to hormonal action even though remote from its original position.

Dr. T. H. Sweetser: I wish to add to the discussion the observation that the ureter is quite liable to damage during operations for endometriosis in the broad ligament. The margins of the endometriosis are ill-defined, hemorrhage is liable to be quite troublesome, and in dissecting down to the lower margin of the hemorrhagic tissue one reaches the plexus of veins at the side of the cervix and is quite liable to clamp the ureter. I have recently been asked to examine urologically one patient whose ureter had been thus damaged with resultant suprapubic urinary fistula. Nephrectomy was finally necessary to obtain a cure.

TERATOMA OF THE TESTICLE: HINMAN OPERATION

Report of a Patient Cured Four and One-half Years Following Radical Surgery Removal

Lawrence M. Larson, M.D., Ph.D., F.A.C.S.

IN the treatment of malignant tumors of the testicle, one has at his disposal three methods. These are as follows:

1. Simple castration.

2. Radical operation in which the testis and its lymphoglandular drainage areas are removed.

3. Roentgen therapy either alone or in combination with the above described methods.

Regarding the first possibility, namely simple castration, it is evident that this method of treatment is not in accordance with the principles of surgery of cancer as applied to other parts of the body. No account is taken of the fact that these tumors commonly metastasize early into the retroperitoneal and aortic region and cure of this lesion cannot be expected in any large percentage of cases without removal of these lymph-bearing tissues.

The second method, radical operation in which the testicular tumor along with the lympho-glandular drainage area is removed at the same time, is a procedure which should and does give much better end results. This has proved to be the case, according to statistics, in a large number of individuals who have been operated for this disease. Furthermore, radical operation such as that recommended by Hinman is not much more dangerous than simple castration and experience has likewise shown that the technical difficulties are not great. The lymphatic drainage area of the testicle has been carefully worked out so that it is possible to excise with anatomical accuracy the region in which metastases are known to occur.

The third possible method of treatment has probably the most to recommend it of any of the other methods. Roentgen therapy in combination with surgical excision of the tumor has proved to be unusually efficacious in a certain group of these tumors, since it is a well-known fact that some of them are highly radio-sensitive. Roentgen therapy alone should probably be reserved for those cases in which it is possible to demonstrate clinically the presence of metastases in the regional lymph nodes. At any rate it is no doubt better to use this combined method in most cases.

Hinman, in 1933, reviewed a large number of cases of malignant testicular tumors with the purpose in mind of determining end results and found that approximately 15 per cent were cured by simple castration, and there were 30 per cent cured by the radical excision of the tumor with its lymph drainage area. The most favorable group of cases he found were those in which no metastases were demonstrable and in whom radical operation was done. Of this group of thirty-six cases, eighteen were living and well four years after the operation. Thus it is evident that even if no metastases are demonstrable clinically, radical removal of the lymph-bearing fascias is certainly worth while.

Pathologically, tumors of the testis are usually divided into two types, the seminoma and the teratoma. Both are highly malignant. They metastasize early to the primary lymphatics as well as to the lungs, liver and other organs. The immediate type of cell in these tumors still remains uncertain although the origin may be the connective tissue, the epithelial tissues or there may be a mixed type of tumor having components of both. Regardless of the origin of these tumors they must all be regarded as malignant. Clinically they all act similarly. The seminomas have been said to be more radio-sensitive than the teratomas, but this is not a constant observation so that roentgen therapy should be used in most of them either alone or in combination with surgical excision.

This patient was nineteen years of age when first seen in May 1933. He had always been in excellent health and had had no operations except for tonsillectomy in childhood. The history of his present illness goes back three or four months when he first

noticed enlargement and pain in his left testicle. These symptoms gradually increased in severity although at no time did he notice any loss of strength. He had had no loss of weight and by wearing a suspensory he has been entirely comfortable. During this four months period he thinks the left testicle had slowly and gradually enlarged but he paid little attention to it.

Physical examination: He is in apparent good health. He is five feet eleven inches tall, weighs 170 pounds, his color is good, and his muscles were all in unusual excellent condition. His entire physical examination was negative except for the left testicle. The latter was two to three times normal size and was surrounded by a fluctuant sac which apparently contained a small amount of fluid. Through this sac could be felt an ovoid tumor which involved the entire testis. The outline of the tumor could be distinctly made out and it was quite smooth with the exception of a few irregular areas in the upper and medial portions. The consistency of the mass was very hard and it was freely movable within the sac. It was not especially tender. The mass did not transmit light and no fluctuation could be made out. The epididymis could be distinctly made out in its usual position and the spermatic cord with the vas deferens could be readily palpated. The skin of the scrotum was freely movable throughout.

June 3, 1933 operation was done under gas anesthesia. A high left inguinal incision was made, the testicle delivered from the scrotum and simple castration was done. The spermatic cord was divided between clamps by cautery after it was dissected free, and the clamp was left on the proximal portion of the cord for traction. Immediate frozen section of the tumor mass was made and the report by the pathologist showed it to be a highly malignant teratoma. The patient was then placed partially on his right side and partially on his back, somewhat similar to the position for exploration of the kidney except the position was a bent dorsal-lateral one. A pad was placed under the left costal margin and the left knee and hip were slightly flexed with the right leg straight. The incision was then extended upward so as to follow the course of the iliohypogastric and ilioinguinal nerves, thus avoiding cutting them. It was carried as high as the tip of the 12th rib to which it ran somewhat parallel. The fascia of the external oblique muscle was next divided starting from the external ring and the muscle bundles then split as they paralleled the course of the incision. The internal oblique, the transversalis, and the latissimus dorsi muscles were divided also in the line of the incision. The ilioinguinal and iliohypogastric nerves were carefully avoided. The peritoneum was next encountered. Beginning in the iliac fossa this was retracted medially stripping it as far as the iliac vessels and the bladder. Here it was necessary to carefully avoid carrying the spermatic vessels and the ureter along with the peritoneum. These structures should be left behind on the surface of the psoas muscle. The spermatic cord was isolated and traction put on it so as to facilitate this dissection.

The vas deferens was then divided where it disappears behind the bladder. Next the peritoneum was further stripped back so that the iliac vessels and the aortic bifurcation identified, thus further exposing the retro-peritoneal tissues. The ureter was carefully avoided overlying the psoas muscle and the peritoneum stripped away as high up as the renal pedicle. The peritoneum was then pulled laterally and maintained in this position by retractors. The lymphatic tissues were then removed from the iliac vessels about the aortic bifurcation and along the pre-aortic area. There was a considerable mass of lymph tissue in this region extending up as high as the kidney

ney pedicle. A few small metastatic glands were encountered along the aorta and trauma to these tissues was avoided. The spermatic cord along with the lymph-bearing tissues described were then removed in one piece. Traction on the clamp attached to the spermatic cord was of considerable help in identifying the tissues to be dissected. Drainage of this large lymphatic area was then made by means of several Penrose soft rubber drains through the lower angle of the wound. Closure of the muscles in the lower part of the incision were made as for hernia.

The tumor measured 8x7x4 centimeters in diameter and it was solid yellowish in color with a few small cystic areas. The tunica vaginalis and the epididymis were not involved and could be identified. There was a small amount of compressed testicular tissue at the lower pole of the tumor and a number of hemorrhagic areas throughout the mass. Microscopically the cells resembled those of carcinoma interspersed with lymphoid stroma. There were many areas of necrosis and hemorrhage and a few smooth muscle bundles could be identified. The diagnosis was teratoma of the testis.

The postoperative course was uneventful. The incision drained considerable serum for about ten days and on the fourteenth day the patient was allowed to go home. As an additional therapeutic measure roentgen therapy was instituted three weeks postoperatively by Drs. Allison and Hanson, who gave him large doses over the entire lower abdomen. About six months after the operation he joined the Civilian Conservation Corps where he stayed in a camp in Northern Minnesota for a year and did all the hard work that was required of him. His strength since the operation has returned to normal. After leaving the CCC's he obtained work as a mechanic and has continued this work since without interruption. He has been examined about twice yearly since the operation, the last time two weeks ago, and at no time has there been evidence of recurrence or metastasis of the tumor.

Discussion

DR. GILBERT COTTAM : Dr. Larson has entered into the technic of the operation so thoroughly that it is unnecessary to deal with that phase of the subject. I would like to say a few things about the incidence of these tumors. The experience that any one of us has is so slight we cannot talk of any statistics derived from our own work. Probably only a half dozen men in this room have ever seen a teratoma of the testicle but any one of us may see one tomorrow morning. There are two things that I think we might consider in regard to the matter of the rarity of them and the only way we can get at it, of course, is by the aggregate experience of others. Hamilton Bailey of London has recently published a monograph which is highly valuable in this connection; it is a compact little work in which he has dealt quite freely with the statistical side of this subject. I will take the liberty of quoting one or two things that he mentions which are very interesting. From a large number of assembled individual cases he has arrived at the conclusion that 58 per cent of all malignant tumors in the male are of the testicle but, on the other hand, the Mayos have seen, in nine years, 155 cases so you see in a large volume of work like theirs one runs against a fairly large number of cases.

Teratomas, according to another set of statistical figures, constitute about one-half of the malignant tumors of the testicle. The other half are carcinomatous seminomas which the French observer, Chevassu, has described and named; and one per cent are sarcomas.

In the diagnostic field there is one feature that is dwelt on particularly and that is the early rapid growth of teratomas as compared with carcinomas. The estimate is made by Bailey that when a man develops a teratoma, he is apt to come in for medical advice within six months after he has first noticed it, whereas in a carcinoma the interval is apt to be a year.

As regards metastasis, an American observer, Ferguson, has collected sixty-nine cases and he has found metastases in the supraclavicular nodes in six, in the mediastinum in eleven, in the pulmonary lymph nodes in thirteen and in the epigastric in thirty-nine. The operated percentage, Dr. Larson mentioned. Hinman had 100 cases but in the case of that one patient who died, it really was not an operative death. He died on the tenth day of pneumonia.

Now, what is the prognosis? Here again we come back to Hinman and we find, of the radical cases, his own operation, out of eighty traced cases, seventeen were alive after five years. In simple orchidectomy, with or without irradiation, 258 cases have been collected. Of these, only seventeen were alive after five years, so you see the percentage of good results appears much greater in the Hinman operation. Yet, I am told, Hinman himself is now lukewarm about his own operation, in view of the early and unpredictable metastasis to the opposite side in so many cases.

DR. KENNETH BULKLEY : At fairly regular intervals this question of malignancy of the testicle comes up and I never miss the opportunity to get up and bring up to date a case which I think has finally become rather well known in medical literature.

This case I reported originally in 1911 in Surgery, Gynecology and Obstetrics. It was that of an individual in the early forties whose wife had been repeatedly examined for sterility. No one had ever thought to examine him, although it turned out that he was a double cryptorchid. The man accidentally, while bathing, discovered a lump in his left lower abdomen. He was seen by Dr. Joseph A. Blake, recently deceased, and was operated upon by him in 1911, a large malignant intra-abdominal testicle adherent to small gut being found. A simple orchidectomy was done with removal of about a foot of small intestine with end-to-end anastomosis. No radical gland dissection was done, yet this man remained alive without further difficulty of any sort until about three years ago when he died from other causes. In those days deep x-ray therapy was unknown and this individual received no treatment whatsoever other than local excision. The excised testicle was pronounced by Dr. James Ewing to be a teratoma. In other words, this is a case of a malignant intra-abdominal teratoma of the testicle which received a local excision only, no gland dissection, no deep therapy and yet the patient lived for some thirty years.

There are a number of points in regard to intra-scrotal masses which I believe should be brought out in this discussion. The diagnosis is, of course, important and is not always easy, inasmuch as in a case I operated on only a few days ago, the mass may prove not to represent a testicular malignancy but an old hydrocele with walls so thick that transillumination is impossible. Tuberculosis also must be thought of and of course syphilis of the testicle. As far as the type of malignancy is concerned, I cannot help but be convinced that all malignant tumors of the testicle represent teratomas. This was first brought out by Ewing. In the particular case to which I referred at the beginning of this discussion, some ten or a dozen blocks were made, all of them showing apparently a pure sarcoma. However, with the cutting of more blocks different types of malignancy were encountered showing the case to be one of a teratoma.

There is just one other point which I would like to emphasize, chiefly because it sustains the thesis that radical gland dissection is inadvisable and unnecessary.

It is not uncommon for an individual to present himself for examination totally unconscious that anything wrong within his scrotum is the cause of the mass in the left supraclavicular region. When the man so presents himself always examine carefully the contents of the scrotum. Sooner or later the vast majority of cases of a malignancy of either testicle present a metastatic node above the left clavicle. I have never seen or heard of one appearing on the right side. It is probably due to lymphatic drainage and the position of the thoracic duct on the left.

Summarizing this discussion I would like to emphasize, first, the importance of diagnosis; second, the high radio-sensitivity of these tumors, rendering gland dissection unnecessary, and third, the fact that they probably are 100 per cent teratomas.

Dr. S. R. Maxeiner: I would like to add one more report of a case treated by the Hinman operation for embryoma of the testicle more than three years ago. The patient to date is apparently entirely well.

I would like to call attention to the research done by the Veterans Administration Facility at Hines, Illinois, with reference to the Prolan "A", and Prolan "B" as demonstrated in the urine by the Friedman test, and from a bulletin of January, 1934, I wish to quote as follows:

"While urine from normal males does not contain Prolan 'A' and/or 'B', urine from patients affected with teratoma contained from 50 to 50,000 mouse units per liter, depending upon the embryonic type of the tumor and the extent of the disease.

"Negative test results indicate: (1) No teratoma type tumor; (2) No active metastases of teratoma tumor; (3) That irradiation or surgical treatment of such cases has proven effective.

"Positive test results indicate: (1) Presence of a teratoma type tumor; (2) A recurrence of such a tumor; (3) Metastases from such tumor, whether the original tumor was removed or not; (4) The extent of the disease and the status in regard to treatment; (5) Serial tests at frequent intervals show the effectiveness of the treatment employed."

Our patient showed positive Friedman test before his operation. He has been given postoperative x-rays and although he has been checked regularly at intervals, the Friedman test became negative postoperatively and has remained negative to date.

TUMOR OF THE PARATHYROID WITHIN THE THYROID CAPSULE

J. M. HAYES, MD.

IN presenting this case I want to apologize to the Society for not having more definite information to confirm our suspicions. This was very interesting to me and I think I learned something from it, and hope some of you may profit by our mistakes.

The clinical symptoms, both before and after operation gave a picture which I wish I had the ability to present to you. Now I feel that we had a combination of hyperthyroidism and hyperparathyroidism present. We made a diagnosis of hyperthyroidism before operation but felt we were missing something.

The patient was a female, sixty-one years old. She had been treated for heart trouble, and a suggestion of hyperthyroidism had been made. She had tachycardia, marked tremor and all the symptoms that accompany exophthalmic goiter. She had a basal metabolic rate of plus 35 per cent.

On Lugol's solution she improved very much and her basal metabolism came to normal. Dr. Graves said her blood study would suggest Hodgkin's disease or glandular fever, but no other symptoms of these diseases were present. Even after taking Lugol's solution for three or four weeks she still had extreme exhaustion and pain all over her body, and especially in the long bones. Before operation the patient was extremely depressed, got around with much difficulty, had a stooped, rapidly aging appearance. The slightest trauma on any of her bones gave extreme pain. In addition to these symptoms, she had typical signs and symptoms of exophthalmic goiter.

The pain in her bones and extreme exhaustion ever after taking Lugol's solution puzzled us even when we were ready to operate. We should have x-rayed the bones before operation but did not. In fact, it is rare that a diagnosis of hyperparathyroidism is made before the bone begins to break down.

I did a thyroidectomy on her in June, 1935. At operation the gland generally gave the typical appearance of hyperplasia. The pathologist said the gland was one of hyperplasia with some small adenomata about 1 cm. in diameter. At operation I noticed one small nodule at about the level of the entrance of the inferior thyroid artery. I didn't think much of it at the time but later I recalled this did appear much the same as parathyroid tumors I had seen. Unfortunately I had just recently listened to a surgeon of considerable experience say that parathyroid bodies did not occur within the thyroid capsule.

The sudden and remarkable change in the symptoms after operation surprised every one who saw her. On the second day after operation she said she couldn't imagine so great a change taking place in any one in so short a time. The whole picture seemed to change very rapidly. She appeared cheerful and said the pain in her bones had all gone. She said she thought she could get up then and go to work. She did go to the polls and vote just one week after operation.

I have seen this sudden change take place after removing toxic adenomata but never after operating on an exophthalmic goiter. The adenomata were small and gave no evidence of degeneration, so we did not think they could account for the toxicity. We were therefore at a loss to account for this unusual, sudden change. About six months later when Dr. Lahey published his paper dealing with hyperparathyroidism and cited a case very similar to this, I came to the conclusion we had missed something here. I went back to find the specimen but it had been thrown away. The patient was perfectly normal by this time so x-ray of her bones revealed nothing. I know have not proven to you yet that we did have a parathyroid tumor here, but I do know if I get another patient with similar symptoms I will at least think of a parathyroid tumor. Perhaps many of our degenerative bone conditions would be picked up if we recognized these symptoms earlier.

Discussion

Dr. E. C. Robitshek: I am very happy to have heard Dr. Hayes' report of this case, because it gives me an opportunity to bring out that which I think should be emphasized regarding the early diagnosis and treatment of parathyroid tumors. I dare say there are only a few of us who have had much experience with the diagnosis and treatment of this condition. If you will recall, it is only about ten eleven years ago that the first operation on the para-thyroid glands was undertaken, and thus you will realize that only a short time has elapsed in which any great amount of work could have been accomplished and much further study of tumors of these glands made. Only last year Dr. Frank Lahey of Boston stated that he had seen five cases of para-thyroid hyperplasia or tumors and he cited the fact that he thought he had missed the diagnosis in many cases and felt sure that many others also have had such cases pass through their hands unrecognized. Personally, I believe that one of the reasons for this lies in the fact that we, as surgeons, do not begin to think of parathyroid pathology until we meet a patient with a palpable or visible tumor or nodule in the neck, or until we find what I term the end symptoms, rather than the beginning or initial ones, and, unfortunately, it is not until we see a patient with a pathological fracture, or a bone cyst, or a Von Recklinghausen lesion that our attention is attracted to the possibility of parathyroid pathology. Therefore, I have listed a few of the initial symptoms, in accordance with their percentage, as found by Gutman, Swenson and Parsons, who, in an analysis of 115 such cases, found the initial symptoms to be pain in the back or extremities in 72 per cent, pathological fractures in 28 per cent, bone swellings in 26 per cent, disturbances of gait in 24 per cent, muscle weakness in 22 per cent, gross deformities in 19 per cent, poly-uria, polydypsia and marked loss of weight in 10 per cent, renal colic in 9 per cent, and nausea and vomiting in 8 per cent. Lahey also calls attention to possible hyperparathyroidism in any patient showing progressively developing round back, so often due to de-calcification of the vertebral bodies. X-ray examination of the bones, especially of the skull, the spine, sacrum and the femora, is important and helpful in arriving at an early diagnosis. The only certain criterion, however, upon which a diagnosis of hyper-thyroidism can be made at the present time is a demonstration of a disturbance in calcium and phos-phorus metabolism, (hypercalcemia and hypophos-phatemia).

Now, as regards to the treatment of parathyroid tumors, I wish to state that there is only one accepted treatment and that is removal. No treatment with diet, no treatment with calcium, no treatment with hormones or with X-rays or any other known treat-ment is of any lasting benefit. Surgical treatment, however, should not be undertaken lightly, as it is not always as simple as one might expect. One reason for this is, as Dr. Hayes has pointed out in his case, that parathyroids vary. They vary in their size, from that of a green pea to a plum, they vary in number (normally there are four), they vary in their color, having been found of a pinkish hue, of a yellowish color as that of fat, to a dark color as that of liver, or the color of the thyroid itself, and they also vary in their location. Usually they may be found on the posterial and lateral aspects of the thyroid gland outside the capsule of this gland. They may, however, be found and frequently are, near and about the branches of the inferior thyroid arteries, and also about the superior arteries and their branches, or they may be found in the sulcus between the esophagus and the trachea, or found up as high as the pharynx, or as low as under the clavicle, or found deep in the anterior or posterior mediastinal spaces, which means that one must split or remove the manubrium in order to locate and remove them and besides they may be found within and part of the thyroid gland itself. With such variations in color and appearance, in size and location, plus the fact that one may mistake an aberrant or an accessory thyroid, a piece of thymus, or a hemolymph gland for a parathyroid one, it is essential that a competent patholo-gist be present at the operating table, in every oper-ation undertaken for this condition, in order that a frozen section of a portion of the removed tissue may be immediately examined and accurately diagnosed.

To emphasize all of what I have said, and to pre-sent it in a much clearer manner than I could hope to express, I will conclude by reading you the sum-mary of an article by E. D. Churchill and Oliver Cope, taken from a paper read by them at the last International Congress of Surgery, reporting their re-sults in thirty cases of parathyroid disease, and pub-lished by them in the *Annals of Surgery*, 1936:

1. The corner stone of successful surgery of the parathyroids is a positive diagnosis.

2. An "exploratory operation" to confirm or dis-prove a doubtful diagnosis has little or no place in this field.

3. The findings of the laboratory are more exact than the dissection of the surgeon, and there is no point in the operation at which the operator may lay down his scalpel and find comfort in having disproved the diagnosis. Even the demonstration of four normal parathyroid bodies is not adequate because there re-mains the possibility that a small adenoma of a fifth gland lies tucked away in some inaccessible region of the mediastinum. A positive diagnosis is therefore a challenge to the skill and patience of the surgeon and when these have been exhausted in a fruitless search for an adenoma, the operator is privileged to say "the tumor cannot be found," but not "the tumor does not exist."

As to tumors of the parathyroid, I am sure you are familiar with the fact that adenomas are the most frequent type, cysts much less frequent and carcinomas rare.

DR. R. C. WEBB: A parathyroid tumor so closely resembles a thyroid adenoma that one should not apologize for not recognizing a parathyroid tumor. The case of hyperparathyroidism which I operated upon in January, 1934, and later presented before this society, I had scheduled for operation as hyperpara-thyroidism and there were several surgeons present, all of whom were experienced in thyroid surgery. When the tumor was exposed we were unable to as-sure ourselves that it was the source of the patient's disease until we saw the microscopic section. I am sure that Dr. Hayes should not feel apologetic for not recognizing the tumor in his case of suspected hyperparathyroidism. In my case the tumor was palpable preoperatively. Although the tumors are fre-quently located within the thyroid gland, they are usually situated outside the thyroid gland and are frequently palpable.

For several years it has been known that para-thyroid tumors may be found within the thyroid gland. When Dr. F. H. Lahey discussed my paper at the 1934 meeting of the Western Surgical Association he called attention to eight cases in his own experience in which the parathyroid adenoma was discovered within the thyroid itself. (MINNESOTA MEDICINE, October 1935, page 669.)

The first case of hyperparathyroidism reported in 1926 by Mandl has reappeared in the literature due to a recurrence eight years later. I still have my patient under observation, and there is at this time no evi-dence of recurrence. She is in healthy appearance and has none of the symptoms of hyperparathyroidism. She has a nephritis which may have no relation to the parathyroid disturbance.

DR. J. M. HAYES: In answer to Dr. Webb, I will repeat that the patient had typical symptoms of hyperthyroidism and it was only accidentally that the parathyroid tumor, if it was such, was removed.

I have presented this with the hope that sometime

we might make a diagnosis of parathyroid tumor before the patient sustains a pathological fracture and the x ray must be brought in to make a diagnosis for us.

BENIGN TUMOR OF THE STOMACH

MARTIN NORDLAND, M.D.,

THIS case is presented because of its rare surgical incidence. According to Hunt, the incidence of benign tumors of the stomach depends on whether the material is determined from autopsy or surgically. Surgical incidence is about .5 per cent to 5 per cent.

Of the latter group, those arising from the muscular structures are the most frequent and account for 60 per cent of all benign tumors of the stomach. Thirty per cent of this class of tumors have an epithelial origin. In a series of Judd and Hoerner, including 50 cases, 72 per cent were of muscular origin.

Most benign tumors of the stomach are symptomless and when symptoms occur, they are bizarre. There may be bleeding, massive or otherwise, with tarry stools and anemia and intermittent pyloric obstructions.

There are no clinical characteristics of benign tumors of the stomach. Usually they are not palpable. They

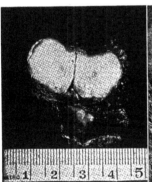 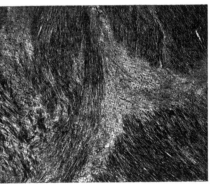

Fig. 1. Specimen of fibroma resected from the stomach wall.

Fig. 2. High power microphotographs of benign fibroma of the stomach.

In autopsy material, about 5 years ago, in the Department of Pathology, University of Minnesota, Rigler and Erickson, in investigating the records of 6,742 autopsies, found 187 gastric neoplasms of which 138 were malignant and 47 benign, an incidence of benign tumors of 26 per cent of all gastric neoplasms. Therefore, while benign tumors of the stomach are not uncommon, those that cause clinical manifestations are infrequent.

Hunt has further classified the origin of benign tumors of the stomach from three sources:

1. The epithelium.
   (a) Papilloma.
   (b) Adenoma.
2. Those from the connected tissues and vascular structures.
   (a) Lipoma.
   (b) Fibroma.
   (c) Myxoma.
   (d) Angioma.
3. Those from the muscular structures.
   (a) Myomas.
   (b) Neuromas.

can be confused with gastroduodenal disease because of anemia, bleeding and gastric motility. They are usually recognized by x-ray.

1. The filling defect is usually central rather than marginal.
2. The outline of the gastric shadow is usually preserved.
3. Spasm as in ulcer and cancer is absent.
4. Peristalsis is uninterrupted.

Case Report

The patient was a married woman, fifty-eight years of age, who presented herself with a typical history of recurrent cholecystitis and cholelithiasis. She had had several spells of gallstone colic over a period of four years with intervals varying from two weeks to six months. She complained that most of this time she had had varying degrees of indigestion. The last attack occurred about three weeks before admission to the hospital. X-ray study of the gallbladder revealed a non-functioning gallbladder but no evidence of stones. Because of the typical history of gallbladder trouble no preoperative x-ray examination of the stomach was made. There was nothing important in the history concerning the patient's past illnesses.

The patient was operated upon on March 26, 1936. The abdomen was opened through a high right rectus

76

incision and exploration of the abdominal contents revealed a thin walled gallbladder which emptied rapidly. The organ was apparently normal. On examination of the stomach a mass the size of a walnut was revealed on the anterior wall near the pylorus and close to the greater curvature. The mass was firm and seemed to be in the wall of the stomach proper. The pylorus was partially obliterated. The appendix was relatively normal with a few adhesions to the cecum near the base of the appendix. The mass described was excised and a pyloroplasty was performed. The wound was closed in three layers of sutures using interrupted linen sutures in the serosa. This procedure was followed by a typical appendectomy and the abdomen was closed in the usual manner.

The laboratory report by Dr. M. I. Smith, Pathologist, Northwestern Hospital: Specimen is an encapsulated tumor from the wall of the pylorus, 2.5x2 cm.; it is slightly yellowish and moderately soft. Microscopic sections show a leiomyoma with some chronic inflammation. The center is rather cellular.

The patient made an uneventful recovery. She was seen on two occasions since the operation and, as far as I know, she is well at the present time.

Dr. Hunt, in a discussion of benign tumors of the stomach at the meeting of the Western Surgical Association at Kansas City in 1936, concluded that most of the cases are undiagnosed. He stated that 60 per cent of the tumors were removed by partial gastrectomy or pyloric resection. Because of difficulty of differentiating a benign from a malignant tumor, and because of hemorrhage, all benign tumors should be operated upon.

Discussion

Dr. E. A. Regnier: As Dr. Nordland mentioned, these tumors are more frequently found coincident with other abdominal diseases. The reports from the radiologists show a more frequent occurrence than would be indicated from surgical reports because many of these tumors are found in routine gastrointestinal studies. Likewise, autopsy specimens reveal a great many small leiomyomata that are of no clinical significance. If these small tumors, as well as polypae of the stomach, are included, the number of these tumors becomes increasingly high.

In a series of cases reported by Judd and Hoerner, 65 per cent of these tumors occurred in the prepyloric area in the stomach and 30 per cent in the mid-gastric region. The importance of these tumors lies in the fact that they may cause very severe symptoms, the chief of which is hemorrhage, and that they may degenerate into malignant growths. It is significant that in Judd's cases 46 per cent of these benign tumors were associated with peptic ulcer. In three cases the tumors consisted of pancreatic tissue.

The x-ray which you see before you shows a tumor in the pre-pyloric region which was diagnosed carcinoma by one of our radiologists. This man, sixty years old, complained of gastric distress for eighteen months. He had moderate secondary anemia with total achlorhydria. There had been a loss of weight of ten pounds in the last six months with gradual failing appetite. The physical findings were essentially negative. With the above history and the diagnosis of carcinoma of the stomach this man was explored. A tumor, 2 cm. in diameter, was found just above the pylorus. The tumor was excised and on the mucosal side there was a small crater ulcer. The pathologist reported it as a benign ulcer with a small tumor mass of pancreatic tissue above it. A pyloroplasty was

done. The man made an uneventful recovery and is well today.

These benign tumors lend themselves to surgical removal by conservative surgery such as resection of the tumor with pyloroplasty or by sleeve resection or some other form of partial gastric resection. Their early removal should be encouraged because of the incidence of malignancy associated with them.

PROSTATITIS WITH CALCULI

T. H. Sweetser, M.D.

THE patient, a male veteran of the World War, forty-two years old, came to the hospital with complete retention of urine of twenty-four hours duration and with high fever and chills. He previously had had several attacks of complete retention and at other times had voided freely. He had been wounded during the war and also had contracted gonorrhea and syphilis at that time.

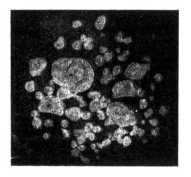

Rectal examination demonstrated a hard prostate containing stones which crepitated. The leukocyte count was 19,600, but the blood urea nitrogen was normal, the Wassermann was four plus, the urine contained some albumin, much pus, and a few erythrocytes. I had considerable difficulty passing the catheter even after passing bougies, but the intern had earlier passed a catheter without any difficulty. X-ray showed calculi filling the prostate and the prostatic urethra. A catheter was tied in place and preliminary treatment of his urinary tract and his syphilis was instituted.

Perirenal cystotomy was planned but finally a suprapubic cystotomy was performed instead. There was almost no trebeculation or thickening of the bladder wall. The bladder outlet admitted the finger. The prostatic urethra contained some small stones. The prostate, itself, was almost completely replaced by numerous stones, two of them being fairly large, and the mass of stones extended quite far back under the bladder trigone. The bladder outlet was dilated with the finger and the stones were removed. The shelf of remaining tissue between the prostate and the bladder was trimmed away and the prostatic space

BOOK REVIEWS

packed with gauze. The wound was closed, the bladder being drained with a Feyer tube.

The stones were smooth and of a brilliant bronze color. On splitting some of them open this bronze shell was translucent and on microscopic examination apparently consisted of compressed prostatic substance (desquamated and disintegrated epithelium?). Within this shell was an inner zone of dense stone inside of which was a softer material of various colors. Microscopically the fragments of prostatic tissue removed showed chronic prostatitis. At several points minute calculi were seen in acini or ducts from which the epithelial lining had disappeared.

The man made a good recovery and had no further prostatic or urinary trouble. About eight or nine months later he suffered an acute decompensation of his heart and died with evidence of luetic aortitis and probably aneurysm.

* * *

The meeting adjourned.

HARVEY NELSON, M.D., *Secretary*.

PROCEEDINGS—MINNESOTA ACADEMY OF MEDICINE

(Continued from page 66)

process, appear to be quite uniformly better in the conservatively treated group, in which only a short cutaneous incision is made when a subcutaneous abscess is demonstrable.

The gynecologist was the first surgical specialist in the field to recognize the great virtues of conservatism in the management of acute infections. When its values are more generally appreciated, our results in the management of acute infections will be better. Were it not that the patient with a sore throat must swallow saliva, if not food and drink, several hundred times a day; or that patients with empyema, lung abscess or peritonitis must inhale and exhale some 25,000 times a day—if means were available to circumvent such necessary motion—undoubtedly the results of treatment of such infections would be much better. In the extremities, however, we have with the employment of plaster casts a satisfactory means of reducing motion to a minimum. The role of the surgeon is such infections is to provide as absolute physical and physiologic rest as he possibly can; to elevate the extremity concerned, in order to reduce filtration in the damaged capillary bed and to diminish existing edema. Only when pus is present should incision be made. Until specific immunologic or pharmacologic means are available with which to deal with pyogenic infections, we must continue to use those agents which we have learned from our own experience affect the issue most favorably.

The meeting adjourned.

A. G. SCHULZE, M.D.

Secretary.

Learning without thought is labor lost,
Thought without learning is perilous.

—CONFUCIUS.

78

BOOK REVIEWS

Books listed here become the property of the Ramsey and Hennepin County Medical libraries when reviewed. Members, however, are urged to write reviews of any or every recent book which may be of interest to physicians.

SURGICAL PATHOLOGY OF THE DISEASES OF THE NECK Arthur E. Hertzler, M.D. Surgeon to the Agne Hertzler Memorial Hospital, Halstead, Kansas; Pro fessor of Surgery, University of Kansas. 237 pages Illus. Cloth binding. Philadelphia: J. B. Lippincot Company, 1937.

PRIMARY CARCINOMA OF THE LUNG. By Ed win J. Simons, M.D. Pp. 263; 30 illus., 2 col. plates $5.00. Chicago: Year Book Publishers, 1937.

The purpose of this book is to provide the genera practitioner with a compendium of the existing knowl edge of a most important subject, for the sake of stimu lating earlier recognition of the disease and thereby offering the patient his one and only opportunity fo relief and cure by early, radical operation. To do thi the author has literally combed the literature on th subject and has consulted freely with those of acknowl edged standing who have given specialized attention t the various phases of the subject, added to his own personal observations and well grounded experience The result is an amazing product of well directed in dustry and a keen example of the most useful type o textbook extant: a practical, scientific monograph.

This book should be on the desk of every practicing physician in the English-speaking countries. It contain the meat of the subject and nothing more. It is an ear nest, honest effort to furnish much needed informatio on a very serious problem in clinical medicine; one tha is becoming increasingly menacing with its known wide ing incidence. The author has done his work und circumstances of unusual difficulty and deserves war commendation for the way in which he has surmounte every handicap. We hope to see the book become wid ly known—and read.

G. C.

PHYSIOLOGY IN HEALTH AND DISEASE, ed. Carl J. Wiggers, Professor of Physiology, West Reserve University. 1122 pages. Illus. Price, $9. Philadelphia: Lea & Febiger, 1937.

A book on physiology that is authoritative, and at same time written in an interesting style, is not co mon. Wiggers' "Physiology in Health and Disea fulfills all the requirements of a handy reference b which one can consult when the question of the ph ologic disturbance underlying any condition arises. is a storehouse of physiological facts, and the rea is not led through a maze of controversial discuss that only makes for confusion. The reputation of author lends great weight to statements made in book. It should be on the book shelf of every p tising physician.

MAX H. HOFFMAN, M.

MINNESOTA MEDIC

MINNESOTA MEDICINE

Journal of the Minnesota State Medical Association, Southern Minnesota Medical Association, Northern Minnesota Medical Association, Minnesota Academy of Medicine and Minneapolis Surgical Society.

| Volume 21 | FEBRUARY, 1938. | Number 2 |

RADIATION THERAPY OF TUMORS WITH A CONSIDERATION OF THE POSSIBLE ADVANTAGES OF SUPERVOLTAGE X-RAYS*

ROBERT S. STONE, M.D.

San Francisco, California

UNTIL recent years malignant new growths were considered to be purely surgical problems. The term "surgical problem" includes not only the technical procedure of removing a tumor, but also the care of the patient with the tumor. The surgeon is expected to see that the patient has the proper preoperative care and the management after operation that will restore him to the best possible health. Such a conception of the surgeon's duties was not always held. For a long period extending into the nineteenth century surgeons were simply technicians who did not dare to stay too long in one community. With the advent of antisepsis and asepsis, operations were made more safe and new operations were made possible. In this period surgeons were so engrossed in developing new technics that they had little time to consider the patients upon whom they were operating. Now the technic of surgical procedures is standardized to such a degree that surgeons have been able to turn their attention to the problem of the patient as a whole.

Radiologists are passing through the same evolution as did the surgeons, but a little more rapidly. It is about forty-two years since the x-ray was discovered. Those physicians who have specialized in the use of these x-rays have been, like the surgeons of the immediate past, so intensely interested in the technical problems involved that some have lost sight of the patient as

a whole. Surgery could not have advanced to its present high state if surgeons had not realized that the patient was involved as well as that part of his anatomy containing a new growth. Now radiology, too, as a branch of medicine, has come to that stage of its development at which the radiologist must view the patient as a whole. He must be prepared to take temporary charge of that patient and to see that proper care is given before and after irradiation.

Due to the preoccupation of radiologists with their technical problems, many physicians and surgeons have developed the custom of sending their patients for a specified quantity of radiation to a tumor instead of referring them to a radiologist for his management and treatment. It should be evident that such a procedure is not for the good of the patient. A prime problem in radiation therapy is for the radiologist to take charge of the patient who is ill, rather than of a tumor that needs irradiation.

Once the diagnosis has been established and the necessity for irradiation therapy jointly decided, it is assumed too frequently by both doctors and laity that all that is needed is an x-ray apparatus and a technician to operate it. A knife never cured a patient of cancer, but a surgeon with a knife has cured many. Similarly, an x-ray machine has never controlled a cancer, but a radiologist using an x-ray machine has controlled many. To such a radiologist each patient is a particular problem, and many factors have to be considered which require a thorough medical appreciation of the constitution of the patient

*From the Department of Surgery, Division of Roentgenology, University of California Medical School. This study of supervoltage x-rays has been aided by a grant from the Christine Breon Fund for medical research. Citizens' Aid Society Memorial Address presented before the annual meeting of the Minnesota State Medical Association, Saint Paul, Minnesota, May 3, 1937.

and the type, size and location of the tumor, as well as a thorough knowledge of the handling of the x-ray apparatus so as to produce the most effective radiation.

The size and number of the areas which are to be treated must be considered in the light of the extent of the tumor, and the condition of the patient. Cachectic and anemic patients are known to stand radiation therapy very poorly, and hence only small areas can be irradiated, or small doses administered. The tumors in such patients respond very poorly. Even patients in the best of health cannot stand irradiation of too extensive areas of the body. With such facts in mind the radiologist must decide how many fields, and of what size, are to be used in applying the radiations.

The total dose desired must be determined in the light of the type of the tumor, its size and location. Some tumors which respond most easily and are called radiosensitive are the least curable. These shrink rapidly with the application of rather mild doses, but may require prolonged treatment if a cure is to be achieved. Other tumors are curable but are very resistant and require extremely large total doses which must be given in such a manner that the patient's normal tissues can stand them.

A decision on the total amount of radiation to be given requires a consideration of the number of days to be consumed in giving it. The total number of roentgens—the unit of exposure of x-rays—means little unless the total elapsed time and the daily distribution are considered. Some tumors respond best to a relatively small total dose given in a few days, while others require a larger total dose given in three or more weeks. The division of the desired irradiation into multiple daily sittings is necessary to preserve the integrity of normal tissues while delivering to the tumor a number of roentgens sufficient to destroy it. This question of the protraction of the dose is one that is only beginning to be understood. Not alone has the total number of days, and the amount of radiation to be given on each day, to be considered, but also the rate at which the radiation is to be given during each sitting.

It is a popular conception that the powerful machines which can deliver large amounts of radiation in short periods of time are the most effective. This may or may not be true. There is

some evidence to show that radiation delivered in small amounts per minute is more effective in many cases than the same total quantity delivered in large amounts per minute. If this is found to be true, the trend will be toward the use of less powerful apparatus for longer periods of time, rather than toward more and more powerful machines.

The distance of the x-ray tube from the patient must also be considered. If a large area is to be treated as a single field, this distance must be great in order to obtain a uniform irradiation of the whole surface. Short distances can be used when a small field is to be treated. This target skin distance also controls to a certain extent the amount of radiation that penetrates to the depths. The greater the distance, the greater is the dose at any given depth. Skin lesions can be treated at short distances but deep-seated lesions require long distances.

Last, but not least, come the problems of the filter and the voltage to be used. These two factors control the quality of the radiation. With regard to the filter, the only statement to be made at present is that increasing the filter, either in thickness or in the density of the material used, cuts down the number of soft x-rays which reach the patient. No amount of filter can give harder rays than the hardest produced by the particular voltage being used. It is common knowledge that soft (or long wave-length) x-rays are absorbed in the skin and the subcutaneous tissues, while a greater proportion of harder (short wave-length) x-rays penetrate to the depths. Hence, the choice of filters is governed by the depth to which we wish the radiation to penetrate before being too greatly absorbed.

The problem of voltage is probably the most vexatious one at the present time. There is a common belief, held by both the medical profession and the laity, that higher and higher voltages are synonymous with better and better treatments, and more and more cures of cancer. This popular feeling is stampeding radiologists into procuring apparatus capable of producing higher and higher voltages. Let us carefully consider the facts which are known at the present time. At the University of California Hospital we have an apparatus which, since 1934, has run at supervoltages for treatment purposes. For the past year it has been operating continuously at one million volts. In adjacent rooms we have machines capable of producing 200 and 100 kv. radiations and we have endeavored to compare the physical and clinical observations on the various voltages as accurately as possible.

Radiations act on cancer cells and the surrounding tissues by means of the ionization which they produce in them. Within the range of x-rays available, the amount of ionization depends on the quantity of radiation that reaches and is absorbed by the tissues which we desire to affect. The voltage used regulates the energy of the x-rays produced, and is therefore the determining factor, up to a certain point, as to the depth to which the rays will penetrate before being largely absorbed. It was long ago conceived, therefore, that if x-rays could be produced by higher and still higher voltages, they would penetrate farther and farther into the tissues before being absorbed. When the advance was made from 100 to 200 kv. radiations, it was found that the rays could and did penetrate farther, and that more marked effects were produced in the depths.

It must be kept in mind that the increase in the quantity of effective radiation at a given depth must be in greater proportion than the increase in that quantity on the surface if the radiation is to be of value. A method of expressing the amount of effective radiation at depths in percentages of the amount on the surface was devised. These percentage figures are called depth doses. We have compared the depth doses produced by 1,000 kv. radiations with those produced by 200 kv. radiations.

It was found soon that the 1,000 kv. radiations penetrate better than the 200 kv. radiations. There is very little difference in the depth doses at from 4 to 6 cm., but, as greater depths are reached, the difference between the two becomes great. Using a field 20 by 20 cm. we found the depth dose at 10 cm. to be 46 per cent for 200 kv. and 55 per cent for 1,000 kv. radiations. It would seem until we look further into the problem, that higher voltage is very much better.

Since it is necessary to administer 100 per cent or greater depth doses to most tumors, it is obvious that more than one field of entry for the radiation is necessary. If the depth dose at 10 cm. is 50 per cent, and it is desired to give a dose of 100 per cent at a depth of 10 cm., the irradia-

tion would have to be applied through two surfaces, 100 per cent to each. The accumulation of the two 50 per cent doses would give 100 per cent at the center point. The two portals of entry of the radiations would probably have to be directly opposite to each other. Some of the x-rays pass through the body and affect the skin on the opposite side. This is called the "exit dose." This exit dose is much greater for 1,000 kv. than for 200 kv. radiations, because of their greater penetration. In calculating how much the skin will get, the exit dose must be added to that directly applied. Hence the amount applied directly must be reduced more for the 1,000 kv. than for the 200 kv. radiations if the skin dose is to be kept at a total of 100 per cent. The smaller amount directly applied reduces in proportion the amount reaching the depth, and we find that the depth dose at the center of a body treated from directly opposite sides is not nearly as much greater as would be expected on a superficial consideration of the subject. In fact, we found that when thin parts of the body, such as the neck, are treated, a greater "center" dose can be given with 200 kv. than with 1,000 kv. radiations. The actual amount of the depth dose depends on the size of the fields irradiated. We found that if fields 10 by 10 cm. were used in parts up to 12 cm. thick, doses could be given by 200 kv. radiation as large as, or even larger than, those supplied by 1,000 kv. With large fields such as may be used on an abdomen, 20 by 20 cm., a thickness of more than 18 cm. was reached before any improvement in the center dose could be found with the higher voltage. Hence, from the aspect of physical measurement, it would appear that 1,000 kv. radiations are of increased value only when the parts to be radiated are thick, or the fields to be used are small, or direct cross-fire can be avoided.

Clinically, other facts are found. It is a very common belief that the effect on the skin is the sole factor limiting the amount of radiation which a patient can receive. This is not true. While treating lesions of the abdomen or pelvis it has been found frequently that the effect on the bowel, i.e., the erythema produced in the mucous membrane, is the limiting factor. When we have used 200 kv. heavily filtered radiations, applied from a distance of 80 cm., the intestinal reaction has frequently become so severe that treatments had to be interrupted or altered before the skin had received its maximum dose. The effect on the lungs when treating over the chest, and the effect on the mucous membrane of the throat when treating over the neck are known to limit treatments in those regions. It

The 1,000 kv. apparatus has been in operation only since May, 1934. Five-year "cures" are therefore not yet in existence. We have, however, compiled some statistics for various lesions which show the unfortunate fact that, with the

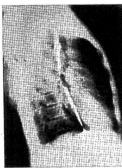
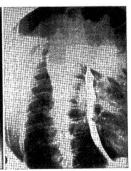
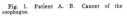

Fig. 1. Patient A. B. Cancer of the esophagus.

Fig. 2. Same patient as Figure 1, eight months after x-ray therapy to the cancer of the esophagus.

would seem that with 200 kv. radiations we are able to get as great a dose into the depths of the body as can be tolerated by the normal tissue in many cases. One thousand kv. radiations can do no better than this. Some other method of differentially affecting the tumor more than the normal tissue around it must be found.

Without further discussing the points involved, our general conclusions may be stated. First, supervoltage delivers greater depth doses from a single field, the differences being more marked the smaller the field and the greater the depth considered. Secondly, with supervoltage radiations there is less scattering into the adjacent tissues. Thirdly, the amount of x-ray in a supervoltage beam does not fall off so markedly on the edge as it passes through the body. This results in a more uniform dose to all points at a given depth. Fourthly, when using cross-fire technic, the large exit doses offset to some extent the practical value of the larger depth doses, the supervoltage being advantageous only if (a) direct cross fire can be avoided, (b) the part is thick, (c) multiple small fields can be used without excessive overlapping of the exit skin fields.

number of patients already dead, we cannot expect any great improvement in the five-year results when the necessary time has elapsed. It should be remembered that the same technic, except for voltage, has been used on the 200 and 1,000 kv. machines. Let us now consider what has been accomplished with specific lesions.

Cancer of the esophagus is recognized as a hopeless disease. Eight patients suffering from it have been treated, six are dead. Of the two alive, one has survived a year, and the other nine months, since the beginning of treatments. Both are comfortable at the present time.

Figure 1 shows the lesion in the middle third of the esophagus of patient A. B. as seen on July 6, 1936. Following this examination he was given 250 r per day to a total of 2,500 r per field to four fields in a period of 23 days. Figure 2 shows the same patient eight months later. Preceding the first examination a biopsy was taken by means of an esophagoscope. Following the second examination another esophagoscopy was performed and no evidence of the previous cancer could be found. The patient is at present enjoying very good health.

82

Figure 3 shows the biopsy specimen of a second patient, G. S., who had a similar lesion in a similar place. This patient received a prolonged course of therapy, following which his ability to swallow was improved. The treatment ended on

twenty-one were dead, eighteen alive with some evidence of cancer, and twenty-four alive with no evidence of cancer. In this series there were four patients with cancer in the first stage, while in the 1,000 kv. series there were none with the

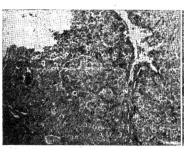 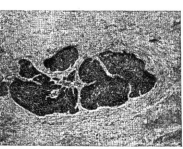

Fig. 3. Biopsy specimen of cancer of the esophagus. Patient G. S.

Fig. 4. Specimen from autopsy of patient G. S. showing encapsulated islands of cancer tissue one month after x-ray therapy.

January 22. On February 28 the patient died and an autopsy was obtained. Scarcely any evidence of the carcinoma of the esophagus could be found, but there were evidences of fibrosis of the lung. The patient also had pernicious anemia, generalized arteriosclerosis, mild diabetes and terminal bronchopneumonia. Figure 4 shows one of the few small islands of cancer cells which were demonstrated after making serial sections of the esophagus. It is easily seen that, whereas the cells in the specimen taken before treatment appear to be growing wildly and invading widely, those in the section made after irradiation appear to be adult in type with no evidence of growth and to be encapsulated. It is evident that in this case the x-rays had almost eradicated the tumor.

In treating cancer of the uterus we have cooperated closely with the Department of Obstetrics and gynecology, headed by Dr. Frank Lynch. Most of the patients were given local radium treatments by members of that department, followed at once by external irradiation. Sixty patients have been so treated. Of these, twenty are dead, twenty-one are alive with some evidence of cancer, and nineteen are alive without evidence of cancer. During the immediately preceding period of two years and seven months, during which 200 kv. radiations were used, 63 patients were treated. At the end of that period,

disease in that early stage. Even taking this fact into consideration, it is obvious that the 1,000 kv. radiations have produced no better results than the 200 kv. radiations.

Several of the uteri that had been irradiated thoroughly were removed by Dr. Lynch at varying intervals after the treatments. A very radical Wertheim procedure was performed. This was done in order to see what happened to the irradiated tumors and the surrounding tissues. He found that foci of tumor cells which appeared to be alive were found frequently and that the surrounding tissues showed a considerable amount of unfavorable change. Such findings as these give us a new conception of what happens after irradiation. In deciding on a practical course to follow in treating patients with cancer of the cervix, we must still rely on the fact, shown by so many authorities, that radiation produces as high a percentage of five year survivals as any other method, and a much lower mortality than surgery. The patient is interested in living as long as possible, even if she has a few foci of cancer cells encapsulated in the pelvis.

The patients having cancer of the breast have had such varied combinations of treatment that little can be concluded from our statistics. All of the patients with early cancers were operated on, and either received no radiation or only a

TABLE I. PATIENTS TREATED WITH 1,000 KV. RADIATIONS DURING TWO YEARS AND SEVEN MONTHS

Location	Alive Without Evidence of Cancer	Alive with Cancer	Dead	Total
Brain	1	3	13	17
Breast	8	12	17	37
Larynx	4	4	6	14
Lung	0	4	18	22
Esophagus	0	2	6	8
Ovary	3	4	7	14
Pharynx	2	4	5	11
Prostate	0	7	9	16
Testicle	6	2	4	12
Thyroid	5	2	1	8
Uterine Cervix	19	21	20	60
Uterine Fundus	4	1	4	9

postoperative course. Thirty-seven patients in all were treated. Of these, seventeen are dead, twelve are alive with evidence of the disease, and eight are alive with no evidence of cancer. Of these eight, seven received only post-operative irradiation and were probably cured of cancer by the surgery. Ten patients were treated by x-ray alone. They had either extensive axillary metastases or some complicating disease. Six are alive and comfortable, but still have evidence of cancer. Three are dead. Only one is alive with no evidence of malignancy.

An examination of some breasts removed solely for study after thorough irradiation showed that most of them had some cancer tissue persisting, but always altered considerably by the treatments. This finding is the same as reported above for esophageal and uterine carcinomata.

The problem of deciding the most practical method of treating cancer of the breast is solved by analyzing the statistics of the results of surgical treatment. In our clinic, Dr. E. I. Bartlett did this some years ago and found that the only patients with a high percentage of cures by surgery alone were those with a small movable tumor in the outer half of the breast and no palpable axillary metastases. In all other cases the percentage of cures was so low that other meth-

ods of treatment should be tried. As a result this I recommend that all patients except th with lesions of the type noted above be give thorough course of radiation, followed by radical operation if there is no spread beyond axilla, and if it seems practically possible to move all the axillary lymph nodes after the action to irradiation has subsided.

Space does not permit a discussion of all ty of cancer treated, nor would it be profitable. ble I shows the statistics for many of the ca treated between May, 1934, and December, 19 by 1,000 kv. radiations. These patients were all treated by irradiation alone. From the ta we can gather the significant and disappoint fact that there are so many patients already d that few will be living at the end of five yea

I have not tried to deal with the results radiation therapy as a whole, but I have tried show that very little improvement in results is be expected from 1,000 kv. radiations. It wo not be doing justice to radiation therapy to c clude this discussion on such a pessimistic no Every physician knows of some patients v have been cured by this means. They are ones who have presented themselves with very calized cancers. The statistics and the mic scopic evidence of persisting cancer in trea patients do not tell the complete story. A g many patients who come in suffering seve from cancer can be relieved of a large part their suffering. Their tumors can be reduced size, and an attitude of depression changed to of hope. The older textbooks are filled with tures of emaciated, suffering patients in advar stages of cancer. By our radiation methods are able to keep many such patients comfort until they die of internal metastases, suc those to the liver, and their deaths are much painful.

Summary

1. The status of the radiation therapist is sidered and it is shown that, if he is to b the greatest value to those suffering from ca he must take his place beside the surgical th pist as a well-rounded physician. He car longer remain a "technician," interested onl administering a dose of x-ray to a tumor, out concerning himself with the patient who the tumor.

2. The method of giving x-ray therapy

not yet become standardized. There are many factors to be considered. Each patient is a new problem, and a great deal more depends on the clinical judgment and technical knowledge of the physician administering the x-ray therapy than on the particular apparatus he uses.

3. Many factors have to be considered before giving x-ray therapy:
   (a) The size of the area to be irradiated depends on the extent of the primary tumor and its spread; and on the condition of the patient.
   (b) The total dose to be applied depends on the type, size and location of the tumor. The number of days required for giving the treatment, and the rate at which the x-ray is applied at each sitting are of great importance.
   (c) The voltage to be used is the most pressing question at the present time. The popular conception that higher voltage means better treatment is not generally true. More powerful machines are not necessarily more useful. A comparison is made between the physical measurements obtained by using 200 kilovolt and 1,000

kilovolt apparatuses. For thicknesses corresponding to many parts of the body, as large a dose can be given to internal parts by 200 kilovolt radiations as by 1,000 kilovolt radiations. Clinically it is unnecessary to go above 200 kilovolts in order to get as large a depth dose as can be tolerated. Advances in x-ray therapy are as likely to result from a better use of the apparatus we now have as from new kinds of apparatus.

4. Various specific tumors are discussed as to the method of treatment and the effect of the supervoltage x-rays on them. The number of patients who have died in the two and a half year period during which the million volt therapy machine has been in use indicates clearly that no very appreciable advance has been made by increasing the voltage.

5. The number dead or the number cured does not tell the whole story. Many of the patients treated were made much more comfortable and their remaining years of life more enjoyable.

THE ENERGY METABOLISM OF THE HEART IN FAILURE*

MAURICE B. VISSCHER, Ph.D., M.D.

Professor of Physiology, University of Minnesota

Minneapolis, Minnesota

THE failing heart is, in general terms, one that is unable to pump sufficient blood to meet the needs of the body. From the point of view of etiology there are many kinds of heart failure, but to focus attention on a single phase of the problem, only myocardial failure will be considered, without reference to the complicating factors of disturbances of rhythm and conduction, and disturbances in coronary blood flow. It is not implied that the principles to be discussed do not apply in the presence of complications due to the aforementioned factors, but the case is simpler when these conditions are excluded.

In the experimental animal, one can study either acute or chronic failure by experiments. To simulate most closely the more common types of failure it would be desirable to do experiments of the chronic type. Unfortunately, methods for study of the more important factors in long-time experiments are not available and therefore experiments have had to be limited, for the most part, to acute situations. Reasons will be advanced for believing that the results so obtained may be applied to the solution of the clinical problem.

A reduction in the ability of any machine to do work might conceivably be due to either one of two factors. Either the amount of energy available may be diminished or the ability of the machine to convert available energy into work may be impaired. Without experimenta-

*Read before the annual meeting of the Minnesota State Medical Association, Saint Paul, Minnesota, May 4, 1937. The work on digitalis glucosides reported in this paper was subsidized partly by funds from the Graduate School of the University of Minnesota and by a grant from the Sandoz Company.

tion it would be impossible to, decide which of these two mechanisms were responsible for the failure of the heart to do its work when it deteriorates.

There are several chemical processes involved in the liberation of energy in muscle contraction. According to the best evidence available at the present time, contraction is associated with a breakdown and subsequent resynthesis of creatine phosphate and adenyl-pyrophosphate, and with the formation of lactic acid from glycogen through several intermediate steps. In the ultimate recovery from contraction there is an oxidation of carbohydrate and fat, liberating energy for the restoration of the system. The stores of creatine phosphate and glycogen might possibly be depleted in the failing heart and thus there might be a lack of the materials which provide the immediate source of energy for the contractile process.

Experiments conducted in collaboration with Mulder[14] showed that so long as the heart was supplied with adequate oxygen there was no significant decrease in glycogen stores. Therefore, it seems very unlikely that failure should be due to the lack of carbohydrate in the heart.

The question of a possible lack of creatine compounds in the failing heart has been attacked from several angles and the results indicate, as will be seen below, that this factor is probably not the critical one in most types of failure. Several investigators have measured the creatine content of hearts in relation to failure. Seecof, Linegar, and Myers[10] made the first extensive investigation. Hermann, Decherd and Oliver[5] studied the creatine content of human heart muscle in 105 cases. They found a 30 per cent decrease in creatine in the congestive failure cases as compared with the normal. Bodansky and Pilcher[1] studied the creatine content of the human heart at autopsy in 310 cases. The hearts from patients dying from congestive heart failure showed somewhat less creatine than did the hearts of normal individuals. There were some failing hearts, however, wich had a creatine content well within the normal range and the average depletion was only a little more than 20 per cent. In view of the finding of high creatine values in some of the congestive failure cases and particularly in view of the fact that terminal anoxemia is apt to be present

longer in patients dying of congestive failure than from other diseases, particularly than in the case of accidental death, it seems that these results must be taken to indicate that the decrease in heart muscle creatine is not the main causative factor in this type of failure. The work of Hermann and Decherd[4] would seem to indicate quite clearly that when the blood flow, and consequently the oxygen supply to tissues are interfered with as in the case of infarction, the creatine content of heart muscle does drop abruptly. The changes that occur in infarction, however, have no particular bearing upon our present problem. Furthermore, there is no significant accumulation of creatine in the blood of the heart-lung preparation when the heart fails. Previously unpublished experiments show that the creatine content of the blood in the heart-lung preparation varies between 3.4 and 7.3 mg. per cent. In two out of five experiments there was an increase of 0.5 mg. per cent in three hours of progressive failure and in three experiments there was no change. If creatine phosphate were to have been lost from the heart it might have been expected that one would find an increase in creatine in the blood. Since this did not occur it may be inferred that there was no loss of creatine phosphate from the muscle during these periods.

Further evidence concerning the availability of energy in the failing heart is to be found in observations on the total oxygen consumption. When recovery from contraction is occurring in a normal way the oxygen consumption of muscle is an index of its total energy expenditure. This is true because the muscle is restored to its resting state by oxidation processes, and in the last analysis all the energy of contraction must come from the oxidation of either carbohydrate or fat. Thus a determination of oxygen consumption should provide a means of measuring the total energy output of the heart in contraction under various circumstances. The only requirement that must be satisfied in order that this may be a valid procedure is that the heart b adequately supplied with oxygen. This can b accomplished readily in the heart-lung preparation, which has been used for studies on thi question.

As an introduction to what will be said concerning the metabolism of the heart in failure certain general principles regarding the dynamics of heart muscle should be reviewed. First one should consider the normal mechanisms of response of the heart to changes in its load. Starling[11] formulated as the Law of the Heart,

The ability of the heart to do larger amounts of work at greater diastolic volume results from the fact that the amount of energy liberated in contraction is dependent upon the diastolic volume or fiber length.[12] Regardless of whether

Adjustment of Ventricles to Load

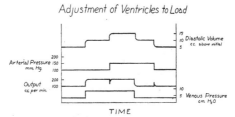

TIME

Fig. 1. Schematic, composite diagram showing mechanism of adjustment of mammalian heart to increases and decreases in load.

the rule that in order to do increased work the ventricles of the heart must dilate. In Figure 1 is presented a composite and somewhat schematic diagram of the results of many experiments on this question. When the work that the heart is made to do is increased by raising the venous pressure, thus increasing the filling, the diastolic volume of the ventricles rises. Again, when the arterial resistance is increased, producing a hypertension, the heart is able, after a few beats to eject the same amount of blood as before, but from a greater diastolic volume. When the inverse changes in filling pressure and arterial resistance are made, the diastolic ventricular volume diminishes. In every case, unless the heart is failing, or excessive loads are imposed, the heart arrives shortly at a constant diastolic volume, which it maintains until a change is made in the filling, or in the peripheral resistance. The general rule may be derived from such observations that when the heart is called upon to do increased work of any type, it adjusts itself by virtue of the fact that the residual blood increases to the requisite quantities so that the diastolic volume will be great enough to permit the heart to eject a quantity of blood equal to that delivered to it during each cardiac cycle. Or, stated more simply, if somewhat less completely, the heart responds to the imposition of more work by diastolic dilatation. The process, moreover, is reversible.

the increase in diastolic fiber length is brought about by increased arterial pressure or increased filling, the oxygen consumption or total energy liberation is the same at any diastolic volume. It becomes apparent that the diastolic volume law is valid because energy liberation depends upon diastolic volume. The heart is able to do more work when it dilates under increased pressure or increased filling because at the greater diastolic fiber length more energy is liberated.

It has long been known that the amount of work the isolated heart is able to do, contracting from a particular diastolic volume, diminishes with time. This phenomenon has been referred to as spontaneous failure in the isolated heart. At least superficially, and it is believed fundamentally as well, this phenomenon is not dissimilar to failure in the clinical sense, which is also associated with cardiac dilatation. In clinical heart failure the heart dilates even though it is called upon to do a minimal amount of work. Transferring the results from the heart-lung preparation to the case of the human heart, we would say further that in failure the heart dilates in order to do a constant minimal amount of work. From the point of view of the pathologic physiology of the heart this point is of prime importance. Dilatation is a mechanism of adaptation and is not in itself an unfavorable, but rather a desirable reaction. It is only the underlying conditions which make dilatation necessary which are unfortunate. The ability of the heart to dilate in failure is actually a life saving compensatory mechanism.

The important question arises as to whether the necessity for dilatation in failure in order to carry a constant load is occasioned by a decrease in the total energy liberation or by a decline in the efficiency of utilization of energy by the contracting muscle. This problem has been attacked experimentally in the mammalian and the amphibian heart. In the simplest case, that is, in the single ventricle of the turtle, the work performed and the oxygen consumption were measured[3] and it was found that the latter was constant when the diastolic ventricular volume was held constant over three hours of beating, but the work that could be done fell off markedly. This finding means that the proportion of the total energy used which was put to useful work decreased. In other words the efficiency of the ventricle as a machine decreased as the heart muscle failed. The efficiency which was originally 17.5 per cent or thereabouts in most fresh hearts, fell to as low as 5 per cent in three hours.

In the mammalian heart this general principle has been confirmed.[7] The heart-lung preparation removed from the dog's body and placed in a closed chamber immersed in a constant temperature bath was employed. The ventricular volume was measured by placing the heart in a cardiometer, the work was controlled by altering the venous inflow, and the energy expenditure was calculated from the oxygen consumption. It was found that except when massive edema of the heart or lungs occurred, the diastolic volume law was valid even when the heart failed badly. It is possible to induce or accelerate failure in the heart-lung preparation by the administration of histamine or by adding anesthetics to the blood. It was found that histamine tended to diminish the energy output at constant external diastolic volume but it could not be definitely ascertained whether the histamine effect in this regard might not have been due to the massive edema which it produces. Anesthetics such as amytal and alcohol decreased the work that the heart was able to do without correspondingly influencing the total energy liberation. In other words their effect was specifically upon the efficiency of the heart

muscle. In spontaneous and induced failure, therefore, the heart is seen to be a less efficient machine than it is when normal. The energy that can be put into contraction is as great as before, but a smaller fraction of it is usefully employed.

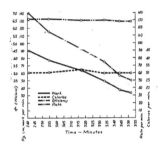

Fig. 2. Spontaneous failure in the heart-lung preparation (dog). The external work expressed in kg. cm. per minute, the total energy liberation measured by oxygen consumption and expressed in calories per minute, the efficiency calculated from these two quantities and the heart rate plotted against time.

In Figure II are presented the results of an experiment performed in the present study, illustrating the decreased efficiency which occurs in spontaneous failure in the heart-lung preparation when the diastolic volume of the ventricles is maintained constant over the course of an hour. It will be noted that the work which the heart could do at constant diastolic volume diminished so greatly over this period of time that the efficiency of the heart declined about 60 per cent.

In all, more than 100 experiments have been performed in which spontaneous failure has been observed and in none of the cases, unless massive edema has developed, has there been any significant deviation from the findings presented above as typical.

Various factors alter the rate at which failure occurs in the heart-lung preparation. It was found[15] that the addition of a small amount of insulin would improve the condition of the heart when it is first added to the perfusion fluid. After the first injection of insulin in a given preparation, subsequent injections have no further effect. Furthermore, the improvement is only temporary and progressive failure super-

88

venes after a short time. Likewise the addition of glucose to the circulating blood improves the condition of the heart muscle with respect to its efficiency. In spite of high blood sugar levels, however, the heart eventually fails as it does when the blood sugar is allowed to fall. These factors, although important, do not prevent myocardial failure for any length of time. Increasing the calcium content of the blood was found to increase both the energy liberation and the efficiency of the dog's heart.[5]

The only agents so far investigated capable of permanently increasing the work and the efficiency of the heart in the preparations we have employed are the glucosides of the digitalis series. This fact seems to be not without importance in understanding the physiological mechanisms by which the digitalis glucosides act. There has been great confusion in the literature regarding the mechanism of the therapeutic action of digitalis. The monographs of Cushny[2] and Luten[6] may be consulted in connection with the history of the subject. It is sufficient for our purposes to say that there has been no clear evidence of a therapeutically useful effect of digitalis upon the heart muscle itself, until recently. The most obvious effects of digitalis upon the heart of experimental animals are upon excitation and conduction. The occurrence of increased tonus, so-called, in the ventricle has long been known, but there is no necessary relationship between increased tonus and increased work capacity. Several investigators have performed inconclusive experiments on the effect of digitalis glucosides in the heart-lung preparation, failing in general to control the diastolic ventricular volume, and no consistent results were obtained until the problem of the work capacity of the failing heart was investigated at constant diastolic fiber length.[7] It was found that strophanthin, scillaren-B, ouabain and the digilanids of Stoll[18] all had a beneficial effect on cardiac efficiency, producing an increase of as much as 200 per cent in this factor.

A further study has been made of the action of the three components of the digilanids in digitalis lanata. These purified, crystalline, natural glucosides have been studied separately.* As might have been anticipated their activities

*I am indebted to the Sandoz company for a supply of the separate digilanids A, B, and C.

are quite different. Digilanid C is from five to ten times as potent in producing an increase in efficiency as is digilanid A. An example is given in Figure 3 of an experiment in which 2 mg. of digilanid A was administered after

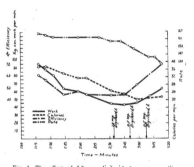

Fig. 3. The effect of 2.0 mg. digilanid A on energy liberation, work, efficiency, and heart rate in the heart-lung preparation.

a period of failure and the resulting change in efficiency was from 4.5 to 7.0 per cent. In a comparable experiment, Figure 4, 0.2 mg. of digilanid C increased the efficiency from 5.3 to 10.0 per cent. The effects of digilanid C come on somewhat more rapidly than do those of digilanid A. This seems not to be due to differential solubility, because the C is less soluble that the A. Rothlin[9] has reported that by the ordinary cat assay method, digilanid C is only slightly more active than digilanid A. By the frog's heart method digilanids A and D have identical activity according to Rothlin. These methods really measure the toxicity of digitalis bodies, giving the dose necessary to kill the animal or to stop the heart. It is quite evident that the toxic dose method does not give evidence concerning the efficiency-increasing power of digitalis glucosides. The classical methods of assay may give useful information in indicating the fatal dose of a glucoside preparation but since equally toxic substances may have ten-fold differences in their therapeutic actions it is obvious that one should not expect such methods of assay to give reliable information as to the more important actions of the drugs, assuming for the purpose of this argument that the increase in the ability to do work is the therapeutically desirable action of digitalis. Only two experiments have been performed up to this time on digilanid B and it is therefore impossible to make any statement as to its actions

that in the chronic failing human heart. is, however, much collateral evidence to : the view that the principles involved : same in the two cases. In both instan

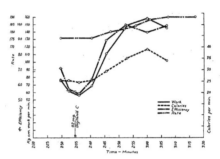

Fig. 4. The effect of 0.2 mg. digilanid C on energy liberation, work, efficiency, and heart rate in the heart-lung preparation.

other than to say that it is very much less active than the digilanid C.

In connection with other reputed cardiac tonics, the action of coramine should be mentioned. The effect of this widely used drug upon cardiac efficiency was studied[7] and it was found that its action upon the heart muscle was deleterious, in the sense that it resulted in a decreased efficiency. It would, of course, be inappropriate to condemn this drug generally because it has one undesirable action, inasmuch as it might be useful in producing a peripheral vaso-constriction or in stimulating respiration, in spite of an unfavorable direct action on cardiac muscle. However, there are many circumstances which might arise in which such a drug as coramine might be employed, and in which the efficiency of the heart muscle might be the critical factor in determining the life or death of a patient. Under such circumstances the employment of an agent which decreases the amount of work the heart can do with a given expenditure of energy is definitely contraindicated.

Finally, the justifiability of the use of the acutely failing heart-lung preparation in such studies as these should be considered. It must be recognized that one is unable to prove that the situation in the dog's heart is comparable to

heart has to dilate in order to do the amount of work. In both, a decrease load results in a decrease in diastolic v Moreover, in both, the therapeutically digitalis glucosides result in a decrease i tricular volume. There is no evident disci between the situation in the two cases burden of proof would therefore seem upon those who would deny the legitim the transference of conclusions drawn fr periments on failure in the dog heart situation in uncomplicated myocardial fa man. As noted above, disturbances in tion, rhythm and coronary circulation cor the situation, and also, it may be added hypertrophy is involved the problem is of less simple. It is beyond the scope of thi to enter into a full discussion of these co tions but it is the author's opinion that w tain minor reservations, the general pi described still hold.

Summary

1. The inability of the heart to mai work output in failure has been show associated with a decrease of the me efficiency of the heart muscle.

2. The efficiency of the failing heart increased temporarily by the administr

glucose, insulin or calcium salts. It is profoundly improved by the administration of glucosides of the digitalis series. It is suggested that the major factor in the beneficial effect of digitalis in myocardial failure is the improvement in mechanical efficiency.

3. The several glucosides from digitalis are not equal in their potency in this regard nor is the effect on efficiency parallel with the toxic properties measured by the usual assay methods. There is as much as a ten-fold discrepancy between therapeutic efficiency and toxicity determination by the frog's heart and the cat method.

Bibliography

1. Bodansky, M., and Pilcher, J. F.: Clinical significance of the creatine reserve of the human heart. Arch. Inst. Med., 59:232, 1937.
2. Cushny, A. R.: The Action and Uses in Medicine of Digitalis and its Allies. London: Longmann, Green and Co., 1925.
3. Decherd, George, and Visscher, M. B.: Energy metabolism of the failing heart. Jour. Exper. Med., 59:195, 1934.
4. Hermann, George, and Decherd, George: Creatine and glycogen content of normal and infarcted heart muscle of the dog. Proc. Soc. Exper. Biol. and Med., 32:1304, 1935.
5. Hermann, George; Decherd, George M., and Oliver, Tom: Creatine content of human hearts. Proc. Soc. Exper. Biol. and Med., 34:827, 1936.
6. Luten, Drew: The Clinical Use of Digitalis, Springfield, Illinois: C. C. Thomas, 1936.
7. Peters, Howard C., and Visscher, M. B.: The energy metabolism of the heart in failure and the influence of drugs upon it. Am. Heart Jour., 11:273, 1936.
8. Peters, Howard C.; Rea, Charles E., and Visscher, M. B.: Influence of calcium ions upon energy metabolism of the mammalian heart. Proc. Soc. Exper. Biol. and Med., 32:268, 1934.
9. Rothlin: Über die Resorption und die Verteilung der herzwirksamen Glykoside, Verhandl. der Schweiz. Naturforsch. Gesellschaft, p. 437, 1932; Ibid: Münch. med. Wchnschr., 80:726, 1933.
10. Seecof, D. P., Linegar, C. R., and Myers, V. C.: The difference in creatine concentration of the left and right ventricular cardiac muscles. Arch. Int. Med., 53:574, 1934.
11. Starling, E. H.: Linacre Lecture on the Law of the Heart, 1915, London: Longmann, Green and Co., 1918.
12. Starling, E. H., and Visscher, M. B.: The regulation of the energy output of the heart. Jour. Physiol., 62:16, 1927.
13. Stoll, Arthur: Neuerer Untersuchungen über Digitalis Glucoside. Chemiken-Zeitung, 76:773, 1935.
14. Visscher, M. B., and Mulder, A. G.: The carbohydrate metabolism of the heart. Am. Jour. Physiol., 94:630, 1930.
15. Visscher, M. B., and Müller, Erich A.: The influence of insulin upon the mammalian heart. Jour. Physiol., 62:341, 1927.

CONSERVATIVE RENAL SURGERY*

ROLAND G. SCHERER, M.D.

Bozeman, Montana

THE term, conservative renal surgery, has taken on a new meaning in recent years. Plastic operations on the renal pelvis and the ureter may become truly radical when they cause long illness, great renal damage or necessitate secondary nephrectomy. Küster made the prediction, many years ago, that plastic operations would become the accepted method of treatment for hydronephrosis. To the present time this prediction has not been fulfilled, and the multitude of surgical procedures used in its treatment serves to indicate in a large measure the lack of general success in the use of plastic renal surgery.

Küster was probably the first to reimplant the sectioned ureter into the renal pelvis as a treatment for ureteral stricture. Fenger first applied the Heineke-Mikulicz principle of gastric surgery to ureteral strictures by incising the stricture longitudinally and suturing the incision transversely. Since these pioneering efforts, many modifications and original procedures have been used. Unfortunately success did not always crown their efforts, and it is my belief that

disaster of one degree or another has occurred more frequently than the literature would lead us to believe. Ormond has recently written a paper entitled "Unsuccessful Plastic Operations for Hydronephrosis"; and, aside from its general excellence, it is unique in that it stresses the pitfalls attendant upon plastic renal surgery. The glowing reports of several years ago on plastic renal surgery will not, I believe, present as glowing a picture after the lapse of sufficient time for the declaration of all the surgical dividends.

The cause of pelviectasis is a failure of the renal pelvis to properly empty itself. This may be secondary to an obstruction at the ureteropelvic junction by a fibrosis in or about the ureter, an accessory blood vessel adversely situated with relation to the pelvis and ureter, a neurogenic dysfunction of the pelvis, an incorrect attachment of the ureter to the pelvis or an obstruction within the ureter. The problem of obstructive renal pelvis surgery is a problem of correct drainage. The renal pelvis is a relatively inelastic structure relying to a large extent upon dependent drainage. Any interference with this drainage causes a retention of fluid with its resultant enlargement of the pelvis due partially to

*Read before the annual meeting of the Medical Association of Montana, Great Falls, Mont., July 14, 1937.

excretory pressure, but, largely, to the weight of the retained urine. This is especially true of the extra-renal pelvis. Thus the great distortion of a large hydronephrosis shows the ureter attached high on the pelvis in a position making drainage

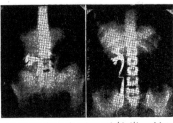

Fig. 1 *(left)*. Retrograde pyelogram of right kidney of forty-eight year old female patient. Complained of severe back and genital pain and recurrent attacks of chills and fever. Renal ptosis, grade 2, with marked ureterectasis.
Fig. 2 *(right)*. Two-months postoperative retrograde pyelogram of same patient. Clinically cured. Operative procedure—nephropexy. Marked improvement in the ureterectasis.

impossible. This non-dependent attachment is a result of the hydronephrosis rather than the cause of it. This is definitely shown in the return of the pelvis to normal or near normal size shortly after the restitution of proper drainage. All of you have seen the prompt reduction in size of a huge hydronephrosis by a properly placed nephrostomy tube. This can be duplicated by any other type of drainage. The important fact is adequate drainage, not the type of drainage. This is a fact that many surgeons have lost sight of in their treatment of hydronephrosis. They have reduced the size of the renal pelvis by resection or by plication, have reimplanted the ureter into the pelvis or have operated upon the uretero-pelvic junction and have neglected the associated or primary cause of the hydronephrosis, e.g., the malposition of the kidney. Many surgeons, on the other hand, have fixed the kidney in a good position in addition to their pelvic surgery but have attributed their good results to the plastic pelvis surgery when it should in a large part, if not entirely, have been attributed to the improved position of the kidney.

Figure 1 shows the pyelogram of a forty-eight year old female patient with renal ptosis of a moderately severe grade having back pains, pain into the genitals and attacks of chills and fever.

Figure 2 shows the same patient two months later. The kidney is held in good position by

nephropexy, the calices and pelvis not much changed but the ureter is greatly improved and the patient has no symptoms.

Careful analysis of the good results from plastic operations upon the renal pelvis will show that nephropexy has also been performed in practically all cases. The state of flux which still prevails in renal pelvis surgery is ample evidence of the rather indifferent results the many complicated procedures have had. A few years ago Walters made this statement, "The conservative treatment of hydronephrosis centers around the surgical principle that adequate relief of the obstruction at the uretero-pelvic junction be consummated with a minimal disturbance of renal and ureteral tissue." This becomes increasingly evident to the surgeon as he gains experience in renal surgery. There are, however, many points of renal surgery lost sight of by the individual surgeon in his enthusiasm for a certain type of operation. It is thus most important for the surgeon to first fit his procedure to each case and then to truly evaluate the results on the basis of the procedure or procedures used.

The obstruction of the urinary tract at the bladder neck or at the uretero-vesical junction is a very frequently encountered condition and, while not a part of this paper, must be mentioned because it so frequently complicates the diagnosis. Because unrelieved obstruction anywhere in the urinary tract will ultimately cause ureterectasis, pelviectasis and caliectasis alone or together, the surgeon must be most careful of his diagnosis so as not to operate on a false premise. Careful diagnosis will practically always necessitate retrograde pyelography. Excretory urography alone may be misleading and one may find varying degrees of function even to apparent total nonfunction of one kidney at one examination only to find an apparently normal functioning kidney at a later examination. When the diagnosis has been made, it is well to reserve judgment as to the exact type of operation to be used until the kidney has been carefully exposed and examined. The final decision as to the procedure to be used must depend upon four factors:

1. The condition of the patient.
2. The condition of the opposite kidney.
3. The condition of the renal parenchyma of the kidney being operated upon.
4. The type of obstruction.

The condition of the patient and of the opposite kidney must both be determined prior to operation through a study of the blood chemistry and the individual kidney functions. Frequently the presence of an excellent kidney on the opposite side may prejudice one to nephrectomy of the involved kidney. This is especially true in the case of an elderly patient unable to stand the financial drain of a long hospitalization and a long convalescence or of an elderly patient in rather poor physical condition. Under such circumstances nephrectomy may be rightly termed the most conservative procedure. In case the kidney is largely destroyed, we are forced to do a nephrectomy unless the opposite kidney is so poor as to demand the saving of all possible renal tissue. Before condemning a kidney as beyond repair, one should remember the tremendous recovery a kidney is capable of making once adequate drainage has been established. A kidney with as little as one-third of its parenchyma intact will recover a life-sustaining function. Two years ago I operated upon a patient with a calculus-obstructed solitary kidney after thirty-six hours of complete anuria. The day following the operation at which the calculus was removed and a nephrostomy performed, the phenolsulphonphthalein excretion was practically nil, the blood urea value was 234 mg. per 100 c.c. of blood and the creatinin value was 9.2 mg. per 100 c.c. of blood. These are usually considered fatal blood chemistry values. In spite of this the patient had only a moderately stormy convalescence and six months later had only slightly elevated blood urea and creatinin values, a phenolsulphonphthalein excretion of over 50 per cent in two hours and was leading an active life. This merely demonstrates what a kidney is capable of doing under the proper conditions of drainage. When the kidney has been exposed and the decision has been made to save it, then the type of procedure will depend upon the type of obstruction present. May I repeat that all good results follow adequate drainage and that, therefore, the simplest method of instituting such drainage must be the method of choice. We must, of course, remove any obstruction which may be present. Frequently, in the case of an aberrant renal blood vessel or a fibrous band of scar tissue, simple excision will suffice. Especially is this true in an early, small hydronephrosis.

Figure 3 is the retrograde pyelogram of a twenty-eight year old female patient with a history of three attacks of severe renal area pain, chills and fever in the past twelve months. Definite obstruction at the uretero-pelvic junction was diagnosed as an aberrant blood vessel prior to

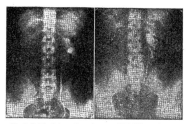

Fig. 3 (left). Retrograde pyelogram of left kidney of twenty-eight year old female patient. Three attacks in past year of severe back pain, chills and fever. Pre-operative diagnosis of aberrant blood vessel obstructing uretero-pelvic junction.
Fig. 4 (right). Fourteen-month postoperative retrograde pyelogram of same patient. Clinical cure. Operative procedure—section of aberrant vessel and nephropexy. Great improvement in the caliectasis and pelviectasis.

operation and was confirmed at operation. Simple excision with nephropexy was performed.

Figure 4 is a retrograde pyelogram of the same patient made fourteen months later, showing the tremendous improvement of the kidney. The patient is now completely symptom-free.

In deciding to divide an aberrant blood vessel, one must be certain that the vessel to be severed is not the sole blood supply of a sufficient area to cause necrosis. Obstruction of the vessel for a few minutes will demonstrate, by the change in color of the involved renal tissue, the area supplied by the vessel. The size of this area will determine the procedure to be followed. Hugh Young has said that impairment or serious injury to the kidney produced by ligation of the vessels to the lower pole and the occasionally very imperfect results obtained by ureteral transplantation have brought forcibly to his attention the fact that both of these procedures are far from ideal. He has, therefore, devised an operation in which the pelvis is plicated in such a manner as to draw the ureter away from the aberrant vessel and thus relieve the obstruction. The decision in the presence of large vessels will, of course, vary with the surgeon and must be either this procedure or reimplantation of the ureter. Nephropexy used in conjunction with simple removal of the obstructing mechanism is so simple as to be almost mandatory. There are many types of nephropexy. One which I described last year is very simple and very efficient in that it permanently fixes the kidney in a high position.

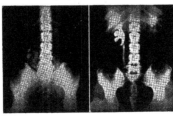

Fig. 5 *(left)*. Retrograde pyelogram of thirty-nine year old patient. Complained of severe back pain relieved on lying down. Renal ptosis, grade 2 plus, with definite callectasis and ureterectasis.
Fig. 6 *(right)*. Twelve-month postoperative retrograde pyelogram of same patient. Clinical cure. Operative procedure—nephropexy. Marked improvement in caliectasis, especially so in the ureterectasis.

Figures 1, 2 and 5, 6 show the remarkable results simple nephropexy will obtain when no obstructing mechanism is present.

The large hydronephrosis will necessitate a nephrostomy in its treatment. Often in the case of great pelviectasis the uretero-pelvic junction will be attached far up on the pelvic wall. This will frequently influence the surgeon to a pelvic resection or a reimplantation of the ureter; but given a properly fixed kidney, a sufficiently patent uretero-pelvic opening and a well-placed and long-retained nephrostomy tube, and very nearly 100 per cent will drain more perfectly than kidneys that have had reimplanted ureters or a resected pelvis. Should the surgeon feel that the pelvis cannot possibly return to a near normal state without better drainage, then the use of Foley's Y incision and suture of the uretero-pelvic junction will be more efficient than resection and reimplantation of the ureter with its attendant dangers. In all but the most simple cases, nephrostomy is a most important part of the surgical procedure; and in cases involving plastic surgery on the uretero-pelvic junction, it is necessary to use a ureteral catheter as a splint passed into the ureter from above and retained for a long period, as Ormond and Hugh Cabot have recently pointed out.

Obstruction of the ureter may be due to cal-

culus or calculi, to strictures or to fixed kink The removal of the calculi is, of course, impera tive although associated conditions must also b treated.

Figures 7 and 8 are of a very interesting cas Figure 7 is the ten-minute excretory urogram c a twenty year old girl. She had complained c chills and fever with intense left-sided pain. Th left kidney shows marked caliectasis with litt or no pelvic or ureteral shadow. The calcifie shadows in the lower ureter region are confusin because of the presence of many shadows in th course of the right ureter which with its kidne is normal. A diagnosis of calculi in the lowe ureter was made especially as I was unable, be cause of obstruction, to catheterize the urete beyond the intravesical portion. At operatic the upper shadow was found to be a calculus an was removed. The lower shadow was also calculus but could not be grasped and remove nor could it be forced into the bladder. Th ureter was greatly inflamed and very friable the wound was closed without removing th lower stone. Eight days later the patient wa cystoscoped using a McCarthy panendoscope an the ureteral orifice incised with a Collings knif The calculus was exposed and flipped into th bladder with the electrode tip. A ureteral cath ter was passed to the renal pelvis and left in pla two days. An uneventful convalescence o curred. Figure 8 is a retrograde pyelogra eleven months later. The patient is symptor free, and the pyelogram is quite normal, consi ering its prior condition.

Strictures of the lower ureter yield themselv very* well to dilation. Fixed kinks below t uretero-pelvic junction are rather rare. Liber tion of the kinks with nephropexy is usua conducive of good results. Strictures which ca not be dilated must be either incised or excis Fenger's procedure is moderately successful, though in strictures at the uretero-pelvic jur tion, Foley's modification of Schwyzer's Y in sion will be more satisfactory. Excision of stricture with resuture using one of several me ods of re-establishment of continuity has been uniformly successful. Von Lichtenberg never resected a ureteral stricture and repai it with end-to-end anastomosis because of his f of later stricture formation. Splinting the ure with a ureteral catheter drawn through a phrostomy opening and kept in place an unusu

94

long time gives the best chance of success and the prevention of secondary stricture formation. In such cases postoperative dilation of the ureter may be necessary.

Uretero-pelvic juncture obstruction requiring surgery is relatively more frequent than ureteral obstructions of similar magnitude. There have been many operations devised for the relief of this obstruction. Many of the originators, as I have stated, ignored the cardinal principles of drainage in their enthusiasm for surgical reconstruction and thus many failures have resulted. Ormond has divided failures into four divisions:

1. Death.
2. Immediate failure of function or immediate complication requiring further treatment, usually nephrectomy.
3. Delayed failure of function necessitating further treatment; again usually nephrectomy.
4. Lack of symptomatic relief.

The causes of failures may be many and varied, but may usually be avoided by proper diagnosis, proper choice of procedure and proper postoperative management. Having performed the plastic procedure upon the renal pelvis, it is well to recognize the fact that dense adhesions will form and that it is, therefore, necessary to prevent ureteral kinking. For this prevention the following procedures are absolutely necessary:

1. Nephrostomy—the correct drainage of the pelvis through the lower portion of the renal cortex with a self-retaining catheter after the method of Cabot and Holland—is greatly superior to pyelostomy.
2. Nephropexy, giving positive fixation in a high position with an unkinked ureter.
3. Adequate perirenal drainage.
4. Splinting of ureter with ureteral catheter drawn out alongside of nephrostomy tube in all cases of reconstruction of the uretero-pelvic junction.

The nephrostomy tube gives perfect drainage and thus promotes shrinkage of the dilated pelvis to a size more closely approaching the normal. It also aids in combating infection by both the improved drainage and by allowing the mechanical flushing of the renal pelvis with antiseptic

solution. This reduces the frequency and severity of cortical abscesses, which are one of the great postoperative dangers.

The nephropexy insures the continuance of this adequate drainage through the ureter when

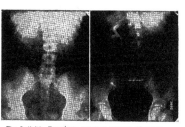

Fig. 7 (left). Ten-minute excretory urogram of twenty year old female patient. Complained of six months' symptoms of pain in left back and side, genital pain, fever, loss of weight. Diagnosis: two calculi in lower left ureter with obstructive hydronephrosis.
Fig. 8 (right). Eleven-month postoperative retrograde pyelogram of same patient. Clinical cure. Operative procedure—removal of calculi. Marked improvement in the callectasis and pelviectasis with diminution in size of the kidney shadow.

the nephrostomy tube has been removed. Failure to remove the uretero-pelvic junction obstruction will be manifested on removal or clamping of the nephrostomy tube by the symptoms of acute pyelonephritis. This condition necessitates further treatment, usually a reestablishment of drainage or nephrectomy.

The perirenal drainage is a most necessary procedure because of the frequency, in fact almost constancy, of extravasation of urine about the kidney when the pelvis has been incised. Failure to properly drain may endanger the patient's life and most certainly detract from the beneficial results of the operation. Cabot has mentioned that one of the fundamental precepts of plastic surgery is to prevent scar tissue contracting for three months. After that period it will not contract. He has applied this to plastic work on the uretero-pelvic junction by keeping a ureteral catheter splint in place for a similar period and has succeeded in cases where at a previous operation he failed without this long period of splinting.

There has been a great deal of work done upon the sympathetic nerve supply to the kidney and ureter. Caporale concluded a recent paper with the statement, "Segmentary sympathectomy of the ureter will produce primarily an atony in the tract itself, and secondarily, a gradual periureteral atony which culminates in a progessive hydro-ureteronephrosis." Sympathectomy also gives the surgeon a temporary false result in that the patient is symptom-free until such times as the increasing hydro-ureteronephrosis, as Caporale names it, becomes of sufficient size or becomes infected sufficiently to cause grave symptoms.

The contentions I have made in this paper were not made to belittle any certain type of operation, but rather to accentuate the need of mature judgment in renal surgery and also in the belief that these contentions are especially applicable to the surgeon of limited experience in renal pelvis surgery. In conclusion, then, conservative renal surgery is dependent upon:

1. Complete and proper diagnosis.
2. Unbiased choice of procedure, determined by individual needs of each case, with the sole idea of instituting proper renal

drainage at a minimum of tissue trauma.

3. Nephrostomy in all infected cases, in all large hydronephroses and in all plastic surgery of the renal pelvis.
4. Nephropexy in all cases.
5. Ureteral splinting in all plastic operations of the uretero-pelvic junction and of the ureter proper.

References

1. Cabot, Hugh: Proc. Staff Meetings Mayo Clinic, 12:282, (May 5) 1937.
2. Cabot, Hugh, and Holland, W. W.: Nephrostomy: indications and technic. Surg., Gyn. and Obst., 54:817, 1932.
3. Caporale, Luigi: The dynamic hydronephroses and sympathectomy of the ureter. Jour. Urol., 33:84, (Feb.) 1935.
4. Ormond, J. K.: Unsuccessful plastic operations for hydronephrosis. Jour. Urol., 36:512-531, (Nov.) 1936.
5. Von Lichtenberg, A.: Plastic surgery of renal pelvis and ureter. Jour. Am. Med. Assn., 93:1706, 1929.
6. Walters, W.: Resections of renal pelvis and other plastic operations for hydronephrosis; and results in thirteen cases. Surg., Gyn. and Obst., 55:508-517, (Oct.) 1932.
7. Woodruff, Stanley R., and Scherer, Roland G.: Renal ptosis. Jour. Urol., 35:125, (Feb.) 1936.
8. Young, H. H.: Obstructions of ureter produced by aberrant blood vessels; a plastic repair without ligation of vessels or transplantation of ureters. Surg., Gyn. and Obst., 55:26, (Jan.) 1932.

RADIUM TREATMENT OF RARE FORMS OF LEUKEMIA*

ROBERT E. FRICKE, M.D., and CHARLES H. WATKINS, M.D.

Rochester, Minnesota

EVER since the original description of leukemia from the postmortem findings by Bennet and Virchow in 1845 and its clinical recognition by Vogel, a satisfactory method of treating the condition has been anxiously sought. Described as an excessive proliferation of the leukopoietic tissues of the body, either myeloid or lymphoid, with the presence of abnormal leukocytes in the circulating blood, the precise etiology is unknown although the condition may follow malaria or severe pyogenic infection. Certain of the lower animals, such as dogs, horses, cattle and chickens, are susceptible.

Before the advent of irradiation, a large number of remedies were tried. Most of them were toxic and dangerous and few afforded much palliation. Iron and arsenic have been given to combat the anemia, and benzol, quinine, tuberculin, and nuclein have been used to

reduce the excessive number of leukocytes. Splenectomy has also been carried out.

These measures were empirical, however, as the true cause of the disease, as has been said, awaits discovery. Hence the therapeutic search has been for methods to afford palliation and relief from the distressing symptoms. In fact, to this day, no palliative treatment has been found for the occasional acute forms of myelogenous or lymphatic leukemia; the disease runs the rapid course of a fulminating overwhelming infection and the outcome is fatal.

In 1903, Nicholas Senn[5] reported gratifying results in the treatment of a patient with chronic myelogenous leukemia by roentgen rays. Rénon, Degrais and Desbouis[4] used radium therapy, and in 1913 reported five cases in which patients were treated by this method. One of the earlier reports in this country (1917) was by Giffin,[3] who reported thirty cases in which radium treatment was employed.

Since this early work, roentgen and radium

*From the Section on Therapeutic Radiology and Division of Medicine, The Mayo Clinic, Rochester, Minn. Read before the annual meeting of the American Therapeutic Society, Atlantic City, New Jersey, June 4-5, 1937.

TABLE I. RADIUM TREATMENT OF RARE FORMS OF LEUKEMIA
Symptoms, diagnosis and results

Case	Age, years, and sex	Admitted	Diagnosis	Symptoms	Results
1	41 F	4-18-35	Subleukemic splenic reticulo-endotheliosis	Nosebleeds (6 mos.). Mass ULQ (6 wks.). Tired easily (2 mos.)	Dismissed 12-10-36. Good general condition
2	50 M	4-25-35	Chronic leukopenic myelogenous leukemia	Swelling left abdomen (3 mos.). Shortness of breath after meals	Fair palliation. Returned 2-37 with enlarged spleen. Condition fair
3	46 F	5-20-35	Subleukemic splenic reticulo-endotheliosis	Tired, weak (5 years.). Enlarged spleen (2 yrs.). Anemia. Spleen 3*	Excellent response and palliation to date
4	49 F	7- 8-36	Chronic leukopenic myelogenous leukemia	Mass ULQ (3 mos.). Discomfort	Much palliation. Improved blood count. Seen 12-4-36, no treatment needed
5	57 F	11-23-36	Subacute lymphatic leukemia	Weak, tired, short of breath, edema of ankles (4 mos.). Spleen 3+,* general glandular enlargement	Remarkable remission. Count practically normal. Dismissed 12-18-36
6	37 M	1- 6-36	Subacute lymphatic leukemia	Weakness, dyspnea (2 yrs.). Spleen 3+*	Spleen reduced, WBC 7,800. Dismissed 1-16-36
7	70 M	6- 4-36	Chronic leukopenic myelogenous leukemia	Anemia (5 to 6 yrs.). Weak, short of breath, lost weight (1 yr.). Spleen 3*	Letter (9-2-36):"Reached home comfortably"
8	47 M	5- 7-36	Chronic leukopenic myelogenous leukemia	Chills, fever, cough, "flu," vertigo, pain in bones (6 mos.). Spleen 3*	Spleen softened and reduced
9	39 M	10-22-36	Acute leukemic reticulo-endotheliosis	Acute tonsilitis. Acute cerv. adenitis (4 wks.); became generalized	Course rapidly downhill. Dismissed 10-29-36. Died 11-1-36
10	61 M	6-18-36	Monocytic leukemia, Naegeli type, sub-acute	Weakness, loss of weight, inability to work (6 mos.)	Dismissed November, 1936; several transfusions elsewhere
11	58 M	11- 2-35	Subleukemic splenic reticulo-endotheliosis	Splenomegaly, petechiae, asthenia following erysipelas	Dismissed 11-20-35, 3-26-36: patient up and around, much improved
12	40 F	6-24-35	Chronic myelogenous leukemia, leukopenic type	Pain and swelling of joints (1 yr.). Vertigo and weakness (7 mos.).	Re-examined 3-4-36. Much better. Arthritis improved
13	3 M	11- 2-36	Leukemic reticulo-endotheliosis	Age 5 mos.: extensive skin infiltration, WBC 300,000, spleen 3.* On admission: swelling right eye, spleen palpable, general glandular involvement	Improved. Letter (12-8-36): doing well, residual pain in ankle and knee joints
14	33 M	3-26-34	Chronic myelogenous leukemia (leukopenic type), low grade	Spring 1933, operated on for appendicitis and cholecystitis. Spleen 2.* Diarrhea and bleeding rectum (8 mos.)	Letter (11-13-36): Much better spleen smaller
15	61 M	11- 5-35	Leukemic reticulo-endotheliosis	Short of breath, weak (1 mo.)	Indeterminate
16	64 M	6-21-35	Chronic leukopenic myelogenous leukemia	Weakness (2 yrs.). Mass abdomen (6 mos.). Dizziness, pallor and dyspnea	Good palliation. Dismissed 4-14-36. Died 8-7-36

*Grade of enlargement.

TABLE II. RADIUM TREATMENT OF RARE FORMS OF LEUKEMIA
Treatment and blood count

| | | TREATMENT | | | | | BLOOD COUNT | | | | | | | | |
| | | Radium* | | | | | | | | Cells, Per Cent | | | | | |
Case	X-ray date of †	Date	Blocks	Hours each	Total Mc. hours	Date	Leuko-cytes, thousands	Erythro-cytes, millions	Hemo-globin, per cent	Lympho-cytes	Poly-morpho-nuclears	Mono-cytes	Retic-ular cells‡	Imma-ture myeloid cells	Stem cells
1	4-27-35	8- 7-35 12-30-35 6-19-36	1 2 1	8 10 12 10	1200 2200 2500	4-19-35 6-18-35	31.1 5.4	3.8	73	84 58.5	11.5 27.5	3.5	13.0		
2	4-27-35 6-27-35	9- 5-35 4-14-36 11-10-36 2-14-37	1 1 1 1	12 12 12 12	2400 1200 1200 2400	4-25-35 9- 5-35	19.6 3.7	4.06	83	18	53.0	3.0		8.0	1.5
3	6-17-35	12-30-35 5-12-36 12-14-36	1 1 1	10 10 12	1500 1000 1200	5-20-35 11-16-36	10.5 2.9	2.84 4.04	50	45.5 32.5	4.5 24.5		49 36.0		
4		7-13-36	8	10	4000	7- 8-36 12- 3-36	10.1 18.3	3.78 3.6	84 77	18.5 9.5	74.5 81.5	2.0 5.0		2.5 0.5	0.5 0.5
5		12-10-36 3 transfu-sions	3	12	1800	11-23-36 12-12-36	7.8 5.5	1.96	43.8	Smears suggest chronic lymphatic leukemia					
6		1- 8-36	4	14	2800	1- 7-36	13.6	3.96	57	43.5 Immature lymphocytes	20		34.0		
7	Else-where Feb. 1936	6-13-36 12 trans-fusions	2 6	8 10	3800	6- 4-36 8- 5-36	1.15 3.7	1.65 3.24	40	"Myeloid immaturity to stem cells"					

Case	Radium dates	No.	No.	Dosage	Count dates	6.1	3.96	78	13.0	67.5	11.5		4.0	0.5	Notes
8	5-15-36, 6-30-36	2, 5	12, 12	1200, 3000	5-8-36	6.1	3.96	78	13.0	67.5	11.5		4.0	0.5	
9	10-27-36	1	12	600	10-23-36, 10-28-36	39.2, 108.0	3.14, 2.11	70	23	25.5 (Metamyelocytes, Promyelocytes)	29.5 (Myelocytes, Metamyelocytes)		3.5, 3.5, 6.0	3.5	
10	6-22-36	4	10	2000	6-18-36	7.5	3.48	59	77.5	18.5	3.5				
11	11-13-35, 5 transfusions	2	10	1000	11-4-35, 11-20-36	3.0, 3			24, 16.5, 25.5	53.5, 68, 59	17, 13, 12.5		0.5, 1.0		
12	7-10-35	5	10	2500	6-21-35, 7-13-35, 3-4-36	7.8, 5.6, 7.8	3.53	68	58.5	32.5	3.5				7-2-35
13	11-3-36	19	12	11,400	11-2-36	6.1	4.4	83							At 5 mos. elsewhere. Elsewhere 6 mos. prev. adm.
14	7-21-36	2, 4	10, 10	3000	3-27-34	7.5	3.94 (Neutro., Eosino., Basophils)	68	25.5	68	3.0		0.5		
15	11-14-35	1	10	500	11-6-35	10.1			48.5, 29.5, 5.0, 4.5		5.0	3.0	4.5		
16	6-25-35, 9-15-35, 4-14-36	6, 3, 9	8, 8, 8	2400, 1200, 3600	6-22-35, 9-19-35	5.9, 3.9	3.6 (Neutrophils, Basophils)	50	34.0, 57.0, 0.5		2.0		6.5	1.0	

To spleen (case 9, neck only; case 13, spleen and all glands).
*Moderate voltage.
‡Reticular cells = reticular endothelial cells. Not to be confused with reticulated erythrocytes.

therapy have been universally accepted as the preferable form of treatment for chronic myeloid or lymphatic leukemia. The beneficial effect, however, has been entirely in the realm of palliation. Exact evaluation of this is difficult because of the natural spontaneous remissions which occur in a very small percentage of cases in which patients are untreated. We have observed no permanent cures following irradiation. One of us (Fricke[1]) reported the results of the radium treatment of 157 patients with leukemia and found no prolongation of life of those treated as contrasted with those who were not treated; the palliation secured, however, was definite and impressive. In nearly all cases the symptoms disappeared completely and the patients were able to resume their normal activities for months at a time.

Typical leukemia is a relatively infrequent disease, Barker having said that there were only one or two leukemic patients in every thousand admissions in general hospital practice. The disease occurs at any age, although it is more frequent in middle life. Males are more often affected than females. The chronic forms of the disease are, fortunately, more common than the acute forms, and chronic myelogenous leukemia is more frequently seen than lymphatic leukemia. Irradiation affords slightly more pronounced palliation in cases of chronic myelogenous leukemia.

In this study we are considering the more unusual or borderline types of this rare disease, and these demand, for their detection, a careful study of the history, physical examination, blood studies, and particularly, care in the recognition of immature blood cells. Many of these aleukemic or leukopenic types of leukemia present as their initial symptom, anemia with a leukocyte count within normal limits or even low, which, in association with splenomegaly, may be confused with splenic anemia or Banti's syndrome. Many times purpuric manifestations will appear relatively early in the disease, and in the presence of an unexplained anemia with purpuric manifestations and a normal leukocyte count, one should make a thorough search for immature cells in the blood. One of us (Watkins[6]) has called attention to the differential diagnosis of these conditions. In our experience these atypical leukemias have frequently been

confused with Banti's syndrome and ap locytosis.

If the incidence of ordinary leukemia or two in every thousand general hospit; missions, there will be found one or tv these borderline types to every hundred of leukemia. The diagnosis of these rarer is improving and more cases are being rej each year. These unusual types of leu may be classed as aleukemic phases of r genous, lymphatic, monocytic or leukemic lo-endotheliosis.

One type of particular interest is subleu splenic reticulo-endotheliosis, which wa scribed by Giffin and Watkins[8] in 1934. : two cases reported at that time, splenectom performed, with only temporary improv in the patients' condition. Since then six cases of this type have been recognized ai patients treated by radium, with quite sa tory results. The longest duration of 1 date, in this group of patients treated by ra has been two years, and the patients ha mained in very good condition. It seems in most of these cases, radium decrease size of the spleen, enables the patient to ma a more nearly normal leukocyte count, ar duces the number of immature cells i blood. It is not the purpose of this paper, ever, to discuss in detail the diagnosis condition except to say that it is finally lished by the finding of monocytes sh characteristics of reticular origin in the lating blood. For detailed discussion, referred to the article just mentioned.

During 1935 and 1936 we have treatec radium, sixteen patients with these atypic kemias (Tables I and II). Of these : patients, ten were males and six females. ranged in age from three to seventy yea average age being forty-seven. Eight; were diagnosed as having aleukemic ph; chronic myelogenous or lymphatic leuker only two of these eight cases was it lymphatic type). One patient had a mc leukemia of the Naegeli type, and sever of reticulo-endotheliosis. We believe th the diagnosis is established in these cases with low leukocyte counts, radiun treatment of choice in order to obtain : tory palliation. Roentgen therapy covers er portal and the effect of treatment is usually too sudden and drastic. Our best results have been obtained by the very cautious and well-controlled use of radium.

At a distance of 1 inch (2.5 cm.) from the skin, 50 mg. of radium sulphate (element), filtered through 2 mm. of lead, was applied for a period of eight to twelve hours, depending on the leukocyte count, the size of the spleen and the general condition of the patient. In addition to daily blood counts, blood smears were studied in detail and the amount of destruction of immature cells was noted. Should there be evidence of a decrease in the leukocyte count or an increase in the degree of anemia, radium treatment is stopped for a while until the blood count returns to its previous level. It is quite the rule that in most of these cases of low leukocyte count there is an increase in the erythrocyte count following treatment with radium. The anemia is practically corrected within a relatively short time and the immature cells of the leukocytes series are gradually eliminated. The differential count usually approaches a more nearly normal level.

The patients were then sent home for three or four months. Treatments varied from one to nine areas over the spleen in one treatment series, and from eight to twelve hours of treatment per area, all carefully controlled by blood counts.

Fifteen of the sixteen patients showed improvement in the condition of their blood and amelioration in their symptoms (Table I). The one exception was a man, aged thirty-nine years, who suffered from an acute reticulo-endotheliosis following a severe attack of acute tonsillitis four weeks previously. Radium treatment was begun, but was abandoned after twelve hours, as the patient was failing rapidly. He died two days later. Too little treatment was applied to have affected the disease one way or another.

Summary and Conclusions

The ability to recognize immature cells is the first requisite in establishing the diagnosis of these rare forms of leukemia. These cases are seldom seen, but they are important and better diagnosis will increase the number that are recognized.

In the differential diagnosis many diseases have to be ruled out, such as aplastic anemia, purpura hemorrhagica, agranulocytosis, Banti's syndrome and hemolytic jaundice. In these conditions, irradiation is not only contraindicated but likely to prove decidedly injurious.

In the treatment of these rare types of leukemia, splenectomy, which has been occasionally performed, does not help. Roentgen therapy, often covering portals which are too large and including too much of the blood-forming apparatus, is too drastic and may prove harmful. The best therapeutic agent seems to be cautious, limited radium treatment. It has, in our experience, proved of great value in producing effectual palliation.

References

1. Fricke, R. E.: Discussion. Am. Jour. Roentgenol. and Radium Therap., 19:19, (Jan.) 1928.
2. Giffin, H. Z.: Observations on the treatment of myelocytic leukemia by radium. Boston Med. and Surg. Jour., 177:686-691, (Nov. 15) 1917.
3. Giffin, H. Z., and Watkins, C. H.: The distinction between splenic anemia and subleukemic splenic reticulo-endotheliosis. Am. Jour. Med. Sc., 188:761-767, (Dec.); Trans. Assn. Am. Phys., 49:318-325, 1934.
4. Rénon, Louis, Degrais and Desbouis: Radiumthérapie de la leucémie myéloide (présentation de malades). Bull. et mém. Soc. méd. d. hôp. de Paris, 36:54-66; 649-651, 1913.
5. Senn, Nicholas: Case of splenomedullary leukemia successfully treated by the use of the röntgen ray. Med. Rec., 64:281-282, (Aug. 22) 1903.
6. Watkins, C. H.: Acute leukopenic leukemia and its differential diagnosis. Wisconsin Med. Jour., 32:156-160, (March) 1933.

TUBERCULOUS INFECTION AND MORBIDITY AMONG MEDICAL STUDENTS AND PHYSICIANS*

FRANK L. JENNINGS, M.D., F.A.C.P.

Oak Terrace, Minnesota

TUBERCULOSIS is still so prevalent a disease that it is encountered by every physician and medical student whether he is aware of the contact or not. Whether this contact can be considered an occupational hazard is a question that has been of great interest to us at Glen Lake Sanatorium because medical students from the University of Minnesota come here for their instruction in tuberculosis. In examining these students upon entrance, we were at first chiefly interested in the study of pathological lesions of tuberculous origin and their clinical activity, but more recently we have included the study of tuberculous infection.

Infection

Fourth year medical students have each spent two weeks as clinical clerks in this sanatorium since 1925. In 1929, we first began to question them in regard to tuberculin tests† given them before they came to us. We found that of the first eighty-seven students questioned, fifty-seven (65 per cent) had reacted positively when tested at the Students' Health Service at the University to 1:1000 dilution of old tuberculin. We felt, however, that more exact information could be obtained if we tested all students the day they came to the Sanatorium. Therefore, beginning in the middle of November, 1930, the next 184 students were tested and 122 (66.3 per cent) were found to be positive to the intradermic test.

Because our percentages in these two groups were so close, we decided in June, 1932, to question the students and test only those who gave a history of not reacting to tuberculin. We felt

this method would give us very satisfactory results because the medical students of the University of Minnesota have been made intelligently aware of the importance of present day methods of detection, prevention and treatment of tuberculous disease through the interest in this subject of Dr. J. A. Myers and Dr. H. S. Diehl. Our findings by the year are shown in Table I.

TABLE I. THE INCIDENCE OF POSITIVE AND NEGATIVE TUBERCULIN REACTIONS

(Among students entering the Sanatorium for study)

Year	Negative	Positive	Question-able or no Record	Per Cent Positive
1930	36	80	4	66.6
1931	38	71	1	64.5
1932	53	90	--	62.9
1933	56	64	2	52.5
1934	39	85	2	67.4
1935	55	62	1	52.5
1936	36	76	--	67.8
	313	528	10	62.04

It will be noted from this table that the range of positive reactors to tuberculin varies for the different years from 52.5 to 67.8 per cent. The average of 62.04 per cent among our 851 fourth year medical students is less than that reported among fourth year medical students in the eastern part of the country. At the University of Pennsylvania,[3] it was found that the number of positive reactors among their medical students increased in each year of the course until in their fourth year 98 per cent of them reacted positively. It was observed that this steady increase in the number of reactors (noticed also at Yale) is not necessarily confined to medical schools, but is probably true of any school where the students' opportunities for infection must increase with continued residence among a large

*From the Department of Medicine, University of Minnesota, Minneapolis, and Glen Lake Sanatorium, Oak Terrace, Minnesota.
†These students had for the most part been examined at the Students' Health Service within a year prior to coming to the Sanatorium and all students who had been negative to tuberculin at this Health Service examination were re-tested. Old tuberculin was the substance used at the University. At Glen Lake, we used from November, 1930, to March, 1932, Dorset's Old Tuberculin, .01 mg. on one arm and MA 100 Human Tuberculin .0005 mg. on the other arm. Those who reacted negatively to the above doses were given a double dose of MA 100. Beginning in March of 1932, only MA 100 Tuberculin was given until December, 1934, when PPD was started and we have continued to use the latter to date. When we first started using PPD, we used both strengths, but during the past year only the second strength (0.005 mg.) has been given.

group of people. Similarly, 91 per cent of the fourth year students at Johns Hopkins[2] had positive reactions, as did 94.1 per cent among the three upper classes in medical school at Yale.[6] It is probable that the lower incidence among our students as compared with that of these other schools lies in the fact that our sudents, for the most part, come from communities less densely settled than do the students attending eastern schools. This lower incidence of tuberculous infection among college students (mostly nonmedical) in the Middle West has recently been observed by Long and Seibert,[4] who also think that the above explanation is the most logical.

Morbidity

The incidence of morbidity among medical students is of equal or greater interest than that of infection. In an effort to obtain facts about the morbidity among our fourth year medical students when they came to the sanatorium, as well as subsequent to their stay here, the following data were accumulated.

Since 1920, medical students from the University of Minnesota have been coming to Glen Lake Sanatorium, an institution caring for 700 patients, for their instruction in the treatment of tuberculosis. Until about 1923, the period of study equalled three months. This time was gradually shortened until it was set at two weeks in 1925. Since then, all the members of each fourth year class have been in residence here for two-week periods of instruction. Their work has consisted of taking histories, making physical examinations, and in helping with various forms of treatment both in the wards and in the treatment rooms. In short, they have been in contact with tuberculous patients during those two weeks to the same degree as have the resident sanatorium physicians.

The possibility of tuberculous disease was taken into consideration from the first, and x-ray films were made of the students' chests the day they started work at the sanatorium. The present study is a review of those films in connection with a questionnaire sent to the former students. The period here covered is the first ten years of this plan, extending from 1920 to September 15, 1930. To the 670 in this group who had been here for training at some time during the ten years, questionnaires were sent early in 1932 in an attempt to ascertain the state of their health

during the interval between receipt of this questionnaire and their sanatorium residence. Replies were received from 526, or 78.6 per cent of the group.

These replies have been classified into two main groups: the normal and the abnormal, depending upon the interpretations of the chest x-rays taken when these people first came to the sanatorium. The normal group, numbering 473, consisted of those whose interpretations were described as any of the following: normal chest, increased bronchial markings, slight thickening of the pleura. The abnormal group consisted of those whose interpretations might constitute possible evidence of tuberculosis or tuberculous infection, such as definite infiltration, primary complex, fibrosis of the parenchyma. There were fifty-three in the latter group.

Normal Group

267 had no subsequent x-rays
206 had subsequent x-rays
—
473 total

The replies to the questionnaire disclosed that 267 of the normal group of 473 had considered themselves in good condition and had not troubled to have subsequent x-rays of their chests. Of the 206 who had had subsequent x-rays, 168 still had normal readings. Thirty others reported abnormal findings consisting of evidence of acute or chronic non-tuberculous conditions variously diagnosed as bronchitis, bronchiectasis, emphysema, et cetera, but no evidence of adult tuberculosis. Briefly there were 465 of this group who had shown no subsequent evidence of tuberculous disease.

The remaining eight in this group whose roentgen findings were considered normal when they were here as students subsequently showed lesions of pulmonary tuberculosis. In two of them, the disease was diagnosed as far advanced, in two others moderately advanced, and in three as minimal. The one remaining case was classed as questionable. Their lesions had all appeared in from one to four years after their training at the sanatorium, but it must be remembered that during that interval they were practicing their profession and had come in contact with all types of patients. Five of these physicians reported at the time of the questionnaire that they were working and a sixth reported that he expected to return to work in a short time.

Abnormal Group

39 had subsequent x-rays
14 had no subsequent x-rays
——
53 total

Ten per cent (fifty-three) of the students who came to the sanatorium showed deviations from the normal that might constitute possible evidence of tuberculosis when their chests were first examined. The answers to the questionnaire that was sent to these students one to ten years after their period of instruction at the sanatorium showed that thirty-nine had had subsequent x-ray examinations. This group of thirty-nine is divided as follows: thirty-three who had shown no clinical evidence of tuberculosis and six who had shown definite evidence of clinical tuberculuosis when they were in residence here. Considering the thirty-three, we find that twenty of them reported that their lesions had shown no change from the examinations made at the sanatorium. Their lesions were divided as follows: two with Ghon tubercles; seventeen with fibroid lesions (six bilateral and eleven unilateral); one with unilateral artificial pneumothorax. Ten of the thirty-three had had subsequent roentgenograms of the chest that had been interpreted as normal. In reviewing the films taken when these ten first came to the sanatorium, we found that eight of them at that time had shown a slight fibroid change in one or both apices and two of them had shown primary complexes. In the three remaining cases of the thirty-three, one showed definite improvement in a bilateral lesion and the two others reported slight fibroid lesions on the opposite side from those found while at the sanatorium.

There were six cases in this abnormal group who had shown specific evidence of tuberculosis when they came to the sanatorium as students. Five of the six had shown definite roentgen changes in the chest. Four of the five had had definite physical findings when first examined. Because of the extent of their disease, two of this group were advised to stop their courses and take up treatment when first seen. The advice was not followed. Four of these five have since shown extension of their lesions and two of them have spent some time in a sanatorium as patients. The fifth case reports malaise but no

extension of his lesion and he has never given up work. Four of the five were working when the questionnaires were returned. The sixth one, who showed clinical evidence of tuberculosis and was therefore put in this group, had a normal chest x-ray when he came here for instruction, and this has remained normal to date. However, tuberculosis of the kidney was first definitely diagnosed when he came here as a student, and careful history revealed that it dated back for a period of about two years. The kidney has since been removed and he is now well and working.

We reviewed the films that were made at this institution of the fourteen doctors in this abnormal group who had had no subsequent films taken and found that ten had slight fibroid lesions (seven unilateral and three bilateral) when they came here as students, and four others had shown Ghon tubercles. Forty-seven of the fifty-three students in this group had shown no evidence of clinical tuberculosis subsequent to their graduation.

We were disappointed in that our questionnaire did not aid us in the question of infection as well as in the problem of morbidity. We found that so few of the doctors had had tuberculin tests after they were graduated that the results were of no material value. It is of interest to note that of the approximate 100 who had had tuberculin tests since leaving the sanatorium, 23 per cent were still negative.

After reviewing the literature of morbidity of tuberculosis, Herman, Baetjer, and Doull[2] stated that in their opinion the proportion of symptomatic tuberculosis in males in the general population between the ages of twenty and twenty-nine years is probably not lower than one or higher than three per cent. Our study of a similar age group (23 to 29) brings out that fourteen students out of a total of 526, or 2.6 per cent, showed definite evidence of tuberculosis. Six showed evidence of advanced tuberculosis when first seen and eight developed tuberculosis from two to twelve years after graduation. Steidl,[7] who in 1932 followed medical students in a manner similar to ours, found that 2.5 per cent of the Harvard medical students developed tuberculosis; about half of these developed the disease before graduation, and in a similar follow-up study on the law students found that 2.08 per cent developed tuberculosis. The incidence of pulmonary tuberculosis in various schools in the University of Michigan from 1917 to 1930 is cited by Herman, Baetjer and Doull,[2] who think that from a statistical point of view the incidence of 2.81 per 1,000 student years found in the medical school is not significantly different from that found in literature, law, engineering and the various other schools in the same university. These figures all compare favorably with ours and do not suggest that the possibilities of developing clinical tuberculosis are greatly increased by a training in a tuberculosis sanatorium as might be inferred from an article by Myers.[5]

Mortality

At the conclusion of this study, there had been no deaths from tuberculosis among the 526 who trained here. Tuberculosis has never caused a proportionately large number of deaths among physicians. Emerson and Hughes[1] found that the tuberculosis death rate among physicians was 39.5 per 100,000 as compared with 133.5 among all white males in the United States. I believe

that it is safe to assume that physicians have always been more or less exposed to tuberculosis, but statistics do not show a high death rate among them, which seems to support the assumption that there is a relatively low morbidity rate.

This study reveals: (1) That 62.04 per cent of our fourth year medical students have been infected with tubercle bacilli prior to coming into known contact with tuberculous patients; (2) that the morbidity over a one to ten year period was 2.6 per cent; (3) that there were no deaths among the 526 students who had been here for a period of study. It does not suggest that tuberculosis can be considered an occupation hazard for medical students and doctors.

Bibliography

1. Emerson, H., and Hughes, H. E.: Am. Jour. Pub. Health, 16:1088, 1926.
2. Herman, N, B.; Baetjer, F. H., and Doull, J. A.: Bull. Johns Hopkins Hosp., 51:41, 1932.
3. Hetherington, H. W.: McPhedran, F. M.; Landis, H. R. M., and Opie, E. L.: Arch. Int. Med., 55:709, 1935.
4. Long, E. R., and Seibert, F. B.: Jour. Am. Med. Assn., 108:1761, 1937.
5. Myers, J. A.: Jour. Am. Med. Assn., 97:316, 1931.
6. Soper, W. B., and Wilson, J. L.: Amer. Rev. Tuberc., 26:548, 1932.
7. Steidl, John: Am. Rev. Tuberc., 26:98, 1932.

CLINICAL NOTES ON THE RESULTS OF FEVER THERAPY*

Report of the First International Conference on Fever Therapy
New York City, March 29-31, 1937

FRANK H. KRUSEN, M.D.

Rochester, Minnesota

ON MARCH 29, 1937, a group of approximately 250 physicians, including representatives from twenty-nine foreign countries, gathered together at Columbia University Medical School to discuss the present status of fever therapy. During the ensuing three days approximately sixty papers on various phases of fever therapy were presented.

In opening the session, Whipple, of New York, expressed the opinion that fever therapy, although young, still had had an astonishing growth, that hazards might be connected with this remarkable growth, but that he was certain fever therapy had established "new standards in medicine." In reply, Abrami, of Paris, who was Chairman of the French Delegation, extended

felicitations and reviewed the early developments in the field with special reference to the original work of Wagner-Jauregg on malaria. A message from D'Arsonval, of Paris, described his early studies on electric heating of the human body that led to the development of physical devices for producing fever. He stated he was proud to have written in 1882 "that the therapeutics of the future will employ as a curative means the physical modificators, heat, light, electricity, and other agents still unknown."

A message was also sent to the Congress by Wagner-Jauregg, of Vienna. He stated that he started his first attempts to treat diseases by means of artificial fever in 1891, when he used injections of tuberculin in the treatment of mental diseases. Since 1900, his studies have been primarily concerned with the treatment of gen-

---

*From the Section on Physical Therapy, The Mayo Clinic, Rochester, Minnesota.

eral paralysis of the insane. He expressed the opinion that high temperatures, per se, do not produce the beneficial effects in dementia paralytica and he urged that malarial therapy always be combined with chemotherapy in the treatment of this disease. He concluded: "It should not be the aim of these combined therapeutic methods to destroy the pathogenic organism in the human body, but to improve the resistance of the organism and tissues against the pathogenic agents."

Abrami compared the effects produced by the two distinctly different methods of production of artificial fever (injections of foreign proteins and production by physical means). He felt that it was remarkable that two methods so different in nature could produce similar therapeutic results. He felt that physically induced fevers had the advantage of less danger "owing to the fact that the temperature can be controlled and measured accurately."

Richet, of Paris, like Abrami, compared the two chief forms of production of fever. Fevers produced by inoculations with infectious organisms or injections of foreign proteins he called "active fevers" while those produced by various physical means he termed "passive fevers." He felt that the effects were not entirely the same.

Hardy, of New York, studied the mechanism of heat loss from the human body in a calorimeter and concluded that "the mechanism for heat loss is adequate to care for twelve times the basal heat production" and that "spontaneous fever is due almost entirely to malfunction of the mechanism for heat loss."

Halphen and Auclair, of Paris, reported on the treatment of 3,000 patients suffering from various diseases. They produced fever by means of short radio waves and expressed the opinion that "it is regrettable that the American authors should have abandoned short waves in fever treatment without having drawn from it all that it could give." They suggested that the technic which they had developed would prove ideal for the production of fever.

Binet, of Paris, and Gernez of Lille, in studies on the physiology of fever, found great modifications in the antibodies of normal and syphilitic individuals following fever.

Gibson, Kopp and Evans, of Boston, studied the changes in plasma and total blood volume

during the course of fever treatment. They concluded that fever unaccompanied by sweating does not, in itself, bring about any considerable changes in blood volume but that when fever is accompanied by profuse perspiration, the reduction in blood plasma may be so great as to produce peripheral vascular collapse. Absorption of fluid from the intestinal tract may be retarded during high fever but intravenous administration of fluids permits rapid restoration of blood volume.

Pijoan, Kopp and Gibson, of Boston, studied the acid-base balance during therapeutic fever and concluded that fever characterized by severe dehydration and hyperventilation brought about a pronounced alkalosis; the degree of alkalosis, which approached critical levels, is dependent primarily on the severity of the dehydration and secondarily on the extent of hyperventilation.

Warren, of Rochester, New York, in seven cases noted the development of jaundice following prolonged fever therapy. He found two significant facts common to each case: (1) the rise in icteric index was accompanied by low value for the serum chloride and diminished excretion of urinary chlorides, and (2) the jaundice was relieved *only* by the administration of large amounts of sodium chloride (as much as 20 gm. in twenty-four hours) and not by the administration of carbohydrates. Proper attention to chloride and water balance "is apparently the most important factor in the technic of administering prolonged fevers."

Doan, of Columbus, Ohio, in an exhaustive study of the differential reaction of bone marrow, connective tissue and lymph nodes to hyperpyrexia, concluded that "hyperthermia by physical means not only provides the thermal factor of importance for the inactivation of the treponema pallidum and the gonococcus but has now been demonstrated to exert a profound effect on the cellular equilibria of the body in the directions which we believe at the present time to be the most effective in the mobilization of the defense forces of the body against these diseases."

Hartman, of Detroit, pointed out that untoward results of fever therapy are "always preceded by cyanosis and vascular collapse" and that it seems justifiable to place anoxemia as the underlying cause of the lesions found at necropsy following deaths from fever therapy.

Ebaugh, Barnacle and Ewalt, of Denver, concluded that most delirium, seen during fever therapy, could be handled by simple psychotherapeutic and physical procedures. They felt that the administration of sedatives contributed largely to the production of delirious episodes. They concluded that schizophrenia was not benefited by fever therapy. They reported on eighty-seven cases of general paresis; 71 per cent of the patients who were treated with combined physical fever and tryparsamide were benefited while 58 per cent of those who were treated with malarial therapy likewise were helped. As to the cerebrospinal fluid, 52 per cent of the patients who were treated with physical fever and tryparsamide were improved or reversed while 39.5 per cent of those who were treated with malarial fever were affected in the same manner.

Dowdy and Hartman, of Detroit, found that in fever therapy carbamide sedatives were more satisfactory for basic sedation than the barbituric acid group of drugs. They also recommended the prescribing of a high carbohydrate meal on the night before fever treatment and the intravenous injection of 500 c.c. of 10 per cent solution of dextrose in physiologic saline solution on the morning of treatment.

Pamboukis, of Athens, Greece, proposed the use of dengue fever as a therapeutic agent.

Simmons and Dunn, of Omaha, Nebraska, reported fifteen cases of acute rheumatic fever in which fever therapy was employed. Thirteen patients obtained complete relief of pain and swelling of the joints; two patients had relapses within two weeks to two months and one patient had a recurrence of chorea twenty-one months after treatment. In many of the cases, leukocyte counts and sedimentation times became normal after fever therapy.

Osborne, Blatt and Neymann, of Chicago, treated twenty-five children, who had chorea, by means of electropyrexia. Choreiform movements ceased in 88 per cent of the cases. The presence of rheumatic carditis did not preclude the use of fever therapy.

Sutton and Dodge, of New York, reported on the treatment of more than 400 attacks of chorea by means of fever therapy. Sixteen patients who had associated rheumatic carditis

were all benefited. A comparative analysis of ninety-five cases in which fever therapy was used and seventy-five cases in which fever therapy was not used showed a definitely lower incidence of rheumatic manifestations in the cases in which fever therapy was used. Fever therapy was capable of cutting short an attack of chorea; the presence of active carditis was not a contraindication to its use but carditis was perhaps benefited by it. Barnacle, Ewalt and Ebaugh, of Denver, during a two-year study, treated forty-five patients who had chorea. Immediate results were excellent and recovery occurred in the majority of cases. There were three recurrences. The incidence of carditis was 42 per cent (nineteen cases). Its presence did not interfere with treatment and two-thirds of the patients who had carditis showed at least an improvement in cardiac function.

Alajouanine and Maruiac, of Paris, concluded that in neurologic practice fever therapy was most beneficial in the treatment of syphilitic disease of the nervous system.

Claude and Rubenovitch, of Paris, advised malarial inoculations followed by prolonged chemotherapy in most cases of general paralysis. They suggested that electropyrexia should be preferred in cases in which Wassermann-fast reactions were present, in cases in which malarial therapy was either contraindicated or had failed, and finally, to reinforce the effect of postmalarial chemotherapy.

Bennett and Cash, of Omaha, Nebraska, recommended fevers at low temperatures as a safe and efficient means of treating neuritic and radicular pains. Hambresin, of Brussels, recommended fever therapy particularly in the treatment of syphilitic optic atrophy as well as in keratitis, iritis and iridocyclitis.

McGavic, of Cincinnati, reported on forty-two cases in which various ocular diseases were treated with fever therapy. Best results were obtained in syphilitic interstitial keratitis while good results also were obtained in gonorrheal ophthalmia and syphilitic iridocyclitis.

Moench, of New York, found that at temperatures ranging from 40° to 42° C. all strains of the meningococcus studied, except one, showed reduction of growth within five to seven hours. Five strains were either destroyed or greatly reduced in five hours or less. She concluded that fever therapy seems worthy of trial in selected cases of meningococcic infection.

Lardennois, of Paris, thought that fever therapy might benefit localized acute infections.

Major, Doub, and Hartman, of Detroit, studied the effect of fever therapy upon dogs which had been subjected to experimental tuberculosis. Temporary improvement was noted and, as compared with control dogs, life was prolonged.

Jares, of Rochester, New York, studied the thermal death time of animal tumor cells in vitro. He concluded that the combined effects of fever and roentgen rays are superior to the effect of either alone. The most destructive combination was simple fractional roentgen ray dosage (about 300 r. daily) plus heat treatment immediately afterward. Stecher and Solomon, of Cleveland, reported that of twenty patients who had acute nonspecific infectious arthritis, twelve obtained prompt relief and apparent cure while eight were partially relieved.

Walthard, of Geneva, Switzerland, observed the effect of short wave fever therapy in twelve cases of multiple sclerosis. He noted temporary diminution of spastic symptoms during and after treatment. The spasticity reappeared in all cases three or four months after treatment.

Russell, of London, reported fifteen cases in which disseminated sclerosis was treated by fever therapy. In four cases the gait became worse, in five cases there was no change and in six cases there was improvement.

Schroeder, of Copenhagen, recommended the use of intramuscular injections of 0.5 to 2 per cent sulphurated oil as a fever-creating agent.

Bessemans, of Ghent, Belgium, concluded that the best antisyphilitic hyperthermic methods are those which present at the sites of infection for the longest possible time to the highest possible temperature.

Hinsie and Blalock, of New York, reported the results of a twelve-year serologic study of general paralysis. They treated patients by four methods: (1) malarial therapy alone, (2) malarial therapy plus chemotherapy, (3) physical fever alone, and (4) physical fever plus chemotherapy. They concluded that physical fever plus chemotherapy gave the best results in their series of 326 cases. Ten years after treatment the Wassermann reaction on the serum was

negative in 75 per cent of twenty-eight cases; in 89.3 per cent of twenty-eight cases the Wassermann reaction on the cerebrospinal fluid was negative; in 100 per cent of twenty-six cases the cell count of the spinal fluid was normal; in 75 per cent of twenty-four cases the globulin reaction was normal, and in 73.1 per cent of twenty-six cases the gold sol curves were normal.

Gourgerot and Durel, of Paris, said that in cutaneous syphilis clinical experiments made thus far have given indisputable evidence of beneficial results with fever therapy, especially when combined with chemotherapy.

Menagh, of Detroit, reported on six months' experience with a mixed group of ninety-nine syphilitics treated with hyperpyrexia combined with chemotherapy. Fifty-four per cent showed improvement, 43 per cent were unimproved and two were not followed. Artificial fever by physical means showed a superiority over malarial therapy only when a satisfactory degree of fever could not be produced with malaria.

Simpson and Kendell, of Dayton, Ohio, in an experimental study of the treatment of thirty-four patients who had early syphilis, by means of artificial fever combined with chemotherapy, said that their observations appeared to indicate that artificial fever fortifies and intensifies the curative action of chemotherapeutic agents and that the time required for treatment can be greatly reduced.

Neymann, of Chicago, in a comparison of 3,000 collected cases in which general paralysis was treated with malarial therapy and nearly 1,000 collected cases in which general paralysis was treated with physical fever, concluded that physical fever has increased the total rate of improvement by 21 per cent and decreased the death rate from between 10 and 30 per cent to a degree which rendered it "no longer a problem." Neymann recommended the use of fever therapy as an adjunct in the treatment of early syphilis.

Kitchevatz, of Belgrade, Jugoslavia, recommended the use of fever therapy produced by means of antistreptobacillary vaccine in the treatment of soft chancre. He felt that it caused improvement and healing of the local manifestations and shortened the duration of the disease.

Ducoste, of Villejuif, France, recommended intracerebral malarial injections in the treatment of general paralysis. Of 435 paralytics treated by this method in the last ten years, 353 (80 per cent) "have been cured." Failures occurred in 12.8 per cent of cases and there were twenty-six deaths (6 per cent).

Janet and Dreyfus, of Paris, concluded that in gonorrhea the main characteristics of regional hyperthermic treatment were: (1) the striking rapidity of the cure, and (2) the easy management and innocuousness of this therapy. Carpenter and Boak, of Rochester, New York reported on the thermal death time of 250 strains of Neisseria gonorrhœæ at a temperature of 41.5° C. The heat resistance of the gonococcus varied between six and thirty-four hours; the mean was sixteen and one-tenth hours with a standard deviation of four and eight-tenths hours.

Warren, of Rochester, New York, presented an analysis of 163 cases in which gonorrheal infections were treated with fever for periods of time less than the thermal death time of the infecting strain of gonococcus. The length of treatment at 41.5° C. might be as long as 85 per cent of the thermal death time and still fail to result in a cure, while, on the other hand, treatments as short as 10 per cent of the thermal death time occasionally result in cure. Warren concluded that the variation is probably influenced by the defensive mechanism of the body.

Bierman and Horowitz, of New York, have devised a combined local and general heating technic for the treatment of gonorrhea in women. They reported that, during the past six years, of 121 women who were treated by this method the results proved successful in 113 (93 per cent).

Krusen, Stuhler and Randall, of Rochester, Minnesota, reported that of 361 patients who had gonorrhea and were given six to twelve hours fever at 106.7° F., 68 per cent obtained negative cultures and 74 per cent showed improvement. Of 266 patients who had positive cultures and completed treatment satisfactorily, 246 (92.5 per cent) obtained negative cultures. Of forty-one patients subjected to a single ten-hour session of fever, thirty-six (87.8 per cent)

obtained negative cultures and three more patients obtained negative cultures after an additional treatment.

Belt and Folkenberg, of Los Angeles, reported on the treatment of sixty-four patients who had gonorrhea, with a single ten-hour fever at 106.8° F. Fifty-nine, or 92.2 per cent, were found to have been constantly free from organisms following the ten-hour session of fever.

Parsons, Bowman and Plummer, of Denver, reported on eighty-seven soldiers who had acute gonorrhea and were treated with fevers of 106.6° to 107° F. for five-hour periods every third day. The patients were divided into treated and control groups. The percentage of cure was the same (72.7 per cent) in both groups but the patients who were treated with fever showed no residual symptoms and the results were accomplished in a third of the time required in the control group.

Trautmen, Stroupe and Devlin, of New Orleans, reported on the treatment of 278 men suffering from gonorrhea. Eighty-seven per cent of the men who had acute gonorrheal infections and 70.5 per cent of those who had chronic infections "were apparently free of gonococcic infection after completion of fever therapy."

Schnabel and Fetter, of Philadelphia, reported on the treatment of 136 patients with gonococcal infections. Seventy of the patients had acute gonorrheal arthritis and twenty had chronic gonorrheal arthritis. Forty-eight of those who had acute gonorrheal arthritis were cured and the remaining twenty-two were improved. Six of those who had chronic gonorrheal arthritis were cured and the other seventeen were unimproved.

Freund and Anderson, of Detroit, reported recovery in a case of gonorrheal endocarditis, following administration of artificial fever at 106.4° F. for thirty hours divided into five periods.

Hazel and Snow, of New York, reported on the successful treatment in one case of gonorrheal septicemia in which two treatments of five hours each at a temperature of 106° to 107.8° F. were used.

TRENDS IN MODERN PEDIATRICS*

· F. C. RODDA,. M.D.

Minneapolis, Minnesota

ALL successful business concerns find it necessary, at times, to take stock of supply, demand and obsolescence. It is quite as logical for doctors occasionally to evaluate medical practices. With such an appraisal, one is impressed with some very striking changes in the medical care of infants and children. Some diseases have almost disappeared, certain procedures are now obsolete, while our services are needed in new fields.

With such a survey one notes:

1. The practical disappearance of his chief "stock in trade" of thirty years ago, namely, smallpox, typhoid, diphtheria, fatal diarrheas, florid rickets and scurvy.

2. Infant feeding has been reduced to such simple routine that little medical supervision is now necessary.

3. The knowledge of hygiene of heating, ventilation, clothing and contagion has cut down the incidence of upper respiratory infections. A general practice of putting a child with an incipient cold to bed in an equable temperature, forcing fluids and providing a light diet, has cut off many grave complications, formerly necessitating medical attendance.

Now, all of these changes have been to the advantage of the infant and child but result in a sharp economic loss in pediatric practice.

However, to replace these losses, there are newly developing fields of endeavor wherein the child can be greatly benefited and the pediatrician may demonstrate he is still a useful citizen in his community. We are cognizant of much important research in cellular chemistry, studies on glands of internal secretion, chemotherapy, search for new curative and preventive sera and inoculations, as yet not practicable, but we are in possession of other facts, which permit of generalization and daily application. Of numerous advances, there are four which I wish to discuss briefly: (1) preventive medicine; (2) better knowledge of nutrition and growth; (3) promotion of health habits; and (4) prevention and early correction of behavior problems.

Preventive Medicine

Now, all four of these problems are preventive measures, but I refer especially to the avoidance of certain specific infections. You know successful vaccination will prevent smallpox. Through immunization against it, diphtheria is on the way out. Employment of the Dick technic against scarlet fever or some modification of it, may win general acceptance. Experience with Sauer's vaccine in preventing whooping cough is encouraging and certainly worth a trial. Military experience, throughout the world, testifies to the efficiency of typhoid vaccine against typhoid fever. But wistful wishing will not prevent these diseases. Procedures of active immunization must be carried out. They present no technical difficulties. A reasonable routine would be to begin protection against smallpox, diphtheria and pertussis at about six months of age, or even earlier; against scarlet fever before entering school, and against typhoid in the face of any threatened outbreak and for our transient, widely traveled, trailer population. One might ask how willing are parents to accept this regime? From my own experience I would say they are most cooperative. It is routine with us, well up to 100 per cent, and, moreover, parents are willing to pay reasonable fees for this work.

Growth and Nutrition

Workable standards of growth and development are in our possession; our knowledge of nutrition is increasing; most of the fundamentals are known. Mineral metabolism is on a scientific basis; the necessary amino-acids and their protein sources are known; knowledge of the metabolism of starches and fats, though not final is serviceable; the chemical structures of four important vitamins are known, three of which can be synthesized. All this knowledge now replaces much which was theory and conjecture twenty-five years ago. But you say it is all so technical. This is not so. Height and weight

*Read before the annual meeting of the Minnesota State Medical Association, Saint Paul, Minnesota, May 3, 1937.

determinations compared with standard tables at once inform us of the deviation from the norm. Of course, we can not standardize the human family, and reasonable allowance must be made for familial tendencies and types of body build. An inspection of bone development and the state of dentition gives us information as to skeletal nutrition. A simple blood examination will determine if anemia is present. With a knowledge of the normal, which we should have if we attempt anything in medicine, we now try to correct deviations from the normal in our patients. By referring to memory or simple tables, we can approximate the nutritional demands of our patients and proceed to outline a diet. It is not well known that the science of diet has been reduced to a simple, practical basis. Any recent text on diet will present understandable tables from which a sensible diet can easily be compiled. Too much detail may lead to confusion. In a gross way, one may state the minimal daily diet for a healthy growing child should include:

One and one-half pints of milk.
A generous supply of vegetables.
A generous supply of fruits and fruit juices, especially orange or tomato.
An egg or two.
A moderate amount of meat.
A moderate amount of cereal and breadstuffs.
Water to maintain balance.
Cod liver oil or its equivalent.

A simple anemia will respond to an iron salt. Only a prolonged deficiency diet will require other specific vitamin therapy. Experience and familiarity breed speed and efficiency so that nutritional management can become a pleasant task rather than a bugbear.

Promotion of Good Health Habits

It will be accepted as axiomatic that the health, accomplishments and happiness of an individual depend greatly on habits established in infancy and childhood. In spite of this, they are sadly neglected. By health habits, we mean regular schedules for eating, for bodily evacuations, regular times for play, rest and sleep, bodily cleanliness, care of the teeth, training in obedience and coöperation, social adjustments and numerous other details of living. It is of little value to outline a proper diet if the child will not take it. Undue fatigue may set up a whole train of bad habits, leading to serious problems. An unenlightened mother, in spite of best intentions, may wreck her child's health. Yet, too often, health habits are ignored by the physicians, and the layman often feels that these problems are aside from medicine. From intensive child study, it has been determined how much play, rest and sleep the average child, at a given age, requires. Contributions have also been made in methods of overcoming many problems in child training. All this, again, has been reduced to a practical basis. This, most assuredly, falls within the province of the physician, who should be in position to add just the right amount of common sense necessary to all rules as applied to children.

Behavior Problems

Behavior problems grow out of heredity, faulty health habits and environment. A goodly share of my energy goes into helping parents with behavior problems. I admit many shortcomings on my part, but not a lack of interest. Life is strenuous even for the young. They encounter strains and cross currents quite as much, or more, than the adult. The population of institutions for mentally unbalanced and insane far outruns the capacity to care for them, and the rate is increasing. Students of this situation contend that efforts to correct behavior problems and reduce maladjustments early in life may forestall many of these calamities. Is it strange that Johnny, who is underweight, has severe dental caries, has poor muscle tone, is chronically fatigued, unable to keep pace with his pals, should fall into a whiny, introspective state and become a problem in his home, school and community? Is it strange that Mary, as she approaches puberty and acquires a stepfather, lacking in understanding, should assume the attitude of a rejected child and become delinquent? Who should be in a better position to get a right perspective than the physician who probably brought them into the world and has followed them through their physical tribulations since? Many lesser behavior problems arise which may grow into big ones and eventuate in grave maladjustments. Some of these are thumb sucking, nail biting, head banging, night terrors, temper tantrums, neurotic vomiting and enuresis. These may not be explained away as being caused by teething or worms. A better approach, and one too often overlooked, is that the patient possesses a psyche which is responding peculiarly to environmental influences. A rational technic is now at our disposal in helping to correct most of these problems.

Now, most of these advances or lead lights have originated in medicine, some from clinical studies and some from tedious research. It is an interesting observation, that when facts have been established and brought to practical application, some bureaucratic agency or uplift organization appropriates the knowledge and at once sets itself up as a fountain head of all truth. But the doctor can do the job much better. We should not let others usurp our rightful place.

When I began my practice only certain activities of a doctor commanded a fee, such as setting a broken bone, administration of an anesthetic, the writing of a prescription and especially cutting or sewing. Time spent on examination or in giving advice was gratuitous. But here, too, I am sure there has been a change in the layman's viewpoint. Time spent in investigating a patient to arrive at a diagnosis and in giving advice, even without medicine or surgery, is now considered worthy of its hire.

I wish, however, to make a still more practical application of this discussion. We hear much of the oncoming state or social medicine. Mark Twain said, "Everybody talks about the weather but no one does anything about it." So it is with state medicine. True, we discuss it in our medical meetings, appoint committees, etc., but we do little intrinsically to avert or

lighten the blow. Remember the appeal of th crippled child is universal and provocative. Mec ical neglect of children provides the most powei ful argument for some form of social medicin Let us look close to home. Some day a surve of your village or county will be made, with th startling disclosure that, for instance, only 5 pe cent of the children of school age have been vac cinated against smallpox and perhaps only 3 to per cent against diphtheria. Suddenly som public health organization will come in and clea up this situation. Or again, a survey will sho a large percentage of children under weigh anemic, with dental caries and below norm: standards. Someone will move in a diet kitche and tell your countryside how to feed kids. C again, an uplift association will get excited abou some new idea for training in child health habit and, behold, a shepherdess to lead them. C again, child delinquency will force the settin up of a psychiatric clinic.

It is my contention that the medical profes sion has the knowledge and equipment to car for these problems, but we must show interes and do something about them. Of course, w need state medicine in an economic sense. Ther should be monetary help so that indigent paren may avail themselves of these aids and prote tions for their children, and to provide th laborer a living wage. But we do not need bureaucratic treatment machine to run over th family physician, or reduce him to a clerkshi The choice may lie with us.

SINUSITIS*

K. R. FAWCETT, M.D.

Duluth, Minnesota

THERE is probably no diagnosis which arouses more suspicion in the mind of the average lay person than that of sinus disease. Time after time the patient confronted with such a diagnosis slides out of the examining chair with the remark that he doesn't wish anything done about it because one of his friends who started treatments for sinus trouble never did get through.

*From the Duluth Clinic, Duluth, Minnesota. Read before the annual meeting of the Minnesota State Medical Association, St. Paul Minnesota, May 3, 1937.

This distrust on the part of the public mean only one thing. Something has be wrong, and perhaps still is wrong, with our c cept of sinus disease. It is upon this prem that this paper has been prepared. The subj can be discussed only in general terms. time is too short and the audience too gene for detailed classifications and exhaustive cussions of the individual sinuses.

Sinusitis, in the not too dim and distant p; has been held responsible for most of the that flesh is heir to. It was eagerly pounced upon as another focus of infection when doctors found out, somewhat to their chagrin, that extracting the patient's teeth and tonsils quite often failed to cure his rheumatism, peptic ulcer, asthma, or kidney trouble. We must admit that hundreds and probably thousands of sinuses have been operated upon ill advisedly. May I quote one example: In 225 cases of retrobulbar neuritis seen at the Mayo Clinic, Benedict[1] reported only one as due to sinus disease. Yet among 500 cases of multiple sclerosis, 60 per cent or 300 patients had had intranasal sinus operations because of visual disturbances—one of the common early symptoms of multiple sclerosis. A similar picture, nearly as bleak, could be painted for sinus surgery directed toward the cure of asthma. It is for reasons such as these that the subject of sinus disease is accompanied by a large question mark in the minds of our patients.

Physiology

The anatomy and physiology of the sinuses may be summed up very briefly. Each sinus has an opening into the nasal cavity, and is ventilated with each respiration, the pressure dropping below normal with inspiration and going above normal with expiration. The interior of the nose and sinuses is lined with ciliated epithelium, and the normal mucous secretions are swept in a steadily moving film by the cilia toward the pharynx and down into the stomach. Thus infective particles that gain entrance to the nose or sinuses are promptly swept out again. Most sinuses are normally sterile.

What then, we may ask, causes sinus disease? The causes may be divided into two groups: local and general. Under local we must consider anything which interferes with the normal ventilation and drainage of the sinuses, such as congenitally narrow nasal passages, adenoids, deviations and spurs of the nasal septum, and enlarged, malformed turbinates. Under general causes we must consider factors which lower our resistance, such as exposure to cold, fatigue, improper food, overheated rooms, and lack of proper humidity. In addition, as regards the maxillary sinus, we must remember that the roots of the upper teeth lie in close proximity, and the records of the Lahey Clinic, as reported

by Hoover,[2] show that 10 per cent of antral infections are dental in origin.

Bacteriology

Our knowledge of the bacteriology of sinus disease is, like that of the common cold, not as yet satisfactory. In 166 cases of maxillary sinus disease, acute and chronic, Enlows and Alexander[3] found pure cultures of streptococcus viridans in 43 per cent. The pneumococcus was found alone in 14 per cent. Streptococcus hemolyticus in pure culture was present in 9 per cent, and the remaining third of the cases were made up of various mixtures of streptococci, staphylococci and pneumococci. Interestingly, there were no evidences of micrococcus catarrhalis, and no anerobic organisms. Following the work of Dochez, a filterable virus seems to be pretty definitely established as the primary etiologic agent, but the presence of the virus does not detract from the importance of the accompanying organisms mentioned above which apparently become activated by the virus. It is significant that swine influenza is transferable only by a virus *plus* bacteria.

Symptomatology

Most of the symptoms of sinus disease, such as nasal discharge, local pain, temperature, sensitivity of the upper teeth, et cetera, are too well known to merit discussion. It is my impression that the patient with a chronic cough or bronchitis is occasionally overlooked as a sinus suspect. The symptom complex in children should be reviewed. It consists of chronic cough, anemia, loss of weight, frequent colds, a pasty complexion, nasal discharge, headache, cervical adenitis, and frequent otitis media.

Wherein lies our biggest error in the diagnosis of sinus disease? The question of allergy is approached with considerable trepidation because of its recent popularity in all fields of medicine, and yet there can be no doubt but that allergic states have been the most common cause of incorrect diagnoses of sinus disease. The pallor of the nasal mucous membranes is the first clinical finding that should put us on guard. The family history is all important. The presence of numerous eosinophiles in the smear of the nasal secretion is almost pathognomonic. Do not let the sinus x-ray deceive you. The sinuses may appear cloudy simply because of allergic thickening of the lining mucous membrane, and the roentgenologist must if possible learn to differentiate between this allergic thickening and actual disease.

Brief mention should be made of the complications of sinus disease. Our greatest danger lies in direct extension to the brain in the form of meningitis, brain abscess, or cavernous sinus thrombosis. Sander[4] reviewed the recent reports in the literature and found that 8 per cent of brain abscesses were due to infected frontal sinuses. Orbital abscesses may develop from ethmoid infection, and at times require external drainage in addition to drainage through the nose. Otitis media, especially in children, has already been mentioned. Ferraris[5] discusses the literature on the subject of optic neuritis and advises conservatism as regards sinus surgery. Iwaszkiewicz[6] analyzed 732 cases of sinus disease and found that only 3 per cent showed ocular complications. Farrell[7] reports 86 per cent of 66 cases of bronchiectasis showing roentgen evidence of sinus disease. The question of asthma needs careful analysis. Cooke and Grove[8] studied 248 cases of asthma due to bacterial allergens and found the sinuses to be the etiologic factor in 92 per cent. One hundred and twenty of these patients had radical sinus surgery, and 70 per cent of these were definitely improved. Sinus surgery is *not* indicated in asthmatics whose allergen is *not* bacterial.

Treatment

The treatment of sinus disease can be discussed but briefly. We should consider carefully the question of prophylaxis. In children it is generally accepted that the removal of diseased tonsils and obstructing adenoids is the most effective therapeutic measure. In adults, submucous resection to open up noses blocked by deviations and spurs of the septum is definitely indicated. The study of questionnaires sent to our patients following submucous resection reveals a rather marked diminution in the number of winter colds and sinus complications. General hygiene, including proper diet, rest, ventilation, and humidity can be only mentioned. Large doses of vitamines A and D have *not* decreased the incidence of respiratory infections in children. Vaccines have been used for many

years, but it is the concensus of opinion that most mixed vaccines confer a minimum of protection.

Acute sinusitis should be treated, as a rule, conservatively. Our purpose should be to aid the normal physiologic activity of the nasal membranes. Proetz says, "To my mind the cilia are by far the most potent factor in restoring and maintaining nasal health."

The medicinal agents used in the treatment of sinusitis are too varied to admit of any specificity. Parkinson[9] states, "By no interpretation of physiologic facts can one correlate such different substances as oils, colloids, antiseptics, lysates, electrolytes, adrenalin, cocaine, ephedrin, and their innumerable combinations." A review of the physiologic action of various commonly used nasal medications is extremely illuminating:

Liquid petrolatum, the vehicle of most of the nose drops on the market, causes marked slowing of the ciliary stream.

Argyrol and neosilvol cause a similar slowing.

Adrenalin 1-1000 causes immediate ciliary paralysis.

Cocaine in more than 2.5 per cent concentration causes slowing or paralysis of the cilia.

Merthiolate even in 1-10,000 dilution causes slowing.

Eucalyptol, menthol, thymol, zinc sulfate, and adrenalin all definitely slow or paralyze the cilia.

Tap and distilled water promptly stop all ciliary activity.

Physiologic saline has no effect on the cilia.

Ephedrin from 0.5 to 3 per cent in saline is harmless and may even cause sustained acceleration.

Thus, the only drug for which we have a physiologic indication in the nose is ephedrin, dissolved preferably in normal saline.

Local heat, in the form of moist packs or the infra red lamp, is definitely efficacious. Steam inhalations are helpful in that they render the muco-pus more liquid, making it easier for the cilia to clear the nasal passages.

Operative procedures in acute sinusitis are necessary only when pain and fever indicate obstruction of drainage and should be limited to the evacuation of the pus. Lillie[10] calls attention to the bad effects of frequent, prolonged irrigations of the nose and sinuses because of their tendency to waterlog the mucous membranes.

Chronic sinusitis can often be prevented by recognition and proper treatment of the acute case. In considering surgery we must be governed largely by the condition of the sinuses themselves. The persistence of chronic infection, thickened, hyperplastic mucosa, and polyps call for surgical interference, and the choice between intranasal and radical procedures must depend on the degree and extent of the involvement.

Conclusions

In conclusion, may I emphasize two points:
1. Allergy must always be considered as a primary factor in nasal disturbances, and must be carefully ruled out before a diagnosis of sinusitis is made.

2. We must be much more conservative in advising sinus surgery, particularly to patients with asthma or ocular symptoms, if we are to win back the confidence of the general public regarding the treatment of sinus disease.

Bibliography

1. Benedict, W. L.: Retrobulbar neuritis and disease of the nasal accessory sinuses. Arch. Ophth., (June) 1933.
2. Cooke, R. A., and Grove, R. C.: Relation of asthma to sinusitis. Arch. Int. Med., (Oct.) 1935.
3. Enlows, E. M. A., and Alexander, S. A.: Bacteriologic studies in acute and in chronic maxillary sinusitis. Arch. Otolaryngol., (June) 1936.
4. Farrell, J. T., Jr.: The importance of early diagnosis in bronchiectasis. Jour. Am. Med. Assn., (Jan. 11) 1936.
5. Ferraris: Quoted by Samuel Salinger: The paranasal sinuses. Arch. Otolaryngol., (Aug.) 1936.
6. Hoover, W. B.: Maxillary sinusitis: A brief discussion and a few points in technic. Surg. Clin., No. Am. (Dec.) 1935.
7. Iwaszkiewicz, J.: Quoted by Samuel Salinger: The paranasal sinuses. Arch. Otolaryngol., (Aug.) 1936.
8. Lillie, H. I: Chronic suppurative sinusitis: A point of view as to treatment. Arch, Otolaryngol., (March) 1935.
9. Parkinson, S. M.: Ephedrin in physiologic solution of sodium chloride and lateral head-low posture in treatment of the nose and sinuses. Arch. Otolaryngol., (March) 1936.
10. Sander, P.: Clinical notes on two cases of abscess of the frontal lobe. Jour. Laryngol. and Otolaryngol., (Jan.) 1935.

CONVALESCENT SERUM TREATMENT IN THE PREPARALYTIC STAGE OF POLIOMYELITIS

BURTON ROSENHOLTZ, M.D.

Saint Paul, Minnesota

THIS study of 2,761 clinical and 1,855 control cases was made with the idea of determining statistically the specificity of human convalescent serum in the treatment in the preparalytic stage of anterior poliomyelitis. Such an evaluation is difficult for various reasons. The material comes from different localities and over a period of years and epidemics, of course, vary greatly as to locale and time. The methods of handling material are not standardized. What one observer calls paralysis, another calls a paresis or muscle weakness. In some cases we have definite follow-up observation, and in others none. One of the greatest difficulties comes from the lack of large numbers of scientifically adequate controls. For this study, however, we felt that certain prerequisites were necessary. First, only those cases were included in which the diagnosis, we felt, was unimpeachable. That is, diagnosis depended on spinal fluid counts plus the symptomatology and the course of the disease. Second,

only those cases which were treated in the preparalytic stage are included in this study.

The main considerations in determining the specificity of convalescent serum are three in number: (1) mortality; (2) the amount of paralysis or muscle weakness during the acute stage; and (3) the residual paralysis.

For the sake of exactness, we have divided the cases into three groups: (1) those with no control; (2) those with controls which we felt for one reason or another were not to be relied on as scientifically accurate, and (3) those with controls scientifically sound.

Table I shows the evidence derived from the uncontrolled material. It is interesting to note the extreme differences in results in both the mortality and paralysis or muscle weakness. In this group of 215 cases all treated with human convalescent serum we have an average mortality of 9.4 per cent, paralysis of 8.1 per cent and no residual paralysis in 51.1 per cent.

TABLE I. UNCONTROLLED GROUP

Author	Time	Place	Number Exper. Cases	Number Cases Control	Deaths Control	Exper.	Paralysis or Muscle Weakness Control	Exper.	Residual No Paralysis Control	Exper.
Peabody	1916	Mass.	51	0		10.0%				69.0%
Amoss	1916	Mass.	14	0		14.3%		14.3%		
Silverman	1928	Syracuse	7	0		.0%		14.0%		
Silverman	1929	Syracuse	5	0		40.0%		.0%		
Shaw	1924	San Francisco	5	0		.0%		.0%		
Shaw	1930	California	53	0		1.9%		16.9%		84.4%
Cowie	1931	Michigan	80	0		.0%		3.8%		.0%
			215			9.4% AV.		8.1% AV.		51.1% AV.

TABLE II. INADEQUATELY CONTROLLED GROUP

Author	Time	Place	Number Exper. Cases	Number Cases Control	Deaths Control	Exper.	Paralysis Muscle Weakness Control	Exper.	Residual No Paralysis Control	Exper.
Zingher	1916	N. Y. C.	54	22	4.5%	.0%	33.0%	19.0%	55.0% At 8 weeks	80.0%
Ayer	1921-26	Syracuse	95	31	3.3%	8.0%	25.0%	18.0%	90.0%	86.0%
Silverman	1924	Syracuse	32	14	.0%	3.0%	35.8%	12.0%		
Silverman	1926	Syracuse	27	1	.0%	15.0%	.0%	51.9%		
McEachern	1928	Manitoba	74	54	11.0%	.0%	63.0%	13.0%		
McNamara	1925-31	Australia	133	151	9.0%	.0%		?		
Aycock	1927	Mass.	106	482	14.0%	.9%		64.0%	1.2% 2 mo. later	36.0%
Aycock	1928	Mass.	116	297	18.5%	6.0%	?	61.2%	53.3% About 3 mo.	43.0%
			637	1051	12.0% AV.	3.0% AV.	31.3% AV.	34.1% AV.	49.8% AV.	61.0% AV.

Table II is that of the inadequately controlled group. The controls in most instances in this group were seen after the acute stage, in some cases months after, and the mortality was taken from records. This is not true in the groups of Zingher and Ayer. Zingher's controls include twelve taken from hospital records and ten cases in which horse serum was given. Ayers thirty-one controls were all given pneumococcic serum. In this table, it will be noticed that no figures are available in the last two columns in the groups of Silverman, McEachern and MacNamara, as there was no follow-up recorded in these cases. The finest work in this group was undoubtedly

done by Aycock at the Harvard Medical Sch‹ The muscle examinations in these patients w done with the idea of arriving at figures to s‹ percentage of paralysis per patient. His contr however, were all patients seen after the a‹ stages by the Harvard Committee on Infar Paralysis. One must, however, be especially c ful in comparing the results in a group of tre‹ cases with a group of untreated ones taker large, for the reason that the number of ‹ abortive cases missed. is indeterminate.

To sum up the evidence, from this grou] 637 experimental and 1,051 inadequate cor cases we find that the only significant evid

CONVALESCENT SERUM TREATMENT OF POLIOMYELITIS—ROSENHOLTZ

TABLE III. ADEQUATELY CONTROLLED GROUP

Author	Time	Place	Number Exper. Cases	Number Cases Control	Deaths Control	Deaths Exper.	Paralysis or Muscle Weakness Control	Paralysis or Muscle Weakness Exper.	Residual No Paralysis Control	Residual No Paralysis Exper.
Laidlaw	1931	N. Y.	689	45	4.4%	3.5%	24.4%	19.1%	71.1% (3 wks.:	77.4% 3-4 mo.)
Park	1931	N.Y.C.	519	408	.9%	3.8%	28.0% (3-4 weeks)	27.2%	84.7%	76.6%
Previtali	1931	N.Y.C.	68	181	A- 2.2% Human B-13.0% Horse C- .9% None		20.3% 19.0% 25.0%		77.2% 67.0% 73.0%	
Previtali	1931	N.Y.C.	7	20	.0%	.0%	5.0%	3.0%		
Aycock	1931	Mass.	42?	40	.0%	5.0%	56.4%	46.5%	43.6%	53.5%
Fisher	1931	N.Y.C.	477	102	2.0%	3.8%	27.4%	27.2%	84.7% (6 Mo.)	78.6%
Dennig	1932	Stettin, Germany	7	8	.0%	.0%	13.0%	15.0%	87.0%	84.0%
			1709	804	3.03% AV.	2.6% AV.	42.7% AV.	22.6% AV.	73.0% AV.	74.9% AV.

for the specificity of convalescent serum is to be found in the average mortality. Here we find that there is a 3 per cent mortality in the experimental group as against a 12 per cent mortality in the controls. This, statistically, is a really significant difference. The 34.1 per cent paralysis in the treated and 31.3 per cent in the controls is a difference which is insignificant. As also is the 11 per cent difference in favor of the treated group in the residual.

The next table is the most important, for it is the one in which all controls are adequate and scientific.

It is Park's organization which has made the first three groups possible. Before the epidemic of 1931 the Health Department of New York City was well organized so as to record a large number of bona-fide, unselected controls, seen by physicians of the Academy of Medicine under Park's supervision. Park, realizing that most patients treated at home requested serum, stopped using it on the patients treated at the hospitals. In this group of a rather large number of treated and control cases, there is, as can be seen, no significant statistical difference between the two, except in the mortality, where four times as many patients died among those treated as in the unselected scientific controls.

Laidlaw's material, which came from upper New York State, was gathered in much the same way as Park's, consultants seeing all cases reported from the beginning.

Previtali's first group comes also from Park's organization. The 181 controls marked B and C were given, in some cases, horse serum, and in others, no serum. A is the group treated with human convalescent serum. The differences in each column, between these three groups, are definitely, statistically insignificant with the possible exception of the mortality, which is lower in those untreated than in those in which convalescent serum was used. The next group of Previtali is from his own private practice.

Aycock's group, although smaller than some of the other groups, has been very thoroughly studied. His controls are also unimpeachable, each patient having been studied from the standpoint of per cent paralysis per patient. Again, we find in this most intensive study a significant difference only in the mortality, and that definitely in favor of the controls. At this point it is of interest to note that Aycock's conclusion after the epidemic of 1927 in which inadequate controls were used was most optimistic, whereas he concluded from the work of 1931, using adequate controls, that he "failed to obtain statistical evidence that convalescent serum is effective."

No large well controlled group treated only in the preparalytic stage has been reported since 1932.

The averages in Group 3 or that of adequate controls have not been commented upon before. The lack of significant difference in this, the most important group, is obvious, in all columns

TABLE IV

	Mortality		Paresis		Residual No Paralysis	
	Control	Exper.	Control	Exper.	Control	Exper.
Group 1. No Controls		9.4%		8.1%		51.1%
Group 2. Inadequate Controls	12.0%	3.0%	31.3%	34.1%	49.8%	61.0%
Group 3. Adequate Controls	3.03%	2.6%	42.7%	22.6%	73.0%	74.9%

except that having to do with paralysis, where the treated cases showed an average 22.6 per cent and the control cases 42.7 per cent. However, this difference is not one of statistical significance (Table III).

Table IV shows the averages already given. The group of inadequate controls shows, as we have said, no significant statistical difference except in the mortality, and that is in favor of the treated group.

Conclusion

From this statistical study, especially of the group in which we had 1,709 treated cases and 804 adequate controls, there is no evidence that human convalescent serum is of value, when used in the preparalytic stage of anterior poliomyelitis.

Bibliography

1. Amoss, Harold L., and Chesney, A. M.: A report on serum treatment of 26 cases of epidemic poliomyelitis. Jour. Exper. Med., 25:581-608, 1917.
2. Aycock, W. L., et al: Preparalytic poliomyelitis. Jour. Am. Med. Assn., 91:387-394, (Aug. 11) 1928. Idem: Preparalytic poliomyelitis. Jour. Inf. Dis., 45:175-190, 1929. Idem: Convalescent serum in preparalytic poliomyelitis. New Eng. Med. Jour., 206-432-435, (Mar. 3) 1932.
3. Ayer, W. D.: Poliomyelitis: its preparalytic period with resuults of serum therapy. Am. Jour. Med. Sci., 177:540-555, (April) 1929.
4. Brodie, M.: Comparison of convalescent and non-convalescent serum. Jour. Exper. Med., 56:507-519, (Oct.) 1932.
5. Brodie, M.: Rôle of convalescent serum in preparalytic poliomyelitis. Jour. Immunol., 28:353-361, (May) 1935.
6. Cowie, D. M.: The therapeutic value of convalescent serum, adult blood. Trans. Am. Ped. Assn., 44:52-56, 1932.
7. Dennig, H.: Zur Behandlung der poliomyelitis mit Reconvalescentenserum. Munch. Med. Wchnschr., 80:1367-1368, (Sept. 1) 1933.
8. Fisher, A. E.: Human convalescent serum in treatment of preparalytic poliomyelitis. Comparison of 447 treated and 102 controlled patients in New York City in 1931. Am. Jour. Dis. Child., 48:481, 1934.
9. Flexner, S., and Stewart, Fred W.: Protective action of convalescent poliomyelitis serum. Jour. Am. Med. Assn., 91:383, 1928.
10. Kessel, J. F., Hoyt, A. S., and Fish, R. T.: Use of serum. Am. Jour. Pub. Health, 24;1215-1223, (Dec.) 1934.
11. Landin, J. F., and Pedivin, J.: Clinical studies, serum treatment in preparalytic poliomyelitis. 5:9-15, (July) 1934.
12. Laidlaw, F. W.: Poliomyelitis in New York. Jour. Am. Med. Assn., 99:1053-1057, (Sept. 24) 1932.
13. McEachern, et al: Therapy with convalescent serum in poliomyelitis. Can. Med. Assn. Jour., 20:369, (April) 1929.
14. MacNamara, et al: Poliomyelo-encephalitis, treatment by human immune serum. Lancet, 1:469-472, (Feb. 27) 1932; Ibid, 527-539, (Mar. 5) 1935.
15. Park, Wm. H.: Therapeutic use of anti-poliomyelitis serum in preparalytic cases of poliomyelitis. Jour. Am. Med. Assn., 99:1050-1053, (Sept. 24) 1932.
16. Peabody, F. W.: A report of the Harvard Infantile paralysis commission on the diagnosis and treatment of acute cases of the disease during 1916. Boston Med. and Surg. Jour., 176:637-642, (May) 1917.
17. Pohlen, K.: Die bekampfung der übertvagbaren kinder lahmung in Deutschen Reich. Deutsche Med. Wchnschr., 62:1245-1248 (Aug. 1) 1936.
18. Previtali, G.: Recent epidemic of poliomyelitis. Arch. Pediat., 49:540-547, (Aug.) 1932.
19. Richardson, D. L., and West, E. J.: Treatment of acute poliomyelitis with convalescent serum. Rhode Island Med. Jour., 15:100, (June) 1932.
20. Shaw, E. B., et al: Canvalescent serum in preparalytic cases of poliomyelitis. Jour. Am. Med. Assn., 85:1555-1558, (Nov. 14) 1925.
21. Shaw, E. B., et al: The treatment of poliomyelitis. Jour. Am. Med. Assn., 97:1620-1624, (Nov. 28) 1931.
22. Silverman, A.: Clement: The number of local and imported patients with preparalytic poliomyelitis treated with serum and the results in Syracuse, N. Y., from 1922 to 1929. Am. Jour. Dis. Child., 41:829-861, (April) 1931.
23. Zingher, A.: The diagnosis and serum treatment of anterior poliomyelitis. Jour. Am. Med. Assn., 68:817-823, (March) 1917.

No Sunshine in Soap

During the past year certain brands of soap have been flamboyantly exploited for their vitamin D content; one for the "filtered sunshine" in its lather. The latter product was introduced to the public with double page spreads in national magazines under the caption: "The Dawn of a Great Beauty Discovery." There is evidence that irradiated ergosterol may be absorbed through the skin of rats. This evidence has been an excuse for adding vitamins to various cosmetic preparations. Redgrove points out that the real question at issue is not the ability of the skin to absorb these substances, but "whether when so absorbed the vitamins exercise any beneficial action on the skin—in short, whether they are of any cosmetic value." Even if it

is established that vitamin D exercises any beneficial action on the skin, it still must be proved that it has a beautifying effect. As a matter of fact, there has been some recent evidence which indicates that the alleged beneficial effects mentioned by Redgrove as resulting from the use of cod liver oil in the promotion of healing of wounds and burns were probably due to some other factor than the vitamin D content of the oil. It is not surprising that the Federal Trade Commission has recently published a complaint issued against a manufacturer who has made extraordinary claims about his product. The advertiser who proclaimed the Dawn of a Great Beauty Discovery may soon be worrying about the twilight of the day when the sky was the limit for claims about "sunshine soaps." (Jour. A.M.A., August 14, 1937, p. 509.)

◆ CASE REPOR_T ◆

MALIGNANT HYPERTENSION FOLLOWING BILATERAL LUMBAR SYMPATHECTOMY FOR RAYNAUD'S DISEASE*

BAYARD T. HORTON, M.D., and HAROLD J. BRUMM, M.D.

Rochester, Minnesota

Raynaud's disease and malignant hypertension both are encountered somewhat infrequently in general practice. This case is reported because, as far as we know, it is the first of its kind. Both diseases are characterized by occurrence of vasospasm. Furthermore, surgical treatment of Raynaud's disease of the lower extremities and of essential hypertension is very much alike, consisting in the former case, of performing lumbar sympathetic ganglionectomy and a resection of the sympathetic trunk and, in the latter case, consisting of performance of a more extensive sympathectomy of the Adson-Craig type. In the case reported below, hypertension of the malignant type developed in spite of performance of bilateral lumbar sympathetic ganglionectomy and a resection of the sympathetic trunk for relief of Raynaud's disease.

Report of Case

A white, married woman, aged forty-five years, came to The Mayo Clinic for the first time on April 1, 1932. She complained of color changes of the fingers and of the hands on exposure to cold. Her first symptoms began in May, 1931, when she noticed blanching of the little finger of the left hand; this was promptly followed by symmetrical involvement of all the digits of both hands. The red, white and blue color phases were noted. Pain was not experienced with these early color changes. Similar color changes were noted simultaneously in all the toes in January, 1932. Excitement and exposure to cold always brought on her symptoms. Later, these symptoms were accompanied by numbness of the digits and by generalized weakness. She promptly recovered from her symptoms in a warm room. This patient also stated that occasionally a tired feeling developed in the calf muscles of both legs when walking on a cold day. On two occasions she had to stop walking. Rest gave prompt relief. She had also experienced similar sensations while dancing. She had observed that she could walk farther on a warm day than she could on a cold day. This patient's father and mother were living and were well. Four sisters were alive and were well. Two brothers were considered to be well until they were six years of age at which time both of them developed an insidious paralysis of the legs and became invalids; one brother died at twelve years of age and the other died at nineteen years of age. There was no history of hypertension in the family. The patient had been married fifteen years and had two healthy children. Her menstrual periods were normal, but flow was scant.

At the time of her physical examination the fingers and toes were cold, mottled and cyanotic. Pulsations in the brachial, radial and ulnar arteries, as well as in the femoral, popliteal, dorsalis pedis and posterior tibial arteries were within the normal range. Definite scleroderma was not present. Neurologic examination gave objectively negative results. In a room of which the temperature was 23.8° C., the surface temperature of her fingers ranged from 25.5° C. to 26.1° C., and the surface temperature of her toes ranged from 26.1° C. to 28.1° C. Following oral administration of 1 ounce (30 c.c.) of ethyl alcohol, there was a uniform rise of the surface temperature of her fingers of 10° C. to 10.6° C. The rise of surface temperature of her toes was somewhat less uniform and ranged from 6.9° C. to 10.2° C. Normally, the surface temperature of the feet rises less than that of the hands during this test.

The blood pressure was 132 mm. of mercury systolic and 84 diastolic: the pulse rate was 96 per minute. Examination of the ocular fundi by Dr. Wagener revealed some excess glial tissue on the disks. The retinal arteries had an exaggerated reflex but sclerosis was not present. The specific gravity of the urine was 1.030; the urine was acid in reaction and albumin and sugar were not present; microscopic examination gave negative findings. The concentration of hemoglobin was 14.2 gm. per cent, erythrocytes numbered 4,450,000 and leukocytes numbered 5,700 per cubic millimeter of blood. The serologic test for syphilis and a roentgenogram of the chest gave negative results. Special examination of the urine for lead and arsenic showed that lead was not present, but 200 c.c. of urine contained 12 mg. of arsenic.

On April 8, 1932, Dr. Craig performed a right and left lumbar sympathetic ganglionectomy and a resection of the sympathetic trunk for the Raynaud's disease. The patient had an uneventful recovery and the wound healed by primary intention. The feet were warm, pink and dry at the time of her dismissal. No changes were noted in the hands.

On July 23, 1937, the patient returned to the clinic complaining of blurred vision, of headaches during the past two months and of hypertension for one year. In March, 1934, her blood pressure was 145 mm. of mercury systolic and 90 diastolic.

In July, 1936, her family physician found that she had a severe degree of hypertension. Headaches were severe, but administration of acetylsalicylic acid (aspirin) gave her relief to a slight extent. Her vision had diminished so that it was difficult for her to distinguish people at a distance of 10 feet (3.3 meters).

Approximately four years previously, the skin of the terminal phalanges of the hands and the skin about her mouth, face and neck had become tighter and definite evidence of scleroderma had developed. She had continued to have color changes of the Raynaud type, in the hands but not in the feet.

*From the Division of Medicine, The Mayo Clinic, Rochester, Minnesota.

CASE REPORT

Physical examination revealed a thin, emaciated woman who had a glossy, tightened skin over the face, neck and terminal phalanges of the hands. No scleroderma was present in the feet; she weighed 87 pounds (39.5 kg.). The blood pressure was 234 mm. of mercury systolic and 150 diastolic. When the blood pressure was taken at hourly intervals, there was a systolic range of 190 to 240 mm. of mercury and a diastolic range of 100 to 170. The second aortic sound was accentuated. Examination of the fundi by Dr. Wagener revealed generalized narrowing of the retinal arteries of grade 1 to 1+ (on a basis of 1 to 4), sclerosis of grade 1 to 2 and localized angiospastic narrowing in the smaller and more peripheral arteries. Scattered cotton wool exudates and hemorrhages were present, as well as edema of the disks to an extent of 2 to 3 diopters. Macular stars were not noted. From the appearance of the ocular fundi, Dr. Wagener thought that one should consider the possibility of acute angiospastic retinitis, in contrast with that of frank malignant hypertension. Pulsations could not be detected by palpation of the ulnar arteries or of the left dorsalis pedis artery. Pulsations were present in the other palpable arteries but seemed markedly reduced in force. No definite sclerosis was evident. The surface temperature of the fingers was approximately 27.5° C. and the surface temperature of the toes was approximately 26° C. with the patient in a room of which the temperature was 77° F. (25° C.) and the humidity was 40 per cent. It is interesting to note that the surface temperature of the digits was essentially the same at the time of her second admission to the clinic as it was during her first visit.

Urinalysis revealed albumin grade 2 to 3 on a basis of 1 to 4; the specific gravity was 1.015 to 1.019; microscopic examination gave negative results. The concentration of blood urea and of blood sulphates was 30 mg. and 3.5 mg. per 100 c.c. of blood, respectively. The concentration of hemoglobin was 15.2 gm. per cent; erythrocytes numbered 4,040,000 and leukocytes 5,800 per cubic millimeter of blood. The basal metabolic rate was +32 per cent. A roentgenogram of the thorax gave evidence of cardiac enlargement and of dilatation of the arch of the aorta. The electrocardiographic tracing revealed a cardiac rate of 119 per minute, sinus tachycardia, iso-electric T waves in derivation 3 and QRS complexes that were notched in derivations 2 and 3 and slurred in derivation 1. The serology of the blood was normal. Following intravenous administration of pentothal sodium (565 mg.) the blood pressure decreased from 200 systolic and 135 diastolic to 180 systolic and 124 diastolic. With administration of 9 grains (0.6 gm.) of sodium amytal, the blood pressures dropped from 220 and 160 to 168 and 112. Following administration of 3 grains (0.2 gm.) of sodium nitrite, the blood pressure decreased from 198 and 140 to 180 and 126. It is very obvious from these tests that the patient had a fixed type of hypertension and she was not suitable for performance of extensive sympathectomy such as has been carried out at the clinic by Drs. Adson and Craig. She died about three weeks after leaving the clinic.

Comment

It seems logical to assume that the vasospastic disturbance which was originally present in the hands and feet and which did not give rise to hypertension had finally become generalized and was of such degree that it produced a severe hypertension which explained the final clinical picture. In our experience, in the average case of Raynaud's disease, a normal or a subnormal blood pressure is present.

Development of scleroderma in the hands, face and neck was fairly marked at the time of her second visit but there was no evidence of the presence of scleroderma in the feet. Apparently the operation of sympathectomy for the condition in the lower extremities had prevented development of scleroderma in the feet.

At the time of the patient's first admission to the clinic, she presented all the classical signs and symptoms of Raynaud's disease and yet complained of definite intermittent claudication in the lower extremities. This is the first time we have observed this symptom in a case of Raynaud's disease. In fact, we were previously inclined to think that this symptom did not occur in Raynaud's disease.

The finding of arsenic in the urine was apparently accounted for by the fact that previously she had been taking Fowler's solution.

Even though the basal metabolic rate was +32 per cent there was no other evidence of hyperthyroidism. It is not uncommon, in our experience, to observe metabolic rates of this height in cases of severe malignant hypertension.

It is extremely interesting to note that pulsations in the ulnar arteries as well as in the left dorsalis pedis artery could not be detected at the time of her second admission to the clinic, although these arteries pulsated normally at the time of her first admission. It is most unusual to observe occlusion of peripheral arteries of this caliber in cases of essential hypertension and we have not observed it in cases of frank Raynaud's disease. We cannot give an adequate explanation of this phenomenon.

Antitularemic Serum-Mulford

Sharp & Dohme, Inc., presented for the consideration of the Council on Pharmacy and Chemistry Antitularemic Serum-Mulford prepared by immunizing horses by injecting cultures of B. tularense isolated from human cases of tularemia. On request of the Council, Dr. Lee Foshay of the College of Medicine, University of Cincinnati, kindly submitted comparative data obtained from 334 untreated cases of tularemia and 481 serum treated patients. He gave a separate analysis of 133 patients (included in the treated group) who received Antitularemic Serum on or before the twelfth day of the disease. The Council considered Dr. Foshay's data, and, while finding nothing definitely to criticize, concluded that corroborative data by other investigators are needed before the product can be accepted for inclusion in New and Nonofficial Remedies. The Council therefore voted to postpone consideration of Antitularemic Serum-Mulford (Sharp & Dohme Inc.) to await development of further data. (Jour A.M.A., August 14, 1937, p. 504.)

THE BACKGROUND OF MEDICAL HISTORY FOR NORTHEASTERN MINNESOTA AND THE LAKE SUPERIOR REGION

By RICHARD BARDON, M.D.

A SUMMATION of some of the medical and hospital history of northeastern Minnesota and the region of Lake Superior merits a brief introduction outlining three major epochs. While the present review is not primarily intended to cover the early exploration period of the eighteenth century, the reader will be better oriented by a short reference to this early colorful period. Two relatively recent books, "The Voyageurs," by Grace Lee Nute, and "Early Candle Light," by Lovelace, should be read by all those seeking a background for our present-day commonwealth.

This early period was decidedly French, or rather, French-Canadian, Indian, and ultimately English as they became supreme in the New World. The human side of the transfer of a great wilderness from Indian control to white usurpation is largely a story of the colorful "Voyageurs de Bois." They were the trekkers, the "safari" for the great fur trading companies in a day when transportation was a matter of canoes, portages, fur trading stations or forts for traffic with the Indians. The voyageur was in the beginning scarcely a generation removed from the immigrant—the most spirited and virile of the French when their nation was in the "Golden Age of Louis the Grand." They were sprightly, singing, praying, cursing, incorrigible, adaptable, indefatigable, and left a heritage and an imprint on this region which may not readily be effaced. Fur trading was not so much a means of gaining a livelihood as an excuse to live in a manner so peculiarly adapted to their temperament and physique. It is too easy in retrospect to lose a sense of their moral fiber and religious devotion in the livelier tales of their drinking, carousing and direct eugenic alliance with the natives. They learned from the aborigines the "methods of living off the country"; in return, they left indelible geographic landmarks and racial imprints: the names of cities, capes, promontories, lakes—mostly French translations of old Indian names. As with all primitive contacts, industrial and missionary in character, the doctors and priests, with the Indian medicine men, became something of a blur. The ability to offer healing solace to the sick or injured was the best approach to the matter of weaning a wavering soul away from pagan worship. The doctors who accompanied the fur traders were, for the most part, itinerants, if not adventurers.

The second phase or epoch began when wars among the European peoples ceased for a full century to embroil their compatriots in the New World. The industrial development of this north region came after the enormous agricultural growth in the mid-American continent, when its fertile land, as James J. Hill said, "had the Indian taken out of it." The varied national groups soon demanded lumber in large amounts. The settlers were readily adapted to the land; they had an extraordinary urge for independent thinking and extreme self reliance. They brought their wives and children, and came to remain; to build cities and farms;

to develop direct land transportation, such as railroads, in contrast to laborious seasonal canoeing via circuitous water routes and portages. The demand for lumber inspired an onslaught of unheard-of proportions, and within four decades the great timber belts of Michigan, Wisconsin and Minnesota yielded, to the axe-men and the mills, their centuries of growth. The lumbermen came largely from Maine and Canada, and occupied the timber states—Michigan, Wisconsin and Minnesota—in sequence. In comparatively recent years, after denuding much of Minnesota, they made broader jumps to the far south on the one hand and the Pacific Coast on the other. Scarcely, however, was the timber cut off when iron ore was discovered in large amounts, and offered another inspiring field for industrial exploitation. It had its aegis in the corresponding demand of an era of city and industrial expansion, and was comparable to the agricultural stimulus that speeded up the lumber mills. In any case, industrialism gave the permanent establishment of most of our hospitals that came later. No longer were the doctors itinerants, and a considerable portion of our narrative will deal with the vigorous pioneers who, coming with the above industries, took on, more or less, both the attributes of the times and the atmosphere of their associated industries.

It was not until 1871 that a railroad came from the South (the Northern Pacific, or, as it was known then, the St. Paul and Duluth Line). Up to that time the contacts, medical and otherwise, were far more with the lower lake ports, via water transportation, and to a lesser degree by rail and stage connections with St. Paul. Up until the '90's the medical practitioners came for the most part from eastern Canada, the New England States, or had followed the lumber industry from Michigan up through Wisconsin. Only after 1900 did more and more graduates from our own medical schools settle in northeastern Minnesota.

The early medical history of St. Louis County naturally is the history of the City of Duluth itself, and consequently we shall attempt to sketch the types of hospitals and methods of support devised in the development of the lumber and mining industries. St. Mary's Hospital in Duluth, for example, sold tickets to the men in the lumber industry covering the cost of their hospital and medical care should they be sick or injured. The price of the tickets varied somewhat, but was in the neighborhood of $12 per year, and served a definite purpose in giving the lumberjacks proper medical care and at the same time developing the early hospitals of our city and county. It was something of an outgrowth of this method that led to the development of most of the iron mining hospitals, except that the assessments were levied monthly, depending on the employment. The plan, under various modifications, still exists.

No historical period abruptly ends when another begins; it is so with our empirical and arbitrary divisions given in this introduction.

The third phase of medical and hospital development took form about 1910. There were no obvious changes in the type of management, for example, of the two large hospitals (St. Mary's and St. Luke's) in Duluth, but with the gradual development of agriculture in northern Minnesota and with urban growth commensurate with wider diversification there came the same change in the type of our hospitals characteristic of all in our state. It may suffice to mention that this change coincided with the period in which rampant epidemics, such as typhoid, ceased to recur, and specialism in medicine developed. The profession adapted itself to the gradual division of its labors, and hospitals were built for the expanding needs. This, very shortly, had its influence upon the hospitals: they became very much more complex units, with a service expanding as rapidly in unit cost as in efficiency. They have become, in other words, symbolic of our eager, alert and vigorous times.

The Era of Exploration and Fur Trading

A knowledge of the early medical history of northern Minnesota depends on the records left by the fur traders and the reports of the government expeditions into this part of Minnesota over one hundred years ago. The Northwest Fur Company, in particular, had men in its employ who were physicians, but who were primarily traders, or what were known as "clerks." They kept diaries and made reports to their superiors in Montreal, and it is from these records that we have information as to conditions then existing. The records of the various government expeditions that traveled through our part of Minnesota are of twofold interest in that they usually contain reports of the surgeon of the party pertaining to medical matters, as well as other interesting episodes of early travel in the Northwest. It is from these sources that the following information was obtained:

About the year 1750[7] a war party of more than a hundred young men of the Fond du Lac band of Indians visited Montreal to assist the French in their war with the British. They became infected with smallpox, and but few of the party survived to reach their home. It does not appear, although they made a precipitous retreat to their own country, that the disease was at this time communicated to any others of the tribe.

About the year 1782 smallpox again appeared among the Chippewas of Lake Superior. The circumstances connected with this introduction are interesting. Sometime in the summer of 1781 a trader who had ascended the Mississippi and established himself near Leech Lake was robbed of his goods by the Indians residing at that lake, and in consequence of his exertions in defending his property he died soon after. It is of non-medical interest to note here that even to this date the band of Indians living in the region of Leech Lake are known as the "pillager" band of Indians. The facts concerning the death of the trader became known to the British at Mackinac and requests were sent to the Leech Lake Indians that they should visit Mackinac and make reparation for the goods they had taken. At the same time, they were threatened with punishment in case of refusal to do so.

In the spring of 1782[9] the Indians decided to comply with this request, and a deputation from the band visited Mackinac with a quantity of furs which they considered an equivalent of the goods which had been taken. The delegation was received with politeness by the English and the difficulties were readily adjusted. When this was effected, a cask of liquor and a British flag, closely rolled, were presented to the Indians as a token of friendship. They were at the same time strictly enjoined neither to break the seal of the cask nor to unroll the flag until they had reached the heart of their own country. These directions they promised to observe, but on reaching Fond du Lac, Superior, after many days' travel, they could not resist temptation, and unsealed the cask and unrolled the flag for the gratification of the tribesmen. The Indians drank the liquor and remained in a state of inebriation for several days. The rioting was soon over and they were fast recovering from its effects when several of the party were seized with violent pains. This was attributed to the liquor they had drunk, but the pain increasing they were induced to drink deeper of the liquor, and in this inebriated state several of the party died before the real cause was suspected. Other like cases occurred, and it was not long before one of the party, who had visited Montreal in

1750 and who had narrowly escaped with his life, recognized the disease as the same which had attacked his party at that time. The malady proved to be small-pox, and nearly the whole population of three hundred Indians then at Fond du Lac was wiped out. Although the epidemic did not extend easterly on Lake Superior, it is believed that not a single band of Chippewas north or west of Fond du Lac escaped its ravages. As late as 1832 the Indians were firmly of the opinion that the smallpox had been transmitted by the articles presented to their brothers by the British at Mackinac, as a punishment for their crime against the trader at Leech Lake.

Grand Portage, said to be the oldest permanent white settlement in Minnesota, is located in Cook County, and has a glamorous past, not easily visualized from what remains. There is no actual record of the date when the white men first visited Grand Portage. It is possible that Radisson and Groseilliers were there in 1660, and Du Luth probably in 1679. In 1731, however, Sieur de la Verendrye recorded his visit to Grand Portage. Subsequently the French, and later the English, used Grand Portage as a depot for supplies destined for the fur trade in western Canada, the district north of Lake Superior, and the upper Mississippi region. Jonathan Carver, the associate of the celebrated Major Rogers, arrived at Grand Portage in 1767. The present popular historical novel, "Northwest Passage," mentions such familiar names as the St. Croix and Brule rivers as routes of travel for Carver on his canoe voyage from the Mississippi to Grand Portage. During the Revolution, in 1778, there was on duty at Grand Portage a small detachment of British soldiers, under the command of a Lieut. Thomas Bennett—the sole participation of the present state of Minnesota in the Revolutionary War. With the formation of the Northwest Fur Company in 1783, Grand Portage began an era of activity and importance that continued until about 1801, when the Company moved its headquarters to Fort William. Much has been written about Grand Portage, and an article by Solon J. Buck in the *Minnesota History Bulletin* tells the story well.

The historical background of Grand Portage is of interest to the medical profession of Minnesota because it was here, as an employe of the Northwest Fur Company, that the first physician in what is now Minnesota resided. Dr. Henry Munro[8] was born in 1770, the son of Honorable John Munro, one of the members of the first legislative council of upper Canada. In 1796 he entered the service of the Northwest Fur Company as surgeon, and for several years was stationed at or near Grand Portage, at a salary of "1,200 Grand Portage currency." Dr. Munro apparently acted as both surgeon and trader, and in 1804 or 1805 was sent to succeed J. B. Perrault "at the Pic" on Lake Superior.[2] During the war of 1812, when the Northwest Fur Company raised among its men a corps of Canadian voyageurs to fight the Americans, Dr. Munro was appointed "Surgeon's Mate." This corps, commanded by William McGillivray, a famous "Northwester," served in at least two engagements, and was disbanded at Lachine, near Montreal, on March 14, 1813. It is said that the jovial, carefree voyageur was not temperamentally suited to army life, and apparently the corps was not as successful as anticipated. Dr. Munro died August 20, 1854, at Lachenaie, lower Canada, and is buried in the old Protestant cemetery at Mascouche.

Perhaps the most colorful figure of the early fur traders in this district was Dr. John McLoughlin,[3,4] who was at Grand Portage and Fort William, apparently as an assistant to Dr. Munro. Dr. McLoughlin was an apprentice and student of Dr. James Fisher of Quebec for "four years and 6 mos." (a letter from Dr.

Fisher dated April 30, 1803, certifies to that effect), and he was licensed to practice "Surgery, Pharmacy or Apothecary" on May 3, 1803, and apparently was employed by the Northwest Company shortly thereafter. There is record of his residence at Lake Vermillion (some say it was Crane Lake) during the winter of 1807-08 as a trader and surgeon.

Letters of Dr. McLoughlin written in 1808 and 1810 are interesting, inasmuch as they give some idea of his salary, which was apparently not satisfactory to him. They also, in view of what happened in his later life, are typical of his spirit and outspoken nature.

In a letter from Fort William in 1808 Dr. McLoughlin writes to his uncle:

"You tell me in your letter that they may increase my wages. I think they may as I have been doing Dr. Munro's duty these five years without having any allowance although I recollect your telling me that if required to practice I would have 100 pounds, i.e., Dr. Munro's salary. Now the first year I came here Dr. Munro's time was out and tho I was oblig'd all along to do his duty . . . yet they engag'd him and gave him the salary that was promis'd to me . . . the 2nd year . . . I was requir'd to practice while he was sent to an Indian post . . ."

Again he writes on July 13, 1808, from Fort William that he was offered 150 pounds but rejected it because it was "less than Dr. Munro, although I had served an apprenticeship to them of five years for 100 pounds, whereas Dr. Munro had a hundred a year the first four years and two hundred every year after . . ."

Several years later, on August 2, 1810, he wrote the following from Fort William: " . . . even when Dr. Munro was in the country I act'd always as surgeon . . . he only act'd now and then when he happened to be here."

After the Northwest Company was absorbed by the Hudsons Bay Company in 1821, Dr. McLoughlin became celebrated as a fur trader and pioneer in the Pacific Northwest. He has been called "The Father of Oregon." The story of his life, "The Whiteheaded Eagle—John McLoughlin—Builder of an Empire," is much more interesting when the reader realizes that he got his start as a surgeon and fur trader in the wilds of northern Minnesota.

In 1826 Governor Cass of Michigan territory came to Fond du Lac to complete a treaty with the Indians. In his party were Henry Schoolcraft, Major McKenny, and Dr. Zina Pitcher of the U. S. Army, along with some soldiers and voyageurs.

Major McKenny[5] kept a diary, which was afterwards published, and in it he recorded the first medical case history within the present limits of Duluth. For July 31, 1826, Major McKenny writes: "I visited today, on the island, in company with Dr. Pitcher and our interpreter, an Indian girl who is afflicted with hemiplegia. About four months ago she was taken with a severe pain in the back of the neck, which, in turn, was soon followed by a complete paralysis of the left half of the body and entire loss of sensibility of the optic nerve, a total amaurosis." This liberal use of medical terminology is explained when the author states that these details were given him by Dr. Pitcher, who made a very careful study of the case. Three days later the doctor applied a cup to the back of the neck: "The blood was very sluggish and dark but the pain was somewhat relieved." The same evening there was further cupping to the right temple and on the following morning cupping to the left temple: "Here the blood flowed more freely and was brighter in color." Food, bedding and better care helped to improve the patient so much that, when the expedition left on August tenth, the doctor was able to report that "there was every prospect of the patient recovering completely, except that her blindness must remain." Dr. Pitcher served in the army from

1819 to 1836, when he located in Detroit, and became well known in state medical affairs.

In 1832 Schoolcraft undertook an expedition to find the source of the Mississippi, and was accompanied by Dr. Douglass Houghton and Lieut. Allen of the army, along with a small detachment of soldiers and voyageurs. Dr. Houghton, in addition to his duties as surgeon, was to vaccinate the Indians along the route and make botanical and geologic observations. At Fond du Lac, which is within the present city limits of Duluth, Dr. Houghton vaccinated two hundred and forty-three Indians. He writes: "In nearly every instance the opportunity which was presented for vaccination was embraced with cheerfulness and apparent gratitude. The efficacy of the vaccine was well appreciated even by the most interior of the Chippewa Indians." No doubt the Indians of that period were well aware of the terrible scourge of smallpox which occurred at Fond du Lac in 1782. Dr. Houghton later became well known in Michigan. He was a practising physician in Detroit; the first state geologist; mayor of Detroit in 1842; a professor in the state university. In 1845, while employed on a government survey, he was drowned in Lake Superior.

The expedition of 1832 made two notable contributions: first, it was successful in discovering the source of the Mississippi; second, the report of Lieut. Allen[1] to the War Department contains an episode which is of interest in that it is probably the first "compensation case" recorded in what is now Minnesota.

The portage above Fond du Lac, which was also called "Grand Portage," was a very difficult one. Today, in driving through Jay Cooke Park, one can visualize the hazards in carrying canoes and provisions over the nine miles of rough country. It was on this portage that a soldier named Beemis, while climbing up the steep river bank fell, with a keg of pork on his shoulder, and injured his back. Beemis was kept in the hospital for more than a year after his return to civilization, and subsequently discharged at Fort Dearborn (Chicago) on a surgeon's certificate of disability.

There were, no doubt, many other medical men of this period who traveled in northern Minnesota, but they left no record of their impressions or mark as physicians. On the first expedition of Governor Cass and Schoolcraft in 1820, a Dr. Alexander Wolcott[5] was surgeon. He was also Indian agent at Chicago, but it does not appear that he made any report of his work as surgeon of this expedition. At a later date, there is record of a young clerk, a physician, who was stationed at Leech Lake in 1833-34, in the employ of a fur trader. In "Letters on the Fur Trade"[6] the following is of interest:

"My companion for the winter is a clerk; a hot headed Irishman; who has received a liberal education; and was by profession a physician, but he had turned all these advantages to his disadvantage. His art was used to gain the good will of the Indians, for they generally look up to such with a great deal of respect; and not a day passed without extracting teeth and bleeding, and our having a small quantity of medicine which was freely administered to all who applied for it; and the dread and respect they have for medicine men, naturally drew respect from them, and they formed the opinion that our medicines were combined, the white and Indian together. Everything aided to win the respect and esteem of our Indian friends; and my companion, being an excellent musician, we had the means of soothing their savage breasts, although frequently there was only two strings to the violin."

The last of the doctors of the fur trading period in this locality was Charles William Wulff Borup, who for many years was the only trained physician west of the Sault Ste. Marie and north of Fort Snelling. Dr. Borup was born in 1806 in Copenhagen, Denmark, where he received a thorough classical and medical education. He came to the United States in 1828, and was employed by the American Fur Company in 1834, in which he eventually became chief agent on Lake Superior. His headquarters were at La Pointe, although he traveled extensively along the south shore of Lake Superior, and as far west as Leech Lake. Although primarily engaged in fur trading, as were Munro and McLoughlin, Dr. Borup kept up his interest in the practice of medicine, as the records of the American Fur Company will show. He was a subscriber to the *American Medical Journal,* which was sent to him from Philadelphia via the Erie Canal and the Great Lakes to the Sault, there by canoe to his post on the south shore of Lake Superior or on the St. Croix. His order to the New York office of the American Fur Company for February 28, 1835, called for:

> "1 good tooth drawer
> 1 dz. bougies in set
> 1 lb. camphor
> 2 ounces Quicksilver
> ¼ lb. cantharides in powder
> I ounce sulphur antim. praecepitatum
> 1 pint spiritus Pennyroyal
> ·½ ounce aleum caryophyl
> 1 bottle Carpenter's Compounded Syrup of Liverwort
> 2 Gross vials assorted with corks"
> and other similar items

On May 11, 1841, he writes:

> "I wish to purchase a newly invented instrument (if it may be called so), the intention of which is preventing the cold air from affecting the lungs. It consists in a kind of mouth covering, furnished inside with metallic springs, through which the air is drawn into the lungs. It is to be had in the principal apothecary shops in Broadway . . . there are two kinds, one for ladies and one for gentlemen."

Dr. Borup settled permanently in St. Paul in 1848, where he died of heart disease on July 6, 1859.

Bibliography

1. ALLEN, LT.: Doc. No. 323, 23d Congress, 1st Session, House of Repr., War Dept.
2. COUES: New Light on the Early History of the Greater Northwest. The Henry-Thompson Journals.
3. DYE, EVA EMERY: McLoughlin and Old Oregon. Ithaca, N. Y., 1926.
4. ELLIOTT, T. C.: John McLoughlin, M.D. Oregon Historical Journal, Vol. 36 and 37.
5. MCKENNY: A Tour to the Lakes 1826.
6. SCHOOLCRAFT: Narrature Journal of Travels, 1820.
7. SCHOOLCRAFT, HENRY R.: Narrative of an Expedition through the Upper Mississippi to Itasca Lake in 1832, p. 250.
   WALLACE: Documents relating to the Northwest Company, p. 488.
8. WARREN, WM. W.: History of Ojibways. Minn. Historical Collections, Vol. V, p. 256.

(To be continued in March, 1938 issue)

EDITORIAL

MINNESOTA MEDICINE

OFFICIAL JOURNAL OF THE MINNESOTA STATE MEDICAL
ASSOCIATION

Published by the Association under the direction of its Editing
and Publishing Committee

EDITING AND PUBLISHING COMMITTEE

J. T. CHRISTISON, Saint Paul   C. B. WRIGHT, Minneapolis
E. M. HAMMES, Saint Paul   T. A. PEPPARD, Minneapolis
WALTMAN WALTERS, Rochester

EDITORIAL STAFF

CARL B. DRAKE, Saint Paul, Editor
W. F. BRAASCH, Rochester, Associate Editor
GILBERT COTTAM, Minneapolis, Associate Editor

Annual Subscription—$3.00.   Single Copies—$0.40
Foreign Subscriptions—$3.50.

The right is reserved to reject material submitted for editorial
or advertising columns. The Editing and Publishing Committee
does not hold itself responsible for views expressed either in
editorials or other articles when signed by the author.

Classified advertising—five cents a word; minimum charge,
$1.00. Remittance should accompany order.

Display advertising rates on request.

Address all communications to Minnesota Medicine, 2642 University Avenue, Saint Paul, or Suite 604, National Bldg., Minneapolis. Telephone: Nestor 2641.

BUSINESS MANAGER
J. R. BRUCE

Volume 21   FEBRUARY, 1938   Number 2

Smallpox in Minnesota

MINNESOTA has been experiencing an increase in the usual number of cases of
smallpox, which in the past two months has
reached the status of a mild epidemic in certain quarters. From the fourth of December
until the middle of January, about one-half
(149) the total number of cases reported (286)
had occurred in Saint Paul with Clay, Pine,
Yellow Medicine and Lac qui Parle Counties
suffering next in the order mentioned. Strange
to state, during this six weeks' period no case
was reported from Minneapolis and only one
from Duluth. This is quite the opposite of
what occurred in 1924 when a laborer from
Canada, suffering from malignant smallpox,

started an epidemic in Duluth. Minneapolis
was severely affected that year and Saint Paul
but little. There were 307 deaths from smallpox in the state in 1924, and 198 deaths in 1925.
So far, fortunately, there have been no deaths
in Saint Paul from the disease.

Each year there are a certain number of cases
of smallpox in Minnesota. In 1935 there were
284, in 1936 there were 397, and in 1937 a total
of 665. The increase in 1937 was noticeable
throughout the last nine months of the year, and
particularly in December.

The increase in cases over last year holds true
for the country at large. Reports show that this
increase has taken place for the most part in
the central and north central states and in those
states west of Minnesota as far as the Pacific
Ocean.

Certain states, notably Massachusetts, have
compulsory vaccination laws. Most of our states
are content to await the arrival of an epidemic,
when regulations requiring vaccination for attendance at school act virtually as a compulsory
requirement and stimulates general vaccination.
In the interim between epidemics the public
becomes lax and the soil becomes fertile for
another epidemic.

While smallpox can be almost entirely prevented by vaccination, it is not generally appreciated that a certain number of cases develop in
individuals who have been successfully vaccinated. In 1924, for instance, there were in
Minnesota 327 cases of smallpox with forty-
seven fatalities in individuals who had been successfully vaccinated more than seven years previous to their infection. The importance of revaccination every seven years is therefore demonstrated.

Incidence of Syphilis

AN ACCURATE determination of the prevalence of syphilitic infection is admitted
difficult. However, some of the statements
which have appeared recently in magazine articles are gross exaggerations. In articles which
appeared in the *Readers' Digest* last year, Pari
ran referred to syphilis as our No. 1 American

killer, and Stokes stated that the disease ranks high if not first among causes of death in this country. In the *Pictorial Review*, Maxine Davis referred to syphilis as the greatest killer of the day, and stated that the leading authorities say that three million sufferers stand in need of treatment each year. Certainly statistics, inaccurate though they may be, do not substantiate such statements.

Studies undertaken by the American Social Hygiene Association and the United States Public Health Service have shown that approximately half a million individuals seek treatment each year and that about 68,300 cases of syphilis are under treatment at any one time. This corresponds to the number of new cases tabulated by the various State Boards of Health, which amount to about half a million. Positive Wassermann reports not designated repeats are considered new cases, but we suspect all such cases are not new because of inaccuracy on the part of reporting physicians. On the other hand many individuals contract the disease unwittingly, resort to drug store medication or seek the services of irregular practitioners and are not recorded. One estimate, that this group of unreported cases amounts to double the number recorded, we consider a rash overstatement. This may have been true years ago, but the number of individuals who seek advice as to the presence of the infection needlessly, incline us to believe that the number of undetected cases does not nearly equal those recorded.

Surveys of various groups have shown a variation from 1 to 25 per cent in positive Wassermann reactions. According to Snow, 5 per cent is probably a conservative estimate for the population as a whole. New infections reach their peak in the age group from twenty to twenty-five and half the infections occur between twenty and thirty years of age. According to the Metropolitan Life Insurance Company, their mortality from syphilis is four and a half times as great in colored as in white males, and six times as great in colored as in white females.

What can be said of the incidence of syphilis in Minnesota? A few years ago 5,000 students at the University were examined and only ten positive Wassermann tests were obtained (0.2 per cent). This, of course, was a selected group

and one which had not gone far into the age period when the incidence of infection reaches its peak.

According to the Census Bureau, about six per 100,000 of population died yearly from syphilis in Minnesota during the period of 1932 to 1936. During those same years about 130 died each year from cancer and from 197 to 251 each year from heart disease. To make the comparison more striking, the total deaths in the state of Minnesota in 1936 attributed to syphilis were 162 compared with 3,519 due to cancer, and 6,619 due to heart disease. Allowing considerable leeway for errors in reporting, syphilis is far from heading the list of killers in Minnesota. As a matter of fact, it ranks about eleventh in the nation as a whole.

Minnesota was one of the first states to institute a program to fight venereal disease. In 1918 the activities instituted in connection with the war to control the disease were made permanent. Syphilis was made reportable and free Wassermann testing was provided by the State Board of Health. The foundations laid twenty years ago for what is today considered essential to venereal control. It is safe to conclude that there has been no falling off in the reporting of new cases to the State Board of Health in recent years as the number of Wassermann tests performed by the State has shown a steady increase until 83,000 were made in 1936. That syphilis in Minnesota is on the decline is shown by the fact that in 1925, 5,147 new cases were reported and in 1936 only 3,379. This is in keeping with the steady decline in deaths among white policyholders from 1923 to 1930 reported by the Metropolitan Life Insurance Company, a reduction which has been maintained since 1930.

Syphilis, then, is not so serious as a cause of death, as has been stated. It is, however, among the leaders as a cause of human misery. Syphilis in its congenital form, as the cause of heart disease and central nervous system disease and, fully as important, the rôle it plays as a destroyer of the home, places it in the front ranks of the enemies of mankind. If the recent publicity campaign serves to further early diagnosis and treatment, it will have been worth while.

MEDICAL ECONOMICS

Edited by the Committee on Medical Economics
of the
Minnesota State Medical Association

B. J. Branton, M. D.   W. F. Braasch, M. D., Chairman   J. C. Michael, M. D.
L. H. Rutledge, M. D.   A. N. Collins, M. D.

New Deductions for Doctors

At the request of the State Medical Association, the Minnesota Tax Commission has reviewed the deductions allowed physicians in making out state income tax returns.

The result of this review is a new ruling made by the Commission, Jan. 21, 1938. According to this ruling, physicians may make the same reduction in their state income taxes, for expenses incurred in attendance at medical meetings and in other postgraduate medical education, as are now allowed under the federal income tax.

Concurring in the ruling were H. E. Boyle, chairman; G. E. Wallace and G. F. Gage, members of the Commission, and W. G. Burkman, director.

A Recent Visit to Buenos Aires

Most of us North Americans have a vague idea of what is going on in the other half of our Siamese Twin south of Panama. South America has always seemed so remote that we never have given it much thought. What we know about it has been learned largely from news reels and movies, such as "Flying Down to Rio." A Cuban, Mexican, or South and Central American all looked alike to most of us, and we carelessly put them all in the same group. I am afraid that my idea of their level of culture, including medicine, was none too high before my recent visit to South America.

Comparatively few Americans from the north have visited the southern half of America in the past. In the year 1936, 12,000 tourists left the United States for South America and 250,000 for Europe. The number was increased last year, but even so, there are all too few. The greatest handicaps have been the distance of 5,000 miles

to Rio de Janeiro and 6,000 miles to Buer Aires, and slow, inadequate passenger boa This has been greatly overcome by the high efficient Pan-American Airways, and there v soon be better and faster boats. The number visitors from South America to the Uni States has doubled in recent years and in future will undoubtedly be even greater. Gr interest in the United States has been arous in South America by our movies, autos and dios, and they are bent on knowing us bett This is also true in medical circles.

Tide Has Turned

In the past physicians in the Latin-Americ countries have naturally gone to Europe graduate training. Since the Great War, and a result of the current unrest and disturbance Europe, the tide of graduate medical interest turned to North America. They are aware our advances in many fields of medicine and coming in rapidly increasing numbers to stu and learn. It is up to North American medic to be prepared to offer every opportunity to South American cousins.

Having received an invitation to attend a me ing of the Pan-American Urological Congres: Buenos Aires, after some hesitation I decided go and I am glad that I did. Although much ti is consumed in the voyage, the journey is m pleasant in every way.

When we finally docked one fine sumi morning in December at Buenos Aires, I was for a series of overwhelming surprises. In first place, I was fairly swept off my feet by generous hospitality of our hosts. Argentini are a wonderful people, virile and progress and they will undoubtedly be a large facto: the future development of South America. T are inordinately proud of their great city

Buenos Aires and the vast resources of Argentina, and rightfully so.

Melting Pot

Let us first glance at Argentina, which has an area of one-third that of the United States, extending some 3,000 miles from Terra del Fuego to a few degrees below the equator, having both an antarctic and subtropical climate, at either end. It has some 13,000,000 inhabitants—almost entirely white—made up of Spanish, with some mixture of Irish, Scotch, British and Indian, who were the early inhabitants. In the last twenty years these were augmented by millions of Italians, Germans and other European immigrants. It is even more of a melting pot than the United States. It is surprising to note how quickly most of the immigrants and all of their children adopt the Argentinian ways, speak Spanish, and become intense patriots of Argentina. Their main resources and wealth lie in the millions of acres of pampas lands, with soil so rich that fertilizing is quite unnecessary. The millions of cattle and the great wheat fields are turned to gold, so that Argentina knows no depression and no unemployment.

Their great capital, Buenos Aires, is a vast city of some 3,000,000 people. With its beautiful buildings, great squares and wide boulevards, wonderful parks and playgrounds, it is one of the most beautiful cities in the world. The Paris of South America, it has been called. It might be almost as appropriate to say that Paris is the Buenos Aires of Europe.

Standards are High

As far as the medical status of Buenos Aires is concerned, I was surprised at the high standards of medical care in that great city. The leaders of the medical profession are well informed, progressive, intelligent and alert to recent developments. Among the many outstanding men of medicine who have received international attention may be mentioned Chutro, Arce, Finochietto and Gutierrez in surgery; Castex, Boneo and Roffo in medicine; Valls in orthopedic surgery, and Saraleguy in roentgenology. Among the various scientists engaged in premedical work is Houssay, head of the University Institute of Physiology. This great scientist has done outstanding work in physiological investigation on

the influence of the pituitary on the pancreas and their interrelationship with the hormones of other endocrine glands. Among the honors he has received is an LL.D. from Harvard last year.

The work of Roffo in regard to the cause of cancer has attracted considerable attention. He thinks he has proved that tobacco is a direct cause.

Medicine in Buenos Aires centers around the great medical school. A vast new building with teaching hospitals is in the course of erection, which will cost $10,000,000. It will be the last word in construction to facilitate modern methods of medical instruction. The standards of education are high.

There are three other large medical schools in Argentina, at La Plata, Rosario and Cordova. These, together with the university at Buenos Aires, graduate some 2,000 students annually. Since a large portion of the public is able to pay very little for medical services, the economic opportunities for the recent graduate are none too good.

Vast National Resources

The economic status of the inhabitants of Buenos Aires, as well as of all South America, is somewhat comparable to that observed in France, Italy and other Latin states. Although the natural resources are vast beyond description, they are undeveloped and as a result the opportunities for earning a livelihood are inadequate. Therefore, labor is cheap and there is a large class, in proportion to the population, which is underpaid and living on very little. Fortunately, climatic conditions are favorable and the bare necessities can be obtained for comparatively little. Since the low income group makes up a large proportion of the population, medical practice is necessarily adjusted accordingly. Many of the people are able to pay but little for clinical care and even less for hospitalization, and the government is forced to care for them. As a result, most of the hospitals are charity institutions. Private hospitals, or sanatoria, as they are called, are few in number and inadequate. Although many of the government hospitals are well conducted and the medical services are adequate, the medical and nursing care in most cases would hardly meet the demands of the average citizen of the United States.

Government Medicine

In some of the institutions controlled by the government the service is either inadequate or extravagant. As an illustration of the inefficiency of government control, an institution was erected by the city to take care of roentgenographic diagnosis and radiotherapy for all the hospitals and dispensaries. The institute is controlled by a competent and excellent roentgenographer. However, his assistants, appointed by the government, fail to coöperate with him and as a result there is considerable confusion and the service is often unsatisfactory. On the top floors of the building, which was completed some seven years ago, there are wards with seventy-two beds, fully equipped for radium treatment, but for various reasons means have not been found to employ the two grams of radium which is available. As a result, these wards are taken care of—dusted and cleaned every day, but no patient has ever appeared. On the same floor there is a beautifully equipped room to be used as a library, and the shelves have been bare these seven years because no books have been provided. There could be no more striking illustration of the fallacy of government medicine.

The hospitals are for the most part old and built in the pavilion style. The Rawson Hospital, recently erected, is a fine example of a well equipped hospital, having more than 2,000 beds. Many new hospitals are being planned or are in the course of construction to take the place of those which are old and inadequate. The hospitals are of three types, federal, municipal, and private. The federal hospitals are largely for the care of patients with chronic illness, and, in particular, female patients and children. They are controlled by a national committee composed of fifty women. These institutions are supported largely by proceeds of the Federal Lottery. Fifty per cent of total earnings are devoted to this charitable purpose. This sum is augmented by 10 per cent of the proceeds of the Jockey Club, derived from wagering on the horse races. Since the passion for gambling is prominent in the Latin soul, the Argentinian government believes that it is best controlled by giving it legitimate opportunities for gratification. Since the government derives enormous profits and the public is satisfied, this solution of the problem of hospital support is a very happy one. In fact, one wonders if

it could not be adopted in succoring the financial anemia of some of our hospitals.

Tuberculosis Care Thorough

There is a large neurological institute which has an outstanding staff of scientific investigators. The care of pulmonary tuberculosis is on a large scale and is very thorough. A surprisingly large number of patients are subjected to phrenectomy, pneumothorax and thoracoplasty.

One criticism which I heard several of the clinicians make was that the clinical material in the various hospitals was divided into so many separate services that the amount in each service was limited to such an extent that the possibilities for clinical investigation were scarce.

Although the government has a very paternalistic attitude toward the medical indigent, no definite attempt has been made to set up state medicine as it exists in many of the European countries. The medical profession is not as closely organized as we are in our own country, but they have been able to exert considerable influence in a personal way and do not seem to fear the European form of state medicine. Some of the profession claim that investigation as to the ability of the patient to pay is very lax. There is comparatively little social service work being done there, although plans are being made to develop this field in the future.

The majority of the medical profession as a whole could be said to compare favorably with our own. There is a great desire for graduate training and in the future we will undoubtedly see many Argentinians visiting our clinics and attending medical meetings in North America. We should extend to them every available encouragement and coöperate with them to our fullest ability.

* * *

I have not referred to the short visit I made in Rio de Janeiro and Sao Paulo in Brazil, and to Montevideo in Uruguay. Sufficient time was not available for a thorough study of medical conditions.

In closing I can heartily recommend a trip to South America as being a most enjoyable and interesting one, and in many respects more instructive than a visit to Europe.

W. F. Braasch

132

Malpractice? Supreme Court Says "No"!

The Supreme Court of Minnesota has recently decided a malpractice case that we are sure will interest the medical profession. The opinion was written by the Honorable Harry H. Peterson, Associate Justice, and held that the plaintiff could not recover in that particular case.

The plaintiff sued a number of physicians in Minneapolis for malpractice, following a severe injury sustained in an automobile accident. The plaintiff suffered a fracture of the femur of the right leg which, as the Court pointed out, "is a very severe bone injury." The plaintiff suffered some discomfort and pain and a pressure sore on the heel from the cast. This work was done between December and the following March. Along in June of the same year the plaintiff developed an infection in the great toe on the right foot, resulting in amputation of a part of the toe.

Justice Peterson, in his opinion, stated that it was admitted that the defendants possessed the requisite skill and learning as physicians and surgeons. The question before the Court was whether or not they were negligent in applying their skill and learning in this particular case. The opinion points out that there was a total absence of any evidence that the practice by the defendants was not in accord with the usual and accepted medical standards. The opinion further points out that

"the highest degree of care was exercised in applying the cast and that notwithstanding such care in this case, as often happens in other cases, pressure sores unavoidably develop."

The Court held that a physician is not liable for injuries unavoidably resulting in spite of the exercise of due care, the Court pointing out:

"A physician or surgeon is only required to possess and exercise the degree of skill and learning ordinarily possessed by members of his school of the profession in good standing, and to apply that skill and learning with reasonable care and diligence and his best judgment."

The opinion further states that the defendants are not liable unless the plaintiff proves that the injuries complained of were the proximate result of negligent acts on the part of the physicians. The Court pointed out that the injuries, other than the heel sore and the pain resulting therefrom, and the stiffness in the leg, did not result from the treatment of the bone fracture; that the plaintiff was suffering from arthritis when he was admitted to the hospital. After the plaintiff failed in his proof of the charge of malpractice he advanced the theory of a technical assault and battery because the second cast was not put on the way the plaintiff thought it should be put on. The Court held that where a plaintiff proceeds against a physician on the basis of negligence and the matter is submitted to the Court upon that issue, he cannot thereafter, in a motion for a new trial, raise, for the first time, the question of assault and battery.

The decision of the Supreme Court was unanimous and the opinion written by Justice Peterson shows, very clearly, that the entire matter received the close scrutiny of the Court. The opinion contains many citations of other cases and a thorough discussion of the most minute details of the present case. A careful reading of the opinion indicates that same malpractice suits are instituted even though the facts and the law show, rather definitely, the absence of merit in the law suit.

This case was first tried in the District Court of Hennepin County before the Honorable Arthur W. Selover, Judge, and a jury. After hearing the evidence, Judge Selover was of the opinion that the plaintiff had not proved any malpractice against the defendants and consequently directed the jury to bring in a verdict for the physicians.

NOTE: Justice Peterson will be remembered by many members of the medical profession as an efficient and aggressive Attorney General of the State of Minnesota from 1933 until his appointment to the Supreme Court in December, 1936.

The Lay Demand For Medical Publicity

The medical Box of Pandora has been opened to the prying eyes of the laity and its medical secrets are now making the front page. It is difficult to pick up a magazine today which does not contain an article pertaining to some phase of medicine.

When one reflects on the publicity given by the daily press alone, often in screaming headlines and written in sensational style, with its exaggerations and distortions of half-truths, one wonders if the old way of thinking would not be best for all concerned. While information concerning disease in certain fields may be of benefit to the public welfare, unless the subjects are carefully selected and written up by competent medical authorities, resulting misinformation may to a great extent overcome any good which might come from such publicity.

By Incompetent Writers

Unfortunately, many articles now flooding the periodicals are written by incompetent lay writers and in some instances by an incompetent medico. Under the guise of giving information to the layman, who has been "kept in abysmal ignorance throughout the ages," a choice lot of balderdash is being dished out to the gullible public. By using catch phrases and playing up sex features, popular interest is attracted and much of the misrepresentation and distortion of facts is believed. Some of these articles will have sensational headlines or illustrations which suggest criticism or inadequacy of the present methods of medical care. In some cases the substance of the article will correct this to some extent, but the casual reader will retain only the superficial impression.

Dressed Up to Catch the Eye

As an example of misinformation which is even worse than the secrecy of yore, attention is called to an article on prostatic disease which appears in the current issue of *Pictorial Review*. Written by a layman and dressed up to catch the public eye, it contains many statements which are controversial and far from exact. To give the article an air of authenticity, it quotes liberally from a well known authority on prostatic disease, so editing his remarks as to substantiate the text of the article. This may well serve as a warning to our profession to beware of the magazine interviewer and to inquire as to the purpose and scope of the proposed article. Circumstances may be such that a request by authorized reporters for information regarding

134

medical subjects should be granted.] wise always to insist on editing the c(publication, and not to contribute p oneself in the course of an operation nation.

Many similar articles can be cited. sult of the mass of misinformation, probably will be more confused than fore the campaign was started. should be done about this.

Relief Clients May Choo
Aufderheide

The month of January brought neg(many counties about medical relief fo

In several, commissioners and boar fare disagreed with representatives of as to the meaning of the clause in the] that provides "choice of vendor" to rel providing the vendor lives up to regul qualifications.

The meaning of the law is clear. Relief Administration properly interp refer to vendors of services as well a: and will enforce that interpretation county that receives aid from the sta dle its relief problem.

In complying with this law it make: ence how individual counties allo funds. They may choose to declare tl relief bills are paid out of local fur hope to evade the law; but relief adn do not recognize such distinctions an pared to refuse state aid to offending

To Send Bulletin

A bulletin to this effect will go from Mr. Herman D. Aufderheide, S Administrator.

Unfortunately the relief departmei feel that it can make the same demai ment of the fees called for by the offic fee schedule.

Fees Another Story

Mr. Aufderheide says that funds fees are adequate. The fees should I he cannot enforce payment. In seve certain modifications have been mad

ence between physician representatives of local societies and the county commissioners or welfare boards. In case of disagreement it appears to be a problem that can be settled only in such conferences. Happily the full schedule is being paid without question in many other counties. A questionnaire is going out from the State Office soon to every county in the state to find out exactly how satisfactory relief arrangements are in Minnesota.

Keener Vision

(Monthly Editorial by the Medical Advisory Committee)

An advertisement in a lay magazine advises that squinting, frowning, or scowling when using the eyes is usually an indication that the eyes need attention, better light, or both. Webster defines these words as follows:

To squint: to have the vision distorted.
To frown: to contract the brows in displeasure.
To scowl: to look sullen or angry.

The need of clearer vision and keener insight into the other man's problems has never been more apparent than in the cases reviewed by your Medical Advisory Committee during the last year.

The squint, the frown, the scowl each have a degree of meaning to the observant person. As the dissatisfied patient of another doctor hangs on every word of his present consultant, so he sees and registers every expression of pleasure or displeasure on the consultant's face.

The average consultant before a malpractice suit does not see the patient until several months after the original injury complained of. Therefore, before giving a positive opinion by look or word, would it not be advisable to obtain all the light possible on the case as procured by the first man, even to the point of a telephone call or personal interview with him?

An hour spent in the study of psychology and economics in the handling of patients could well become a part of every medical man's day.

Visiting President

Mrs. Augustus S. Kech of Altoona, Pennsylvania, is national president of the Women's Aux-

iliary and legislative representative and advisor of the Pennsylvania State Medical Society.

She visited the Twin Cities recently, talked to the Ramsey and Hennepin County auxiliaries, to a group of officers of the Minnesota State Medical Association, proved to everybody who met her that she is a person of unique charm, energy and a remarkable grasp of the political and economic problems of medicine.

Pennsylvania's Troubles

What she told the doctors about the difficulties of the Pennsylvania soicety in handling its cult problem was of especial interest to Minnesota.

Said Mrs. Kech in substance:

There is a Medical Practice Act in Pennsylvania; but it is not enforced. The result is that approximately 200 chiropractors are licensed under the Act and 2,700 are practicing without licenses and in defiance of the law.

(Compare these figures with Minnesota figures for chiropractors under the Basic Science Law, 1927 to 1937. In April, 1927, 592 were registered. Since then thirteen have passed the Basic Science examinations and three have registered by previous licensure. In 1937, however, only 398 were registered and any chiropractor who attempts to practice without a license is subject to prompt prosecution for violation of the law.)

The 2,900 chiropractors in Pennsylvania were assessed $100 each for legislation last year.

That produced a fund of approximately $300,-000 for the chiropractors alone last year.

To combat it, the Pennsylvania Medical Society secured the services of twenty lay speakers, trained them and sent them out to talk to every group in the state, from the smallest sewing circle of ten persons to large public gatherings.

Every one of 141 cult bills was killed as a result of this intensive work, and in spite of the fact that the lower house of the Pennsylvania legislature was so organized that it was impossible for the physicians to work with it.

Auxiliary Help

The Auxiliary helped greatly by clipping newspapers and periodicals throughout the state for editorials, news stories, items of interest that bore in any way upon medicine or the legislative situation.

Minnesota State Board of Medical Examiners

Minneapolis Woman Sentenced to Five to Twenty Years at Hard Labor

Re: State of Minnesota vs. Myrtle L. Brandenburg. Myrtle L. Brandenburg, who holds no license to practice any form of healing in the State of Minnesota, entered a plea of guilty on January 6, 1938, in the District Court of Hennepin County to an indictment charging her with manslaughter in the first degree. The defendant was sentenced by the Honorable Levi M. Hall, Judge of the District Court, to a term of five to twenty years at hard labor in the Women's Reformatory at Shakopee.

Mrs. Brandenburg, who stated she was thirty-seven years of age, and the mother of three children, performed a criminal abortion on a twenty-seven years old married woman who died from the effects of the abortion on November 23, 1937. The defendant resided at 664 Fourth Avenue, Northeast, Minneapolis, and has been under suspicion for some time for being in this type of criminal work. She admitted that she had performed other abortions, stating that she received $25.00 apiece for a few of them, but that most of the time she received from $5.00 to $10.00 per abortion. She also was practicing medicine unlawfully by furnishing pills and other medicines to the patients. She used a chromium plated catheter and elm bark as her chief weapons, and these were found by Minneapolis policewomen, hidden in the radio in the Brandenburg home. Mrs. Brandenburg has had no medical training of any kind. This case again illustrates the terrific penalty paid by lay people who go to quacks who have no knowledge of anatomy or of the absolute necessity of sterile conditions. The prompt and effective disposition of the case is due, in great part, to the splendid work done by the Women's Bureau of the Minneapolis Police Department and the coöperation shown by the Coroner's office under Dr. Gilbert Seashore, and the County Attorney's office. The imposition of this sentence by Judge Hall should be a warning to a number of individuals in Minneapolis that the law does catch up to them and that the penalty can be made quite severe.

Distribution of Smallpox Vaccine

So far as very limited funds will permit, smallpox vaccine will be distributed for use in school or other public vaccination projects, the plans for which have been approved by the County or District Medical Society, and particularly in districts where smallpox has appeared. Requests for vaccine should be accompanied with a statement of facts and that the County Society approves the plans. The date on which the vaccinating is to be done and the number of persons to be vaccinated should be given.

It is important for all group immunizations, or in any case where the parents are not present, that the written consent of the parents be first obtained. Cards for such purpose will be furnished by this Department on request. Only as much vaccine as is immediately needed should be asked for and any unused tubes promptly returned.

The funds available for the purchase of vaccine are quite small. Vaccine must be kept at all times in an icebox. Its potency is less than 90 days. This Department cannot get any credit for outdated tubes nor can outdated tubes be exchanged for fresh vaccine. So the purchase price of an unused and outdated tube is a total loss. In consideration of these facts and the money available, it does not seem possible to furnish vaccine to physicians for use in their regular routine private practice.

MINNESOTA STATE DEPARTMENT OF HEALTH.

Jn Memoriam

Charles Patrick Dolan
1858-1937

DR. CHARLES P. DOLAN died at his home in Worthington, December 23, 1937 at the age of eighty.

Dr. Dolan's parents were among the early settlers in Waseca County, having homesteaded there in 1858. On the old farm, where his parents lived continuously to ripe old age, Dr. Dolan was born September 8, 1858. After attending the county grammar schools, Dr. Dolan later graduated from the high school at Waterville.

Beginning with a year in the office of Dr. E. P. Case of Waterville, Dr. Dolan received his medical degree from the University of Iowa, Iowa City, in 1880 and took a year of postgraduate study at Bellevue Hospital, New York City. Beginning practice in Waterville, he moved to Worthington in 1904.

On January 25, 1888, Dr. Dolan married Tillie McElvoy, a native of Illinois. Two children, Leo Dolan of Worthington and Marie (Mrs. Howard Thrush) of East Chicago, Indiana, survive.

Dr. Dolan has been one of the leading physicians of Nobles County since 1904, when he moved to Worthington, taking over the practice of his brother, Dr. Edward Dolan, who died that year. He was the first president and charter member of the local Kiwanis Club, vice president and one of the original members of the Southwestern Minnesota Sanatorium commission, and for many years county coroner and health officer for Worthington. He owned a cabin in northern Minnesota where he loved to seek diversion in hunting and fishing. During his many years of service, he had endeared himself to his many friends and patients.

Frank Benjamin Hicks
1860-1937

THE death of Frank Benjamin Hicks, of Grand Marias, Minnesota, who passed away at University hospital, Minneapolis, August 21, 1937, marks the closing of a pioneer medical career, which has been compared by many to that of Dr. Wilfrid Grenfell of Labrador.

Born May 3, 1861, at Tomah, Wisconsin, the eldest son of Rev. and Mrs. William C. Hicks, he first chose the ministry as his career. Making his own way, he graduated from Beloit Academy and later received his B.A. from Beloit College. From there he went to the Chicago Theological Seminary, graduating with his B.D. degree in 1888.

During summer vacations, he supplied in missions in the then Dakota Territory. While there he met Miss Ethel M. Barnes, a school teacher, whom he married in

IN MEMORIAM

August, 1888. His pastorates were near Chicago, enabling him to study at the University of Chicago, where he took his M.A. and Ph.D. degrees in history.

A man of vision, he was a bit before his time in that he wished to develop reading and recreational centers in the church. All such activities were considered undignified and not a part of a clergyman's affair by most church fathers. Mr. Hicks finally decided he could do more good for humanity in the practice of medicine. So, with his wife and four small children, he gave up his prosperous church and took two small missions outside Chicago, having only $200 in cash assets.

Preaching Sunday mornings at Genoa Junction, Wisconsin, and in the evening at Richmond, his wife taking charge of the evening service in Genoa and the midweek prayer meeting, Mr. Hicks went to Rush Medical College, graduating with honors in June 1898, in debt but a little over one hundred dollars.

In October, 1898, Dr. Hicks moved to Washburn, Wisconsin, where he began the practice of medicine.

In 1906, he moved to Grand Marais, Minnesota, as physician for the lumber camps. At that time there were thousands of men in the lumber camps and he visited each camp once a month unless called oftener. He supplied hospital care for those who needed it. These trips were made with horses and bob sled, or on horseback. A trip to the camps required three days' time.

In 1907, he was appointed government physician for the Indians of that district, a post which he held until his death. Until the last years of his life, he was never off duty for illness but four days and in all those years his only vacation was one of three weeks' duration.

In those days, travel by road in summer time was practically impossible and he made his trips by way of his small motor-boat up and down the shore on treacherous Lake Superior, often having narrow escapes with his life. Trips inland were made as far as possible on horseback or driving himself. Then taking a canoe he would paddle across a lake, and with the canoe on his back, his medicine case in his hand, make a portage of from three-fourths of a mile to three miles, launch the canoe and paddle on. On one of his calls he made fourteen such portages. In the winter, he used dog teams. At another time, he walked fifty-eight miles to the bedside of a very sick and penniless woman. He brought hundreds of children into the world and in spite of the crude conditions he had to work under, never lost a mother. He often had to act as nurse as well as doctor. In a few instances, in the absence of another clergyman, he performed the burial service for those in out-of-the-way places, and on one occasion also during a smallpox epidemic when the clergyman refused to officiate. For twenty-five years he was the only doctor within a radius of ninety miles. The large lumber camps were there but two years and after that the greater part of his work was done for "love of humanity."

In 1913, he was appointed by Governor Eberhardt to the Minnesota State Board of Medical Examiners, a position which he held for several years, acting as president for one year.

When the coast guard was instituted at Grand Marais he was made their physician.

Everything he could do for public good he did gladly. Largely through his efforts a high school was established in Grand Marais. The Congregational Church there was founded by him and later he was an important factor in the "good roads" movement.

He was passionately fond of music and his hospitality was a by-word among all who knew him.

By his side a constant source of help and encouragement through all the years, stood his wife.

Dr. Hicks is survived by his widow and four children: Dr. Harvey R. Hicks of Grand Marais; Mrs. Hester Temple of Blue Earth; Mrs. Celia Valentine of Ely; and Mrs. Elizabeth Roberts of Cleveland, Ohio. Mrs. A. Tymeson, of Minneapolis, is a sister.

It may well be said that here was a life dedicated to "Service," where any who asked might receive.

Mineral Oil in Foods

The Council on Foods reports that it is well known that liquid petrolatum is not absorbed from the gastro-intestinal tract, and that it yields no calories. Because of these properties, mineral oil is extensively used in the treatment of constipation and, to a lesser extent, in replacing fat in certain foods, chiefly mayonnaise and salad dressings, and a few other products. According to published reports mineral oil interferes with the utilization of vitamin A by experimental animals. Later reports indicated that the ingestion of mineral oil resulted in a considerable loss of vitamin A to the animal organism if the oil was administered with the source of vitamin A but not if the mineral oil was given at some other time of the day. It was also brought out that different results could be expected with different sources of vitamin A. It is apparent that liquid petrolatum would be a poor vehicle for vitamin A and particularly for provitamin A, and its use in this connection could not be countenanced. On the other hand, it appears that in the amounts usually prescribed and under the conditions which should be observed (not to be taken at mealtime), the effect of liquid petrolatum on the absorption of vitamin A of the human diet probably is of little consequence. When incorporated in foods, however, so that the mineral oil is taken at mealtime, it is obvious that there is danger of interference with the absorption of the fat soluble vitamins. The Council on Foods therefore advises strongly against any indiscriminate dosage of mineral oil either alone or incorporated in special foods. (Jour. A.M.A., Nov. 27, 1937, p. 1814.)

OF GENERAL INTEREST

Dr. C. A. Scherer, of Duluth, has been reappointed county health officer.

* * *

Dr. A. L. Arends, of Askov, has moved to Sandstone, where he will practice medicine.

* * *

Dr. William L. Wall has opened an office in Anoka for the practice of medicine.

* * *

Dr. William Von Rohr Heise, son of Dr. and Mrs. W. F. C. Heise of Winona, has opened an office for the practice of medicine in Winona.

* * *

Dr. Arthur Neumaier, formerly on the staff of the Raiter Hospital and Clinic in Cloquet, has taken over the practice of Dr. C. P. Truog at Lindstrom.

* * *

Dr. Z. E. House and family, of Cass Lake, have returned from Florida, where they have spent some time. Dr. House will engage in private practice.

* * *

Dr. P. F. Meyer, of Faribault, has been reappointed county physician, health officer and member of the county board of health.

* * *

Dr. T. J. O'Leary, of Duluth, has been appointed president of the St. Mary's Hospital executive committee, by the governing Sister body.

* * *

Dr. J. E. Arnold, formerly of Miles City, Montana, has been appointed school doctor and village health officer of Mountain Iron.

* * *

Dr. E. J. West, who has been associated with the Arrowhead Clinic for the past ten years, has opened offices in Faribault for the general practice of medicine.

* * *

Dr. Kee Wakefield, of Minneapolis, formerly of Hutchinson, celebrated his ninety-fifth birthday on December 28.

* * *

Dr. E. V. Strand of Bayport recently returned from a trip East. Doctor Strand spent about six or seven weeks at the Polyclinic Hospital in New York.

* * *

Dr. C. T. Berger, formerly of Britt, Iowa, has opened an office in Blue Earth for the practice of medicine. Dr. Berger is a graduate of the University of Minnesota School of Medicine.

* * *

Dr. E. M. Jones, of Saint Paul, was the guest speaker at the regular meeting of the Washington County Medical Society on January 11. He spoke on "Abdominal Adhesions."

138

Dr. W. R. Bagley, of Duluth, who has been a ated with movements for the conservation of r resources in Minnesota and the Northwest, w dorsed for the 1937 Duluth American Legion H Fame by the West Duluth Business Men's Clu

* * *

Dr. Paul A. O'Leary, of Rochester, attende meeting of the Coöperative Clinical Group for Re in Syphilis, and a meeting of the syphilis commi National Research council held in Washington, early in January.

* * *

Dr. Ralph T. Knight, Minneapolis, has been app Director of the Division of Anesthesia at the U sity Hospital, and since December 1 has bee supervising the Department of Anesthesia a Charles T. Miller Hospital, Saint Paul.

* * *

Dr. H. I. Lillie, of Rochester, attended the meeting of the American Laryngological, Rhino and Otological Society in New York early in Ja He is president-elect of the Society and will att eastern section meeting of the organization in Ph phia.

* * *

Dr. Maurice B. Visscher, professor of physiol the University of Minnesota, was the principal s at a meeting of the Ramsey County Medical S held on December 27. The question of how phys cal methods and ideas can be applied to the prob a failing heart was discussed.

* * *

At a special meeting of the Wabasha County M Society held at Lake City on the evening of Jan Dr. Rudolph C. Logefiel of Minneapolis delive illustrated address on "Gastric Diseases and the the Gastroscope," with demonstrations of the i instrument.

* * *

There are a few vacancies at present and in p for duty with the CCC in this military district medical service is rendered by Reserve Officers civilian physicians, who enter into contract w Surgeon, Seventh Corps Area, who may be ad at the Federal Building, Omaha, Nebraska.

* * *

The Interurban Academy of Medicine met in on January 19. Dr. Russell Best of Omaha, Ne spoke on "Some Newer Surgical Aspects of the Tract," and motion pictures showing various ph arterial sclerotic heart disease and changes stages of development were presented by Dr Clement and R. L. Nelson, both of Duluth.

* * *

The Milwaukee Sanitarium announces the a ment of Dr. Lloyd H. Ziegler as Associate Med

MINNESOTA M

rector. Dr. Ziegler received his M.D. degree at the University of Minnesota, and was formerly staff consultant in neurology and psychiatry at the Mayo Clinic. He has studied clinical methods extensively in this country and abroad.

* * *

A Division of Neurosurgery in the Department of Surgery was established last summer at the University Medical School with Dr. William T. Peyton, Associate Professor of Surgery, as Director. The other staff members appointed to the Division were: Dr. J. Frank Corbett, clinical professor; Dr. A. A. Zierold, clinical professor; Dr. George R. Dunn, clinical assistant professor, and Dr. Wallace P. Ritchie, clinical assistant.

* * *

Dr. Charles K. Petter, formerly at Glen Lake Sanatorium, Oak Terrace, Minnesota, has moved to Waukegan, Illinois, where he is the Medical Director of the Lake County Tuberculosis Sanatorium Board. The Lake County Tuberculosis Sanatorium Board expects to begin the construction of a new sanatorium in the spring, and Dr. Petter will be the director of that institution.

* * *

Dr. Louis E. Jones, physician in charge at the St. Croixdale Sanatorium, passed away early in January. He was a graduate of Brown University, and received his M.D. degree at the University of Minnesota in 1924. He served his internship at St. Barnabas and University Hospitals. Dr. Jones has practiced continuously at Prescott, Wisconsin, where, in 1925, he opened the hospital which later became known as St. Croixdale Sanatorium. Dr. Jones was thirty-nine years of age, unmarried, and is survived by his mother and sister.

* * *

Dr. and Mrs. H. P. Wagener and Dr. and Mrs. Norman M. Keith, of Rochester, have returned from Europe. Dr. Wagener and Dr. Keith were delegates to the International Congress of Ophthalmology, held in Cairo, Egypt. Because of illness, Dr. Keith was obliged to remain in Amsterdam while Dr. Wagener continued the journey to Cairo, where he presented a paper by himself and Dr. Keith. Dr. Wagener also conducted a symposium on the relation of high blood pressure to the eye, and the general nature and connection between the two. He visited several eye hospitals in Egypt, where the principal problem is the treatment and prevention of trachoma.

* * *

The thirty-fourth annual Congress on Medical Education and Licensure will be held at the Palmer House, Chicago, February 14 and 15. The first day will be devoted to a report of the Council on Medical Education and Hospitals with papers covering general subjects pertaining to licensure, medical examining boards, curricula in medical schools, limitation of student enrolment. On Tuesday morning a symposium on Graduate Medical Education will be presented. At a joint session of the Council on Medical Education and Hospitals and the Federation of State Medical Boards, Tuesday afternoon, a symposium on Promulgation of Regulations Authorized by Law will be presented.

___

Special Convention Tour

The thought that the forthcoming A.M.A. Convention in San Francisco, June 13 to 17, is a splendid opportunity for a tour of the United States both going out and coming back, has inspired definite action. The coöperation of more than twenty-five state medical societies has made it possible to arrange a special train tour which will include the Indian Detour, the Grand Canyon, Los Angeles, Riverside and Santa Catalina Island—on the way out to San Francisco. A choice of two return routes is possible, one of which visits the cities of Portland, Seattle, Victoria and Vancouver and the scenic spots of the Canadian Rockies; the second route travels via Yellowstone National Park, Salt Lake City, Royal Gorge, Colorado Springs, and Denver.

There is an all-inclusive price for this tour which includes transportation from home town to home town, though the tour starts officially at Chicago, on Monday, June 6, from which point an American Express escort will join the group, as this travel company has been appointed transportation agent and the business details of the trip are in their hands.

Further information concerning the tour may be found elsewhere in this issue.

___

Sigma Xi Lecture Series

"Man and His Diet" will be the general subject of the eleventh annual lecture series by members of the University of Minnesota faculty given under the auspices of the Sigma Xi honorary scientific society this month.

The lectures will be given at 8:15 o'clock each Friday evening in Northrop Memorial Auditorium and will include the following speakers:

February 4—"The Fundamentals of Nutrition"
    Dr. LeRoy S. Palmer, Professor of Agricultural Biochemistry, University Minnesota

February 11—"The Feeding of the Child"
    Dr. Chester A. Stewart, Clinical Professor of Pediatrics, University of Minnesota

February 18—"Fads, Fancies and Fallacies in Adult Diets"
    Dr. R. M. Wilder, Professor of Medicine and Chief of Department of Medicine, Mayo Foundation, University of Minnesota

February 25—"The Food Industries of Minnesota"
    Dr. Clyde H. Bailey, Professor of Agricultural Biochemistry, University of Minnesota

Preceding each lecture a half hour's program of music will be given by the University Symphony Orchestra under the direction of Professor Abe Pepinsky.

REPORTS and ANNOUNCEMENTS

MINNESOTA HOSPITAL ASSOCIATION

The 15th Annual Convention of the Minnesota Hospital Association, together with eight allied organizations, will be held at the Nicollet Hotel in Minneapolis on May 19, 20 and 21, 1938. The allied organizations consist of the following:

Minnesota Anesthetists Association
Minnesota Dietetic Association
Minnesota Record Librarians Association
Minnesota Society of Medical Technologists
Minnesota Occupational Therapists Association
Minnesota Chapter of the American Physiotherapy Association
Minnesota District of the American Association of Medical Social Workers
Minnesota Association of Hospital, Medical and Institution Librarians

It is expected that the total attendance at this gathering will be about seven hundred and fifty.

* * *

MEDICAL BROADCAST FOR FEBRUARY

The Minnesota State Medical Association Morning Health Service.

The Minnesota State Medical Association broadcasts weekly at 9:45 o'clock every Saturday morning over Station WCCO, Minneapolis and Saint Paul (810 kilocycles or 370.2 meters).

Speaker: William A. O'Brien, M.D., Associate Professor of Pathology and Preventive Medicine, Medical School, University of Minnesota. The program for the month will be as follows:

February 5—Infant Feeding.
February 12—Scarlet Fever.
February 19—Asthma in Children.
February 26—Gingivitis.

* * *

DOUGLAS COUNTY MEDICAL SOCIETY

The Douglas County Medical Society has elected Dr. J. C. Kyllo president for the coming year. Other officers are Dr. C. W. Mason, vice president, and Dr. S. H. Perrin, secretary-treasurer.

* * *

SCOTT-CARVER COUNTY MEDICAL SOCIETY

The Scott-Carver County Medical Society met at Mudcura Sanitarium, Shakopee, on January 11. Dr. Willard White of Minneapolis spoke on "Treatment of the More Common Fractures." Dr. Owen Robbins of Minneapolis spoke on "Problems in Prenatal Care."

* * *

WASHINGTON COUNTY

The Washington County Medical Society held its regular monthly meeting January 11. The scientific

program was given by E. Mendelssohn Jones, M.D., of St. Paul. The subject was "Abdominal Adhesions" and was very interesting, practical, and well illustrated by x-rays.

Due to the smallpox situation in the state, the Society put a notice in the newspapers advising people to be vaccinated.

* * *

WINONA COUNTY MEDICAL SOCIETY

Dr. Robert B. Tweedy, of Winona, was elected president of the Winona County Medical Society at the annual meeting. Other officers elected are Dr. H. J. Roemer, vice president; Dr. Irving W. Steiner, secretary; and Dr. L. I. Younger, treasurer.

Speakers at the meeting included Dr. Herman E. Hilleboe of Saint Paul, who talked of the work being done in this state for crippled children, and Dr. Morse J. Shapiro of Minneapolis, who spoke on heart disease among children.

CENTER FOR CONTINUATION STUDY, UNIVERSITY OF MINNESOTA

Advance Registration

Advance registrations are now being received for the winter and spring medical institutes. During the past year, medical institutes were held in: Traumatic Surgery, Obstetrics and Gynecology, Pediatrics, Internal Medicine, Roentgenologic Diagnosis, Disease of Heart, Surgical Diagnosis and Treatment, Dermatology and Syphilology and Ophthalmology and Otolaryngology. During the remainder of the scholastic year 1937-1938, institutes will be offered in Medical Diagnosis and Treatment, Traumatic Surgery, including fractures and dislocations, Endocrinology, including disorders of metabolism, Disease of Rectum and Colon and Roentgenologic Diagnosis.

Nearly 230 physicians have attended the institutes. An advance registration sufficient to guarantee a complete program as outlined above has been received. As enrollment in future institutes will be limited, physicians planning to attend should register as soon as possible. It is also helpful in planning programs to know the interests of the group in advance.

Many physicians in Minnesota and the Northwest are still unfamiliar with what the Center for Continuation Study has to offer. Under the directorship of J. N. Nolte, advanced courses of study have been offered in cooperative management, nursery teacher training, pharmacy, probation and parole problems, social welfare administration and supervision, waterworks operation, hospital administration, adult education, photography, international relations, architectural concrete, Scandinavian culture, police training, parent-teacher leadership, traffic safety, structural engineering, educational guidance, general collegiate education, religious and ethical philosophy, trade and industrial coördination in education, technic of writing, family welfare administration and supervision, library practice and problems, Boy Scout executive leadership and medicine. For the future, a list of subjects similarly diverse is under consideration.

The Center has proved an ideal place in which "To live and learn." With accommodation for seventy-eight persons in comfortable, well-furnished rooms, every need of the postgraduate physician is satisfied under one roof. The majority of lectures are given in the Center with clinics in the University of Minnesota and affiliated hospitals. As postgraduate physicians make a personal sacrifice in giving up their practices, the Center for Continuation Study is attempting to do its part by offering full programs of practical instruction and good living at the lowest possible price.

Advance Program

Medical Diagnosis and Treatment. February 7 to 12, 1938. Lectures, clinics, demonstrations and therapeutic conferences on diseases of the gastrointestinal and respiratory tracts, the blood and blood forming organs.

Traumatic Surgery, including fractures and dislocations. March 7 to 12, 1938. Clinics will be held in the hospitals followed by lectures and conferences at the Center. Dr. Wallace H. Cole and associates. Enrollment limited to 25 students.

Endocrinology, including disorders of metabolism. April 4 to 9, 1938. Treatment of obesity, diabetes and the more common disorders of the endocrine glands, including the thyroid, uterus and ovary. Dr. J. C. McKinley and associates. Enrollment limited to 30 students.

Disease of Rectum and Colon. May 2 to 7, 1938. Clinics and demonstrations followed by lectures and conferences. Dr. Walter A. Fansler and associates. Enrollment limited to 15 students.

Roentgenologic Diagnosis. June 6 to 11, 1938. One of the popular institutes of last year. Arranged primarily for physicians who use their own apparatus for roentgenologic diagnosis. Dr. Leo G. Rigler and associates. Enrollment limited to 30 students.

Information

Write at once to J. N. Nolte, Director, Center for Continuation Study, University of Minnesota, for registration details and room reservations.

WOMAN'S AUXILIARY

MRS. J. F. NORMAN, Crookston, *President*
MRS. A. A. PASSER, Olivia, *Editor*

UNDER the direction of the State President, Mrs. J. F. Norman, and the Chairman of Organization, Mrs. W. B. Roberts of Minneapolis, three medical auxiliaries were organized in the fall of 1937. On

October 7, a Woman's Auxiliary for Wabasha County was organized with the following officers elected: President, Mrs. B. A. Flesche, Lake City; vice president, Mrs. J. A. Slocumb, Plainview; secretary, Mrs. G. W. Holt, Wabasha; treasurer, Mrs. D. A. Burlingame, Mazeppa. On November 18 the Winona Auxiliary was organized with the following officers: President, Mrs. C. P. Robbins, Winona; vice president, Mrs. H. W. Satterlee, Lewiston; secretary, Mrs. A. E. Meinert; treasurer, Mrs. L. J. Nilles, Rollingstone. Eighteen members joined this group. On December 9th the medical society of Clay-Becker voted to have an auxiliary and Mrs. Norman organized the auxiliary at that time with six members present. The following officers were elected: President, Mrs. O. O. Larson, Detroit Lakes; vice president, Mrs. E. K. Ingebrigtson, Moorhead; secretary-treasurer, Mrs. L. H. Flancher, Lake Park. We cordially welcome these new units and wish them a happy, active role on the honor roster. We now have twenty-four active women's auxiliaries in the state.

The midwinter board meeting of the State Medical Auxiliary was held at the Woman's Club of Minneapolis, on Friday, January 14, at 10:30 A. M. Mrs. J. F. Norman, Crookston, state president, presided at the business session, at which time a nominating committee was elected, and plans were heard for the state meeting to be held in Duluth June 29, 30, and July 1. Mrs. Augustus S. Kech of Altoona, Pennsylvania, president of the National Women's Medical Auxiliary, was the honor guest of the meeting and was the luncheon speaker to which all members of the Women's Auxiliary were invited. Reservations for the luncheon were in charge of Mrs. W. W. Moir, Minneapolis, former president of Hennepin county. Mrs. Martin Nordland of Minneapolis, a former state president, gave a tea at her home on Saturday, January 15, in honor of Mrs. Kech.

Hennepin County Auxiliary

The regular monthly meeting was held at the Hennepin County Medical Library on January 7. "Community Health Service" was discussed by Miss Laura Draper. Mrs. Edward Kelly, well known Minneapolis artist, gave a talk on "An Artist's Summer in Mexico," at the February meeting. A program of music was furnished by Mrs. H. P. McCrimmon, violinist.

Olmstead-Fillmore-Houston-Dodge Auxiliary

At the auxiliary meeting held in November, Mrs. L. M. Randall of Rochester, president, presided. Miss Priscilla Keely, social service worker at the Mayo Clinic, and Miss Jose Bosly, visiting nurse, spoke. Mrs. W. C. MacCarty of Rochester, district chairman of the Woman's Field Army for the Control of Cancer, also presented a report. Mrs. F. P. Moersch of Rochester was hostess to the auxiliary at her home on January 6. Mrs. L. M. Randall reported on activities of the state auxiliary at the American Medical Association meeting last year.

PROCEEDINGS of the MINNEAPOLIS SURGICAL SOCIETY

Stated Meeting, December 2, 1937

The President, DR. O. W. YOERG, in the Chair

THE OPERATIVE TREATMENT OF HYPOSPADIAS

With a Report of Three Cases in Brothers

C. D. CREEVY, M.D.

Abstract

Dr. Creevy reported three cases of penoscrotal hypospadias in brothers aged six, fourteen and sixteen years; their father stated that two maternal uncles had similar deformities. The three were operated upon successfully in two stages. The first operation straightened the penis, the second constructed the urethra. A urethral fistula resulted in the oldest boy, and was closed by a third operation; in the others healing was by first intention.

The speaker discussed the various operations proposed and used for hypospadias, after pointing out that the glandular variety required no treatment, while the penile, penoscrotal and perineal varieties needed operation to relieve the functional impotence and sterility resulting from the ventral curvature of the penis and the misplacement of the external urinary meatus.

He advocated the Duplay operation for straightening the penis, and doubted whether the more elaborate procedure of Edmunds often required, since satisfactory straightening was secured in twelve cases, while reoperation was needed in the thirteenth. The importance of diverting the urine from the operative field during healing, either by urethrostomy or by cystostomy, was emphasized.

Of the numerous methods advocated for construction of the urethra, that of Thiersch seems most practical, while the methods of Cabot and of McIndoe are useful in certain cases. In the Thiersch operation as modified by Cecil, the new urethra is constructed from the skin of the inferior surface of the penis sutured around a sound, so that the suture line adjoins the corpus cavernosum along the roof of the urethra. The new tube is covered by a flap of penile skin pulled across it so that the external suture line lies at a distance from that in the urethra.

In two of the three cases reported, the urethra was constructed in one stage; the third required a second stage to close a fistula, but most of the other operations regularly require two stages for the construction of the urethra.

Discussion

DR. IVAR SIVERTSEN: I feel as though I bring coal to Newcastle when I try to discuss a paper such as was delivered by Dr. Creevy. Most of us do not see these cases, not very many of them, at least. We probably

see the penile type of hypospadias which, as Dr. Creevy says, is not of much consequence. The only treatment necessary, here, would probably be either a dilatation or even a little incision with a suture of the mucous membrane to the glans penis.

I have seen only one case of the penile type and it had a large roof of mucous membrane which it was possible to dissect away from the side of the penis and bring over a catheter. We obtained in this way a fairly good result except that a small fistula resulted which was later cured.

As to the time of operation in these cases, it seems to me that the best time to operate is before puberty. Some recommend that they be operated upon between the sixth and the tenth year. I don't know that Dr. Creevy mentioned that it makes any difference. Certainly, in the penile type of case where it is necessary to straighten the penis you have to separate the corpora cavernosa from around the urethra. Most men, I think, bring the penis up on the abdominal wall after they have made such a dissection of the corpora cavernosa and then probably do a cystostomy. I don't know which is the better procedure. Dr. Creevy certainly is a master in this work and it is not for me to say. The only cases we have seen we did do that very thing. I have not had any experience with the perineal type but I am sure that it is a very difficult procedure.

There was one operation, however, the Bucknell operation, that he spoke about, that has been modified by an Englishman where they used the prepuce of the penis and split that and brought it down upon the surface of the scrotum after making an incision on the scrotum and using the mucous surface of the prepuce as the floor of the urethra. To me, this appears to be a very satisfactory way. After doing this they wait some weeks and then do a modified Bucknell operation and apparently get good results. I don't know whether Dr. Creevy has seen this operation, the so-called Winsberry-White modification of the Bucknell operation. There, you will get tissue that is without hair and it can be brought up against the roof of the urethra.

Most men feel that unless you have a very definite reason for performing these operations, as in the so-called perineal hypospadias, they had better be left alone unless they can be done by an expert. I don't know but what I would leave them alone unless I could send them to Dr. Creevy. The penile type, of course, can be improved by the so-called Winsberry-White modification of the Bucknell operation.

I certainly want to congratulate Dr. Creevy on his very beautiful demonstration of this procedure, and I am very happy to have had the privilege of listening to his paper.

DR. KENNETH BULKLEY: I would like to know what Dr. Creevy thinks about the most suitable age for the operative procedure on these cases?

DR. C. D. CREEVY: Dr. Sivertsen mentioned an important point that I neglected to speak about in connection with the straightening of the penis. In the extreme degrees of deformity the intact part of the urethra just behind the hypospadiac meatus may also be shortened and in this particular variety it is very helpful to make the urethra completely free from the corpora cavernosa. One then circumscribes the meatus by a circular skin incision, lets the urethra re-

142

tract beneath the skin, and makes a buttonhole in the skin further back for the meatus.

As for the best age for operation, it is usually said that the penis ought to be straightened whenever the patient is first seen, and that the construction of the urethra ought to be put off until the penis has become large enough to make the operation a simple matter. Early correction of the deformity is urged because, as time goes on, the ventral surface of the corpora cavernosa becomes shortened and the deformity may be permanent. However, I have operated on a man of twenty-five, and didn't find it any more difficult to straighten the penis than in very young children. As a matter of fact, because of the size of the structures, it was considerably easier, so that I am not sure that there is any particular advantage in straightening the penis early in life.

HEPATIC CIRRHOSIS

Talma-Drummond-Morrison Operation

R. R. CRANMER, M.D.

Most classifications of liver cirrhosis are not wholly satisfactory. The following classification is based on the condition of the liver and the presence or absence of certain findings as ascites, portal vein obstruction, jaundice, and enlargement of the spleen.

1. Atrophic cirrhosis, hobnail liver, Laennec's cirrhosis, alcoholic cirrhosis.

   In this type the liver is rough and nodular, tends to be smaller than normal, there is marked portal obstruction with ascites and enlarged spleen, and no jaundice.

2. Obstructive biliary cirrhosis.

   Liver enlarged, smooth or granular. Jaundice present with clay colored stools. Usually no ascites but spleen may be enlarged.

3. Hypertrophic or Hanot's cirrhosis.

   Liver large and smooth. Jaundice but bile stained stools. No ascites, splenic enlargement.

4. Tuberculous and syphilitic cirrhosis.

   In addition Banti's disease (splenic anemia) is considered by some to be in reality another form of this condition in which the blood changes are marked, due, in large part, to massive hemorrhages.

Many things have been blamed as the cause of liver cirrhosis. Chronic alcoholism seems to be the thing most generally considered responsible. Arsenic and copper have frequently been mentioned. About 50 per cent of patients with cirrhosis give the history of alcoholic addiction. Perhaps, many of the remaining 50 per cent are users of it but do not admit it. Postmortems done on 134 chronic alcoholics in one large institution showed cirrhosis in only six.

Splenomegaly and ascites, with or without jaundice, depending upon the type, are the outstanding features in the advanced cases. Men present this condition about four times as frequently as women.

Conditions simulating liver cirrhosis and requiring

differential diagnosis are: abdominal carcinoma, cardiac disease, tuberculous peritonitis, and, in women, large ovarian cysts.

The ascites in cirrhosis has been generally considered to be due to portal obstruction within the liver with resulting back pressure and accumulation of a transudate in the peritoneal cavity.

Others believe that following this the ascites is increased by congestion-excited endothelial cells pouring out an exudate.

Many of these cases have a coexisting myocardial insufficiency which may also be an etiological factor.

Toxins generated in the intestinal tract and spleen, when not removed by the liver, are thought by some to be the cause of the endothelial stimulation.

If the ascites is due to portal obstruction and also, in part, to the presence of toxins in the circulation causing stimulation of the endothelial cells of the peritoneum, any operation looking toward a cure should be one that reduces the obstruction and reduces the toxemia. If the toxins have their origin in the spleen its removal or the establishing of collateral circulation through adhesions produced between it and its contact peritoneum should be logical treatment.

The long continued portal obstruction results, in many cases, in dilatation of anastomosing venous systems uniting the portal with general circulation.

These anastomoses occur:

1. Between the coronary veins of the stomach and lower esophageal veins, the later opening into the right azygos and intercostals.

2. Between the branches of the inferior mesenteric vein, the superior hemorrhoidal and the branches of the internal iliac veins, the middle hemorrhoidal.

3. The veins of Retzius which originate in the walls of the intestines, and through a small trunk open into the ascending vena cava.

4. Anastomosis of veins about the umbilicus (caput medusæ).

Surgical procedures are aimed at:

1. Establishing collateral circulation
2. Reducing the portal bed
3. Draining the ascitic fluid.

Omentopexy suggested first by Talma and carried out by many others, including Drummond and Morrison, has been a popular procedure. This, in conjunction with the production of adhesions between the liver and peritoneum and between the spleen and peritoneum, constitutes the more modern operation known as the Talma-Drummond-Morrison operation.

Operations to reduce the portal bed are splenectomy and enterectomy. The last named operation described by M. K. Fuller of Chicago and her associates, in the *Surgery, Gynecology and Obstetrics* of September, 1937, consists of removal of several feet of small bowel. Basis for enterectomy in this condition is the hypothesis that obliteration of part of the portal bed by resection of several feet of small intestine might decrease the returning venous blood to an amount which might pass through the cirrhosed liver, thereby decreasing the pressure in the portal veins and capillaries, and diminishing the transudation from the portal system into the peritoneal cavity.

Operations for the drainage of the ascitic fluid are, of course, palliative in nature.

Paracentesis continues to be the most practical of these. Eck's fistula, while ideal theoretically, is of no practical value because of the technical difficulties of the operation and high mortality associated with it.

Spheno-peritoneal anastomosis has been successfully done with good results in a few cases.

Case Report

The patient, a male, aged fifty-five, entered the hospital on March 1, 1935. His chief complaint was distention of abdomen, anorexia, nausea, general weakness, loss of weight, and pains in calves of legs.

Family history was essentially negative, no member of the family having had a similar condition.

The patient had the usual diseases of childhood. He had pneumonia two years previous to his admission. There was no history of scarlet fever or rheumatic fever. Genito-urinary history was negative except for gonorrhea fifteen years previous. He had been addicted to drinking for a period of thirty years and during the last twenty years averaged a pint of hard liquor daily. He dates the onset of his illness July, 1934, when he first became faint and dizzy upon exertion. Following this there was a loss of appetite and weight. He, then, noticed a distention of the abdomen which was progressive. His weakness increased until six weeks previous to his admission it became necessary for him to stop his work. He noticed that the urine was dark and that the stools were occasionally light yellow. There was no apparent jaundice.

Physical examination revealed that the patient was a moderately well developed man who did not appear acutely ill. There was no appearance of jaundice. Heart and lungs were normal. Abdomen was considerably distended. It was impossible to palpate the liver or spleen satisfactorily. There was no abdominal tenderness and no palpable masses. There was no no edema of ankles. Varicosities of abdominal walls especially noticeable over right side extending into the chest. Blood examination showed hemoglobin 65 per cent; 3,200,000 red blood cells and 5,700 white blood cells per cu. mm.; pmns. 74.8 per cent, lymphocytes 25 per cent. Urinalysis revealed 1015 specific gravity; urobilin, 1 plus; urobilinogen, faint trace; occasional hyalin and granular casts; 2 to 4 pus cells; and no red blood cells. Quantitation urobilinogen test showed .44 mg. in twenty-four hours. Icteric index was 13. Urea nitrogen 7 mg. per 100 c.c. Galactose liver function test showed a total urinary output of 79 per cent of sugar in five hours.

Diagnosis: Cirrhosis of liver with ascites.

The patient remained in the hospital four weeks before operation, during which time abdominal paracentesis was done several times. The amounts of fluid removed ranging from 1,500 to 4,000 c.c. Following paracentesis, the lower edge of the liver could be felt for a distance of three fingers breadth below the costal margin. The spleen was easily palpable. The fluid was amber in color. His condition after a month's rest seemed slightly improved although there was no diminution in the amount of ascitic fluid accumulating. On May 2, following a paracentesis a Talma-Drum-

144

mond-Morrison operation was performed under general anesthesia. The abdomen was opened through an upper left rectus incision and about a liter and a half of straw colored fluid was aspirated. The liver was enlarged to three fingers below the costal margin. Its edge was sharp and the surface was finely granular. The spleen was enlarged about three times the normal size. The upper surface of the liver was roughened by dry gauze spread over the fingers. The under surface of diaphragm was treated in a similar way. A similar procedure was carried out on the outer surface of the spleen and its contacting peritoneum. The anterior surface of the omentum was sacrificed, as was, also, the parietal peritoneum covering the anterior wall, for a distance of about seven centimeters lateral to the wound edges. The entire anterior surface of the omentum was sutured to the anterior abdominal wall and the wound was closed. The patient left the hospital June 4 with a small amount of ascitic fluid present in the abdomen. There was no paracentesis done following operation. Two months after his discharge very little fluid was present in the abdominal cavity and in four months time it had entirely disappeared. He returned to work about six months after the operation.

Discussion

DR. E. A. REGNIER: I think Dr. Cranmer is to be congratulated in presenting a patient with cirrhosis who is apparently in such good health. Our results in treatment of ascites associated with cirrhosis by the Talma-Morrison operation have not been good; in fact, they have been so discouraging that in the event of an apparent recovery one always is inclined to doubt that he was dealing with a true cirrhosis. The cause of the ascites is still very debatable. If it is due to a toxin the progress of the disease is not affected by any surgical operation. The case presented here this evening has obviously been completely relieved of ascites, which has brought him great bodily comfort and this good result certainly justifies the procedure. My own experience in this field has been very limited. I have one case relieved of ascites five years after operation. This was a case of cirrhosis associated with Banti's disease in a young girl, nine years old, in whom a splenectomy was done five years ago. She has remained well following splenectomy and omentopexy for the relief of ascites. One must not lose site of the fact that we are not treating cirrhosis but are operating to relieve a very annoying symptom, namely ascites, and the progress of the disease is not altered by this procedure.

DR. RALPH KNIGHT: I would like to ask Dr. Cranmer if the abdominal veins are now distended?

DR. KENNETH BULKLEY: Has the size of the liver changed any?

DR. R. R. CRANMER: No, the veins are not distended. I would like to say that one of the best papers I have ever read in connection with this type of thing is one written by Dr. Earl Hendrickson. He reviewed all the literature very thoroughly and it was published last year in the Archives of Surgery. I do not believe you can see any dilated veins here now. Here is the incision, a left rectus incision, and here especially is where he had quite a few dilated veins, over the chest and right side of the abdomen.

Replying to Dr. Bulkley's question, we had him on the table a couple of days ago and we could feel the edge of the liver at least two fingers below the costal margin.

In the Talma-Morrison operation the idea is to produce collateral circulation by adhesions between the liver and peritoneum on the under-surface of the diaphragm and between the spleen and peritoneum and if good collateral circulation results in these locations and between the omentum, and the abdominal wall, any dilated veins on surface should disappear.

DR. C. E. MERKERT: I would like to ask whether the formation of adhesions in this operation actually does drain the abdominal cavity by forming new veins or is it through the lymphatics that are connected as in the Kondoleon operation for elephantiasis of the leg?

DR. R. R. CRANMER: I believe it is in the new veins.

OBSCURE RETROPERITONEAL ABSCESS

VERNE CABOT, M.D.

Miss A. O., a school teacher, unmarried and thirty-one years of age, entered the hospital September 11, 1936, with a history of illness for the past five weeks consisting of weakness, abdominal distress and fever, associated with severe anorexia but without nausea or vomiting. She was a rather small woman in moderate state of nutrition though showing the effects of a prolonged and severe illness.

Her previous history was of special import in that fourteen years ago she had undergone surgical intervention for appendiceal disease with abscess which was drained. Her postoperative period was very stormy and during her ninth postoperative week she was again submitted to abdominal incision for secondary abscess and again in her tenth week a deep abscess in the right lower lumbar region was also evacuated. From these surgical procedures she apparently convalesced until her eleventh week, when she suffered a siege of pneumonia, from all of which she recovered and was discharged from the hospital after fifteen weeks. She states that her health has not been robust since this period. She has tired easily and has been subject to backache for which she had been treated under the diagnosis of spinal arthritis (lumbar). The school-year of 1935-1936 she did not teach because of poor general condition. The summer of 1936 was spent in resting until in mid July when she became acutely ill complaining of indefinite abdominal discomfort with weakness and fever which had persisted to the time of our first seeing her when she was admitted to the hospital.

On admission, examinations showed a moderately tender lower right abdomen with greatest intensity along the anterior margin of right ilium downwards from the superior iliac spine for a distance of about 10 cm. and extending mesially for about 2 cm. There was no appreciable muscular rigidly. Other examinations of the abdomen and pelvis were essentially normal. There was slight pain on complete extension of the right thigh, which she attributed to the position she had assumed during her illness and to her chronic arthritis. There was no undue tension or tenderness over her lumbar areas. Her weight had dropped from 116 to 92 pounds the past year.

Temperature 102.6; pulse 78; respirations 18.

Blood studies: Hgb. 76 per cent; r.b.c. 4,250,000; w.b.c. 18,400. Repeated w.b.c. ranged from 12,000 to 22,000 with an average of 80 per cent pmns. Numerous urinalyses were at all times normal. The blood Wassermann and Mantoux tests were negative.

Roentgen studies of chest and urinary tract with pyelograms revealed no abnormalities. Gastrointestinal studies showed normal findings except for a very low lying cecum somewhat fixed and tender. The appendix was not visualized. Detailed x-ray studies of skeletal systems of chest, lumbar and pelvic regions were nega-

tive for osseous changes though there was a slight scoliosis of the lumbar region and a fogginess of the lateral margin of the right psoas magnus, especially, in its lower portion, which was explained as being a result of her previous lumbar suppurative processes both intra- and retroperitoneal.

An attempt was made to obtain records of her earlier operations but the records of both hospital and surgeon had been destroyed. We felt these records were of great importance, thinking that possibly the appendix had not been removed.

Consequently on her sixth day in the hospital she was submitted to abdominal exploration, at which time a few omental adhesions attached to areas of previous drainage sites were separated. The cecum was low and somewhat fixed. The appendix had been removed. There was a definite irregular enlargement of the right psoas muscle with increased tension, especially in its lower or iliac portion. The wound was closed and walled off. Following this, aspiration of the concavity of the right ilium extraperitoneally was attempted without success. Incision was then made just mesial and downwards from the right superior iliac spine. It being carried inwards outside the peritoneal cavity until the mass was entered and drained of heavy yellow pus. Cultures taken showed subsequent growths of staphylococcus only. Her convalescence was definite though her draining sinus persisted despite rest, high protein diet, vitamins, autogenous vaccines, etc. She left the hospital at the end of her second month much improved in health, but with the sinus draining steadily though somewhat less. She continued to drain and was again admitted to the hospital January 11, 1937. Repeated x-ray studies prior to her leaving the hospital and following readmission showed no further abnormalities. Biopsy of the sinus tract showed chronic inflammatory changes with occasional giant cells.

To ascertain the exact location and extent of the abscess and persisting sinus, the tract was injected with lipiodol as shown by the films, following which there was a noticeable diminution of discharge as well as a change from heavy pus to a more serous type. The improvement was so noticeable that four days later lipiodol was again injected. Then sodium ricinoleate 5 per cent and lastly 5 per cent sodium psylliate were injected. Her improvement was so marked that she was discharged three weeks following the first injection, with her sinus rapidly granulating in, which it continued to do until shortly it closed over without further recurrence. In all she received nine injections, three of iodized oil and six of sclerosing solutions. Her general health has been excellent to date as evidenced by her normal temperature readings and weight gain to normal.

Repeated x-ray studies of the involved areas have been taken, the last one of which was taken September 27, 1937.

The diagnosis in this case was: Retroperitoneal abscess involving right psoas and iliac muscles, origin undetermined.

Discussion

DR. DANIEL A. MACDONALD: In studying case histories of retroperitoneal abscess one is impressed with the difficulty of diagnosis and the obscurity of the cause of the abscess. The difficulty of diagnosis is admitted by the fact that on an average about five weeks elapses before a diagnosis is made.

There may be no tenderness in the subcostal angle. Redness and swelling in the lumbar region occur late because the inflammatory mass lies beneath thick muscles and strong fascial planes. Pain may be absent because sensory nerve endings are absent, and, with practically no restriction to the expanse of exudate, tension is lacking till late. There is no irritation or displacement of organs which would help in diagnosis. The kidney varies so much in its mobility that its change of position may be of little significance.

The source of infection in retroperitoneal abscess a great many times comes from intra-abdominal organs. The source of infection in intra-peritoneal subphrenic abscess usually comes from a diseased intra-abdominal organ. Subphrenic abscess is more common than retroperitoneal abscess because when these intra-abdominal organs do perforate, as a rule, they perforate into the free peritoneal space rather than retroperitoneally. The reason for this is because most organs of the abdomen have a more perfect fusion of their posterior peritoneum, or, in other words, a more perfect mesentery. Therefore, we would expect a retroperitoneal abscess to come from a perforation of the colon, posterior duodenal wall, retrocolic appendix, abscess of the head of the pancreas, etc., if the source of infection is from an intra-abdominal organ, because with these organs we do not have as perfect a fusion of their posterior peritoneum.

The peritoneum is more sensitive to irritation and subphrenic abscess develops more quickly unless the great protective powers of the peritoneum destroy the infection, so with less irritation and symptoms developing more slowly the cause of retroperitoneal abscess is more obscure. There may be no urinary findings if a perinephritic abscess originates from the cortical portion of the kidney.

I feel that Dr. Cabot showed considerable ingenuity in treating his case with the sclerosing fluid and one would feel she would remain well after this length of time, with no recanalizing of the sinus or evidence of the infection.

X-RAY TREATMENT OF ACUTE INFECTIONS

M. B. HANSON, M.D. (by invitation).

Roentgen-ray therapy has proven itself a very valuable agent to the surgeon in the treatment of acute infections. With the publicity and propaganda given cancer and other malignancies and the treatment of x-ray, I think we have lost sight of the beneficial effects of x-ray therapy in other conditions. X-rays, shortly after their discovery, in 1895, were used in the treatment of cutaneous infections with varying results. This was due to incomplete knowledge of the output of the machines, filters, and also the biological reaction of the tissues. Since that period there has been a tremendous advance in the application and control of x-ray therapy, selection of cases, and comparative appreciation of results. It is the clinical evaluation of these results which gives us a rationale for this type of therapy.

X-rays per se are not bactericidal in vitro with the doses administered to a patient. However, when these same doses are administered to an infected area there is a complex biological reaction which not only is bactericidal but stimulates tissue repair. There have been many explanations of these processes but today the details of this reaction (which I shall not discuss) are still debatable.

Both acute and chronic infections are amenable to x-ray therapy. Acute infections, with their relative large number of leukocytes and small amount of connective tissue, however, respond more favorably. It is very important that the infected area be treated as early as possible, preferably within eight to twelve hours after the onset. It is within this period that many of these infections may be aborted. Baensch, in reporting over a hundred cases of furuncles of the face, was able to abort a large number and this mortality was less than 2 per cent as compared to a similar series conducted at the same time without roentgen therapy, which had a mortality of 10 per cent.

The clinical response to x-ray consists of:

1. Relief of pain, which occurs quite rapidly, usually within eight hours after treatment.
2. Lower temperature, which in many conditions such as erysipelas, boils, felons, lymphangitis, postoperative parotitis and acute bursitis, may return to normal within twelve to twenty-four hours.
3. Lessened toxicity.
4. Fairly rapid regression of the inflammation, if treated early, or, if treated later, a definite tendency to localize the infection with a resulting decrease of disability and number of hospital days.

In conclusion:

1. The surgeons have a valuable method to add to their armamentarium in the treatment of acute and chronic infections.
2. The earlier an infection is treated the more favorable the results.
3. Roentgen therapy is now well controlled without danger and discomfort to the patient.

Discussion

DR. KENNETH BULKLEY: This paper of Dr. Hanson's has been of interest. I do not believe he has quite covered his field. He spoke of the rapid subsidence of pain. In the fall of 1936 I had the misfortune to contract a tularemia. My primary focus was in my right hand and subsequent to leaving the hospital I developed a large mass of glands in the right side of my neck and right axilla. I would say that for a period of six weeks there was not a night that I did not wake up about one o'clock with a steady ache in my neck and armpit. Previous to this time I had not been cognizant of the value of x-ray therapy in tularemia. Dr. Hanson, however, very kindly gave me two exposures, using, I believe, one-third of an erythema dose on a 200,000 volt machine. The first dose was given one morning at about nine o'clock. Thereafter I slept without pain and had no further difficulty with my glands. They had subsided fully 50 per cent within a week and a week after the second dose were entirely gone. I wonder if anyone has any knowledge as to the early treatment of a fresh case of tularemia by x-ray therapy? It would be interesting to see what would happen if such a case received adequate therapy, certainly over the initial lesion, probably over the spleen, and possibly also over the lungs.

DR. IVAR SIVERTSEN: I would like to ask Dr. Hanson if he would use serum in cases of erysipelas and also of gas gangrene plus x-ray treatment.

DR. M. B. HANSON: In reply to Dr. Bulkley, I realize that this large field has only been scratched in this brief paper. There are so many acute infections which are being treated with x-ray therapy and with good results, that I tried to cover only a few of the most common surgical problems in the ten minutes allotted. X-ray has been used with satisfactory results in the treatment of enlarged nodes associated with tularemia. In these cases there has been a fairly rapid disappearance of pain and a slower regression of the size of the nodes. ·

Dr. Sivertsen's question concerning the use of serum in erysipelas, x-ray or ultra-violet lamp is sufficient for treatment in the average case of erysipelas. However, when the lesion is very extensive, serum may be used as an added weapon.

PRIMARY LOBECTOMY FOR BRONCHIECTASIS

Thos. J. Kinsella, M.D., F.A.C.S.

Abstract

The four patients to be presented this evening were chosen because they illustrate a number of points in the surgical treatment of bronchiectasis. Bronchiectasis is essentially a condition, not a primary disease. It may be congenital in origin or occur secondary to a number of conditions such as intrabronchial foreign bodies, pulmonary abscess, bronchial tumor, tuberculosis and a number of other processes in which the association of infection with bronchial stenosis or some other interference with bronchial drainage leads to weakening of the bronchial wall, dilatation and the production and retention of various amounts of secretion in the involved area. The condition is essentially a chronic one whose early course is frequently mild and characterized by periods of complete or relative absence of symptoms. Intercurrent episodes of pneumonitis or pneumonia are not uncommon. The early symptoms are those of a recurrent chronic bronchitis, but later there occurs more constant cough with expectoration of varying amounts of purulent material which becomes foul if there is retention of secretion. Pulmonary hemorrhage of varying degrees of severity occurs in at least one-half of the patients. In the later stages, cyanosis of the lips, cheeks, and digits is a frequent occurrence and clubbing of the fingers and watch crystal nails are often seen. The condition is compatible with life for long periods of time. In the early stages the cough is more of a nuisance than a handicap, but in the later stages the profuse expectoration, particularly if foul, becomes a serious handicap, interfering with useful work and more or less ostracizing the patient from his associates. Pulmonary hemorrhage and the attacks of pneumonitis may seriously endanger the patient's life.

Conservative measures of treatment, even combined with treatment for sinus infection, postural drainage, bronchoscopic aspiration or lavage, etc., may temporarily relieve symptoms but do not cure the condition. Removal of intrabronchial foreign bodies or tumors or strictures, or the aspiration and drainage of associated abscess, may improve the condition but do not eliminate the damage that has already been done.

The rapid development of thoracic surgery in the

past fifteen or twenty years has now made it possible to relieve a number of these patients, if the condition has not progressed too far. Thanks to the pioneering work of Brumm, Shenstone and others, it is now possible surgically to remove the involved lobe or lobes in certain selected patients without the appalling mortality which attended all earlier attempts to treat this condition. The following four patients will be used to illustrate these points:

The first patient is a little boy upon whom I performed a left lower lobe lobectomy on April 23, 1937, when he was three years ten and one-half months of age. He gave a history of pertussis at the age of one, an attack of pneumonia or pneumonitis of a chronic type in October, 1935, with high fever, sweats, severe cough, choking spells and cyanosis and the expectoration of thick, brownish green sputum with foul odor. In September of 1936 he had cough and small hemoptysis on two occasions. He had been subject to repeated colds, showed evidence of sinus disease and presented clubbed fingers and watch crystal nails. His tonsils and adenoids had been removed in November, 1936, when sinus drainage had also been established. Bronchoscopy revealed cylindrical and saccular bronchiectasis of the left lower lobe with associated atelectasis. The upper lobe and the contralateral lung were apparently free of involvement. The chest was opened by a posterior incision along the seventh interspace and a wide segment of the seventh rib excised and the sixth and eighth ribs sectioned near their angles. The pleural cavity was then opened and found to be almost entirely free of adhesions. The upper lobe was soft and pink, crepitant throughout, and collapsed readily. The lower lobe was purplish blue in color, firm, indurated and somewhat nodular, and collapsed very little when the chest was opened. The inferior pulmonary ligament was sectioned, the interlobar fissure freed and the pedicle of the lower lobe mobilized. A lobectomy tourniquet was placed around this pedicle, which was then transfixed and doubly ligated with braided silk. A second tourniquet was placed distal to the first and the involved lobe resected between the two tourniquets. All protruding vessels and bronchi were then sutured individually, and an attempt was made to close the exposed stump by approximating the adjoining pleural surfaces, but this could only be done incompletely. A second mass ligature was placed in the groove occupied by the tourniquet as it was removed. The chest wound was then closed tightly, leaving three mushroom catheters through stab wounds in the chest wall, and constant negative pressure of approximately 15 to 18 mm. of mercury applied. The postoperative condition was at all times satisfactory. Apparently the upper lobe expanded to fill the whole chest as breath sounds soon became evident throughout and we were left with only a small empyema pocket posteriorly into which a bronchial fistula opened as the stump sloughed off at the end of twelve days. We have been unable to determine just exactly what has happened to the upper lobe on this side. We will note from the x-rays that there is a

147

diffuse shadow occupying this side of the chest, although there are breath sounds present and the percussion note is not markedly altered. Whether this represents thickening of the pleura or whether there has been a thrombosis of the pulmonary vessels on this side or a permanent atelectasis of this lung we have been unable to determine. This boy ran a slight febrile course for several weeks but eventually his temperature returned to normal. He still has a very slight cough, but apparently is raising nothing, although at times, from the sound of his cough, one would suspect that there is a little secretion present. I believe that he still has a small bronchial fistula leading into a very small pocket posteriorly near the hilum. Deep fistulæ of this type eventually close spontaneously and should not be disturbed. His general condition is good. He apparently is developing symmetrically, is gaining weight, running no fever, and is running a normal leukocyte and differential count.

The second patient, a boy eight years three and one-half months old, was subjected to a right lower lobe lobectomy June 7, 1937. He gave a history of a pneumonia at the age of two years, frequent colds, and a productive cough at times. In December, 1933, he apparently had an acute mononucleosis with a leukocyte count of 94,000, with 90 per cent lymphocytes. In January, 1937, he had another attack of pneumonia or pneumonitis, with a temperature of 102.8, at which time he became delirious. Examination revealed bilateral ethmoid and maxillary sinusitis, and bronchoscopic examination revealed a bilateral lower lobe bronchiectasis, much more extensive on the right side. The tonsils and adenoids were removed and sinus windows established on February 18, 1937. Cough and expectoration were present but only very mild finger changes. Because of the extensive involvement in the atelectatic right lower lobe, it was decided to do a right lower lobe lobectomy on this side in spite of the bilateral disease. This was performed June 7, 1937, under cyclopropane anesthesia and was well tolerated. The technic was essentially the same as described previously except that we found the pleural cavity obliterated by filmy adhesions which were easily dissected away. The post-operative convalescence was relatively uneventful. The temperature reached a maximum of 103 on the eleventh post-operative day, but was down to normal at the end of thirty days. The remaining lung expanded rapidly to fill the pleural cavity. No empyema pocket developed and to our knowledge no bronchial fistula resulted. An obliterated pleural cavity before operation undoubtedly reduces the chance of an extensive post-operative empyema. He has no cough or expectoration now. We plan no surgical attack on the left lower lobe unless future progression of the disease renders it imperative.

The third patient is a man thirty-three years of age, who had no pulmonary trouble until 1927, when, soon after the extraction of all his teeth under general anesthesia, he began to cough and expectorate moderate amounts of purulent sputum, which at times was quite

foul. Symptoms continued more or less the same until 1930, when he was bronchoscoped by Dr. Vinson at the Mayo Clinic and a tooth removed from the right lower lobe. Following this he improved somewhat, but continued to have cough and expectoration, frequent colds which always extended to his chest, and was continually below par and unable to work. Bronchoscopy revealed pus from the right lower lobe bronchus, and bronchography an atelectatic right lower lobe with cylindrical bronchiectasis. On September 3, 1937, under intratracheal cyclopropane anesthesia administered by Dr. Ralph Knight, the right pleural cavity was opened through a posterior incision, the adhesions about the lower and middle lobes dissected free, and the atelectatic lower lobe resected. The chest was closed tightly and two catheters inserted through stab wounds and continuous negative pressure applied. Obstructive atelectasis of the right upper and middle lobes followed, but cleared within forty-eight hours. A small empyema pocket developed posteriorly about the lung stump as the bronchus opened at the end of two weeks. This was opened widely and packed, and is healing satisfactorily. He now has practically no sputum, is up and about, and in good condition generally.

The last patient is a physician thirty-nine years of age who has coughed as long as he can remember, always raising varying amounts of sputum which was never foul. Severe pulmonary hemorrhage occurred on numerous occasions. In 1917, following an unusually severe hemorrhage of about 500 c.c., pulmonary tuberculosis was suspected and a left pneumothorax induced and continued until 1920 without controlling either the hemorrhage or sputum. The diagnosis of tuberculosis was never confirmed. Cough and expectoration of purulent sputum in amounts from 4 to 60 c.c. continued with frequent blood-streaked sputum, and occasional frank pulmonary hemorrhage amounting to 300 c.c. in 1930 and again in 1935. In April, 1937, he developed an acute pneumonitis at the left base. Blood-streaked sputum appeared again in July, 1937. Examination revealed elevation of the left diaphragm and displacement of the heart and mediastinum to the left from atelectasis of the lower lobe. Bronchoscopy revealed pus from the left lower lobe bronchus, which was definitely stenosed. There was no evidence of foreign body. Iodized oil visualized a cylindrical bronchiectasis of the left lower lobe.

Through a posterior incision a left lower lobectomy was performed under intratracheal cyclopropane on September 2, 1937. The pleural cavity was completely obliterated by very dense scar tissue containing numerous large blood vessels. The whole operation was very difficult, requiring nearly seven hours of tedious dissection to complete it. Closure was made as in the previous cases. The post-operative convalescence was relatively smooth except for a small area of bronchopneumonia at the right base. A very small abscess about the bronchial stump drained through the bronchus. The wound is completely healed. He now has almost no

148

cough or expectoration, has gained weight, feels fine, nd plans to resume practice very soon.

A more complete report of these and other cases will e made later.

Discussion

Dr. Ralph Knight: Dr. Kinsella is to be congratulated upon his meticulous, exact work and beautiful results. It has been a pleasure to give some of these anesthesias for him.

Recently I saw Dr. Shenstone of Toronto perform chest operations. For his lobectomies two types of nesthesia were employed by his anesthetist, Dr. Harry Shields. On a certain morning, the first case, a woman, was given spinal anesthesia. The dose and the dilution of the novocaine were so calculated that the patient had anesthesia up to the clavicle, but the intercostal muscles were not paralyzed and the patient was able to cough and clear out the secretions, which were rather copious on account of the bronchiectasis for which she was being operated. The second case was a large man and Dr. Shields chose for him general anesthesia by cyclopropane, administered through an intratracheal tube. The surgeon seemed to like the spinal anesthesia fully as well as the other. While spinal anesthesia is very fine, I feel that in these cases the anesthetist has better control over the whole situation if he employs an intratracheal tube. The expansion and ventilation of the lungs and the removal of secretions are accomplished at will.

Our ideas are changing in regard to the use of the intratracheal tube even in rather small children. We find that they can be given a tube very well. If a rather small tube must be used it helps very much to mix about 50 per cent helium with the oxygen. This reduces the specific gravity of the gas mixture very materially and it passes through the small tube with much less resistance than does oxygen alone. Even after 20 per cent or 25 per cent of cyclopropane is added to this mixture to produce anesthesia the percentage of oxygen still remains very high and oxygenation is ample. When an intrabronchial tube is used for the administration of cyclopropane through the good lung, during the removal of the entire opposite lung for bronchiectasis, the tube is necessarily smaller than a tracheal tube and the helium mixture is a great help. The same is true in giving an anesthetic to an asthmatic patient.

It was not necessary to use helium for either of these lobectomy operations on adults for Dr. Kinsella. They both took the cyclopropane very well through an intratracheal tube, their respiration was shallow and quiet throughout and their color very good. Secretions were sucked out at frequent intervals.

I have noticed that in all of these major chest cases there is a tendency to the occurrence of post-operative paresthesias and partial paralysis of the arm on the same side. The position on the table and the need of the operating team for room probably causes the arm to become hyperextended, thus stretching the brachial plexus. The effect is upon the radical and median nerves, not upon the ulnar. Recovery is rather slow but is practically always complete. Every effort should be made to avoid this complication.

Dr. Nathaniel Lufkin (by invitation): As you know, the presence or absence of bronchiectasis is not as a rule difficult to determine at the autopsy table. In most cases where death has resulted from bronchiectasis or its complications, dilatations of the bronchi are very obvious. These are most frequent toward the periphery of the lung and frequently the dilatations have become converted into large abscesses.

The specimens removed by Dr. Kinsella presented a picture quite unlike that customarily seen in the post-mortem specimen. (Here is shown a lantern slide made from the photograph of one of Dr. Kinsella's specimens. Both the external and cut surfaces of the lung are shown.) This is the specimen removed from the first youngster. As you will note, it is much smaller than normal. The entire specimen is not much more than two inches long. This, I believe, is the result of atelectasis, part of which probably occurred during the operation. On the cut surfaces you will note the entire absence of dilated bronchi or abscess cavities. Instead, you have a very striking picture of very white, greatly thickened bronchi standing out in high contrast against the surrounding hemorrhagic and atelectatic lung tissue. This thickening is caused by two fundamental changes. First, there is a tremendous hypertrophy of the bronchial mucosa. Not only the membrane but the individual cells of the membrane are hypertrophic. Fairly frequently the mucosa is so redundant that it might be described as polyoid. Not infrequently a section of bronchus bears a superficial resemblance to a section of fallopian tube because the mucous membrane is thrown into so many irregular folds. The other change which contributes to thickening of the bronchi is bronchial and peribronchial fibrosis and infiltration. The connective tissues surrounding the mucous membrane are densely infiltrated with leukocytes, largely plasma cells and lymphocytes. There is a severe degree of accompanying fibrosis which extends far beyond the muscular coats of the bronchi and to varying degrees involves the air-bearing pulmonary tissue adjacent. Almost invariably the bronchial musculature is altered by this chronic inflammatory process. Frequently, it can hardly be made out. In these places it has evidently been almost completely destroyed.

All four of the specimens removed by Dr. Kinsella showed these changes as the outstanding alterations. There were, of course, minor differences between the specimens and there were also other alterations which were probably not part of the fundamental process. Only one showed cavities. This was the case in which symptoms had lasted for thirty or more years. It is my feeling that the fundamental change shown by these specimens is a severe chronic bronchitis and peribronchitis with destruction of bronchial musculature. This results in the dilatation of the bronchi so well demonstrated by the x-ray films. Probably the atelectasis consequent upon removal has caused a collapse of the saccules so that we can no longer see them except in the case of longest duration. Quite probably in this case many have reached sufficient size and attained a sufficiently thick fibrous tissue wall to keep them from complete collapse.

Harvey Nelson, *Secretary.*

BOOK REVIEWS

Books listed here become the property of the Ramsey and Hennepin County Medical libraries when reviewed. Members, however, are urged to write reviews of any or every recent book which may be of interest to physicians.

FEVER THERAPY. Abstracts and Discussions of Papers Presented at the First International Conference on Fever Therapy. Edited by members of the American Committee. 486 pages. Price, cloth, $5.00. New York: Paul B. Hoeber, Inc., 1937.

THE PHYSICIAN'S BUSINESS. Practical and Economic Aspects of Medicine. George D. Wolf, M.D. Attending Otolaryngologist, Sydenham Hospital, New York City; Attending Laryngologist, Riverside Hospital, New York City, etc. 384 pages. Illus. Price, cloth, $5.00. Philadelphia: J. B. Lippincott Co., 1938.

MACLEOD'S PHYSIOLOGY IN MODERN MEDICINE. Eighth Edition. Edited by Philip Bard, Professor of Physiology, Johns Hopkins University School of Medicine, and Collaborators. 1,051 pages. Illus. Cloth binding. St. Louis: C. V. Mosby Co., 1938.

SIR KENELM DIGBY. Writer, Bibliophile and Protagonist of William Harvey. John F. Fulton, M.D. 75 pages. Illus. Linen binding. New York: Peter and Katharine Oliver, 1937.

ANNUAL REPORT OF THE SURGEON GENERAL, PUBLIC HEALTH SERVICE OF THE UNITED STATES. 164 pages. Illus. Price, paper, 60c. Washington, D. C.: Government Printing Office, 1937.

PROCEEDINGS OF THE THIRTY-FIRST ANNUAL CONVENTION. Association of Life Insurance Presidents. 254 pages. Illus. Paper binding. New York: Association of Life Insurance Presidents, 1938.

CONCEPTS AND PROBLEMS OF PSYCHO-THERAPY. Leland E. Hinsie, M.D., professor of Clinical Psychiatry, College of Physicians and Surgeons, Columbia University; Assistant Director, New York State Psychiatric Institute and Hospital. 199 pages. Price, $2.75. New York, N. Y.: Columbia University Press, 1937.

This book aims to be a preface to psychotherapy. The author asserts that it covers the general principles involved in the several schools of psychotherapy. He believes it undesirable to promote the interests of one school of psychotherapy. The Freudian psychoanalysis as it is applied today has, it is stated, but a limited field; it is usable in a mere fraction of psychoneurotic individuals, and it is of little public service therapeutically. He discusses in his text also the psychotherapies of Adler, Jung and A. Meyer.

With reference to therapeutic results, the lack of control data until very recently is noted. The fifth of the six chapters in the text is devoted to a discussion of "A Statistical Evaluation of Psychotherapeutic Methods" by Carney Landis, Ph.D. In his conclusion the author indicates that he inclines to the belief that "even if we cannot apply the laws of biometrics to our current conceptions of therapy, we can at least meet some of the preliminary requirements upon which the laws are based."

J. C. MICHAEL, M.D.

MATERIA MEDICA TOXICOLOGY AND PHARMACOGNOSY. Wm. Mansfield, A.M., Ph.D. 708 pages. Illus. Price $6.75. St. Louis; C. V. Mosby, 1937.

This book is written by a pharmacist as a text and reference book on the therapeutics, pharmacognosy, toxicology and posology of the official drugs of the United States Pharmacopoeia XI and the National Formulary VI. It has one very interesting and valuable feature: the vegetable drugs are described singly with only one drug on a page and a picture of the crude drug is printed opposite the description. Following this there is a detailed description of the drugs of animal origin. There is a chapter on poisons which is interesting and valuable. This includes ways in which poisons may be taken, types of poisoning, symptoms, antidotes and treatment in general and in particular. The poisons which are used as drugs are described. This section includes most of the ordinary chemicals, such as arsenic, iron, local anesthetics, alcohol, ergot, etc. Finally, there is a large posological table with drugs arranged alphabetically and according to dose of liquids and solids.

There is a tremendous amount of facts in this book, but most physicians will find their more usual sources pharmacopoeia and the larger texts of pharmacology or treatment more serviceable. Pharmacists and perhaps doctors who do their own dispensing will probably find this worthwhile. It will be useful to doctors giving lectures to nurses.

For most physicians, this volume will be of very little value and the reviewer would not recommend its purchase for the personal library.

H. B. SWEETSER, JR.

MINNESOTA MEDICINE

*Journal of the Minnesota State Medical Association, Southern Minnesota Medical Association, Northern Minnesota
Medical Association, Minnesota Academy of Medicine and Minneapolis Surgical Society.*

Volume 21	MARCH, 1938	Number 3

ACUTE LYMPHOCYTIC MENINGITIS*

E. M. HAMMES, M.D.

Professor, Neurology and Psychiatry, Medical School, University of Minnesota
Saint Paul, Minnesota

WALLGREN, in 1925 and 1926, described a new syndrome of central nervous system infection under the title of acute aseptic meningitis. He reviewed the reports of two epidemics which had occurred in France in 1910 and 1913 and which were supposed to have been an abortive type of poliomyelitis, and similar epidemics in Europe in 1922 and 1923 which had been diagnosed mild cases of encephalitis. The characteristic symptoms of these cases were severe headaches with neck rigidity and other evidences of meningeal irritation with ultimate recovery. Wallgren reported several similar cases and emphasized the importance of the typical spinal fluid findings.

Since then other cases have been reported in increasing numbers both in Europe and in this country. Many names have been suggested but the terms, acute lymphocytic meningitis or acute aseptic meningitis, have been most universally adopted. Viets and Watts published the first three cases in this country in 1929. Thorson reported the first case in this state in 1936 and stated that two cases had occurred at the University Hospital and five at the Minneapolis General Hospital.

Although the disease is still considered by some as an abortive form of the meningitic type of epidemic encephalitis, the course of the disease and the characteristic spinal fluid findings make it a distinct clinical entity.

The onset is usually quite sudden, rarely with convulsions. Headache is frequently the first symptom, increasing in intensity, so that the patient becomes bedridden within a few days. This is associated with nausea and vomiting, and occasionally photophobia. About this time neck rigidity manifests itself and the clinical picture is quite suggestive of a tuberculous meningitis with which it is frequently confused.

Repeated spinal fluid studies, however, enable one to arrive at the correct diagnosis. The spinal fluid is usually clear and under normal or slightly increased pressure. The cell count varies from a moderate increase to over 1000, depending on the severity of the disease. Most of the cells are small lymphocytes, in many cases 100 per cent. In the early stage of the disease, although the lymphocytes predominate, one may encounter polymorphonuclear leukocytes. These may be as high as 35 per cent although usually in smaller numbers, and are an index of the severity of the infection. The protein frequently shows a slight increase. The characteristic diagnostic findings, however, are that the spinal fluid sugar remains within normal limits during the entire course of the disease (50 to 75 mgm. per 100 c.c.), as do also the chlorides (720 to 750 mgm. per 100 c.c.). The colloidal gold curve is usually in the meningitic zone. In one of our cases (Case three), however, it gradually shifted from the meningitic to the syphilitic zone and finally gave a definite paretic curve. Viets and Watts and Warren reported similar findings in two of their cases. Although the spinal fluid does not contain clots, several cases have been reported where a delicate fibrin web developed several hours after its removal similar to what occurs so characteristically in tuberculous meningitis. No organisms have been found on smear, culture or guinea pig inoculation. A moderate leukocytosis is frequently found in the blood during the early stage of the disease.

*Read at the annual meeting of the Southern Minnesota Medical Association at Winona, Minnesota, August 11, 1937.

The course is usually a benign one. The temperature gradually subsides, the irritative meningeal signs disappear and the spinal fluid findings gradually return to normal. Repeated spinal drainage favorably influences the course of the disease and should be performed in every case. In the severe cases, delirium and even prolonged psychotic symptoms may manifest themselves, with an ultimate favorable outcome. Cranial nerve palsies or other organic signs are infrequent or only transient when present; choked discs may occur early in the course of the disease.

In contrast to encephalitis, these patients rarely develop any late manifestations or sequelæ. This is considered an important differential diagnostic point. Complete recovery is the rule. Only one death has been reported in the literature. A patient observed by Viets and Warren died on the fourteenth day of his illness, immediately after his second convulsion. Post-mortem studies revealed extensive perivascular infiltration and slight ganglion cell changes throughout the central nervous system, indicative of a marked encephalitis as well as meningitis. Although the nervous tissue reaction was a severe one, the authors felt that the pathologic appearance did not preclude recovery.

Acute lymphocytic meningitis usually develops in isolated cases. However, epidemics have been reported suggesting an infectious origin. Anderson and Wolff think that this disease has become more prevalent since 1920 than epidemic encephalitis. If this is true, it has not been recognized in the majority of instances. Eckstein reported an interesting epidemic of thirteen cases at Dusseldorf in 1930. Toomy reported a group of seventy cases occuring in an orphanage which housed three hundred and sixty male children and sixty-five adults. These cases developed within a period of twenty-one days. The clinical picture, spinal fluid findings and course of the disease were quite typical of acute lymphocytic meningitis. However, the blood picture examined in eighteen cases revealed a leukopenia with a high relative lymphocytosis. In a small percentage, a hemolytic streptococcus was obtained from throat cultures. In his paper Toomy states that twenty-five similar cases had been observed by Currier of Grand Rapids, Michigan, and fourteen cases by Ashton of Beckly, West Virginia. Dummer et al reported a small epidemic occuring

in a group of twenty-two children during 1935.

Although no definite etiologic factors have been found in this type of meningitis, Scott and Rivers reported two cases in which a filtrable virus was obtained. The etiologic agent was isolated from the spinal fluids of these patients, and their serums possessed neutralizing antibodies for at least one hundred lethal doses of the virus from nine to eleven weeks after the clinical onset of the disease. However, in some typical cases this virus could not be demonstrated. Dominick reported three cases, two of which contained antibodies for the virus. He suggests that in those cases of lymphocytic meningitis where the organism is found or when the neutralization tests of the serum have positive results the term lymphocytic choriomeningitis should be employed. Rivers and Scott have further demonstrated that acute lymphocytic meningitis may be caused by etiologic agents other than this virus.

In the differential diagnosis, one must consider:

1. The various types of purulent meningitis which can be readily excluded from spinal fluid studies.

2. The abortive forms of poliomyelitis which may offer considerable difficulty except that in the early stages, polymorphoneuclear cells frequently predominate in the spinal fluid.

3. The cases of meningismus associated with acute otitis media and other acute systemic infections, in which the etiologic factor can readily be determined.

4. Tuberculous meningitis where a decrease in sugar and chlorides in the spinal fluid and the findings of the organism confirm the diagnosis.

5. The meningitic form of epidemic encephalitis which frequently offers the most difficult problem. The presence of localizing signs and lethargy, the sugar increase in the spinal fluid when present, and some manifestations of sequelæ are important diagnostic indications.

6. Syphilitic meningitis, which can be readily diagnosed from the positive spinal fluid findings.

We have observed seven cases during the past year, three of which are reported to illustrate the variations in the severity of the disease. One of our cases referred by Dr. L. N. Bergh of Montevideo, Minnesota, had a typical severe course of acute lymphocytic meningitis of four

152

weeks duration. During this period he had two convulsions. With the improvement in his meningitis, he developed a psychosis associated with delusions and hallucinations. He gradually improved and made a satisfactory recovery after four months.

Case 1.—A woman, aged thirty-nine, was admitted to the neurological service at Ancker Hospital on March 15, 1937. The family and personal history were negative except that the patient has always been mentally deficient. She completed the fifth grade at the age of sixteen. Because of her mentality it was difficult to obtain an accurate history. Apparently she developed a headache on March 12, 1937, which gradually grew worse. The next day she began to vomit. These two symptoms became more pronounced. She complained of vertigo and backache and was admitted to the hospital three days after the onset of her illness. The physical examination was negative. X-ray of sinuses and mastoids and lungs revealed no pathology.

The neurological examination was negative except for a rigid neck, and a moderate increase of all deep reflexes. The Kernig was negative. The blood count was normal, leukocytes 9,750. The urine was normal. The blood Wassermann and Kahn tests were negative. Twenty-five c.c. of clear spinal fluid under normal pressure were removed. The fluid contained a trace of globulin, 269 cells (94 per cent lymphocytes, 6 per cent polymorphonuclear); chlorides 704 mg. per 100 c.c.; sugar 78 mg. The spinal fluid Wassermann was negative; the colloidal gold curve negative; no organisms were found. The temperature and pulse were normal.

A provisional diagnosis of tuberculous meningitis was made. During her stay at the hospital the temperature was normal except on the second day when it was 100.6 for twenty-four hours. Her symptoms gradually subsided and she was discharged as recovered on her twenty-first hospital day.

Five spinal punctures were done.

Date	Cells		Chlorides	Sugar
March 16, 1937	269			
	94 per cent lymphocytes		704 mg.	78 mg.
March 17, 1937	790			
	90 per cent lymphocytes		712 mg.	72 mg.
March 19, 1937	647			
	all lymphocytes		708 mg.	74 mg.
March 25, 1937	172			
	all lymphocytes		706 mg.	78 mg.
March 27, 1937	28			
	all lymphocytes		710 mg.	70 mg.

Two months later she reported to the out-patient department because of a discharging right ear. This cleared up in ten days. There were no other symptoms or complaints.

Case 2.—A laborer, aged twenty-one, was admitted to the neurological service at Ancker Hospital on September 21, 1936. His family and personal history were negative. His present illness began about 10 A. M. on September 20, 1936, while helping a neighbor dig a basement. He developed a severe headache, throbbing in character which rapidly grew worse so that he had to discontinue work after two hours. He went to bed

and two hours later began to have attacks of vomiting of a projectile type. About this time he noticed some neck rigidity. All these symptoms became more pronounced and he was brought to the hospital at 2 A. M. on September 21, 1936. At the time of admission his temperature was 102, pulse 100, respiration 24. The physical examination was negative except for a slightly injected throat. The neurological examination revealed marked neck rigidity and a positive Kernig sign. All cranial nerves were normal. All deep reflexes were moderately decreased, the left Babinski questionably positive. He complained of pain and tenderness in the muscles of both lower extremities.

The urine was normal; blood count normal except for a leukocytosis of 26,000; blood pressure, systolic 120, diastolic 70. A lumbar puncture made at 4 A. M. on September 21, 1936, revealed a slightly cloudy fluid and under slightly increased pressure. Sixty c.c. were withdrawn.

The spinal fluid contained 314 cells, all lymphocytes; chlorides 715 mgs. per 100 c.c.; globulin one plus; spinal sugar 83 mg.; Wassermann and Kahn negative; colloidal gold curve 0000012200, no organisms; protein 46 mg. A tentative diagnosis of acute poliomyelitis was made and 20 c.c. of convalescent polio serum was administered intramuscularly.

Course: Following the spinal drainage his headache and vomiting improved. On September 22, 1936, a cisternal puncture was performed and the spinal fluid contained 251 cells, mostly lymphocytes. His general condition improved. the temperature gradually became lower, was normal on the fifth day and remained so. The rigid neck and Kernig gradually disappeared, his symptoms subsided and he was discharged on October 24, 1936, thirty-four days after his admission to the hospital, apparently recovered. He was seen in the out-patient department three weeks later at which time he had no complaints nor abnormal findings. His leukocytosis dropped to normal after the third day. Eight spinal punctures were done, the last one on October 13, 1936.

Date	Cells		Chlorides	Sugar
September 21, 1936	314	all lymphocytes	715 mg.	73 mg.
September 22, 1936	251,	90% lymphocytes	720 mg.	74 mg.
September 25, 1936	340,	90% lymphocytes	740 mg.	75 mg.
September 28, 1936	462	all lymphocytes	690 mg.	..
October 1, 1936	460	all lymphocytes	710 mg.	72 mg.
October 5, 1936	192,	90% lymphocytes	750 mg.	70 mg.
October 7, 1936	188,	90% lymphocytes	720 mg.	..
October 13, 1936	36,	70% lymphocytes	720 mg.	..

Case 3.—A negro, a Pullman porter, aged thirty-five, was admitted to the neurological service at the Ancker Hospital on July 6, 1936. His family history was negative. His personal history was negative except that he contracted gonorrhea in 1928 and a chancre in 1929 for which he had received four "arm shots" and two "hip shots." His present illness began six days prior to admission to the hospital. On July first he had several severe chills, fever and "ached all over." Soon after he developed severe headache, pain and stiffness in the neck and back and generalized weakness. He had some nausea and had been very constipated since the onset of his illness.

The physical examination was negative. The neurological examination was negative except for a rigid neck, a positive Kernig and generalized tenderness. All cranial nerves, including the pupils, and all reflexes were normal. His temperature was 102.6; pulse 128; urine and blood count were normal except a leukocytosis of 12,450; blood Wassermann negative.

were found on smear, culture or guinea pig inoculation. After the paretic colloidal gold curve developed, the patient was placed on antisyphilitic treatment without any appreciable effect on the serology of the spinal fluid. Clinically he had recovered and left the hospital December 9, 1936.

Date	Cells		Chlorides	Sugar	Colloidal Gold Curve
July 7, 1936	1230		658	72	0000123310
	65 per cent lymphocytes				
July 8, 1936	733		690	70	0001332000
July 9, 1936	807		720	70	....
July 15, 1936	2170		712	67	0023332000
	all lymphocytes				
July 20, 1936	573		695	55	....
	all lymphocytes				
August 20, 1936	331		740	65	0000044550
	all lymphocytes				
September 15, 1936	166		...	..	4555554331
October 7, 1936	65		710	45	4555532100
November 6, 1936	34		...	48	4554432100

The spinal fluid was somewhat cloudy under increased pressure and 30 c.c. were removed. It contained a 2 plus globulin, 1,230 cells, 65 per cent lymphocytes and 35 per cent polymorphonuclears; chlorides 698 mg.; sugar 72 mg.; Wassermann and Kahn negative; colloidal gold curve 0000123310. Smear and cultures were negative for organisms. Immediately following the spinal drainage 30 c.c. of antimeningococcic serum were given intraspinally and intravenously because of the diagnosis of meningitis suspect.

Course: During the first eight days the temperature fluctuated between normal and 102 and pulse around 110. He was semi-delerious, extremely restless, had an occasional involuntary urination and complained of severe pain and neck rigidity. Because of the restlessness and confusion he had to be kept in restraint. All these symptoms gradually subsided as the temperature continued to be normal after July 14. From July 15 to July 27, two weeks after the onset of his illness, he complained of numbness and weakness of the right upper extremity and had some loss of motor strength of the right shoulder girdle muscles. This slowly improved and by August 14 he was up and felt well, but was kept in the hospital because of the continued pleocytosis in the spinal fluid.

Daily spinal drainage was performed during the first ten days and at frequent intervals thereafter. A total of thirty-four lumbar punctures was made, the last one on November 6, 1936. The highest cell count was 2,170 on July 15 and the lowest thirty-four on November 6; the lymphocytes varied from 60 to 95 per cent, while the remaining cells were mostly polymorphonuclear leukocytes. During the first ten days the spinal fluid was slightly cloudy, then became yellowish for a short period and then clear. The colloidal gold curve was in the meningitic zone until September 15, then quite rapidly extended into the syphilitic zone, and on three occasions presented a paretic curve. The Wassermann and Kahn were negative at all times; the sugar and chlorides were normal throughout; no organisms

Although this patient gave a positive syphilitic history, the normal pupillary findings and the negative Wassermann and Kahn, both in the blood and spinal fluid, exclude syphilis as the etiologic agent. However, it may have been a contributing factor in prolonging the pleocytosis in the spinal fluid.

Conclusions

1. Acute lymphocytic meningitis is a definite clinical entity characterized by symptoms of meningeal irritation, typical spinal fluid findings and a favorable outcome with repeated spinal drainage.

2. The etiologic agent evidently is a filtrable virus isolated by Scott and Rivers.

3. Seven cases have been observed by the author. Three are reported in detail.

1125 Medical Arts Building.

References

1. Dominick, D.: Lymphocytic choriomeningitis. Jour. Am. Med. Assn., 109:247-250, (July 24) 1937.
2. Dummer, C. M., Lyon, R. A., and Stevenson, F. E.: Benign lymphocytic meningitis. Jour. Am. Med. Assn., 108:633-636, (Feb. 20) 1937.
3. Eckstein, A.: Epidemische meningitis serosa. Klin. Wchnschr., 10:22-24, 1931.
4. Scott, T. F., and Rivers, T. M.: Meningitis in man caused by a filterable virus. Jour. Exp. Med., 63:397-414, (March) 1936.
5. Scott, T. F., and Rivers, T. M.: Meningitis in man caused by a filterable virus. Jour. Exp. Med., 63:415-432, 1936.
6. Thorson, O. P.: Benign lymphocytic meningitis or acute aseptic meningitis. Minn. Med., 19:664-68, (Oct.) 1936.
7. Toomy, J. A.: Acute lymphocytic meningitis. Jour. Pediat. 8:148-155, (Feb.) 1936.
8. Viets and Warren: Acute lymphocytic meningitis. Jour. Am. Med. Assn., 108:357-61, (Jan. 30) 1937.
9. Viets, H. R., and Watts, J. W.: Acute aseptic meningitis. Jour. Nerv. and Ment. Dis., 80:253-73, (Sept.) 1934.
10. Viets, H. R., and Watts, J. W.: Three cases of aseptic (lymphocytic) meningitis. New England Jour. Med., 200:633-34, (March) 1929.
11. Wallgren, A.: Eine eigenartige Form von epidemische Meningitis. (Meningitis aseptica acuta.) Wien, Arch. f. inn. Med., 12:297-312, (Feb.) 1926.

THE PRESENT STATUS OF THE INSULIN-HYPOGLYCEMIA TREATMENT IN SCHIZOPHRENIA*

EDWARD F. ROSENBERG, M.D., FREDERICK P. MOERSCH, M.D.,
RUSSELL M. WILDER, M.D., and BENJAMIN F. SMITH, M.D.

Rochester, Minnesota

INSULIN-HYPOGLYCEMIA therapy for schizophrenia is in the forefront of medical thought today. As a result of the enthusiastic reports of Sakel and his followers, both here and abroad, and because of the favorable publicity given the treatment in the lay press, public interest has been aroused to a high pitch. Medical men and hospitals are being flooded by requests from anxious relatives to employ the treatment on their beloved ones who have fallen prey to this tragic malady.

In spite of the extraordinary claims for the insulin-shock treatment it appears premature to draw final conclusions regarding the ultimate value of this form of therapy. We have been impressed by the wisdom of the attitude of the Committee on Public Education of the American Psychiatric Association which in February, 1937 issued the following statement: "It is hoped and may prove to be a fact that the so-called insulin-shock treatment for dementia præcox will find a useful place among the forms of treatment for dementia præcox, but its exact value has yet to be determined and it can be definitely stated that it is not a specific, nor by any means a cure for all cases of dementia præcox. It would be a source of regret should the insulin-shock treatment be a means of holding out a false hope to the families of tens of thousands of sufferers from dementia præcox when this hope most certainly cannot be widely realized with the present-day knowledge of insulin therapy."

A survey of the medical literature reveals reports of some very glowing results in the treatment of schizophrenia by insulin-shock therapy. Thus Sakel[17] reported more than 70 per cent of complete remissions in cases of early schizophrenia. Müller's[13, 14] report of more than 300

cases reveals even better results. Berglas and Süsič[1] said that in a total of eighty-five cases 70 per cent of patients who had early schizophrenia obtained complete remission. At the meeting of the American Psychiatric Association in Pittsburgh in May of this year, figures of a very similar nature were reported. Summing up the various figures a fair statement would be about as follows: In cases in which the psychosis is of less than six months' duration, the recovery rate is said to be from 60 to 80 per cent; if the psychosis has been present between six and eighteen months, the recovery rate is 30 to 50 per cent, and in cases of chronic schizophrenia the recovery rate is 10 to 20 per cent.

Thus far but few voices have been raised in protest. Professor Berze,[2] Lichter and Lichter,[11] Langenfeldt[9] of Oslo, Adolf Meyer[12] and a few others have cautioned against accepting the claims of those who have reported so encouragingly on the results of the treatment.

We hold no brief for either side in this controversy. Certainly, any treatment, even if it holds out but slight hope, is worthy of a thorough trial. It may at least open the way to some new avenue of attack and keep up that needed stimulus so necessary in the pursuit of a problem that has seemed so hopeless.

We recently have brought to a conclusion the treatment of thirteen patients who had schizophrenia. We must acknowledge that our material is limited and does not represent patients who were very favorable for treatment. However, we feel that a review of our experiences may be of value to those interested in this problem.

The Method of Treatment

Descriptions of the insulin-shock treatment have been published in Europe by Sakel,[17] Dussik and Sakel,[4] Müller,[13, 14] Braunmühl,[3] Hoff,[6] Larkin,[10] Wilson,[21] and Schaeffer.[19] In this country adequate accounts of Sakel's methods have been given by Glueck,[5] Sakel,[18] Reese,[15]

*Read before the Society of Neurology and Psychiatry, Rochester, Minnesota, May 29, 1937; also before the Southern Minnesota Medical Association, Winona, Minnesota, August 11, 1937.

Since this paper was presented for publication, thirty-three patients have completed their treatment. Of this group, five made complete recoveries, three were moderately improved, and twenty-five showed no improvement. Two of the five patients that recovered have had a recurrence of mental symptoms. One death was attributed to the treatment.

and Wortis.[22][17] We recently made a preliminary report of our work.[16]

In our work we have duplicated the original methods of Sakel as nearly as possible, but it

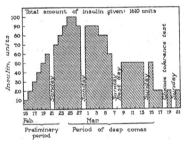

Fig. 1. Dosage of insulin in Case 8.

must be obvious at once that those who apply such a complicated procedure will have to evolve the method of handling numerous details through experience. A prime consideration in the treatment was the selection of patients. For our original group of patients we required that the physical condition of the patient be good. We insisted also that the responsible relatives be aware of the dangers of the treatment and be willing that it be undertaken. The Rochester State Hospital population includes relatively few patients who have schizophrenia of recent onset; consequently our cases have been those in which the psychosis usually extended beyond the critical period of six months.

Our working scheme has permitted us to handle approximately six to ten patients at one time. Breakfast is withheld at 7 a.m., following the recording of the patient's temperature, pulse rate, respiratory rate and blood pressure, the insulin is injected. The pulse rate, respiratory rate and blood pressure are then recorded at intervals of thirty minutes until the morning's treatment is terminated.

The Dose of Insulin.—Our plan for the dosage of insulin is illustrated (Fig. 1) in Case 8, in which the patient improved during treatment. The treatment begins with the injection of ten units of insulin. This amount is increased daily by ten units until the coma dose is reached. This coma dose is repeated several days and

then, if sensitivity to insulin develops, the dose is gradually lowered as a smaller dose becomes sufficient to produce satisfactory coma. When a sufficient number of comas have been induced, the dose of insulin is lowered to twenty units. This last period of small dosage is our equivalent of "Phase IV" of the treatment as outlined by Sakel.

The Termination of the Morning Treatment.—The effect of insulin, if not interrupted, would cause coma to persist an indefinite number of hours. It would, undoubtedly, be dangerous to prolong the coma unduly, and the following active measures are taken to terminate the hypoglycemia. At 11 a.m., four hours after the injection of the insulin, patients who have not become comatose are given by mouth 150 gm. of sucrose in chocolate flavored milk. Patients who have become comatose are allowed to remain in coma as long as one and a half hours (if the general condition permits). A nasal tube then is inserted and 150 gm. of sugar in water is allowed to flow into the stomach by gravity. These measures usually cause the patient to awaken within a few minutes.

Sakel expressed the opinion that short severe shocks are to be preferred to long light episodes of coma. Some workers (James, Freudenberg and Cannon[7]) have gone so far as to administer cardiazol in an effort to produce convulsions in addition to coma, in the belief that the convulsive reactions are of aid in bringing about more speedy improvement.

The Phenomena of Insulin Shock

Much has been written of the phenomena which one observes as cases in which schizophrenia is treated by this method. In our cases the first effect of a coma dose of insulin has been to cause drowsiness. This drowsiness in most instances has persisted for about two hours. During the period of drowsiness, pallor and marked perspiration are frequently but by no means constantly present. Following the stage of drowsiness, some patients exhibit a more or less wild motor and psychic excitement, lasting a variable length of time, after which coma appears. Others pass quietly from drowsiness into coma without excitement. It is during the phase of excitement, when it occurs, and during the early stages of coma that remarkable neurologic phenomena of hypoglycemia occur.

During coma the respirations, the position of the patient in bed and his general condition require constant attention. This, together with frequent observations of the condition of the pulse, respiration, blood pressure and temperature, constitutes the special duties required in the nursing care of these patients (Fig. 2).

The patient in hypoglycemic coma presents a treatment problem which is similar in many respects to the problem of handling a patient during the coma of surgical anesthesia. Both require particular efforts on the part of the attendant to preserve the body heat, to keep the patient warm and dry, and to meet emergencies demanding immediate attention to prevent serious complications.

Subjective Reactions

A visitor observing the insulin treatments may infer from the patient's reactions that he suffers greatly. Powerful muscular contractions, grimacing, grinding of teeth, and extraordinary noises combine to present a picture of unmitigated misery such as accompanies few if any other medical procedures. It is very fortunate that, if this treatment does cause discomfort, the memory of the uncomfortable sensations does not persist. Patients cause no difficulty by refusing or being unwilling to take the treatment, because, they have no recollection of the past treatments and no patient has complained of discomfort. On being questioned, an occasional patient recalls a sensation of intoxication or dizziness as the last thing he remembers before slipping off into coma. One patient has written an excellent description of his sensations during the induction and recovery phases (Case 11). This description is an account of well-known sensations frequently experienced during induction and recovery from general anesthesia.

It is usual for the patient to have a splendid appetite immediately on reacting from the coma and he will usually devour sufficient food at the time of his noon meal so that he will more than make up for the calories missed because of omission of breakfast.

Dangers

Fifteen years of experience in the treatment of diabetes with insulin has proved that the

symptoms of overdosage of insulin are not very dangerous. On the other hand, the degree of overdosage is much greater in the treatment of schizophrenia with insulin and occasionally serious complications may be encountered.

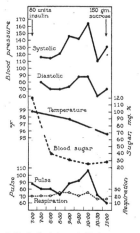

Fig. 2. Usual changes in blood pressure, temperature, blood sugar, pulse and respiration during insulin coma,

The coma initiated by hypoglycemia may persist even after the blood sugar has been restored to a normal level. We have observed two reactions of this type. Two patients failed to awaken promptly from coma after the administration of the usual sucrose by the nasal tube. Both were given dextrose intravenously and more sucrose by nasal tube, which increased the concentration of blood sugar. Coma continued for forty-eight hours in the first instance and then cleared. The second patient remained stuporous four days and Babinski's sign could be elicited on his right foot for thirteen days. In neither case has any evidence of these episodes remained. v. Pap[20] has observed similar incidents.

"After-shock" has occurred in five instances in our series of cases. These reactions are likely to occur in a case in which the patient eats poorly at the time of the noon meal. Rather severe hypoglycemic symptoms, even coma, may

TABLE I. TREATMENT OF SCHIZOPHRENIA (DEMENTIA PRÆCOX) BY INSULIN-HYPOGLYCEMIA

Cases*	Age, Years	Type of Schizophrenia	Duration of Psychosis, Years	Length of stay in Hospital, Months	Prognosis by Usual Treatment	Treatment		Results
						Total Number of days of	Number of Comas	
1	28	Hebephrenic	3	7	Poor	36	20	Unimproved
2	30	Hebephrenic	5	6	Poor	41	24	Unimproved
3	27	Hebephrenic	10	5†	Poor	80	47	‡
4	30	Hebephrenic	2/3	6	Poor	74	38	‡
5	22	Hebephrenic	1 1/2	13	Poor	62	47	Unimproved
6	26	Hebephrenic	1 1/3	5	Poor	64	48	Slightly improved
7	27	Hebephrenic	4 1/2	39	Poor	50	23	Unimproved
8	30	Catatonic	6	6†	Fair	29	17	Marked improvement
9	19	Catatonic	3	5§	Poor	36	21	Unimproved
10	19	Catatonic	3	1 1/4	Poor	41	22	Unimproved
11	22	Catatonic	1/2	2	Fair	31	10	Marked improvement
12	27	Paranoid	1/12	1/2	Poor	40	25	Unimproved
13	34	Catatonic	6 1/2	1/4§	Poor	37	30	Unimproved

*All patients were males.
†Third admission.
‡Some transient improvement.
§Second admission.

appear late in the afternoon. "After-shock" is inconvenient but not dangerous; in cases in which it has occurred the patients have responded promptly to the intravenous administration of glucose. Feeding carbohydrates during the afternoon usually prevents "after-shock." Our routine now includes the administration of 50 to 75 gm. of sucrose in the form of chocolate candy at 3 p.m. and at bedtime to all patients who have received insulin during the morning.

In man, epileptiform attacks occur occasionally during hypoglycemic shock; in dogs, such attacks appear very frequently. These attacks yield promptly to the administration of sugar and epinephrine, and it has been our practice to terminate the hypoglycemic state whenever the attacks become severe. Some writers, as Küppers,[8] do not interrupt the treatment when convulsive attacks appear. This appears to us to be somewhat hazardous and perhaps unnecessary. Symptoms of circulatory failure have not occurred in our cases and records of the pulse and blood pressure do not show any instances of alarming change during treatment.

Young,[23] of Omaha, recently reported one death due to pulmonary edema and one death due to cardiac collapse.

Results

Throughout our work we have adhered to a policy of attempting to make observations as objective as possible. We have made a complete physical, psychiatric and laboratory survey of each patient before treatment was undertaken. We have recorded by photographs and by means of moving pictures the appearance and behavior of each patient before the treatment was begun, as we feel that these data afford valuable evidence in the estimation of any changes which may appear to have occurred as a result of the treatment.

In the thirteen cases which are the basis of this report (Table I), the type of schizophrenia was as follows: hebephrenic in seven cases, catatonic in five cases and paranoid in one case.

Hebephrenic Type.—No improvement was noted in six of the cases in which the schizophrenia was of the hebephrenic type but slight improvement occurred in one case (Case 6). The outstanding features in this case may be found in the following history.

Case 6.—The patient was a man aged twenty-six years. The psychosis had been present for fifteen months before the insulin-shock therapy was started. He was very untidy; he had a fixed expression, and there was no spontaneous speech. His voice was monotonous, his mood was absolutely indifferent, and he collected all sorts of odds and ends in his pockets, including a match box which he usually kept filled with butter or some other food. He could not be induced to do work of any kind.

At the completion of the treatment he was a little more careful of his dress than he had been. He would read papers and magazines, he would help willingly in the ward work and in the occupational therapy pavilion. His movements remained slow and deliberate and his facial expression remained fixed and staring. The general opinion is that the amount of improvement attained in this case would hardly justify the prolonged, difficult and somewhat dangerous treatment, namely forty-eight deep comas in sixty-four treatment days.

In two other cases (Cases 3 and 4) in which the schizophrenia was of the hebephrenic type the patients experienced transitory changes in their psychoses and for a short time it appeared as though they might improve. At the completion of the treatment, which included forty-seven and thirty-eight deep comas respectively, the patients were unimproved.

Catatonic Type.—The two cases (Cases 8 and 11) in which the schizophrenia was of the catatonic type, the patients improved markedly during the course of the treatment. A summary of the events of these two patients follows:

Case 8.—The patient was a man aged thirty years (Fig. 3). His birth and development had been normal. When he was first admitted to the hospital in August, 1930, psychotic symptoms had been present for one month. He remained in the hospital until June 20, 1931; at that time he was markedly improved and was allowed to return to his home. He was readmitted to the hospital in August of 1934; at this time he was negativistic, sullen and uncommunicative. He improved slowly and was paroled in April of 1935. He returned home and later worked on a farm. He was admitted to the hospital, for the third time, August 27, 1936. For two months he had not shown any interest in his work. A few days before this he had struck his sister and had tried to tear the clothes from his brother. He had stood in one position for long periods. Mental examination at the time of admission was impossible because he failed to answer questions. There was

no spontaneous speech but he exhibited marked flexibilitas cerea.

Between August, 1936, and February, 1937, there was no detectable change in his mental condition. At the time the insulin treatment was started it was his habit to sit quietly and apathetically about the ward. At

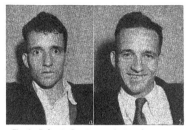

Fig. 3. Patient in Case 8 (catatonic dementia praecox); *a*, before treatment; *b*, after treatment.

times he refused to eat. There was no spontaneous speech and his mental status could not be assessed because he remained mute. The result of general and neurologic examination was negative except that catalepsy was marked.

The insulin treatment was started February 15, 1937 (Fig. 1). On February 18, profuse sweating appeared following the administration of 40 units of insulin. On February 22, 80 units of insulin was administered at 7 a.m. At 11 a.m. a condition of wild motor and psychic excitement was present. The patient made noises, screamed, threw himself around in bed and made powerful forceful thrusts and jumps. After he recovered from the hypoglycemia he spoke freely but was very silly. A half hour later he would no longer respond. Between February 23 and March 6, deep coma was induced daily (except for a rest day on Sundays). On March 6, following the administration of the usual dose of sucrose (150 gm. in 500 c.c. of water) at 11 a.m. he failed to respond and at 1:45 p. m. 25 gm. of a 50 per cent solution of dextrose was administered intravenously. At that time he was in deep coma; salivation and stertorous respirations were present. Ankle clonus and Babinski's signs were present bilaterally. At 2:00 p.m. he had not responded to the intravenous administration of dextrose and 1,000 c.c. of a 20 per cent solution of dextrose was injected slowly into a vein. In addition, 150 gm. of sucrose in water was administered through a nasal tube. At 6:30 p.m. he had not responded to the treatment. His skin was dry and there was urinary incontinence. The value for the blood sugar was 190 mg. per 100 c.c. The pulse rate was 82 beats per minute and there were 24 respirations per minute. The pupils were 2 mm. in diameter and reacted to light. On March 7, his condition continued the same all day. March 8, the stupor had cleared, and the general and gross neurologic examination did not reveal any abnormality.

Deep comas were induced on March 9, 10, 11, 12, 13 and 15. Beginning on March 9, a remarkable change appeared in his condition. His movement seemed gradually to become more free. Flexibilitas cerea dis-

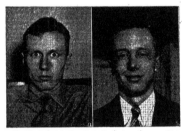

Fig. 4. Patient in Case 11 (catatonic dementia praecox); a, before treatment; b, after treatment.

appeared. The grimacing ceased. He began to speak freely with doctors and attendants. His gait became free and purposeful. He was sent to the occupational therapy pavilion in the afternoons, where he began wood-carving. His speech was silly at times and it occasionally was irrelevant. He did not seem to have much insight into his condition. He did state, however, that he realized he had been "mentally sick." He could describe his former jobs in an upholsterer's shop and in a bowling alley. He spoke freely of his previous earnings and discussed his home conditions intelligently. On March 16, the dose of insulin was decreased to 20 units and this small dosage was continued daily until March 21, after which insulin treatment was discontinued.

On April 26, 1937, he was paroled to the care of his family. He was neat, spontaneous speech was normal and he addressed the physician in an intelligent manner. He smiled and was good humored. He did not have a very good mental grasp of the events of his illness (he thought it might have resulted from smoking, although he had only smoked occasionally, or from drinking, although he had confined his drinking to an occasional glass of wine). He was well oriented as to time, place, and person and his memory for the events of his own life was excellent. His grasp of current events was very poor; he knew nothing of the current Spanish Civil War or of the abdication of the English king. He could calculate accurately and his speech throughout the examination was relevant and logical. He denied hallucinations and no delusions were expressed.

Case 11.—The patient was a man, aged twenty-two years (Fig. 4), who was a senior in a university. The past history was irrelevant. His mother said that he always had been somewhat moody and quiet, but he

had been an average student. The patient was admitted to the Rochester State Hospital on January 27, 1937. During the preceding summer he had seemed unusually preoccupied and very quiet. He had started his senior year at the university in the fall of 1936 and while he had been at home he had spent most of his time studying. About December 1, 1936, his mother had noted that he seemed to be having difficulty in concentrating; he would scowl and keep pressing his forehead with his hand while reading. He had become more peculiar until January 1, 1937, when he had to be removed to a sanitarium because he refused to eat.

On examination prior to treatment he refused to speak and was filthy in his habits. He would protrude his tongue on command and allow the examiner to prick it with a pin, without evidencing any pain. There was marked flexibilitas cerea and he had to be fed almost entirely with a tube. He had lost 24 pounds (10.9 kg.). Routine laboratory procedures including serologic tests for syphilis did not reveal any abnormality.

Insulin treatment was started March 17, 1937. One hundred and twenty units of insulin produced satisfactory coma on April 1. He experienced a rather marked "after-shock" about 6 p. m. on April 8.

On April 9 the usual dose of 120 units of insulin produced a deep, satisfactory coma. This coma was terminated at 11 a.m. by feeding with a nasal tube. At 2 p.m. he was talkative but very peculiar. He answered to "how do you feel" by a long pause and then nodded his head slowly up and down and finally said "pretty good." He talked with the ward attendants about his meal and hummed a song in tune with a nearby radio. At 8 p.m. he refused to answer questions and would not look at the examiner.

The usual morning coma was induced on April 10. At 1 p.m., he was seen washing his face carefully and it was observed that his movements were free, whereas he previously had been very stupid and rigid. When he finished he smiled a greeting and stopped to chat. He was "feeling much better." He knew that he had been ill. He said that he had been unable to eat or talk because a voice told him not to do so.

On April 13, the dosage of insulin was reduced to 20 units daily; sugar was administered two hours later. Two hours after the insulin was injected the patient became comatose and presented a striking instance of insulin sensitization. He was sent to the occupational therapy pavilion this day and began the caning of a chair. He was amenable, polite, quiet and good-natured. He smiled naturally when speaking and was anxious to please. He described the sensations of the insuline treatment as follows: "One feels before unconsciousness comes, not very sleepy but as though one wanted to move or arise from bed. It took much effort to move my arms, legs or body with much deliberation beforehand. When I moved any part of my body my mental condition changed." Concerning his awakening from the insulin coma he said: "Mentally, I felt a space separation between myself and the world. Voices and other sounds came to me clearly but they were considered as coming across space, myself being on the opposite side from where voices and sounds came. My head felt as though it were expanding from within, causing mental pain. The sickening headache which resulted would continue for about two seconds, lessen in degree, then in two seconds become more intense, then lessen." When he was paroled on June 4, he was in excellent condition.

In the three remaining cases in which the schizophrenia was of the catatonic type the patients were not improved.

Paranoid Type.—Only one patient who had the paranoid type of schizophrenia was treated. This patient did not show any improvement.

Summary

Thirteen patients who had schizophrenia have been treated by the method of insulin hypoglycemia. Of these patients, ten were unimproved, one was slightly improved and two were markedly improved. The results of our work in the treatment of schizophrenia by the method of insulin hypoglycemia have not been as encouraging as those reported by Sakel. There may be several reasons for this difference. First, the patients were not treated at the most favorable time, and second, we have been cautious about permitting the continuation of convulsive manifestations which are now looked upon as desirable.

Regarding the two patients who improved markedly, the first had improved spontaneously on two previous occasions from similar attacks and there seems to be no way of assuring ourselves that he might not have recovered spontaneously in this instance. It does seem proper to assume that the treatment hastened the recovery. The second patient who improved was a young man who had catatonic schizophrenia; he feel that he would have been given a fair prognosis with the usual methods of treatment. However, there is little doubt that the treatment brought about his speedy improvement. We believe that the insulin-hypoglycemia treatment is a heroic form of therapy and should not be used haphazardly. Our results, while not too encouraging, justify further work in order to evaluate the results of the treatment and possibly point the way to added therapeutic measures. Accordingly, we have recently placed under treatment a group of twelve female patients who were suffering from schizophrenia.

Undoubtedly, the selection of patients must play an important rôle in determining the usefulness of this type of therapeutic procedure. Rules to be followed in this selection are not apparent from our work. A review of the literature is also unavailing in an attempt to settle this point beyond the fact that the more recent the onset of the psychosis the more favorable is the prognosis.

Uncertainty exists as to how many comas constitute a complete course of treatment. In our work, when improvement has not appeared after the patient has experienced twenty-five to forty satisfactory comas, we have concluded that the treatment is unavailing. Some workers have employed as many as 200 comas without beneficial effect. From our experience we would say that if a patient shows no improvement after forty comas the treatment should be discontinued.

Results obtained by us up to this time suggest that much more work will be required to provide a firm foundation for the extraordinary claims which have been made for this method of treatment.

Insulin treatment of schizophrenia demands of those who attempt it continuous watchfulness and a readiness to act in emergencies, which is based on definite knowledge of the situations at hand. The procedure deals with helpless patients in coma. Violent epileptiform convulsions are an ever-threatening menace. Cardiovascular, respiratory and cerebral calamities have been reported. Other dangers may lurk in regions incompletely explored. Accordingly, this method of treatment should be employed only in hospitals with trained personnel and a physician must always be at hand. The personnel of the insulin treatment ward should be well organized and should be similar to the modern trained operation room force in efficiency and readiness to act. To do less is to expose patients to unjustifiable risks.

We wish to express our appreciation to the Eli Lilly Company for supplying us with insulin for this work.

References

1. Berglas, B., and Susic, Z.: Über die Hypoglykämie-Chock-behandlung der Schizophrenie. Psychiat.-neurol. Wchnschr., 38:599-602, (Nov. 28) 1936.
2. Berze, Josef: Die Insulin-Chockbehandlung der Schizophrenie. Wien. med. Wchnschr., 83:1365-1369, (Dec. 2) 1933.
3. Braunmühl, A. V.: Die Insulinschockbehandlung der

Schizophrenie. München. med. Wchnschr., 84:8-11, (Jan. 1) 1937.
4. Dussik, K. T., and Sakel, Manfred: Ergebnisse der Hypoglykämieshockbehandlung der Schizophrenie. Ztschr. f. d. ges. Neurol. u. Psychiat., 155:351-415, 1936.
5. Glueck, Bernard: The hypoglycemic state in the treatment of schizophrenia. Jour. Am. Med. Assn., 107:1029-1031, (Sept. 26) 1936.
6. Hoff, Hans: Hypoglykämie-Shockbehandlung von Psychosen. Wien. klin. Wchnschr., 49:917-918, (July 17) 1936.
7. James, G. W. B., Freudenberg, Rudolph, and Cannon, A. T.: Insulin shock treatment of schizophrenia. Lancet, 1:1101-1103, (May 8) 1937.
8. Küppers, E.: Die Insulinbehandlung der Schizophrenie. Deutsch. med. Wchnschr., 63:377-383, (Mar. 5) 1937.
9. Langenfeldt, G.: Die Insulin-chok-behandlung der Schizophrenie. Psychiat.-neurol. Wchnschr., 38:483-484, (Sept. 19) 1936.
10. Larkin, E. H.: Insulin shock treatment of schizophrenia. Brit. Med. Jour., 1:745-747, (April 10) 1937.
11. Lichter, C., and Lichter, N.: Vol. Jubilaire en l'honneur du Prof. Dr. C. Parhon., 1934, pp. 281-285.
12. Meyer, Adolph: The origin and nature of the hypoglycemic therapy of the psychoses. Jour. Nerv. and Ment. Dis., 85:578-580, (May) 1937.
13. Müller, M.: Die Insulinschocktherapie der Schizophrenie. Schweiz. med. Wchnschr., 66:929-935, (Sept. 26) 1936.
14. Müller, M.: Die Insulinshockbehandlung der Schizophrenie. Nervenartz., 9:569-580, (Nov.) 1936.
15. Reese, H. H.: Insulin shock therapy of schizophrenia (dementia praecox.) Wisconsin Med. Jour., 36:111, (Feb.) 1937.
16. Rosenberg, E. F., Smith, B. F., Wilder, R. M. and Moersch, F. P.: Treatment of schizophrenia (dementia praecox) by insulin hypoglycemia. Proc. Staff Meet. Mayo Clinic, 12:273-278, (May 5) 1937.
17. Sakel, M.: Schizophreniebehandlung mittels Insulin Hypoglykämie sowie Hypoglykämischer Schocks. Wien. med. Wchnschr., 84:1211, (Nov. 3) 1934; 1265, (Nov. 17) 1934; 1299, (Nov. 24) 1934; 1326, (Dec. 1) 1934; 1353, (Dec. 8) 1934; 1383, (Dec. 15) 1934; 1401, (Dec. 22) 1934; 85:35, (Jan. 5) 1935; 68, (Jan. 12) 1935; 94, (Jan. 19) 1935; 121, (Jan. 26) 1935; 152, (Feb. 2) 1935; 175, (Feb. 9) 1935.
18. Sakel, Manfred: A new treatment of schizophrenia. Am. Jour. Psychiat., 93:829-841, (Jan.) 1937.
19. Schaeffer, Henri: Le traitement de la schizophrénie par le choc insulinique. Presse méd., 44:1566-1569, (Oct. 7) 1936.
20. v. Pap, Zoltan: Erfahrungen mit der Insulinshocktherapie bei Schizophrenen. Monatschr. f. Psychiat. u. Neurol., 94:318-349, (Jan.) 1937.
21. Wilson, Isabel, G. H.: A study of hypoglycaemic shock treatment in schizophrenia. His Majesty's Stationary Office, London, 1936, 74 pp.
22. Wortis, Joseph: On response of schizophrenic subjects to hypoglycemic insulin shocks. Jour. Nerv. and Ment. Dis., 84:497-506, (Nov.) 1936.
23. Young, A. G., and Young, R. H.: Unpublished data.

MEDICINE: A CO-OPERATIVE BUSINESS, A NON-COMPETITIVE PROFESSION*

B. J. BRANTON, M.D., F.A.C.S.

Willmar, Minnesota

DR. ALAN DE F. SMITH in a current issue of *Surgery, Gynecology and Obstetrics* writes a short biographic sketch of Dr. Russell A. Hibbs, and I wish to quote from it as follows:

"To those who knew him best his greatness lay even more in his fine spiritual qualities, in his never failing conviction that the truth must always prevail, in his steadfast adherence to any course that he believed was right, and in that rare gift of leadership which inspired all those who served under him to give the best that was in them and to feel that to work with him was a privilege. He always maintained that any accomplishment that was made in the advancement of medicine must come from a deep sympathy of the doctor for his patient and from his real concern in making him well."

What a privilege it must have been for him to be able to express in such beautiful words his honest opinion regarding a colleague and his worth to society. What a satisfaction to have been associated with a man of such fine accomplishments. What an honor to live so that we may leave behind us such sentiments of love to be expressed by those that we have worked and toiled with. That is the result of work well done, purposes accomplished, a life well spent.

Are we each of us devoting ourselves to our fellow men for the good we can accomplish or purely for selfish reasons? Is the practice of medicine wholly mercenary or purely sentimental? Are we doing our part in the economy of the state and nation, or are we shrugging our shoulders and shifting the burden on the heads of others less able by education or learning to carry it, with the possible regimentation of medicine to the purposes of the State as the penalty for our lack of interest?

Two thousand years ago there was born in Palestine on the banks of the Jordan the greatest Teacher and Physician of all times. He taught the gospel of love and peace to all mankind. He said, "Love your enemies." Men have said His teachings cannot be carried out in this essentially practical and competitive world. Experience, the leveler of all men's thoughts, teaches us that it can and should be as truly practical now as then.

Ambition, the young man's spark plug, gives way gradually to a fuller realization of the need of tolerance in most men's lives in later years. What we need most in America at present is to submerge that mythical ideal of success, the accumulation of wealth, in a development of American standards of just dealing.

If fair dealing for mutual welfare has been found so essential between lawyers, bankers, and business men generally; if friendship is a great and indispensable attribute in business, then

*Presented before the Northern Minnesota Medical Association, Virginia, Minnesota, August 27, 1937.

162

aren't we, as practitioners of the most sacred calling on earth, remiss if we do not develop a sense of mutual understanding of each others' problems, both economic and professional?

Thoreau once wrote, "If you have built castles in the air, your work need not be lost; that is where they should be. Now put foundations under them."

We are in Minnesota, I believe, putting solid foundations under our professional buildings. Nowhere are higher ideals of practice promulgated than here. We have not builded on the shifting sands. The 2,300 members of our State Association are an essentially learned and highly developed type of men. They have to be. The people among whom they work demand the best in service. We have built their demands up to a high plane. We cannot and will not let down this faith.

The standard of work which we have carried on during the late disagreeable depression among the so-called indigents gives the lie to those who say "medicine" has not done its share to make the lot of the people more tolerable. The long hours of service, the worry of nights of vigil have all been the same even though the incomes of physicians have shown a lessened figure from month to month. We have carried on medicine's unswerving traditions with unfaltering devotion. It is my belief that this "carrying on" through troubled times will be rewarded many fold in the future if we do not lose faith in each other. We are our brother's keeper to no small degree. Elbert Hubbard, that inimitable philosopher, said, "Do not lose faith in humanity. There are over ninety million people in America who have never played you a single nasty trick."

Many of us can remember when Dr. So-and-So would not speak to Dr. So-and-So. When to speak of a man's competitor was to bring down wrath and words of vituperation of unmentionable degree. The Hippocratic Oath was a thing forgotten since the day of graduation. The doctor's family were victims of unjustifiable censure. Small towns were divided into two camps, each with their medical man, much after the custom among ancient tribes of aborigines.

Has this changed today? Have organizations such as we have meeting here changed this attitude to a marked enough degree or are we still in the transitional state?

It is my belief that we have changed, at least

to some degree. The change is not marked enough, but surely is gaining ground toward the ideal, a sincerely united profession.

Statistics show that the number of physicians practicing in states such as ours is just about keeping up with the population; that, while good roads and automobiles have made it easier for men to cover larger territories, new modes of treatment of disease, the intricacies of living and even the good roads and automobiles themselves have added to the work of the man of medicine. Industry and its insurance have entered the picture. Public health measures draw their workers from the graduates in medicine, thus lessening the number available for private practice.

There is work for all who seek it. No one needs to loiter at the door of the temple of Æsculapius. He who searches shall find. The workers are many but the opportunities are threefold.

The youth who looks through colored glasses, colored by the present trend of economic thought, into the future and sees no opportunity for him will find that the boy with imagination has passed him and has reached the goal of his desires. He is the master, teacher, and leader of the generation.

The success of coöperative enterprises in this State has placed Minnesota at the head of the states of the Union in this type of business; but back of coöperatives are years of solid thought. History but repeats itself and passing time finds but few changes in the economy of the world's wants. The mountains do not move though the winds and hurricanes harass them with their fury. The vast amount of water in the body of the oceans does not change though the waves roll over them.

In 1879 Roswell Dwight Hitchcock wrote "The Socialist" and in it gave us the picture of communism as we know it today. So every profession and business has found, passing down through the ages, that there is strength in numbers, that concentrated thought does the most good for all, that coöperative organizations with strong leadership are successful and easily survive the ravages of time.

Medicine, to keep its place in the fore of professions and protect its members, must foster the spirit of coöperation, must become a solid unit of economic thought, must forget petty jealousies and bickerings between individuals.

Cicero once said, "Men condemn because they do not understand." To better understand a man is the spirit of better coöperation. Society asks this of the man of medicine. Are we giving it?

While we sit at this meeting we are making resolutions to practice better medicine in the future, to live and forget past differences, to think and speak well of our confreres, to more fully enjoy that abundant life which we hear so much about. Can we and will we carry these same resolutions into effect when we reach our several homes? Why not endeavor to close the gap of unfriendliness between the door of your neighbor's office and your own. If in union there is strength and from fellowship and association come admiration, we can well remember this: "Man's conscious influence, when he is on dress-parade, when he is posing to impress those around him, is wonderfully small. But his unconscious influence—the silent, subtle radiations of his personality, the effect of his words and acts, the trifles he never considers—is tremendous."

From this day forth let our competitor be our coöperator; coöperation, not competition, our motto. An old friend of mine wrote the following after years of sorrow. It made a lasting impression on me. I give it to you:

I've shut the door on yesterday, its sorrows and mis-takes,
I've locked within its gloomy walls past failures and heartaches,
And now I throw the key away to seek another room,
And furnish it with hope and smiles and every spring-time bloom.
No thought shall enter this abode that has a hint of pain,
And every malice and distrust shall never therein reign.
I've shut the door on yesterday and thrown the key away,
Tomorrow holds no doubt for me since I have found today.

Tomorrow will hold no doubt for us if we have found each other today and are determined to extol each man's good qualities above his faults.

Let us make of medicine a coöperative business, a non-competitive profession.

MEDICAL TOUR OF SOUTH AMERICA

O. A. OLSON, M.D.

Minneapolis, Minnesota

UNDER the auspices of the Interstate Post Graduate Association of North America, a party of physicians visited the Universities of South America in the spring of 1937. This association for the past fifteen years has conducted clinical tours to Europe. This is the first visit to South America. There were twenty-six members in our party. The voyage was delightful, the kind one associates with the South Seas. The Neptune party was a new experience to most of us. Continuous pleasant weather banished sea sickness and made weather reports unnecessary.

On the morning of April second we entered the harbor of Rio, the most beautiful in the western hemisphere. As we passed the Sugar Loaf we saw the city spread out along the beautiful beaches. The harbor, twenty-five miles long, offers a beautiful vista as far as the eye can see. Rio is a city in the latitude of the tropic of Capricorn and its climate is similar to

that of Havana. It is the capital of Brazil, a country larger than the United States and abundantly supplied with natural resources. The Amazon Basin, which was once an inland sea, contains rivers, mountains, plains and immense forests.

Many of the hospitals throughout South America are supported by benefit associations whose memberships vary from twenty-five to seventy-five thousand. One Catholic institution in Rio has thirty thousand members. The fee which one pays varies with age. It is approximately one hundred dollars for men and one hundred ten for women. The fee is paid when one joins and entitles the individual to free care for life, hospitalization, physicians, drugs, lawyers, x-rays, burial expenses, grave and grave markings. The reason life care can be given for such a small amount is due to the fact that the institution is endowed. The doctors are not paid.

The old Emergency Hospital at Rio, an efficient institution, has a fleet of ambulances always on call. The doctors are government employees and receive fifty dollars a month for part time and one hundred dollars for full time.

The Beneficencia Portugeza hospital is a beautiful building said to have cost ten thousand dollars per bed. Here we saw Dr. Gudin demonstrate his method of total sterilization. Operating room, dressings, surgical instruments and sponges are sterilized by formalin method. This occurs in a hermetically sealed, air conditioned and air filtered operating room. The amphitheater is above the operating room and one looks down through glass. The operating room is set up and formalin is introduced into the room under a valve control. After a certain time this is neutralized by ammonia and the ammonia neutralized by sulphuric or tartaric acid. Dr. Gudin claims that with care three or four clean operations may be done with one sterilization. At the time of the operation all persons in the room are completely gowned, including the feet. Surgeons are then free to touch anything about the room. If a sponge is dropped on the floor it may be picked up and used within the abdomen without danger of infection. The doctor claimed that by this method wound infection is much less frequent than by the method ordinarily used (Fig. 1).

We visited the Hospital dos Espostos, a hospital for abandoned children. Dr. Jose Martinho da Rocha is the director. Children brought to this hospital are passed through a hole in the wall. Persons leaving the child ring a bell to announce the arrival of the child. Sometimes the name of the child is left, sometimes it is not. The hospital takes care of all children who are left there. At the time of our visit there were seven hundred and fifty children in the institution and two hundred and fifty of them were infants. The children are educated and taught trades in the hospital. There were many cases of lues, tuberculosis and dysentery among the children. Their mortality from syphilis is 30 per cent in babies under one year of age. The diseases most common in children in Brazil are lues, tuberculosis, malaria and worms.

We were invited to a reception at the Brazilian College of Surgeons. Professor Jayme Poggi delivered an address of welcome to the doctors from North America. Membership in the college is limited to forty and is by invitation only.

At the Deutsches Krankenhaus, Dr. Maurity Santos, who is a very skillful surgeon, did a

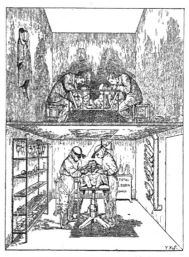

Fig. 1. Gudin's method of total sterilization.

vaginal hysterectomy for cancer of the cervix. No radium is used for cancer of the cervix in this institution. Dr. Santos also did a resection of the rectum for strictures from granuloma inguinale, a very common disease in Brazil. He used his own method, doing a combined abdominal and perineal operation, first liberating the diseased bowel through the abdominal opening, then, by an incision to the side of the rectum, resected the rectum and the diseased bowel, saving the sphincter. The proximal end of the bowel was then pulled through the anal opening and was split for several inches, each half being sutured to the buttock. A small tube was inserted into the bowel and four strips of iodoform gauze were placed into the ischiorectal fossa. The split portion of the protruding bowel was then allowed to slough. Dr. Santos has operated in fifty such cases. All cases showed a positive Frie's test.

Our medical section made the rounds with Professor Annos Dios in the clinic of Professor Clementino Fraga. He showed a variety of medical diseases, also demonstrated studies of bile chemistry pertaining to acidosis and alkalosis. In this hospital the government maintains a meteorologic station and for twenty years they have studied and correlated the effect of atmospheric changes on disease. Professor Dios concludes that certain atmospheric and meteorologic changes are responsible in part for certain complications such as pulmonary hemorrhages, typhoid hemorrhages, post-operative bleeding and shock as it appears following surgery. When the weather is too hot or the humidity is too great, they avoid operating except in emergency.

On April eighth we went by rail to Sao Paulo traveling through interesting mountainous country. Here and there the valleys were studded with ant hills, some as high as a man's head. Sao Paulo, named after the prophet, is situated on a plateau, has a delightful climate and its people are an energetic populace. The city has doubled in the last six years and now has a population of one million two hundred thousand. It is an industrial city, the "Chicago" of Brazil.

At the Santa Casa hospital Professor Ramos demonstrated cases of lipoid nephrosis showing a transition of this disease into parenchymatous nephritis, also aneurysm of the aorta, with erosion of vertebræ and ribs. He showed cases of Ayerza's disease, claiming that this is not a pathological entity and should not be designated nosographically as a disease. It might well be called black cardiac disease characterized by polycythemia. Dr. Ramos presented cardiac cases well worked up; extensive studies of electrocardiographs in cases of bundle branch block.

The Pro-Matre Paulista Hospital is a modern, private maternity hospital of fifty beds, owned by twelve physicians, and has an open staff. They have portable incubators for premature children which are used to bring in cases for hospitalization.

At the Sanitoria Santa Catherina, a private hospital, Professor B. Montenegro did a gastric resection for ulcers of the stomach, using a technic which he developed. The operation was done under spinal anesthesia with one assistant,

one interne and no clean nurse. His technic is used at the University and we saw students doing dog surgery, using his technic, for gastric resections. It is a simplified procedure and enables him to do a resection in one hour. He prefers gastric resection, removing approximately two-thirds of the stomach, in preference to all other operations for both gastric and duodenal ulcers. Dr. Montenegro, who formerly was professor of anatomy, received his surgical training under John B. Deaver in Philadelphia. He has done about twelve hundred gastric resections for ulcers. The mortality in the first 622 cases was 4.5 per cent. He has lowered his mortality in the last series. In his first 500 cases three cases of jejunal ulcers developed; none has developed in the last 700. He thinks this is due to the fact that he now does a more extensive resection. He uses the Van Slyke method of carbon dioxide determination in the blood as an indication for the use of glucose and subcutaneous saline. Glucose is often used pre-operatively but never post-operatively unless there is special indication. Blood transfusions are seldom done.

He thinks that megacolon, megaureters and cardiospasms are all due to deficiency of vitamins B and B[1]. Cardiospasm, called "Ecclasia," is very common on the coffee plantations of Brazil. It is not the same as Hirschsprung's disease, which is congenital. Ecclasia is due to paralysis or inability of the various sphincters in the large bowel to open. The spasm of the various sphincters of the colon, including Cannon's sphincter at the hepatic flexure and including spasm of the voluntary sphincter at the rectum is due to vitamin B deficiency, which is responsible for the lesion in Auerbach's plexus. He believes that the spasm of the internal sphincters could be cured by dilatation if the sphincters could be reached, but there is no way of reaching them except surgically, by doing an open stripping operation, cutting the muscular layer down to the mucosa similar to the Ramstad operation. He also believes these cases should be treated postoperatively with a general high vitamin diet. We were shown a case of common duct drainage in which the duct contracted under the influence of morphine. Lipiodol was injected into the common duct. When morphine was given, the lipiodol was forced back into the pancreatic ducts showing that morphine caused contraction of the sphincter of Oddi.

On the afternoon of April eighth we visited the Butantan Institute where Professor Alfrania Amaral, a graduate of the Harvard School of

The department of records has been adopted from the United States. Bi-weekly meetings are held in which all departments exchange information. Practically all papers are published in Portuguese.

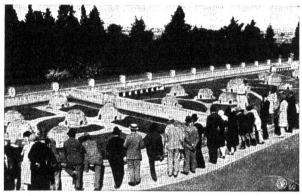

Fig. 2. The Butantan snake farm.

Hygiene in 1924, is director. Fifty years ago this was a private institution for the study of smallpox and plague. It has now been taken over by the state, and it is practically self-supporting. The institution, consisting of many buildings and large grounds, is divided into twelve departments and research is conducted in a variety of scientific problems pertaining to Brazil. Smallpox vaccine is made which can be injected under the skin and does not cause a sore. This was first developed at the Rockefeller Institute. In the department for the study of fertilization, they are trying to develop better fodder, grain, etc. They grow oats from Australia, crossing it with Brazilian oats to improve its yield. A school is also conducted for the children of the employees. They provide a general education for the children and also educate them in special fields of work of the institution with the idea of thereby training future workers for the institute. Professor Amaral stated that it may well be that a child of the laboring man of the institute may become its director. The department of propaganada spreads knowledge of their findings among the people of Brazil.

The Butantan snake farm (Fig. 2) comes under the department of biology. There are three types of poisonous snakes: rattlers, vipers and cobras. The rattlers and vipers are found in Brazil. Three types of antivenom are made: one for the rattler family, one for the viper and one that is polyvalent. When not certain of the reptile the polyvalent serum is used until the symptoms show which type is indicated. An injection should be given every two to three hours until the patient shows definite symptoms of recovery. One of the striking symptoms is blindness; another ptosis of the upper eyelid. As the toxins are neutralized these symptoms improve.

Professor Amaral has succeeded in crystallizing the toxin but so far has been unable to synthesize it. He knows that it contains carbon, hydrogen, oxygen and zinc. The poison is very complex in structure. In one species of snake Professor Amaral claims to have isolated twelve different poisons, each having an affinity for certain structures of the body. One affects the cardiac muscles, one causes lysis of the white blood cells, one of the red blood cells, another causes smooth muscle poisoning, one paralysis of the phrenic nerve, one affects the brain and nervous system and one coagulates the blood, et cetera. This coagulation factor is used in the treatment of purpuric diseases. The snakes are obtained from ranches in the interior in exchange for antivenom. The snakes will not eat while in captivity and die in one or two months. More snakes are received at the institute than can be used.

The use of alcohol is not helpful but is injurious in treatment of snake bites as it reduces the resistance of the victim. The bite of a venomous snake seldom causes bleeding because it is a deep puncture of the fangs and the venom coagulates the blood. Non-poisonous snake bites cause bleeding because these snakes have many teeth and they tear the tissues. The black snake is immune to snake bites and will destroy the poisonous snake if in the same enclosure. A poisonous snake will not attack people but non-poisonous snakes do.

The venom is comparable to the parotid secretion of man, it is proteolytic for the carnivorous food of the snake and for the tissues of man. The dose of the antivenom is inversely proportionate to the weight of the patient. Smaller individuals receive the larger doses. Success also depends on the time factor, the earlier the antivenom is given the better. The laity can administer the serum. Only 30 per cent of persons bitten need antiserum but there is no way of selecting this group. The mortality has been lowered from 20 to 2 per cent by treatment. It is very difficult to immunize against snake bites, for it takes three months to produce an immunity which lasts only a few weeks.

The guinea pig is very susceptible to snake poison. A guinea pig is now being crossed with a native pig called "Kova" which is resistant to venom. It is found that the hybrid animal produced by this crossing develops skull changes resembling the "Kova." Dr. Amaral said this indicates that immunity laws apparently follow the Mendelian laws of heredity. He does not recommend the use of South American serum in other countries because of the necessity of strict specificity.

In Brazil the Japanese inhabitants eat snakes as a delicacy. Professor Amaral is doing some research work upon a worm infestation which occurs in Brazil. These worms occur in re eaten by snakes and the snakes are eaten l Japanese. He believes this worm will be in the Japanese immigrants.

They also have several species of large p ous toads from which they have extrac toxin that resembles digitalis in action. parotid gland secretion of toads is alkalin its alkaloid is Buffotoxin.

The institute is doing research on the bean. Professor Amaral has demonstrate the harmful effect of coffee is not that of c but another alkaloid which is not yet isola

They are conducting research in virus di and other infections, such as Rocky Mo fever and typhus in relation to Brazil.

In the laboratory of Endocrinology, Pro Amaral demonstrated two rats, a male female, whose peritoneal cavities had anastomosed. The male had been cas The experiment showed that the excess of tary hormone from the castrated male was ing an enlargement of the uterus and a in the female. The uterus occupied both itoneal cavities. In the eye of the femal had transplanted a piece of the ovary and able to see with an ordinary magnifying this ovary form follicles in the cavity of th He showed a second animal in which the cinereum had been destroyed by cauteri This animal showed a profuse growth of teeth which had become so long they h appearance of tusks curled upon them This demonstrated the factor of growth the tuber cinereum which may be related growth factors of the body in general.

In the laboratories we also saw mo phagedenic ulcers which had been cured application of plain horse serum, dried an dered, which is very stimulating for growth. This dried serum may be used i cose ulcers.

Professor Dr. Joao de Aguiar Pupo, D Professor of Syphilology and Derm; showed us through the medical center Paulo. It is a new building finance $2,000,000 grant from the Rockefeller F tion matched by the State of Sao Pau teaching facilities are modern in every w; medical school could ask for finer eq or better facilities for study. The depa of Embryology and Physiology are very complete, having models, drawings and actual specimens projected and artificially lighted. A lecture room designed by Professor Edmundo Vasconcelos was the last word in equipment. The entire room was artificially lighted. There were illuminated glass boards which could be used in a dark room. The projecting apparatus was controlled from the operating table and the seats were individually lighted.

The medical course at the University is six years and the requirements for entry are two years pre-medical and competitive examination. Three hundred and fifty apply; only seventy are accepted. Students pay no tuition. Only graduates of this University are admitted to practice. Foreign doctors must take the last three years at the school and also must take the examination in Portuguese. Only naturalized citizens may take the examination.

We traveled by cable railroad to Santos, a town of about fifty thousand and the seaport of Sao Paulo. It was formerly called the white man's graveyard due to ravages of yellow fever and typhus. Modern sanitation has changed all this. A paved road has just been completed connecting Santos with Sao Paulo. Ninety per cent of the world's coffee is transported over the cable railway from Sao Paulo to Santos. This is considered the most remarkable railroad in the world. Trains are taken up and down by counterbalanced cables, three cars up and three down every seven minutes. The construction of this road is a great engineering feat, not only on account of the steep incline but because of the annual rainfall of one hundred and eighty inches which necessitates elaborate watercourses to prevent washouts.

The Orchid Park at Santos has four thousand of the forty thousand varieties of orchids found in Brazil. There were rare varieties of orchids most strange and beautiful.

At Montevideo, the capital of Uruguay, we were received by Dr. J. A. Whitelaw at the Department of Health. He explained their public health set-up, which is most advanced. They have public health stations in all parts of the country where laboratory work and serology examinations are at the disposal of practicing physicians. Tuberculosis and syphilis are under complete control. Formerly 25 per cent of the

population were luetic. Since control measures were adopted this has been much reduced. The cost of the program has been defrayed by a one per cent land tax.

The medical societies of Uruguay are organized in a federation of medico-scientific societies. Twenty-three medical journals are sent to all its branches for dissemination of medical literature, of which twenty-one are from the United States. Its own reports and transactions are sent to thirty-five medical institutions in the United States.

The incidence of echinococcus is high. As one doctor expressed it, "A man who comes from the country, wears high boots and has a large liver, may be safely diagnosed hydatid cyst." In treatment of echinococcus cysts of the lung the choice is for a two-stage operation. Daughter cysts occur in the liver but not in the lung. At the Pasteur hospital Professor Alfredo Navarro performed a one-stage operation on echinococcus.

Professor P. Lasnier, at the school of medicine, was experimenting with the possibility of diagnosing carcinoma of the lung from cells found in the sputum. At the University School of Medicine several clinical presentations and papers were given. One advocated the use of folliculin ointment for acne vulgaris and for hypertrichosis with a report of ten cases treated effectively by folliculin ointment 25,000 to 50,-000 units.

Cases were demonstrated showing a coincidence of hyperthyroidism with hypopituitarism in undergrowth with delayed ossification, slow dentition, mental retardation and delayed speaking. They discussed the relation of thyroid to ossification while Americans who follow Engelbach believe that the thyroid is responsible. A case shown was a patient with hypothyroidism who received large doses of thyroid and showed premature ossification. This case throws much weight in favor of the American viewpoint.

On the evening of April eighteenth we boarded a river steamer for Buenos Aires, a city of two million people located on the Plate river. The Plate river is forty miles wide at its mouth. The harbor at Buenos Aires is not deep enough to accommodate the largest ocean-going vessels. Buenos Aires is a busy place which has caught the modern trend. Nowhere else have I seen so many wide boulevards being cut through the business section. When these are completed they will rival the Boulevards of Paris. They have three subway systems. Buenos Aires, as a city, has favorable health conditions. There is no dysentery or malaria. They have one medical center and ten general hospitals, all assisted by the government. We were welcomed by Dr. R. Castex and his associates. Professor Castex in general chairman, holds the chair of internal medicine and is in charge of clinics for all of South America.

We were treated to an array of medical clinics. There were twenty-six papers and demonstrations covering a variety of medical subjects. There was a demonstration of cisternal puncture and encephalography; paper by Dr. Dowling on tumors of the central nervous system; paper by Lanari on the dangers of thorium oxide medication for diagnosis of liver disease; demonstration (Jacobeus's method) of pleural blebs which comes with acute idiopathic pneumothorax; cataract removal by pneumatic forceps; a case of progeria, premature senility with senile type of loss of teeth in a congenital syphilitic boy; bronchographic demonstration of cancer of the lung; lung puncture for diagnostic removal of tissue cells; and a case of obesity whose underlying condition was due to suboxidation due to faulty breathing with improvement from breathing exercises. In a discussion of black cardiacs, x-ray demonstration of bronchial changes in black cardiacs showed they do not suffer from a lack of oxygen in the blood. There is polycythemia and they are worse in the winter. The chief pathological finding is a chronic bronchitis with emphysema. X-ray gives the appearance of: (1) winter tree; (2) spring tree; (3) summer tree, according to the stage of the disease.

Dr. Pollitzer demonstrated his "Diagraphia" which visualizes in the x-ray film respiratory excursion in normal and abnormal lungs, heart, mediastinum and diaphragm. These films were put into a machine which gave them the appearance of a normal expansion and contraction of these organs. Dr. Pollitzer was able to show some lung cavities which contracted and others that expanded while still others showed no change. Its scientific value is not determined.

170

The intra-arterial injection of acetylcholine for therapeutic uses was demonstrated.

The recommended treatment of intermittent claudication and thrombo-angiitis obliterans is the subcutaneous injection daily of 250 to 750 c.c. of oxygen 95% plus carbon dioxide 5%, twenty days in succession. The injection requires ten to fifteen minutes, under moderate pressure. It is not painful and the gas is absorbed completely in twelve to sixty hours. Body movement facilitates absorption. A patient who could walk one or two blocks now walks sixty blocks without claudication.

We were shown the use of a single large dose of sodium salicylate in acute rheumatic fever when a liter containing 23.5 grams was administered per rectum, 40 drops per minute by Murphy drip.

A lecture on parasitology in Argentina was given by Dr. Greenway. Fifty per cent of digestive disturbances in Buenos Aires is due to tenia saginata which travels from cow to man to cow. Raw meat is the medium. Hookworm and trichinosis are common.

We were shown the use of paper x-ray films for diagnosis of tuberculosis in a general population. Demonstration was given of a method for taking a large number of x-rays in rapid succession. This apparatus can be taken from place to place and chest plates of large groups of people taken in a very short time. In one year 80,000 x-rays of the general population were taken by this method. Thirteen thousand showed tuberculosis, 71 per cent with lesions, and 61 per cent of the 71 per cent with cavitation.

Our medical group visited the municipal hospital, Hospital Muniz. It is a large hospital equipped to segregate contagious diseases. The tuberculosis building is new and beautiful. There is a new department of pathology in which research on leprosy is to be carried on. The chief prepared slides of leprosy bacilli. Diagnostic points on leprosy are: anesthesia to pin prick, falling of eyebrows, alopecia, mask face, bulbous nose and face, pocked skin, etc. In the wards we saw medium and advanced cases, varying from lesions which consisted of atrophy of the subcutaneous tissue to peripheral neuritis to diffuse skin lesions with ulceration and destruction of extremities.

Dr. Biassoti, assistant to Professor Houssey, is a co-discoverer of the importance of the pituitary in diabetes. His experiments on hypophysectomized dogs led to the knowledge that the anterior lobe of the hypophysis is the source of many hormones, among which are those that control carbohydrates, protein. and fat metabolism, as well as those that govern growth, gonads, secondary sex characters, et cetera. Biassoti holds that insulin is glycolytic and thyróxin proteolytic.

Biassoti and his colleagues have produced histine insulin to replace protamine insulin. His curves show that its effects are completely comparable to protamine insulin. Chemically it is crystalline insulin plus histine.

Professor Houssey after conducting us through his laboratory gave us a lecture on the hypophysis. Though a very modest individual, he is one of the outstanding men in medicine today. His laboratories are well organized and he is making real progress in his field of research. He has added such to our knowledge of the pituitary gland. He showed us pictures and graphs showing the effect of pituitary on experimental animals. Many of his experiments on the pituitary are carried out in frogs. He stated, "It is easier to operate upon the pituitary in the frog as it can be reached through the mouth and besides the reactions that occur seem to be exaggerated, making it easier to study."

Some of our members visited the clinic of Dr. Gutierrez. He is chief surgeon at the Spanish hospital, an institute supported by a benefit society of 70,000 members, each paying two pesos and up per month. They have free beds, second class and first class rooms. The first class pay ten pesos a day, have a private bath and a bed for relatives in the same room.

Dr. Gutierrez demonstrated the use of epidural anesthesia. He has used this anesthesia in 3,400 cases without a fatality. It is injected into the epidural space, 40 c.c. of a 2 per cent solution of novocaine. This anesthesia is based on the physiologic fact that the epidural space has a negative manometric pressure. This space can hold as much as 200 c.c. of fluid. The dura being attached to the foramen magnum prevents the anesthetic from reaching the brain. The anesthesia extends from the clavicle to the feet,

lasts from one and one-half to three hours. The method was first presented by Dr. Pages, a Spaniard, in 1921. He reported forty-one cases. Soon after, he was killed in an automobile accident. In 1931 an Italian surgeon claimed the invention. When Dr. Gutierrez published his report he gave credit to Dr. Pages. Dr. Pages used a 1 per cent solution, which is not strong enough. One must use 2 per cent. Dr. Gutierrez uses it in selected cases, preferably when blood pressure is high. It is a good anesthetic. There is no drop in blood pressure, no headache and no vomiting; it also lasts longer and is safer than the subdural. It requires skill in administration. The needle is introduced slowly; a drop of water is placed in the head of the needle. When the epidural space is entered the negative pressure disturbs the drop. One can also test by trying to inject the anesthetic. If one meets resistance the needle is not in the proper place. When the epidural space is entered the fluid can be injected without any resistance. If one enters the subdural space the needle is withdrawn and the next interspace is tried. Dr. Gutierrez usually injects in the first or second lumbar space. For the new beginner he recommends a small manometer attached to the needle, as this makes it easier to find the space. At first 5 c.c. are injected, then after a five-minute interval, 10 c.c. are injected followed by 20 c.c. a few minutes later. This gives enough anesthesia for a breast amputation or resection of the stomach. Hernia can be done with 25 to 30 c.c.

Dr. Gutierrez has also devised an operation for nephropexy. Most floating kidneys occur on the right side. He stated that the kidney has a space of its own and when this space is deformed you have ptosis. It is possible to demonstrate this space by liberating the hepatic flexure of the colon and turning it toward the midline. The kidney is then shoved back into position. A transverse incision into this space just below the kidney is made. The upper edge of this incision is stitched to the psoas muscle with three or four silk sutures, thus reducing the space to normal size. In ptosis of the kidney the hepatic flexure is usually too low on the colon so he selects a point higher up on the colon, fastening this new flexure by silk sutures through the white band of the colon to the parietal wall. This is a successful operation. He operated on one case for us and showed us x-rays of several successful cases taken years after the operation showing the kidney in normal position.

Dr. Gutierrez also devised an operation for difficult inguinal herniæ where he transplants the sartorius muscle under the cord and attaches it to the rectus muscle. The muscle is cut through a separate incision at the middle of the thigh, taking care to preserve the nerve and blood supply, bringing it under the cord and fastening it to the external oblique. Two incisions are necessary.

He used Delbet's plaster splints for fractured ankles. They consist of two strips of plaster, one on each side, from below the knee to the sole of the foot, then a figure-of-8 plaster from the lower end of the lateral splints up and crossing the back of the ankle just above the tendo Achillis, then forward over the front of the leg a circular plaster unites the upper ends of the splints. This allows free use of the ankle joint and is a good ambulatory splint.

The BCG is used quite extensively in Buenos Aires as a prophylactic against tuberculosis. American doctors are afraid of this vaccine. It is used extensively in France; about 600 packages are sent out daily from the Pasteur Institute. It is given in milk by mouth at birth.

On April twentieth we visited the Institute of the Benevolent Society of the capital. Professor Ramos did a cesarean section on a patient with contracted pelvis. The patient, a primipara, had been in labor two days. Ether anesthesia was used. The patient was placed in a unique position, the legs being spread and held over stirrups. This allowed the second assistant to stand between the legs. Professor Ramos has good technic. He sutured the peritoneum to the skin before opening the uterus. Dry towels were used within the abdomen. A transverse low incision was made through the visceral peritoneum of the uterus which was reflected up, then a midline incision of the muscle was made. After delivering the fetus with forceps, he injected pituitrin intravenously and allowed the placenta to deliver spontaneously, which it did in ten minutes without much bleeding. The suture line in the wall of the uterus was covered by the reflected peritoneum.

Professor Ramos also operated on a case of multiple fibroids in a young woman twenty-six years of age. She had many large fibroids and several small ones. The uterus was split in the midline and half a dozen fibroids the size of one's fist were enucleated. The uterus was reconstructed using the Reverdin needle. He said she would be able to bear children after this procedure.

There were clinics at the University of La Platte, which is a one hour ride from Buenos Aires. Of special interest was the museum of La Platte. There one finds the most complete collection of early Indian relics found anywhere. They have an enormous fossil collection containing the largest dinosaur skeleton ever discovered.

The hospital, Sanatorio de Llanura e Vincente Lopez y Planes, is located forty miles from Buenos Aires. After a visit to this wonderful institution we were impressed with the prevalence of tuberculosis in South America. The hospital has eight hundred beds and a waiting list of five thousand. Dr. Florencio E. Boneo and staff showed us through the hospital. It is a clean, orderly, efficient institution. Eighteen cases of extrapleural thoracoplasty were lined up before us, all showing splendid results. They showed us fine x-ray studies, a splendid hall of pathologic specimens, long wards of fifty to sixty beds with overhead canopies and spotless white linens. We noted the perfect coiffures of the girls in the beds, their bright eyes, sunburnt complexions and pleasing faces. All of these features together with perfect military discipline made this a model tuberculosis sanatorium. The discipline was perfect, with certain hours relegated to rest, exercise, diet, hygiene, etc. This place is a great credit to Buenos Aires and Argentina. Dr. Boneo demonstrated his own saddle chair for thoracoplasty (Fig. 3).

Our receptions at the American Embassy at Montevideo and at Buenos Aires were particularly pleasant. At Buenos Aires the Embassy overlooks the park system. The buildings, grounds and view makes the White House at Washington look cheap by comparison. The Embassy, formerly the home of a private citizen of Buenos Aires, is owned by the United

States Government. It cost the government one and one-half million dollars.

On April twenty-third we left Buenos Aires by train and arrived at Mendoza, the grape center of South America, the next morning. The trip over the Pampas was most interesting. It is a flat country with grass knee-high and cattle everywhere. No other country can produce cattle with so little effort as Argentina with thousands of miles of good pasture, wide open ranges and plenty of water. The owner has to see his animals only twice, once when the calves have their ears clipped for identification and again when they go to market.

The trip across the Andes is one never to be forgotten. The Christ Monument is in a pass about 13,000 feet high and the descent on the West slope is very steep. I counted one hundred thirty-two hairpin turns from the monument to the river below. Some of our party felt the effect of the altitude and we were all glad to get down. It is a very dangerous trip. We traveled by automobile on a one way road, starting at 5:00 A. M. and reaching Santiago at 10:00 P. M., a long, hard, interesting journey.

Santiago is a beautiful city situated in a valley at the foot of the Andes. The medical work is of high grade. Buildings and operating rooms are antiquated. Coal stoves were used for heat while ether was being administered nearby. At the Institute of Cancer we saw exceptionally high-class work by Dr. Leonard Guzman. They have one and one-half grams of radium and use it to the exclusion of surgery in carcinoma of the cervix. His cures run from 25 per cent to 65 per cent according to the degree of involvement. They follow the French school and apply small doses over a long period of time, rather than massive doses for short time as is the usual practice in the United States. Ten or fifteen milligrams are left in the uterus for as long as three weeks, being taken out every other day, cleansed and re-applied. Dr. Mardonez is director of the medical school, which was established one hundred years ago.

We went by train to Valparaiso, the seaport of Santiago. It was formerly the largest city of Chile but now Santiago is twice the size of Valparaiso. The medical work of Valparaiso is of high character in spite of dilapidated build-

ings and poor equipment. As Dr. Munich expressed it, "We have stopped apologizing for the looks of the buildings and call attention only to our work. After seeing the old ampitheater in Vienna where Billroth and Von Eiselberg did

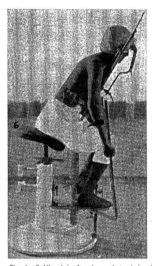

Fig. 3. Saddle chair for thoracoplasty designed by Dr. Florencio E. Boneo.

such brilliant work we have decided that it is not the buildings that are important."

Dr. Munich and staff had a full morning of surgical cases, including cervical rib, diverticulum of esophagus, acute hemorrhagic pancreatitis, goiter, thoracoplasty and gastroenterostomy for hourglass stomach due to stricture. Teratoma of the testicles in which a positive Aschheim-Zondek test proved the diagnosis.

The prevalence of lues can be judged by the statement of Dr. Reed, who said, "With every clinic of ten patients there are eleven cases of syphilis, if you include the professor."

Dr. Marrianna's test for Addison's disease is based on the fact that morphine plus glucose alters the blood sugar curves. In Addison's after morphine, the blood sugar falls; in normal cases the blood sugar rises.

The San Agustin and Vina del Mar Hospitals

were erected sixty-four years after Columbus discovered America. Acute infectious hepatitis is a very common disease in Chile. They had fifty cases at the hospital this spring. Twelve per cent of all admissions are affected with this disease, the cause of which is unknown, but may be a spirillum. Asthma is treated by intravenous injections of 20 per cent 90 proof alcohol in glucose water solution, first dose of 5 c.c. being later increased to 10 or 20 c.c.

After a delightful banquet given by the medical profession and city of Valparaiso, we boarded the Grace line, Santa Clara, and sailed up the west coast of South America. The captain said he was always glad to leave the harbor of Valparaiso on account of his fear of earthquakes. The voyage up the west coast was the most interesting of our journey.

The west coast is influenced by the Humboldt current as much as England and the Scandinavian countries are influenced by the gulf stream except that the Humboldt current is cold, coming from the Antarctics, while the gulf stream is warm, coming from the Equator. The Humboldt current strikes the west coast of Brazil south of Valparaiso and follows the coast up as far as the middle of Peru where it turns toward Hawaii and is joined by the Japanese current. This cold current causes the moisture from the trade winds to fall several hundred miles out to sea, and on the coast of Chile and Peru they only have rains about three times a century. This happens only when the current for some reason changes its course. On account of the Humboldt current the west coast is dry and cool in spite of the blazing tropical sun. The average temperature of Lima, Peru, is from 65 to 75 degrees the year around.

The bird life along this coast is most interesting. There were millions of guana birds resting on the water, and the sea was alive with fish which came to the surface so that one could see their fins churning the water. Thousands of birds feeding upon these fish would drop like spears into the water. We also sailed among many schools of seal and porpoise.

At Lima we saw ruins of the old ancient Aztec civilization. Their capital city is Cuzco, located on a plateau in the Andes.

On May eighth we visited Guayaquil, a city without rain. It is the principal center for panama hats, which, contrary to the popular belief, come from Ecuador. We were courteously received by the President of the University and several members of the faculty. The buildings are quite antiquated and evidence of their economic limitations is visible on all sides. We were driven to the city hospital, which is also the University hospital. There were more than one hundred patients and visitors at the entrance waiting admittance to the out-patient department. They filled the entrance corridor. The hospital wards contained about fifty to sixty beds. I asked one of the doctors what kind of diseases they treated. He promptly replied, "Syphilis." We learned that they also had cases of bubonic plague and a few cases of yellow fever at the time of our visit. A doctor from the United States Health Service had just been there to make the diagnosis. Some of our doctors were shown bacillus pestis out of a fresh case.

From Guayaquil we sailed to Panama city. As we passed through the canal this interesting project was explained to us by a professional lecturer furnished by the Grace Line. Colon on the Atlantic side is a free port and enormous cargoes from all parts of the world were being transferred there. We spent one day in Havana and then journeyed back to New York.

The South American trip was very interesting and well worth the time and money spent.

* * *

In addition to the doctors mentioned, hosts of other distinguished physicians gave us clinics and demonstrations, for which we are grateful We were received by the public officials of all countries visited and we appreciate this honor.

I am indebted to the members of the party for the use of their notes, particularly to Dr. J. H. Barach, who consolidated them.

CONGENITAL MEGACOLON TREATED BY DAILY HOT IRRIGATIONS
OF NORMAL SALINE SOLUTION AT 115 DEGREES*

AARON FRIEDELL, M.D.

Minneapolis, Minnesota

ACCORDING to Ruhrah,[16] Billard in 1820 described a case of congenital megacolon and called it sclerosis of the colon; Parry reported a case in an adult in 1825; Hirschsprung gave this malady the name megacolon in 1880 and published his classical description in 1888. Since then many cases and summaries of reported cases have been published. The summary by Judd and Thompson[10] in 1928 includes sixty-five reported cases.

According to Rankin, Bargen and Buie,[18] Hirschsprung defined the disease as "congenital, high grade dilatation of the colon with thickening of all its tunics, especially the tunica muscularis, and retention of large quantities of fecal matter." To date this definition is accepted as it was when it was first published.

Rankin, Bargen and Buie[18] list twenty-two hypotheses concerning the etiology of megacolon. They reduce these hypotheses to a summary under three headings, namely: congenital defects, obstructive processes (due to either anatomic conditions or to disturbances in the nervous mechanisms), and infectious processes. In most cases the pathogenesis is mixed with the several etiologic factors often combining to produce the condition of megacolon.

In the realm of treatment many recommendations are made by various authors. The most successful form to date is sympathectomy, first reported by Wade and Royle[18] in 1927. However, in this paper a suggestion is made for treatment employing mechanical and thermal stimuli in a simple form. Although this form of treatment is slow in achieving its results, yet because it carries none of the risks and complications of a sympathectomy, it deserves further study and trial.

The following three cases were so treated with good results.

Case Reports

Case 1.—R. F.,* male, three and a half years old, was diagnosed congenital megacolon when but five months old. He had medical care at various times, dietary regime, and hospitalization, but up to the time of this last admission he had little or no relief.

On admission to the University Hospital on May 16, 1931, his constipation was quite marked, more so than at any previous time. At irregular intervals he had attacks of nausea and vomiting, accompanied by marked abdominal distention. He was rather pale and weak. His abdomen protruded and was unusually large. It measured 64 cm. in circumference. His weight was 14,500 gm. The physical examination was essentially negative except for his very large abdomen. The urine was normal. The blood showed an anemia: hgb. 55 per cent, r.b.c. 3,800,000. The differential was normal. The blood calcium was normal. The Wassermann was negative. During the first three weeks he was given an abundant diet, also iron and cod-liver oil, enemas and purgatives and blood transfusions, but there was no improvement.

At the time this form of treatment was instituted, this boy was actually failing. He was pale and weak and could not sit up to take nourishment. Even though he was fed he could not take much nourishment and he had emesis frequently.

Sympathectomy was considered during the first three weeks, but as the patient's condition was becoming more and more serious this could not be done. On June 9, treatment consisting of a hot daily colon irrigation through a specially designed rectal instrument (Fig. 1) permitting a controlled inflow and outflow, was instituted. Normal saline solution was used at 115° F. The treatment lasted from thirty to ninety minutes at first, depending upon the response of the patient. It never lasted less than twenty minutes, but it lasted longer if necessary, until the saline returned clear repeatedly. Several gallons of solution were used at one time. The solution was prepared at the bedside by dissolving the required amount of salt in a gallon of hot water. These irrigations were given slowly in order to avoid distention. In a few days this patient showed signs of recovery and improvement. His listlessness became less marked, he started to take an interest in things about him, and to take food. In ten days he

*From the Department of Pediatrics, University of Minnesota.

*A report of this case was presented to the American Academy of Pediatrics at its annual meeting in Minneapolis in October, 1934 (Jour. Pediatrics, 5:733, 1935).

started to sit up and later to stand up. On August 17 he was allowed to be up and around.

The following excerpts from the x-ray reports by Dr. L. Rigler indicate the improvement in the condition and size of the colon,

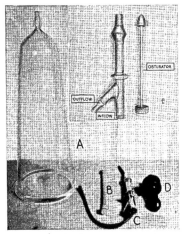

Fig. 1. Apparatus including (*A*) two gallon flask; (*B*) longer irrigator; (*C*) catheter, large size; (*D*) Austin irrigator, small size; (*E*) rectal irrigator.

May 22, 1931 (before treatment) . . . "Enormous colon. On account of the marked distention, only the rectum and part of the sigmoid were filled with 1,500 c.c. of barium sulfate. Conclusion—congenital megacolon." (Fig. 2.)

September 25, 1931 (after four months' treatment) . . . "Marked diminution in size. Caliber is two-thirds to one-half of what it was previously, peristalsis well demonstrated and much more marked than normal. Conclusion—megacolon diminishing." (Fig. 3.)

November 4, 1931. . . . "Further decrease in the size of the colon." (Fig. 4.)

This patient was discharged on December 9, 1931, his mother being instructed how to continue the irrigations at home if needed. The mother continued to give him irrigations at irregular intervals for eight months. On June 29, 1937, this boy was fine, had no more treatments and was having normal stools. He was as normal and as active as other boys nine years old, but his abdomen was still larger than the normal.

Certain observations were made on this first case and checked several times. After but a few minutes of treatment, marked evidence of peri-staltic activity was frequently noticeable through the abdominal wall. These waves were very well shown by motion pictures (Fig. 5). To the palpating hand at such times the sensation was similar to that of the contracting uterus during a pain. We noticed at the same time that the outflow had ceased and yet frequently the outflow tube pulsated or jerked. This suggested that possibly the rectum in this case contracted in a region somewhat higher than the sphincter. To the palpating finger this was rather vague, though we were inclined to interpret the muscle rigidity that was felt high up in the rectum as probably capable of preventing an outflow with the outflow tube pulsating. We, therefore, made up a longer irrigator (Fig. 1) and with its use the outflow was better.

Case 2.—Anthony W., male, aged five, was recognized as having congenital megacolon in early infancy, and was admitted to the Minneapolis General Hospital three times. His first admission was on March 21, 1933, when he was fourteen months old. X-ray on March 23rd corroborated the diagnosis of megacolon. He had marked constipation and abdominal distention. The bowels did not move without enemas and he had frequent attacks of pain in his abdomen usually accompanied by listlessness, nausea and vomiting. Repeated x-ray studies corroborated the diagnosis of megacolon. All other findings were negative. The last hospital admission was on August 23, 1936.

X-ray studies on September 9, 30, October 9, and 19, all taken before this method of treatment was instituted, showed no improvement. X-rays January 6, February 10, March 12, 1937, during this treatment, show improvement.

General improvement was noticed a few days after treatment was instituted and was continuous. His general appearance became better, his appetite improved, pain disappeared, the abdominal distention became less marked and he became much more active.

After four months of this treatment a complication became apparent in that his sphincter became gradually more and more spastic though apparently quite normal at the beginning. This spasticity increased and even caused pain on the passage of the rectal irrigator. Dr. W. A. Fansler dilated the sphincter manually under gas anesthesia and relieved the spasticity. His stools have been normal for over ten months.

Case 3.—Emmett C., male, three and one-half years of age, was diagnosed as having congenital megacolon in early infancy. He had marked constipation with frequent attacks of pain, nausea, and vomiting. His abdomen was large and the distention became aggravated quite often. At the time of admission to the Minneapolis General Hospital, January 13, 1937, his complaint was an upper respiratory disturbance with middle ear involvement. After that cleared up a complete study was made of his case. The diagnosis of megacolon was corroborated by x-ray examination. He was treated by hot saline irrigations with good results. His stools

intracolonic tension." The importance of gentleness and taking plenty of time cannot be overemphasized.

The work of Kappers[11] and Alvarez[1] further

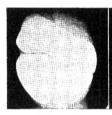 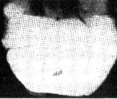 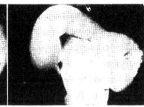

Fig. 2. Large colon.   Fig. 3. Colon size reduced.   Fig. 4. Colon size more reduced.

became normal early in May, and he was discharged May 21, 1937, as improved.

The last two patients were taught abdominal exercises after the stools started to become voluntary; the exercises probably contributed some benefit.

Treatment of megacolon by hot irrigations must not be hurried. It might be better to suspend the treatment entirely than to hurry it. This method of therapy attempts to establish a better coördination between the sympathetic and parasympathetic nervous mechanisms of the colon which have been out of harmony or have probably never been established. But this mechanism has a tempo of its own which cannot be speeded up suddenly. Hurry or rough handling will frustrate our efforts, aggravate the condition and may even produce shock. We have observed more or less reaction every time we tried to rush the treatment or allow over-distention. At one time our first patient actually showed symptoms of shock when we produced marked distention by allowing a great deal of fluid to be retained. The need for gentle handling of the colon can well be corroborated by the physiologist,[8] surgeon[9] and internist.[7] Erlanger[8] showed experimentally how rough handling of the intestines produces shock. Homans[9] states that "shock is caused principally by prolonged handling and mishandling of tissues . . . particularly within the abdomen or thorax." Gardner[7] states that "the giving of a large test enema may reproduce the patient's symptoms by increasing

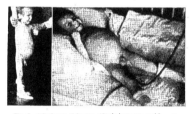

Fig. 5. (A) Large abdomen; (B) irrigator in position, showing peristaltic waves.

emphasizes the importance of the time element in the stimulation of the various parts of the alimentary canal, that the rate of conduction is slowest in the lower intestinal canal. Both of the above mentioned authors state that "the visceral regions keep a primitive type of nervous organization; that the plexuses of Meisner and Auerbach have a conduction rate similar to that in the ganglionic plexus of Coelenterates (20 cm. per sec.)."

The three patients here reported have responded to our efforts to establish normal bowel function. The rationale of this treatment can probably be explained as based on the following considerations:

1. Biologists have observed that tropical heat affords the organism a better opportunity for readjustment and evolutionary changes, as noted by Harold H. Plough and Phillip L. Ives.[14] One wonders, therefore, if under the influence of this heat treatment the colon may not be afforded

a more favorable opportunity for peristaltic activity and in time even reduce in size because of such activity.

2. Garbat and Jacobi[6] show that hot saline in the upper rectum stimulates the liver, an important detoxifying organ, to greater activity. They have demonstrated that 150 c.c. of one of several hot solutions start the flow of bile in a very few minutes and the flow may last over one hour.

3. Okay[13] found direct relationship between peristalsis and increased circulation of the blood in the bowel wall.

4. Freyer and Gellhorn[5] show that high temperature above 104° F. stops parasympathetic action and suspends the production of acetyl choline, but it does not stop sympathetic action.

5. Sir Thomas Lewis[12] shows that the sympathetics are relaxed at a temperature between 43° and 45° C. or 110° and 113° F. and that the response to the above mentioned heat is similar to the response of a local anesthetic. By using hot saline raised to 115° F. we probably overcome the undue tension that may be present in both the sympathetic and parasympathetic control of the colon. Under this comfortable heat both factors are probably afforded a period for activity with its handicaps temporarily allayed.

6. Gardner[7] showed that mechanical distention of the upper rectum may produce symptoms of severe intoxication, which immediately disappear as the pressure is released. We observed similar occurrences in our cases whenever distention occurred. On one occasion in particular, as mentioned above, there was marked reaction, almost shock, and that was relieved with the gradual emptying of the lower bowel.

Conclusions

1. Three cases of congenital megacolon were treated with hot daily irrigation of saline at 115° F. with good results.

2. The method above described, because of its simplicity and absence of risk, is worthy of further study and trial.

3. From this small series no claim can be made that all patients with megacolon can be cured by hot colon irrigation. No damage, however, can be done by trying this method first, and those ultimately requiring a sympathectomy will be benefited and be better prepared by such irrigations.

Bibliography

1. Alvarez, Walter C.: The Mechanics of the Digestive Tract, New York: Paul B. Hoeber, 1922, p. 13.
2. Counseller, V. S.: Treatment of chronic infection of the pelvis. Jour. Am. Med. Assn., 101:916-920, (Sept.) 1933.
3. Erlanger et al: Studies in secondary traumatic shock. Am. Jour. Physiol., 49:90-116, 151-173, 1919; 50:31, 104, 119, 1919.
4. Feller, W.: Gonococcemia with recovery. Jour. Am. Med. Assn., 100:1149-1150, (Apr. 15), 1933.
5. Freyer, A. L., and Gellhorn, E.: Heat principle of autonomic nervous action; observations on the resistance to temperature of the endings of vagus and sympathetic in heart. Am. Jour. Physiol., 103:392-399, (Feb.) 1933.
6. Garbat, A. L., and Jacobi, H. G.: Secretion of bile in response to rectal instillations. Arch. Int. Med., 44:455-464, (Sept.) 1929.
7. Gardner, E. L.: The indications for and examination of the colon. Minn. Med., 14:992-995, 1931.
8. Holden, F. C.: The Elliott treatment, a new method of applying vaginal heat. Am. Jour. Obst. and Gynec., 22:87, (July) 1931.
9. Homans, John: Textbook of Surgery. Springfield, Ill.: Charles C. Thomas, 1936, p. 131.
10. Judd, E. S., and Thompson, H. L.: Megacolon: an analysis of sixty-five cases. Minn. Med., 11:439-448, (July) 1928.
11. Kappers, C. U. Ariens: The evolution of the nervous system. Haarlem, Holland: DeErven F. Bohn, 1929, p. 15.
12. Lewis, Thomas: The Blood Vessels of the Human Skin and Their Responses. London: Shaw and Sons, 1927, p. 143.
13. Okay, K.: Quoted by Charles E. Pope. Trans. Am. Proctolog. Soc., 1936, p. 48.
14. Plough, H. H., and Ives, P. T.: Heat induced mutations in orosophilia. Nat. Acad. Soc. Proc., 20:268-273, (May) 1934.
15. Rankin, F. W., Bargen, J. A., and Buie, L. A.: The Colon, Rectum and Anus. Philadelphia: W. B. Saunders Co., 1932, p. 83-84.
16. Ruhrah, John: A note on history of hypertrophy of the colon. Charles Michell Billard. Am. Jour. Dis. Child., 49: 736-738, (Mar.) 1935.
17. Rumph, Wm. H.: Treatment of salpingitis. Minn. Med., 14:1028-1030, 1931.
18. Wade, R. B., and Royle, N. D.: Operative treatment of Hirschsprung's disease; a new method Med. Jour. Australia, 1:137-141, (Jan.) 1927.

COMPRESSION FRACTURES OF THE SPINE*

W. W. NAUTH, M.D., and P. A. MATTISON, M.D.

Winona, Minnesota

THIS paper is presented from the experience and observation of the general surgeon rather than that of an orthopedist and we hope that it will be so considered during the discussion which may follow.

Of a total of 886 fractures of all kinds taken care of in our group since 1933, thirty-four or approximately 4 per cent were compression fractures of the vertebral bodies. Of these, two involved the cervical, twelve the dorsal and twenty the lumbar vertebræ.

This 4 per cent is somewhat lower than the 6 per cent reported by other surgeons who take care of more than the average number of fractures encountered in general practice.

Due consideration has been taken in the series of vertebral body anomalies and abnormalities, in order that such may be ruled out. Among these changes in shapes and contour of the vertebral bodies, which are apt to confuse the surgeon and roentgenologist, may be mentioned the following:

1. Normal variations
2. Postural changes
3. Anomolies of development
4. Inflammatory changes
5. Changes in bodies due to intervertebral disc injuries
6. Metabolic changes
7. Malignancy

The diagnosis in all of our cases has been based on the history of a definite injury, with definite symptoms, x-rays before and after reduction, and follow-up x-ray studies.

Until a few years ago perhaps 75 per cent of compression fractures of the spine were overlooked by the average practitioner unless the patient complained severely of his back following injury, or had an associated paralysis which prompted x-ray studies. Many of these patients were left with permanent back disabilities.

In many instances no x-ray studies of any kind were made or when made were taken only in the anterior-posterior position. Anterior-posterior and principally lateral studies are essential in the diagnosis of compression fractures, even following trivial injuries.

While the most important part in the diagnosis rests upon x-ray findings, it is also true that a carefully taken history of the modus operandi of the injury is equally important. Jack-knifing injuries such as falling backwards, landing in a sitting position, or driving under a low bridge while sitting on a wagon, or landing in an upright position with knees extended, are definite reasons to suspect vertebral body fracture, which call for thorough x-ray study of the entire spinal column regardless of the location of pain.

Four of our cases were fractures in patients taken care of in other well appointed hospitals within one week to six months following their original injury, in which only anterior-posterior x-rays were taken and the fractures missed. Several of our cases have been associated with fractures of the os calcis. Because fracture of the os calcis is frequently produced by the individual landing in an upright position, compression fracture of the spine is always a possible complication and should be suspected and investigated.

A case in point is that of a man who walked into an open pit, landing, after a drop of about 20 feet, in an upright position, with knees extended. When brought to the hospital he was in severe shock, with a fracture of the humerus, radius and ulna, a badly comminuted fracture of the upper end of the tibia and fibula, and a fractured os calcis. Owing to his complaints of these severe injuries, he complained very little about his back. Not until months after, when he was allowed to be on his feet, did he complain to any great extent about his back. X-rays taken at this time revealed severe compression fractures of the first and second lumbar. Results of treatment for his other fractures were satisfactory, but the man will always be unable to work because we had overlooked a compression fracture of his spine which, without question, if diagnosed

*From the Winona Clinic, Winona, Minnesota. Read before the annual meeting of the Southern Minnesota Medical Association at Winona, Minnesota, August 11, 1937.

and properly treated at the time of injury would have made him a useful member of society. The modus operandi of his injury should have prompted us to look for a compression fracture of the vertebra.

ity. In none of our cases have we failed to note this symptom commensurate in degree to the severity of the injury to the vertebra involved. Visceral injuries following an accident have symptoms similar to those found in compression

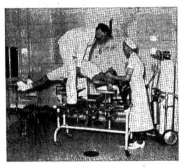

Fig. 1. Method of reduction.

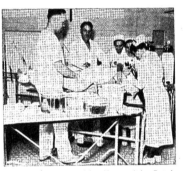

Fig. 2. Patient hyperextended on Magnusen jack. Buttocks and shoulders supported by table. Plaster cast applied.

Another case in point was that of a man who dropped into a river bed in a standing position, then falling against some piling sustained five rib fractures and a fracture of the lower end of the tibia. He was in severe shock when brought to the hospital. Within twelve hours, he developed a traumatic pneumonia and was desperately ill. An anterior-posterior plate was taken of his chest to corroborate our diagnosis of pneumonia and chest injuries. This plate revealed what was reported by the hospital roentgenologist as an arthritic process of the twelfth dorsal vertebra. No lateral studies were made at this time in spite of this report, because following his recovery from pneumonia and other injuries, he made no complaint about his back. [Subsequent x-ray studies, however, did reveal a definite fracture.]

· These were early cases which taught us important lessons, and I dare say that we have missed no compression fractures since that time. Multiple injuries to an individual should always call for x-ray studies of the spine.

In our experience and observation besides x-ray findings and the modus operandi of the injury, one of the most important symptoms and points of diagnosis is abdominal pain and rigid-

fractures, namely, abdominal pain and rigidity. However, in visceral injuries there is also localized tenderness over the organ involved. In compression fractures with abdominal pain and rigid.ity, there is as a rule no localized tenderness.

In our series of thirty-four cases, we had two cases of complete lower extremity and visceral paralysis with full recovery. These cases were treated by hyperextension, body cast, and traction followed by braces. Two patients with paralysis, prior to this series, on whom we did laminectomies, did not do so well. One died without recovering, about one year later, the other, while he recovered somewhat, is a wheelchair case for the rest of his life.

It is our belief from our experience that, since the average surgeon is not a neurologist, he is unable, when a back injury with paralysis presents itself, to make a diagnosis as to whether the cord is merely compressed or actually severed. We have not used the Quackenstedt test, therefore, do not know its relative value in settling the question. Edema and hemorrhage in and around the cord rather than a true blocking by bony displacement may confuse and render valueless the Quackenstedt test, except to those who have had considerable experience in its interpretation. Key and Conwell recommend reduction by manipulation and hyperextension in all cases before making the Quackenstedt test. According to the experience of surgeons relying principally on the extension methods for reduc-

the patients difficulty in the breathing. Both became cyanotic and had to be turned before the application of the cast was completed. We, therefore, adopted the following method which we have not seen described: The patient is

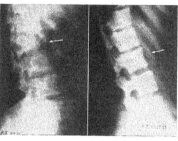

Fig. 3. Compression fracture of second lumbar vertebra with visceral and lower extremity paralysis. (a) Before reduction. (b) Eleven months later.

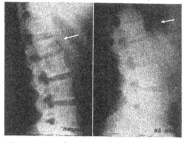

Fig. 4. Compression fracture of first lumbar vertebra. (a) Before reduction. (b) Eleven months later.

tion and recovery, there is only a small percentage of cases in which laminectomy is indicated.

One of our patients with a fracture of the second lumbar, developed, on the day following his injury and reduction, a paralysis of the entire left arm. X-ray studies revealed no injury to any of the cervical vertebræ. We assumed that this paralysis was caused by hemorrhage and pressure in the cord, described as hematomyelia by Dr. Hammes. This patient obtained full recovery of his arm within three months. We had one case of cervical body fracture with paralysis of the left shoulder and arm with full recovery following traction and cervical brace.

Treatment.—Many methods of reduction and treatment have been used successfully as long as hyperextension was the main factor in reduction and retention. Among these methods are the Magnusen jack, the Allen reduction table, the hammock suspension method, and the symphysis chest position with the patient face down. Manipulation in this position by a sudden sharp thrust downward at the point of injury is often attended by an audible sound when the impaction is reduced. This treatment is followed by a carefully applied body cast, with the patient in the hyperextended position.

In two of our cases with the chest-symphysis position we had considerable worry, because of

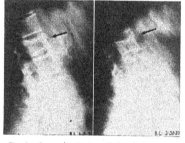

Fig. 5. Compression fracture of first lumbar vertebra. (a) Before reduction. (b) Ten months later.

anesthetized lying flat on his back, the table is straddled by the operator who places his arms with locked fingers under the patient's back at the point of injury, slowly suspending the patient until the buttox and shoulders are free from the table. He then gives a sudden sharp upward thrust of the body, then by dropping his locked hands he intercepts the drop of the patient and holds him in this position until the Magnusen jack is placed under him. The cast is then applied. We have had no respiratory complications with this procedure and have had equally good results. All of our non-paralyzed cases, regardless of the degree of compression, if reduced, are permitted to be up and about in from one to two weeks. The cast is kept on for three months. Then a well-fitting Taylor brace is applied, made always from a plaster model of the patient in the hyperextended position. Such braces always fit perfectly.

Prognosis.—Prognosis is essentially very satisfactory if properly treated. All of the patients in this series, including the two with paralysis, are well without major complaints, able to work and carry on practically as well as before injury. We think this justifies a good prognosis for the majority of patients who sustain a compression fracture of the vertebræ. Both compensation and private cases as a matter of fact have given us less trouble than other fractures as a whole.

A CLINICAL TEST FOR PREGNANCY*

D. E. MOREHEAD, M.D., F.A.C.S.

Owatonna, Minnesota

INTEREST in the possibility of securing an accurate intradermal test for the diagnosis of pregnancy has again been stimulated by the recent report of Gilfillen and Gregg[4] on the intradermal use of Antuitrin-S. The advantages of such a test, if accurate, are self-evident.

Zondek[8] and Aschheim[1] showed that there was present in pregnancy urine a large amount of gonad stimulating hormones. It is not known who originated the idea to utilize this substance in some way for the diagnosis of pregnancy; however, Porges and Pollatschek[6] were probably the first to report work of this kind.

The pregnancy urine gonadotrope was originally considered to be of pituitary origin, so that it is not surprising to find the above investigators as well as subsequent workers using anterior hypophyseal extracts for the same purpose. Deutsch[2] in 1929 and Strauss[7] in 1930 reopened the study, as did Dowell[3] in this country in 1934. The results from all these sources were considered to be of no value, due to the high percentage of error. Gruskin[5] in 1936 attempted to solve the problem by using a placental extract as an intracutaneous test. This was similarly found to be inaccurate.

It is not surprising, however, that failure followed these attempts since pituitary extracts containing the gonadotropic hormone also contain large amounts of extraneous matter. This would be true also of placental extracts.

Antuitrin-S was used by Gilfillen and Gregg[4] in their work. They reasoned much the same as their predecessors that the pregnant subject having a high concentration of the anterior pituitary-like hormone present should be "desensitized" or "immune" to its intradermal administration; further, that the reverse should obtain in the non-pregnant state.

Antuitrin-S contains two milligrams of solids per cubic centimeter. One milligram is the active hormone and the remainder is extraneous, inactive material of a non-protein nature. The potency is adjusted so that one milligram in 1 c.c. of solution contains 175 rat units of the hormone. The solution is adjusted to a pH of 7.1 or 7.2, this being the pH of optimal preservation of the hormone. The only protein in solution found by test is that directly attributable to the anterior pituitary-like hormone. That this hormone is protein in nature is undoubted although total nitrogen runs around 0.9 per cent. (The average protein is from 14 to 16 per cent nitrogen). Furthermore, Antuitrin-S varies negligibly in solid content, that is to say, the protein content is constant. If we may now theorize we might suspect that the hormone is an aggregation of complex protein molecules possibly resembling the polypeptides.

In this paper I am reporting pregnancy tests in 100 cases, not all of pregnancy, made with Antuitrin-S manufactured by Parke, Davis and Co., and Follutin manufactured by E. R. Squibb and Co. Sixty-one of these cases are my own and thirty-nine were run by Dr. James Morrow of Austin, Minnesota. Neither one knew the other was making similar tests. Dr. Morrow was kind enough to turn over his cases to me to be reported at this time.

Dr. Morrow's series includes two post-partem cases, two cases where the menopause had set in,

*Read before the annual meeting of the Minnesota State Medical Association, Saint Paul, Minnesota, May 4, 1937.

and several questionable cases of pregnancy which were checked with the Friedman test. In his series Antuitrin-S affirmed the presence of pregnancy in four cases in which the Friedman test was negative. There were eleven cases of pregnancy positive both with Antuitrin-S, and the Friedman test. Six cases affirmed the absence of pregnancy while the Friedman test was positive. Two patients past the menopause gave negative results with both the Antuitrin-S and Friedman tests. Two patients sixteen and twenty-seven days post-partem respectively gave a positive Antuitrin-S reaction. Antuitrin-S was positive for pregnancy in three patients who were not pregnant.

In my own series I tried to adhere to the rules laid down by Gilfillen and Gregg, that is, to read the test in one-half hour and again in one hour. I found that I could not depend on the test to react in one hour's time. I found that the test might require six or eight hours to react, showing an absence of pregnancy, so that a reading in a shorter period of time would lead to an erroneous diagnosis. Antuitrin-S and Follutein were used, one to check against the other. There was one case of ectopic pregnancy where Antuitrin-S and Follutein both showed pregnancy present. Operation confirmed this diagnosis. In one case where an ectopic pregnancy was suspected the test showed pregnancy absent after six hours. The patient was not

operated upon and time has proved that pregnancy was absent. In six patients known to be pregnant, both Follutein and Antuitrin-S showed an absence of pregnancy. On repeated tests they both showed pregnancy absent. The remainder of the known pregnancy cases were confirmed with both Follutein and Antuitrin-S. In thirty non-pregnant patients the test showed an absence of pregnancy and none of the tests showed pregnancy when it did not exist.

Summary

From my observations I would say the test is more accurate if used to diagnose the absence of pregnancy. Further study must be made to determine why some reactions fail to confirm the presence of pregnancy.

Bibliography

1. Aschheim, S.: Die Schwangerschaftsdiagnose aus dem Harn durch nachweis des Hypophysenvorderlaffen-hormons; praktische und theorestische Ergebnisse aus den Hornunter-suchungen. Klin. Wchnschr., 7:1453-1457, (July 29) 1928.
2. Deutsch, Alfred: Uber die Verwendbarkeit der Porges-Pollatschek'schem Schwangerschaftsprobe. Zentralbl, F. Gynak., 53:2920-2921, 1929.
3. Dowell, D. M.: Preliminary observations on menstrual cycle and pregnancy with simple pregnancy diagnostic test. Jour. Missouri Med. Assn., 30:275-277, (July) 1933.
4. Gilfillen, G. C., and Gregg, W. K.: New, rapid, economical test for pregnancy and certain gynecologic conditions. Am. Jour. Obst. and Gynec., 32:498-501, (Sept.) 1936.
5. Gruskin, B.: Intradermal test for pregnancy. Am. Jour. Surg., 31:59-61, (Jan.) 1936.
6. Porges, R., and Pollatschek, O.: Foreign letters-Vienna. Jour. Am. Med. Assn., 93:559, 1929.
7. Strauss, H.: The Porges Pollatschek skin test for pregnancy. Am. Jour. Surg., 8:1271-1272, 1930.
8. Zondek, B.: Darstellung des weiblichen Sexualhormons aus dem Harn, insbesondere dem Harn von Schwangeren. Klin. Wchnschr., 7:485-486, (March 11) 1928.

 # CASE REPORT

CHYLURIA*

GEORGE B. EUSTERMAN, M.D.

Rochester, Minnesota

A WHITE, married woman, fifty-nine years of age, entered The Mayo Clinic on November 16, 1936, with the complaint that one morning while she had been collecting a specimen of urine for periodic urinalysis by her family physician she had noticed that it had the appearance of milk. The patient had had the urine examined on an average of four times a year for the past ten or twelve years but this was the first urine of abnormal appearance, to her knowledge. On four successive days before admission at the clinic the urine first voided, usually about 6:30 a. m., was milky, but all urine passed thereafter remained clear. Exclusive of chronic senescent arthritis of low grade, affecting one knee, and mild digestive disturbances after eating too heartily of rich foods, the patient made no other

complaint. Recently she had lost 8 pounds (3.6 kg.) as the result of voluntary dietary restrictions.

Physical examination gave essentially negative results. The blood pressure and temperature were within normal limits. The urine had a decidedly milky appearance. It was necessary to convince the laboratory technician that it was not milk before she would undertake examination, for a week previously a young mother mistakenly had sent a small bottle of milk for examination instead of the child's urine which had been collected in a similar bottle. The specific gravity was 1.023; albumin and sugar were absent. Microscopic examination disclosed a few erythrocytes and about 20 leukocytes per low power field. The presence of chyle was determined by further chemical and microscopic examination. A catheterized specimen, obtained the same day, was free of erythrocytes and leukocytes. The concentration of blood urea was within normal

*From the Division of Medicine, The Mayo Clinic, Rochester, Minnesota. Read before the meeting of the Southern Minnesota Medical Association, Winona, Minnesota, August 11, 1937.

CASE REPORT

limits. There were no significant changes in the ocular fundi. Roentgenographic examination of the urinary tract, including an intravenous urogram, roentgenographic examination of the organs of the thorax, as well as roentgenoscopic examination of the stomach and duodenum, failed to disclose evidence of any abnormality.

The patient returned a month later for further examination of the urinary tract in order to determine whether the chyle issued from one or from both kidneys, or from a lower level, and whether there was a fistulous communication with the lumbar lymphatic structures. Whether or not such communication was demonstrable, it also was decided at this examination to inject the contrast media under pressure while doing retrograde pyelography because this procedure had been known to interrupt such a fistulous communication, with permanent disappearance of chyle from the urine. Cystoscopic examination was carried out early in the morning, before the patient had voided or had assumed an erect position. Clear urine was found to issue from the meatuses on both sides. The first catheterized specimen from the left renal pelvis appeared to be clear but the second one was slightly turbid and milky in appearance. This specimen also clotted soon after its collection. Chemical and microscopic examination of this milky specimen revealed the presence of chyle but absence of filaria and bacteria. Retrograde pyelography disclosed that the outlines of the right renal pelvis, calices and ureter were normal. The pelvis of the left kidney and ureter also appeared to be normal. Beyond the tip of the lower calix apparently there was some small extravasation but evidence of a lymphatic communication was lacking. The contrast media was injected under pressure and there has been no recurrence of the chyluria up to the present time.

Under the title "nonparasitic chyluria" two previous communications dealing with cases encountered in the clinic have been made. The first one was made by Allen in 1933, who reported two cases, and the second by Wakefield and Thompson, whose article appeared July, 1937, in the *Journal of Urology*. This latter article dealt with five cases encountered in the clinic up to January, 1937, and included the cases reported by Allen and the case presented herewith, briefly summarized. More than 100 cases of nonparasitic chyluria have been reported so far in the literature.

A few features of clinical interest, as they pertain to this case, may be discussed. In the first place, the possibility of parasitic origin of the chyluria cannot be ignored; neither can it be definitely proved. The patient had traveled extensively at home and abroad and in former years had sojourned for long periods in areas where filariasis was endemic, such as Charleston and Camden, South Carolina, and Cairo, Egypt. However, repeated examinations after the patient entered the clinic, of concentrated specimens of venous blood, failed to disclose the presence of filaria. Their absence would not exclude parasitic origin of the condition because they could cause lymphatic blockage by their dead bodies or by inflammatory fibrosis of the lymphatic vessels. Cookson and Pullar maintained that "if the patient has been at any time resident in a district in which filariasis is endemic, the chyluria may be assumed to be filarial unless convincing evidence of another etiologic factor is forthcoming." Another fea-

ture of clinical interest is the fact that the urine was milky only when first voided in the morning. This feature also was characteristic of one of the cases reported by Allen. Apparently the horizontal position favors retrograde lymphatic flow to the renal pelvis. The patient also noticed that rich, fatty meals tended to aggravate or precipitate the chyluria. Such meals possibly would be sufficient to cause a fresh discharge of chyle by increasing the flow of lymph in the vessels of the mesentery. The chylous urine seems to be the only symptom in the majority of the cases reported and this feature was exemplified in this case. Colic or discomfort, the result of coagulation of the urine before it is voided, sometimes occurs but it was not observed in the case here reported. In the interval of one month between the first and second examinations, the patient complained of some loss of weight and energy but this was attributed to a state of anxiety rather than to the loss of fat. Authorities are agreed that loss of fat which does not exceed 400 calories daily is negligible and does not account for the malnutrition and weakness of some of these patients.

In the presence of a milky urine one must exclude such possibilities as pyuria from any cause, phosphaturia, lipuria, and artificial or purposeful additions to the urine. The most elementary chemical and microscopic examinations should suffice to make a satisfactory identification of the causative substance from the laboratory standpoint. The obvious absence of those serious conditions which usually give rise to lipuria (advanced diabetes mellitus, tuberculosis, pancreatic disease, fracture of the bone, fat embolism and so forth), in the presence of fat in a molecular form, and other laboratory criteria, fairly definitely exclude lipuria. Of course it was felt that lipuria should be excluded because the patient tended to be a gourmet. Schöndorff has observed increased amounts of urinary fat after hearty eating of fatty food and after the use of fat-containing medicaments. Moreover, according to the secretory hypothesis of the genesis of chyluria, fat exists in the blood in excess and is passed by the renal epithelium. The first of these two possibilities was dismissed because chyluria occurred in the absence of dietary indiscretions and disappeared after treatment in spite of the patient's eating rich meals. The secretory hypothesis, in contrast to the mechanical one, does not rest on any secure foundation and now has few supporters. Moreover, the recent investigations of Elkan, on blood fat in cases of nonparasitic chyluria, seem definitely to nullify the secretory hypothesis.

References

1. Allen, E. V.: Nonparasitic chyluria. Proc. Staff Meet. Mayo Clinic, 8:477-480, (Aug. 9) 1933.
2. Cookson, H. A., and Pullar, T. H.: True nonparasitic chyluria associated with menstruation: report of a case. Arch. Int. Med., 53:878-884, (June) 1934.
3. Elkan, O. T.: Die nichtparasitäre Chylurie mit besonderer Berucksichtigung fortlaufender Blutfettbestimmungen. Zentralbl. f. inn. Med., 57:697-713, (Aug. 29) 1936.
4. Schöndorff, B.: Quoted by Strauss, Ludwig: Über passagere Chylurie. Ztschr. f. urol. Chir., 38:347-352, 1933.
5. Wakefield, E. G., and Thompson, Gershom: Nonparasitic chyluria. Jour. Urol., 38:102-110, (July) 1937.

HISTORY OF MEDICINE IN MINNESOTA

ORGANIZATION OF THE ST. LOUIS COUNTY
MEDICAL SOCIETY

By RICHARD BARDON, M.D.

IN a preceding account of the medical history of Northern Minnesota, an introduction explained the historical background of the early practitioners who were fur traders and explorers as well as doctors. This period ended with Dr. Borup, who eventually located in St. Paul in 1848.

The period from 1854 to 1886 is of vital importance, not only to Duluth but to St. Louis County as well. Up to 1854 Northern Minnesota was Indian country. In that year a treaty was negotiated with the Chippewas at La Pointe, Wisconsin, and as a result Northeastern Minnesota was open to settlement by the whites. No settlement within the present confines of Duluth was made until about 1855 or 1856, and that was very scattered. The settlement in Oneota (now West Duluth) and the present site of Duluth hardly got under way when the depression of 1857 came along, and, with the Civil War impending, settlement was entirely given up for the time being. During the Civil War and up until 1869, there was no doctor permanently located in what is now Duluth or St. Louis County. Previous to this a few pioneers who lived in the present Duluth were attended by the doctors from Superior, who, during the same period, were not very numerous. It may be of interest here to state that the chairman of the first board of county commissioners was Dr. W. W. Mayo, who was the medical officer with the Territorial Survey which laid out the northern counties of the state. There were few inhabitants in this territory. At Rice's Point, where Duluth now stands, there was one cabin, but the trapper who lived there was away, and Dr. Mayo was made temporary chairman of the board of county commissioners, an office which he held for about six weeks, until someone who lived in the county could be found to take his place. The records of the county auditor's office do not throw any light on this early appointment, but inasmuch as the office was temporary, doubtless no record was ever made. However, St. Louis County and the City of Duluth are proud to have the name of Dr. Mayo listed among their pioneers.

The earliest mention of the medical profession in the present City of Duluth is taken from the diary of the Reverend Mr. Pietezl, who spent much time among the Indians as a missionary along the south shore of Lake Superior. In 1859 he was located in the village of Oneota, and mentions that at that time one of his children was ill with a severe cold that he thought might be scarlet fever, and when the second child became much more seriously sick he called in Dr. John A. Thomson from the village of Superior, across the bay. Dr. Thomson confirmed the diagnosis. As there is no record of the child's death it may be assumed that the doctor's ministrations were successful. Dr. Thomson located in Superior in the fall of 1859, and on November 13, 1860, married Helen Rowena Abbott, daughter of Dwight and Jane Abbott, at Oneota. Shortly afterward Dr. Thomson moved to Hastings, Minnesota, and in a list of physicians and surgeons in Merwin's Business Directory of Minnesota for 1869-1870 his address was given as "Ramsey Street, Hastings, Minnesota." Dr. Thomson died in Philadelphia on March 19, 1869, while on a visit to his father.

Dr. Thomson, born July 11, 1830, at Wilmington, Delaware, was descended of Colonial stock. His ancestors were prominently identified in civil and military capacities during the American Revolution, and received many honors for this participation. His father, Dr. James William Thomson, was a Virginian, related to many prominent Virginia families, including the Washington, Lewis, Warner, and Throckmorton families. Dr. Thomson was a man of considerable education and refinement. He graduated from Jefferson Medical College in 1851. Thereafter he did post-graduate study in Vienna, and traveled extensively abroad in Italy and Palestine.

It will be seen, then, that during the period of 1855 to 1869, Duluth had no resident physicians, and whenever necessary the doctors came from Superior. It was during this period that the pioneers had to make use of the remedies that were at hand. There are the usual stories of the midwives, the "bone setters," and the various people who had a natural bent for treating sickness. There is also the story concerning the occasional Indian who, with "tea" made from various herbs, could cure dropsy and other allied conditions. Stories are told of the treatment of gangrene by amputation and searing the stumps with red-hot frying pans! True, the people were hardy and vigorous, and possibly needed little medical attention.

Probably the first physician to locate permanently in Duluth was Dr. Edward Erastus Collins, who arrived in May, 1869. Dr. Collins was born July 26, 1833. He attended public schools in New York state, and the Brookfield Academy in New York City. After graduating from the medical college of New York in 1857, he practiced medicine in that state for a number of years, and was a contract surgeon in Washington, D. C., during the Civil War. In the winter of 1868-1869 he attended a series of lectures at the Chicago Medical College, after which he moved to Duluth. Dr. Collins practiced here until 1874, when he removed to Minneapolis, where he remained for four years. He next moved to Stoughton, Wisconsin, but returned to Duluth in 1881, where he lived until his death in 1912. Dr. Collins was a charter-member of the county medical· society. Later he also engaged in the real estate business. He is best remembered as the kindly pioneer type of physician.

About the same time there were other doctors who located in Duluth, but how long they remained is unknown. In the *Duluth-Minnesotian* there appear the business cards of professional men recently located in the city. On May 19, 1869, is the name of "Guy M. Daly, Physician and Surgeon"; for June 19, 1869, "D. G. Saivy, Physician and Surgeon"; and on July 3, 1869, "T. R. Potts, Physician and Surgeon." Very little is known about these men, except that Dr. Daly practiced in Superior before coming to Duluth. Dr. Potts was graduated from the University of Pennsylvania in 1831, and was a relative of H. H. Sibley and Franklin Steele, who were well known in early Minnesota affairs. Dr. Samuel Carson McCormick arrived in Duluth in·April, 1870. The reason for this sudden increase in the medical profession was the advent of the railroad connecting St. Paul and Duluth. With the completion of .the railroad in 1870 Duluth began to grow. Dr. McCormick was born in Union County, Pennsylvania, September 8, 1837. He graduated from Jefferson Medical College at the outbreak of the Civil War, and immediately joined the Union forces as an army surgeon. He served with distinction throughout the war. His desire for adventure still unsatisfied, he went West as a surgeon on the Union Pacific Survey, where he met the famous characters of the Wild West. Subsequently he located in Duluth. Dr. McCormick was married in 1871 to Miss Louise Smith of Superior. Her father, Dr. Vespasian Smith, had been a resident of Superior since 1857. The name of Dr. McCormick figures very prominently in the early annals of medical history in Duluth and St. Louis County. A news item for November, 1872, is interesting: "Dr. S. C. McCormick has just received a fine horse from St. Paul. Dr. Collins' purchase of a fine buggy horse seems to be contagious." A previous item stated that Dr. E. E. Collins "exhibits a fine horse, which receives the encomiums of all judges of horseflesh" In 1872 a further notice states: "Dr. McCormick has removed his office from the Bloomer Block on the Foster Lot to the building opposite—the new Hayes Brick Block, upstairs next in the rear of Col. Gow's Northern Pacific Office. The doctor has a beautiful room and his patients will no doubt want to be sick on purpose to have a prescription written from such a pleasant locality."

During the period from 1870 to 1873 Duluth increased in population, and other doctors located there, among whom were Dr. O. B. Bird, a homeopath, a Dr. Hanley and the Doctors Tanner, who came in 1871 but moved to Hudson, Wisconsin, in 1873. Their professional announcement read:

H. S. TANNER, M.D.   MRS. M. J. TANNER, M.D.

Eclectic and Homeopathic Physicians offer their professional services to the citizens of Duluth and vicinity. The diseases of women and children made a specialty. Office and residence First Ave. West opp. Clark House.

Office hours from 10 to 12 A. M. and 1-3 P. M.

Carefully prepared Homeopathic medicines for family use kept for sale at our offices.

Later, Dr. Tanner achieved considerable publicity on account of his lengthy fasts. In January, 1881, the following note appeared: "Dr. H. S. Tanner began his 40 day fast yesterday at the Clarendon Hotel."

Dr. S. S. Walbank moved from Superior in 1871, and made his home in Duluth until his death in 1890. A newspaper clipping for May 4, 1890, reports his death:

"After a three weeks' illness, Dr. S. S. Walbank, one of the oldest and best known citizens of Duluth, passed into the great beyond. His death occurred yesterday afternoon, caused by pneumonia.

"Dr. Walbank was born April 30, 1823, at Morton Homestead, Devonshire, England. His medical education was received at Toronto University in 1848. He came to Superior in 1869, and cast his lot with Duluthians three years afterwards, and has since remained here. Dr. Walbank has since been identified with many of the leading projects for the upbuilding of the city. Himself and Dr. S. C. McCormick were, for a long time, the only medical practitioners in Duluth. His sterling worth and integrity as a business man, his uniform kindness and courtesy to all, has endeared him to all who knew him."

Dr. Vespasian Smith, who had lived in Superior since 1857, moved to Duluth in 1871 or shortly afterward. Dr. Smith figures frequently in the early civic and medical development of Duluth, and was mayor for two terms (1873 and 1874).

In the "History of St. Louis County," page 472, there is an episode worth recording:

"Dr. Vespasian Smith was a staunch, sterling old character, that builded well with his great common sense, while enlivening his fellows, as they went, with his kindly humor. He became mayor of the city in April, 1873, and he got 226 votes, but one being cast against him. When his term was out he was again elected, but he was not so fortunate this time, for there were three votes cast against him. He used to say that the only vote against him the first time was his own, but that during his second term he made two enemies, so there were three votes against him on his second election."

Dr. Smith was born in Mount Vernon, Ohio, October 23, 1818, of old Virginia stock. He first showed an inclination to become a trader among the Indians, but after only a year took up the study of medicine under a preceptor, later attending the medical department of Western Reserve University, from which he was graduated in 1851. After practicing for several years in smaller Ohio towns he came to Superior in 1857. Evidently he was quite a politician, for he was soon appointed physician to the Chippewas at the Bayfield agency. Thereafter he held some political appointment continuously, from his first under Buchanan until the time of his death, with the exception of the Cleveland administration. He was a member of the Minnesota State Board of Health for twenty years. Inasmuch as Dr. Smith figures frequently later on in this narrative, his activities will not be further enumerated at this point. He died in 1897. His son, Frank Smith, owned and operated one of the earliest drug stores in Duluth.

One of the early medical pioneers of Duluth, who was not actively engaged in medical practice, so far as could be ascertained, was Dr. Thomas Foster. He came to Duluth in 1868 from St. Paul. Dr. Foster published the first newspaper in Duluth, the *Duluth-Minnesotian,* which appeared on April 23, 1869. Dr. Foster was a unique character, and a biographical sketch of his life is interesting, not because of his work as a physician but because of his political activities. He was born May 18, 1818, in a southern suburb of Philadelphia. He studied medicine for a time under the preceptorship of Dr. Ord of Lewistown, Pennsylvania, but gave it up to enter the newspaper business and engage in politics. While in Uniontown, Pennsylvania, he again took up the study of medicine, and probably practiced for a short time, when he returned to the newspaper business and politics. In 1848 he became secretary of the Whig State Committee of Pennsylvania, of which Alexander Ramsey was chairman. Dr. Foster accompanied Ramsey to Minnesota as his secretary when Ramsey was appointed territorial governor. When Ramsey became state governor Dr. Foster was again appointed his secretary. For a time previous to 1860 he published the *Daily Minnesotian* in St. Paul. He served in the commissary department of the army during the Civil War, with the rank of captain. In 1867 Dr. Foster was chairman of the Republican state committee of Minnesota. The same year he edited the first daily paper in Minneapolis, *The Chronicle.* In 1868 he arrived in Duluth. Just how long he remained there is difficult to state, as the paper soon passed out of his control. He eventually obtained a clerkship in the postoffice department in Washington, and in 1902 moved to San Francisco, where he died shortly thereafter.

During the early seventies epidemics of scarlet fever were frequent. In a column of the *Daily Minnesotian,* under the caption "Local Rip-Raps," was the statement pertaining to "that terrible epidemic to children of scarlet fever, which still continues to linger in our city, and many of the little ones are lying under its dreadful scourge." In subsequent issues it appears that the epidemic continued to afflict the city until the spring of 1876, with consequent mortality to many children. During the winter, records show that schools were closed in an effort to control the spread of infection. In 1876 it was reported that Dr. S. C. McCormick was health officer and Dr. Vespasian Smith was appointed "a private member of the board of health." About this time Drs. J. L. Graham and C. H. Graff arrived in Duluth.

The coming of the railroad and the cutting of the canal in the early seventies was a great stimulation to the struggling village. In the panic of 1873 Jay Cooke, who financed the Northern Pacific, failed and the city was at a standstill. However, with the discovery of iron ore on the Vermillion Range in the early eighties, and with the development of the lumbering industry, the city began to grow rapidly. Throughout this period the medical profession was unorganized. Hospital facilities were lacking until the establishment of St. Luke's in 1882. There is mention of a "temporary hospital" in 1871, but evidently it did not grow into a permanent institution. St. Mary's Hospital was not founded until 1888.

The newspaper reported for February 2, 1882, that "Dr. Bowman had a telephone put in his office in the Hayes Block yesterday."

The Board of Health was created in 1884, and "the streets and alleys of the Village were thoroughly inspected and several old timers were deprived of their almost immemorial privileges of keeping pig-pens underneath their neighbors' windows and of maintaining other nuisances to the neighborhood, much to their indignation."

This was Duluth at the time the St. Louis County Medical Society was proposed.

The exact date of the formation of the St. Louis County Medical Society was unknown until December, 1936, when on checking through some of the old newspaper files it was ascertained that the year of the founding was 1886 instead of 1887 as recalled by Dr. McComb. The early records of the Society have been lost or misplaced, and there are various theories as to just what happened to them. There is the story that they were burned when fire destroyed an office building. However, this is somewhat questionable and no doubt they were thrown out, as so many historical records have been in the past. In the newspaper files for June 26, 1886, this item appears:

A CALL
To the Physicians of St. Louis County
Notice is hereby given that a meeting will be held for the organization of a County Medical Society of St. Louis County, Thursday next, July 16, 1886, at 8 p. m., at Dr. McComb's office.

This is interesting, because Dr. McComb stated that the first meeting was in the office of Dr. S. C. McComb in the Norris-McDougall Block, which at that time was a popular building for doctors. On the following day there was a notice in the paper reporting that

"The St. Louis County Medical Society met in council on Thursday night, July 16, to form a county association for mutual protection and improvement, and after the preliminary business a committee was appointed to draft a table of fees and report thereon at the next meeting. The following well-known medical men were elected as officers for the ensuing year:

President .... Dr. V. Smith
First Vice President...................... Dr. A. F. Ritchie
Second Vice President........ :........ Dr. S. C. McCormick
Secretary .... Dr. Stocker
Treasurer .... Dr. McComb
Censors .... Drs. Sherwin, Magie and Speier

"The elections being decided, the meeting adjourned, to meet on the second Thursday in August, and will meet on the second Thursday in each and every month."

There is very little known about the early meetings of the society except that Dr. McComb states that the meetings were rather informal and discussions were always in order. Dr. Stocker apparently was a very careful secretary, and it is certainly a calamity that his records have not been preserved so that we might have first hand information as to just what went on. Those who saw the early minutes always recall the perfection of the handwriting and the great detail and exactness of Dr. Stocker's reports.

During the year 1886, in coöperation with the Duluth Chamber of Commerce or its predecessor, an attempt was made to get the State Medical Society to meet in Duluth the following year. This was successful. Dr. McComb recalled that the meeting was successful in many ways, inasmuch as he was elected president of the state society and was introduced to the members by the late Dr. W. W. Mayo. At that time Dr. McComb was only twenty-nine years of age, and had been a resident of Duluth since 1883. Subsequently he had been president of the county society on two occasions the second time during a state meeting there, but he was unable to supply the exact dates.

In a newspaper file for September 10, 1887, there is a note on a meeting of the St. Louis County Medical Society, and it is of sufficient interest to have it reproduced:

"A meeting of the St. Louis Medical Society was held in the office of Dr. Magie on Thursday evening, at which the following members of the profession were present: Drs. Ritchie, McComb, McCormick, McAuliffe, Judd, Speier, Sherwin, Davis, Magie, Stocker and Dr. Specht of West Superior. Pres. Ritchie occupied the chair and Secretary Stocker recorded the minutes. The first paper on 'The Ophthalmoscope as One of the Main Factors in Diagnosing Obscure Diseases,' was read by Dr. McAuliffe. A discussion followed, in which various members gave their experiences on the subject. An oral debate opened by Dr. Stocker was quite interesting. It was in regard to 'The Treatment and Causes of Summer Complaint and Intestinal Catarrh.' Another discussion was participated in by several regarding 'Contraction of the Pupil and Affection of the Eyesight Resulting from Injuries to the Spine.' Dr. Stocker led this discussion also."

The calibre of this program is remarkable, and is an indication of the progressiveness of the young society.

There is another notation in the newspaper for June 16, 1887, which stated:

"The Medical Association will commence tomorrow morning at 10 o'clock. Dr. S. C. McCormick, Chairman of the committee of arrangements, requests 'The News' to say that, owing to the unavoidable absence of Dr. H. H. Kimball, Pres. of Minnesota State Medical Society, Dr. W. L. Beebe of St. Cloud, 1st Vice Pres., will be the acting President. The Society will be divided into two sections. Dr. R. D. Barber of Washington, 2nd Vice Pres., will preside over the first section and Dr. A. Holmes of Oronocco, 3rd Vice Pres., will preside over the 2nd section."

It is of interest to note that at the very first meeting of the county society there was some question regarding a standardization of the medical fees. Dr. McComb states that it was customary at that time to get $1.50 for a day call and $1.00 for an office call, or, as he calls it, "a prescription." After considerable debate the society decided to raise the day calls from $1.50 to $2.00. This, according to some of the members, was not entirely sufficient, but it eventually became the standard fee for a good many years.

The first annual banquet of the society was held at the Spalding Hotel in 1895, and it was customary during those years not only to have a sumptuous repast but plenty of liquid refreshments as well! In 1895 the state society again met in Duluth and the local committee in charge of arrangements was Dr. W. H. Magie, chairman, Dr. C. F. McComb, Dr. C. A. Stewart, Dr. S. C. McCormick. At that time Dr. Justus Ohage of St. Paul was president, and the meeting was on June 19.

The decade from 1880 to 1890 saw many changes in the medical profession, and Duluth as well. The hospitals were being developed, the Board of Health set up, and the medical society organized. Sanitary conditions in the city, however, continued to be a source of dissatisfaction, with typhoid an ever present menace.

The "Mortuary Report" for September, 1888, furnishes an interesting sidelight on vital statistics of the period:

```
"Total Number of deaths reported.............................48
    "Cause  1 Railroad accident
            1 Drowning
            1 Capillary Bronchitis
            6 Cholera Infantum
            1 Convulsions
            2 Diarrhea
            2 Dysentery
            1 Enteritis
            1 Entero-colitis
            2 Heart disease
            1 Pulmonary hemorrhage
            1 Indigestion
            1 Marasmus
            1 Chronic nephritis
            2 Phthisis pneumonia
            1 Traumatic peritonitis
           17 Typhoid Fever
            7 (Not reported)
```
                                            Dr. Sherwin,
                                                Health Officer."

The population of the county was increasing rapidly, and many physicians whose names are now familiar appeared in the news of the times.

(To be continued in April, 1938, issue)

EDITORIAL

MINNESOTA MEDICINE

Official Journal of the Minnesota State Medical
Association

Published by the Association under the direction of its Editing
and Publishing Committee

EDITING AND PUBLISHING COMMITTEE

J. T. Christison, Saint Paul   C. B. Wright, Minneapolis
E. M. Hammes, Saint Paul   T. A. Peppard, Minneapolis
Waltman Walters, Rochester

EDITORIAL STAFF

Carl B. Drake, Saint Paul, Editor
W. F. Braasch, Rochester, Associate Editor
Gilbert Cottam, Minneapolis, Associate Editor

Annual Subscription—$3.00.   Single Copies—$0.40
Foreign Subscriptions—$3.50.

The right is reserved to reject material submitted for editorial
or advertising columns. The Editing and Publishing Committee
does not hold itself responsible for views expressed either in
editorials or other articles when signed by the author.

Classified advertising—five cents a word; minimum, charge,
$1.00. Remittance should accompany order.

Display advertising rates on request.

Address all communications to Minnesota Medicine, 2642 University Avenue, Saint Paul, or Suite 604, National Bldg., Minneapolis. Telephone: Nestor 2641.

BUSINESS MANAGER

J. R. Bruce

Volume 21   MARCH, 1938   Number 3

Social Scientists and Medical Care

MICHAEL DAVIS, Ph.D.,* of New York,
has recently circularized the profession
quite generally and has codified the "Social Scientists' " viewpoint in regard to "organized medical care." These two final sentences in his summary deserve impartial scrutiny: "Medical
service must be judged from the point of view
of the people who receive and pay for it, as

*Facts and issues regarding public medical care, New England
Jour. Med., 218:143-47, (Jan. 27) 1938.

192

well as from the standpoint of the physicians
and institutions that furnish it. The participation of medical and social scientists is therefore
needed in appraisal as well as in planning, and
the rate and smoothness of progress will depend
largely upon ungrudging coöperation between
physicians and the public."

It would appear that the *science* in *social*
achievement is on a par with that which obtains
in Medicine, if we are to accept the author's
thesis. It is not for us to acclaim that we
represent science in all our medical achievement.
Much of what we individually accomplish may
well be grouped under priestly or even less dig-
nified effort to appease the unrest inherent in
man's conflict with his consciousness.

We may go a considerable distance with the
social propagandists and lend them recognition, and even example (should they seek to
follow it), in seeking to utilize science in their
economic and humanitarian efforts, but at this
time it is only reasonable to ask them how
far they have gotten. Some ten years ago I
overheard in Switzerland a distinguished Con-
tinental economist remark that social economics
and political government were at the stage of scientific attainment that Astronomy held when
Copernicus announced his theory of the universe! It is said that one of the major causes
for wreckage in the recent German Republic
was the attempt to acccomplish social and economic security by edicts. Many of these dealt
with matters of health, unemployment, old age,
and the usual penalties of circumstance. Idealistic efforts no doubt added to the immediate
popularity of a socialistic regime. It all looked
very promising on paper. Within a comparatively short time, however, these measures lent
disaster, not only to organized medicine but to
the economic stability of a country tested far
beyond its capacity. Reform had outrun itself.

Missionaries have long resorted to approaching the heathen's soul via the route of caring
for his bodily ailments. There is a subtle compliment to our profession in that observation.
These social and economic reformers would en-

joy teaming up with us in order to make more palatable a re-deal of the cards in a game in which they establish most of the rules and base all of them upon experiment. "The public medical care" is indeed a problem. However, the success in the Twin Cities, in Minnesota, of the hospital insurance plan for employed groups, would indicate that the hospitals at least are far from ready to turn over their management to governmental bureaucratic guidance. Movements of this order point the way for tying up our scientific heritage with such portions of social advancement as are workable and judicious. We have come a long way in a muddling world; and for the most part independent of Government subsidies or entanglements. Whatever socialization we absorb should be like the dosage of our drugs—"quantum suffict," and no more.

E. L. T.

Marihuana

THE rumors that have been growing more insistent the past few years about the increasing use of marihuana in our country, evidently have some basis in fact. Marihuana, also spelled marijuana, is the term used for that portion of the plant Cannabis Sativa, a species of Indian hemp, containing the drug. Although all but one of the states have had laws governing the raising and use of Indian hemp, last summer the Federal government took cognizance of the growing evil and passed the Marihuana Tax Act. An article* written from information furnished by H. J. Anslinger, United States Commissioner of Narcotics, and abstracted in the *Reader's Digest* for February, emphasizes, perhaps with overemphasis, the enormity of the growing evil.

Indian hemp grows wild in all parts of the United States and is cultivated in the east. Its stalk has commercial value, while Cannabis Indica preparations are obtained from the flowering tops of the plant and its resin.

The drug may be taken by mouth or can be incorporated in a cigarette, which method is said to have originated in Mexico and to have spread into this country rapidly the past two or three

*Anslinger, H. J., with Cooper, Courtney Ryley: Marijuana—Assassin of youth. American Magazine, July, 1937.

years. These cigarettes, known as reefers, are being peddled particularly to the youth of the country.

The drug and its psychic effects are not new. Homer described how it made the victims forget their families and turned them into swine. It is the hashish of Oriental reputation. While its action is unpredictable it usually causes hilarity at first, loss of judgment and eventually somnolence. During stimulation the mind acts so nimbly that the passing of time seems slowed. Most atrocious crimes have been committed following the use of the drug. Our word "assassin" is derived from this Arabic word "hashish."

The Federal Marihuana Tax Act requires registration of all those who grow or handle the plant. The mature stalks of the plant are excepted. In an effort to control marihuana, physicians wishing to prescribe Cannabis Indica preparations are required to pay a special tax of one dollar yearly and keep a record of their prescriptions. Needless to say, few physicians will wish to prescribe the drug, for its narcotic effect for which it is mentioned in pharmacopœias is far surpassed by many safer drugs.

The widespread wild growth of Indian hemp will make its control difficult. The very fact that it is so available, however, has prevented marihuana from coming under the control of gangster syndicates. Publicity and emphatic warning of the grave danger incident to the use of the weed will, it is to be hoped, nip in the bud the spread of the traffic in the weed.

Mea Culpa and Its Author

EVER since the days of Tobias Smollett (1721-1771) and Oliver Goldsmith (1728-1774), both of whom were rank failures as physicians, the pursuit of literature as an auxiliary to the profession for which they were originally trained has appealed to medical men. Many who were wholly unknown in medicine have become famous as writers. Some, like Oliver Wendell Holmes and S. Weir Mitchell, made substantial contributions both to medical and general literature and were eminent in both professional fields, but that is unusual. Gen-

erally speaking, when a man has made his mark
as a writer he has abandoned medicine; there
have been very few exceptions to this rule and
the two last named were not among them, in
their later years.

Contemporary writers who began as physicians, like Deeping, Maugham and Cronin in
England, Léon Daudet and Georges Duhamel
in France and others in this country, have been
mentioned in some detail in these columns by
the present writer (MINNESOTA MEDICINE, December, 1935) and further reference to them
at this time is unnecessary. But another French
physician-author was referred to casually and
it is to his later efforts and his own peculiar
life and personality that brief consideration is
now being given.

Louis-Ferdinand Destouches was born in
1894 in Asnières, a small pleasure-resort suburb
on the left bank of the Seine, three miles north
of Paris. After a boyhood of poverty and misery he found himself, at twenty, sent to the
front in the first stresses of the World War,
out of which he came with a brain injury, a
definite psychosis and functional cerebral disturbances which have never disappeared. He
studied medicine, with intermissions for economic reasons in which he went first to the
French colonies in Africa, later finishing his
studies and writing the doctorate thesis which
gained him his degree in 1924. Then he went to
the Ford factories and filled a medical post at
Dearborn, afterwards going to Africa under the
auspices of the Rockfeller Institute to investigate
tropical sleeping sickness.

Back in Paris, finally, he secured an outpatient connection with a hospital in the Montmartre district, picked up some practice among
the poor and then began writing. His first effort was a laborious affair, immensely bulky
and so fantastic and radical that he refused to
allow it to be published as his own. Our comment on it at the time was that "in form it resembles closely a very prolonged example of
what our psychiatric friends would call a 'flight
of ideas.'" Destouches said that its publication
over his own name would indicate that he was
not merely exposing himself to mockery but
also making the whole literary profession appear
foolish. This was his *Journey to the End of the
Night* and he ultimately allowed it to appear, in

194

MEDICAL ECONOMICS

Edited by the Committee on Medical Economics
of the
Minnesota State Medical Association

B. J. Branton, M. D.   W. F. Braasch, M. D., Chairman   J. C. Michael, M. D.
L. H. Rutledge, M. D.   A. N. Collins, M. D.

President's Message

T THE Northwest Regional Conference held recently in Chicago, the general theme ɔr discussion was: "Medical Care for All the eople." The discussions were led by officers f the national, state and county societies. The onsensus of opinion seemed quite well crystalized about the fact that the county must be the responsible unit for the care of the sick. Climatic conditions, the variable types of citizenship, economic conditions, and many other factors make it impossible to establish a plan for the medical care of all the people which would be applicable to all parts of the country. To a lesser degree the same holds true in attempting to formulate a state-wide plan. Of the eighty-seven counties in Minnesota, perhaps the same plan may be applicable to about one-third this number. Many are able to take care of their own indigent and other medical problems. Some are sparsely settled and financially low. It is necessary for the state to come to their rescue. To determine which counties should have outside assistance and just how much is no small task. Our State Board of Control and State Relief Department, in conjunction with the Local County Welfare Boards and local committees of the County Medical Societies, are doing excellent work in formulating workable plans for these various needy counties. To coördinate these various agencies a central authority is necessary. Our State Association has done well in this capacity. At our Regional Conference, seventeen states were represented. So far as I could ascertain, no state represented at this conference had a better set-up for the care of the sick than has Minnesota, and few have as good.

Our State Board of Health, Public Health Association and Medical Society have the coöperation of the state and federal relief groups in every move to improve the care of the needy

sick. We all acknowledge the need for improvement and all are striving for such improvement. In former years duplication of effort was confusing and wasteful. Today this seems to be eliminated to a high degree.

While all our various state and county organizations are doing their best to work in unison and care for the sick to their best ability, we hope we all may learn and improve our methods from our contact with those from other states and counties. A study of their various plans and experiences should help us in our attempts to formulate workable plans throughout the state.

To me one of the most attractive parts of the program put on in Chicago was the outline of the Health Program in the state of Indiana. Such a program means much work, but I believe it is worthwhile in making the public medically conscious. I hope some day we may have such a program in Minnesota.

J. M. HAYES, M.D.

New Call to Action

For several years the American Medical Association has been urging county and state medical associations to experiment with new plans for the care of the indigent and low income groups.

The result has been a considerable amount of healthy activity in many parts of the United States.

It was not the type of activity that catches the public eye or fires the public imagination, however, and it has clearly become desirable, now, for organized medicine to take action on a large scale. Furthermore, a nation-wide, organized effort on the part of organized medicine promises to be more effective, now, than ever before.

The action taken recently by the Board of Trustees calls first for a thorough study of the medical needs of their own communities on the part of all state and county medical societies. A comprehensive outline of the two phases which such a study must cover—the demand for services on the one hand, and the supply available—has already been sent to all State societies.

Time is Ripe

The time is ripe for a new study of medical services in the United States and it is right and proper that this study should be under medical auspices.

Several years have passed since the Committee on Costs of Medical Care made its report and times have greatly changed. The studies made recently by the United States Public Health Service on the amount of chronic illness in this country have filled in some parts of the

current health picture; but new and authoritative data are needed on the actual condition of medical services and the need for extended care.

The next step will be, of course, to work out some practical plan in every community where it may be needed, to meet that individual community need.

Acts of Congress and heavy appropriations are not necessary for practical action of this sort. For medical men this is the time and opportunity to show that medicine can and will make any needed adjustments that it may uncover without outside aid.

Council Will Act

The outline for the study, prepared by Dr. R. G. Leland, director of the Bureau of Medical Economics, will be presented shortly to the Council for decision as to Minnesota's participation in this nation-wide study.

Northwest Conference

The Northwest Regional Conference originated in Minnesota in 1927 when Dr. W. F. Braasch was president of the Minnesota State Medical Association and it was held in Saint Paul under the auspices of the Minnesota Association for many years.

At the meeting held February 12 in Chicago, President J. M. Hayes, Dr. Braasch and Mr. R. R. Rosell, executive secretary, represented the Association.

Following are some interesting highlights on public welfare work carried on by a few of the seventeen state societies participating. They furnish evidence of a fact that was strikingly evident to those who were present at the 1938 meeting: Organized Medicine has moved rapidly in the last few years along the road to efficient handling of relief and welfare problems that involve care of the sick in their own communities.

Preventing Disease

Indiana.—A general public health education program is carried on by all the county societies in the state, according to a definite schedule that changes monthly. For example, February was devoted to syphilis education; March is to be devoted to the pneumonia program; April to cancer. News stories sent out from the state

196

office follow the program throughout the state. Special talks, health exhibits, demonstrations, mark each campaign.

Roving Committee

Wisconsin.—As a result of last year's long fight in the legislature to defeat the Beimiller bills (for sickness insurance, state subsidies, et cetera) the Wisconsin State Medical Society is now engaged in what is perhaps the most thoroughgoing study ever made in any state as to medical care, adequacy of facilities, costs. A roving committee, so-called, goes into each community, meets with representative groups including representatives of all leading service organizations, Rotary and Kiwanis clubs, churches, carefully studies the local situation, makes notes of findings. A permanent committee is left behind which will study the problem further and report to the state society. The committee is still assembling information and no reports have been issued to date. It will be remembered, in this connection, that the Wisconsin Society is also sending its executive secretary, Mr. George Crownhart, to Europe this spring to make a first-hand study of sickness insurance systems in European countries.

Rehabilitating Sick Men

West Virginia.—The West Virginia State Medical Society is carrying on a significant demonstration of the value in money to the state of the medical rehabilitation of otherwise unemployable relief clients. The society started with a trial of appropriation of $1,000 to be used for the rehabilitation of ten men. This cost was determined on the basis of a survey by which they also showed to the state that it was costing an average of $224 to maintain the same unemployables on relief. At the end of the first year the medical men returned each of the ten men to regular jobs. The accomplishment so impressed relief authorities of the state that a large appropriation is now set aside each year for the rehabilitation of unemployables. It is estimated that the state saved $169,120 during the last year.

Cutting Red Tape

Oakland County, Michigan.—The Oakland County Medical Society has developed a working alliance with county relief authorities whereby any relief client may apply at any time to the doctor of his choice, without any preliminary authorization whatever, for needed medical service. The procedure is this: the relief client calls the doctor or visits his office; the doctor gives him whatever care or advice may be immediately needed and signs the patient's own identification card; *subsequently,* within seven days from the date of the first visit, the doctor sends to the relief office a statement on a simple form as to the call, name and identification of the patient, diagnosis, need, if any, for further service. Further care is given as needed on the basis of a fee schedule determined by an advisory committee of the medical society and the medical director of the relief administration. Discipline of physicians who might chisel is the responsibility of the advisory committee. The plan has worked, with additions and notable developments, in Oakland County (population about 200,000, largest city, Pontiac) since 1934.

County Society Clinic

Sedgwick County, Wichita, Kansas.—The Sedgwick County Medical Society has formed a clinic for the handling of medical care for relief patients. A lump sum of $500 is paid to the society for the service and all relief patients apply to the clinic for medical aid. The society also operates a credit bureau and collection agency for its members. Low income patients who are unable to pay regular fees are referred to the bureau, their needs and bills budgeted and the care administered at costs within their ability to pay.

Government Medicine

Statements frequently have been made to the effect that the government institutes postgraduate training for members of the panel in the countries where compulsory sickness insurance is in force.

In a recent issue of the *British Medical Journal* it was announced that arrangements had been made to give a course of postgraduate instruction to some forty-five members of the panel over a period of two weeks. One cannot help but compare this with the opportunities for graduate instruction available to members of the medical profession in this country,—and this under the spur of individual initiative.

There is a great variety of opportunities here. For instance, in Michigan practically all the doctors go to school at least two months out of a year. Instead of giving up their entire practice, the graduate lectures and demonstrations are brought to various parts of the state so that the physicians will have to sacrifice but two or three hours a day two or three times a week. So-called refresher courses are given by many state universities in regular centers ·over a period of a week or two. The annual meetings of the state, as well as national medical societies, are made centers for graduate education. There are many other agencies for graduate instruction, such as the College of Surgeons, the Inter-State Assembly, hospital clinics, beside the courses which are arranged by the various county societies in the larger medical centers. Opportunities are continually being increased so as to reach the majority of the practitioners.

Many of these activities are now being described in detail in the Economic Columns of *The Journal of the American Medical Association.*

One would hesitate to predict what might happen to these manifold opportunities if American medicine should ever be controlled by the state. There would be but little incentive to maintain the present facilities and those which might be developed undoubtedly would be restricted and stereotyped by governmental control. This is only one more of the calamities which would befall medicine if our socialistic friends had their way.

"Forewarnings"

(Monthly Editorial by the Medical Advisory Committee)

Four cases in four days, each with a potential warning to the members of our Association, were reviewed by the Medical Advisory Committee the first week in February.

1. A case of alleged unauthorized autopsy.

In no case should an autopsy be performed except by the duly constituted authority authorized by law to perform such autopsies unless written permission which has been signed by the next of kin and notarized or witnessed is in your hands.

2. A case of alleged negligence.

Never fail to examine a case thoroughly even though you do not feel it necessary. If you haven't time, make a future date or send the patient to someone else who has the time. If the patient will not do as you wish, refuse to treat him until he will. Better to lose the patient than to lose a malpractice suit.

3. A case of giving unauthorized information.

Information obtained from a patient should be kept confidential. There is no finer relationship than the patient-physician relationship. Lawyers and others are not entitled to information unless the patient signs the request. Be sure again that the request is notarized or witnessed. It may save you trouble.

4. A case where an assistant talked out of turn.

When cases are referred to associates or assistants for care, see that they are fully aware of their responsibility to you or to the surgeon who formerly treated the case. A derogatory word spoken by an unthinking or irresponsible assistant caused the last case reviewed.

If foresight is better than hindsight, then forewarning, if heeded, will save disaster in many a case. Take heed to the "mariner who watches the thin clouds and takes a reef in his sails, before the storm breaks."

Remember

Deductions for expenses incurred in attendance at medical meetings and in postgraduate study may now be made by physicians in making state income tax returns.

This new ruling made by the Minnesota Tax Commission brings the state regulations into conformity with federal income tax regulations in this matter. Physicians who have not yet made returns should remember this ruling.

"Sorry for Their Patients"

"I cannot understand why so few men attend their county and state medical society meetings. It is not because they are so busy, as the busiest doctors are always found where there is a chance to learn. After years of observation I have reached the conclusion that there are three kinds of physicians who don't attend meetings: the

198

person who has not the ability to plan his work so that he can have an evening for recreation at the meeting; second, the man who thinks he knows it all, has not read a new book since leaving school, and has no time for reading the journal or other publication; and third, the man who is afraid he might lose a patient should he leave his office. These three types form the fault finding group, complaining, but will not come to the meetings and put their shoulders to the wheel, clarify their visions, help remove the faults they see and become what is most needed by the society and always welcomed by its officers—a worker instead of a drone or complainer.

"Yes, the opportunity for the present-day doctor to be an up-to-date doctor is right at one's door, and I am not only sorry for those who are missing these opportunities, but for their patients."—*Pittsburgh Medical Bulletin.*

Minnesota State Board of Medical Examiners

Self-Styled Health Expert Loses in Supreme Court

Re State of Minnesota vs. Vivi Ann Mielke, also known as Vivi Ann Wyntor.

On February 4, 1938, the Supreme Court of Minnesota, in a unanimous decision, held that the above defendant, who represented herself in Minnesota as a health expert, had brought herself "squarely within the basic science law" by her conduct. The opinion of the Supreme Court, which is printed in full at the end of this article, was written by the Honorable Charles Loring, Associate Justice. The opinion is clear and concise and should go a long ways to effectively demonstrate that quackery will not be tolerated in Minnesota through any such attempted evasion of the law.

Following the decision of the Supreme Court, the defendant appeared in the District Court of Ramsey County, and entered a plea of guilty on February 14, 1938, to the amended information charging her with practicing healing without a basic science certificate. The plea of guilty was entered before the Honorable Richard A. Walsh, Judge of the District Court, who, after hearing the facts and questioning the defendant, imposed a fine of $100.00 or thirty days in the Saint Paul Workhouse. The fine was paid. The disposition of the case was recommended by the County Attorney's office of Ramsey County, and the Minnesota State Board of Medical Examiners because the defendant was also obliged to pay the expense of the appeal to the Supreme Court. Judge Walsh, in passing sentence, remarked that, in view of the Supreme Court's decision, the defendant had clearly violated the law; Judge Walsh also stated that the basic science law was enacted to protect the people against such things.

The defendant, who is twenty-five years of age, was arrested at the Lowry Hotel in Saint Paul, on April 23, 1937, following an investigation conducted by the State Board of Medical Examiners and the Saint Paul Police Department. At that time the defendant was

released upon $500.00 bail, waived her preliminary hearing when arraigned in Municipal Court on April 24, and was held to the District Court, where she was arraigned on April 26. The case was continued to May 10, 1937, and reset for trial on May 18, on which date an amended information was filed setting forth the charge in considerable detail. A demurrer was interposed by the defendant and on July 12, 1937, the Honorable Richard D. O'Brien, Judge of the District Court, made an order overruling the demurrer and certified the case to the Supreme Court of Minnesota for a decision as to whether or not the amended information charged the defendant with a public offense. The information alleged that the defendant had advertised herself as an assistant and staff lecturer for one R. A. Richardson, an osteopath of Kansas City, Missouri, who holds no license to practice any form of healing in the State of Minnesota. It also charged her with giving free lectures at the Lowry Hotel in Saint Paul, following which she gave a lecture course on health matters for which she charged a fee of $5.50; that during these lectures she advertised certain products including pills, tablets and other preparations which she had for sale. These concoctions were represented as being used in the treatment of anemia, thyroid disturbances and a multitude of other conditions.

The defendant, at the time of her arrest, maintained an office in the Lyceum Building at Duluth. She also operated in Virginia, Hibbing and St. Cloud. She admitted that she had never studied medicine and that her only training for this type of work was supplied by Richardson.

The defendant was represented by George H. Lommen, State Senator from Eveleth, Minnesota, who devoted a great deal of his time and argument in a futile attempt to divert attention from the real issue by attacking the medical profession. The State was represented by the Honorable William S. Ervin, Attorney General of Minnesota; Mr. Roy C. Frank, Assistant Attorney General; Mr. M. F. Kinkead, County Attorney of Ramsey County, and his assistants, Mr. James F. Lynch and Mr. Horace R. Hansen.

No. 4   Ramsey County   Loring, J.
State of Minnesota, Plaintiff,
         31501 vs.
Vivi Ann Mielke, also known as
   Vivi Ann Wyntor, Defendant.
         Endorsed:
      Filed February 4, 1938.
      Russell O. Gunderson, Clerk.
         Minn. Supreme Court.

SYLLABUS

An information examined and found to charge defendant with practicing healing without a certificate under the Basic Science Act. The requirements of that act are germane to the protection of the public as applied to the acts charged against the defendant. The question certified to us is properly answered in the affirmative.

OPINION

LORING, Justice.

The trial court has certified to this court the question: "Does the amended information as filed charge a public offense under the Basic Science Act of the State of Minnesota as set out in Section 5705 of Mason's Minnesota Statutes for the year 1927?" The amended information charges the defendant with practicing healing as defined by law without a valid existing certificate of registration in the basic sciences. As amended the information charges the defendant with advertising herself as an assistant and staff lecturer for Dr. R. A. Richardson of Kansas City, and that she would give free daily lectures commencing April 13, 1937, to and including April 15 of that year; that she gave the lectures at the Lowry Hotel in Saint Paul, and during the lectures solicited women present to attend a lecture course which would follow immediately, for which a fee was charged; that a number of women attended and paid the fee, and during the lectures certain products or concoctions were described and their uses and values discussed and certain circulars were distributed by and under the direction of the defendant, which circulars further described such products; that during the lectures it was announced that she had such products for sale, and she suggested and recommended their purchase by her hearers, who actually bought them from her at the Lowry Hotel; that from these sales she derived a commission of 55 per cent, the remainder going to Dr. Richardson, who was an osteopath holding no license to practice healing in the state of Minnesota; that one of the paragraphs in the circulars distributed by her was entitled: "How to Improve Your Health and Personal Appearance," and that it stated further:

"An anemia condition of the blood may mean either a deficiency of the blood itself or a deficiency of its red blood corpuscles.

"Recent scientific discoveries have proved the effectiveness of powdered bone marrow and spleen in the symptomatic treatment of anemia. This treatment offers greater promise of success than previous treatments, and it is endorsed by physicians.

"The effect of red bone marrow and spleen is shown in several ways. It has been found that these substances increase the formation of red blood corpuscles and their hemoglobin content. They also serve as an increased resistance to the process of hemolysis. By this process the hemoglobin or iron content of the blood is separated from the corpuscles and appears in the blood serum. Red bone marrow and spleen has a tendency to make the blood coagulate more quickly, and in this connection it has been used very effectively in the treatment of abnormally profuse menstruation."

She offered for sale tablets claimed to contain red bone marrow and spleen and labeled: "Useful in Secondary Anemia." Circulars which she distributed contained the following paragraphs:

"Women may become excessively fat or unusually thin, or have other physical disturbances. For instance, the young woman whose female organs are not functioning properly, and whose menstrual periods are irregular, practically always has a deficiency of glandular secretions. The thyroid gland as well as the ovarian glands, is practically always involved.

"The reason we feel so certain that both the thyroid and ovarian glands are concerned is because when thyroid and ovarian substances are supplied, the condition invariably improves. Not only does the patient feel better, but she is more alive and alert, and her complex, the light in her eyes, and the cheerfulness of her expression, all prove that the very thing she needed was glandular food, or female hormones."

Defendant is also charged with having sold female hormone tablets in connection with the lecture.

The Basic Science Law, Sec. 5705-1 et seq., Mason Minn. St., forbids the practice of healing without first having obtained a certificate of having passed an examination by the state board of examiners in the basic sciences. By the terms of the act, the basic sciences are defined to include the following: anatomy, physiology, pathology, bacteriology, hygiene, and chemistry insofar as the same relates to the human system or mind as generally treated in each or all of said subjects. The practice of healing is defined by the act as including any persons who shall in any manner for fee, gift, compensation or reward, or in expectation thereof, engage in the diagnosis, analysis, treatment, correction or cure of any disease, injury, defect, deformity, infirmity, ailment or affliction of human beings or who for any fee suggests, recommends or prescribes any medicine or cure thereof.

The defendant does not attack the constitutionality of the basic science law, but asserts that as it applies to her or to the acts charged against her it infringes upon her constitutional rights and that there is no relation between the requirements of the basic science law and the protection of the public as applied to her situation.

With the defendant's contention we cannot agree. It is essential to the public health and safety that persons who, for compensation, are suggesting, recommending, or prescribing medicine or treatment for the correction or cure of human ailments have a basic understanding of the subjects required by the basic science law. In our opinion it is within the police power of the state to so require. According to the information lodged against her, the defendant induced women to come to lectures for which she charged a fee and for those who had menstrual troubles she suggested and recommended tablets which she had for sale for correction and cure of their affliction. It is our view that her conduct came squarely within the basic science law and that the requirements of that law are germane to the safety and health of the public in the treatment

of such ailments as those for which she sold and recommended her tablets and medicines. Such being the case, no constitutional right of the defendant is infringed upon.

It is our opinion that the question certified to us by the trial court should be answered in the affirmative and that the court properly overruled the demurrer to the information.

Olivia Chiropractor Pleads Guilty

State of Minnesota vs. Hans C. Hanson

On January 29, 1938, Hans C. Hanson, sixty-two years of age, entered a plea of guilty to an information charging him with practicing healing without a basic science certificate. Hanson's plea of guilty was entered before the Honorable G. E. Qvale, Judge of the District Court at Willmar. The Court, upon being advised that Hanson had closed his office and taken his signs, sentenced the defendant to pay a fine of $50.00 plus court costs of $11.00.

The investigation made by the Minnesota State Board of Medical Examiners disclosed that Hanson opened an office at Olivia in October, 1937, for the practice of chiropractic. Hanson has no license to practice any form of healing in the State of Minnesota or elsewhere. He had a diploma on his office wall dated December 5, 1914, from the Palmer School at Davenport, Iowa. He admitted, however, that he had only taken a one-year course to obtain the diploma and that his preliminary education was limited to the eighth grade. He stated that after his graduation from the Palmer School, he practiced chiropractic for fifteen months at Sydney, Montana, and returned to his home at Hutchinson, Minnesota. He also stated that in 1919, when the Minnesota chiropractic law was passed, he was farming. Shortly before opening his office at Olivia, Hanson stated that he took a one month postgraduate course at the National College in Chicago. Hanson used no pretext about practicing, having the chiropractic sign on his door and also one on the outside of the building where he was located. He also ran a card in the Olivia Times.

The Medical Board wishes to acknowledge fine cooperation from Mr. Russell L. Frazee, County Attorney of Renville County.

The Zinc Sulfate Spray for the Prevention of Poliomyelitis

The successful use of a zinc sulfate spray in the prevention of experimental poliomyelitis in monkeys by Armstrong, Sabin, Schultz and their co-workers has stimulated much interest in its effectiveness as a preventive of the disease in human beings. Schultz demonstrated at Stanford University that in the experimental infection a solution containing 1 per cent of zinc sulfate, 1 per cent of pontocaine and 0.5 per cent of sodium chloride in distilled water is most effective in the monkey. The use of this technic in the human being has been too variable and uncontrolled to permit even an approximate estimate of its value. Dr. J. C. Geiger, the director of public health of San Francisco, and his distinguished committee have recommended that the use of this spray must be strictly limited until the proper technic has been worked out. (J.A.M.A., Sept. 18, 1937, p. 958)

Dr. W. A. Brand of Redwood Falls has been reapinted to the State Board of Health.

* * *

Dr. Walter P. Gardner has assumed charge as supertendent of the Anoka State Hospital.

* * *

Dr. R. R. Hendrickson of Wadena has been named sident physician of the St. Cloud reformatory, effecve February 1.

* * *

Dr. G. H. Olds of Waseca was elected chairman of e Waseca County District Scout Committee for 1938 t the district annual meeting held on January 27.

* * *

Dr. E. H. Rynearson of Rochester was elected chairan of the Zumbro Valley District Boy Scout Comittee at the recent annual meeting of the group.

* * *

Dr. Z. E. House, who recently retired from government service, has returned to Cass Lake after a three onths' vacation in Florida, and will enter private ractice.

* * *

Dr. Walter S. Neff, who has been practicing medicine n Boston, has joined the staff of the Lenont-Peterson Clinic, Virginia, Minnesota, as head of the division of internal medicine.

* * *

Dr. Olga S. Hansen of Minneapolis spoke on "The Medical Profession as a Career for Women" at a ecture-tea for women students of Gustavus Adolphus College at St. Peter recently.

* * *

Dr. Leo Hilger of Saint Paul was elected president of the advisory board of St. Joseph's Hospital at its annual meeting, succeeding Dr. W. C. Carroll. Dr. William Kennedy was named to the board for a five-year term.

* * *

Dr. Joseph F. Malloy, associated with the Bratrud Clinic of Thief River Falls, was recently appointed Soo Line surgeon. Dr. Edward Bratrud also will continue to serve as surgeon for the company as he has for a number of years.

* * *

Dr. and Mrs. A. R. Ellingson of Detroit Lakes have gone to New Orleans, where Dr. Ellingson is taking a six weeks' course in surgery and x-ray diagnosis at the University of Tulane. They expect to return to Detroit Lakes about April 1.

* * *

Dr. Henry Porter Johnson of Fairmont celebrated his eighty-third birthday on February 3. Dr. Johnson has practiced medicine for fifty-nine years, thirty-eight

of which have been spent in Fairmont, and is still actively engaged in the practice of his profession.

* * *

A special program of lectures and demonstrations in surgery and medicine will be held in Rochester under the direction of The Mayo Foundation from March 28 to April 1, inclusive. Symposiums on gastric diseases, diseases of children, cardiology, urology and backache, and conferences on roentgen, radium and physical therapy will be included. Visiting physicians are invited to attend.

* * *

The Foundation Prize of the American Association of Obstetricians, Gynecologists and Abdominal Surgeons, consisting of $500, is open to internes, residents, graduate students and doctors of medicine practicing or teaching the specialty. Manuscripts limited to 5,000 words should be submitted before June 1, 1938, to the secretary, Dr. James R. Bloss, 418 Eleventh Street, Huntington, West Virginia.

* * *

Dr. Paul O'Leary and Dr. G. B. New of Rochester, attended the International Postgraduate Medical Assembly of Southwest Texas in San Antonio in January. Dr. O'Leary spoke on the treatment of syphilis and dermatological conditions. Dr. New also attended the meeting of American Association of Plastic Surgeons in Dallas and Houston, and a sectional meeting of the American College of Surgeons in Houston. He appeared on the program at each of these meetings.

* * *

Dr. J. C. Litzenberg, Professor of Obstetrics and Gynecology at the University of Minnesota, presented a paper on "What is Good Care for Mothers and Babies" before the Conference on Better Care for Mothers and Babies held by the Children's Bureau of the United States Department of Labor, in Washington, January 17, 1938. Others from Minnesota who attended were Dr. Ruth Boynton, Director of the Student Health Service, University of Minnesota, Dr. E. C. Hartley, Clinical Instructor of Obstetrics and Gynecology, University of Minnesota, and Dr. A. J. Chesley, secretary of the Minnesota State Board of Health.

* * *

The Third Annual Postgraduate Institute, offering an intensive and interesting study of the Diseases of the Digestive Tract, will be conducted by The Philadelphia County Medical Society from March 28 to April 1, inclusive. The program to be held in the Bellevue-Stratford Hotel, Philadelphia, has been designed to meet the needs of all members of the profession, but particularly those in general practice.

Physicians from fourteen states having attended last year's institute, an invitation to attend the 1938 session has been extended to the members of all county societies. The only charge is a $5.00 registration fee to cover the Institute's expenses. Additional information may be secured from your County Society or from the Philadelphia County Medical Society, 21st and Spruce Streets, Philadelphia, Pa.

* * *

The medical staff of the Menninger Clinic will conduct its fourth annual Postgraduate Course on *Neuropsychiatry in General Practice,* April 25 to 30, inclusive, at the Menninger Clinic, Topeka, Kansas. The course this year will include a brief introduction to the fields of neurology and psychiatry and a specific application of this knowledge to the large group of cases of psychoneuroses, psychoses and psychogenic and neurological disorders which every physician meets in his daily practice. Suggestions made by those who took the course last year have been embodied in this year's program in order to make it applicable to the most common practical problems of the physician.

As in previous years, several guest speakers, prominent in the fields of neurology and psychiatry, will appear at the evening sessions of the course.

* * *

The American Physiotherapy Association has announced a Vocational Service in providing trained physiotherapists for hospital and office positions. The Association was organized very soon after the close of the World War, the charter members being former Reconstruction Aides in service. Since then the membership has increased to more than 800. The present requirements for membership are: 1. One year's practice in physical therapy within two years of graduation from an approved school of physical therapy. 2. An approved course in physical therapy of not less than nine months, following graduation from a school of nursing or physical education which meets the requirements of the individual states. These requirements have been approved by the Council on Medical Education and Hospitals of the American Medical Association. The object in having these qualifications for membership is to provide for the hospitals, schools for crippled children, and offices of physicians, trained physiotherapists who are able to follow the physicians' orders intelligently and thoroughly.

One of the purposes of the American Physiotherapy Association is to "coöperate with and work only under the prescription of members of the medical profession."

Further information may be obtained by writing to Miss Edith Monro, 483 Beacon Street, Boston, Massachusetts.

* * *

The A.M.A. Convention Tour

According to latest reports physicians and their families are evincing a keen interest in the arrangements made for a convention tour of America en route to and returning from the San Francisco convention.

The "See America" movement by deluxe special trains is endorsed by approximately twenty-five State medical societies. It presents an opportunity for members and their families to join with their colleagues from other states, and enjoy the facilities and service of deluxe special trains, and at the same time visit the many scenic attractions of our western states.

Many physicians, completely immersed in their practices, have hesitated to take such an extended vacation heretofore but now the fact of the A.M.A. convention and the attractiveness and economical features of this travel program have brought such a trip within the realm of desirable possibilities.

The all-inclusive price is unusually low because of the coöperation of so many medical societies. An attractive folder, describing these travel arrangements, may be obtained through the secretary's office or the Transportation Agents, The American Express Travel Service, 723 Marquette Avenue, Minneapolis, Minnesota.

*

State Meeting

The fine program arranged for the 85th Annual Meeting of the Minnesota State Medical Association at the Hotel Duluth in Duluth is prompting several special societies to hold their own annual gatherings in conjunction with the state meeting. Dates for the assembly are June 29 and 30 and July 1.

The Northwest Pediatric Society, which is bringing one of the distinguished speakers scheduled for the regular program, will adopt the program of the pediatrics session for its own annual session. Dr. C. Anderson Aldrich of Winnetka, Illinois, is the speaker to be sponsored by the pediatricians. His subject will be, "Some Practical Points in the Management of Nephritic Children."

Other special societies and sectional groups who will finance speakers for this meeting include the Society of Internal Medicine, the Radiological Society and the Northern Minnesota Medical Association. Their speakers are respectively Dr. E. K. Marshall of Johns Hopkins, Dr. Hollis Potter of Chicago and Dr. Philip Lewin of Chicago. The Minnesota Society of Ophthalmology and Otolaryngology was of assistance in securing Dr. Edward Jackson of Denver for the program. Dr. Roland Cron of Milwaukee, Dr. Irvin Abell of Louisville, Kentucky, president-elect of the American Medical Association, Dr. Carl Meyer of Chicago, and Dr. Howard Haggard, noted writer and lecturer of Yale, were secured by the Committee on Scientific Assembly.

The completed program provides for extensive exhibits and demonstrations during morning and afternoon exhibit periods. Otherwise all sessions will be held in one lecture hall, the ballroom of the hotel, with guest speakers as features of each morning and afternoon session.

Doctor Haggard will talk to the doctors at the banquet Thursday night and he will also be principal speaker at a meeting to which the public will be invited at the Lyceum Theater in Duluth.

HOSPITAL NEWS

Dr. C. H. Schroder of Duluth was chosen chief of staff of St. Luke's Hospital at the recent annual meeting of the hospital staff.

Other staff officers named are: Dr. A. G. Athens, vice-chief of staff; Dr. S. H. Boyer, Jr., secretary; Dr. W. N. Graves, chief of surgery; Dr. R. L. Nelson, chief of medicine; Dr. R. J. Moe, chief of obstetrics; Dr. M. F. Fellows, chief of eye, ear, nose, and throat; Dr. R. E. Nutting, chief of pediatrics; Dr. A. H. Wells, chief of staff, laboratory section, and Dr. R. M. Mayne, chief of staff, x-ray section.

* * *

The Minnesota Association of Hospital, Medical and Institution Librarians held a luncheon meeting Saturday, February 5, 1938, at the Women's City Club in Saint Paul with thirty-three people present. Elizabeth Jensen of the St. Peter State Hospital and Mildred Schumacher of the Rochester State Hospital reported on the usability of the books of Temple Bailey and Mary Roberts Rhinehart respectively. Mary Heenan of the School for the Blind at Faribault described her work and dwelt in some detail upon the "Talking Books" and the government arrangements for the use of them by the blind people in this district. Mrs. Stella H. Amass, Director of Psychiatric Nursing in Minnesota, spoke upon the various types of patients to be found in hospitals and institutions, using as her title "The Librarian's Approach to the Patient." The next meeting will be at the time of the meeting of the Minnesota Hospital Association in May.

* * *

Drs. Edward Schons and J. P. Medelman announce the completion of the installation of a 1,200,000-volt, constant potential roentgen therapy apparatus which took nearly two years to construct in the Charles T. Miller Hospital of Saint Paul. This equipment was built especially for the hospital, and is considered the largest and the most advanced of its kind. It will be used primarily for the more adequate and efficient treatment of deep-seated tumors. The high voltage and filtration used will yield a radiation of high quality and penetrating power, permitting homogeneous irradiation of deeply situated tumors. Lower voltage equipment has also been installed and will be used as heretofore where that type of irradiation is indicated, as will also radium.

The Charles T. Miller Hospital has constructed a special building and made alterations in the adjacent wing, in order to accommodate the equipment and provide for needs incidental to the treatment of patients. The giant steel and porcelain tube is surrounded by lead 4 inches thick to prevent escape of radiation into the treatment room except through the treatment portals. Adequate protection of the personnel has been provided for with concrete walls 3 feet thick. Provision has been made for measuring equipment, indicating the quality and quantity of the radiation used.

In Memoriam

De Witt Clinton Jones
1868-1937

DR. D. C. JONES, Saint Paul, was born January 19, 1868, in Saint Paul, his parents having been early settlers. His aunt, Cleopatra Irvine, born in 1844, is said to have been the first white female child born in Saint Paul, at which time Minnesota was part of Wisconsin Territory.

Dr. Jones received his primary education in Saint Paul, and later attended De Vaux University, Toronto. In 1890 he was granted a degree in midwifery by the Toronto General Hospital, and the following year passed written examinations entitling him to diplomas from the Toronto, Victoria and Queen's Universities and the Trinity Medical College.

Returning to Saint Paul, Dr. Jones served his internship at the City and County Hospital in 1891 and 1892. Granted his license to practice in Minnesota in 1892, he opened an office at Seven Corners.

During the Spanish-American war, Dr. Jones served as contract surgeon at Fort Snelling and in 1911 was made First Lieutenant in the Medical Reserve.

For ten years he was coroner of Ramsey County. During this period he organized the Minnesota Coroners Association and was instrumental in revising laws relating to the duties of coroners.

Always active in politics, Dr. Jones was a founder and organizer, in 1895, of the first Democratic Club in Saint Paul. He was a member of the Ramsey County Medical Society, the Minnesota State and American Medical Associations. He was a member of the Masonic order, the Modern Woodmen and the Odd Fellows. He was also a member of the Episcopal Church. At Norwood, Minnesota, on August 22, 1908, Dr. Jones married Fannie Trocke, a well known business woman of Saint Paul. He is survived by his widow.

John Thomas Rogers
1867-1938

DR. JOHN T. ROGERS, for many years one of the outstanding surgeons of Saint Paul, died very suddenly at his home on January 2, 1938, at the age of seventy.

Born in Woodford County, Kentucky, July 18, 1867, of Kentucky stock, he received his academic education at Transylvania University. He moved to Saint Paul with his parents in 1886, and was temporarily employed in a haberdashery shop soon after his arrival. His ambition to become a doctor was made possible by his acquaintance with Dr. Charles A. Wheaton, who was then one of the leading surgeons in Saint Paul. Employment in Dr. Wheaton's office enabled him to attend the medical school at the University of Minnesota and during his student days he assisted Dr. Wheaton at emergency operations performed in outlying districts. Following his graduation from the University Medical School in 1890, Dr. Rogers continued his association with Dr. Wheaton and became what might have been termed a resident surgeon at the City and County Hospital in Saint Paul.

Upon Dr. Wheaton's retirement from practice in 1906, Dr. Rogers' became associated with Dr. A. R. Colvin until 1915, when this partnership was dissolved and he took Dr. Harry B. Zimmermann into partnership.

Dr. Rogers was largely responsible for persuading Mrs. Charles T. Miller, the widow of Charles T. Miller of Saint Paul, to donate funds for the construction of a hospital in memory of her husband. Permission was obtained during our participation in the World War to begin construction of the hospital now known as 'he **Charles T. Miller Hospital** with the idea that the hospital would, upon completion, be temporarily used by the United States government. The government never used the hospital and it was necessary to obtain additional funds for equipment. This was accomplished partly by the assistance of a group of St. Paul physicians who formed the Miller Clinic in 1919. Dr. Rogers was a member of this clinic group until it dissolved in 1934. During the early days Dr. Rogers did most of his work at St. Luke's Hospital, being frequently called to operate in outlying cities. With the establishment of the Miller Hospital he became chairman of the Board of Trustees and Chief of Staff of the hospital, positions he held until his death.

Dr. Rogers was a younger member of a group of surgeons who, in the eighties and nineties, made Saint Paul a surgical center of the Northwest. A most lovable character, who inspired immediate confidence, Dr. Rogers enjoyed an enviable reputation and practice. A student rather than a scholar, he did not make numerous contributions to surgical literature. He had an almost uncanny ability to absorb minute details of operative technic by observation. He made many visits to clinics in this country and abroad for self-betterment.

During Dr. Rogers' more than forty-seven years of practice, he served as president of the Minnesota Academy of Medicine in 1901 and as president of the Minnesota State Medical Association in 1915. He was also a member of the American College of Surgeons and of the Ramsey County Medical Society and the Minnesota State and American Medical Associations.

Dr. Rogers is survived by his daughter Mrs. Jerome Helpern of Saint Paul, having been preceded in death a few years ago by his wife.

Philemon Roy
1869-1938

D R. PHILEMON ROY, Saint Paul, died of coronary disease, January 21, 1938, while on vacation in McAllan, Texas.

Dr. Roy was born at St. Anaclet, Quebec, December 13, 1869, of French parents, the third of a family of fifteen children. He received his primary education at the College of Remouski in the Province of

Quebec. He received his M.D. from the University of Minnesota in 1896.

After practicing a few years at Pierz, Minnesota, he took three years of postgraduate study in Paris, Vienna and Berlin. Upon returning to the United States he served one year as assistant to the chief surgeon in the French Hospital at San Francisco. In 1902 he began general practice in Saint Paul with offices in the Grand Opera House Building, in 1919 moving to the Hamm Building.

In 1907, Dr. Roy married Ada Cheverton of Rich Hill, Missouri. He is survived by his widow, a daughter Germaine, and a son, Dr. Philemon C. Roy, who has been associated with him the past two years.

Dr. Roy was a member of the Elks, the Maccabees, L'Union Francois, the Woodmen of the World and a life member of the Saint Paul Athletic Club. He was a member of the medical staffs of Bethseda, St. Joseph's and St. John's Hospitals. He was a member of the Ramsey County Medical Society, of which he was vice president in 1937, and of the Minnesota State and American Medical Associations.

Gonorrhea and Sulfanilamide

In view of the widespread interest in sulfanilamide and related compounds in the treatment of gonorrhea, the work of Johnson and Pepper (Weekly Roster and M. Digest, 33:465, (Dec. 11) 1937) on this subject is of interest. Twenty-four patients were given a benzyl sulfanilamide (*p*-benzylamino-benzene-sulfonamide), a drug as yet not on the market in this country, and seventy-five were given sulfanilamide (thirteen were given courses of both drugs). Of the twenty-four patients given this benzyl sulfanilamide, fourteen were treated for ten consecutive days with a minimum ten-day dosage of 600 grains. Only two of the entire group seemed to be improved. Of the seventy-five patients given oral daily divided doses of sulfanilamide, sixty-four were seen sufficiently long to analyze the results. Of this group more than half represented failures, based on an arbitrary ten-day standard. Fifty-five per cent of the sulfanilamide group and 50 per cent of the benzyl sulfanilamide group showed toxic symptoms. As a result of the somewhat disappointing observations the authors feel this type of therapy should not be employed in the routine treatment of outpatient gonorrhea. This work represents an additional argument for the careful administration of this group of drugs, since they appear to be of considerable value in some cases of the disease. (Jour. A.M.A., Jan. 1, 1938, p. 51.)

Crystalline Vitamin A.

The actual isolation of vitamin A in crystalline form appeared desirable chiefly for definite confirmation of the mass of circumstantial evidence pointing to its actual chemical configuration. This isolation has now been attained as a result of a series of noteworthy investigations by Holmes and Corbert at Oberlin College. By the use of purified solvents, low temperatures and special technical precautions, it has been possible to isolate the vitamin in crystalline form from the liver oils of three different species of fish. Biologic assay indicates that the crystalline preparation has a value of approximately 3,000,000 international units per grain. The molecular weight determinations and elementary analyses of the compound correspond to a formula already suggested for the vitamin. Thus, a dietary essential which has been known for a quarter of a century has finally been obtained in a crystalline, probably pure, form. (Jour. A.M.A., Dec. 11, 1937, p. 1992.)

◆ REPORTS and ANNOUNCEMENTS ◆

AMERICAN BOARD OF OBSTETRICS AND GYNECOLOGY

The general oral, clinical and pathological examinations for all candidates (Groups A and B) will be conducted by the entire Board, meeting in San Francisco, California, on June 13 and 14, 1938, immediately prior to the meeting of the American Medical Association.

Application for admission to the June 1938 Group A examinations must be on an official form and filed in the Secretary's Office before April 1, 1938.

The annual informal Dinner and General Meeting of the Board will be held at the Palace Hotel, San Francisco, on Wednesday evening, June 15, 1938, at seven o'clock. Dr. William D. Cutter, Secretary of the Council on Medical Education and Hospitals of the American Medical Association, will be the guest speaker, and the Diplomates certified at the preceding days' examinations will be introduced individually. All Diplomates are invited to attend the dinner meeting, and to bring as guests their wives and any persons interested in the work of the Board.

For further information and application blanks address Dr. Paul Titus, Secretary, 1015 Highland Building, Pittsburgh (6), Pennsylvania.

AMERICAN COLLEGE OF SURGEONS MID-WEST SECTIONAL MEETING

The Mid-West Sectional Meeting of the American College of Surgeons, including the states of Wisconsin, Minnesota, Iowa, Illinois, and Upper Michigan, will be held in Milwaukee, Wisconsin, on March 29, 30, and 31. The headquarters will be at the Schroeder Hotel. A most active Committee on Local Arrangements, headed by Dr. Carl W. Eberbach, is making excellent plans for this meeting. There will be an exceptionally interesting program consisting of clinics, scientific sessions, hospital conferences, medical motion pictures, and other features during the meeting. A visiting group of ten or twelve outstanding surgeons will be present to participate in this program.

The three-day session will be devoted to clinics, conferences and the inspection of scientific exhibits.

This meeting will be of interest not only to Fellows of the College but to the medical profession at large, as well as to hospital trustees, superintendents, nurses, and hospital personnel. Members of State Medical Associations are most cordially invited to attend. There will be no registration fee.

ASSOCIATION OF MILITARY SURGEONS

The Association of Military Surgeons of the United States will meet in Rochester for its annual convention October 13, 14 and 15, 1938. Dr. F. L. Smith of Rochester, a member of the Association, has been ap-

pointed by the Mayo Foundation to be chairman of local arrangements.

Headquarters of the Association are in the Army Medical Museum in Washington, D. C., with Major General H. L. Gilchrist, United States Army, retired, acting as national secretary.

It is expected that approximately 500 persons will attend the convention. Programs for the meetings usually include physicians from foreign countries and officials of the Army and Navy departments.

UPPER MISSISSIPPI SOCIETY

The following officers were elected at the annual meeting of the Upper Mississippi Medical Society, January 29, at Brainerd, Minnesota:

President..............Dr. H. L. Lamb, Little Falls
First Vice President........Dr. Z. E. Kerlan, Aitkin
Second Vice President........Dr. O. Ringle, Walker
Secretary................Dr. G. I. Badeaux, Brainerd

WASHINGTON COUNTY

At the regular meeting of the Washington County Medical Society, February 8, two county commissioners and S. E. Gilkey, M.D., Medical Advisor to the State Relief Administration, met with us to discuss the various problems of relief.

The county commissioners were asked to state their position, inasmuch as there had been some dissatisfaction, which they did briefly. The doctors presented their problems and difficulties. The commissioners asked for questions—which were not slow in coming. After the pros and cons were gone over, it was evident that some progress toward a better understanding was undoubtedly made. After the county commissioners left, Doctor Gilkey analyzed the situation from the State Relief Administration's point of view.

Viosterol and Psoriasis

Cedar and Zon (Pub. Health Rep., 52:1580, (Nov. 5) 1937) administered massive doses of viosterol without local treatment of the lesions, dietary adjustment or any other therapeutic measure. A series of fifteen patients from 30 to 50 years of age with chronic widespread psoriasis were given from 300,000 to 400,000 units of vitamin D as viosterol. Eleven of the fifteen subjects showed complete involution of the psoriasis within six to twelve weeks' time. At the end of the period of treatment, three patients showed incipient symptoms of excessive vitamin D dosage. All the subjects exhibited an elevation in the level of blood calcium. There was a recurrence in some of the patients, though the degree of severity was much less than originally observed. Although the proposed treatment would appear to be safe, the authors suggest not only that there may be a smaller effective dose of viosterol but also that certain accompanying products of the irradiation of the ergosterol may be the potent factor. (Jour. A.M.A., Jan. 8, 1938, p. 133.)

The regular monthly meeting of the Minnesota Academy of Medicine was held at the Town and Country Club on Wednesday evening, December 8, 1937. Dinner was served at 7 o'clock and the meeting was called to order at 8:10 by the president, Dr. E. M. Jones.

There were forty-nine members present.

Minutes of the November meeting were read and approved as read.

The following officers were elected for the year 1938:
President..................R. T. LaVake, Minneapolis
Vice President...............Carl B. Drake, St. Paul
Secretary-Treasurer........A. G. Schultze (reëlected)

The scientific program consisted of a symposium on Syphilis, and the following papers were presented:
1. Syphilis as a Social Problem....Dr. S. E. Sweitzer
2. Immunobiology of Syphilis....Dr. H. E. Michelson
3. Primary Syphilis ....Dr. John Butler
4. Visceral Syphilis.................Dr. H. L. Ulrich
5. Asymptomatic Neurosyphilis.....Dr. Paul O'Leary
6. Syphilis as Seen in the Human Clinic Thirty-five Years Ago ....Dr. Frank Wright

---

SYPHILIS AS A SOCIAL PROBLEM*

S. E. SWEITZER, M.D.
Minneapolis

It may seem superfluous to discuss syphilis as a social problem before a medical group, but recently Dr. Thomas Parran, Surgeon General of the United States Public Health Service, started a campaign against syphilis and the social diseases and has asked for coöperation from the various states. Here in Minnesota the President of the State Medical Society appointed a committee to coöperate in this work with the United States Public Health Service.

The difficulty of the control of a disease like syphilis can be shown by the success that we have in this country in eradicating smallpox. Van Etten[1] in a recent article mentions that we still have 40,000 cases of smallpox annually and this is a preventable disease. Vaccination and revaccination could eradicate it in a few years. We have no vaccine for syphilis and must endeavor to work on different lines. No one will deny that syphilis presents a tremendous problem and an endeavor will be made to examine this problem and to suggest how we can aid here in Minnesota.

With the publicity given the Surgeon General's attack on syphilis it has become popular to mention this disease in the newspapers and magazines and over the radio. For a time the public may become syphilis

minded but a warning must be given in regard to syphilis control, for when the fanfare of publicity ceases, any permanent and effective control of the disease must be accomplished by steady and continuous efforts of the medical profession.

From reading many of these news and magazine articles and from some of the statements made by men interested in the subject, one might assume that syphilis is on the increase. Let us see what has happened here in Minnesota in regard to the incidence of syphilis. .

The first concerted attack upon syphilis was as a war measure. Minnesota was up among the leaders at that time and after the War this anti-syphilis campaign never was dropped. In most states, due to lack of funds or other causes, the war on syphilis was allowed either to be dropped entirely or was greatly limited in scope. As a result of our efforts here there has been a steady decrease in the incidence of syphilis in Minnesota. Many of you have read articles recently in which the incidence of syphilis is given as high as 10 per cent of the population. This is not true in Minnesota.

The following table will show a steady decrease from a high in 1925. The year 1918, being the first year, of course did not show many cases reported.

TABLE I. VENEREAL DISEASE CASE REPORTS—
State Department of Health, Division of Preventable Diseases Minnesota—1918-1936

Year	Syphilis
1918	1801
1919	3551
1920	4422
1921	4814
1922	4291
1923	4779
1924	4809
1925	5147
1926	4871
1927	4938
1928	4438
1929	3983
1930	4104
1931	4199
1932	4033
1933	3824
1934	4071
1935	4224
1936	3379

The latest comparison is shown in Table II, where there is a slight increase this year in reported cases. This is more than likely due to the recently inaugurated campaign against syphilis with its attendant publicity. As a result, while in the first half of 1936 there were 39,713 Wassermanns sent in, in the same period of 1937 there were 50,570 sent in. No wonder a few more cases were discovered and most of these were from Minneapolis.

Dr. H. G. Irvine, in a personal communication, stated that in 1936 out of over 83,000 Wassermanns only about 6 per cent were positive. Diehl[1] over a two-year

---

*From the Department of Dermatology and Syphilology, Minneapolis General Hospital, Dr. S. E. Sweitzer, Chief.

period of observation of 5,000 students at the University of Minnesota was able to find only ten cases of syphilis.

TABLE II. VENEREAL DISEASE—CASE REPORTS

First Two Quarters 1936

	Syphilis		
State	Minneapolis	Duluth	Total
1089	466	161	1716

First Two Quarters 1937

State	Minneapolis	Duluth	Total
1103	513	138	1754

In our neighboring state of Wisconsin, Lorenz[2] recently stated that the incidence of syphilis in the general sick does not exceed 3 per cent and that the admission rate of late syphilis to State Hospitals has been reduced over 60 per cent in the last ten years.

Syphilis for many years has been decreasing. It is becoming increasingly difficult to obtain sufficient active cases for teaching purposes in many of our Universities. Syphilis also has decreased tremendously in private practice and especially so among men who specialized in the disease.

Table III, below, will show the decrease at the Minneapolis General Hospital where we treat more cases than are treated in any clinic in the state.

TABLE III.

	Primary	Secondary	Tertiary	Pre-natal	Total
*1937	10	19	174	13	216
1936	15	32	217	11	275
1935	27	66	297	7	397
1934	31	78	268	26	303
1933	29	113	269	33	444

*Over a ten months period.

With these figures from our own state and from Wisconsin it seems that we are making a successful attack upon syphilis and have been doing so for many years. This success by no means should cause us to lessen our efforts but should spur us on to a greater and more effective attack upon the disease.

Suggestions for Further Efforts

1. The more widespread use of the Wassermann reaction as a routine in general medicine.
2. Early and routine Wassermanns upon all pregnant women. An early discovery of syphilis in a pregnancy can practically eliminate prenatal syphilis.
3. Greater facilities for dark field examinations.
4. Better social service work in looking up sources and contacts.
5. Special attention and close follow-up as to continuous treatment should be given to food handlers, pregnant women, prenatal syphilitics and prostitutes.
6. Continued education of the medical profession in regard to long and continuous treatment of syphilis.

References

1. Diehl, H. S.: Wassermann, reactions in college students. Am. Jour. Pub. Health, 21:1131, (Oct.) 1931.
2. Lorenz, W. F.: Syphilis in Wisconsin. Wis. Med. Jour., 36:188, (March) 1937.
3. Van Etten, N. B.: Medical service for all Americans. Minn. Med., 20:411, (July) 1937.

PRIMARY SYPHILIS

JOHN BUTLER, M.D.
Minneapolis

After inoculation of the broken skin or mucous membrane with the spirochete pallida, a syphilitic incubation period begins which lasts approximately seven weeks. During this incubation period there is a gradually increasing general spirochetal invasion of the tissues through the blood stream. One to two weeks later (eighth or ninth week of the disease) the reaction in the tissue caused by localized foci of spirochetes produces the eruptive manifestations of the disease.

During the first three weeks of the incubation period there is no evidence to the patient or the physician of the impending disease. Between the third and fourth weeks the primary lesion or chancre appears.

A week or ten days after the appearance of the chancre, the regional lymph glands enlarge and show the characteristic pea- to nut-sized round, hard, freely movable, painless, nodular swellings. During the ensuing three weeks the lymph glands in distant parts of the body become involved.

The systemic symptoms in primary syphilis are usually slight or absent and are of no diagnostic import. More frequently they are present and intensified in the secondary or eruptive stage of the disease. When present, they may show as anemia, fever, headache, insomnia, arthritic pains, etc.

Our conception of the course of early syphilis has been changed as a result of the discovery that the lymph and blood of animals and humans infected with syphilis may contain the spirochetes a few hours after infection and may be found in the blood stream for an indefinite time—months or years—in latent Wassermann-negative cases. This brings to the fore the potential danger of transfusion syphilis from latent syphilitic donors.

A clinical diagnosis of the incipient primary lesion is generally impossible and uncertain and the fully-developed chancre, to the unpracticed eye, is often undiagnosed.

The chancre, like other manifestations of syphilis, varies in appearance according to the location, the structure and reaction of the tissue in which it is situated. It may assume different appearances as to shape and size, surface secretions, and multiplicity. It may, or may not, be indurated. We read in many current textbooks on syphilis that the primary lesion presents a fairly definite appearance, the induration of the sore receiving special consideration in formulating a positive diagnosis. As a matter of fact, there are clinical varieties of the chancre that show no appreciable induration on the most careful examination.

Prior to the discovery of the spirocheta in the initial lesion of primary syphilis, the clinician's attitude was that of watchful waiting and observation.

An early diagnosis of primary syphilis depends on finding the spirocheta pallida in the early chancre before the organisms have been disseminated and localized in large numbers in the denser tissues throughout the body, before profound pathological changes have taken place. The Wassermann test is of no diagnostic value during the first five weeks of the disease, as it is usually negative then.

If the chancre has been treated locally with antiseptics, especially mercurials, it is a waste of time to attempt to recover the spirocheta pallida from the lesion. By stopping the local treatment, they may or may not be demonstrated after a week or ten days. In such cases, aspiration of the adjacent lymph nodes may be successful. The dark field method should be used instead of the India ink or staining method.

The possibility of aborting or curing a large percentage of primary syphilis by early diagnosis (before the sixth week of the disease) when the Wassermann is usually negative, should not be overlooked; and immediate intensive treatment should be a matter of persuasive interest to the physician of today. Every day lost in diagnosis and treatment is of vital importance to the patient. The patient receiving early treatment, when the primary lesion is not more than a week or ten days old and with a negative Wassermann, has a 25 per cent better chance for a cure than a patient with secondary syphilis.

VISCERAL SYPHILIS

HENRY L. ULRICH, M.D.
Minneapolis

I am detailed to speak on visceral syphilis. With the limited time at my disposal, I would like to confine myself to one type of visceral syphilis—namely aortitis and its sequences. Syphilis of the stomach is rather rare and more or less problematic. Syphilis of the liver is likewise not so common and perhaps not so problematic. There is no organ in the body exempt from syphilitic invasion except the ovary. Wartin claims he has never seen the ovary involved.

It is thirty-two years since the Treponema palida was discovered. It is thirty years since salvarsan was first used. The curative effect of standard syphilitic therapy is as high if not higher than any other treatment for any other disease, surgical or medical. Why is it there is so much visceral syphilis in our population today? Let me just hint at several factors which may be involved in the explanation of this paradox. There is the psychology of our people who still cling to the attitude that syphilis is a disgrace rather than misfortune. This is a cause for a lag in getting early treatment. The high cost of therapy and the time element hinder the result. That leads me to the statement that the treatment of 60 per cent of all venereal disease is in the hands of 5 per cent of the physicians. In other words, the treatment has become highly specialized. Students of this phase of the problem are beginning to think that this is a mistake. The treatment of syphilis should be in the hands of the family physician and general practitioner. I am aware the last

statement has its controversial point. I have stated it merely to show the trend of things in the larger problem.

Potentially speaking, every syphilitic may develop aortitis. It usually manifests itself in the most efficient years. It is the commonest lesion found at the post mortem table. It is the most deadly visceral lesion. It is one of the most avoidable complications if proper treatment is instituted and carried out in the primary stage. In its uncomplicated state, it is extremely difficult to diagnose. It is this last feature I wish to elaborate and emphasize.

In 1885 Dohle definitely established the difference between syphilis and atherosclerosis of the aorta. It took some eighteen years before it was definitely accepted by his German colleagues. It is only in recent years that some semblance of order is establishing itself regarding aortitis as a clinical problem. Langer in Germany reports 23,105 necropsies on syphilitics of which 70 to 80 per cent showed evidence of involvement of the aorta.

The clinical grouping is seen in Table I. The standard of diagnosis usually given is that by Carter and Baker (Table II). A year later Moore, Danglade and Reisinger modified this as shown in Table III.

TABLE I. CLINICAL CLASSIFICATION

1. Uncomplicated Aortitis. Latent 4.9 to 49.5 per cent in all types of aortitis (living).
2. Aneurysm. Latent syphilis 1.2 per cent, active 11.8 per cent, postmortem 27.7 per cent.
3. Aortic Valvulitis. Living 2.7 per cent to 4.1 per cent, postmortem 24.7 per cent to 36.5 per cent.
4. Coronary osteal involvement. Postmortem 19.9 per cent to 33.3 per cent.
5. Combinations of 1 with either 2 or 3 or 4.
6. Aortitis or its complications associated with lesions of the heart unrelated to syphilis, i.e., hypertension (essential or renal), coronary disease (atherosclerosis), valvulitis due to rheumatism; subacute bacterial endocarditis (rare); pericarditis (rare).

The standard for the diagnosis of aortitis in general is usually that given by Carter and Baker.[1]

TABLE II. STANDARD FOR DIAGNOSIS OF AORTITIS
(Carter and Baker)

1. The history of a relative abrupt and unexpected onset of circulatory embarrassment.
2. The presence of a positive Wassermann reaction.
3. A demonstrable increase in the retromanubrial dullness in the second interspace and a change in the tonal qualities of the second aortic sound. The fluoroscopic evidence of aortic dilatation.
4. An absence of the signs of mitral disease connating rheumatic infection.
5. The history of paroxysmal dyspnea, often nocturnal.
6. The history of pain, particularly paroxysmal pain.
7. Progress in cardiac failure.
   If any five of these seven criteria are present, a diagnosis of cardiovascular syphilis can be made.

Moore, Danglade and Reisinger[2] give as criteria for an uncomplicated aortitis diagnosis any three of the following seven criteria.

TABLE III. STANDARD FOR DIAGNOSIS OF AORTITIS
(Moore, Danglade and Reisinger)

1. Teleroentgenographic and fluoroscopic evidence of aortic dilatation.
2. Increased manubrial dullness.
3. A history of circulatory embarrassment.
4. A tympanitic, bell like, tambour, accentuation of the second aortic sound.
5. Progressive cardiac failure.
6. Substernal pain.
7. Paroxysmal dyspnea.

TABLE IV. A COMPARISON OF THE CORRECTNESS OF THE CLINICAL AND PATHOLOGICAL DIAGNOSIS OF SYPHILITIC AORTITIS IN ONE HUNDRED AND FIVE CASES SO DIAGNOSED AT NECROPSY[2]

| | Total Cases | Syphilitic Aortitis | | Diagnosis could have been suspected on basis of physical findings | | | Diagnosis obscured by other cardio-vascular lesions | Heart and aorta thought clinically normal | Patient too ill for adequate examination |
		Definitely diagnosed	Suspected	Signs	Symptoms	Both			
Medical Service	63	4	12	12	2	9	9	11	4
Surgical Service	42	0	1	5	4	3	3	23	3
	105	4	13	17	6	12	12	34	7
Percentage of of Total	16.2				33.3		11.4	32.3	

TABLE V. THE CORRECTNESS OF THE CLINICAL DIAGNOSIS OF SYPHILITIC AORTITIS AS INFLUENCED BY THE CAUSE OF THE FATAL ILLNESS[2]

	Total Cases	Diagnosis correctly made or suspected	Diagnosis might have been made	Diagnosis obscured by other cardiac findings	Diagnosis missed (Impossible to make. ?)
Fatal illness related to syphilis	24	6 (25%)	7 (29%)	5 (20%)	6 (24%)
Fatal illnesses unrelated to syphilis which if diagnosed was an incidental finding	81	10 (12%)	29 (35%)	7 (8%)	35 (43%)

Moore et al[2] made a study of 105 cases of aortitis uncomplicated by aortic regurgitation or aneurysm. They worked backward from the postmortem material to the clinical findings (Table IV). From a study of this chart only four of the 105 were definitely diagnosed and thirteen were suspected, making a total of 16.2 per cent. There were twenty-three cases where the diagnosis could have been suspected on the bases of physical signs, and incidence of 33 per cent. There were 12 cases where the diagnosis was obscured by other cardiovascular lesions—11.4 per cent. There were thirty-four in which the heart was considered normal clinically—32 per cent, and there were seven cases in which the patient was too ill for adequate examination.

In the cases which were correctly diagnosed or suspected, either the classical signs of widened manubrial dullness, pulsation in the suprasternal notch, an aortic systolic murmur or an altered tympanitic, bell-like quality of the second sound, or the symptoms of substernal pain, dyspnea on exertion or paroxysmal nocturnal dyspnea, or both signs and symptoms were present. In the thirty-five cases which could have been diagnosed, these symptoms and signs were present in some degree.

The significance of these findings were entirely disregarded by the clinicians. The majority of these patients were admitted for an acute illness unrelated to syphilis. Judging, however, from the extent of the

lesions at autopsy, they suggest that the clinical diagnosis was not necessarily impossible.

Table V gives the correctness of the clinical diagnosis of syphilitic aortitis as influenced by the cause of the fatal illness.

Curiously enough hypertension which can confuse the picture did not make the diagnosis more difficult. In fact, more cases of aortitis with hypertension were correctly diagnosed than without hypertension.

The most recent study of uncomplicated aortitis is that by Wilson.[3] He too worked backward from the postmortem table to the clinical findings. His material consisted of 106 cases. Extensive pathological changes were found in twelve, moderate in twenty-seven and only slight in twenty-one cases. Three cases showed marked dilation; there was moderate dilation in seven, slight in ten and there was a normal sized aorta in forty cases. He agrees the physical signs adopted in the above criteria are without a doubt dependent on aortic dilation. The symptoms, however, "are by no means indisputable and the validity of ascribing certain of these symptoms to purely uncomplicated aortitis has been seriously questioned."

He quotes Keefer and Resnik who in twenty-four cases of uncomplicated aortitis never found dyspnea on exertion, nor paroxysmal dyspnea, nor signs of myocardial insufficiency. In every case where such symptoms supervened, there was some additional factor, aortic insufficiency, aneurysm, myocarditis, hyper-

TABLE VI. INCIDENCE OF SYMPTOMS IN SYPHILITIC AORTITIS[3]

	Total* Cases	Dyspnea on exertion	Paroxysmal dyspnea	Precordial pain	Con; h fa
With aortic insufficiency	49	49	14	10	
With thoracic aneurysm	31	24	5	7	
With narrowing of coronary ostia	21	20	5	8	
Uncomplicated syphilitic aortitis	106	44	4	5	
Inadequate history	17				

*Th,rteen patients had more than one of the complications of syphilitic aortitis, i.e., aortic insufficiency, aneurysm, o: involvement.

TABLE VII. ANALYSIS OF SYMPTOMS IN CONDITIONS ASSOCIATED WITH UNCOMPLICATED SYI AORTITIS[3]

	Total Cases	Dyspnea on exertion	Paroxysmal dyspnea	Precordial pain	Co: heart
Hypertensive heart disease	29	29	2	4	
Chronic nephritis	7	5	1	0	
Coronary heart disease	5	5	1	1	
Chronic myocardial degeneration	2	1	0	0	
Tuberculous pericarditis	1	1	0	0	
Obstructive lesions	2	2	0	0	
Without other cardiovascular disease*	60	1	0	0	
Totals	106	44	4	5	

*The one patient showing dyspnea had leukemia.

tension or organic obstructive lesions. He cites Maynard, Curran and Rosen who conclude myocardial failure only ensues after some complication develops. Adequate explanation of the story of circulatory embarrassment, progressive heart failure, substernal pain, and paroxysmal dyspnea, long considered as typical of pure aortitis, has not been given. In other words, when symptoms of circulatory embarrassment occurs, the case has gone beyond the stage of simple aortic involvement, or there are complications unrelated to syphilitic aortitis which explain the symptoms. He cites sixty cases of the 106 in which an analysis of the symptoms were possible. In only one was there a record of dyspnea, and that patient had leukemia (Tables VI and VII).

Wilson's analyses which reveals that uncomplicated aortitis is an asymptomatic disease is quite correct, which leaves for our diagnosis of this condition only the physical signs. These signs must depend entirely on weakness dilatation of the aorta. If this is present, increased manubrial dullness in the second interspace, a systolic bruit at the base, or a second sound having bell-like qualities should put us on our guard. These with a history of syphilis, or a scar on the penis, or a positive Wassermann reaction makes the diagnosis fairly reliable. With the growth of x-ray technic, our finger-tips, our eyes and ears are losing their sense of accuracy. Few men will accept a diagnosis of a chest condition on the data which inspection, palpation, percussion and auscultation afford. Without the x-ray check, as it is called, our physical signs are not complete. The x-ray criterion for aortitis uncomplicated by aneurysm is usually considered either an increased

density of the aorta or an increase in the the aortic arch. In a six-foot plate of the the anterior-posterior direction two measuren computed in estimating the diameter of the a first is the distance from the widest part of th ing aorta to the midsternal line. The secor distance from the farthest lateral point on to the midsternal line. The sum of these t arbitrary diameter of the aortic arch. There i computation. The width of the aorta is me the right oblique. The inability to visualize quently makes its value less than the arbitrary of the arch. Between the ages of seventeen nine in the male, this figure gradually incre 4.6 to 6.1 cm.; in the female from 4.3 to 5.6 variation above these figures of 0.5 cm. can l ered abnormal within 80 per cent of accura conditions, as a rule, may produce a chan silhouette of the arch either by dilation o placement of the aorta. They are syphiliti aortic insufficiency, hypertension and arteri With such an array of causes the x-ray is qu in its usefulness. It can tell us there is a the aorta. To sift out these components, resort to the history, physical findings and data. In uncomplicated aortitis this is an difficult task. Since it is the stage in which of aneurysm or valvulitis or both is poss most important that it be recognized. Stati that very few cases treated at this period g symptomatic phases of aortitis. Furthermor show that uncomplicated aortitis rarely is persons given the proper antisyphilitic treat

chancre stage. Better still would be the eradication of the scourge of syphilis itself. This is a public health problem. What has been done in the Scandinavian countries can be done in our own.

References

1. Carter and Baker: Certain aspects of cardiac disease, Johns Hopkins Bulletin, 48:315, 1931.
2. Moore, J. E., Danglade, J. H., Reisinger, J. E.: Arch. Int. Med., 49:753, 1932.
3. Wilson, Robert, Jr.: Am. Jour. Med. Sci., 194:180.

ASYMPTOMATIC NEUROSYPHILIS*

PAUL A. O'LEARY, M.D.

Rochester, Minnesota

Asymptomatic neurosyphilis is the most significant manifestation of syphilis of the central nervous system. This somewhat inclusive statement is based on the following facts: (1) asymptomatic neurosyphilis becomes clinical neurosyphilis if not sufficiently treated; (2) in the great majority of cases of asymptomatic neurosyphilis, the response to treatment is exceedingly good if treatment is adequately and intensively given; (3) by the early recognition and thorough treatment of asymptomatic neurosyphilis the development of the late forms of neurosyphilis, such as tabes dorsalis, paresis, and so forth, may be avoided, a fact which emphasizes the preventive value of adequate treatment of this complication of the disease. Accordingly, it is my purpose in this paper to discuss the incidence, the prognosis and the results of various types of treatment of asymptomatic neurosyphilis.

As the name implies, asymptomatic neurosyphilis is recognized by the finding of a positive spinal fluid test in a case in which neither clinical signs nor symptoms of neurosyphilis are present. The complication is a manifestation of syphilis in any of its various phases; and for reasons to be discussed shortly, it is divided into two groups, early and late. Early asymptomatic neurosyphilis is seen among those patients whose syphilis is of four years' duration or less, while among patients who have late asymptomatic neurosyphilis are those whose disease has been present for four years or more. As has been said, asymptomatic neurosyphilis is recognized by the obtaining of positive tests of the spinal fluid. In testing the fluid it is essential to do not only the Wassermann or flocculation procedure, but also to count the lymphocytes and other cells which may be present, to do a colloidal benzoin or colloidal gold test, and to estimate the globulin and protein content. The analysis of these five factors of the fluid permits classification of the type of invasion or involvement existing in the nervous system at the time the examination is made. Such classification is essential to an intelligent program of treatment. For example, if a patient has acute syphilis, the finding of 30 lymphocytes (normal 1 to 6) per cubic millimeter of spinal fluid with negative flocculation, globulin and colloidal tests indicates that invasion of the central nervous system has taken place. In such a

case, if the Wassermann or flocculation test on the blood does not revert to negative and remain so after treatment is completed, or if it continues to remain positive during treatment, presumptive evidence is at hand that the treatment has not controlled the complication and that what was merely an invasion has now become, or is in the process of becoming, an involvement of the central nervous system. Another significant reason why all the tests of the spinal fluid are essential is that patients are encountered who have acute syphilis, and examination of their spinal fluids discloses the following: strongly positive Wassermann tests, positive globulin tests, 60 to 80 mg. or more of protein per 100 c.c., a cell count of 50 or more lymphocytes per cubic millimeter, and a Zone I or paretic type of colloidal test.* A spinal fluid which gives these findings is interpreted as a paretic type of fluid, and its presence indicates that the treatment must be carried not only beyond that given to the average patient, but also that the spinal fluid must be examined frequently during the course of treatment and several times after the fluid has become negative. This last is urged as a precaution against neurorelapse because this type of fluid is especially prone to relapse to positive.

In the late type of asymptomatic neurosyphilis, appraisal of all the factors referable to the spinal fluid is also essential for adequate management of the case, not only because examinations of the spinal fluid permit a classification which prognosticates the eventual outcome of the case, but particularly because it enables the physician, by repeated testing of the fluid, to estimate intelligently the effect of treatment on the course of the disease. As will be shown subsequently, a patient who has late asymptomatic neurosyphilis, with a spinal fluid of paretic formula, which does not lose its paretic characteristics under two or more intensive courses of treatment with arsphenamine and bismuth or mercury, should be considered a candidate for more radical therapeutic measures, such as intraspinal or fever therapy. If all of the named diagnostic tests are not done on the first examination of the spinal fluid, subsequent efforts to estimate changes in the fluid, either favorable or otherwise, will be impossible. Attention is also called to the fact that in tests of spinal fluid the cell count is the first indicator of a return to normal, and that the colloidal test is the second in order of frequency to revert to the normal side; the globulin and protein tests follow, and the Wassermann test, as a rule, is the last to become negative. Accordingly, it is recommended, in fact it is urged, that all these tests be considered each time the spinal fluid is examined, and that repeated examinations of the spinal fluid of patients with asymptomatic neurosyphilis be made during the treatment if

*In a normal spinal fluid the colloidal gold or benzoin test is reported as follows: 0 0 0 0 0 0 0 0 0 for the gold, or 000 000 110 000 000 for the benzoin. With a paretic patient the curve for gold will be reported as 5 5 5 5 5 4 2 1 0 0, whereas that for benzoin will be reported as 333 333 333 321 000. The syphilitic or tabetic curve, which is considered a favorable type of report for the neurosyphilitic patient, is recorded 0 1 2 3 3 2 1 0 0 0 for the gold, and 000 000 333 000 000 for the benzoin.

*From the Section on Dermatology and Syphilology, The Mayo Clinic, Rochester, Minn.

the result is to be appraised adequately. Examination of the spinal fluid should also be made at least twice yearly after the fluid has become negative. Apropos of this last statement it is acknowledged that the flocculation tests, such as the Kahn, Kline, and Hinton, are so much more valuable than the older Wassermann technics that repeated examinations of a spinal fluid which has become negative are not essential if flocculation tests of the blood are repeatedly negative.

I have already commented on the fact that asymptomatic neurosyphilis is a manifestation of acute syphilis. In the coöperative clinical studies,[1] evidence has been accumulated which shows that among 30 per cent of patients who have primary syphilis the central nervous system has already become invaded. A study of the later manifestations of the disease revealed that in secondary syphilis 35 per cent, and in 56 per cent of the patients with recurrent secondary syphilis manifestations of neurosyphilis in one or the other of its many forms were noted. This incidence in a group of patients who were not treated is highly significant, as it demonstrates that a half to a third of those who acquire syphilis are potentially neurosyphilitics. Moore[2] carried this type of study further in that he appraised the incidence of asymptomatic neurosyphilis according to the yearly duration of the disease and found that the lowest incidence occurred in cases in which the disease was of four years' duration. From the fourth year on, the incidence of the disease remains the same, about 10 per cent, while the incidence of the clinical forms of neurosyphilis steadily increases after the fourth year. This effort to control the disease by development of the defensive mechanism during the first four years of infection is to be noted in other manifestations of syphilis, and it is the reason for classifying asymptomatic neurosyphilis as the early type, which includes cases in which patients are in the first four years of the disease, and the late type, or those who have had the infection more than four years.

A discussion such as this would be incomplete without calling attention to the influence of treatment of acute syphilis on the incidence of asymptomatic neurosyphilis, as it particularly emphasizes the value of certain methods of treating the disease in its early manifestations. Among patients who received more than twenty-four injections of mercury or bismuth given by the so-called continuous system, I found asymptomatic neurosyphilis in 7.5 per cent. Among those whose treatment was inadequate, consisting of less than twenty-four injections of arsphenamine and a metal, 22 per cent had a positive spinal fluid test. If the treatment was given at irregular intervals, and with no thought to system or persistence, the incidence increased practically to 30 per cent. These data are significant in that they illustrate the fact that a sufficient amount of treatment during the acute phase of syphilis, if given intensively and by the continuous system, will cut the incidence of asymptomatic involvement of the central nervous system in late syphilis in half.

The prognosis of asymptomatic neurosyphilis is, on the whole, quite satisfactory if treatment is adequate and sufficiently intensive. My observations indicate that if both the specific and the nonspecific therapeutic measures are employed, satisfactory serologic reversal may be obtained in more than 65 per cent of these cases, and that in less than 3 per cent of the cases in which asymptomatic neurosyphilis was treated adequately by all the therapeutic measures at our command today, did clinical manifestations of neurosyphilis develop. These figures illustrate the value of adequate treatment in the prevention of serious sequelæ in the nervous system, and in the discussion on treatment attention will be called to the different methods or systems of treatment which have been proved of value.

The earlier in the course of the disease, invasion of the central nervous system is noted, the more satisfactory are the results of treatment. In the early type, of syphilis, of less than four years' duration, most of the cases in which examination of the spinal fluid reveals a mild form of the disease will give evidence of a complete serologic reversal following three courses of arsphenamine and mercury. I have shown that it is the normal tendency for the fluid to revert to negative by the fourth year of the disease, so that treatment should be directed to the encouragement of this phenomenon. In those cases in which the findings on examination of the spinal fluid are of the paretic type, the incidence of favorable response is lower in both the early and late types of asymptomatic neurosyphilis, and it is in these cases that the application of the more intensive systems of treatment is warranted. In a case in which the findings on examinations of the spinal fluid are of the paretic type, and the patient has failed to give evidence of improvement following the first course of arsphenamine and bismuth or mercury, the use of intraspinal therapy of the Swift-Ellis type will double the number of cases of successful serologic reversals.

My experience with the Swift-Ellis technic has impressed me repeatedly with its outstanding value for this type of neurosyphilis, and it is to be regretted that so valuable a measure is not used more liberally in the treatment of asymptomatic neurosyphilis. One of the reasons that the method is not used more universally is perhaps attributable to its inefficiency in the treatment of tabes dorsalis and general paresis, as the accumulated evidence indicates that its value in these manifestations of syphilis is best in the early cases. In the advanced forms of tabes dorsalis or general paresis, the results of treatment of this type are unfavorable.

Patients who have received three or four regular courses of arsphenamine and bismuth or mercury, augmented by several combined intraspinal courses, and whose spinal fluid has not been materially influenced, are those among whom parenchymatous neurosyphilis is prone to develop. Before continuing further with a discussion of methods of treating such patients, I will digress for a brief but fundamental discussion of neurosyphilis. There are three possible explanations

212

of the development of neurosyphilis: (1) Spirocheta pallida may be of the neurotropic strain; (2) treatment received during the acute phase of the disease may have been insufficient, irregularly given, or even inefficient in its effect, and (3) the "soil" may be predisposed to the development of neurosyphilis, a conception which includes the elusive factors of resistance or immunity. An analysis of these three explanations indicates that although a neurotropic strain of the organism is demonstrable in the laboratory animal, evidence is still lacking that a specific strain with particular affinity for the nervous system attacks man. That inadequate treatment predisposes to neurosyphilis has been demonstrated in this statistical study. An explanation has not been advanced, however, as to why neurosyphilis eventually develops in certain cases even though the patients were treated thoroughly during the early stages of syphilis. It is possible that the treatment, although adequate as to amount and intensity, was inefficient. The third conception involves the factor of lack of resistance, and it seems the most plausible explanation for the failures in treatment. This is evidenced by the frequency with which neurosyphilis develops in the early case in which treatment was adequate. An experience with nonspecific therapy, especially malaria therapy, during the past ten years has repeatedly emphasized the superiority of fever therapy in the treatment of neurosyphilis when the so-called specific remedies have failed. Accordingly, when the patient with asymptomatic neurosyphilis has received arsphenamine and mercury or bismuth in adequate amounts and in an intensive manner, and when intraspinal therapy has been added and tests of the spinal fluid continue to remain positive and to indicate the malignant nature of the condition, it is advisable to adopt a different therapeutic program. When a fair trial with the specific agents fails to produce the desired serologic result in a given case, it is logical to adopt measures that are directed toward stimulation of the patient's resistance and to drop those which have been inadequate in the destruction of the invading organisms. This is the rationale for the use of malaria therapy in neurosyphilitics who have failed to secure serologic reversal.

In several other reports I have called attention to the value of malaria therapy in the prevention of general paresis. When the use of specific remedies fails to influence satisfactorily the course of the disease, application of intensive nonspecific measures will completely reverse the course of the disease in many of the cases. The mechanics by which this is accomplished is still not understood and the method continues to be used empirically. Treatment with typhoid vaccine produces a lower incidence of serologic reversals than malaria therapy, and my experience with electric units that produce fever is still too limited to permit me to pass judgment on their value. Tryparsamide has been proved to be inefficient in the control of asymptomatic neurosyphilis, as the highest incidences of progression to clinical neurosyphilis were noted following its use and the use of silver arsphenamine.

Summary and Conclusions

Asymptomatic neurosyphilis is to be anticipated in approximately a fifth of all cases of syphilis, and it must be eliminated by examination of the spinal fluid in all cases of acute syphilis in which the Wassermann or flocculation tests on the blood remain positive; likewise, if serologic tests on the blood remain positive when treatment is stopped, invasion of the nervous system should be suspected. Eighteen per cent of patients with latent syphilis who are "Wassermann fast" will be found to have asymptomatic neurosyphilis. The results of treatment in cases of early asymptomatic neurosyphilis are decidedly better than those cases in which the disease is of four years' duration or more. Accordingly, the spinal fluid should be examined early in order that the complication may be handled intelligently. The fact that the patient develops the maximal amount of resistance against invasion of the central nervous system during the first four years should also be kept in mind in treating syphilis of longer duration. Routine measures are successful in the majority of cases, but when they fail the addition of intraspinal therapy may satisfactorily reverse the serologic reaction. The fact that five or more courses of arsphenamine and bismuth or mercury, and intraspinal therapy in addition, fail to produce serologic reversal is indicative not only of a malignant type of involvement of the central nervous system, but also suggests that an adequate defensive mechanism is lacking against such involvement. The use of malaria therapy in such cases apparently supplies the necessary stimulus to the mechanism by which immunity is obtained. Fever therapy is therefore of value in the treatment of parenchymatous neurosyphilis, and in the treatment of asymptomatic neurosyphilis in cases in which satisfactory serologic reversals have not been produced following the use of arsphenamine, bismuth and mercury.

References

1. Clark, Taliaferro, Parran, Thomas, Cole, Harold, Moore, J. E., O'Leary, P. A., Stokes, J. H., and Wile, U. J.: Coöperative clinical studies in the treatment of syphilis. From Venereal Disease Information, Reprint No. 41, vol. 13, Nos. 4, 5, 6, 7, (April, May, June, and July) 1932.
2. Moore, J. E.: The modern treatment of syphilis. Baltimore: Thomas. p. 535, 1933.
3. O'Leary, P. A.: Treatment by malaria in asymptomatic neurosyphilis. Jour. Am. Med. Assn., 97:1585-1586, (Nov. 28) 1931.
4. O'Leary, P. A.: Malaria therapy in asymptomatic neurosyphilis. Ann. Int. Med., 7:1513-1522, (June) 1934.

SYPHILIS AS SEEN IN THE NEUMANN CLINIC THIRTY-FIVE YEARS AGO

F. R. WRIGHT, M.D.

Minneapolis

What I have to say tonight is a memory sketch of thirty-five years ago. Incidentally I might say that of the 1,500 men who are practicing medicine in Minneapolis and Saint Paul I do not believe that there are fifty who know syphilis clinically when they see it; their diagnosis depends entirely on whether or not a patient has a positive Wassermann.

I arrived in Vienna in January of 1900. At that time there were two rival clinics, Kaposi Clinic known as Dermatology and Syphilis, and the Neumann Clinic known as Syphilis and Dermatology. The rivalry between these two goes back quite a little farther. In the early days Hebra, who is known as the father of Dermatology, had two assistants, Cohn and Neumann, both Jewish. He also had a charming daughter. Cohn and Neumann both wanted to marry the girl but Hebra, who was a German, said that he would not have a Jew in his family. A few weeks later Hebra had a heart-to-heart talk with Cohn, who went down to Hungary to the village where he was born and paid one gulden to have his name changed to that of the village, then came back to Vienna and, as assistant, Kaposi married the girl. If any of you are so fortunate as to have a copy of the first edition of Kaposi's Haut Krankheiten you will find at the foot of the first page of the tenth or twelfth chapter a footnote which states "at this point J. Cohn changed his name to Kaposi."

The teaching in those days was purely clinical. The spirochæta and the Wassermann reaction had never been heard of. Teachers at that time believed that each different variety of syphilis was due to a different virus. Professor Neumann taught in 1900 that syphilis was due to a specific cause. He felt that there were three types of this virus: one which attacked the skin, one the bones, and the third the nervous system.

In those days syphilis was not considered as a constitutional disease, it was simply dermatology. We were taught that eruptions developed on the flexor surfaces of the body; that all lesions on the skin were round and painless; all ulcerative lesions were necrotic, not granulating; that the chancre instead of being covered by a granulating surface is covered by necrotic tissue. It is only when the chancre has begun to heal that it presents a granulating surface.

We were taught that syphilis had two incubation periods, one from the time of the infection to the appearance of the initial lesion, twenty-one days; the second period was from that time until the general eruption appears on the body. They traced the age of the infection by the clinical skin condition. If there was a sore on the penis, round with a sloping edge and a necrotic base, it was an initial lesion, infection twenty-one days old. If the base of the sore has become indurated, infection is twenty-eight days. By the thirty-fifth day lymphatic glands on one groin have become enlarged and by the forty-second day, glands of the opposite groin. If the glands in the posterior triangle of the neck and the epitrochlear glands were palpable the condition was forty-nine days old. The eruption came out on the body on the fifty-sixth day. We were taught that the normal course of syphilis, if left untreated, was a relapse every three months. For example, if a man was infected the first of April he would develop an eruption on his body approximately the first of June. This eruption would remain bright for a few weeks and then gradually fade, to disappear partially or completely until about the first of September, when a new eruption would appear. We were taught that the lesions of the new eruption

would be the same as those of the primary; that is, a macular eruption would follow a macular eruption and the papular follow a papular. The relapsing eruptions were different from the primary by the fact that they were larger and showed a more or less well-defined tendency to grouping. It was taught that certain eruptions were characteristc of certain ages of the disease, as, for instance, the loss of the hair on the side of the head never occurred before the first relapse, which would be at the fifth month, and was not a part of late syphilis; that the condylomata, or moist papules which develop at points of irritation, as between the buttocks, about the genitals, or under the pendulous breasts of women, never occurred before the ninth month. Every man was taught to know symptoms so that he could tell the age of a given case up to a year.

The teaching was entirely clinical. Professor Neumann lectured from nine to ten o'clock, Professor Kaposi from eleven to twelve o'clock. During the hour from ten to eleven their clinics for ambulatory patients were held. The daily visit in the Neumann wards was made at eight in the morning. I think that I am the only American who was ever invited by Professor Neumann to make the visits with him. I made this morning visit with him for fourteen months. At this visit all patients in the hospital were reviewed. The men came before the Professor wearing a mantle or linen duster, and a pair of slippers. This mantle was removed, the slippers kicked off. Every patient was examined stark naked although the only lesion on his body might be a spot on his face. If the patient was syphilitic he was required to show the palms and the soles.

In the female wards the girls wore a loose blouse short skirt and slippers. When they came up before the Professor the blouse was removed, they then dropped their slippers and were then put up on the table. The skirt was pulled up and the lower half of the body and genitals examined.

The treatment of syphilis at that time was entirely by mercury. The Kaposi Clinic used hypodermic solutions of salicylate, bichloride or succinamide of mercury. The Neumann Clinic used the inunctions of mercurial ointment exclusively. Both clinics agreed that it was a mistake to begin treatment in a case of syphilis before the constitutional symptoms had appeared that no matter how early it was begun it would not prevent, simply delay, the appearance of the eruption. They were also sure that the cases treated early, that is, before the eruption appeared, did not run a normal course. In the Kaposi Clinic the hypodermics were given intramuscularly in the gluteal region, the soluble salts given every day and the insoluble salicylate given once a week. In the Neumann Clinic the inunctions were carried out by the patients themselves. Six men were placed astride a narrow bench, each rubbed the mercurial ointment into the back of the man in front of him. Every day the man in the front of the row took his place at the foot so that in a week each man had six days' treatment and one day's rest.

214

a routine, the course of treatment inunction was kept up until all symptoms disappeared and then continued half again as long. The average course was about six weeks, and under no circumstances continued longer than eight weeks whether symptoms had disappeared or not. It had been clinically observed that at the end of eight weeks patients became satiated with mercury and the treatment was no longer effective. Following this routine course of treatment a patient got four courses of mercury the first year, the second year he was given three courses, in the third year one or two depending on the number of clinical relapses he had developed. After that no further treatment was given. If at the end of the fourth year the patient had been without clinical symptoms for a year he was considered cured and was allowed to marry.

Syphilis was known to them as a disease of the skin. They believed and taught that nerve syphilis, which they called parasyphilis, was not due to the syphilis virus but to the toxin which had been produced and had remained in the body.

At my last visit to Vienna in 1906 the spirochæta had been discovered and I saw in the laboratory of Professor Ehrmann the first spirochæta that was ever stained in nerve tissue. Some years later Noguchi stained the spirochæta in the spinal cord, proving that locomotor ataxia is due to a direct invasion of the cord by the parasite.

Discussion

DR. C. D. FREEMAN, St. Paul: Syphilis has been discussed this evening from A to Z. As you have probably noticed, there have been no recent advances in its treatment. The real messages as regards syphilis are all history and some of them have been very important. Whether any new discoveries are to be made remains to be seen.

Off-hand, I would say there have been about six messages pertaining to syphilis that stand out prominently:

1. Discovery of causative factor.
2. Ehrlich's salvarsan therapy.
3. The Wassermann blood test.
4. Noguchi's finding of the spirocheta pallida in the brain and cord tissue.
5. Malarial inoculation for paresis.
6. Bismuth and tryparsamide therapy.

Twenty-five years ago, or before Schaudin and Hoffman discovered the spirocheta pallida as the causative factor of syphilis, we were taught not to treat the primary lesion of syphilis until the secondaries appeared, with the result that the patient carried an infectious lesion for six weeks, and then, when the secondaries appeared with mucous patches, etc., he became doubly infectious; and this was followed by several weeks more of transmission until the patient was under control with mercurial rubs or salicylate of mercury injections. It is easy to understand how difficult it was to control a disease under these circumstances.

At present, when a patient with a primary lesion presents himself, a dark-field examination is made and he is given a salvarsan at once. Twenty-four to forty-eight hours after his first salvarsan injection it is difficult to find any organisms in the lesion; and, personally, I believe after the second or third salvarsan he is not infectious and will remain so providing he continues his treatment.

As to the Wassermann reaction, it has been a great

aid when there is any doubt as to diagnosis. In every general examination by any medical man, a Wassermann test should always be included. In this way, cases of syphilis are picked up which would otherwise be overlooked. A four plus Wassermann reaction does not by any means prove conclusively that a patient is infectious, but it indicates that treatment should be given, especially to ward off late visceral manifestations.

Noguchi's discovery of the spirocheta pallida in the brain and cord tissue put general paralysis and locomotor ataxia 100 per cent in the syphilis category. Malarial treatment for paresis, while not 100 per cent perfect in any sense, offered us a method in treating a previously fatal condition, and in which we now obtain in some cases very good results.

Bismuth and tryparsamide have also been adjuncts in our therapy.

The above methods have reduced syphilis to a minimum, especially in Minnesota, which is the only region I personally know about. In my office, a primary lesion is a rarity; and, in talking with other dermatologists, their experience seems about the same. At the Ancker Hospital in St. Paul, there have been two primary lesions in the out-patient department in the last six months; and at the University Hospital there have been about ten during the last year.

Wassermann tests on 5,000 University students gave five positives, three of which were congenital, one extragenital, and only one contracted by sexual intercourse. Dr. Cole told me that, at the Shriners' Hospital for Crippled Children, a positive Wassermann is a rare occurrence. And I received the same report from Dr. Hedenstrom at the Baby Welfare Clinic in St. Paul.

Syphilis is, and always has been, a social problem; but it is definitely under control and is disappearing rapidly; this, in my opinion, is due to the above discoveries which I have mentioned, and not by "educating the public," which, to me, is more or less of a myth pertaining to things medical.

DR. GORDON KAMMAN, St. Paul: I was glad to hear Dr. O'Leary say that, in the treatment of neurosyphilis, he feels that malaria is more effective than any other forms of pyrotherapy. Walter Freeman, of St. Elizabeth's in Washington, D. C., has shown that malaria produces a reaction in the reticulo-endothelial system that does not appear in other forms of fever therapy. I suspect that the participation of the reticuloendothelial system has something to do with the resorption of the perivascular exudates that we see in neurosyphilis. In Von Jauregg's Clinic in Vienna, I recall seeing sections in which the actual passage was shown of perivascular exudates through the walls of the capillaries. This connotes a change in the permeability of the endothelium that is produced by the dynamic action of the malarial parasite. This action cannot be produced by the various other methods of artificial fever production. Malaria seems to be the only agent that causes this type of reaction. This undoubtedly has a bearing on the relative merits of malarial therapy and other forms of fever therapy. I think statistical studies tend to show that malarial treatment produces a higher percentage of remissions than other forms of fever therapy.

I would like to ask Dr. O'Leary whether or not insufficient early treatment is worse than no treatment, or whether insufficient early treatment really does help.

DR. F. R. WRIGHT, Minneapolis: Regarding the treatment of late syphilis, it is not the temperature at all which does the work. It so happens that in malaria an immunizing agent is produced which, at certain stages, produces a positive Wassermann. Instead of the temperature, it is the theory that malaria produces some immunizing body which kills the spirochete.

'Dr. S. E. Sweitzer, Minneapolis: In general we find that the neurologists feel that these patients who have no active symptoms should not be actively treated. But I feel that we should treat the so-called preparetics with malaria and intensive post-malarial treatment with arsenic and bismuth so that they will not get paresis. The figures which Dr. O'Leary has given us tonight show that very well.

Dr. H. L. Ulrich, Minneapolis: The only vector for syphilis is the human body. We cannot kill the vector, so we must destroy the treponema pallidum. The acceleration of this destruction lies in the improvement of our arsenicals. My criticism of the specialists is due to the fact that in the last thirty years they have fallen down. The only benefit I can see in a campaign is not one of education but one of propaganda which would emphasize the early treatment of syphilis.

Dr. Paul O'Leary, Rochester: The people of Minnesota are indeed fortunate in having had, back in 1921, two men interested enough and with sufficient vision to have created a venereal disease program that has become a model for this country. I refer, of course, to Dr. H. G. Irvine and Dr. A. J. Chesley of the State Board of Health. Even when the funds which were originally set aside by the state legislature were discontinued, Dr. Chesley and Dr. Irvine were able to carry on a campaign that has maintained a state serologic laboratory of the highest type, that has supplied drugs to physicians for the treatment of indigent patients with gonorrhea and syphilis, and that has maintained a consultation service for the physicians of the community. The adoption of the Minnesota plan by the national health officers as a model type of program should indeed be a source of satisfaction and encouragement to these two pioneers in the venereal disease campaign.

In answer to Dr. Kamman's question, I believe very decidedly that the modern treatment of syphilis does not produce neurosyphilis but rather that it actually prevents its development. The basis for this assertion is that, of a group of 500 patients with clinical neurosyphilis, 72 per cent had not been treated for syphilis when the neurologic disease was recognized. Of those who received treatment, even though it was insufficient in amount according to our present-day standards, only 8 per cent developed clinical neurosyphilis. Likewise, when we studied those patients who were given the recommended amount of treatment, only 4 per cent showed either invasion or involvement of the central nervous system. The statistical evidence is decidedly in favor of the modern treatment of syphilis as the best "preventer" of neurosyphilis we now have at our disposal.

The successful serologic and clinical results that follow malarial therapy are apparently not due to any symbiotic reaction between the plasmodium vivax and the spirocheta pallida, as Dr. Wright mentioned. The reason for this is that other types of organism, spirochetal and bacterial, as well as the by-products of these organisms, have produced equally satisfactory results in the patient with syphilis; but there use has not become popular because of controllable complications or the inability to control the disease produced.

Dr. F. R. Wright: Answering Dr. O'Leary, I might say that the spirocheta does not live in the blood stream; it lives in the tissue fluids. Fever alters the character of these fluids. That is what happens when you treat gonorrhea with heat. Forty years ago they taught at the clinic in Vienna that only 2 per cent of the cases treated by mercury for over three years would develop neurosyphilis; so, if the figures Dr. O'Leary just gave are correct, and these old figures in Vienna are correct, from a neurological standpoint the end-

216

results have not improved much in the treatmen syphilis.

The meeting adjourned.

Albert G. Schulze, M.D.,
Secreta

BOOK REVIEWS

Books listed here become the property of Ramsey and Hennepin County Medical librar when reviewed. Members, however, are urged write reviews of any or every recent book wh may be of interest to physicians.

MENTAL THERAPY. Studies in Fifty Cases. I S. London, M.D., formerly Assistant Sur (R) United States Public Health Service; Me Officer United States Veterans Bureau; Assi Physician, Central Islip State Hospital, Central New York, and Manhattan State Hospital, W Island, New York. Cloth. Price, $12.50. Two umes, pp. 774, with 22 diagrams. New Y Covici, Friede, 1937.

These two volumes present fifty case historie various types of neuroses and psychoses. The la part of this work is taken up with cases of so neuroses. The author is a student of Freud's so of psychoanalysis and uses Freud's interpretatio his analyses. Is is very questionable that this will, as the publishers aver, displace Krafft-Eb "Psychopathia Sexualis," mainly because only a paratively few types of sexual perversion are disc The title, "Mental Therapy," is misleading for a proportion of the case histories have no menti therapy. A more accurate title would be "A Fre Interpretation of Fifty Cases of Neurosis, S Perversion and Psychoses, with Emphasis on S Perversion." For those who cannot stomach ps analysis this contribution is not recommended. those who do believe in psychoanalysis it offers n essentially new.

N. J. Berkwitz,

MANUAL OF DISEASES OF THE EYE. C H. May, M.D. 498 pages. Illus. Price $4.00. W Wood and Company, 1937.

This work first published in 1900 has now through fifteen editions and while it contains 500 pages it is still of convenient size.

For the undergradute and general practitione perhaps the most ideal work of its kind. Dia and treatment have been brought up to date; s operations for the respective fields have beer chosen, clearly described and illustrated; an colored plates are especially illuminating al former editions had similiar plates.

That the work has great merit is evident by t that it has been translated and printed in sever tions in eight foreign tongues.

George C. Dittman, M

PROCEEDINGS of the MINNEAPOLIS SURGICAL SOCIETY

Stated Meeting, Thursday, January 6, 1938

President, Dr. O. W. Yoerg, in the Chair

THE USE OF FASCIAL TRANSPLANTS IN HERNIOPLASTY*

Stanley R. Maxeiner, M.D., F.A.C.S.

Erdman, in a follow-up of 978 herniotomies on patients over sixty years of age, found 10 per cent recurrences after operations for oblique hernias and per cent recurrences after operations for direct rnias. The regular gut suture method of hernioplasty followed by 15-25 per cent recurrences, in direct rnia and 40-50 per cent failures after operation for current hernias. This is not due to faulty technic nen all the surgical indications have been complied ith, namely, removal of the sac, proper approxima- n of tissues, primary healing, and an adequate heal- g period.

Reoperation reveals that the tissues have not re- ained as they were approximated surgically, but have parated and returned to their original position with e formation of a new sac. The answer must be und in the deficiency of the healing process.

Healing takes place first by the advent of inflamma- on followed by new fiber cells and blood vessels :sembling granulations which eventually become scar. wo edges of fascia sutured together become united y scar whether approximated edge to edge or over- ipped. Union of fascia to muscle takes place by the ormation of new scar joining the fascia to the fibrous overing of the muscle bundles. It naturally implies, rerefore, that approximation must be maintained un- l adequate scar is formed to insure against stretch- ig and separation under stress. Absorbable sutures ften fail to accomplish this objective. Non-absorbable utures, on the other hand, if they do not cut out under :nsion are found to be incorporated in a strong bed f scar. Experimentally, Mootz, Selig and others ound that removal of intervening areolar tissue and :arification of approximated surfaces aids the security f the healing process.

Gallie in 1921 reported his work, experimental and linical, on the use of living fascial sutures and grafts. 'ree grafts were found to shrink and became joined ɔ hernial rings by wide areas of scar tissue. This ras overcome by the use of grafts resembling the 1any tail binder, the tails being sewed into the sur- ounding tissues. Fascial strips cut from fascia lata nd used as sutures were found to be stronger than atgut or kangaroo tendon and were less irritating o the tissues, producing little or no reaction. They ecame incorporated in the healing scar and were emonstrated two to five years later as persistent fibrous

cords of equal tensile strength and unshrunk as demon- strated by spacing silk markers along the sutures. McArthur in 1901 described the use of a fascial suture procured from the medial cut edge of the external oblique and left attached at the pubes. We used his method successfully in the early days of my associa- tion with Dr. Farr but it was later only seldom em- ployed. Recently, however, popularity seems to have returned it to its just place in surgery. Our own ex- perience based on 383 hernias repaired by the Mc- Arthur fascial suture has reduced our recurrences three and a half times when used in the repair of direct hernia. We have reserved the McArthur operation for the milder type of direct hernia, some selected recurrent hernias, and certain indirect hernias in older persons.

The Gallie operation is more radical and has been reserved for post-operative incisional hernias where the edges can not be brought together without too much tension or where a gap actually remains between the edges. This gap is darned with fascial strips as one might mend a sock. We have recently repaired all recurrent inguinal hernias by this method. Large umbilical hernias, selected femoral and epigastric hernias and certain large long-standing indirect hernias where tissues are weak lend themselves best to the Gallie method of closure.

Gallie in 100 herniotomies, most of which were for direct or recurrent hernias, had no recurrences although three wounds suppurated. Burdick in 163 cases, twen- ty-nine of which were for recurrence, had four recur- rences only. Behrend performed 125 operations with three recurrences and recommends the use of fascial sutures in practically all herniotomies. Burdick, Gil- lespie and Higinbotham (Am. Surg., 1937) report the only adverse criticism found in the literature reviewed by the writer. However, they report 133 infected wounds in 1,485 cases, 7.9 per cent of the wounds with autogenous sutures and 12 per cent with ox fascia being infected. Of 975 followed operations of all types of hernia 284 failures occurred. They report 15.4 per cent recurrences in indirect hernias with the use of fascia and now employ silk sutures almost ex- clusively. These statistics are not as good as those obtained by the use of catgut and their percentage of infections is very high.

In discussing sutures Koontz remarks as follows:

A (1) Catgut is uncertain as to its duration and may disappear before the healing process is complete; (2) in the presence of collected serum it softens and often unties; (3) unfavorable reaction to the tissues about the sutures is common.

B. Silk is not absorbed and is more dependable and there is very little reaction in the surrounding tissues.

*From the Department of Surgery, University of Minnesota.

The objection to silk is based on the grounds that it is a foreign body and often leaves a sinus or it may cut through.

C. Animal fascia preserved in alcohol (70 per cent) still has collagen fibers undestroyed and live cells penetrate and incorporate the sutures as in a graft of autogenous fascia.

Autogenous fascial sutures do not absorb but continue to function for all time. They are strong and easily procured. Fascia may be used as a graft, pedunculated flap or as a suture. Fascial sutures may be mounted on a Gallie needle or may be pulled through by small forceps which penetrate the layers to be united. The strip should be anchored at regular intervals, preferably with silk, as fascia is very slippery. Defects may be darned by strips or the layers may be brought together by the ordinary running suture if there is no undue tension.

Personal cases from our own private practice consist of twenty-eight hernias repaired by fascia; fourteen by the McArthur method and fourteen by the Gallie technic.

At the Veterans Hospital at Ft. Snelling, Dr. Sedgeley, Dr. Culligan and I have performed 405 herniotomies by using fascial transplants. There have been 372 operations of the McArthur type and thirty-three operations of the Gallie type.

Among the writer's twenty-eight patients there has been one infected wound with prompt failure. This was a strangulated hernia recurrent seven times in which we ill-advisedly attempted to do a Gallie suture to obtain permanent relief. The infection in this instance was unquestionably due to the presence of bacteria from the incarcerated bowel. None of the other twenty-seven cases became infected and there have been no recurrences to date.

In order to completely clarify my stand on the use of fascia I would state that I am not recommending the use of fascia for the ordinary indirect hernia, especially in young people, where even the removal of the sac alone may be adequate, but I am advocating its use as stated in the text and in the report of the following cases where, in my judgment, catgut closure is apt to be followed by failure. Occasionally one hears the statement that removal of fascia lata strips from the thigh may be followed by muscle hernia. We have not experienced this condition as yet in forty-seven cases in which we have removed strips of fascia lata. Following the rendering of the above paper, ten cases treated by the Gallie and McArthur operations were personally shown as a clinic. Six of the most interesting ones are herewith reported.

Case 1—Mr. F., aged sixty-five, has had two herniotomies on the left side in 1911 and 1919 and one herniotomy on the right side in 1919, all of which recurred. The patient has been treated by hernia injections on both sides for a nine-month period without improvement. In August, 1936, the right (which is giving the most symptoms) twice-recurrent hernia was repaired by the Gallie technic using three strips of fascia lata one-fourth to one-third inch wide. One and a half years later the closure is entirely satisfactory. The

by approaching it from the rear of the right thigh. The inguinal wound suppurated and necessitated removal of slough and fragments of bone. A hernia subsequently developed from which the patient has been operated upon subsequently nine times. At the last preceding operation the surgeon ingeniously withdrew the testicle from the scrotum, passed it behind the right rectus muscle, out the midline and back again into the scrotum and then closed the inguinal canal. This was followed not only by hernia in the inguinal region but likewise one in the midline where the cord emerged from behind the rectus. In October, 1937, the patient agreed that we might remove the testicle or resect the cord if we thought it would give him a better chance of a permanent cure. Operation: a long oblique incision was carried downward over the inguinal canal into the midline over the pubis. The cord was exposed in the inguinal canal following beneath the rectus muscle and to the midline as described. Under the circumstances we reasoned that the testicle having been delivered from the scrotum must have developed a new collateral circulation from adhesions to the surrounding tissue. For that reason the testicle was not removed but the cord was doubly ligated and completely excised to the peritoneum. The midline hernia, the rectus sheath, and the inguinal canal were now closed tightly, using three, more than ordinarily wide fascial strips. The layers were imbricated and deep bites were taken into the normal tissue on both sides of the approximated tissues. It is now only four months since the last repair which was done by the Gallie fascial strip technic and it is altogether too early to report the result of this operation. However, we believe that we have given this patient his best chance for a permanent cure. It is interesting to note that there was no swelling of the testicle following the division of the entire cord and it remains the same size as the testicle on the opposite side.

Motion pictures in color of fascial operations performed by both Drs. Culligan and Maxeiner were shown demonstrating the technic of the two types of fascial strip operations.

Discussion

DR. LEO CULLIGAN: In 1931 when we first started using fascia in the repair of hernia at the Veterans' Hospital, we limited its use to large ventral hernias, the larger recurrent hernias, and those recurrent hernias which had come back more than once. For that reason, during the next three years, we used it in only nine cases, all by the Gallie technic. In February, 1934, we became interested in the old McArthur operation originated by him in 1901. The use of this simple and effective means has so widened the scope of the use of fascia that up to the present time we have used it in 406 cases, thirty-three of these by the Gallie technic, and the remainder by the McArthur technic.

From the experimental work of many men we know that fascia as a suture material persists and does not absorb. Some men say that it continues to live much like transplanted skin lives. Others say that it persists as an inert tendinous structure which becomes infiltrated from the surrounding tissues. However, all agree that it is not absorbed, and that it will continue to hold tissues together in place where one sutures them.

From our own experience at the Veterans' Hospital we know that fascia is an innocuous kind of suture material. The wounds in which it is used heal readily without irritation and without any undue formation of serum. We have had a low incidence of infection, somewhat higher percentage in the Gallie than in the McArthur operation, yet the series using the Gallie technic is so much smaller that the comparison is hardly accurate. In the Gallie we have had four in-

fections in thirty-three cases (12 per cent), while in the McArthur herniotomies done during the last year, amounting to 132 operations, we have had only two infections (1.5 per cent). In all our cases, even those which have become infected, we have never had a fascial strip slough. A year ago in a paper before this society I compared the results of the use of catgut and fascia in the repair of the direct hernia. At that time I showed that we had approximately three and one-half times the recurrence rate using catgut that we had had using fascia.

In view of this satisfactory experience I now use fascia almost as a routine in the direct hernia, the large indirect hernias, sliding hernias, the ventral hernias, and the recurrent hernias. Whenever possible I use the McArthur technic.

Because I prefer this simpler McArthur technic in repairing the recurrent inguinal hernia I do not use the suggestion of Gallie to take the fascial strips from the thigh before opening the herniotomy wound, for I have found that in the majority of these cases one can get sufficient fascia locally to make a satisfactory repair. Possibly it is just that I have a weakness for the method of McArthur. However, it has been my experience that in most recurrent inguinal hernias the defect is a small one, often not larger than two or three centimeters in diameter, and for that reason one does not need a great deal of fascia to make a good repair. Moreover, the repair of the recurrent hernia using fascia, can be different from that using catgut in that it is not necessary to break down the floor of the canal in order to get sufficient tissue to overlap and make our closure in that way. All we have to do is to pull the edges of the defect together with fascia and they will hold where we put them.

So in repairing the recurrent inguinal hernia, after dissecting out the defect, I have been taking a strip of fascia from the adjacent aponeurosis of the external oblique, leaving it attached near the fascial defect and using it as suture material. I have been able to use this method in the last thirty-two consecutive recurrent inguinal hernias upon which I have operated and as yet none of them have returned for reoperation. On the other hand when the defect is large, and I cannot get sufficient fascia locally to make the repair, I go to the thigh and take enough fascia to make a firm closure.

On the whole, our experience with fascia has been so satisfactory that now whenever I operate any hernia, especially in a patient over the age of thirty-five or forty, I ask myself the question, "Why not use fascia?" As time goes on it is becoming increasingly difficult to find sufficiently good reasons for not using it.

DR. FRANK R. SEDGLEY (by invitation): This would be a wonderful opportunity to review the history of the surgical treatment of hernia from prehistoric times, but I will refrain owing to the length of the program this evening. Until the advent of modern surgery no real progress was made in the treatment or the understanding of hernia. The subject remained in the same status as during the Dark Ages.

There were three factors that changed the situation. These were the principles of antisepsis and asepsis, improved surgical suture material and a better understanding of the anatomical relations to the lines of intra-abdominal force, intra-abdominal pressure and especially the stresses that occur upon the operated structures. The Bassini and Halstead operations, as well as a number of others that bear proper names, reflect the progress of development of a better anatomical understanding.

The first two factors preceded and were necessary to the development and application of the anatomical principle in the same degree that they were and still are fundamental to the development and progress of modern surgery. Asepsis is an absolute term and implies, naturally, a perfection in that particular direction, but it is a perfection that is practically obtainable. Surgical sutures nowadays are excellent and for wide general uses are near to perfection but in the special field of hernial surgery with its transposed anatomy, the three factors do not combine as effectively as in many other circumstances. The use of living, autoplastic fascia, I believe, represents, if not perfection, at least a distinct improvement in the suture factor. It may be thought of as bearing the same relation to other sutures as vital staining of the blood and other tissues does to ordinary staining methods. Whether there is anything essentially vital in it or not, one warning should be borne in mind: the fascial strip, whether free or pedicled, remains a suture still and as such must be carefully applied. It has such a smoothly sliding, sleek quality that it must be firmly anchored in its position at several points to insure its fixation and later incorporation where desired. This is done with accessory sutures of plain and chromic gut, or silk as may be preferred.

I want to express my appreciation of Dr. Culligan's laborious and painstaking efforts in going over our large number of cases at the Veterans' Hospital and I anticipate that his analysis of our present practice continued over a longer period will show a definite improvement in our own recurrence rate, and especially in results of operative procedures on recurrent hernias.

Dr. Willard D. White: In these cases that have to be operated on for bilateral hernias, do you do them both in the same sitting or do you do one and allow it to heal and then do the other side?

I would also like to add that Dr. MacArthur had described this operation in 1901 and then somewhere around 1904 he showed, at a meeting, a patient who had been operated upon in 1901 with this McArthur operation of fascial suture. Then, this patient died from some other cause somewhere about 1904 and he had the specimen removed at autopsy and it showed that the fascial strips that had been placed in the wound nearly four years previously still remained* and you could trace the course of these strips, showing that the strips do actually live.

Dr. Hamlin Mattson: There is still another possible use for fascia transplants which I tried recently. A primipara, aged thirty-two, suffered a third degree laceration following breech delivery August 21, 1934. Two extensive procedures performed elsewhere had failed. The patient had complete fecal incontinence and absence of the rectovaginal septum for a distance of 6 cm. proximal to the anal sphincter. The tissues showed extensive scarification. On April 22, 1935, the rectum was freed and drawn downward and the remnants of the levator ani muscles sutured. The wound healed well with the exception of the ends of the sphincter, which did not unite. On May 7, 1937, the ends of the anal sphincter were freed and sutured with three strips from the fascia lata. Apparently fascia transplants when buried in poorly vascularized scar tissue are transformed into scar and when in better vascularized tissues remain in as fascia indefinitely. Nevertheless, this patient obtained complete functional control of her bowels.

Dr. R. Hultkrans: Dr. Dunn had a case when I was with him. A man of considerable weight fell and ruptured both quadriceps tendons. They were completely ruptured because he had no power of extension at either knee. Repair was done with fascia lata. Dr. Dunn is here and can probably tell us about it.

*This statement was made in a discussion, by Dr. E. S. Murphy, of a paper on fascial sutures in the repair of inguinal hernia by W. J. Pickett, Illinois Medical Journal—Vol. 59, p. 227, March, 1931.

Dr. George R. Dunn: This was a rather heavy chap and he evulsed the quadriceps tendon at the top of each patella. We used fascia lata in restoring them. He got practically a perfect result on one side and a fairly good result on the other side. He weighed, after considerable reducing, about 265 pounds. The use of the fascia was about the only way we had of restoring the continuity of the tendons. There was no fracture, simply an evulsion of both quadriceps tendons from the patella on the right and left sides.

Dr. Stanley R. Maxeiner: With reference to Dr. White's question, I personally have not done a double hernia at one sitting for several years. The man who had a bilateral hernia had a three weeks interval between the two operations. I personally think it is wise to have an interval of probably two to four weeks as the closure of the two hernias undoubtedly exerts additional tension on both lines of sutures and one or both are more likely to give way.

With reference to Dr. Mattson's remarks, I wish to add that they are using fascial strips for almost everything and they have been repeatedly using them in the repair of extensive laceration of the perineum where the tissue is inadequate. At the last meeting of the Western Surgical Association, Dr. Charles Mayo, Jr., showed motion pictures of a new technic in which he used fascia lata for building up the pelvic floor to cure prolapse of the rectum. The exposure is through an incision similar to that used in operation for carcinoma of the rectum. The peritoneum is opened and the rectum and sigmoid is tucked up into the abdomen. Fascial strips are then woven in such a manner that a new internal pelvic floor is made which fits around the rectum. They had a very successful result in the one case which he reported.

FEMORO-ILIAC THROMBOSIS AND THROMBOPHLEBITIS

H. O. McPHEETERS, M.D.

Much has been written on the subject of thrombosis and thrombophlebitis. The importance of its prophylaxis, care at the time of onset and the treatment of the sequelæ that may often follow, has not yet received proper attention. This is well borne out by the splendid presentations the past year. The paper by Homans[1] is a most complete thesis on the subject, while Edwards[2] has given evidence as to the destruction of the venous valves in severe cases.

Pathologists and clinicians agree that the first and most important factor in the development of a thrombophlebitis is a slowing of the blood stream. An injury to the intima of the vessel, either traumatic or infectious, furnishes a focus for its development. Blood platelets are then deposited at that area in the slowly moving blood stream. Thrombocytes appear and then fibrin is deposited which enmeshes the blood cells. The process may terminate with only a slight local involvement or it may close the vein lumen and extend in both directions. The extension of the process terminates at the inflowing of collateral veins with a good current. It is the thrombus attached to only a portion of the vein wall and only partially filling the vein lumen that is provocative of most of the emboli. There may be sufficient current present at times to carry a portion of the poorly attached thrombus, which may become loosened by exercise, in a proximal direction.

The infection is hematogenous, and may arise from some distant focus, or may be by way of the lymphatics. In the latter case it is thought to be carried in the perivenous lymphatics and then to involve the vein wall from the outside by direct extension. It then penetrates the wall and causes an inflammation of the intima to initiate the thrombophlebitis. Barker[2] has discussed primary idiopathic thrombophlebitis and cites cases in which no probable source of the infection was ever found.

Homans[3] has divided thrombophlebitis of the lower extremity as follows: deep femoro-iliac thrombophlebitis commonly called "phlegmasia alba dolens"; deep peripheral thrombophlebitis involving the deep cavernous viens of the calf; thrombophlebitis of varicose veins; thrombophlegitis of non-varicose veins.

At this time I wish to discuss only the deep femoro-iliac thrombosis and phlebitis and present three case reports of patients who, I believe, had this condition. In each case the symptoms were so acute and severe as to leave no doubt but that the pathology was initiated in the femoro-iliac segment of the vein. The onset of the condition in each case was rapid and the symptoms of thrombosis were more prominent than those of phlebitis. The condition is most dramatic for both the doctor and the patient. In one case the onset and pain was similar to that of an arterial embolus.

Case 1.—Mrs. T., aged forty-eight, a housewife in good general health, three years previously had stumbled on the steps and bruised her left knee and leg over its outer and middle surface. Following this she recovered with bed rest. One year later and more than a year before I saw her, she complained much of a pain along the crest of the left tibia and the outer middle third of her left leg. There was also a sharp pain at times in the left mid-thigh. This was along the distribution of the left femoro-cutaneous nerve. Both she and her home physician associated both these pains with the fall of three years previously and with some small varicose veins that had developed since.

Careful examination showed the patient in good general health and with no complaints other than the above described pains and the few varicose veins. I advised both her doctor and the patient that I did not think the varicose veins were the cause of the pains but suggested that we inject them to rule them out. The varicose veins were injected with sodium morruhate 5 per cent with good results and the usual local reaction. The original pains still persisted.

Five days after the injections the reaction was rapidly subsiding. The patient was sitting waiting for her husband planning to return home when she felt a pain in the left groin which rapidly became worse. Following this she said the entire leg seemed to feel "full." She came to my office at once, a distance of two blocks, crying with pain. The pain was principally in the groin and upper thigh but also somewhat throughout the entire leg.

Examination showed the entire left leg very cyanotic and swollen. The skin was tense. The cyanosis showed a sharp line of demarcation at the groin which passed outward even with the greater trochanter. It was not more than 3 inches from the normal pink skin above to the deeply cyanotic skin below. The pulsation in the femoral and popliteal arteries was

good. The foot was too badly swollen to permit palpation of the dorsalis pedis. The temperature was normal.

The patient was sent to the hospital. The leg was put in high elevation and hot magnesium sulphate packs were applied. Four hours after onset the temperature was 99; at the end of the twenty-four hours 99.4; and at the end of forty-eight hours it was 100.4. It rose to 100 daily for four days and then dropped to 99 for the rest of her stay in the hospital.

During her stay in the hospital the hot packs were removed for 1 hour at a time twice a day and the electric baker was applied over the entire leg.

There was no medication given directly for the condition itself as I did not think the patient had a true infectious phlebitis. The patient had a great deal of pain and she was kept under sedatives all the time.

She went home by ambulance on the eleventh day and continued the hot wet packs four hours twice a day followed by the electric baker. She continued this treatment for eight weeks. The pain through the entire leg gradually lessened but the original pain in the external thigh and lower leg continued. The leg was painful when held dependent but the patient was urged to be up and about with an Ace bandage on the lower leg. This gave her much relief.

Six months after the onset of her complication she returned and Dr. R. P. Caron injected the painful areas with novocaine and later with quinine and urea hydrochloride 1—600. This was repeated one month later. Today the patient has recovered almost completely. She has no pain but does wear an elastic stocking which easily controls the swelling.

In this case the thrombosis must have been either the result of an idiopathic phlebitis, as suggested by Barker, or the delayed result of the injections, a condition such as I have never seen before, even though the reaction from the injections was only the usual amount and that was rapidly subsiding.

Case 2.—Mrs. W., a housewife, aged forty-four, had an attack of influenza in February, 1937, and was bedfast for three weeks. In bed, while convalescing, she suddenly developed severe pains through the left inguinal region and throughout the entire left leg. Four hours later, by daylight, she noticed that the entire left thigh and lower leg was of a greenish, cyanotic color. Both pain and cyanosis were aggravated on standing. The patient did not have a chill and the doctor said her temperature was normal.

She was sent to the hospital for five weeks, where two blood cultures were negative. There was only a moderate swelling of the leg during that time, while in bed, but it did swell and the pain was worse as soon as she would get up and about.

After another four weeks in bed at home she began to get up and about with an Ace bandage on the lower leg. Without it the lower leg to the knee would become dark, cyanotic and swollen.

The attending physician at that time diagnosed the condition as a femoro-iliac thrombosis and not a thrombophlebitis.

The patient was first seen by me on September 1, 1937 at my office. The entire left leg, from the groin to the toes, was larger by actual measurement than the right leg. The skin was definitely cyanotic in relation to that of the right leg and the abdomen. The patient was wearing an Ace bandage on the lower leg. When this was removed there was but slight edema and the color was good. The femoral, popliteal and dorsalis pedis arteries were normal. The left great saphenous vein was palpable and only half an inch in size, not at all large enough to be considered a compensatory vein. Tests proved it was not. After the bandage was removed the leg became discolored and there seemed to be a definite line of demarcation of the cyanosis about the level of the knee. After a forced walk of four hours without the bandage the swelling was only moderately increased and the color was good. The leg rapidly became cyanosed on standing. I advised her to continue wearing a Lastex stocking and go about her work.

On November 18, 1937, the patient reported that she had led a normal life, including dancing, and felt fine. She was not handicapped by the leg. There was still some cyanosis and swelling of the lower leg to the lower thigh when going without the supportive stocking.

Case 3.—Mr. S., aged fifty, a millwright, had an injury to the left ankle and foot many years previously. Two years before the present illness I treated him for a bad varicose ulcer and injected a large group of varicose veins. The patient was last seen one year previously. On December 30, 1936, he presented himself at the office with the history of having had the varicose ulcer recur two weeks previously but stated that it was rapidly getting worse. He also had had a severe pain develop in the left groin the day before, following which the left leg became cyanotic and badly swollen.

In his case, examination of the left leg showed the same line of cyanotic demarcation at the groin as described in Case 1, but he also showed an extensive fungous or ringworm infection over the entire inner ankle and lower leg. There was much inflammation in the tissues in this area. This case was thought to be a definite infectious thrombophlebitis and the patient was given four intravenous injections of gentian violet 0.5 per cent, six of Creohex and six doses of Edwenil subcutaneously.

In spite of all treatment and consultation the condition spread upward into the iliac veins, with an involvement of the right iliac and femoral veins and a septic lung embolus with later abscess formation. The patient finally died of a rupture of the lung abscess into the bronchus and an acute pneumothorax. At the autopsy a thrombus was found to be completely plugging the inferior vena cava, four inches above the bifurcation at the pelvic brim. This thrombus was firm and was of at least several days, duration.

The most important phase of the treatment of thrombophlebitis is its prophylaxis. This is accomplished by exercise and doing all those things in the individual case that will aid venous drainage. Tight abdominal postoperative binders should be avoided as much as possible. The patient should be urged to move the legs actively as early as possible and several times a day. Thyroid gland given before and after operation increases the circulatory rate. The patient should walk immediately after an injection treatment of varicose veins and be up and about the house every two hours after the preliminary ligation and injection of veins. This avoids the stasis in the deep veins of the calf which could be injured by the injected solution. In Sweden[9] a mortality rate of 0.33 per cent following the combined ligation and injection treatment has been reported. This is higher than for the former resection operation of years ago which was given as 0.26 per cent. This I am satisfied is due to the surgeon demanding bed rest for his ligation cases.

For the active treatment of the individual case, elevation of the extremity and hot packs from toes to abdomen with the electric light baker at hour intervals four times daily seem to give the best results. Medication has been of little help. Sulfanilamide should be tried and in some cases the intravenous use of 0.5 per cent aqueous solution of gentian violet does seem to help.[7] Murphy[4] claims excellent results with mecholyl iontophoresis in the treatment of the

222

chronically indurated and inflamed lower leg so commonly seen after phlebitis.

Summary

Thrombophlebitis of this particular type is in my experience very rare. The three cases presented were, however, seen this past year. Though radical surgery has been advised in the way of ligation of the vein above the thrombus,[5,6,8] I believe that the above method of expectant treatment is to be recommended.

Bibliography

1. Bancroft, F. W.: Proximal ligation and excision of viens for septic phlebitis. Ann. Surg., 106:308, 1937.
2. Barker, Nelson W.: Idiopathic thrombophlebitis. Arch. Int. Med., 58:147, 1936.
3. Edwards, E. A.: The effect of thrombophlebitis on the venous valve. Surg., Gynec. and Obst., 65:310, 1937.
4. Fontaine, R., and Pereira, A.: Obliterations et resections veineuses expérimentales. Contribution a l'etude de la circulation collatérale veineuse. Rev. de chir., 56:161, 1937. (Abstr.) Internat. Abstr. Surg., 65:347, 1937.
5. Homans, John: Venous thrombosis in the lower limbs; its relation to pulmonary embolism. Am. Jour. Surg., 38:316, 1937.
6. Murphy, H. L.: The treatment of thrombophlebitis with acetyl-betamethyl choline chloride iontophoresis. Surg., Gynec. and Obst., 65:100, 1937.
7. Neuhof, Harold: Excision of vein for suppurative thrombophlebitis. Ann. Surg., 106:308, 1937.
8. Stanley-Brown, M.: Intravenous injections of gentian violet in the treatment of phlebitis. Surg. Clin. No. Am., 8:1031, (Oct.) 1928.
9. Westerborn, A.: Ueber die Emboliegefahr bei Injektionsbehandlung von Varizen nebst einem Bericht ueber die in Schweden vorgekommenen Emboliefaelle. Acta chirurg. Scand., 79:321, 1937. (Abstr.) Intern. Abstr. Surg., 65:349, 1937.

Discussion

DR. CARL O. RICE: Dr. McPheeters has described three very interesting cases. In view of the fact that this condition is relatively so uncommon, it is difficult to say a great deal about it.

It appears that these cases are a bit different from the ordinary milk leg, or infectious thrombophlebitis, which is not infrequently observed postpartum. The report of these cases suggests that at least two of them were not initiated on an infectious basis.

The first case seems to suggest that the thrombophlebitis was the result of the chemical irritation from the injected sodium morrhuate. On the other hand, one is inclined to speculate as to why it should occur in this case and not in thousands of others similarly.

When we investigate the causes of venous thrombosis, we find that they may be classified into three different groups.

1. These may be disorders in the vein wall (injuries, inflammation, etc.). Homans states that in large veins the initial change in the intima of the vein may not necessarily be present. He has described exploratory operations in cases with iliofemoral thrombophlebitis in which he found a definite exudative reaction about the common and external iliac arteries. This, he believes, might be considered a deep perivascular lymphangitis—the etiology of which he has not determined.

2. Disorders of the blood, chiefly in the form of dehydration, have been described as another cause for thrombophlebitis. Dehydrated and debilitated individuals more frequently develop thrombophlebitis than comparatively healthy persons.

3. Disorders of the venous return may be due to general circulatory failure, or to factors which cause the blood flow to be slowed up. Among these are, postoperative inactivity, immobilization of extremities, pelvic masses, etc. The anatomical position of the external iliac and the common iliac veins in passing behind their corresponding arteries may also be a

factor, in the inactive bed patient, in causing the delay in the venous return.

Homans has described the following different varieties of thrombophlebitis:

1. Deep (femoroiliac) thrombophlebitis, sometimes described as phlegmasia abladolens. This is a not uncommon type of thrombophlebitis. If it produces a great deal of swelling it indicates greater extensiveness. There may be instances in which a thrombus may exist and may break off, causing a pulmonary embolus without having given any evidence of its previous existence.

2. Deep peripheral thrombophlebitis, which involves the veins in the muscles of the leg.

3. Traumatic and infectious thrombophlebitis, which does not have its origin in varicose veins.

4. Thrombophlebitis in varicose veins.

5. Migrating thrombophlebitis. This is a condition in which the thrombus extends toward the heart within the vein, and lies attached at only one point. In endeavoring to explain these three cases which Dr. McPheeters has reported, it seems possible that in the first case this may have been a factor, with the migrating thrombus having taken its origin from the chemical thrombus below.

In the other two cases, it is difficult to state what might have been the origin. The second case may have been similar to those which Homans has described as having a perivascular lymphangitis. The third case in which there had been a varicose ulcer and infection, may have been an infectious thrombophlebitis.

I agree that the best treatment for these cases is that which Dr. McPheeters has described: elevation, dry heat and early graduated exercises.

* * *

Dr. H. O. McPheeters: In conclusion I wish to emphasize one point. The relief from the peripheral neuralgic pain was so complete and so easily obtained that next time I will inject the painful areas first and the varicose veins later.

THE THERAPEUTIC EXPEDIENTS IN THE MANAGEMENT OF ACUTE INFECTIONS OF THE EXTREMITIES

Owen H. Wangensteen, M.D.

Abstract

Immobilization and elevation are of the greatest importance in the treatment of acute infections of the extremities. The most rigid immobilization is best achieved by placing the extremity concerned in a plaster of paris cast including the body trunk. Immobilization reduces muscle movement to a minimum. It also decreases the risk of dissemination of infection via the lymphatics; in addition it also reduces lymph production.

Accompanying all infections of the soft tissues swelling occurs, in consequence of the capillary injury. The extent of the swelling is limited by the occurrence of a high tissue pressure or tension which tends to delimit filtration from the capillary bed. Elevation of an infected extremity in a fixed position as high above the heart level as can conveniently be done with comfort to the patient, succeeds in early reduction of the swelling. Swollen tissues favor spread of the infection.

Bier's hyperemia in the treatment of acute infections of the extremities is physiologically unsound in that it increases venous pressure and consequently capillary pressure and augments filtration of fluid from the capillaries into the tissues. Heat also accentuates capillary permeability and is not to be used with an infected extremity in a dependent position.

The relief which has attended elevation of an inflamed member in an elevated position has been striking. The essayist has the impression that less extensive surgery need be done if immobilization and elevation are employed early in the treatment of infection. In acute osteomyelitis a body plaster is applied with a window over the tender area. When evidence of a subcutaneous abscess is present, an incision is made. Joints are similarly immobilized but incisions are made early and drainage secured by positioning. Fresh burns are treated in plaster with vaselinized shirting over the burned area.

Discussion

Dr. J. M. Hayes: As Dr. Wangensteen has said, one important factor in the treatment of all acute infections is immobilization. I am going to confine my discussion to these very acute infections, in which you have a severe lymphangitis and adenitis, from fifteen to twenty hours after a small wound on the extremities becomes infected.

Many years ago after spending a year in the University Hospital, I went out to practice in the country. In one particular town, not far from where I was located, it seemed that an epidemic of severe streptococcus infections developed. In a short period of time a large number of these cases came in with severe infections. It seemed that almost every one who got a slight pin prick got an infection. This took place during harvesting and threshing. These patients were mostly farmers and you usually couldn't get one of them into the hospital, until he was ready to drop. We used all the hot applications we had ever heard of but our results were not good.

About this time I read a statement in Ochsner's textbook of surgery, stating that he never had a crippled or deformed hand or loss of life, not even had to amputate a finger, since he learned of this method of treating acute infections of the extremities. I went to Chicago and went out to the Augustana Hospital. Here the late Dr. A. J. Ochsner was just putting one of these dressings on a leg. He told us at that time that his brother, Dr. Ed. Ochsner, had many years ago before observed the application of this dressing in the out-patient department of Cook County Hospital. He didn't even mention the name of the man who applied it. This man only used a saturated solution of boric acid on the dressing but obtained results that attracted Dr. Ochsner. Together with Dr. Kahlenberg, more recently of the University of Wisconsin, he determined to find out more about the use of this dressing. They found with this dressing applied to the extremity, boric acid appeared in the urine in a very short time. Later A. J. Ochsner suggested the addition of alcohol and phenol, much the same as the solution we use now.

Before application of this dressing with this latter solution they took material from the infected wound and injected it into the peritoneal cavity of a guinea pig and killed him in twenty-four hours. After the application of this dressing for forty-eight hours, they again took material from the wound and injected it into the peritoneal cavity of a guinea pig and it didn't even make him sick. We have verified these experiments to a small degree and have obtained the same results.

The solution we use now we call Modified Ochsner Solution. There is a formula for a solution dispensed by druggists called Ochsner Solution. This solution apparently was put in there by mistake. It is dangerous and should not be used. The Modified Ochsner Solution may be used on the skin of an infant

for forty-eight hours with no bad results.

I have talked about this dressing for many years in the out-patient department of the University. Dr. Hirshfelder has repeatedly said this solution would not penetrate the tissues more than one-half a centimeter. He is right in the way he applied it but with this dressing the resistant part of the skin is soon mascerated to such a high degree that the solution readily penetrates the tissues. This has been definitely proven. I know this seems like an extravagant statement to some, but when we get one of these cases within the first forty-eight hours of the onset of infection, we promise the patient definitely that we can stop the spread of the infection by the application of this dressing for forty-eight hours.

For the details of the treatment I refer you to MINNESOTA MEDICINE, volume 16, page 255 (April) 1933.

CLASSIFIED ADVERTISING

MINNESOTA MEDICINE

Journal of the Minnesota State Medical Association, Southern Minnesota Medical Association, Northern Minnesota Medical Association, Minnesota Academy of Medicine and Minneapolis Surgical Society.

Volume 21   APRIL, 1938   Number 4

THE IMPORTANCE OF IMMOBILIZATION AND POSTURE IN THE TREATMENT OF ACUTE INFECTIONS OF THE EXTREMITIES*

OWEN H. WANGENSTEEN, M.D.

Minneapolis, Minnesota

IN THE management of acute pyogenic infections, the objective is plain, but by what ends that purpose is best served is not so obvious. Experience has suggested certain expedients which have become generally adopted in practice. It has been difficult to evaluate critically what the virtues of these tried remedial agents are. Surgeons individually have continued especially those therapeutic measures which have appeared to effect the end-result most favorably.

Rest, hot packs, incision and drainage have constituted the essentials of the usual surgical treatment of acute pyogenic infections of the extremities. Biers' hyperemia and roentgen treatment have their enthusiastic supporters. Surgeons generally have become considerably more withholding in the employment of incisions in the treatment of infections, limiting their use almost entirely to the evacuation of localized pus. Time was not so long ago when incisions were used freely in the treatment of cellulitis. Surgeons have learned from their own experience that these often did harm and rarely accomplished any good.

During the period of the World War, surgeons reverted again to the employment of antiseptics in wound management. Aseptic surgery, which followed so closely upon the Listerian scheme, displaced largely the use of antiseptic agents in the treatment of infected wounds. Like the use of ill-timed incisions, they often did more harm than good. With the development of Dakin's solution and the Carrel technic of its

employment, it appeared that the chemical Messiah had been discovered. Surgeons in high places who spoke with authority acclaimed its accomplishments. Said the late W. W. Keen: "Lister taught us above all how to *prevent* infection; Dakin and Carrel, following Lister's principle, have taught us how to conquer even rampant infection. . . . Prevention and cure both are now ours." Such statements are now only of interest as a matter of record but serve to indicate how even the best oriented may be deceived by new things. Most surgeons have learned that Dakin's solution, like incisions, will not accomplish localization of infection; only the natural defense mechanism of the body can do that. To be certain, Dakin's solution has real value, but chiefly in accelerating clearing up of an infection which the tissues have conquered already.

Anyone who reads the literature of infection of the early decade of this century, cannot escape the impression that an immunologic specific would soon be available for every bacterial disease. This hope which seemed practically assured never materialized. After a few triumphant exploits, the new science of bacteriology, which in a relatively short period of time revolutionized the practice of medicine, seemed to have become therapeutically sterile and no further conquests were forthcoming. Yet to the development of specific immunologic or pharmacologic aids, surgeons, whose office it is to deal with acute pyogenic infections, look with anxiety and hope; for we know that our accomplishment in the management of spreading infections is not great. Our task is essentially to help the natural de-

*From the Department of Surgery, University of Minnesota, Minneapolis, Minnesota. Presented before the Minnesota Academy of Medicine, November 10, 1937.

fense mechanism of the body in its conflict with the infection and to evacuate pus when localized suppuration has occurred.

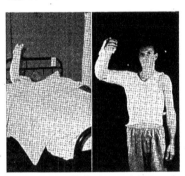

Fig. 1. (*left*) Immobilization of arm in a body plaster spica for phlegmonous inflammation of the hand. (*right*) Same patient ambulant. It is important that the extremity be placed in such a position that the hand will have maximum elevation in both recumbent and erect postures.

Immobilization

About four years ago, a young woman came under my observation who had sustained a compound fracture and a virulent phlegmon of the left thigh. After many consultations, short incisions for drainage were replaced by extensive incisions. These measures and employment of the Carrel-Dakin technic of wound irrigation all proved fruitless. Hectic fever continued and it appeared that we had lost our opportunity to save the woman's life by an earlier amputation. As a last gesture, a plaster spica cast, extending as high as the nipples and including both lower extremities, was applied—windows being left in for drainage. Despite adequate skeletal traction which had satisfactorily reduced the fracture, the relief from pain upon the application of plaster was striking. In ten days the patient was afebrile and made a satisfactory recovery.

This experience was startling, and on occasion, when unsatisfactory results were had with orthodox methods of treating infections, as a matter of last resort, encasement in plaster was tried. The improvement attending its use suggested trial with the method as the initial mode of treatment. During the past two years, I have treated a large variety of acute infections in this manner,

with windowed plaster casts. Among these are spreading infections of the soft tissues of the hands and feet including phlegmons, lymphangitis, phlebitis, acute osteomyelitis and suppurative arthritis. It has come in our clinic to be the standard method of treatment. In tenosynovitis, the necessity for early opening by incision of the tendon sheath still appears necessary. In established felons and paronychias, we have not employed immobilization in plaster. However, in all other varieties of hand infections immobilization of the hand and arm in a body plaster, in as great elevation as can be obtained conveniently, is regularly done. Latterly a severe burn of the trunk and lower limbs in a young child has been treated also in this manner. Vaselinized shirting was pulled over the burned lower extremities and trunk and a body plaster applied over all. The remarkable relief of pain was very pleasing to everyone. The child could be turned without discomfort and on the first change of plaster about three weeks later, the appearance of the burned area was very satisfactory—much of it had healed.

Immobilization in plaster, though it does not obliterate tonus or voluntary motion, does reduce movement to a minimum. The immobilization obtained by splints or traction does not begin to approximate the security and rigidity lent by adequate immobilization in plaster. The lymphatics, it is to be remembered, ramify in the fascias overlying the muscles. The importance of keeping muscles as quiet as is physically possible in phlegmonous inflammations is therefore understandable.

John Hilton, of Guy's Hospital in London, wrote a fascinating and informative treatise on Rest and Pain during the period of the Civil War in this country. Langenbeck suggested employment of windowed or bridged plaster casts in war wounds, and in the Franco-Prussian war, closed plaster casts were used by Ernst V. Bergmann in the treatment of gunshot wounds of joints, leaving the plasters on usually for about a period of a week. A short time later Dennis of New York (1884) pointed out the great value of immobilization in plaster in the treatment of compound fractures. With the advent of general acceptance of antiseptic and aseptic practices, this conservative plan fell largely into disuse, being replaced by more energetic technics (irrigations, et cetera), by the sur-

226

geon. Impressed with the futility of chemical wound management in localizing infection, Orr of Lincoln adopted rigid immobilization in plaster as a constant sequel to sequestrectomy for chronic osteomyelitis, shortly thereafter employing closed plaster casts and the massive vaseline pack together with extensive osteotomy as well, in the management of acute osteomyelitis.

Elevation

It soon became apparent that employment of elevation was a valuable addition to this mode of treatment of acute infections—particularly when the inflammation concerned the soft tissues. Increased relief of pain and quicker reduction of swelling were noted. Institution of rigid immobilization in a body cast with the extremity concerned in marked elevation occasionally made incision for the evacuation of exudate in soft tissues superfluous. Not uncommonly a single short incision sufficed in instances where one had anticipated doing considerably more. In paronychias where there is no hazard of dissemination of the infection, continuous steep elevation of the arm and hand on a suitable bed-side splint has been carried out with encouraging evidence of subsidence of the infection.

It is apparent that the patient must lie upon his back in order to secure the greatest elevation. If he sits up in bed, elevation of the lower extremity can not be obtained. (Incidentally, Fowler's position is much over-used by surgeons. I rarely employ it.) Raising the foot of the bed on a shock frame is a helpful means of obtaining elevation for the lower extremity when a body plaster is applied. For the thigh and leg the placement of staples in the cast permit it to be suspended at a steep angle by means of an overhead bed frame.* The upper extremity can be positioned easily in a condition favorable for lymph flow.

Hot Packs and Bier's Hyperemia

It is apparent that encasement of an extremity

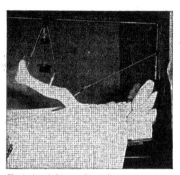

Fig. 2. A method for securing maximum elevation for an infection in the lower leg. When a body plaster cast is applied it is apparent that effectual elevation of the lower extremity can only be obtained by elevation of the foot of the bed.

therapeutic expedient has been lost thereby. The application of heat and employment of Bier's hyperemia are measures which increase swelling —objectives which, I have come to feel, are to be avoided in the treatment of acute pyogenic infections.

The experiments of Landis on capillary filtration throw considerable light on these matters. He has made direct measurements on capillary blood pressure and finds that a gradient in pressure obtains from the arterial to the venous end of the capillary. Mean capillary pressures at the base of the nail in man he found to be 45 cm. of water at the arterial end of the capillary loop and 22 cm. at the venous end. The ordinary colloid osmotic pressure of the blood in man is of the order of magnitude of 36 cms. of water. Measures which elevate capillary blood pressure therefore increase filtration into the tissues. Increases of venous pressure are directly reflected in the same degree in the capillary pressure. The swelling which occurs with dependency of an extremity or with the employment of heat or Bier's hyperemia is, therefore, readily understandable. The capillary injury which attends infection also results in increased permeability and augmented filtration of fluid. The only manner in which the tissues can limit filtration is through sufficient accumulation of

in plaster affords little opportunity for the application of heat. In consequence, I have come to neglect its use and can not feel that a worthwhile

*I do not believe that maximum elevation of the lower extremity should be employed for long periods of time, particularly in older people. In the erect posture a patient with normal vessels has a blood pressure in his dorsalis pedis artery of 100 mm. Hg or more over that of the arm at heart level. The lower extremity therefore is not well accommodated to the lowering of systolic pressure which attends great elevation. However, fairly steep elevation is well tolerated and the warmth of the toes is a good indication of an adequate circulation. Elevation decreases venous pressure as well as systolic pressure—both of which in turn lower capillary pressure and decrease filtration. Parenthetically, I might add here, that it may prove that free use of the erect posture (which increases the hydrostatic force of systolic blood pressure) may be the best means of forcing blood through arteriosclerotic vessels before circulatory inadequacy sets in.

fluid to produce a high tissue tension which tends to keep the fluid in the vessels.

Agencies such as Bier's hyperemia, which

extends to the knee on the opposite leg. A window is cut in the plaster over the tender area. Only when there is evidence of a subcutaneous

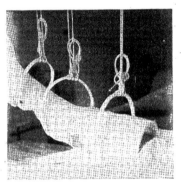

Fig. 3. This patient had a swelling of long standing attending a compound fracture. The reduction in swelling following elevation of the swollen member is evidenced in the separation evident between cast and upper surface of the thigh.

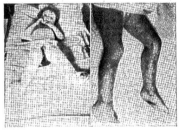

Fig. 4. (*left*) Second degree burn of the extremities encased in a plaster cast with sterile vaselinized shirting over the burned areas. (*right*) The situation one month later on removal of the cast; the burned area is nicely healed. Before the application of the cast the patient complained considerably of pain; following encasement in plaster the patient could be turned and managed without difficulty.

cause increases in venous pressure, probably abet the infectious process for it is well known that areas of swelling are predisposed to inflammation. Under increases of venous pressure lymph production is also increased. Great elevation of an injured or infected member above heart level will not suffice to prevent increased filtration in a damaged capillary bed. Yet with lymph outflow being favored by steep elevation it is apparent that swelling will be minimal unless the increased filtration is great. In the reduction of swellings of long standing in extremities as occur in malunited fracture and chronic inflammations of many varieties, I have come to feel that an inch of gravity operating for three days, will accomplish as much as three weeks of heat and massage.

Technic

I have elsewhere described in some detail' the mode of management. Here, for purposes of clarity, I only wish to mention briefly the manner in which instances of acute osteomyelitis and suppurative arthritis have been treated.

A patient with an acute osteomyelitis of the tibia is encased in a body plaster with a long leg cast on the side of the lesion. A short leg cast

abscess is an incision made. In one instance (lower femur) because of persistence of severe pain despite immobilization and elevation, a single hole was made in the bone with a small gimlet before evidence of a subcutaneous abscess became apparent. Plasters are worn for a variable period, but usually until the skin is healed or drainage is minimal. As soon as the patient is afebrile, he is encouraged to move his extremity.

In suppurative arthritis, a body cast is applied similarly. A window of appropriate size is cut to permit aspiration of the joint (knee). If the temperature is not favorably influenced by daily aspiration of the exudate, short vertical incisions are made on either side of the patella after two or three days. A small rubber tube drain is placed down to the capsule. In order to secure the benefit of gravity drainage, the patient must lie on his face for several hours a day. Drainage is established for suppurative arthritis of the hip joint as soon as pus is obtained by aspiration. (Ober's posterior incision). Positioning in the cast to facilitate drainage is also important. Sulphanilamide may be given to advantage, for a large proportion of joint infections are streptococcal. The patient is encouraged to move his extremity as soon as he is afebrile. When movement in the plaster causes no pain and does not

228

produce fever, the cast should be removed and a wider range of motion encouraged.

Conclusions

The rôle of the surgeon in the management of acute infections of the extremities has been reviewed. It is pointed out that his chief objective should be to assist the natural defense mechanism of the body in overcoming or localizing the infection. Other than that his function is that of a pus evacuator—to incise an abscess when suppuration occurs.

The great virtue of rigid immobilization and elevation of the affected member in infection is described. It should be the aim of the surgeon to keep the infected extremity as quiet as physically possible; in addition he should, through

employment of elevation, strive to keep swelling at a minimum. The attainment of these objectives serve the natural defense mechanism of the body in a most helpful manner.

Bibliography

1. Bergmann, E.: Die Resultate der Gelenkrescetionen im Krieg nach Eigenen Erfahrungen. St. Petersburg: Carl Ricker, 1874.
2. Dennis, F. S.: Treatment of compound fractures; 154 cases without a death from septic infection, and 100 cases with no death from any cause. Jour. A.M.A., 2:673, 1884.
3. Hilton, J.: Rest and Pain. A course of lectures on the influence of mechanical and physiological rest in the treatment of accidents and surgical diseases and the diagnostic value of pain. Second edition. New York: Wm. Wood and Co., 1879.
4. Keen, W. W.: The Treatment of War Wounds. Second edition. Philadelphia: Wm. B. Saunders Co., 1918.
5. Landis, E. M.: Capillary pressure and capillary permeability. Physiol. Rev., 14:404, 1934.
6. Orr, H. W.: The treatment of osteomyelitis and other infected wounds by drainage and rest. Surg., Gyn. and Obst., 45:446, 1927.
7. Wangensteen, O. H.: The rôle of the surgeon in the treatment of acute pyogenic infection. Wisc. Med. Jour., (In press).

THE IMMEDIATE AND SUBSEQUENT TREATMENT OF BURNS

RAYMOND F. HEDIN, M.D.[†]

Chicago, Illinois

IN THE past twelve years much progress has been made in the treatment of burns. Davidson's[12] discovery that tannic acid applied to burns formed a crust was outstanding in this field of surgery. Since then, the treatment of burns has been based on the surgical principle of making a "closed surface out of an open surface," without injury to tissue and consistent with early functional and cosmetic results.

In reviewing the literature on burns one finds the articles divided into two groups: those dealing with the factors involving the mortality and morbidity and those dealing with the treatment and care of burns. One is impressed with the controversy as to whether or not the morbidity and mortality in burns are due to toxic absorption or to the loss of vital body fluids. Robertson and Boyd[24] showed that toxic symptoms would be produced in eight hours if a normal animal were grafted with burned skin. Other investigators[20] have found that iodides are absorbed through burned surfaces. Rosenthal[25] reports that following burns there is a histamine-like substance in the blood stream capable of lowering blood pressure and causing a guinea pig's uterus to contract in Ringer's solution.

Kapsinow[16] doubts that toxins can be absorbed through burned surfaces, as he was unable to find such evidence when phenolsulphonphthalein or strychnine was applied to the burned site. Blalock,[11] Underhill, Kapsinow, and Fiske[26] have shown that body fluids are lost through burned surfaces and that there is a concentration of fluids in the tissue surrounding burns. They point out that the so-called primary and secondary shocks following burns are due respectively to alteration in the relative and actual blood volume. The most convincing evidence seems to militate against the toxic absorption theory, although both factors may be involved. In this paper an attempt will be made to outline the immediate and subsequent treatment of burns as practiced in the Children's Surgical Ward of the Cook County Hospital.

Tannic acid was used during the years 1934-1936 inclusive. During this period 395 patients were admitted for burns. Twelve of these died within twenty-four hours after the accident; eight died in the second twenty-four hour period and nineteen died after forty-eight hours, making a total of thirty-nine deaths or a mortality rate of approximately 10 per cent. It is obvious that statistics on burns are difficult to evaluate because of the many factors involved,

[†]Former Resident in Surgery, Cook County Hospital, and at present Resident in Surgery, Wesley Memorial Hospital, Chicago, Illinois.

namely: the cause, location, extent, degree, and the time the treatment is begun. The above figures are given to show the number of cases treated and the accompanying high mortality rate rather than to offer anything of statistical value.

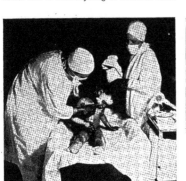

Fig. 1. Method of debridement and careful, thorough cleansing prior to application of tannic acid-silver nitrate.

The deaths from burns as well as the cases requiring protracted hospitalization resulted chiefly from matches, coffee-pot and tea-kettle accidents. Many of these pitiful and tragic results, no doubt, could have been avoided if only a few precautions had been taken and if there had been a greater realization of the consequences of burns. From an economic standpoint it is easy to conceive how the financial status of a family with a moderate income could be completely shattered by such an accident requiring sometimes months of hospitalization.

Gentian violet has not been used because it has the disadvantage of staining everything with which it comes in contact and so adds to the nursing problem. Furthermore, the coagulum often cracks, thus allowing organisms to enter the burned area.

Picric acid preparations produce toxic symptoms when absorbed from extensive burned surfaces. Like gentian violet, it fails to form a firm, adherent crust. These objections prompted our use of tannic acid for the treatment of burns on our service.

From January, 1937, until October, 1937, the tannic acid-silver nitrate treatment of Bettman[2] was used in eighty-two consecutive cases. Two

patients died during the first twenty-four period; one died in the second twenty-four hours and three died after forty-eight hours, making a total of six deaths in eighty-two cases, or a mortality rate of 7.3 per cent.

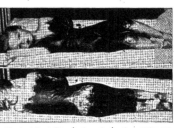

Fig. 2. (Above) Extensive burn showing the coagulum produced by the application of tannic acid-silver nitrate. Photograph taken two hours after accident. Note the apparent comfort of the patient. (Below) Posterior view of the patient.

It is the writer's opinion that the claims made by Bettman[2,3,4,5] are correct and the treatment should enjoy more widespread use. The important claims which have been substantiated by our own observations are:

1. The patient is safely carried over the critical first twenty-four hour period by the rapid tanning of the burned area which prevents the loss of body fluids.

2. Infection is prevented by the rapid drying of the tanned tissues.

3. The patient is made more comfortable.

4. The nursing problem is simplified, especially in the first twenty-four hours.

5. A thin, flexible coagulum is formed (Fig. 2a, 2b).

6. The kidneys and other organs are saved from the effects of fluid concentration and the absorption of toxins and infection.

7. The burned areas heal quickly, thereby shortening the period of hospitalization.

Immediate Treatment

Whether or not the patient is in a state of shock is of primary concern. The treatment of shock supersedes the treatment of the burns. Shock following burns is best treated by the judicious use of morphine, maintenance of body temperature, the administration of oral and parenteral fluids, and blood transfusion. Following

236

the improvement in the patient's general condition, the treatment to be used on the burned areas depends chiefly on the time that has elapsed since the accident and the gross contamination of the burned surface. If eight or ten hours have elapsed and the surface is so contaminated with grease, dirt, and clothing that it is likely that infection will result, then the burned areas had best be treated with moist saline dressings in an endeavor to promote drainage and sterilize the surface so that an early skin graft may be instituted. If the patient responds quickly to shock therapy and it is felt that the burned surface can be rendered clean, the treatment then is the same as if the patient had been seen immediately following the accident.

If the patient does not have symptoms or findings of shock, morphine is given in sufficient quantity to control pain and restlessness. In this regard, the respiratory rate serves as a reliable guide as to the dosage. The thorough cleansing of the patient at this time is of vital concern and negligence in this important step of the care predisposes to failure. To best attain this end, the disrobed patient is placed in a bath-tub which has a suspended false bottom (Fig. 1), which allows the escape of contaminated water into the tub drain. With this arrangement sterile sheets are placed under the patient, replacing soiled ones when necessary. In carrying out this cleansing bath, the surgeon and assistants wear caps, masks, gowns and gloves. Every effort is made to prevent the further contamination of an already contaminated field.

Benzine or other fat solvents are used to remove grease that usually has been applied to the burns before the patient enters the hospital. The patient is then given a thorough cleansing with white soap and sterile water. White soap has the advantage over green soap in being less irritating to the tissues (Koch).[18] The loose burned tissue is carefully removed and blebs are opened. The controversy[27] on the rationale of opening blebs is of long standing. We believe that to open the blebs and tan the underlying surface precludes the danger of future rupture and infection of blebs incident to nursing care. This cleansing process often requires an hour of meticulous care and patience to render the unfortunate victim grossly clean. Much depends upon this detail in the successful treatment of burns.

Following the thorough cleansing, the patient is placed in bed on a sterile sheet. The burned areas are then dried with an ordinary electric hair dryer in preparation for the tanning. At this time it is well to inspect carefully the sur-

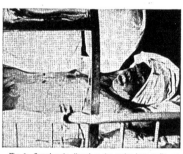

Fig. 3. Coagulum is allowed to dry under heat cradle covered by sterile sheet.

faces because a definite idea may be gained as to the depths of the burns. A dull, grayish surface usually means destruction below the dermal layer which foretells a long hospitalization. However, as Davidson[12] pointed out, because of the loss of fluids the surface area involved is of more importance than the depth in the immediate treatment of burns. Berkow[1] has computed the surface area of the body as follows:

a. Trunk 40%
b. Lower extremities 38%
c. Upper extremities 16%
d. Head 6%

Underhill and his co-workers have shown that a patient weighing 150 pounds with one-sixth of the surface burned, may lose 3500 c.c. of blood serum in the first twenty-four hours. For this reason the quicker the "open surface can be made into a closed surface" the better for the patient. With the use of tannic acid followed by silver nitrate, as described by Bettman, this end may be accomplished in a few minutes.

When the surface is dried, a freshly made aqueous solution of 5 per cent tannic acid is sprayed on the surface by means of an atomizer. Immediately after the single spray, silver nitrate in 10 per cent solution is applied to the surface by means of cotton pledgets. There is very little pain during this procedure. A firm, adherent, flexible crust results almost immediately. The patient is then placed under a heat cradle (Fig. 3), covered by a sterile sheet and taken to his room. Light bulbs may be added to the heat

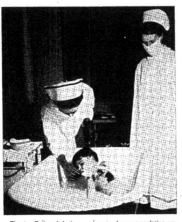

Fig. 4. Daily tub baths are given to cleanse granulating surfaces of pus and débris in preparing them for skin grafts.

cradle to maintain the temperature at a constant level. Occasionally the patient is placed on a Bradford frame to facilitate subsequent nursing. In this event the frame is covered with sterile sheets.

If there is a widespread surface area burned, a substantial blood transfusion is given routinely. Like Gunn and Hillsman,[15] we believe that when there has been any oozing prior to the tanning, whole blood offers the patient the greatest benefit. The taking of oral fluids is encouraged and parenteral fluids are given as indicated. The most reliable criterion as to the adequate fluid intake is the urinary output. In a child if the output is 500 c.c. to 750 c.c. daily, the intake is adequate. In an adult 750 c.c. to 1000 c.c. usually indicates sufficient fluid intake. Of value in this regard is the erythrocyte count and hemoglobin reading, which may be elevated due to the relative or actual blood concentration.

Shortly after the crust is formed, the patient is comfortable (Fig. 2a, 2b) and will need no further medication to control pain and restless-

ness. It is indeed a pleasure to see patients in such comfort and tranquillity of mind in contrast to the agonies shown prior to being treated. The most amazing thing is that the transition has taken place in such a short space of time. The necessary nursing care is reduced to a minimum and is in direct contrast with the treatment required when tannic acid is used alone and when spraying is needed every fifteen minutes for twelve hours.

It has been suggested that argyria may result from absorption but it has not been observed in our series of cases.

The eyelids are the only region not treated with tannic acid and silver nitrate. It would be impractical to splint the eyelids with the coagulum and in these regions bland ointments are best.

Minor burns lend themselves well to the tannic acid-silver nitrate treatment and can effectively be treated in the home or office.

Subsequent Treatment

Daily urine examinations are made in all burn cases. Albuminuria is rarely found even in the most extensive burns. A careful examination of the crust is made daily to ascertain any retention of pus. The temperature chart and leukocyte count forewarn of infection. If no infection develops, the crusts loosen and may be removed in two or three weeks, leaving behind a completely healed surface. If pus is found along the edges or anywhere under the crust, the overlying covering is immediately cut away, in order to prevent the undermining of the entire coagulum. Moist saline dressings are applied to these areas to promote adequate drainage. These dressings are moistened and changed as often as necessary. Care at this stage may save the remainder of the covered areas from becoming infected.

Should the entire surface become infected, in spite of all the previously mentioned precautions, the patient (Fig. 4) is placed in a clean bathtub and the crusts are gently removed by soaking in warm water to which soda has been added. When this unfortunate and not infrequent complication occurs, an attempt is made to get the surface in a suitable condition for an early skin graft. This objective is gained by giving the patient daily soaks in a bath-tub, at which time the dressings are soaked off less painfully, and the infected areas are carefully cleansed of pus and debris. Moist saline dressings are then applied. Blair and Brown[8] have stated that they arouse the fighting forces of the surrounding tissue, provide adequate drainage and allay pain. Great care is taken in applying these dressings. Moistened strips of fine meshed gauze are placed next to the infected surface. The fine pattern of this gauze prevents granulations from growing up through the mesh.[17] In this way the granulations are preserved rather than traumatized and there is no bleeding encountered when the dressings are changed. This smooth covering of fine meshed gauze is then covered by dressings moistened with saline. They are evenly applied and are thick enough to prevent soiling. Rubber tubing in which holes have been cut may be incorporated in the dressing and sterile saline may be instilled. Care is taken to see that the dressings do not dry in place. They should be moistened sufficiently to be absorbent. Excessively wet dressings cause the surrounding tissues to become macerated. Firm, even pressure is maintained by moistened soft, sea sponges which are held in place by wide bandages. Adhesive tape and safety pins are so placed that the dressings are comfortable and will remain firm and stationary. Where a moving part is involved, such as the back, chest and abdomen, a wide elastic bandage tends to hold the dressing well in place.

Antiseptics are not used on granulating surfaces because they are irritating and tend to destroy the tissue. However, when necrotic tissue covers the infected area, freshly made Dakin's solution is used in place of saline for a few days. This results in a rapid separation of the necrotic tissues.[19] Vaseline and other ointments are not used on granulating surfaces because they do not give the stimulation afforded by a moist saline dressing. Vaseline dressings prevent adequate drainage by allowing pus to accumulate on the infected surface.

Whenever dressings are changed great care is exercised in not introducing new organisms on the surface. It was our experience during March, 1937, that five out of seven burn cases developed fever and pus on relatively clean surfaces. All of these cases had been cared for by an attendant who was suffering from a pharyngitis. The importance of adequate masking has been properly stressed by Meleney,[21] Davis,[14] and others.

Throughout the period that the granulation tissues are being prepared for a skin graft, every effort is made to build up the patient's general physical condition. Precautions should be taken against exposure to upper respiratory infections which are so prevalent during winter and spring months.[21] A palatable, nourishing diet is beneficial. When the healing powers of the patient seem to be at a stand-still, blood transfusions[23] often provide the necessary impetus to hasten recovery.

As Blair and Brown[7] have so excellently stated, "skin grafting must be early, quick, permanent and conserve health, comfort, function, time and money." The proper time to cover the granulation surfaces with a skin graft is based on the patient's general physical condition and the condition of the site to be grafted. The patient must be able to withstand a short, general anesthetic. It should be felt that the healing potentialities will, with a degree of certainty, assure a "take" of the graft. The granulation surfaces should appear bright red, indicating their splendid vascularity. They should be flat and firm.[22] Bacterial counts are not made because such procedures are indefinite and offer little clinical information. The surrounding tissue should not be red and indurated. When granulations are dull, grayish red in color and appear to be exuberant, jelly-like, with a large amount of drainage, they do not lend themselves to successful skin grafting and had best be further prepared.

Type of Graft

The best type of graft to employ should be one that will most quickly convert the open granulating surface into a closed surface with the best functional and cosmetic results. The graft that best fulfills these requirements, in the majority of cases, is the Blair split-graft of intermediate thickness. This type of graft is easily and quickly obtained in sizes large enough to cover completely the granulating surfaces. It is of uniform thickness, which adds to the cosmetic results. The fact that this type of graft includes a substantial portion of the corium prevents it from contracting, thereby giving a good functional result. The donor site heals readily without scarring. With this graft the "take" is remarkably good on surfaces that are only relatively clean.

Ollier-Thiersch grafts include a very small portion of the corium and although the "take" is usually excellent, because of their thinness, they offer little protection. Also, on a movable surface they may contract up to as much as 60 per cent of their original size. Then too, they are not any easier nor any quicker to obtain than the split-graft of intermediate thickness.

Reverdin grafts include the epidermis with a very small portion of the corium. They are placed on the granulating surface as islands with the hope that epithelization will take place and connect them. They fail to close the surface completely.

Davis'[18] small, thick grafts include varying thicknesses in each graft. Because of the technic by which they are obtained (cutting the base of a piece of skin that has been elevated by a needle) they are of full thickness in the center and thin at the periphery. Like the Reverdin graft, they are but islands on the site to be grafted and fail to make a complete covering. To place the islands on a large, granulating surface by this type of graft is time-consuming. This type of graft, when healed, gives a spotty appearance because of the uneven thickness. The donor site, from which these grafts are taken, is left with punched-out scars which also give an unsightly appearance.

"Seed" grafts almost invariably become smothered by exuberant granulation tissue.

Full thickness grafts and pedunculated flaps[10] are not suitable for granulating surfaces. They are best utilized in reconstructive surgery, as in freeing contractions, where fresh, raw surfaces are made.

The split graft of intermediate thickness with its advantages, as stated above, has, in our hands, been the most effective in covering defects resulting from burns. The technic of the use of this type of graft on our service at Cook County Hospital is outlined as follows:

A general anesthetic is given.

Selection of Donor Site

A site is chosen that will provide the adequate amount of skin to cover the defect. The skin is usually taken from the outer or inner surfaces of the thighs. When these surfaces are unavailable the buttocks or abdomen are used. The skin on the back does not lend itself well for grafting. It should be borne in mind that hair may continue to grow if the grafts are taken from a region containing hair. The donor site must be free of any infection. Furuncles, paronychia and other infections, even some distance removed from the field of surgery, may cause infection and destroy the hope for a successful graft.

Preparation of Donor Site

The surface is gently washed with white soap and water, using coarse cotton to cleanse mechanically the site. This preparation requires ten minutes or longer and care is taken not to traumatize the skin by too vigorous rubbing. Antiseptics are not used in this preparation as they destroy tissue.

Preparation of Receptor Site

The receptor site is also prepared with white soap and sterile water. When the surrounding tissues are washed, the granulations are covered so as not to submit them to undue contamination. The granulations are gently washed, care being taken not to cause trauma. The granulations down to the capillary layer, as well as indurated edges immediately around the site, are removed by means of a razor. In this way the granulations are made flat and even. Firm pressure applied to a saline dressing controls hemostasis until the graft is applied. When persistent bleeders are encountered, they are ligated with fine silk. Curretting[9] of granulations to freshen the surface should not be done as the resulting surface is left ragged and uneven.

Skin Grafting

A thin film of xeroform ointment is spread over the donor site. A Blair knife and suction traction are used to remove the skin. Firm tension on both sides facilitates the cutting of the grafts (Fig. 5). An endeavor is made to cut grafts which will completely cover the defect and slightly overlap its borders. When the site to be covered is of such magnitude that many grafts are required, they are placed so that each graft is overlapped by its neighbor, making complete covering. A continuous horsehair suture is used to baste the graft down and hold it in place. When the surface is completely covered, several small holes are made in the graft by means of a sharp, pointed knife. This allows blood and serum to escape which might otherwise undermine the grafts. The entire graft

2. The tannic acid treatment of burns was used in 395 cases admitted to the Children's Surgical Ward at Cook County Hospital during the period 1934-1936 inclusive. There were thirty-nine deaths or a mortality rate of 10 per

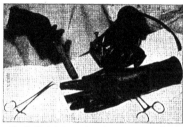

Fig. 5, Method of removing skin by means of Blair knife and suction traction.

cent, showing the disastrous consequences of burns.

3. In the nine month period beginning January 1, 1937, eighty-two consecutive cases of burns were treated by the tannic acid-silver nitrate method of Bettman. Our clinical observations confirm the claims made by Bettman for this therapy.

4. The importance of the initial cleansing with white soap and sterile water is stressed. When properly done this lessens the chances of subsequent infection.

5. Infection frequently complicates the treatment of burns. This is best dealt with by daily cleansing baths and moist dressings. The point is made that granulations are not traumatized when covered by a layer of fine meshed gauze. Sea sponges serve as the best means of applying mechanical pressure. With the intelligent use of these agents, infected granulations are quickly and effectively prepared for skin grafting.

6. The various types of skin grafts are briefly outlined. On our service the use of the split-graft of intermediate thickness, described by Blair and Brown, has proven to be the quickest and most effective method of providing a permanent and complete covering to a granulating surface.

7. The technic for using this type of graft is given. The importance of a firm pressure dressing over the area grafted is discussed.

.I wish to thank Dr. Sumner L. Koch, Dr. Gatewood, and Dr. E. M. Miller for their co-operation and instruction given me regarding the treatment of burns.

References

1. Berkow, S. G.: A method of estimating the extensiveness of lesions (burns and scalds) based on surface area proportions. Arch. Surg., 8:138, 1924.
2. Bettman, A. G.: The tannic acid-silver nitrate treatment of burns. Northwest Med., 34:46-51, 1935.
3. Idem. Tannic acid and silver nitrate in burns. Surg., Gynec. and Obst., 62, 2a:458-463, 1936.
4. Idem. The rationale of the tannic acid-silver nitrate treatment of burns. Jour. A.M.A., 108:1490-1494, 1937.
5. Idem. A simpler technic for promoting epithelization and protecting skin grafts. Jour. A.M.A., 97:1879-1881, 1931.
6. Blair, V. P.: The influence of mechanical pressure on wound healing. Ill. Med. Jour., 46:249-252, 1924.
7. Blair, V. P., and Brown, J. B.: Use and uses of large split-skin grafts of intermediate thicknesses. Tr. South. Surg. Assn., 41:409-424, 1928.
8. Idem. Use and uses of large split-skin grafts of intermediate thicknesses. Surg., Gynec. and Obst., 49:82-97, 1929.
9. Idem. The early care of burns and the repair of their defects. Jour. A.M.A., 98:1355, 1932.
10. Blair, V. P., and Brown, J. B., and Hamm, W. G.: The release of axillary and brachial scar fixation. Surg., Gynec. and Obst., 56:790-798, 1933.
11. Blalock, Alfred: Experimental shock vii. The importance of the local loss of fluid in the production of the low pressure after burns. Arch. Surg., 22:610-616, 1931.
12. Davidson, E. C.: Tannic acid in the treatment of burns. Surg., Gynec. and Obst., 41:202-221, 1925.
13. Davis, John S.: The small deep graft; development; relationship to the true Reverdin graft; technic. Tr. South. Surg. Assn., 41:395-408, 1928.
14. Idem. Is adequate masking essential for the patient's protection? Ann. Surg., 105:990-997, 1937.
15. Gunn, J., and Hillsman, J. A.: Thermal burns. Ann. Surg., 102:429-443, 1935.
16. Kapsinow, Robert: Poor absorption from burns, burn toxins doubtful. New Orleans Med. and Surg. Jour., 85:597, 1933.
17. Koch, Sumner L.: Injuries of the hand. Ky. State Med. Jour., 34:101-109, 1936.
18. Koch, Sumner L.: Personal communication.
19. Martin, J. D., and Fowler, C. D.: The germicidal effects of tannic acid. Ann. Surg., 99:993-996, 1934.
20. Mason, E. C., and Paxton, P., and Shoemaker, H. A.: A comparison of the rate of absorption from normal and burned tissues. Ann. Int. Med., 9:850-853, 1936.
21. Meleney, Frank L.: Infections in clean operative wounds, a nine year study. Surg., Gynec. and Obst., 60:264, 1935.
22. Orr, T. G.: Pressure as a factor in skin grafting. Ann. Surg., 76:799-800, 1922.
23. Robertson, B.: Blood transfusion in severe burns in infants and young children. Canadian M. A. Jour., 11:744, 1921.
24. Robertson, B., and Boyd, Gladys L.: The toxemia of severe superficial burns. Jour. Lab. and Clin. Med., 19:1-14, 1943.
25. Rosenthal, S. R.: Neutralization of histamine and burn toxin. Ann. Surg., 106:257-265, 1937.
26. Underhill, F. P., and Kapsinow, R., and Fiske, M. E.: Studies on mechanism of water exchange in animal organisms. Amer. Jour. Physiol., 95:315, 1930.
27. Willis, A., Murat: Value of debridement in treatment of burns. Jour. A.M.A., 84:655-658, 1925.

ERRORS IN THE DIAGNOSIS AND TREATMENT OF HYPERTHYROIDISM

ARNOLD S. JACKSON, M.D.

Madison, Wisconsin

THE basis of this paper is a study of one hundred cases incorrectly diagnosed as hyperthyroidism previous to our examination. In every instance, thyroidectomy had been advised for relief of symptoms, but in no case was it possible for us to corroborate the diagnosis of toxic goiter. In none of the one hundred patients was surgery performed nor has the need for such ever been established. This study was begun in 1929 so that in many cases at least five years have elapsed since the error in diagnosis was determined. Recently a follow-up letter showed that many had completely recovered and that none was suffering from hyperthyroidism. Most of the patients were cases of nervous and physical exhaustion.

Not long ago the reverse of this error in diagnosis was true. Advanced cases of hyperthyroidism long overlooked and long treated as cardiac, gastro-intestinal disorders and other conditions were brought to the surgeon for cure. Within two decades a goiter-ignorant profession has become very goiter-conscious in contrast to

the situation a few years ago when the textbooks and medical schools were vaguely informative on this subject. They variously classified goiter as outward, inward, cystic, calcareous, nodular, irregular, physiological, et cetera. It was generally believed and taught that iodine was contraindicated in exophthalmic goiter. This notion had become popular because Kocher reported ill effects from the widespread use of iodine in the treatment of goiter in Switzerland. The resulting condition was termed Iodine Basedow and since the latter's name and exophthalmic goiter were synonymous, it was felt that iodine might initiate or aggravate the disease.

Today we know that this is not the case and that iodine in the presence of adenomatous goiter may precipitate hyperthyroidism but not exophthalmic goiter, although some still refuse to admit it. When I presented this idea before the American Association for the Study of Goiter in 1924,[3,4] the subject was debated and the term "iodine hyperthyroidism" was criticized. Now, however, the literature generally supports this contention. In a recent study,[1] it was shown by Freeman and the writer that ir

*From the Jackson Clinic, Madison, Wisconsin. Presented before the Hennepin County Medical Society, Minneapolis, Minnesota, November 1, 1937.

236

a series of 279 cases of toxic adenoma, the disease was aggravated in 38 per cent by the use of iodine.

Much of this early confusion regarding the diagnosis and treatment of goiter has been clarified by the work of the American Association for the Study of Goiter, by Henry Plummer and others. Whereas twenty years ago there was not a satisfactory text on goiter, today there are several. Metabolism machines were unknown before the World War except in the scientific laboratory; today their use is widespread throughout the profession.

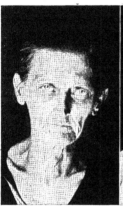 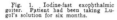 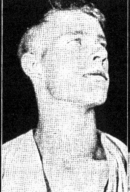 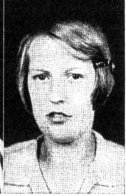

Fig. 1. Iodine-fast exophthalmic goiter. Patient had been taking Lugol's solution for six months.

Fig. 2. Colloid goiter diagnosed as hyperthyroidism elsewhere and thyroidectomy advised.

Fig. 3. Colloid goiter shows symmetrical enlargement of the thyroid gland. Thyroidectomy had been advised because of elevation of basal metabolic rate, nervousness and tremor.

As a result of this great increase in knowledge of thyroid disease, our diagnostic sense has become attuned to the point that long standing hyperthyroidism is becoming a rarity. The same is true of pronounced exophthalmos, thyroid crises, huge goiters, and other manifestations of neglect. Unfortunately, the pendulum is swinging too far and patients with possible incipient hyperthyroidism, nervous and physical exhaustion, and the menopause, are advised to have a thyroidectomy. Has not the time arrived to stop this? If one department of an institution can report one hundred such cases observed over a short period of time, the number sub-jected to needless thyroid surgery throughout the country each year must be considerable.

From a study of these one hundred cases, I would place the source of error in diagnosis on the following factors: inadequate knowledge of the differential diagnosis of true and pseudo-hyperthyroidism; failure to elicit essential facts in the history; inaccuracy of the metabolism test or its interpretation; neglect in observing important physical findings; failure to try the iodine test; and the mistake of considering thyroidectomy an emergency operation.

If the important facts in the history such as weight loss together with an increased appetite, weakness in the knees on climbing stairs, pounding of the heart even at rest, heat intolerance, and emotionalism are not obtained, one should hesitate to make a diagnosis of hyperthyroidism. If physical examination reveals a normal appearing thyroid gland, and the absence of a thrill or bruit, together with a normal pulse pressure, hyperthyroidism should be excluded. Yet the mere complaint of tightness in the neck, so typical of nervous and physical exhaustion, large eyes, a full neck, a coffee or nicotine tremor of the hands, and a history of palpitation and insomnia, often seem to be sufficient to warrant a diagnosis of hyperthyroidism. Various remedies such as thyroid therapy, iodine, salves, x-ray, radium, beads, injections, massage, and thyroidectomy are advised.

If doubt exists as to diagnosis final judgment is often reserved pending the outcome of the metabolism test. Such evidently was the case in fifty-seven of one hundred patients in this study since the rate had been reported above normal. In one instance, the rate was said to have been plus 94 per cent. In another it was reported to have been plus 55 per cent, yet our metabolism studies in all these cases indicated a normal condition of the thyroid gland.

The metabolism test is responsible for many errors in diagnosis. The test may be inaccurate because the machine is obsolete or has leaks, or because the technician errs, or, most important, its interpretation may be incorrect. Food, rapid breathing, fever, and nervousness are other factors which lead to error. If the patient's nose is tightly pinched with a clip, he will breathe too rapidly and the test will register higher than it would under normal conditions. This frequent source of error is generally overlooked.

One should not allow his judgment to be misled by any metabolic report. Last week I saw a middle aged woman who had recorded a test of over plus 25 per cent on three occasions. This was similar to her record at another laboratory, yet I feel certain that the patient is not hyperthyroid. Certainly surgery is not indicated on the mere basis of these reports. This patient was sent home for a month's rest. If she is hyperthyroid, it will soon become evidenced by a loss of weight, increase in the pulse pressure and elevation of the metabolic rate. That will be sufficient time to think of surgery.

Two years ago a patient came from New York City to consult about a goiter operation which he had been advised to have. Much to his surprise and apparent disappointment, his thyroid gland was found to be normal and he was told that he did not need an operation, but was advised to have more recreation such as golf. Recently he wrote, "Following your advice, I have taken up golf, feeling at the time that I was more or less swapping goiter for golf. After the game I played today, I am not so sure I wouldn't just as soon have the goiter."

Before seeing a patient, certain points in the history are helpful in determining a diagnosis.

test is plus 30 per cent or more, what should be done? The patient may be given an iodine test for ten days and if exophthalmic goiter is present, there should be a gain in weight and a lowering of the rate. As a further check, the iodine may be stopped, thereby aggravating the symptoms. That should be sufficient evidence to warrant a diagnosis of hyperthyroidism and surgical treatment.

Unfortunately our errors in the diagnosis of hyperthroidism are not easily detected by the pathologist. In looking through his microscope, he is unable to tell us whether or not an adenomatous goiter is toxic or non-toxic. Moreover since the advent of Lugol's solution, an exophthalmic goiter which has been saturated with iodine may have all the gross and microscopic appearances of a colloid goiter. Careful search will usually reveal small areas of hyperplasia and infolding of the epithelium.

Errors in the treatment of hyperthyroidism are frequently attended with diastrous consequences. In spite of everything that has been said and written about the danger of the prolonged use of iodine in exophthalmic goiter, iodine-fast cases are still coming to surgery. The risk of operation is such that I seldom attempt anything but a two-stage thyroidectomy on these patients. Recently I had occasion to regret attempting even this much and, if given a second choice, would resort to a ligation, a procedure which I abandoned in 1925.

Since two out of three cases of toxic adenoma will improve on iodine, it should be given preoperatively as a routine. The cases not benefited will be only slightly affected in the short period of preparation.

Operative and postoperative complications such as laryngeal nerve paralysis, tetany, hemorrhage, pneumonia, and tracheitis will be lessened by the use of superficial cervical nerve block anesthesia. I have seen several fatalities which occurred following thyroidectomy for exophthalmic goiter where either through ignorance or mistake the patient was given insufficient amounts of iodine or none at all. This statement is made despite a recent article to the contrary by Davison and Aries.[1] A study of this treatise will show that they were apparently dealing in several instances with cases of toxic adenoma rather than exophthalmic

goiter. The postoperative use of iodine is of but small consequence in toxic adenomas. In 1923 I showed that iodine in considerable amounts was important in the immediate postoperative treatment of exophthalmic goiter in order to combat hyperthyroidism. In the treatment of a considerable group of cases since that time I have seen nothing to alter this opinion.

Toxic adenomas rarely recur following subtotal thyroidectomy, but the average rate of recurrence for exophthalmic goiter throughout the country is probably about 10 per cent. This is largely due to failure to remove sufficient hyperplastic tissue at the time of operation and lack of proper postoperative care. Iodine should be continued in small amounts for three months; coffee and other stimulants should be prohibited; there should be a return to normal weight within three months after thyroidectomy; activity should be somewhat restricted, and relaxation should be stressed. The progress of recovery should be gauged by metabolic tests. Observance of these factors will tend to curtail the number of disappointing end-results of surgery.

In conclusion, I believe that this report of one hundred cases of error in diagnosis emphasizes the importance of a careful study of patients suspected of having hyperthyroidism. Thyroidectomy should not be considered until such conditions as nervous and physical exhaustion have been eliminated, and hyperthyroidism has been proved to exist. Possible errors in metabolism studies must not be overlooked, and the iodine test should be tried in doubtful cases. Finally, I believe that the diagnosis of hyperthyroidism is a continual challenge to us as physicians and surgeons, and, in order to maintain our highest ideals, thyroid surgery should be performed only when it is truly indicated.

References

1. Davison, M., and Aries, L. J.: The fallacy of the use of iodine immediately after bilateral subtotal thyroidectomy. Surg., Gynec. and Obst., 64:999-1001, (June) 1937.
2. Jackson, Arnold S., and Freeman, H. E.: The effect of iodine in adenomatous goiter. Jour. Am. Med. Assn., 106: 1261-1263, (April 11) 1936.
3. Jackson, Arnold S.: Preoperative treatment of patients with exophthalmic goiter with special reference to Lugol's solution of iodine. Am. Jour. Surg., 37:315-316, (Dec.) 1923.
4. Jackson, Arnold S.: Lugol's solution of iodine in exophthalmic goiter. Internatl. Jour. Med. and Surg., 37.:131-134, (Apr.) 1924.

SOME ATTEMPTED LEGISLATIVE SOLUTIONS TO THE PROBLEMS OF MEDICAL CARE*

THOMAS V. McDAVITT

Bureau of Legal Medicine and Legislation, American Medical Association

Chicago, Illinois

I T IS apparent that concerted efforts are being made in the United States to establish forms of medical practice totally at variance with the individualized practice of medicine, which has produced in this country a system of medical care unmatched elsewhere—unmatched not only in its scientific excellence but also in the universality of its distribution.

Some of the particular factors to which American medicine owes its eminence are obvious. We know, for instance, that individual initiative, unhampered by bureaucratic or political control, together with a reasonable prospect for making a decent livelihood for self and dependents, is an essential of scientific achievement in medicine as in all other fields of service. We know, also, that the relation of physician and patient has played a part of incalculable value because the practice of medicine is, and probably always will be, an art as well as a science. It will not, it can not, render its greatest benefit if it becomes merely a cold, calculating, impersonal application of scientific truths or half truths. Yet the legislative proposals made to change the form of medical practice would do away with these very essentials.

Let no one assume, because of the variety of proposals advanced, that American medicine has failed, that a vast proportion of our people are without adequate care, and that even an appreciable portion of the people are dissatisfied with the job American medicine has done and is doing. The fact, however, that there is really no public demand for change and that the revolutionary proposals emanate from a numerically insignificant, interested minority does not mean that there is no possibility of change occurring. Most unfortunately, in some respects, we are passing through such a tumultuous period of change in social concepts that legislative panaceas are advanced and accepted almost blindly without the consideration and the finer weighing of values that attend more normal times.

*Read before the County Officers' meeting, Saint Paul, Minnesota, February 26, 1938.

The proposals of change are so numerous and varied in type that only a few of the apparently more important can be discussed. This discussion, therefore, will be limited to a consideration of three general types of proposals or activities, contemplated or initiated: (1) compulsory health insurance; (2) legislation to permit corporations or other lay groups or individuals to engage in the practice of medicine; and (3) what for want of a better phrase may be termed invasion of the field of the private practice of medicine by governmental agencies.

Compulsory Health Insurance

Notwithstanding the agitation for compulsory health insurance by some students of the social welfare problem for the past twenty-five years or so, no state legislature was presented with a concrete proposal until after the Association for Social Security, Inc., Abraham Epstein, Secretary, brought forth late in 1934 a so-called model state bill for health insurance. This bill is believed to embody the general outline, at least, of any scheme for compulsory health insurance that will be pressed for consideration in state legislatures, for some time to come.

This bill, with certain minor amendments, was introduced but failed of enactment in 1935 in the legislatures of five states, in 1936 in two states, in 1937 in five states and the United States Senate, and so far in 1938 in three states.

Bills proposing systems of compulsory health insurance, founded largely on the Epstein philosophy but differing somewhat on details, were considered and killed in two states both in 1935 and 1937.

The so-called model health insurance bill in short proposes to create in each state a health insurance fund, to which all employees to whom the compulsory features of the bill apply, together with their employers and the state, would pay a total of 6 per cent of the wages paid and received. A person electing voluntarily to come under the act and the state would contribute a sum equal up to 6 per cent of the person's income, the percentage varying according to the benefits desired. The fund thus created would be used to supply to the worker and his dependents all manner of medical, hospital, dental and nursing services and the services of specialists, laboratories and clinics for preventive, diagnostic and therapeutic care.

The bill also provides for other benefits, such as the payment of cash during disability, but these will not be here discussed.

The compulsory features of the bill apply to *all* employees *except* (1) persons employed at other than manual labor and receiving in excess of $60 a week in *wages;* (2) farm laborers, and (3) domestic servants. Almost any person whose net *income* is not over $100 weekly and who is not covered by the compulsory provisions may for himself and dependents elect to come under the Act. The medical benefits may also be available to persons receiving old age or unemployment benefits.

Estimates as to what percentage of the population all of the groups just enumerated would constitute run from 70 to 95 per cent.

Some reference must be made to the administrative set-up of the bill for it ignores organized medicine and would seem to leave the individual physician and even the medical profession in a most impotent position without any authority in the administration of the law and powerless against the dictates and encroachments of political caprice.

The supreme administrative authority is a State Health Insurance Commission of five members, only one of whom would be representative of what the bill designates as the "Professions" and this representative, appointed by a political governor, might as well within the terms of the bill be a nurse, a pharmacist, a dentist, a hospital manager, as a physician. Acting in only an advisory capacity to this commission are a State General Advisory Council and a State Medical Advisory Council, on neither of which is the medical profession afforded adequate representation.

The act would be administered in local areas through local councils consisting of seven members, one of whom would be a local medical manager (an M.D.), the local health officer, and one representative of "the professions." With the exception of the local health officer, all members of the local council are to be appointed by

the lay-controlled State Health Insurance Commission.

A person entitled to medical benefits theoretically has the right to choose the general medical or dental practitioner he desires provided that practitioner is on a list of eligible practitioners compiled by the local council. The general practitioner chosen has the right to prescribe the specialist or laboratory or clinic services necessary for further treatment and the general practitioner or the specialist has the right to prescribe the necessary hospital treatment and nursing care, provided the persons or agencies selected are on the eligible list compiled by the local council. Every practitioner has the right to be included on such list. Names on the eligible list may be removed by the local council or by the State Health Insurance Commission, after written notice and hearing, "when in its operation continued inclusion in the list" would be prejudicial to the adequate, proper or efficient furnishing of the medical benefits." Whether the presence of this provision would prevent the arbitrary removal of a physician from the eligible list is debatable. A physician after a number of years of such practice and with a negligible private practice might well be at the mercy of political schemers.

The manner in which and extent to which persons and agencies on the eligible list would be recompensed could be fixed in each local area by the appropriate local council. In remunerating general medical and dental practitioners the local councils would be authorized to adopt either a salary system, a per capita system, a fee system, or any combination of the systems just enumerated. However, no system of remuneration could be inaugurated for any one local area unless a majority of the eligible general medical or dental practitioners, respectively, in that locality consented. This language means nothing, however, for it could be construed to mean a majority at the time the plan was adopted when a very few were on the eligible list and all subsequent additions would take subject to the existing plan.

The foregoing has been but a brief summary of such provisions of the Epstein bill as affect physicians. Without indulging in argument, it seems obvious that the long range effect of the enactment of such a measure would be to dilute and debase medical services to the public and eventually to eliminate the high caliber and high purpose of an independent medical profession, leaving in its stead a group of practitioners, not physicians in any connotation the word bears today. Whether or not this bill or any one founded on a similar philosophy will ever become law in any state is debatable. Compulsory health insurance bills, however, will appear before legislatures for some time to come.

Practice of Medicine by Corporations and Other Lay Associations and Persons

Another threat to the quality of medical services has been legislative proposals, the effect of which would be to permit corporations and other lay associations and persons to exploit the services of physicians in the distribution of medical services to the public.

The past ten years have seen the rise of proposals ostensibly endeavoring to utilize the insurance principle in the distribution of medical services. Presumably so long as these proposals contemplate cash payments to the beneficiaries in the event of sickness or disability in order that they may themselves pay physicians they themselves have selected free from outside dictation the medical profession faces no apparent danger. However, when the proposal is for the insurance company or the medical service association, or whatever it may be called, to undertake, in case of sickness or disability, to supply the services of physicians of their own choosing, the situation is radically different.

Almost unnoticed, beginning in 1934, nine states have enacted laws authorizing the formation of corporations to operate on a so-called non-profit basis hospital service plans. Generally, these laws authorize such corporations to accept periodical premiums from subscribers and in the event the subscriber becomes sick or disabled to supply, either themselves or through hospitals with whom they have contracted, necessary hospital services. Some danger is inherent in such laws unless the term "hospital services" is limited to actual hospital services and the law as so limited enforced. In actual operation some of the plans authorized by these laws have infringed on the practice of medicine to varying degrees. Such laws have been enacted in New York, Alabama, California, Illinois, Maryland, Massachusetts, Mississippi, Georgia, and Pennsylvania. Similar bills were before the Minne-

sota legislature in 1937* but failed of enac

Bills which expanded on the theory by posing to permit designated types of co tions and associations to operate hospita medical service plans, were before six stat islatures in 1937.† None of them was er

In some of our western states many similar to those just referred to have be operation for years. The plans have beer erally available only to workers in the e of stated corporations, industries, or g mental agencies and not to the public gen In some sections, medical societies hav tempted to operate similar plans because presence of commercial ventures in the On the whole, however, with a few notab ceptions, it would seem that even where plans are in operation, by commercial in or by medical societies, the public has not p ized them in appreciable numbers.

One of the most widely publicized attem a corporation to offer medical, surgical an pital services on an insurance basis is no curring in Washington, D. C., in the act of the Group Health Assn., Inc., which w recipient of an outright gift of $40,000 fr agency of the Federal Government, the Owners Loan Corporation.

According to its certificate of incorpo the corporation will render medical, surgic hospital services to every subscribing em and his dependents, of every branch United States government other than th sonnel of the army and navy. It began t pensing of medical care November 1, 193 by December 18, 1937, about 900 perso subscribed to the plan.

Responsible officials of the Home C Loan Corporation say officially that a gr its employees organized the corporation a the HOLC approved the scheme, believi the HOLC would stand to benefit by sick leaves if a complete so-called health could be arranged for its employees on of monthly pay deductions. Now as a of fact, the plan as it evolved embraced articles of incorporation are any criteri only employees of HOLC but all other mental agencies with the exceptions note

---

*S. 962, H. 1142.
†Calif. S. 121, A. 1283; S. 605, A. 1491; Ohio S. 20 Oklahoma H. 335; Ore. H. 281, H. 283; Wash. H. 38 Wis. A. 850.

s a matter of fact, the HOLC did considerably ore than approve the plan. It coöperated, if actually it did not instigate the whole business, and without the aid of the HOLC it probably could not have come into being.

In March, 1937, shortly after the corporation was organized, the HOLC entered into a contract with the Group Health Association by which the HOLC agreed to give $40,000 spread over more than a two year period to the association and the association agreed to operate a medical service plan that would include employees of HOLC and would provide by-laws satisfactory to HOLC, which by-laws would provide that two of the association's directors be named by the Federal Home Loan Bank Board and that those two directors would be members of an executive committee of five of the association's directors. Rather active approval. Now while the association did not begin to dispense its medical care until November 1, 1937, all the $40,000 had been handed over to the association prior to that time. This haste was due probably, at least in part, to a premonition that the appropriate Congressional committee which would pass on appropriations to the HOLC might not feel favorable to diversions of public funds of that sort. And so it developed. The theory by which the HOLC sought to justify this diversion of public funds met strong criticism from members of the subcommittee of the Committee of Appropriations, House of Representatives, in a hearing held on December 18, 1937, on the Independent Offices Appropriation bill for 1939, when this whole matter was under discussion.

In any event, it would seem that the activities of GHA are illegal for two reasons: (1) they constitute the practice of medicine by a corporation, which the law forbids; and (2) they constitute the doing of an insurance business without complying with the laws of the District of Columbia which permit insurance companies to operate only when licensed by the Superintendent of Insurance after complying with certain requirements of law, among which is a requirement of a deposit of certain funds. This conclusion was reached by the corporation counsel and by the district attorney of the District of Columbia. Furthermore, the Acting Comptroller General of the United States, Richard N. Elliott, on December 17, 1937, ruled that the HOLC

acted without authority of law in disbursing the $40,000 to the GHA.

There the matter now rests. Nevertheless the Group Health Association continues to operate in open defiance of law. Unless curbed, it can, if it expands to include all eligible persons, practically destroy the private practice of medicine in the District of Columbia. Whether it will do so and whether its activities will eventually encompass the United States, as they well can are questions that only the future can answer.

Practice of Medicine by Governmental Agencies

A third, and possibly the most menacing, threat to the private practice of medicine are proposals for the governmental assumption of some or all of the functions of the practice of medicine and the rendering to some or all of its citizens necessary medical care free of charge or at such reduced rates as will preclude the coexistence of an independent body of medical practitioners.

In the past we have seen the development of state medicine to a limited extent. Probably the expansion of state health departments in the field of preventive medicine, and the care afforded mental incompetents, the tuberculous, and to some of the poor can be so classified. In many states, also, state or county general hospitals are in operation and there has been a constant effort to expand such facilities and to enlarge on the classes of population eligible for treatment therein.

Proposals put to the legislatures and the Congress in the last few years and the actions sought to be authorized by governmental agencies are continually going further and further into the field of the practice of medicine. Consider, for instance, the Lewis bill introduced in the U. S. Senate July 22, 1937,* which sought to make all physicians civil officers of the Federal Government, to require them to attend any "impoverished individual" on request and to authorize them to make such charges as "are just and reasonable," which charges were to be paid by the Social Security Board. That bill is still pending but is believed to have no chance whatsoever of enactment.

Reference should be made here to the rendition of the services contemplated by the Federal

*S. J. Res. 188.

Social Security Act, namely, care for crippled children, maternal and child health services, and state and public health services. Fortunately the services contemplated have been rendered to date in a most ethical manner, after consultation with and in accordance with the advice of the organized medical profession. But the possibility of abuse is always present so long as any portion of those services is subject to lay control. In this connection, too, vigilance must be unremitting in the enactment or enforcement of state laws designed to enable a State to avail itself of the federal subventions preferred in the Social Security Act. There have been isolated proposals—I believe one was pending before the Minnesota House in 1937—to permit a lay agency to supervise or administer the distribution of the medical services called for by the act.

The administration of medical aid to the clients of the Rural Resettlement Administration, now the Farm Security Administration, has aroused considerable comment. The practice varied from State to State. It almost seemed that in those States in which the state medical society was alert no objectionable practices were instituted and the plans that were put into operation were often the result of consultation with the medical society. Elsewhere attempts were made to care for the medical needs of the relief clients on a contract basis with individual physicians or groups of physicians. This, obviously, would deprive the patient of free choice of physician. In several States attempts were made to set up medical coöperatives which seemed objectionable because the terminology employed in the articles of incorporation of some of these coöperatives was so broad that (1) it would permit a much greater group of the inhabitants of the State in question than the relief clients to avail themselves of the medical care it offered and (2) it would enable the coöperative to *supply* the services of physicians rather than pay for them. Whether the coöperatives actually will do more than pay for medical services rendered FSA clients is a question for the future to determine.

In some states repeated efforts have been made to enact legislation to permit the admittance to various types of governmental hospitals of all persons needing medical care, regardless of indigency or non-indigency, on the payment of fees determined by the governing board.†

†1937 Calif. SCA 5, A. 1196; Nev. A. 187; Idaho S. 169.

244

The possible consequences of the enact such legislation are not hard to imagine. the very recent past in one county in a State the county general hospital became ical football. Certain members of the county commissioners, which appointed pital board, stood for re-election on a of free medical and hospital services fo. a campaign of vituperation was c against the county medical society, wh naturally opposed the scheme. The ma eventually settled in the courts and the board was enjoined from caring for oth indigents.

Bills have been considered recently in States, which, if enacted, would have socialized the practice of medicine an under governmental domination more than any proposal heretofore alluded to of these bills contemplated nothing mor than the creation of a separate depart state government to render free medica and hospital care to all residents.* Tw bills proposed† that all physicians in t treat patients under the direction of the d State department, each physician being monthly salary based on the number of had been licensed. A bill recently cons South Dakota‡ sought to authorize cou missioners to levy a tax sufficient to necessary medical, surgical and hospital all residents of their counties. A resi to be at liberty to choose any physician pital he desired and the county would bill in accordance with a definite fee which made none of the distinctions prevailing medical charges are made.

There is an increasing tendency to c state to arrange for and supply the maintenance, medical and surgical treat hospitalization for indigent expectant Such a law was enacted in Nevada in 171) and was considered and killed i states in 1937. Such a law is not obje of course, if it provides free choice of affords reasonable compensation to the chosen, and if its administration is I indigents.

Falling in the category of legislative

*Wash. (1935) H. 583, H. 580; Mass. (1930) H (1938) A. 2143.
†Wash. (1935) H. 583; N. Y. (1938) A. 2143.
‡H. 201 (1935).

discussed in this paper are a series of bills introduced in the Wisconsin Assembly in 1937 by Assemblyman Andrew J. Biemiller of Milwaukee. One bill so introduced (661A) sought to create an interim committee "to investigate the general subject of medical care and the ways and means of lightening the burden thereof." Another bill (662A) sought to authorize the formation of non-profit corporations to operate group hospitalization plans. Another bill (740A) proposed to make it the duty of the county boards of supervisors in each county to provide "medical, dental and hospital services and treatment for all poor persons receiving relief in said county." Still another bill (747A) proposed to authorize the common council or board of any political subdivision to "subsidize wholly or partially a physician or physicians whenever there shall be an insufficient number of competent physicians in their respective communities." Such physicians were to "work under the direction and rules of the common council or boards affected." Another bill (850A) would have permitted the creation and operation of so-called medical coöperatives and proposed to prohibit medical societies from disciplining such of their members as supplied services to a coöperative and to forbid hospitals from discriminating in any way against physicians coöperating with

such groups. Finally, one bill (852A) embraced a compulsory health insurance scheme based largely on the Epstein philosophy but which did not propose to confer anything but medical, dental and hospital benefits. None of these bills was enacted.

These, in brief, are a few* of what may be termed preferred legislative solutions to the problems of medical care. Not one of them, it is submitted, even approaches a partial solution to that problem. No solution, it can be asserted confidently, will be found in any plan that in any way debases the medical profession, for the quality of medical services is of primary importance. The medical profession, it would seem, must fight not only to maintain its own independence, integrity, and high standards, but also to see to it that the public is not cajoled into accepting a form of medical practice that in destroying an independent and capable profession will leave in its place an incompetent group of servile practitioners bringing with them a retrogression in medical progress and medical care. The American public must not be placed in the situation Æsop depicts in the fable of the dog which dropped his bone for a seemingly larger and more delectable one reflected in the water below him.

FOOD SENSITIVITY SIMULATING GASTRO-INTESTINAL DISEASE*

CLEMENT T. KRANTZ, M.D.

Duluth, Minnesota

DURING the past several years the medical profession and even to some degree the lay public have become conscious of the fact that food idiosyncrasies may be at the basis of some of the ill defined, indefinite symptoms referable to the gastro-intestinal tract. Great advances have been made in the field of allergy, since the observations on anaphylaxis by Richet of France. The proof that hay fever was caused by the protein fraction of pollen soon followed and, in the natural course of investigation, the food proteins came in for consideration so that the cause for many obscure cases of food poisoning was now found. Under the leadership of Coca, Duke, Rackemann, Vaughan, and many others, the treatment of these cases of allergy

was soon started, so that today the sufferer may in a large percentage of cases acquire some and even complete relief from his distressing symptoms.

The diagnosis of food sensitivity is not always easy. Perhaps the earliest and certainly one of the most reliable tests has been the patient's own experience with the production of symptoms on eating the offending food. This has been most apparent in those cases where eruptions on the body or urticaria have resulted after the ingestion of, or contact with, the material at fault. However, when asthma, eczema, or similar allergic manifestations are present, it is rare that the individual himself recognizes the importance of foods as the causative factor. Moreover, this is even more true in cases where

*Read before the Northern Minnesota Medical Association at Virginia, Minnesota, August 27, 1937.

foodstuffs have been found to be the offending material in the production of gastro-intestinal symptoms and so often the symptoms are ascribed to other, non-allergic, often vague diseases of the digestive apparatus.

The value of the scratch and intradermal tests in searching for the cause of the underlying sensitivity is at present open to some question. Care should be used in their interpretation, because a positive reaction may not mean clinical allergy and, by the same token, a negative test may be present when the offending material may produce clinical symptoms. Alexander[1] and Vaughan[11] have thrown some light on this subject and state that the gastro-intestinal tract, bronchi, or other reacting tissues of the body may alone contain reagins, whereas the skin may contain none, and hence negative tests result. Furthemore, the age of the patient and the technic of testing as well as the site of application may cause variations in the test.

The skin test, however, should not be disregarded, for in some instances at least, it may give a lead to further study. The trial by diet, the so-called elimination diet, has assumed a greater importance in the diagnosis of this problem. Rowe[8, 9] in several reports has gone into detail discussing its value, which has since been corroborated by many writers. There are further means of diagnosis, namely the passive transfer test, and the leukopenic index as presented by Vaughan.[12] The latter test is of definite value in some cases[7, 10, 12, 13] though the results must be interpreted with caution.[5]

In the present report, a study has been made of individuals giving evidence of food allergy with symptoms referred to the gastro-intestinal tract. Many of these cases had been previously studied and treatment instituted, often without relief. These symptoms were such as to simulate other conditions, viz., duodenal ulcer, gallbladder disease, acute gastro-intestinal disturbances, spastic or irritable colon, etc. For convenience in illustrating these symptoms, the following case reports are presented:

Cases Simulating Upper Gastro-Intestinal Disease

Case 1.—J. B., male, aged forty-five years. His chief complaint was discomfort in his abdomen, particularly a few hours after meals. In 1927, he was informed that he had a duodenal ulcer, though several roentgen-

ray studies failed to reveal any ulceration of the upper gastro-intestinal tract. His diet was varied, though he had abstained from fatty foods. Vegetables caused no discomfort, but highly seasoned foods did. The principal foods were quantities of milk, eggs, beef, and bread. The usual powdered medication used in the treatment of ulcer gave no relief from symptoms.

For many years past he had had mild attacks of hay fever and there was a history of allergic disease in his family.

The physical examination was essentially negative except for moderate tenderness upon palpation of the epigastrium.

Scratch and intradermal tests were given and showed markedly positive reactions to milk and eggs and a two plus reaction to beef and black pepper. The articles were then eliminated from his diet with complete relief of symptoms. When eggs and milk were again restored to the diet, the symptoms of abdominal distress returned, and since then these have been entirely withdrawn from his food intake.

Case 2.—Mrs. F. H., female, aged thirty-six years, complained of an acute onset of nausea, vomiting and acute upper abdominal distress, which she believed resulted from taking a small amount of fermented liquor the evening previous. Further investigation revealed that she had never taken milk or eggs except mixed with other cooked foods, but that during the past few days she had taken a glass of milk each evening.

In the past she had had several spells of less severity on rare occasions. There was no history of allergic disease in her family.

Physical examination revealed nothing except some abdominal distention. Intradermal tests were made with extracts of various foods and a three plus reaction to milk and a two plus to eggs resulted. These substances were accordingly eliminated from her diet.

She recovered promptly from her illness and found also that fermented liquor did not cause return of any symptom. On one occasion she was ordered to take milk with her diet and then had a return of epigastric discomfort. Since avoiding these food materials she has since been free from any gastro-intestinal symptoms.

Case 3.—Mrs. A. H., aged thirty years. The chief complaint was vomiting, epigastric discomfort and headaches of the migraine type, which would disable her for three days at a time every few weeks. These had been present for years, and the headaches relieved only temporarily by medication. There was no history of allergic disease in the family, but her mother had suffered from headaches.

The physical examination was entirely negative. Elimination diets were tried after intradermal tests had shown a markedly positive test for milk, and lesser reactions (two plus) to bananas, cabbage, and black pepper. Milk elimination stopped the above mentioned symptoms. An oral desensitization diet for milk according to Kesten and Hopkins[4] was tried, but when this was half completed, she had a return of headaches and gastro-intestinal distress. Complete elimination of milk alleviated all symptoms.

In January, 1937, she was delivered of a child, which she began to nurse. Headaches and nausea of milder degree returned, lasting only one day. She last reported that these seemed to lessen slightly, but it is probable that they will not be completely eliminated until she has stopped nursing her child.

Cases Simulating Acute or Chronic Disease of the Colon

Case 4.—Miss E. C., female, aged twenty-five years. Her chief complaint was pain in the right and mid-epigastrium, alternating spells of diarrhea and constipation. She had been chronically ill for many years. In 1932 a retrocecal appendix was removed and in 1935 a gallbladder without stones but with a few adhesions was taken out. Symptoms still persisted despite the many varied forms of medication given. There was no family history of allergic disease.

Examination showed a somewhat undernourished young woman. There was tenderness on pressure in the right epigastrium and along the descending colon on the left side. Roentgen-ray films revealed a moderate degree of visceroptosis and a spastic colon.

Scratch and intradermal tests showed a positive reaction to many foods, particularly tomato, pork, and carrots (three plus). The reaction to milk was only one plus. Because of the severity of the symptoms, elimination diets were tried. Among the first foods eliminated was milk. During this period, the symptoms of pain in the epigastrium were greatly alleviated and the bowel function returned to normal. However, because she was not gaining in weight, goat's milk was added to her food intake. For a period of two months she was fairly comfortable, but in June, 1936, diarrhea again set in with fifteen to twenty movements per day. Hospital treatment was instituted and goat's milk was removed from the diet. The diarrhea subsided within a few days and since then she has not been troubled in this way. Tomatoes and citrus fruits caused return of epigastric distress, but elimination of these alleviated the symptoms to a great degree. Soy bean milk has been used to replace milk and she has regained six pounds in weight. At present she is comfortable unless she experiences mental strain, when a mild diarrhea sets in for a few days.

Case 5.—Mrs. R. MacG., aged thirty-one years. For years this patient had been troubled with gastro-intestinal distress and she stated she had to be "fussy" with her diet. She had spells of what she called colitis, with pain particularly over the descending colon. In 1934 symptoms of pain in the pelvis were complained of and examination revealed a mass in the left culdesac. At operation endometrial tumors were found and removed and a chronically inflamed appendix was taken out. However, she still complained of food difficulties and roentgen-ray studies revealed a spastic colon. She did not receive much relief from treatment.

In May, 1937, she complained of discomfort after eating, stating that she believed her trouble was due to poisoning from food stuffs. She always felt tired and at times had much distention of her abdomen. At these times palpitation of her heart would set in and the pulse rate increase to 140 or 150 beats per minute. Her stools were watery and loose, but sometimes stringy with much mucus. She believed meat and eggs caused most of her trouble.

Examination was negative except for tenderness in the epigastrium and left flank of the abdomen. Scratch and intradermal tests revealed a three plus reaction to milk, two plus to wheat, rye and white potatoes. These were removed from her diet with complete relief of symptoms. Oral desensitization diets were given and after a few months she was able to eat small amounts of bread without discomfort. She has never been able to partake of milk without return of symptoms.

Discussion

The symptoms presented by these patients are common in many non-allergic diseases of the gastro-intestinal tract. In determining the underlying etiological factor causing these complaints, careful attention to the history is essential. Often there is a history of hay fever, as in Case 1; or a familial history of allergic disease may be obtained, which will give a clue to the diagnosis. A careful evaluation of the diet list may reveal some new food recently added to the list and may be the material at fault as in Case 2. Moreover, it is not uncommon for these sufferers to have widely varied medical treatment, even undergoing operation without relief of symptoms. In cases suggestive of ulcer or cholecystic disease, the absence of positive roentgen-ray findings may be the determining factor in stimulating the physician to resort to the study of possible allergic factors.

The dislike for foods very often has no relation to the allergic food factor at fault and even the patient's own statement that certain foods are disliked or cause distress may or may not be contribute to finding the cause, as in Case 2. So often the offending food comes as a complete surprise not only to the patient himself, but also to the physician. The foods that are most commonly used, such as milk, eggs, wheat, or tomatoes, are most often the causative factors in a series of cases studied. Alvarez[2, 3] has discussed this problem at length with a careful analysis of symptoms and their relation to food sensitivity and has come to the same conclusions.

These selected cases also show that too much reliance should not be placed on one method of diagnosis alone, but that the elimination diet or diary diet of Alvarez should be resorted to in these individuals. This is well illustrated in Case 4 where the intradermal test was only very slightly positive, but there was clinical evidence of severe sensitivity to milk as proven by the test diets. Here the gastro-intestinal tract was the shock organ, so to speak, and the skin showed only slight sensitivity. Thus it is evident that the patient should be given the benefit of the test diets, for with those sensitive to many food stuffs, the diet list may be cut down too much for the patient's own welfare, even to the extent of making his food intake lack both in the amounts and kinds of food material necessary for well-being.

Patients 3 and 4 present an interesting study in antigenically related substances, in this case milk. Ratner[6] has studied this problem and suggests that milk derived from the various species of animals may be antigenically related. In patient 3, there is a probability that the symptoms of nausea, vomiting, and migraine headaches may be due to her own milk. Patient 4 did well after the removal of cow's milk from her diet. However, she used goat's milk for two months and then severe gastro-intestinal symptoms appeared. They were relieved only by removal of this article of food from her diet. In this case we can assume that there was a relation between cow's and goat's milk to produce allergic symptoms.

Summary and Conclusions

1. Case reports have been presented to illustrate that food sensitivity may often simulate organic gastro-intestinal disease.

2. Too much reliance should not be placed on a single method of diagnosis, such as the scratch test, but a careful history of previous allergic disease should be obtained and then the elimination or diary diets together with other methods of diagnosis should be used.

3. This is even more necessary in those individuals positive to many substances by the scratch test, because too limited a diet may deprive the patient of food elements necessary to the proper sustenance of life and well-being.

Bibliography

1. Alexander, H. L.: An evaluation of the skin test in allergy. Ann. Int. Med., 5:52, 1931.
2. Alvarez, W. C.: Specific food sensitiveness. Am. Jour. Digest Dis. and Nutrition, 3:693, 1936.
3. Alvarez, W. C., and Hinshaw, H. C.: Foods that commonly disagree with people. Jour. Am. Med. Assn., 104:2053, 1935.
4. Kesten, B. M., and Hopkins, J. G.: Oral desensitization to common foods. Jour. Allergy, 6:431, 1935.
5. Loveless, M., Downing L., and Dorfman, R.: Leukopenic index, Jour. Allergy, 8:276, 1937.
6. Ratner, B.: The treatment of milk allergy and its basic principles. Jour. Am. Med. Assn., 105:934, 1935.
7. Rinkel, H. J.: The leukopenic index in allergic diseases, Jour. Allergy, 7:356, 1936.
8. Rowe, A. H.: Food allergy. Its manifestations, diagnosis, and treatment. Jour. Am. Med. Assn., 91:1623, 1928.
9. Rowe, A. H.: An evaluation of skin reactions in food-sensitive patients. Jour. Allergy, 5:135, 1934.
10. Sullivan, C. J.: A statistical analysis of the leukopenic index. Jour. Allergy, 8:491, 1937.
11. Vaughan, W. T.: Food allergens, II, Trial diets in the elimination of allergenic foods. Jour. Immunol., 20:313, 1931.
12. Vaughan, W. T.: Food allergens, III, The leukopenic index, Preliminary report. Jour. Allergy, 5:601, 1934.
13. Vaughan, W. T.: Further studies on the leucopenic index in food allergy. Jour. Allergy, 6:78, 1934.

THE DANGERS OF LATE DIAGNOSIS OF INTESTINAL DISEASES*

J. ARNOLD BARGEN, M.D.

Rochester, Minnesota

SOME of the most serious lesions of the human body are found in the large intestine. Their early diagnosis, therefore, is imperative. It is my purpose in this paper to call attention to some of the more common symptoms, signs, and methods of early diagnosis of intestinal disorders.

Any change in bowel function should suggest

*From the Division of Medicine, The Mayo Clinic, Rochester, Minnesota. Read before the Northern Minnesota Medical Association, Virginia, Minnesota, August 27-28, 1937.

the possibility of intestinal disease. Sometimes such a change may be very slight, for when one considers the nature and contour of the large intestine, a lesion may grow to considerable dimensions before it produces a change in the intestinal habits. In an individual whose bowel movements have always occurred at a regular time of day, therefore, any irregularity in going to stool may be an early symptom of intrinsic disease. Another common early complaint is fragmentation of the stools, and where formerly an individual may have had one normal, formed stool, he may suddenly have three or four small ones, and he may not seem to be able to empty his bowel completely except after repeated small passages.

Gaseous dyspepsia and bloating are common complaints, and indefinite abdominal discomfort, which may or may not follow the line of the large intestine, occurs frequently. The passage of intestinal mucus may or may not signify a lesion in the intestine. Without doubt much too much attention has been paid to mucous discharge from the rectum. Too often it has been called evidence of colitis without a thorough investigation. More often than not it is simply the result of a type of systemic irritation in which the intestine is affected reflexly. However, it is not possible to establish this fact without proper objective investigation. Hence, when unnatural quantities of mucus are passed, a thorough study of the intestine should be made to establish the possibility of an early organic lesion. The passage of pus is indicative of some type of inflammatory disease.

Blood in the stools should always be considered of serious moment until proved otherwise. It is easy to blame the passage of blood in the stools on the presence of hemorrhoids. It is much safer to consider the presence of blood as due to a neoplastic lesion until proof to the contrary is available.

The development of constipation in an individual who has otherwise had normal bowel function should also be considered of significance. Constipation, of course, is more often due to functional disorders than to actual organic disease, but one should never be satisfied to say that the constipation is of a functional nature unless every effort has been made to prove the contrary. Unexplained loss of weight may be associated with early intestinal disease. The pallor seen in individuals with slowly progressing anemia is rather characteristic, particularly in cases in which the lesion is in the right half of the colon. Then, too, among patients who have had chronic ulcerative colitis (colitis gravis) for some time there develops a peculiar pallor which was originally described by Logan as that of "visceral degeneration." Innumerable nervous disturbances may also be associated with intestinal disorders, often to the point of depression, and the old saying of Osler that "disease above the diaphragm makes for optimism and that below the diaphragm for pessimism" well expresses the situation. These and many other symptoms may be taken as early expressions of intrinsic intestinal disease.

When satisfied that a patient's complaints point to a disturbed function of the intestine, a very careful physical examination should be made, and this in detail often gives valuable information. Probably the most important part of the physical examination is a careful examination of the rectum. A general examination of the chest and abdomen often gives valuable and sometimes unexpected information. A well-planned and well-ordered set of objective tests, including examination of the stools, x-ray studies of the large intestine, and the direct inspection of the bowel lining through the proctoscope, has the greatest value.

If this plan of study is followed, many of the serious lesions found in the intestine will be diagnosed early and at a time when their complete eradication is possible.

Vitamin D Milk Produced by Feeding Cows Irradiated Yeast

In 1929 Wachtel reported that the feeding of irradiated dried yeast to cows resulted in the secretion of vitamin D in the milk. This report was confirmed and amplified by the observations of Hart and Steenbock and their associates at the University of Wisconsin. Since 1932 this type of vitamin D milk has been made commercially available. The product is sometimes referred to as "metabolized" vitamin D milk. Numerous investigators have reported on the clinical effectiveness of metabolized vitamin D milk. These investigators have shown that, if there is any difference, unit for unit, between different types of vitamin D milk, the difference is too small to be of practical significance. Metabolized vitamin D milk is produced under the joint sponsorship of Standard Brands, Incorporated, and the Wisconsin Alumni Research Foundation. The irradiated dried yeast intended for use in the feeding of cows may be sold by Standard Brands, Incorporated, only to dairymen licensed by the Wisconsin Alumni Research Foundation. The vitamin D content of the milk produced, as shown by repeated bioassays, is not less than 400 units of vitamin D per quart. The Council on Foods voted to accept pasteurized metabolized vitamin D milk and to grant the use of the seal of acceptance to licensed dairies that conform to the Rules and Decision of the Council. (Jour. A.M.A., Nov. 27, 1937, p. 1814.)

COMPARATIVE VALUES OF INJECTION AND SURGICAL
TREATMENT OF HERNIA*

GEORGE EARL, M.D.

Saint Paul, Minnesota

PREVIOUS to the last decade, injections for the cure of hernia attracted little attention. The solutions of Pina Maestræ of Spain were handled with great secrecy and in this country sold at such high prices that they had been little used. Mayer of Detroit was using the injection method long before he gave medical publicity to it. Bratrud of Minneapolis, together with McKiney, Rice, and Larson, deserve credit for taking the matter up in a clinical teaching way and giving the profession solutions, methods, and the results of their experience.

It is estimated that 10 per cent of the population have herniæ in some form or other. The majority, influenced by economic considerations, necessity of hospitalization, objections to surgery and recurrences after operation, prefer to wear trusses. The tendency now is for active treatment to be sought earlier.

Inguinal hernia comprises most of the cases selected for injection because trusses are fitted more easily, and, anatomically, the injections are simpler. The direct inguinal type gives more difficulty than the indirect because of gravity and also because the structures of the internal and external oblique muscles are often frayed out or almost absent. Evidences of this are the many surgical devices used, such as fascia lata strips from the thigh, turning down of fascia from the rectus muscle or incision of the fascia of the internal oblique near its attachment to the rectus muscle so as to free the internal oblique for approximation to Poupart's ligament. Direct hernia becomes more frequent in later life. Age presents poorer reacting qualities, hernia of longer duration, degenerative changes, often increased fat, and the protruding abdomen placing the inguinal hernia more at the bottom of a sack. The number of injections needed increases with each decade of life, and many more are usually needed with direct than with indirect inguinal hernia. The same factors necessitate more careful surgical procedure with direct hernia.

Is injection likely to damage the spermatic cord or the circulation of the testicle? Before any treatment, surgical or injection, the status of the cord and testicles should be carefully noted. Variation in size may be developmental or due to illness, such as mumps, or it may follow operations. I am injecting a dentist who suffered marked testicular atrophy following an operation and, with hernial occurrence on the other side, he has selected the injection method. The spermatic cord is very resistant to any needle implantation. The younger the individual, the more resistant the elements of the cord are. The thickness of the wall of the cord on section is many times greater than the lumen. Records of potency, semen examinations, findings at such operations as may be necessary following failure of the injection method, and post-mortem examinations in operated and injected individuals will ultimately determine comparative risks.

Femoral hernia, if reducible, may lend itself to injections. Femoral hernia occurs jointly with inguinal hernia more frequently than is usually suspected. Sometimes it is not noticeable until the inguinal hernia has been corrected by operation or injection.

Umbilical hernia, if small and free from any abdominal contents, may be treated by injections.

Post-incisional abdominal hernia, if small, may occasionally be closed by injections. One difficulty is that often this type of hernia may have multiple points of weakness. In the upper abdomen, because of the presence of the mesentery and liver, there is less chance of the development of bowel adhesions and hence injections are safer above the navel than below. Unless very minute and treated early, post-incisional rectus muscle and midline herniæ below the navel are positively surgical.

Recurrences in inguinal hernia following operation often lend themselves to control from injections. Previous operation has rearranged the tissues so that injections may fill in weak spots more readily.

Before injections are made, a satisfactory truss must be fitted. No one type fits every kind of hernia. A spring bar is most efficient in the in-

*Read before the Northern Minnesota Medical Association, Virginia, Minnesota, August 27, 1937.

guinal type. In umbilical and incisional hernia, trusses with attachments encircling the body are used. The truss may have to be adjusted repeatedly. The surgeon should fit and closely observe the truss. The truss must function positively to hold the hernia. For the discomfort and chafing present at times, a buffer cloth between the truss and skin is helpful. Toughening of the skin with alcohol and dusting powder is useful. The truss is worn night and day to begin with and preferably so during the injection period. After apparent cure, it should still be worn two to six months longer, depending upon the type of hernia and the difficulty in securing healing. Then it is left off at night only and later during the day unless special strain or activities are undertaken.

Next comes the choice of the irritant to produce a foreign body granuloma—microscopically, a proliferation of endothelial and connective tissue cells forming scar tissue. Many solutions are being used, and this fact in itself is evidence of the still unsettled question as to which solution is best. Of the many in use, I have had experience with five.

1. Thuja Mixture

Phenol, 50 parts.
Alcohol, 25 parts.
Lloyds Specific Tincture of Thuja, 25 parts.
Allow to stand two days and then either decant or filter.

Except for a half dose at the internal ring, an average of eight minims is injected at each treatment. A tuberculin syringe is used. With such a small quantity of solution only a small area is affected, necessitating a greater number of injections. The Thuja mixture is its own sterilizing agent and needs no preliminary novocain for anesthesia.

2. Mayer Formula

Zinc Sulphate, 1 dram.
Glycerin, 4 fluid drams.
Fluid Extract Pinus Canadensis (dark), 5 fluid drams.
Phenol Crystals, 6 drams.
Aqua Cinnamomi, 1 fluid dram.
Sterlized chemically pure redistilled water, 2 fluid ounces.

The solution must be brought to boil each time before it is used. The average dose is eight minims.

3. Bratrud Formula

Tannic Acid 0.50
Benzyl Alcohol 3.00.
Thymol 0.50
Alcohol (95%) 100.0

This product is suggested by Dr. A. Bratrud of Minneapolis. The tannic acid may be increased to 1 per cent in selected cases. Its advantage is that a larger amount can be used, probably on the average of 2 c.c. It is preceded by 1 c.c. of 2 per cent novocain. Bratrud adds two minims of Thuja mixture. All solutions are given through the same needle with change of syringes. The larger amount of solution gives a reaction over a larger area.

4. Sodium Morrhuate

This solution was suggested by Dr. D. D. Turnacliff of Minneapolis. I have used 2 c.c. of the solution preceded by 2 c.c. of 2 per cent novocain and followed by 1 c.c. of novocain. I have limited its use to the above dosage in difficult cases in which other solutions had previously been used. In my experience, with the dose mentioned, it gave the most marked reaction of all and therefore should be used with caution. I have seen no other reports regarding its use.

5. Sodium Psylliate

Of late I have used a sodium psylliate preparation. It causes no damage if spilled on the skin, the reactions are certainly less marked and, experimentally on animals, the reaction even on the peritoneum is reported mild. In cases which are difficult to close, I am inclined to return more frequently to solutions of greater reaction, such as Bratrud's formula, sodium morrhuate, or Thuja mixture.

For injection of an inguinal hernia, the patient is placed on a table with the hips elevated. Alcohol (70 per cent) is applied to the skin area. The approach to the region of weakness is through skin, fat, and fascia. The resistance of the fascia is definite. When the needle is passed through the fascia, freedom of motion of the needle is evident. An attempt should always be made to withdraw the piston of the syringe, to insure avoidance of vessels. The patient's reaction to pain also guides in the placement of the needle. The injection should be immediately stopped with any unusual reaction. It should be given slowly. Repeated injections are placed in various areas of the inguinal canal according to the reaction obtained and points of greatest weakness. The nearer the internal ring, the more need for caution.

The frequency of injection depends upon the reaction, upon the number of areas needing injection and, to some degree, upon the convenience of the patient, particularly an out-of-town patient. The injections range from daily to weekly injection, usually allowing a week to elapse between injection of each area. Reaction in the form of swelling is encountered. I have seen none that has not subsided. I have not encountered infection.

In umbilical hernia, the defect is approached from all sides, dosage at any point being from one-quarter to one-eighth of that used in inguinal hernia. The peritoneum should not be penetrated. In femoral hernia, the dosage is about one-quarter and the approach is made with great care. Incisional herniæ, except in the inguinal region, are approached with much caution.

There are many interesting reports in literature. Pina Maestrae of Spain reports favorably on 8,000 cases.

Mayer of Detroit states that in his work a census of 2,100 cases of inguinal, femoral and umbilical hernia by subcutaneous injection showed complete relief without recurrence after a period of years in 98 per cent of the cases. Furthermore, more than 200 cases of hernia recurring after operation were subsequently completely relieved by the subcutaneous injection method.

Bratrud and McKinney at the University of Minnesota Hospital, and Rice and Larson at the Minneapolis General Hospital have given favorable reports on large series. This work at the University of Minnesota is especially to be commended because of the spirit of open-mindedness shown, and also because of the scientific approach and willingness to teach. Samuel W. Fowler of New York City has recently reported several hundred cases. Total reports now from all sources are large.

During the years 1933 and 1934 in a private practice trial, I operated upon thirty-eight patients and injected forty-two. Since then over two years have elapsed. Patients treated since 1934 are too recent for evaluation. Of the in-

jection cases, thirty-seven were inguinal hernia, two were incisional, one umbilical, and two femoral. Of the thirty-seven inguinal, four had, in addition, femoral ring impulse; hence, both areas were injected. Two of the inguinal group had marked hydroceles which were treated also. Three of the injected cases were surgical recurrences, one of which had had three operations, and another two operations. These operated cases reacted well as the operations had left smaller areas of weakness for closure.

Of the operated patients, two had undescended testicles, two had marked testicle atrophy from mumps (one unilateral and one bilateral), five had femoral herniæ and six had post-incisional herniæ. The remaining twenty-three of the surgical group were inguinal herniæ.

Certain difficulties were encountered.

1. Severe enough reactions to cause the patient to lay off from work. The first was a laborer doing exceptionally heavy lifting and to whom I gave the largest dose of sodium morrhuate I ever used at one injection. He had the most marked reaction of my series. His lay-off lasted one week. He had a closure of the hernia following the severe reaction and has since referred a patient to me. The second was an older man who complained much of the character of his work. Besides compensation, he had other sources of insurance income and had it not been for the character of his work and also for his insurance, I feel that he would not have laid off at various times for a total of several weeks. Three other patients laid off, missing part or all of a day from work. Since using sodium psylliate, none has laid off from work. Reactions have been much reduced, but I am of the opinion that more injections are required than with the other solutions.

2. The most difficult herniæ to close were in four patients, all old men with long standing, large, direct herniæ. Two I have operated upon after prolonged injections. Adhesions were marked from the injections, but operation was not more difficult than expected. One of the two tired of injections and suggested operation himself. Another I apparently closed with forty-four injections but the hernia reopened. I have advised operation, which he may accept, although he still comes for injections. Another

has had thirty-nine injections and progress is very slow. He comes occasionally for injections. The advice I would give generally for hernia of this type is plastic repair. Others of this type, which apparently closed, will have to be injected again from time to time for recurrences or they may come to operation by me or drift into other hands, if they have not already done so. Observance for recurrence should be repeated regularly. Extra injections after apparent closure are necessary to improve results.

3. Swelling in the tissues accompanying the cord does occur at times with all the solutions mentioned except sodium psylliate. It has always subsided, however, in my experience. Twice I removed fluid from the center of the reacting mass. Patients become somewhat disturbed over such swellings and must be reassured.

4. Pain results from proximity to the nerves or to the peritoneum. In such cases the needle must be reinserted.

5. Influx of blood with a preliminary withdrawal of the piston, previous to injection, has occurred several times. The needle was promptly withdrawn and no complications followed. If the withdrawal had not been made promptly, trouble might have followed.

6. With patients who are unusually temperamental and highly sensitive to any manipulations, bromides or phenobarbital reduce the sensitiveness.

7. Difficulties with operation due to adhesions following injections. I have operated on two patients whom I myself have injected. Further, I have operated upon two others who had been treated elsewhere. Recently I removed an acute appendix in a patient who had had injections previously by a very competent man. I found the cecum markedly adherent, which made the operation for an acute, beginning gangrenous appendix located postcecally most difficult. Of course, at times, we find marked adhesions of the cecum without the patient ever having had injections, but in this case the adhesions were directly in line where the injections had been placed. Unquestionably, patients whom I have injected will have some adhesions which will come to light at operation or postmortem.

The cases reported on were injections begun in 1933 and 1934, and during those years, taking

in all types of herniæ, I injected a few more than I operated upon, the ratio having been surgical 47.5 per cent, and injection 52.5 per cent. Of the cases of hernia I have seen in 1935, 1936, and 1937 and have not reported because they are too recent to evaluate, I have operated upon more than I have injected, the ratio being surgical 57 per cent and injection 43 per cent—a distinct shift toward surgery. Just where the pendulum between surgery and injections will come to rest will probably depend upon the individual surgeon. Some surgeons will operate only, others will tend toward injection. The majority of surgeons will probably do both injection and operation, depending upon the indications, upon the surgeon's inclination and experience, and somewhat upon the patient's economic circumstances and acceptance of, or objection to, surgery. A factor to be considered is that in the future patients with herniæ will come earlier for treatment due to compensation insurance, better health education, and the interest aroused by the chemical injection method.

Conclusion

Herniæ to be injected must be reducible and satisfactorily held in position with a truss. The large percentage of injections will be made in inguinal hernia, a few in femoral and umbilical. Only the smallest postoperative abdominal herniæ above the umbilicus lend themselves to the injection treatment. Below the navel the small bowel is more commonly directly adjacent to the peritoneum. If surgical recurrences are found early enough, the injection method may prevent reoperation, particularly in inguinal hernia.

Of the solutions used in my experience, sodium psylliate has been less accompanied by pain and swelling. Proliferal and sodium morrhuate produce greater reaction but, in spite of that, may be indicated. Thuja mixture and Mayer formula are useful at times. Other solutions with which I have had no experience may have equal or greater merit. Study of injection material will be continued and widened.

Because many injections are being given to older men who are succumbing to the degenerative diseases, postmortems should be increasingly available. Study should be made of the question of semen and potency in patients operated and in those injected. The grouping of complications from either operation or injection should be increasingly recorded.

More accurate observation of the condition of the testicle and cord, previous both to operation and injection, should be recorded. It is natural that great interest should be aroused with any change in these organs, but too often an unfair and unjustifiable attitude of complaint is taken and hence every precaution is needed to record previous abnormalities.

Precautions always to be remembered are: Complete replacement of protruding tissues, which should positively be held in place with truss; withdrawal of the piston of the syringe to avoid injecting into a blood vessel; slow injection to try out the location and patient's reaction; careful follow-up and extra injections to secure sufficient strength in the holding tissues.

In selecting cases and advising patients concerning results with either operation or injection, ease of cure is in proportion to the decade of

life, size and character of the hernia, general condition of patient's health, patient's coöperation, and the doctor's interest, knowledge, and experience in the procedure. A simple, indirect inguinal hernia is relatively easy of closure by the chemical injection method. All other types of hernia deserve careful study before treatment, other than operation, is advised. In the aged or decrepit, injections may bring relief without cure.

A qualified enthusiasm for the injection method will, of course, secure better results than half-hearted interest and less experience. To secure results with the injection method takes more persistence, close attention to detail and study of the individual case than some are willing to give when operation offers satisfactory results.

Because of recurrences and realizing that, after all, only scar tissue is secured from injections and this tends to give way, and because of the other difficulties discussed, I tend increasingly to advise operation more often than when first I began the trial of the injection method of treatment.

THE PRESENT STATUS OF INFESTATION OF FISHES OF LONG LAKE, ELY, MINNESOTA, WITH THE LARVAE OF DIPHYLLOBOTHRIUM LATUM*

HIRAM E. ESSEX, Ph.D.

Rochester, Minnesota

IN previous papers[1,2] it has been shown that susceptible fishes of Long Lake, also known as Shagawa Lake, at Ely, Minnesota, were more heavily infested with the plerocercoid larvæ of Diphyllobothrium latum than were fishes of any other body of water studied in this state. During the past summer (July, 1937) another series of fishes was examined to determine whether any changes in the incidence of infestation had occurred. The number and species of fishes examined were as follows: fifteen Stizostedion vitreum (walleyed pike); four Esox lucius (pickerel); two Perca flavescens (yellow perch). Both the musculature and viscera were inspected. The walleyed pike measured from 21.2 to 28.8 cm. in length and harbored from one to twenty-six larvæ. The average infestation was more than six larvæ for each fish.

The pickerel varied from 38.7 to 45 cm. in length and each harbored from four to twenty-six larvæ. The average number of larvæ for each fish was more than fifteen. The two small yellow perch examined were not infested (Table I). The number of larvæ found in the different species of fishes examined prior to 1930 was approximately the same as found in the present survey (Table II). These data indicate very clearly that there has not been a change in the infestation of fishes of Long Lake, at Ely, Minnesota, since the previous investigations.

I wish to thank Dr. T. Surber for his coöperation and Wardens Hanson and Carlson for valuable assistance in obtaining fish for examination and Dr. J. E. Thompson for the use of his laboratories. I wish also to express appreciation to Donald C. Balfour, Jr., who assisted in all phases of the investigation.

*From the Division of Experimental Medicine, The Mayo Foundation, Rochester, Minnesota.

TABLE I. THE INFESTATION OF FISHES OF LONG LAKE WITH LARVÆ OF
DIPHYLLOBOTHRIUM LATUM IN 1937

	Species	Common Name	Length, cm.	Diphyllobothrium latum larvae
1.	Stizostedion vitreum	Walleyed pike	25.6	7
2.	Stizostedion vitreum	Walleyed pike	25.6	10
3.	Stizostedion vitreum	Walleyed pike	28.1	2
4.	Stizostedion vitreum	Walleyed pike	26.9	10
5.	Stizostedion vitreum	Walleyed pike	27.5	4
6.	Stizostedion vitreum	Walleyed pike	25.0	2
7.	Stizostedion vitreum	Walleyed pike	28.1	4
8.	Stizostedion vitreum	Walleyed pike	38.0	26
9.	Stizostedion vitreum	Walleyed pike	21.25	4
10.	Stizostedion vitreum	Walleyed pike	37.5	6
11.	Stizostedion vitreum	Walleyed pike	28.8	4
12.	Stizostedion vitreum	Walleyed pike	28.8	1
13.	Stizostedion vitreum	Walleyed pike	28.1	5
14.	Stizostedion vitreum	Walleyed pike	26.2	4
15.	Stizostedion vitreum	Walleyed pike	23.1	3
1.	Esox lucius	Pickerel	45.0	4
2.	Esox lucius	Pickerel	43.1	17
3.	Esox lucius	Pickerel	46.2	26
4.	Esox lucius	Pickerel	38.7	16
1.	Perca flavescens	Yellow perch	12.5	0
2.	Perca flavescens	Yellow perch	15.0	0

TABLE II. THE INFESTATION OF FISHES WITH LARVÆ OF DIPHYLLOBOTHRIUM
LATUM PRIOR TO 1930 COMPARED WITH INFESTATION IN 1937

Species	Prior to 1930		1937	
	Examined	Positive	Examined	Positive
Esox lucius	12	12	4	4
Stizostedion vitreum	6	6	15	15
Perca flavescens	10	6	2	0
Total	28	24	21	19

References

1. Essex, H. E.: A report on fishes from the Mississippi River and other waters with respect to infestation by Diphyllobothrium latum. Minnesota Med. 12:149-150, (March) 1929.

2. Magath, T. B., and Essex, H. E.: Concerning the distribution of Diphyllobothrium latum in North America. Jour. Prev. Med. 5:227-242, (July) 1931.

OVARIAN TUMORS AMONG YOUNG GIRLS

CHARLES W. MAYO.† M.D., and WINFIELD L. BUTSCH.‡ M.D.

Rochester, Minnesota

W HILE comparatively rare, ovarian tumors occur with sufficient frequency among young girls to make it essential to keep the possibility in mind when dealing with abdominal symptoms. The diagnosis can be made preoperatively in most instances.

Mayo and Fauster, in 1932, reviewed the cases in which ovarian tumors were found among young girls at The Mayo Clinic. This report deals with the subsequent cases in which this condition was encountered. Hubert recorded 175 cases in which solid and cystic tumors of the ovary were found among children up to seventeen years of age. Of these, sixty were malignant and 115 benign. Of the malignant tumors, thirty-two were sarcomas and twenty-eight were carcinomas. Of the benign tumors, fifty-three were cysts, thirty-nine were dermoids, nineteen were cystadenomas and four were hematomas.

This clearly brings to mind the serious import of the diagnosis of an ovarian tumor in childhood as the occurrence of malignant tumors at this age is relatively much more frequent than it is in adult life.

Since the report by Mayo and Fauster, nine young girls who had ovarian tumors have undergone operations at the clinic. A study of the clinical history in these cases and a review of the cases reported in the literature revealed certain important facts. While these facts cannot be made to fit every case, yet they are sufficiently common to all the cases to permit one to be suspicious of ovarian tumors when they are encountered.

The first fact that is significant is the history of the pain and its nature. It is usually a mild, dull type of pain which is situated in the right or left lower portion of the abdomen; it persists twenty-four to forty-eight hours and then recurs at short intervals of a week or two. It frequently is related to an enema relieves the

pain and this leads to another characteristic, namely, that the pain commonly is not associated with any digestive disturbance. There is no nausea, vomiting or diarrhea. The child may be slightly constipated. When the pain is sharp it is often brought on by active play or by riding in an automobile; it completely disappears in a few minutes to a half hour. The child may then wish to go out and play again.

Sudden attacks of agonizing abdominal pain which are associated with vomiting and much abdominal tenderness do, however, occur infrequently. Wakeley ascribed this to a sudden rising of the cyst out of the pelvis, which causes shock. Twisting of the pedicle, as is well known, may cause the same acute symptoms. In only one of the nine cases in this report was any nausea or vomiting associated with the pain. Girls may have symptomless abdominal tumors.

The physical findings are dependent on the size of the tumor. If the tumor is sufficiently large to enter the abdominal cavity, it is palpable, usually, as a freely movable mass and there is slight associated tenderness. Should the tumor remain in the pelvis and its presence not be suspected, the lesion may be erroneously considered appendicitis. However, rectal examination affords very definite information because if it is made the tumor can be palpated. Because of the small size of the pelvis of a young girl, the pelvis can be very completely explored by bimanual palpation with one finger in the rectum.

As pointed out in the paper by Mayo and Fauster, the acute abdominal symptoms caused by a twisted ovarian cyst may very easily be confused with those caused by an appendiceal abscess. The physical findings of abdominal tenderness and a pelvic mass are likewise confusing. The preoperative diagnosis in one of our nine cases was appendiceal abscess.

Roentgenograms of the abdomen, taken to exclude the possibility of stones in the urinary tract, showed definite soft tissue shadows in the pelvis in three of our cases. In one instance the pres-

†With the Division of Surgery, The Mayo Clinic, Rochester, Minnesota.
‡Fellow in Surgery, The Mayo Foundation, Rochester, Minnesota.

ence of multiple smaller shadows within the soft tissue mass enabled the roentgenologist to surmise correctly that the tumor was a dermoid.

The total leukocyte count and the percentage of neutrophils are of no value in the diagnosis as they may either be elevated or normal.

Report of Cases

Case 1.—A girl, aged twelve years, had had a few mild pains in the right lower abdominal quadrant for six weeks. She had noted that riding in a car would bring them on. The pains had been sharp at times and of short duration; they had lasted about a half hour. There had not been any associated digestive or urinary symptoms. For two days before the patient came to the clinic the pain had been constant and more severe. Examination of the abdomen did not reveal any abnormality but rectal examination disclosed a tender mass in the right side of the pelvis. A diagnosis of appendiceal abscess was made and the abdomen was explored. A hemorrhagic dermoid, which had a twisted pedicle, was found and removed. Convalescence was uneventful.

Case 2.—A girl, aged thirteen years, had darting pain in the right lower abdominal quadrant for four months; the pain had lasted only a few minutes. There had not been any radiation of the pain. The patient had not had any symptoms which were referable to the gastro-intestinal or urinary systems. Examination of the abdomen revealed a large mass which on rectal examination was found to be pelvic in origin. A diagnosis of pelvic tumor, probably a cyst, was made and exploratory laparotomy was performed. The mass was found to consist of a simple hematocyst, 5 cm. in diameter, and a hematocolpos caused by a diaphragm-like occlusion just behind the hymen.

Case 3.—A girl, aged thirteen years, came to the clinic because of sharp attacks of pain in the left lower abdominal quadrant; the attacks had lasted about six hours. In the three weeks before the patient came to the clinic, she had had five such attacks; the last one had been accompanied by vomiting. The pain had extended down the anteromedial aspect of the left leg. A tender mass was found in the left lower quadrant of the abdomen, both by abdominal and rectal examination. A roentgenogram of the kidneys, ureters and bladder did not reveal any abnormality and the urine was normal. A diagnosis of twisted ovarian cyst was made. Operation revealed that the left fallopian tube and ovary were twisted on the mesosalpinx with a double twist. A gangrenous fallopian tube and a simple cyst of the ovary, 9 cm. in diameter, were removed.

Case 4.—A girl, aged twelve years, had had a strangulated necrotic right fallopian tube and ovary removed five years before she came to the clinic. In

the year before the patient came to the clinic she had had six attacks of pain in the left lower abdominal quadrant; the pain had been relieved by enemas and the passage of gas. On examination, a mass the size

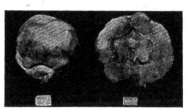

Fig. 1. Gross appearance and cut surface of dermoid cyst removed in Case 8.

of a grapefruit was palpable in the left lower abdominal quadrant; rectal examination confirmed the presence of the mass. A roentgenogram showed a mass of soft tissue in the same region. A roentgenogram of the kidneys, ureters and bladder was normal. A hemorrhagic gangrenous ovary was removed from the left side; it consisted almost entirely of a blood clot.

Case 5.—A girl, aged eleven years, had had frequent attacks of headache, vomiting and abdominal pain for a month before her admission to the clinic. A large abdominal tumor the size of a grapefruit was palpated. A roentgenogram of the abdomen did not reveal any abnormality except a mass of soft tissue. The preoperative diagnosis was ovarian tumor. Exploratory laparotomy revealed a simple hemorrhagic cyst of the left ovary, 14 cm. in diameter; the cyst was removed. The right ovary was 10 cm. in diameter and contained one large cyst and numerous bean-sized cysts. It was removed, but a small strip of ovarian tissue was left. The uterus was congenitally absent; only a stump of the cervix was present. When the patient returned to the clinic four years later she was in good general health and was menstruating from the cervical stump.

Case 6.—A twelve-year-old girl presented herself complaining of left-sided abdominal pain which had begun eight months before she came to the clinic and had continued intermittently. She had had no nausea or vomiting or any intestinal symptoms except slight constipation. Examination revealed a tender pelvio-abdominal mass. A diagnosis of pelvic tumor was made and exploratory laparotomy revealed a hemorrhagic par-ovarian cyst on the left side and a markedly engorged fallopian tube which had resulted from a twisted pedicle. Both of these were removed.

Case 7.—A girl, aged eight years, had been operated on four months before she came to the clinic. She had had an attack of pain in the right lower quadrant of the abdomen and the right thigh. There had been some abdominal tenderness and rigidity and a fever of 101° F. Part of a tumor and the appendix had been removed. The same attacks had continued intermittently ever since the operation. The tumor was found to form a mass which completely filled the lower part of the abdomen and was adherent to the small bowel, cecum and sigmoid colon. It originated in the right ovary. The tumor was removed, together with the left ovary, fallopian tube and the uterus, because of their dense attachment. It proved to be a teratoma which contained hair, cartilage, sebaceous material and a multitlocular papillary cystadenocarcinoma, grade 1.

Case 8.—A girl, aged seven years, came to the clinic complaining of dull pain in the lower left side which had lasted one to two days. It had been relieved by an enema and had not been accompanied by nausea or vomiting. These attacks had recurred every one or two months. Three months before the patient came to the clinic, abdominal tenderness, fever and some vomiting had occurred. A diagnosis of streptococcus peritonitis had been made. She was hospitalized for three weeks. Examination showed tenderness in the left lower abdominal quadrant and a large mass which was connected with the uterus. A roentgenogram of the abdomen revealed soft tissue shadows which suggested a dermoid. Accordingly, she was operated on and a dermoid cyst the size of a lemon, which arose from the left ovary, was removed (Fig. 1). It was lying in the cul-de-sac of Douglas and was attached to the uterus and sigmoid colon.

Case 9.—A girl, aged fourteen years, was admitted to the clinic because of sharp pains in the right lower quadrant of the abdomen. The pains had lasted only a few minutes and then had disappeared. These attacks even had awakened her from sleep. She had had no nausea or vomiting. The attacks first had occurred two weeks before her admission to the clinic. Examination revealed tenderness in the right lower abdominal quadrant and some rectal tenderness on the right side.

On exploration a tumor the size of a golf ba... was filled with clotted blood, was found in t ovary. The tumor and adjacent ovarian tiss removed; the remainder of the ovary, which : normal, was left. The tumor proved to be : luteum cyst.

Comment

The technical problem in the removal (tumors is usually not difficult. Davidso... gestion of the use of extreme care in m... a twisted cyst and the placing of a clam... pedicle well below the twist before any m... tion is valuable in the prevention of pu... embolism following operation.

Summary

We have added eight more cases, whic... a total of sixteen cases in which ovarian... have been found among young girls at th... The majority (seven) of these tumor... simple ovarian cysts; four were dermoi... three were carcinomatous cysts; one wa... ovarian cyst, and one was a sarcoma. Thi... to emphasize the importance of keeping... the possibility of ovarian tumors in your... as a fourth of the tumors in this series w... ignant.

References

1. Davidson, C. L.: Twisted ovarian cyst; a pr... prevent fatality from embolism. Am. Jour. ... 27:79, (Jan.) 1935.
2. Hubert: Quoted by Findley, Palmer: Chapt... Diseases of the Female Genital Organs in Chil... Abt. I.A.: Pediatrics. Philadelphia: W. B. Co., 4:1207-1242, 1924.
3. Mayo, C. W., and Fauster, J. U., Jr.: Ovari... of children. Surg. Clin. N. Amer., 12:1047-105... 1932.
4. Wakeley, C. P. G.: Ovarian teratomatous cyst... in children. Surg., Gynec. and Obst., 56:692-695... 1933.

COEXISTING PERNICIOUS ANEMIA AND CHRONIC PULMONARY TUBERCULOSIS*

DAVID V. SHARP, M.D.

Oak Terrace, Minnesota

NUMEROUS theories have been advanced to explain the rarity with which pernicious anemia and chronic pulmonary tuberculosis have been associated. Mathias[4,5] believed that a lack of hydrochloric acid in the stomach produced an unfavorable medium in the tissues for the

growth of the tubercle bacilli. This ... proven by Neuberger,[7] who reported a... with deficient acid secretion as well as ... ent hemolytic jaundice and chronic pu... tuberculosis. Neuberger, Meisner,[6] and ... believed that the toxic substances cause... tubercle bacilli stimulated the bone marr... way comparable with those produced

*From Glen Lake Sanatorium, Oak Terrace, Minnesota, and Minneapolis, Minnesota.

258

and gastric mucosa. Quarnström,[8] Scheidel,[10] Shandel[11] and Wilkinson[12] explain the rare association of these two diseases in the following way: "Tuberculosis occurs chiefly in young people while pernicious anemia has its incidence in older people, and the association of these two diseases would therefore be rare, and is of no special significance in so far as actual antagonism is concerned."

The material for this study was obtained from the records of Glen Lake Sanatorium and Nopeming Sanatorium, the State Board of Vital Statistics for the year of 1934 and reviews of current medical literature. Since pernicious anemia is not a reportable disease, I have borrowed heavily from the works of Scheidel and of Shandel, who reviewed 269 and 1,127 cases of pernicious anemia respectively. The age incidence tabulated here represents the average of these two similar series (chart).

The age incidence of chronic pulmonary tuberculosis at Glen Lake Sanatorium for the year 1934 begins its rise at the 10-19 year level (5.5 per cent) and climbs rapidly to 32.9 per cent at 20-29 years, from which point it recedes gradually to 9.5 per cent at sixty plus years.

The age incidence of pernicious anemia begins its slow climb at 0-29 years (2.7 per cent) and rises to its maximum point of 33.5 per cent at 50-59 years, from which point it declines to a low point of 6.8 per cent at 70 plus years.[9] The morbidity and mortality rates of pulmonary tuberculosis in Minnesota for the year 1934 are 118 and 30.5 per 100,000 population; a ratio of about 4:1. The incidence and death rate are strikingly similar in pernicious anemia; e.g., 4.9 and 4.4 respectively. Approximately three out of four cases of pulmonary tuberculosis recover. In the event that healing occurs under the age of fifty years, one can well appreciate this factor in the rare co-existence of these two diseases.

Case Report

W. S., a white man, sixty-seven years of age, was admitted to Glen Lake Sanatorium on August 10, 1934, with a history of cough and expectoration of five years' duration, increasing in severity until upon admission he raised two drams of muco-purulent sputum in twenty-four hours. The sputum contained tubercle bacilli which could be seen on stained preparations and which were pathogenic for guinea pigs. For three years, dyspnea had been present to such an extent that it was audibly evident at absolute rest; weakness and weight loss had been present for the same length of

time. In November, 1933, he was hospitalized for this complaint, and at that time he had a lemon yellow skin and sclera, pale mucous membrane and atrophic mucosa on the tongue. Numbness and tingling of the

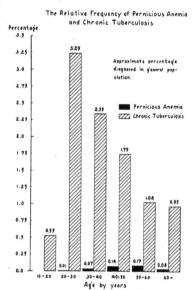

The Relative Frequency of Pernicious Anemia and Chronic Tuberculosis

hands was noted. Blood studies, and gastric analysis confirmed the diagnosis of pernicious anemia.

	Nov.1933	Jan. 1934	Aug. 1934	Admitted Glen Lake
Red Blood Count	1,950,000		3,350,000	
White Blood Count	5,300		5,500	
Hemoglobin	48%	90%	78%	
Morphology	anisocytosis macrocytosis polychromasia neutrophiles shifted to rt. poikilocytosis		anisocytosis macrocytosis polychromasia poikilocytosis shifted to rt. reticulocyte .8%	
Gastric Expression	Free HCl 0 degree Combined 10-15 degrees Total 10-15 degrees		Free HCl 0 degree (after Histamine) Free HCl 0 degree Combined 0 degree Total 2 degree	

During 1933 and 1934 the patient responded well to liver, iron citrate, and dilute hydrochloric acid, and was discharged in January, 1934, with a hemoglobin of 90 per cent. He reported to the Out-Patient Department of the hospital for liver therapy intramuscularly.

On admission to Glen Lake Sanatorium this patient had far advanced pulmonary tuberculosis of chronic fibroid type as well as cavitation in the left upper lobe. The sclerae were yellow, and the face red; a small easily reducible inguinal hernia was present; the liver and spleen were not palpable. Vibratory sense was completely absent from ankles to iliac crests and markedly reduced at the wrists; other neurological examinations showed nothing of note. Intensive intramuscular liver therapy was instituted, and the reticulocytes increased temporarily from 0.8 to 2.9 per cent; the hemoglobin from 78 per cent to a level ranging from 85 to 95 per cent (Sahli). The patient thought the numbness and tingling of his fingers had diminished somewhat since admission.

The pulmonary tuberculosis has been practically without change over a fourteen month period of observation. His ultimate prognosis is rather poor and his tuberculosis does not seem to have been aggravated by the associated pernicious anemia.

Discussion

In Shandel's series of 117 cases of pernicious anemia, 69, or 59.6 per cent, are above fifty years of age. Two cases had associated pulmonary tuberculosis to which no special significance was attributed by the author.

From a study of 370 cases of pernicious anemia, Wilkinson feels that many conditions may co-exist with pernicious anemia without apparent causal relationship. Of this series eighty-six (23.3 per cent) had signs or symptoms of other conditions distinct from Addisonian anemia and one (0.27 per cent) showed a co-existence of acute pulmonary tuberculosis. There were no cases of chronic pulmonary tuberculosis.

In an extensive review of the literature, Wilkinson was able to collect only nine cases of chronic pulmonary tuberculosis associated with pernicious anemia before 1933. Of these, four cases were reported between 1903 and 1910 and some doubt may exist as to the diagnosis of pernicious anemia in these patients. Miliary tuberculosis was not mentioned.

In this study of 7,983 admissions to sanatoria for tuberculosis, only one patient was found to have these two conditions. In a series of 16,600 autopsies, Barron[1] found ninety-six cases of pernicious anemia, two accompanied by miliary tuberculosis, and three arrested or healed tuberculosis. He reports two cases of pernicius anemia associated with active pulmonary tuberculosis.

This is the first recognized case of chronic tuberculosis in association with pernicious anemia in 6,600 cases admitted to Glen Lake Sanatorium and 1,383 admissions to Nopeming Sanatorium. There is a marked difference in the incidence of pernicious anemia and chronic pulmonary tuberculosis. This study reveals that the coexistence of these two diseases is extremely rare, and apparently the presence of one has no inhibitory effect on the other.

References

1. Barron, M.: Pernicious anemia and tuberculosis; is there antagonism? Review of occurrence of tuberculosis in 93 cases of pernicious anemia as found in 16,600 postmortem examinations, with report of 2 clinical cases. Jour. A. M. A., 100:1590-1592, (May 20) 1933.
2. Freeman, W.: Pernicious anemia complicated by acute miliary tuberculosis; report of case. Jour. A. M. A., 97:996-998, (Oct. 3) 1931.
3. Levin, N.: Anaemia perniciosa und Lungentuberkulose, Med. Klin., 28:261-264, (Feb. 19) 1932.
4. Mathias, E.: Ueber das freibleiben perniziöser Anamien von der Tuberkulose der Kachektischen. Deutsche Med. Wchnschr., 52:2190-2191, (Dec. 24) 1926.
5. Mathias, E.: Zur Frage des Ausschliessungsverhaltnisses zwischen perniziöser Anamie und aktiver Tuberkulose. Frankfurt. Ztschr. f. Path., 46:376-384, 1934.
6. Meissner, R.: Anaemia perniciosa und perniciosa-ahnliche Zustande (auch bei Lungentuberkulose). Klin. Wchnschr., 9:1066-1068, (June 7) 1930.
7. Neuberger, J.: Die Beziehung der Tuberkulose zum hamolytischen Ikterus und zur perniziosen Anamie. Deutsche Med. Wchnschr., 53:997, (June 10) 1927.
8. Quarnström, E.: Pernicious anemia and tuberculosis. Finska lak.-sallsk. handl., 71:849-855, (Oct.) 1929.
9. Sajous: Analytic Cyclopedia of Practical Medicine. 12: Supp., p. 52, 1932.
10. Scheidel, H.: Ueber das Vorkommen, die Aetiologie die Symptomatologie und den Verlauf der perniziosen Anamie. Munchen. Med. Wchnschr., 80:302-305, (Feb. 24) 1933.
11. Shandel, Burger: Study of 117 cases of pernicious anemia from 1913-1930. A. C. T. A. Med. Scandenavica Supp., 30-41;1-121, 1931.
12. Wilkinson, J. F.: Diseases associated with pernicious anemia in study of 370 cases. Quart. Jour. Med., 2:281-309, (July) 1933.

CENTRAL FRACTURES OF THE NECK OF THE FEMUR TREATED BY INTERNAL FIXATION*

WILLIS C. CAMPBELL, M.D.

Memphis, Tennessee

IN AN analysis of 495 fresh fractures of the neck and trochanter of the femur, the distribution as to location was as follows:

Trochanteric 229
Complete central 214
Impacted central 52

*Abstract of paper read before the Southern Minnesota Medical Association, Winona, Minnesota, August 11, 1937.

Of those occuring in elderly individuals over seventy, the average age of 108 trochanteric fractures was 78.1; of seventy-eight complete central fractures, 74.6; and of nineteen impacted central fractures, 79.5 years.

Thus, impacted fractures of the neck of the femur and intertrochanteric fractures constitute more than half (56.7 per cent) of these fractures, and in this half, union may be expected in practically 100 per cent, if only approximate anatomic apposition is maintained.

Consequently, in any discussion of fractures of the neck of the femur it is most important that differentiation as to location and characteristics be made. Central fractures of the neck of the femur constituted only 43.3 per cent of fractures in and about the neck and trochanter of the femur; only in this group is there any doubt as to securing osseous union. Prior to 1904, it was considered that central or intracapsular fractures did not unite by osseous union.

No one has been a stronger advocate of the Whitman procedure than I, but after seeing the results of Smith-Petersen and others, I have come to the conclusion that internal fixation not only gives a higher percentage of excellent functional results and firm osseous union, but also materially decreases the time in which union is secured, so that weight bearing and walking without support is obtained in from four to six months as compared to six to twelve months by the Whitman method. Also function in the knee and hip is materially conserved, and permanently restricted motion is exceedingly rare. The mortality has been materially decreased by the less extensive means of immobilization and the shorter time of confinement to bed.

My colleagues and I have employed the three-flanged nail in forty-nine cases of complete, central or intracapsular fractures of the neck of the femur. In eleven, the procedure as described by Smith-Petersen was employed, which consisted in a complete exposure of the hip joint and trochanter; in thirty-eight, the nail was inserted through a lateral incision with "blind nailing." The Smith-Petersen technic has been entirely discarded, as so-called "blind nailing" is a less extensive surgical procedure.

The present technic of insertion may be described as follows: Reduction is uniformly accomplished by the well-known Whitman abduction method, so that usually no roentgenogram is made at this time. After reduction, abduction is reduced to about 120 degrees so as to facilitate insertion of the nail. An incision approximately four inches in length is now made over the lateral aspect of the greater trochanter and upper two inches of the shaft exposing the lower half of the greater trochanter and upper two inches of the shaft. A 3 mm. steel wire peg is then placed into an ordinary chuck drill, and the sharp end of the wire inserted into the center of the shaft about three-quarters of an inch below the trochanter. Great care must be taken that the wire drill makes an angle with the shaft of about 45 degrees and is angulated forward about 10 to 15 degrees to conform to the normal anterior deviation of the neck. The wire is now drilled about two inches in this direction, after which roent-

genograms are made in both planes which will confirm reduction and the exact direction of the wire drill. If reduction has not been accomplished, a second attempt can be made, but this has not been necessary in any case; also if the wire is not accurately placed, other attempts can be made until the desired direction is obtained. If reduction and direction of the wire are satisfactory, the wire is drilled into the head of the bone to within one-quarter to one-half inch of the joint, depending on the length of the proximal fragment. This is confirmed by the roentgenogram. The protruding portion of the wire is now measured by placing a wire drill of the same length parallel with the protruding portion, and a nail of the exact length selected. I employ a modification of the three-flanged steel Smith-Petersen nail with a tunnel through the center, which is slightly larger than the wire. The nail is then threaded on the wire. A driver with a tunnel in the center is now threaded over the wire and the nail driven through the neck and head by the aid of a heavy mallet. The wire is removed and the driver placed over the trochanter, and the instrument tapped a few times with a mallet so as to closely approximate the fragments. Roentgenograms should not consume more than fifteen minutes, and should be developed and returned to the operating room in five minutes. The entire procedure requires not more than thirty to forty minutes.

After operation, the limb is placed in a Hodgens' splint. At the end of three weeks, roentgenograms are made in order to confirm the position, which we have always found undisturbed. Motion in the knee is instituted at the end of four weeks, when the patient may be removed to his home. At the end of three months, walking is instituted without weight bearing, and at the end of four months, weight is borne on crutches. At the end of five to six months, crutches are discarded if union is firm, as demonstrated by the roentgenogram, which should show trabeculae transversing the line of fracture. Undoubtedly, it is possible that function may be resumed earlier, but the physiologic status in this location is such that firm union is always slow.

In this series, twenty-one cases have been followed for over one year with 88 per cent solid union; however, nine per cent of these have degenerative changes indicative of a devitalized head with an ultimate prognosis of very poor function. With improvement in technic and further experience, 80 to 85 per cent solid osseous union with a good functional result can be anticipated.

CASE REPORT

POISONING WITH CICUTA MACULATA OR WATER HEMLOCK

CLYDE A. UNDINE, M.D.

Minneapolis, Minnesota

CICUTA is a highly toxic plant. Many deaths amongst men and animals have been traced to this plant. This plant is also known as Wild Parsnips, Water Hemlock, Cowbane, Beaver or Muskrat poisoning, Children's Death, et cetera. This is one of our most common swampweeds, growing abundantly along streams, ponds, ditches and wet meadows, throughout the Eastern and Central portions of the United States.

Since the middle of the sixteenth century, Cicuta has been recognized definitely in the United States. It has sometimes been confused with Conium which was a poisonous hemlock given to Grecian and Roman criminals. The poison was probably Conium or extracts and mixtures of several other poisonous plants. It was this plant which was probably similar to Cicuta. The symptoms of Socrates' death which were recorded in detail bore no resemblance to those of Cicuta poisoning.

Conium was studied in 1541 very accurately by Konrad Gesner. He gave the name Cicuta Aquatica to Water Hemlock.

Cicuta Maculata is a perennial and a member of the parsnip family. The Cicuta plant has a hollow green, jointed stem which grows from three to six feet high, and has narrow leaves divided several times. It has a small green-white flower with dense clusters. The root has a bunch of spindle shaped shoots which give forth a yellow, gummy secretion similar to that of the parsnip. This secretion is sweetish, and not disagreeable to the taste, so that adults and children have eaten quantities sufficient to prove fatal.

From other umbelliferous plants, the roots are differentiated by the presence of numerous transverse chambers which are seen in a section. Cicuta differs also from garden parsnips with which it is sometimes confused in that the parsnip has yellow flowers, one single root, a leaflet which has a broader stem and which is rough, and the plant is not necessarily grown in wet places.

In 1679 Wepfer recorded the symptoms of Cicuta poisoning, giving a detailed account of five children who were fatally poisoned. He dwelt particularly on the non-coagulation of the blood. Later in 1723 Weimann described the poisoning of two students. In 1756 Schwenke recorded the poisoning of four children in the village of Overschie. A New Englander, Stockbridge, in 1814, gave the first public account in this country of Cicuta poisoning. He described the poison-

ing of three patients, one dying in violent convulsions. M. R. Stratton published an account of the poisoning of eleven boys in Denver, two proving fatal. This is the greatest number of cases of Cicuta poisoning reported by any one observer up to the present time. In a review of the literature of this subject, Egdahl included a total of 47 cases, but it doesn't seem possible that this represents the entire number of poisonings due to Cicuta.

Toxicology

The poisonous resin of this plant was first isolated in 1876 by Bachm who named it cicutoxin. An aromatic, yellowish, oil like-substance exudes when the root stock is cut and the odor is similar to parsnip. The toxin has been described as a clear plant resin, which is sticky and soluble in either chloroform or alcohol. The leaves and stems are less toxic than the root stocks. This plant is most poisonous during the spring. During the growing season, the stored material is absorbed in the development of the plant and is of course then less virulent.

Necropsy examinations have reported the following findings:

1. Emphysema and edema of the lungs.
2. Non-coagulation of the blood after twenty-four hours.
3. Multiple hemorrhages.
4. Generalized congestion of the central nervous system.
5. Widely dilated pupils.
6. Glomerular nephritis.

Report of Cases

On June 14, 1924, I was called to attend two boys nine and thirteen years of age who had been taken suddenly ill. They had been dismissed from their classes at 3:30 P. M. apparently well, and immediately went to play. At 5:15 the boys were eating their evening meal. The parents observed that they appeared pale and sickly and that they refused their supper. One of the boys asked permission to leave the room, complaining of nausea, but before going very far, fell to the floor with violent convulsions. When I arrived, twenty minutes later, the older child was in a convulsion and the other was vomiting and appeared seriously ill. The children were evidently suffering from some sort of poison. I soon found out they had eaten of a plant, the nature of which was unknown to me at the time. There was a plot of swamp land adjoining their home in which water hemlock grew

(Continued on Page 296)

SURVEY OF PIONEER MEMBERS OF THE ST. LOUIS COUNTY MEDICAL SOCIETY

By RICHARD BARDON, M.D.

IN TWO previous chapters an attempt has been made to trace the development of the medical profession in Duluth and St. Louis County, and to record the contribution of the men who practiced during that period. These men are well known to the older members of the society; some are still living and in active practice. It is not possible, in this narrative, to include detailed biographies of all the pioneer practitioners. The selection has been made somewhat arbitrarily on the basis of available data. The choice casts no reflection on the records of those who are mentioned by a few lines or paragraphs only. They were all pioneers in the civic and medical development of the county, and many will go down as "unsung heroes," who played their part in serving the community.

It is not the scope of this chapter to mention in detail the records of the surviving members of this early group, although it is difficult to pass by some names without giving them a salute. Such recognition is fitting not only because of their seniority in membership but because of their unselfish labors in the field of medicine, and the honors they have brought to the profession.

The appended list includes the names of the practitioners from 1883 to 1900, as appearing in the city directories. Doubtless, this list is incomplete, and it is to be hoped that the material presented in this brief series of papers will serve as a framework for future definitive research.

Acknowledgment is made to many who contributed data or suggestions used in this compilation: Dr. J. M. Armstrong of St. Paul, Dr. E. L. Tuohy, Dr. D. L. Tilderquist, Dr. C. A. Scherer, Dr. S. H. Boyer, Sr., Dr. W. A. Coventry, Dr. C. F. McComb, and Dr. A. E. Walker of Duluth.

William H. Magie

Duluth had a population of about 10,000 when Dr. Magie arrived there in 1884. William Henry Magie was born at Madison, New Jersey, September 30, 1854. When he was three years of age his parents moved to Henderson County, Illinois, and from the time he was about seven until he was fifteen he lived with the family in Chicago. Dr. Magie acquired his early education in the public schools in Chicago and Abingdon College at Abingdon, Illinois. In 1874, the family moved to Kansas, then recently freed from Indian occupation. The family settled on a ranch, and the father became an extensive rancher and a man of prominence in Kansas affairs during the seventies and eighties, being elected to the state legislature. Dr. Magie lived on the Kansas farm and ranch for several years, and previous to his medical training spent a year in a drugstore at Pittsburg, Kansas, and in 1882 entered the College of Physicians and Surgeons at St. Louis. He was graduated in 1884, and after a brief practice at Pittsburg, Kansas, arrived in Duluth, September 10, 1884. During the first fifteen years of his life in Duluth, he devoted himself to the arduous work of the general practitioner, but subsequently confined his work to surgery. Dr. Magie was for twenty-eight years official surgeon of St. Mary's Hospital. He was president of the Minnesota State Medical Association in 1908. He was also a Fellow of the American College of Surgeons, and a Fellow of the Western Surgical Association.

Dr. Magie died in 1932. The following tribute, written by Dr. E. L. Tuohy, is of unusual interest:

Tribute by Dr. Tuohy

The safe exhibition of ether anesthesia in anybody's hands; high pressure sterilization, with proper ligatures and instruments for hemostasis; hospital beds and twenty-four-hour nursing—these and many other developments skyrocketed surgery into unexampled prominence after 1880. However, none of these developments could have come without the direction and intuitive judgment of men who, though not to be classed either as pioneers or researchers, became the great operating surgeons of that epoch. They were not the McDowells, the Rushes, the Beaumonts, or even McBurneys. They developed independently here and there, usually in association with a hospital backed either by a nationalistic group or a religious order. Thus did Dr. J. B. Deaver advance with the German hospital in Philadelphia, J. B. Murphy with Mercy Hospital in Chicago, W. W. Mayo and his celebrated sons with St. Mary's in Rochester.

In like manner, but obviously in a lesser orbit, did William H. Magie advance himself to prestige and position in connection with St. Mary's Hospital in Duluth. The very distinguished daughters in the St. Paul family of Kerst (Mother Scholastica and Sister Alexia) put their lives and their considerable fortune at the disposal of the Benedictine Order in Duluth. Their present hospital was opened in 1898. Few investments of soul and money have ever produced better dividends. To Dr. Magie goes the honor of having been the surgical standard bearer who did for Duluth and vicinity what others were doing in something of the same tempo throughout our Middle West.

He left his impress in countless ways. He was honored by the profession at home and respected abroad. He was one of the earliest industrial surgeons, and under him many young men secured a first-hand introduction to the realities of practice that made them very successful men. His manner was not ingratiating. He was given to rather grandiloquent criticism of his fellows, and particularly his later competitors. This led no one to fail to appreciate his great diagnostic powers and technical competence. At a time when few laboratory and no x-ray aids were available, fancy what men of his type and essential isolation were pitted against. Malpractice suits threatened even as now, and without office or hospital records of any consequence such men relied upon their judgment and memory to a degree few of us may appreciate.

Dr. Magie performed the first appendectomy in this region at the old St. Mary's Hospital (now St. Ann's Home for the Aged) in the year 1891. He performed the first gastro-enterostomy done here in 1895. For some years, I recall his use of the McGraw ligature type of anastomosis. He was a tireless visitor to medical sessions and surgical amphitheatres here and there. He was prone to retail the exploits of men like Ochsner, Deaver, Charles A. Wheaton of St. Paul, and Bernays of St. Louis (one of his early teachers). He handled fractures as cleverly as he supervised typhoids. With a twinkling eye he enjoyed nothing better than to regale the operating room troupe with gossipy comments of the day. For example, "I saw a new sign on our building today. A recent addition to our profession announces that he is to treat 'Diseases of Women and Children.' That's a fine idea. For years I've specialized in 'diseases of men, women and children.'"

Behind all the banter, however, was a devoutly keen appreciation of the duties and privileges of those who find themselves the masters in our guild. It was his way to discipline and teach, and be it said to his very great credit—he played no favorites.

When the Steel Corporation built the new plant at Gary, on the St. Louis River, a fine unit hospital was built, and to it he transferred his work. In addition, he was medical consultant for several railroads and industrial plants. As his health failed, however, he returned to St. Mary's Hospital, where, after a lingering illness, he died. His early devotion to the interests of the Benedictine Sisters when his faculties were at their zenith brought him peace and surcease, as well as loving care, in his long, racking, final illness, with the tragic discomforts of myocardial weakness from coronary decay.

It may be said, without disparaging the work of any other men, that Dr. Magie, above all others, set the goal of honest and square dealing for this area as between doctor and patient; and he who was critical to a degree, at times, of others was equally severe with himself where he felt judgment had failed him. He was generous to a fault, and had the feeling of many who went through the panic of ninety-three that it was absurd to store up any savings. This thought may well obtrude at a time when history in the repetition may well be in enactment.

Apropos of Dr. Bardon's comments upon styles in horses and buggies for St. Louis County doctors, Dr. Magie had a spanking pair of bays, that vied for pre-eminence with the very exceptional equipages that were the pride of the Head of the Lakes at that time. The musk-ozen robes and beplumed cutter-like droshky are well recalled. He joined with many men of prominence in establishing hunting and fishing lodges on Isle Royale and elsewhere. The old guard in the State Medical Association knew him well. They elected him president at a Duluth meeting in 1908.

John J. Eklund

By E. L. Tuohy, M.D.

Dr. John J. Eklund practiced in Duluth from 1885 to the time of his death in 1922. Born in Hälsingland, Sweden, March 13, 1861, he came with his parents and family to Taylors Falls, Minnesota, at the age of five. He became ultimately the leading Scandinavian surgeon at the Head of the Lakes.

It is both impossible and improper to attempt to evaluate his useful career apart from the great migration to Minnesota of Swedes, Norwegians and Danes, which began shortly after our war between the States. The virile, individualistic and intelligent immigrants truly made great portions of Minnesota a new Viking stronghold. They came with their ministers, teachers, doctors, and other qualified artisans. Dr. Eklund typified the best among them to such a degree that these items may well become a part of a discussion of his life. These men and women held very closely to their home traditions and religion. It is conspicuous, for example, how many of our present-day Minnesota physicians are sons of Scandinavian ministers. While Dr. Eklund was not a minister's son, he early fell under the influence of the Church in his formative adolescence, and lived with an uncle, Reverend Engdahl, at Cambridge, Minnesota. He never forsook nor forgot this native religious guidance. It was one of his attributes, coupled with his sturdy body and honest mind, which led him directly into the confidence and esteem of thousands of his like-thinking compatriots.

He continued his education, still under Swedish guidance, at Gustavus Adolphus College in St. Peter, Minnesota. For a number of years after 1893 he was a director of the College. It would appear that it was in St. Peter that he met Miss Nannie Asp, whom he later married in Duluth in 1888.

He received his medical training at the old Minnesota Hospital College, which later became the Medical Department of the University of Minnesota. Thus, it appears that he came under the tutelage of doctors who not only introduced him to American Medicine but American life as well. This was likely important, for Scandinavian doctors, trained before coming to America, often found great difficulty in adjusting their attitudes to the obvious novelties inherent in the development of the new land. Dr. Eklund suffered none of the restrictions upon manner, personality, approach or conduct imposed by a transfer so late in life. His was the great combination of deep traditional, religious and intellectual certainty gleaned from his clear-thinking Swedish forebears, upon which was engrafted an outlook and political urge, the product of living in a fertile and at that time unfettered land.

It is easy to see, therefore, in retrospect, how he developed along so many lines. A worthily religious man, he liberally supported his own church, not condemning other denominations; he acquired a high degree of surgical judgment and technic without in any way disparging the work of others; he became almost a political seer and prophet, without ever asking for himself any conspicuous position; his business judgment led him to relative financial affluence, untrammeled by the envy of anyone, or leaving the evidence of wreckage, so often the obvious result of competitive ruthlessness.

It is true that he was elected Coroner for St. Louis County in 1898; he served on the first charter commission of Duluth, and was chairman of the Board of Health Committee of the Duluth Water and Light Board. Later, he was Presidential Elector at large for Minnesota in 1908. However, these and many other responsible and honorary positions he took in his stride. They did not keep him from successive visits for graduate courses and instruction in New York, Baltimore, Chicago, and elsewhere. In later years, he was associated in the management of two important Duluth banks, but maintained the keenest interest in all medical activities, and assisted greatly in the development of the Duluth hospitals.

Few men were ever more beloved among the profession for what they actually were. The writer best recalls certain personal attributes that memory retains of the period of about 1905: He had a very black Vandyke beard, always well trimmed. At the same time, he had a very heavy, black horse. This horse had acquired the faculty of lying down gracefully while harnessed and within the traces and tethered to a hitching post, the while he awaited the convenience of his master. After long days of calls and hospital duties the doctor's meals were likely rarely on time. Then, as was the custom, he had interminable evening office hours. Just across from his office was a theater which ran two evening shows. On occasion, the genial Dr. Charles F. McComb and his wife were planning to attend the second show. "Isn't it fine," remarked Mrs. McComb, "see, the crowd is just leaving the first show: the street is full of people." "You are wrong, my dear," Charles F. replied, "that is not the theatre crowd—Eklund is just closing up his office!" In those same offices, where he saw so much of life and granted its furtherance to many, came also his death. A demented man took his life and his own under some awful twist of the human consciousness which no one may ever understand.

Mrs. Eklund died in 1905. Their son, Dr. William J. Eklund, born in 1890, is now a member of the Minnesota House of Representatives, and president of the Duluth National Bank, which his father helped to organize.

Charles Adams Stewart

In 1887, Dr. Charles Adams Stewart arrived in Duluth. Dr. Stewart was born in Sandusky, Ohio, on June 23, 1848. He was educated in the public schools of Sandusky, took a course at the Western Reserve Normal School, and graduated from the Medical Department of the University of Iowa, at Keokuk, in 1870, with a degree of M.D. He then returned to Ohio and practiced a while before entering the Medical Department of Western Reserve University, from which he was graduated in 1877. He then practiced in Marinette, Wisconsin, for about six years, later moved to Chicago, where he was in practice for about four years; and finally located in Duluth.

Dr. Stewart was one of the pioneer surgeons of the city, and the following description, written by Dr. E. L. Tuohy, who knew him well, is most interesting:

Dr. Stewart—The Man

By E. L. Tuohy, M.D.

As will be seen by this recital of his activities, medical and otherwise, he came to Duluth with "great expectations." Eighty-seven was not long before Ninety-three—the depression period that all those who passed away before 1929 looked back to as a chapter of despair that would never be repeated. Charles A. Stewart was one who stood in line for hours at the old Land Office in Duluth ready, when the minute and hour arrived, to make certain "filings" on the property near the upper St. Louis basin near Spirit Lake. With visions of an amplified Chicago in Minnesota, this land near the future docks had exceeding potential value, at least in the minds of those who at the same time swarmed into East Superior and laid out a city that fifty years later was said to have "usurped a lot of fairly good farm land." In any case, Dr. Stewart later said, when he sold his acreage to the Steel Company for part of its present site, "I received for it almost exactly what I paid for it, and had the honor of paying taxes on it yearly in the quarter-century interim."

Nevertheless, while his speculative ventures wound up in the conventional way, the failure to amass a fortune likely saved him for an extraordinarily useful and successful medical life. Among those who practiced in Duluth at the turn of the century none more decisively exemplified the doctor of poise, alertness, polish and resourcefulness. Endowed with indomitable will and self control, he held a rigid rein on his patients. So long as they obeyed him faultlessly he was their abject slave, calling on them at any and all hours, with total disregard for his own convenience and comfort. If they questioned his judgment or ventured to seek counsel elsewhere he maintained his equanimity if he could, and if he couldn't his sarcasm and irony were as superb as any of Voltaire's. Said a fluttery grand dame to him on occasion: "But Doctor, I am only going to get their opinion." "Yes,' he replied, as he characteristically nodded his head and drew up the corners of his mouth sardonically, "and when you return you will have their opinion in a bottle."

He practiced in some four medical decades when it was all right to specialize in the eye or maybe at times the ear . . . but for the most part, every he-man doctor should be equal to the care of anything at any time. The growth of specialism in later years distressed him, as it did many others who saw the "family' stepping out and choosing their own type of doctor, even as they did their political party or religion. Some of us, today, could have learned much from him, and not a few did. He believed in therapeutics, and had a polished sequence of vehicles and adjuvants that were only exceeded by his extraordinary finesse in getting about among his patients. On occasion he told the writer, "You must enter a house; examine the patient, doing all that is essential for his comfort and outlook; speak to the family and give full reassurance; gain access to the hall and hat rack; leave as if in no hurry whatsoever, and be in your buggy and on your way in five minutes." Please remember, those were the days when "contagion" and "typhoid" bulked large in practice; when hospitals housed emergencies and transients; and when the doctor was supposed to be able to forecast the exact hour when crises, like comets, were to appear. A consultation was no casual affair, and to a young man it was a brilliant lesson in dignity. It was particularly awe inspiring when men like Drs. Stewart and Magie appeared in consultation and showed each other that courtesy of approach and expression that was most exalting; but when they foregathered singly and candidly gave their real opinions it was indeed a sorry reflection of how discordant personal competitive attitudes could so widely separate such truly gifted men.

They lived through the beginning of a period when our territory turned from lumbering to mining. Saddle-bag medicine had gone, but the "Horse and Buggy Age" was producing a coterie of independent folk in all lines who, at least, had their "feet on the ground' a goodly portion of the time. The highways and cars had not as yet despoiled the hamlets and assembled the urban pack of people who seem to serve mass service as well in Medicine as in Politics. So, when Dr. Stewart suffered a hemiplegia, sudden and permanent, he was in no mood to quit. To the writer he actually said, "Cut the damn leg off and I'll get down and sit in my office all day." He knew that if he had been able to get there a lot of old patients who worshipped him would come to see him.

A man wonderfully read, his mind was stored richly with wisdom, and he had the great gift to illustrate it with anecdote and reminiscence. It is not likely that he left any published papers, but he read many before local and state societies. Fate dealt kindly with Medicine, as it often does, when his trip to the Head of the Lakes, in search of fortune, ended his finding instead fame and friends.

A. J. Braden

The following résumé of Dr. A. J. Braden's activities was taken from the records of the Society:

Dr. Braden was born in New London, Ontario. He sprang from the sturdy Revolutionary stock of the state of Maine. While still a boy, his parents migrated across the line to the small town of Climax, Michigan, and here the Doctor received his grade school education, high school at Battle Creek College, and his college education at the University of Michigan. At the age of twenty, from 1880 to 1884, he served in the United States Army, most of the service on the Texas border. The urge for further training took him back to the University of Michigan, where he graduated from the Medical School in 1888. He must have loved this North Country for he went directly from his medical course to the shore of Lake Superior and practiced his profession at Munising from the time of his graduation until he changed location to come to Duluth in 1893. The work in upper Michigan must have been strenuous. He frequently related tales of the hardships of the practitioner in the earlier days of the upper Peninsula.

While in Duluth, he carried on as a general practitioner, acquiring a reputation as a keen diagnostician and a careful surgeon. Several postgraduate courses in surgery led him to closely limit himself in this field. In recognition of his work, he was admitted to fellowship in the American College of Surgeons among the earliest of the Duluth members. During his later years of practice he did much orthopedic and industrial surgery. He introduced various younger men to the practice in Duluth and several of our outstanding physicians thank Dr. Braden for the training received from him. The doctor was very assiduous in attending all local medical meetings, and was always prepared to discuss scientific papers. While never pushing himself he was always active in medical and civic affairs and held many offices. During the late war he served on the draft examining board. He was also the examining physician for the Shrine Hospital for Crippled Children for Duluth from its foundation.

Other Early Practitioners

Among the many early practitioners, A. F. Ritchie may be mentioned. He was a graduate of McGill in 1876, a charter member of the Society; a man of wide training, and of unusual skill in his profession.

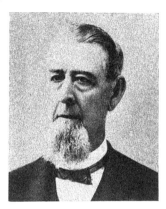

DR. VESPASIAN SMITH

Dr. Smith figured frequently in the early civic and medical development of Duluth. An account of his life may be found in the preceding chapter on "Organization of the St. Louis County Medical Society."

Frank O. Sherwin, also a charter member, a graduate of Rush in 1878, was Health Officer for many years.

George W. Davis, a graduate of the University of Detroit in 1879—a pioneer physician and obstetrician—built up a large practice. He died May 4, 1923.

Jonas M. O. Tufty, a Norwegian by birth and medical training, was probably the first of his nationality to practice in St. Louis County.

Frank N. Phelan received his training in Wooster, Ohio, in 1884, and achieved a large following.

Horace Davis was graduated from Dartmouth in 1884; arrived in Duluth in 1888.

A. C. Taylor arrived in Duluth in 1889. Dr. Taylor was born in Michigan, May 4, 1848. He graduated from the University of Michigan in 1874, and practiced in Manchester, Michigan, for fourteen years, coming to Duluth in 1889. Dr. Taylor was actively identified with the organization and operation of the Training School for Nurses at St. Mary's Hospital. Although he engaged in general practice, he was particularly interested in Surgery, and at one time was local and consulting surgeon for the Duluth and Iron Range Railroad. He died suddenly on April 21, 1926.

J. A. McCuen was born January 27, 1864, at Guelph, Ontario. He was graduated from Toronto University in 1891, arrived in Duluth the same year, later serving as Mayor of the City in 1912-1913. He died in November, 1927.

Pioneers Still in Active Practice

There are some twelve men whose arrival in Duluth places them in the pioneer period, although most of them are still in active practice. Among these are Dr. F. C. Bowman, born March 26, 1849; graduated from Hahnemann, Philadelphia, in 1881; located in Duluth the same year. Dr. D. C. Rood arrived in Duluth in 1888. A detailed sketch of his life is included in a paper by Dr. O. W. Parker, "Pioneer Physician of the Vermillion and Missabe Ranges of Minnesota," to be published subsequently. Dr. A. E. Walker, a graduate of Bellevue Hospital Medical College in 1890, has practiced continuously in Duluth since June, 1890. Dr. Mary McCoy, Michigan 1890, arrived in Duluth, July 8, 1890. Dr. Homer Collins practiced first in Rochester, Minnesota, for five years; then located here in September, 1890. He was graduated from Physicians and Surgeons, New York, in 1884. Dr. S. H. Boyer, Sr., arrived in Duluth on New Year's Day, 1891, and opened his office January 20, 1891, in the Norris-McDougall Block at No. 7 West Superior Street. In 1896, he was elected president of the County Medical Society, with the following slate: "President, Dr. S. H. Boyer; Vice President, Dr. Mary McCoy; Second Vice President, Dr. A. J. Braden; Treasurer, Dr. S. C. McCormick; and Secretary, Dr. C. R. Keyes." In 1930, Dr. Boyer was elected president of the State Society. He is in active practice, and has aided materially in the preparation of this paper.

Dr. C. R. Keyes graduated from Vermont in 1881; located in Duluth in 1891, after practicing in Olmsted County for nine years. Dr. Robert Graham graduated from Detroit Medical College in 1893, and has practiced in Duluth ever since. Dr. Peter Kraft took his medical work in Munich, 1892, coming to Duluth in 1893. Dr. J. M. Robinson, a graduate of Pennsylvania in 1891, came to Duluth in 1893; was a general practitioner, later specializing in Eye, Ear, Nose and Throat. Dr. William R. Bagley is a graduate of Michigan, and has practiced in Duluth since June 30, 1898; he is a past president of the County Society.

Charles Frederick McComb has been in continuous practice in Duluth since 1883. He was born at Stillwater, Minnesota, August 7, 1857, the son of James G. and Eliza Jane McComb. His father, a native of Pennsylvania, lived in Iowa, and subsequently became a territorial pioneer in Minnesota, and for many years was in business at Stillwater. Dr. McComb grew up in Stillwater, and spent two years at the State University, and after beginning his studies under Dr. P. H. Millard at Stillwater, entered Rush Medical College in Chicago in 1877, graduating in 1879. For three and one-half years he practiced in Rush City, Minnesota; then, following a postgraduate course in New York City, he located in Duluth.

Dr. McComb has twice been president of the St. Louis County Medical Society. He was the first president of the Interurban Academy of Medicine, and was president of the State Medical Society in 1887, being the first physician of Duluth to be so recognized. He was also a member of the State Board of Health under three governors. He served as Coroner of St. Louis County for two terms in the eighties, and in 1912 was appointed County Coroner, and has held that office continuously by election. During the World War, Dr. McComb was a medical officer on board the battleship Iowa, and was discharged from the Navy with the rank of Lieutenant Commander. Dr. McComb is the only living charter member of the St. Louis County Medical Society, and it is peculiarly fitting that an account of his life should bring to a close this "Survey of Pioneer Physicians of Duluth and St. Louis County."

(To be continued in May issue)

EDITORIAL

MINNESOTA MEDICINE

OFFICIAL JOURNAL OF THE MINNESOTA STATE MEDICAL
ASSOCIATION

Published by the Association under the direction of its Editing
and Publishing Committee

EDITING AND PUBLISHING COMMITTEE
J. T. CHRISTISON, Saint Paul   C. D. WRIGHT, Minneapolis
E. M. HAMMES, Saint Paul   T. A. PEPPARD, Minneapolis
WALTMAN WALTERS, Rochester

EDITORIAL STAFF
CARL B. DRAKE, Saint Paul, Editor
W. F. BRAASCH, Rochester, Associate Editor
GILBERT COTTAM, Minneapolis, Associate Editor

Annual Subscription—$3.00.   Single Copies—$0.40
Foreign Subscriptions—$3.50.

The right is reserved to reject material submitted for editorial
or advertising columns. The Editing and Publishing Committee
does not hold itself responsible for views expressed either in
editorials or other articles when signed by the author.

Classified advertising—five cents a word; minimum charge,
$1.00. Remittance should accompany order.

Display advertising rates on request.

Address all communications to Minnesota Medicine, 2642 University Avenue, Saint Paul, or Suite 604, National Bldg., Minneapolis. Telephone: Nestor 2641.

BUSINESS MANAGER
J. R. BRUCE

Volume 21   APRIL, 1938   Number 4

Cancer Control Campaign

CANCER today is one of the outstanding problems of medicine and public health. Because of its rapid advance as a cause of death in the past few years, cancer has aroused considerable interest. It is fortunate that the American Society for the Control of Cancer has, as its managing director at this time, such an able leader as Dr. Clarence C. Little of Bar Harbor, Maine. Dr. Little, a former president of the University of Michigan, who was recently appointed to the National Advisory Board on Cancer by Mr. Morgenthau, did much to stimulate and assist the State Committee and those

interested in the local control of cancer by his recent visit to the Twin Cities.

While here, he addressed professional groups and a large lay audience. He emphasized that cancer is an individual problem and that the control of cancer lies with the cancer patient and his physician. *What* is done and *when* it is done largely determines the outcome of every case. He called attention to the fact that there are no community aspects to the cancer problem. Improvement of housing, protection of foods, purification of milk, water, and sewage, have no effect on cancer incidence.

The unwillingness of the layman to hear about cancer is being rapidly broken down. Daily it is becoming easier to enlist the interest and co-operation of laymen in the educational program. This fact makes it important to control and direct this lay interest into proper channels. This is the job of the medical profession, individually as well as a group.

While the fundamental research into the cancer problem is now focused more on the fields of chemistry, physics and biology, than on clinical fields, it remains for the clinician to apply these findings to the saving of lives and to the prevention of the disease. This means that he must keep abreast of the knowledge in these related fields.

The cancer death rate in Minnesota is much higher than for the country as a whole. Today, approximately every eighth death in the state is due to some form of malignant disease.

By coöperating fully in the cancer educational campaign being sponsored by the Women's Field Army of the American Society for the Control of Cancer, especially the campaign for periodic examination to detect the beginning of cancer, the medical profession can create an influential body of opinion favorable to the ideals for which the profession stands, thus strengthening its stand against the encroachment of destructive forces. It is believed that from one-third to one-half of the 150,000 annual cancer deaths in the United States could be prevented if existing knowledge about the control of cancer would be utilized by the medical profession and the public. It is known that cancer in some sites, such as the skin, mouth, breast, and uterus, offers from 75 to 95 per cent chance of a five-year cure if treated before metastasis occurs.

That early cancer is curable is shown from the latest report of the American College of Surgeons, which has reported more than 29,000 five-year or longer cures of authenticated cases.

M. N.

Pulmonary Embolism

NOT much progress has been made in the control of pulmonary embolism since the true nature of embolisms in general was first disclosed by Virchow in the middle of the last century. Three types are readily apparent: those in which death occurs immediately, those in which death is delayed for a few hours at most and those which recover spontaneously. Obviously, for those in the first class, nothing curative can be done, for they are dead before a finger can be raised. Preventive measures have accomplished very little. Various drugs which delay the coagulation time of the blood have been used, without definite benefit. Increasing the patient's bodily activity while convalescing in bed from surgical operations, parturition, accidental injuries, et cetera, in the hope of stimulating the peripheral circulation and preventing the stagnation and thrombosis in the lower extremities, which so often is found to be the basis of these emboli, has come into general use and is undoubtedly useful, but as yet the incidence of pulmonary embolism has not shown any material reduction. Patients continue to die sudden, tragic deaths just as they are about to leave the hospital, or have reached a point in their convalescence when everyone concerned is looking forward to their complete recovery in a short time. It is the most catastrophic calamity in all professional experience and few practitioners escape meeting it, sooner or later. In the present state of our knowledge we are very helpless when it happens.

In the third class, where recovery occurs spontaneously, it is questionable whether treatment of any kind makes much difference. Sedatives and vasodilators are generally used, likewise oxygen inhalation, and when the patient recovers these agents receive the credit, but it is difficult to believe that such medication can

have any direct influence on a mechanical situation like this, where at least one fairly large embolus, or a "shower" of smaller ones, is plugging branches of the pulmonary artery.

It is in the second, or intermediate, class that the most definite advance has been made in curative treatment and where the greatest opportunity for further improvement is being anticipated. It was for this type, where the patient survives the onset of profoundly serious symptoms long enough for something to be done, that Trendelenburg devised his operation of pulmonary embolectomy, in 1907. Although he and his assistants tried it a number of times the attempts were always unsuccessful and it was not until the year of Trendelenburg's death, in 1924, that Kirschner had the first case of recovery. In all, there have been nine fully successful operations, all performed by Swedish or German surgeons. This would lend more encouragement, if there were not so many barriers to be surmounted. One of the greatest of these is the possibility of spontaneous recovery without operation and this has led Nystrom, who has had two successes, to postulate that only the obviously dying should be subjected to the operative treatment. Other obstacles are readily seen, especially in this country, where the surroundings and the medico-legal aspects are not nearly so well adapted to quick and effective action in these highly emergent situations as they are in the older countries.

The recent work of Leriche and his associates in the infiltration of the stellate ganglion with procaine solution invites serious attention. It is based on the hypothesis that the vasomotor reflexes play an important part in the mechanism of death in pulmonary embolism. At least the suggestion contains the merit of a simple technic and an absence of operative risk, but whether it will accomplish anything remains to be seen, for the experience of its progenitors is far too scanty, as yet, to warrant forming any definite conclusions.

G. C.

Nazi Persecution in Vienna

THE tragic events which followed the "anschluss" of Austria last month have involved not only political figures in Austria but prominent members of the medical profession in Vienna. That so many physicians, most of them

272

Jews, should have preferred death to certain persecution under Nazi rule is an indication of what has been taking place in Germany.

Among those who have already committed suicide are Professors Wolfgang Dent, Gabor Nobl, Edmund Nobel, Arnold Baumgarten, Moritz Oppenheim and Jonas Borak of Vienna and Gustav Bayer of Innsbruch. Professor Sigmund Freud, of international fame, despite his eighty years and recent illness, is reported to have been robbed and prevented from leaving Austria. The fate of Professor Heinrich Neumann, the outstanding ear and throat specialist of Europe, hangs in the balance. It was he who got "in Dutch" two years ago by his refusal to operate on Hitler for a supposed cancer of the throat, on the ground that his nationality would be blamed in case of an unsuccessful outcome.

Hitler's usurpation of power which is an outstanding political phenomenon of all ages was made possible and in the eyes of many was essential because of the lawlessness and political chaos in Germany following the war. The same train of events came to pass in Italy and the situation in Russia is different only in that the dictator calls himself a communist instead of its foe. One man is the law maker, judge and executive and to maintain his position must also be the executioner.

While we do not for a moment believe that all Germans approve of the ruthlessness of Nazi methods, those who voluntarily support the Nazi régime give their approval to the present German political philosophy which has shown itself paganistic in its attitude to Christianity, not only unchristian but barbarous in its treatment of political opponents and Jews and has for the time being at least suppressed all ideas of individual rights and freedom for which democratic countries have fought for centuries.

"The Birth of a Baby"

THE American Committee on Maternal Welfare has prepared an educational film entitled "The Birth of a Baby" which is now being shown in regular moving picture theaters with an admission charge. Health leaders have used the printed page, radio, exhibits, and to some extent moving pictures as educational media. The chief drawback of most of these methods has been the limitation of audiences to indivi-

duals of certain types. A public moving picture with sufficient dramatic interest should be an ideal method of reaching all types of people. "The Birth of a Baby" shows this to be true.

The functions of health education are to allay fear through understanding of the body, to emphasize the importance of preventive measures, and to stress the value of early diagnosis and treatment. Since the chief interest of most people is their health, the demand for such information is very great. To be effective it must originate from reliable medical sources. The moving picture entitled "The Birth of a Baby" was supervised in its making by five eminent obstetricians connected with leading universities and hospitals. The committee's effort has the endorsement of such organizations as the American Medical Association, United States Public Health Service, American College of Surgeons, and American Public Health Association.

For some time motion picture producers have known of the public interest in medical subjects. Hampered by tradition in producing other types of pictures, medical films with a few exceptions have left much to be desired. Many of the productions have been marred by sensational advertising, exaggeration, distortion, overemphasis of unimportant details and the inevitable love interest. In order to avoid this, the American Committee on Maternal Welfare assumed complete charge of production and distribution of "The Birth of a Baby." They were able to do this because of a gift from Meade Johnson and Company, which defrayed the expenses of making the picture, and an arrangement with a moving picture organization for distribution in an ethical way. The company is under contract to carry out rigid provision in regard to advertising and exhibition. The picture cannot be shown with any other picture which might be objectionable.

The first public showing in the United States was made in Minneapolis where it has just finished a run of three weeks. It was witnessed by 85,524 individuals. As the majority of those who saw it were between fifteen and forty-five years of age, it apparently reached one-third the population of Minneapolis in this age group. Before public exhibition it had been endorsed by the Minnesota State Medical Association, Hennepin County Medical Society, Ramsey County

Medical Society, and the Minnesota State Association of Obstetricians and Gynecologists. Early in December, 1937, it was seen at Northrop Memorial Auditorium, University of Minnesota, by a crowd of more than 4,000 members of the medical, nursing and allied professions. This audience voted 98 per cent in favor of public exhibition.

The story is simply told. A young married woman tells her husband's mother that she thinks she is pregnant. She is advised to consult a physician at once. The audience witnesses her prenatal care through a series of examinations, sympathetic explanations, illustrated charts, and animated drawings. For contrast, a woman who desires an abortion, an inconsiderate husband of a pregnant woman who had borne many children, and a patient with toxemia who did not consult her physician, are seen. The climax of the educational picture is a carefully screened view of the final stage of birth. This is such a logical conclusion that it does not offend anyone.

The audiences in Minneapolis reacted in a wholesome fashion. Sensation seekers were disappointed, as the film is not a sex picture. There was no age limit at the box office which enabled families to come together. High school students were admitted without question as sex is developing during this age period. Many parents wisely concluded that it was much better for their children to get reliable information in a much better way than they were able to give it. If the children seemed too young, their parents were called to learn their wishes in the matter. During the entire three weeks' exhibition of the picture, no complaints were received. On the contrary, many people went out of their way to thank those responsible for its production.

In some states the film has met with official disapproval. When civic officials realize the value of wholesome information on prenatal care, the film will undoubtedly be shown. In 1936, 12,000 mothers died in childbirth in the United States, and 70,000 babies died between birth and one month of age. This is a desperate situation which should be corrected if possible. Ordinary educational channels have been tried without apparent success. The film brings the message home to those who need it most as it attracts mainly younger people of childbearing age. Much of the confusion in regard to the

MEDICAL ECONOMICS

Edited by the Committee on Medical Economics
of the
Minnesota State Medical Association

B. J. Branton, M. D.
L. H. Rutledge, M. D.

W. F. Braasch, M. D., Chairman

J. C. Michael, M. D.
A. N. Collins, M. D.

Future of Medicine

The importance of the American Medical Association survey of medical care in the United States cannot be over-stated.

It is up to every physician, through his county society, to furnish data requested and to coöperate in every respect with this survey.

The Minnesota State Medical Association is aware that the survey, to be of value, must be accurate and complete and will do everything in its power to make it so.

Instructions and plans will be available soon to all county officers. In the meantime committees should be appointed by every county society to carry on this work.

Action in Minnesota

"The technical committee on medical care, without mentioning 'socialized medicine,' tonight informed President Roosevelt that the effective distribution and use of health and medical services requires a national plan for economic application of our resources in maintaining and improving health."

This paragraph is quoted from a United Press dispatch printed February 26, in the *Minneapolis Journal*.

The committee mentioned is said to be an interdepartmental committee set up by the President to coördinate health and welfare activities.

Possibly one-half the population is unable to pay for medical services, the committee estimated in this newspaper report of its study submitted to the Administration; and "health and sickness services must be made more extensively available through measures that will lighten the . . . costs."

The importance of the American Medical Association study mentioned above in these columns is clear. It is clear also, that the study must be started promptly and pursued vigorously in every quarter of the United States.

Not even lack of funds can prevent damaging action by Congress or the legislatures on the basis of such alarmist reports, unless a sane, comprehensive and absolutely unassailable study of fact can also be put in the hands of the President and Congressional leaders *before* and *not after* laws have been passed.

Study outlines and blanks for the study have already been printed and are in the hands of state medical societies.

It remains now for each society to see the acute need and go to work. A meeting of the Committee on Medical Economics has been called by Chairman W. F. Braasch (also chairman of the Advisory Committee of the American Medical Association for this study) for April 3 in Saint Paul. Every effort will be made to make a prompt, accurate and honest study in Minnesota.

Replying to *Survey Graphic*

A series of articles on the English panel system of medicine have appeared in the last four issues of Survey Graphic. Like so many articles appearing in magazines of this type, they are inexact and biased and contain many superficial observations and half truths. However, they fulfill the mission for which they were intended in attracting a misguided and uninformed public. The purport of these articles is to emphasize that medical care in America is in crying need of reform and that it is much inferior to that given the lower economic group in England. The articles are written by a young physician just out of his medical school in collaboration with his wife, a social worker whose observations apparently form the bulk of the contributions. The authors were sent to England for this purpose, with funds given them by a social welfare organization.

Might Spoil Story

Typical of writers of this kind, no attempt was made to obtain the wealth of data concerning the actual working of the panel system which has been accumulated over the course of years by various American investigators. Such data could have been procured for the asking right in Chicago, at the headquarters of the American Medical Association—but they would, of course, have spoiled the articles.

To the average layman who might read these articles, the case would seem to be closed and proven. One might easily infer from some of the statements made that the only reason socialized medicine has not been instituted in this country is because of opposition from a group of retroactive, narrow-minded officials at the headquarters of the American Medical Association. It would also be inferred that the physicians who compose the A.M.A. are ignorant of the results and the workings of the panel system, have no ideas of their own, and stand dumbly by while the aforesaid officials tell them what to do.

They Do Not Know

The authors apparently do not know that many members of the American medical profession have either personally studied the panel system, discussed the matter fully with various types of English physicians, or have heard innumerable arguments on both sides of the question, so that they are able to form a fair idea of the situation for themselves.

The main argument set forth in favor of the panel system is the fact that most of the English laborers on the panel who were interviewed are satisfied with the medical treatment received. It should be remembered that prior to the establishment of the panel system the laborer had little or no medical care whatever, so that the treatment he receives now is undoubtedly, by comparison, a great improvement. Whether or not such standards of medical care would equal that received by the American laboring man is open to question.

System Admitted Incomplete

The authors admit that the panel system is incomplete in its scope and that the cost of laboratory diagnosis, examination and treatment by specialists, special medication, hospital fees, nursing care and surgery is all extra. These items,

Medical Association is at present making a nation-wide survey of the exact needs for medical care and most of us believe that American medicine can be trusted to work out a plan which will prove best for our country's needs.

With County Society Officials

The County Officers' Meeting affords the best opportunity of the year for county officers to compare notes, air grievances, get assistance.

More than eighty county officers, state officers and members took advantage of it at the 1938 session in Saint Paul, February 26. Proceedings and discussions are briefly reflected in the following highlights of the program.†

J. M. HAYES, Minneapolis, president of the Minnesota State Medical Association: On the basis of a recently conducted survey we may congratulate ourselves on Minnesota's system for handling medical relief. The plan is satisfactory in the majority of counties, a state of affairs which is in striking contrast to many other states where the right to choice of physician on the part of the relief patient is not recognized in the law. Fees for medical relief are unsatisfactory in some instances and require further negotiations between physicians and local county welfare boards for a better adjustment in others. The right of the patient to his choice of doctor is generally recognized, however, with only a few conspicuous exceptions where other difficulties exist also to cloud the issue.

For Revised Constitutions

J. C. HULTKRANS, Minneapolis: Every county society should review its constitution with a view to bringing it into conformity with present needs. A few societies are without written constitutions; this lack should be remedied at once. Disciplinary problems and questions arising out of requirements for admission to membership demand a written constitution for settlement. The state association *cannot* determine for the county society who shall and who shall not be admitted to membership. That is the most important single function of the county or district society.

GORDON C. MACRAE, Duluth: The St. Louis County Society revised its constitution recently; but has had to amend it since the revision. The

†The paper by T. V. McDavitt, American Medical Association, is printed in full elsewhere in this issue. The interesting address by Attorney General W. S. Ervin on the duties of his office is not included in this report.

President's Message

The recent action of the Board of Trustees of the American Medical Association in instituting the study, by state and county medical societies, of the prevailing need for medical and preventive medical services where such may be insufficient or inavailable, seems very timely.

This body occupies the key position for the supervision of such a study. Many other organizations with lofty ideals but equipped with improper armamentaria have attempted somewhat similar studies. No one can deny the usefulness of any of these studies. We may not like them nor agree with them. They may have done nothing but force out into the open controversial subjects. They may have done nothing but put us in the light as others see us. They may have uncovered only minor deficiencies in the practice of medicine. But we must admit they have aroused the medical profession to action. The profession must prove that it still maintains the high ideals handed down to it by our predecessors. It must prove that it still is true to the precedent long established. Probably no profession or group can look to a more favorable precedent than can the medical profession. Our knowledge and facts have been gained mostly from the work of those who have gone before us. A very superficial study readily reveals the marked scientific advancement in the recent past. Sometimes in our struggle to reach our goal in the more important side of medical practice, as well as in any other walk of life, we are likely to overlook other quite essential factors. No doubt, the practicing physician has to some extent, in the past, overlooked preventive medicine. The study of the relation of the practice of medicine to our general social program, especially from the economic side, has been left largely to those outside our profession.

These surveys and investigations of outside organizations at least serve to make us aware of these deficiencies. They serve to arouse us to the fact that we must devote more attention to these factors or allow those not so well trained to take charge of these angles of practical and preventive medicine. This study suggested by the National Board of Trustees should supplant all other medical surveys in the state. While much of the information will necessarily be only approximate, yet it is not conceivable that any other organization can obtain more definite information.

This study should result in giving us a fair estimate of the proportion of indigent to pay cases; how and where they are being cared for and the efficiency of our preventive medical program. Possibly, also, it will serve to eliminate any duplication of effort, either in the medical care or our preventive medical program.

J. M. HAYES, M.D.

new constitution provides for a president-elect who serves on an advisory committee for one year previous to taking office. An amendment providing for a nominating committee (to replace nominations from the floor) is now in process of passage. Balloting is done by mail in advance of our annual meeting.

Unsung Physicians

M. C. PIPER, Rochester: For the sake of adequate records; for the sake of medical history; for the sake of the unsung doctor about whom, otherwise, little will be known when his family and friends are gone, the new application blanks should be filled in by members and applicants to membership alike. The new blanks call for a minimum of genealogical and biographical data; but they will serve as the basis for a general biographical file in the State Office. This data should be extended by some regular system such as a detailed questionnaire sent to all members each five years. The Woman's Auxiliary could help (see "The Council Meets," page 282) both by clipping information in publications and by actually interviewing members to secure the important data.

Health Records Included

These records might include not only scientific accomplishments, and progress but civic interests, hobbies, recreations. Also they should contain information concerning physical condition and general health. The large number of doctors who die prematurely of heart disease points to the importance of securing regular health records of many physicians over a long period of time.

Physicians did not object to filling out repeated records in the years of their preparation for practice. They should not object to keeping a regular record of their progress in life.

G. H. OLDS, Waseca: The county secretary could keep track of his members, act as their agent, to some extent, in keeping a record of achievement.

W. F. WILSON, Lake City: We should apologize for having started so late this effort to keep accurate biographical records of all our members.

Informal Meetings

GEORGE EARL, Saint Paul: Our relations with the other professional groups who are concerned in the care of the sick are important and should be as close and friendly as possible. They should not take the form of a formal interpro-

permits lay officials to come between patient and doctor.

The first step then, is to make an honest and exhaustive survey with the coöperation of every county society in Minnesota and throughout the United States.

Armed with facts we can then go to Washington and say: These are the conditions in the United States and here are our recommendations based upon them.

It has been reported that some thirty to sixty per cent of our people are not getting medical care because they have no money to pay for it. We as doctors know that a large percentage of people do not get medical care because they do not want medical care whether they have money or not. With this survey we hope to get a real picture of the problem in America and analyze it sanely.

Emphasis on "Medical Indigent"

The interest in this survey will center among the so-called "medically indigent" more than upon definitely indigent. There is no doubt in the minds of anyone about the need for outside help in the care of the indigent. The question of medical care for low income groups on the other hand, is the subject of much difference of opinion and misinformation. It is to clarify the situation with respect to these groups and to determine upon plans suited to individual localities if they are needed that the American Medical Association has embarked upon this study.

A statistician and other expert assistance has been added for purposes of this study to the Bureau of Economics of which Dr. R. G. Leland is director. An advisory committee of representative persons from all over the country has been appointed to guide the bureau. The chairman of this committee is Dr. W. F. Braasch, Rochester, chairman of our Committee on Medical Economics. Dr. A. J. Chesley, secretary of the Minnesota Department of Health, is a member of the committee.

The Board of Trustees is determined to make this study complete and significant. They mean business. It remains now for our county societies to help them.

MR. C. R. CARLGREN, Saint Paul, Chairman, State Board of Control: It is important for the future of this state and nation and for the future of civilization, I believe, that socialists and economists should be as effective in their own fields as the medical profession has been in its special field.

Personally, I cannot imagine a society so benevolent or so completely regimented that individual initiative can be eliminated. I firmly believe that we must plan our social order on a basis which allows freedom of initiative to the capable individual.

In the Right Direction

I should like to express to the organization of physicians our appreciation for the fine coöperation and the constructive suggestions given our department. It is my belief that in our Minnesota welfare program, at least, we are proceeding along sane and sound lines of development. The enactment of the County Welfare Board legislation last year was a tremendous step in the right direction because it retains to the individual county local responsibility and initiative.

There has been a tremendous increase in the appropriation to the State Board of Control; but it is chiefly due to the new social security activity which has placed Old Age Assistance, Aid to Dependent Children, Aid to the Blind, Services to Crippled Children under the direction of the Board's Division of Public Assistance. A little more than one out of every three persons of 65 or over in Minnesota is receiving Old Age Assistance.

New Hospital

The increase in the populations of our state institutions has been rather staggering in the last few years, especially in the hospitals for mental ailments. The seventh institution for the mentally ill with a capacity of 200 beds has just been completed at Moose Lake and, I believe, with the leveling off in commitments that seems to be going on now, it should be a long time before Minnesota will be obliged to add any more beds of this type.

There has been very little increase, since the so-called depression, in the correctional institutions. The programs for these institutions is important and the best possible program is the most economical one in the long run. Our training schools at Red Wing, for boys, and at Sauk Center, for girls, are purely training schools. The inmates are of a normal mental level, and for the most part, they have been more sinned against than sinning. Out of 250 paroled from Red Wing last year, seventy-four had no parents and almost none of the rest have normal home conditions. We have arranged a fine vocational program for these institutions and we now have fine medical care for them. At Red Wing this care is furnished by two local Red Wing clinics.

Qualified Staff

The penal institution for men is self-supporting by the work of the inmate population and the industries established have been of benefit to the farmers of the state. The inmates retain one-third of what they earn and two-thirds goes to their families. Those who have no families retain the whole amount and some are making considerable savings.

I contend that we cannot have proper correctional or disciplinary institutions without a properly qualified staff to participate in every part of the program. That means that we must have vocational experts, qualified medical men, psychologists and psychiatrists to guide in the improvement of mental as well as physical condition of our wards.

J. F. DuBois, Sauk Center, Secretary, State Board of Medical Examiners: The title of this paper—"The Public's Basic Science Law"—is used with a purpose. The Basic Science Law is a Public Health Law, for the public and not for the physicians. In fact, all of the medical laws on our statutes since the territorial days have been placed there for the benefit of the public and the sooner physicians make this fact known, the sooner our legislative problems will be reduced.

All the basic science law tries to do is to raise the standards of all the people caring for the sick. Can any of you think of a more altruistic law than that? Of necessity, it has curtailed cultists; but until cultists are adequately trained, they should be curtailed.

In the six years prior to 1938, Minnesota averaged 39 new chiropractors a year and in ten years under the basic science law we have averaged 1.4 per year. A good many states are now asking for Minnesota's set-up and wanting to know how we got it.

fifty members responded to the call for volunteers to participate. These volunteers met weekly, discussed material for their talks, submitted specimen speeches. By the time the campaign arrangements were all made, some 35 to 40 talks had been prepared, approved and typewritten. Both speakers and audiences were enthusiastic about the success of the campaign. Requests are still coming in for talks and engagements are booked up, now, until April.

The campaign began very fortunately with a large luncheon meeting addressed by Dr. Morris Fishbein. Everything went with remarkable smoothness. The Speakers' Bureau received considerable publicity and the demand for medical speakers on all subjects has increased.

We now have the organization, experience and machinery to undertake other public health campaigns as they may be needed in Saint Paul.

H. E. HILLEBOE, Saint Paul: There are approximately 1,000,000 children under twenty-one years of age in Minnesota and there are records in the State Board of Control at the present time of approximately 9,000 crippled children among them, the majority of whom are unable to pay for private medical care.

With Medical Advice

The State Board of Control is continuing to hospitalize a certain number of crippled children in private hospitals, to be cared for by private orthopedic surgeons. This will continue as long as there are waiting lists at the public hospitals in Minnesota. The orthopedic surgeons are paid for this service on a fee basis which was set up by the Minnesota-Dakota Orthopedic Club. For the year ending June 30, 1937, 20.5 per cent of our total budget of $82,847.36 was paid out for physicians' fees and 42.8 per cent for hospital costs.

The majority of the members of the advisory committee for our service are eminent physicians of our state and it may be said, definitely, that the program is being carried out according to the most ethical standards of medical care.

MRS. HARLOW HANSON, Minneapolis, State Commander Women's Field Army: The Women's Field Army was created to fill the need for a connecting link so far as education is concerned, between the medical profession and the lay public. There has been no lag in the scientific attack on cancer, certainly, and yet, there

are still three times as many deaths from cancer as from tuberculosis. I asked the doctors why and they told me, "We think because we do not see the patient soon enough."

Want to be of Use

I have talked to the women in the women's clubs and I find that fear is the principal reason why women hesitate to consult a doctor early about symptoms that might mean cancer. That fear has its source in ignorance. When women have an opportunity to learn the scientific facts about cancer the fear lessens. Intelligent women will listen when we tell them that there is a cure for early cancer; that there are now 25,000 cases on record with the American Surgical Society showing five-year cures for cancer. I am convinced that the death rate from cancer can be cut if we can reach the women with this message. The Women's Field Army is under the direction of the medical profession. We want to be of use to the doctor and we welcome your suggestions.

W. A. O'BRIEN, University of Minnesota: To date, ten postgraduate medical institutes have been held in a little more than a year at the Center for Continuation Study with a total attendance of 256 physicians. There has been a total of 252 men on the teaching staff of the institutes. The courses have included sixty hours of instruction and 400 hours of intensive clinical and practical work. Thirty-two members of our faculty have come from the full-time teaching staff of the University; 115 from the part-time staff; twenty-four from the Mayo Clinic; sixteen from elsewhere in the state and three from out of the state. Students have come from Minnesota, North Dakota, Wisconsin, Iowa, Montana, California, Nebraska, Persia, China. Of the Minnesota men, twenty-one were from the twin cities, four from Duluth, 101 from elsewhere in the state. It is interesting to note that 40 per cent were in the age period between thirty-five and forty.

E. C. HARTLEY, Saint Paul: The so-called "Refresher Course," the name of which is going to be changed to something like "postgraduate study course," has just completed its first year. Last year there were courses in six centers throughout the state held at intervals over a period of six weeks. Average attendance ranged from nineteen to thirty-seven.

This spring the course will be given in eight centers and it will last one full day, only. We are picking out instruction centers and making our plans in consultation with the office of the State Medical Association. We learned a great deal last year and hope to learn more this year to the end that these courses may justify the expenditure made for them out of social security funds.

The Council Meets

New Committee

Further evidence of the close and friendly relationship between the Division of Public Assistance and the State Association—a new committee has been appointed by the Council to confer informally with division officials. Many difficulties are encountered by these officials in interpretation of regulations involving health and physical condition. For help, they requested appointment of the medical committee. Dr. A. W. Adson, chairman, Dr. T. H. Sweetser, Dr. George Earl and Dr. J. M. Hayes (ex-officio) will serve.

Transients Again

A new survey of medical needs of transients is to be made in Minneapolis by the United States Public Health Service, Dr. Hayes reported to the Council. Nurses and social workers will question the transients.

Continuous After-Care

Tuberculous patients of state and county institutions will have continuous after-care and supervision if the plan reported to the Council for approval by Dr. H. E. Hilleboe works out as outlined.

Each patient will be reported to his family doctor at home a month before he leaves the sanatorium. The doctor will have all the case history and the recommendations for future care made by the sanatorium superintendent so that there will be no break in medical supervision. At the same time, if necessary, the relief office will receive an advance notice of the return of the patient to his home. If relief is needed, the worker can make necessary arrangements, visit the home and see that necessities of life are provided. The Council approved the plan.

Community Doctor?

Some of the residents of Puposky and the Pleasant Valley believe they need a doctor nearer than Bemidji medical men. They have written to the State Office for advice and assistance.

In 1934 a careful study was made by the Committee to Study Medical Care in Isolated Communities under President Savage's chairmanship. It was found, then, that roads were good and doctors were available. The greatest need appeared to be for public health education to persuade people to seek attention early.

The new complaint was discussed by the Council and referred for study to Beltrami county medical men with the suggestion that any plan for retaining a government doctor be discouraged as unwise and unnecessary.

Aid from the Auxiliary

The suggestion by officers of the Women's Auxiliary that Auxiliary members in Minnesota be asked to follow the lead of Pennsylvania women and clip all local papers carefully for news with any bearing upon doctors or medicine, was applauded by the Council.

Such clippings will be useful to keep up the biographical file on members; to keep committee chairmen informed on lay opinion; and to check use of legitimate newspaper material on health and medicine.

The aid of the women will be accepted with thanks.

Disposing of Samples

Many philanthropic organizations petition doctors for samples from pharmaceutical houses to distribute to their clients. The result is often the administration of remedies to the sick by unqualified if well intentioned lay persons. This practice was disapproved by the Council and should be discouraged. It was suggested that physicians save their samples to administer at their discretion to their own needy patients.

Rehabilitating Unemployables

In West Virginia the State Medical Association is directing a profitable program of rehabilitating otherwise unemployable relief clients and so removing them from relief rolls (See March issue, page 197). The program was outlined in detail to the Council and referred by that body to the Committee on Low Income and Indigent

Problems for study with a view to the possibility of a similar project in Minnesota.

Protest

There are a few quirks in federal regulations that work hardships upon recipients of Social Security Aids and upon physicians also. Members of the Council discussed them, suggested that further inquiry be made of the American Medical Association as to the origin of the regulations and the advisability of protesting them.

One is the regulation of the Comptroller General which makes it impossible to budget for recipients of Old Age Assistance except on a current monthly basis. Another is the regulation which makes it impossible to pay physicians for initial examinations for eligibility required for recipients of some other Aids. The question of failure to pay physicians who care for the needy in their final illnesses was also discussed in view of the fact that undertakers' funds are provided.

Memorial Fund Complete

The final $80.00 needed to make the $2,000 goal set for the Herman M. Johnson Memorial Fund was subscribed by the Council members. The fund will now be invested according to the resolution passed by the House of Delegates and only interest will be used for the lectures on medical economics that will bear his name.

The first lecture in the annual lectureship will be given by Governor Benson Friday, July 1, in connection with the 85th annual meeting in Duluth.

Facts and Figures

A few copies of a pamphlet called "Facts and Figures on Medical Relief in Minnesota" are still available at the state office.

This pamphlet was prepared for the benefit of officers and contact committeemen of county and district societies and contains the latest available information on welfare and relief services in each county, also on the funds spent for these services. There is also a map showing how medical care for relief clients is handled in virtually every county in the state.

The material has proved to be of such interest to others besides the county society officials that Washington, Chicago and some of the official agencies are rapidly exhausting the supply.

There is information, in the pamphlet, conveniently arranged for comparison and study

that cannot be secured in this form from any official source of fact and figures. For this reason anyone who has a special interest in welfare and relief matters from the medical point in Minnesota should see a copy. Physicians who attended the County Officers' Meeting in Saint Paul have copies and will lend them, perhaps, since only a handful still remain at headquarters.

Sound Public Policy

Monthly Editorial Prepared by the Medical Advisory Committee

Today, as never before, professional groups are being scrutinized by lay people, and every opportunity is taken to deride and break down the time-tested ethics of these groups.

Your Medical Advisory Committee believes that perhaps we, the members of the medical profession, are at fault to a great extent in this loss of confidence, that the dignity of our calling is being lost sight of by us in the search for the "pot of gold." Especially is this true when we find doctors testifying in court on a contingent basis, their fees depending on the winning or losing of the case at hand. Will their testimony be unbiased and for the best interest in a court of justic under this arrangement? Does it not bring disrepute on all medical testimony to sell our knowledge for a "mess of pottage"? Why not be honest with ourselves and the lawyers in the case—an honest fee for an honest opinion.

The Principles of Medical Ethics, Article VI, Section 5, reads as follows:

"It is unprofessional for a physician to dispose of his professional attainments or services to any lay body, organization, group or individual, by whatever name called, or however organized, under terms or conditions which permit a direct profit from the fees, salary or compensation received to accrue to the lay body or individual employing him. Such a procedure is beneath the dignity of professional practice, is unfair competition with the profession at large, is harmful alike to the profession of medicine and the welfare of the people, and is against sound public policy."

This means that entangling alignments between doctors and lawyers are against sound public policy, and no member of our association should be guilty of such conduct. Remember, "As ye sow, so shall ye reap." If we are going to elevate our standing in the eyes of our communities, we must do it ourselves. "Honesty is the best policy" in court as well as in other types of consultation.

Minnesota State Board of Medical Examiners

Minneapolis Quack Sought by Sheriff

Re: State of Minnesota vs. Francis Howard Punchard, Sr., alias J. Francis Clark.

Sheriff John P. Wall of Minneapolis holds an order for the arrest and commitment of Francis Howard Punchard, Sr., alias J. Francis Clark, fifty-eight years of age. On February 17, 1938, the Honorable Arthur W. Selover, Judge of the District Court of Hennepin County, issued an order vacating the stay of sentence previously given Punchard on October 5, 1936, by Judge Leary. Punchard, at that time, was sentenced to six months in the Minneapolis Work House and a stay given him on the condition that he leave the State of Minnesota and remain out of it for a period of not less than five years. Punchard was seen in the Lowry Medical Arts Building, St. Paul, on February 16, 1938, by a representative of the Minnesota State Board of Medical Examiners. He stated at that time that he had been teaching at the Minnesota Chiropractic College, 1824 15th Avenue South, Minneapolis. He was ordered to report to the County Attorney's office the following morning but failed to show up. The order of Judge Selover followed. At the time this article was written the Sheriff's office had been unable to locate Punchard. It has been reported, however, that Punchard was again in the Lowry Medical Arts Building on Monday, February 21.

Punchard is a rather well known quack, having been convicted in Chicago in 1932, on a charge of practicing medicine without a license. He makes rather elaborate representations as to who he is and where he has obtained his education. He has represented himself, on occasion, as being a graduate of Oxford, the University of Maryland, and as having taught at the University of Minnesota. Punchard holds no diploma from any recognized medical school, nor is he licensed to practice medicine anywhere in the United States.

The Medical Board respectfully requests that it be immediately notified by telephone, Cedar 2064, Saint Paul, if Punchard comes to the attention of any members of the medical profession in this state.

Dakota County Janitor Pleads Guilty to Abortion

Re: State of Minnesota vs. Kish.

On March 1, 1938, Frank Kish, forty years of age, entered a plea of guilty to an information charging him with the crime of abortion. The plea of guilty was entered before the Honorable Richard A. Walsh, Judge of the District Court for Ramsey County. After hearing the facts, Judge Walsh sentenced the defendant to a term of eighteen months at hard labor in a state penal institution.

Kish, who stated he was born in 1897 at Coaldale, Virginia, and who has resided in Minnesota since 1916, was arrested on February 24, 1938, following a joint investigation made by the Minnesota State Board of Medical Examiners, the County Attorney's office and the Sheriff's office of Ramsey and Dakota Counties. Kish was employed as a janitor at School District Number 5 of Dakota County. For the past three years he has been performing an occasional criminal abortion, admitting some twenty to twenty-five abortions. Some of these were performed at the school in Dakota County, and others at the homes of the women in Saint Paul. Upon being questioned by Judge Walsh, Kish stated that he had only an eighth grade education and no medical training whatsoever. He used a catheter in his work and in some cases administered ergot. He charged whatever he could get, the fee varying from $5.00 to $30.00 per case. The defendant is married and the father of four children.

List of Physicians Licensed by the Minnesc Board of Medical Examiners on February 11, 1938

January Examination

Bagley, Charles Miller, Stanford U., M.D., 1937 Minn.

Bagwell, John Spurgeon, Jr., Baylor U., M.] Rochester, Minn.

Bailey, Allan Archibald, U. of Toronto, M.] Rochester, Minn.

Baumgartner, Florian Herman, U: of Minn., M Saint Paul, Minn.

Caspers, Carl Gerald, U. of Minn., M.B., 19: Paul, Minn.

Cochrane, Byron Barlow, U. of Minn., M.] Saint Paul, Minn.

Code, Charles Frederick, U. of Manitoba, M. Rochester, Minn.

Davis, Luther Forest, U. of Minn., M.B., 1937 apolis, Minn.

Doss, Alexander Keller, Tulane U., M.D., 193 ester, Minn.

Ferris, Deward Olmstead, Queen's U., M.I Rochester, Minn.

Fisher, Herbert Calvin, Cornell U., M.D., 193 ester, Minn.

Fitzsimons, William Edmund, U. of Minn., M. Saint Paul, Minn.

Giffin, Herbert Martin, Johns Hopkins, M.I Rochester, Minn.

Giffin, Lewis Albee, Harvard U., M.D., 1935, R Minn.

Gilman, Lloyd C., U. of Minn., M.B., 1937, Mir Minn.

Glabe, Robert Alfred, U. of Minn., M.B., 1 luth, Minn.

Hackie, Edward Anthony, U. of Manitoba, M Minneapolis, Minn.

Hargis, William Huard, Jr., U. of Texas, M. Rochester, Minn.

Harris, Leon Dunham, U. of Minn., M.B., 193 apolis, Minn.

Howard, E. Graham, U. of Minn., M.B. and M Minneapolis, Minn.

Jenovese, Joseph Francis, U. of Pa., M.D., 19 ester, Minn.

Jones, Orville Hugh, U. of Minn., M.B., 193 apolis, Minn.

Kindschi, Leslie George, Harvard, M.D., 19 ester, Minn.

Lauer, Dolor John, U. of Minn., M.B., 1937 Minn.

Lovering, Joseph, U. of Pa., M.D., 1934, I Minn.

Marshall, Mary Emily, U. of Toronto, M Rochester, Minn.

Martin, Dwight Lewis, U. of Minn., M.B., 1 Paul, Minn.

Meller, Charlotte Louise, U. of Minn., M.B., 1 Paul, Minn.

Meller, Robert Louis, U. of Minn., M.B., 1 Paul, Minn.

Pansch, Frank Norman, Northwestern, M M.D., 1937, Rochester, Minn.

Quill, Thomas H., Georgetown U., M.D., 19 ester, Minn.

Randall, Karl Chandler, II, U. of Pittsburgh, M.D., 1935, Rochester, Minn.

Roxburgh, Douglas Brant, U. of Alberta, M.D., 1932, Rochester, Minn.

Sako, Wallace Saburo, U. of Minn., M.B., 1935; M.D., 1936, Minneapolis, Minn.

Schamber, Walter Fred, Rush Med. Col., M.D., 1937, Duluth, Minn.

Schlicke, Carl Paul, Johns Hopkins, M.D., 1935, Rochester, Minn.

Schulte, Thomas Lacoste, Stanford U., M.D., 1936, Rochester, Minn.

Schunke, Gustave Bernard, Stanford U., M.D., 1936, Rochester, Minn.

Schwartz, Eleazer Robert, U. of Minn., M.B., 1936; M.D., 1937, Minneapolis, Minn.

Sharpe, Wendell Smith, Johns Hopkins U., M.D., 1935, Rochester, Minn.

Smith, James John, St. Louis U., M.D., 1937, Saint Paul, Minn.

Smith, Kendrick Adelbert, U. of Chicago, M.D., 1937, Rochester, Minn.

Sommers, Ben, U. of Minn., M.B., 1937, Saint Paul, Minn.

Tesch, Gordon Harrison, U. of Minn., M.B., 1937, Saint Paul, Minn.

Tessmer, Carl Frederick, U. of Pittsburgh, M.D., 1935, Rochester, Minn.

Textor, Jerome D., U. of Minn., M.B., 1936; M.D., 1937, Minneapolis, Minn.

Thigpen, Francis Marion, Tulane U., M.D., 1934, Rochester, Minn.

Tooke, Thomas Bell, Jr., Tulane U., M.D., 1936, Rochester, Minn.

Usher, Francis Cowgill, U. of Pa., M.D., 1935, Rochester, Minn.

Wadd, Clifford Theodore, U. of Minn., M.B., 1937, Minneapolis, Minn.

Waggoner, Richard Perham, U. of Ore., M.D., 1935, Rochester, Minn.

Wilcox, Leigh Edgar, U. of Louisville, M.D., 1933, Rochester, Minn.

Willson, Donald Maclean, U. of Pa., M.D., 1935, Rochester, Minn.

Wittels, Theodore Saul, U. of Minn., M.B., 1936, Minneapolis, Minn.

By Reciprocity

Baker, Ellis Ellsworth, U. of Neb., M.D., 1932, Gillette, Wyo.

Gillesby, William James, U. of Ill., M.D., 1932, Chisholm, Minn.

Puumala, Marie Bepko, U. of Ill., M.D., 1935, Cloquet, Minn.

National Board Credentials

Buirge, Raymond E., Duke U., M.D., 1934, Minneapolis, Minn.

Derbyshire, Robert Cushing, Johns Hopkins, M.D., 1936, Rochester, Minn.

Limbert, Edwin Manning, U. of Toronto, M.D., 1934, Rochester, Minn.

Mueller, Roland Frederick, Wash. U., M.D., 1929, Two Harbors, Minn.

Nesbitt, Samuel, Harvard U., M.D., 1935, Rochester, Minn.

In Memoriam

George Sheryl Cabot
1899-1937

DR. GEORGE S. CABOT, of Jamestown, North Dakota, died on December 16, 1937, following an emergency operation. Dr. Cabot was associated in practice with his brother Dr. Verne S. Cabot, and his brother-in-law, Dr. Arthur A. Wohlrabe, in Minneapolis, from 1925 until 1935, when he moved to Jamestown.

Born August 2, 1899, in Minneapolis, Dr. Cabot attended the elementary and high schools in Minneapolis and received his M.D. from the University of Minnesota medical school in 1923.

Dr. Cabot was a member of the Hennepin County Medical Society and the Minnesota State Medical Association while residing in Minneapolis, and transferred his membership to the North Dakota State Medical Association upon moving to North Dakota. He was a member of the Alpha Kappa Kappa medical fraternity, and of the Masonic order.

Dr. Cabot is survived by his widow, whose maiden name was Grace McCrum, and two sons, Hugh, aged nine, and Allyn, aged six. Besides a brother, Dr. Verne S. Cabot, and a sister, Mrs. Arthur A. Wohlrabe, both of Minneapolis, Dr. Cabot is survived by another brother, Dr. Clyde N. Cabot of Calgary, Canada.

Joseph Edward Honore Garand
1874-1937

DR. J. E. H. GARAND, for the past forty years a practicing physician of Dayton, Minnesota, passed away on December 12, 1937, at the age of sixty-three, from pneumonia.

Born at Sherbrooke, Quebec, February 14, 1874, Dr. Garand attended local schools and received his medical degree from Laval University, Montreal, where he graduated with honors.

Arriving in Dayton in 1900, Dr. Garand was active in local affairs. At different times he was mayor of Dayton, clerk of the village and a member of the school board.

Dr. Garand is survived by his widow and a daughter, Mrs. Honorine Dupont, of Minneapolis.

The Cornell Cancer Treatment

Recently newspapers contained an announcement to the effect that Dr. Beaumont Cornell of Fort Wayne, Ind., had discovered an amazing treatment for cancer. Briefly the treatment consists of the injection into patients with cancer of a product which he has labeled Anomin and which represents extracts made from the testicular and ovarian tissues of cattle. It was claimed for this new extract that it prevented the formation of metastases, that pain ceased and that tumors liquefied. The only evidence is the unsupported statement of the author. The work is all recent; time is required to determine whether or not cancer is really cured in any patient. The methods of promotion and the publicity associated with the announcement of this method would seem to be wholly outside the usual accepted scientific procedures. (J. A. M. A., Feb. 26, 1938, p. 656.)

◆ OF GENERAL INTEREST ◆

Dr. L. M. Roberts, of Little Falls, has retired after forty-eight years of active practice.

* * *

Dr. V. J. Telford has returned to Litchfield from Denver, and has resumed practice.

* * *

Dr. and Mrs. E. G. Bannick, of Rochester, are moving to Seattle, where they plan to make their home.

* * *

The *Journal of School Health* for March, 1938, announces Dr. Lillian L. Nye's Fellowship in the American School Health Association.

* * *

Dr. W. L. Sibley, formerly located at Rochester, Minnesota, has moved to Roanoke, Virginia, where he is affiliated with the Lewis-Gale Hospital.

* * *

Dr. P. O'Hair, pioneer Waverly physician, celebrated his ninetieth birthday on February 24. He retired from active practice in 1930.

* * *

Dr. and Mrs. Robert J. Hill, formerly of Saint Paul, have moved to Anoka, where Dr. Hill has established his practice.

* * *

Dr. and Mrs. William A. O'Brien, of Saint Paul, are receiving congratulations on the birth of a son, Patrick, born March 17.

* * *

Dr. C. G. Ochsner, of Wabasha, was elected president of the Chamber of Commerce at the organization meeting held recently.

* * *

Dr. and Mrs. L. C. Culligan, Sibley Highway, are receiving congratulations on the birth of a daughter, born March 3.

* * *

Dr. L. B. Wilson, of Rochester, addressed the Hi-Y club there early in March on the subject of "How to Spend Leisure Time."

* * *

Drs. W. E. Johnson and E. W. Wahlberg, of Morgan, have moved into new quarters in the former Farmers and Merchants Bank Building.

* * *

Dr. F. Schleinitz has settled in Avon, where he will engage in the practice of medicine. His office and residence are located in the new hospital building there.

* * *

Dr. Julian F. Du Bois, secretary of the Minnesota State Board of Medical Examiners, was elected vice president of the Federation of State Medical Boards of the United States at its annual meeting held in Chicago in February.

* * *

Dr. F. N. Solsem, of Sacred Heart, has sold his practice to Dr. R. Erickson, a graduate of the Medical School of the University of Minnesota. Dr. Solsem

plans to take up graduate work at the Medical School of the University of Colorado, after a visit with his daughter and son-in-law in Denver.

* * *

Dr. S. A. Slater, of Worthington, has been appointed on a national committee of five to study the coordination of federal, state and local programs against tuberculosis, and recommend a workable plan. The appointment was made by Dr. J. A. Myers of Minneapolis, president of the National Tuberculosis Association.

* * *

Dr. W. P. Olson, of the Gaylord Hospital, has announced that his son, Dr. Duane Olson, will soon become associated with him in the conduct of the Gaylord Hospital, and in general practice. Dr. Duane Olson is a graduate of the University of Minnesota and is just completing his internship at General Hospital, Minneapolis.

* * *

Dr. S. A. Forestiere will return to Pine River from New York City about April 1 to take over the St. Matthew Hospital, which he has purchased from Dr. A. J. Button. Dr. Button opened the hospital January 1, 1934 and has operated it since that time. It was first known as the Holman Hospital, but was recently incorporated as St. Matthew Hospital.

* * *

Dr. and Mrs. John S. Lundy of Rochester sailed for Europe late in March. Dr. Lundy expects to visit clinics in Vienna and other medical centers in Germany, France, Switzerland, Holland and England. They will return to Rochester about June 1.

Before sailing, Dr. Lundy will address a meeting of the American Society of Anesthetists in New York, his topic being "Intravenous Barbiturate Anesthesia."

* * *

Dr. and Mrs. P. S. Hench, of Rochester, have sailed for Europe. Dr. Hench attended the meeting of the International Congress on Rheumatism and Hydrology at Oxford, March 26 to 31, and will address the International Conference on Rheumatic Disease which is being held in Bath, England. His topic will be "The Effect of Spontaneous and Induced Jaundice on Rheumatoid Arthritis and Fibrositis."

Dr. Hench will also visit clinics in England and Scotland.

* * *

Dr. Edgar H. Norris, for the past four years a teaching fellow in the Department of Pathology at the University of Minnesota Medical School, during which period he has made a number of important contributions to medical literature, has been appointed Head of the Department and Professor of Pathology in Wayne University College of Medicine, Detroit, Michigan. He will assume his duties in the early fall. Dr. Norris graduated from the University of Minnesota Medical School in 1919. He practiced surgery for a number of years in Saint Paul before devoting himself to Pathology.

DICAL BROADCAST FOR APRIL

he Minnesota State Medical Association Morning Health Service.

he Minnesota State Medical Association broadcasts kly at 9:45 o'clock every Saturday morning over tion WCCO, Minneapolis and Saint Paul (810 kiloles or 370.2 meters).

peaker: William A. O'Brien, M.D., Associate Prosor of Pathology and Preventive Medicine, Medical ool, University of Minnesota. The program for the nth will be as follows:

pril 2—10th Anniversary.
pril 9—Arteriosclerosis.
pril 16—Glaucoma.
pril 23—Brain Tumors.
pril 30—Dental Research.

ERICAN ASSOCIATION FOR E STUDY OF GOITER

he third international goiter conference will convene Washington, D. C., September 12 to 14, 1938. Engwill be the official language, but interpreters will furnished for papers read in a foreign tongue. Furr information may be obtained from Dr. Allen aham, chairman of the Program Committee, 2020 st 93rd Street, Cleveland, Ohio.

MERICAN BOARD OF OPHTHALMOLOGY

The American Board of Ophthalmology announces at in 1938 it will hold examinations in San Francisco, ne 13, during the American Medical Association :eting; Washington, D. C., October 8, during the nerican Academy of Ophthalmology and Oto-Laryng->gy meeting; Oklahoma City, November 14, during ∶ Southern Medical Association meeting.

The American Board of Ophthalmology has estabhed a Preparatory Group of prospective candidates r its certificate. The purpose of this Group is to rnish such information and advice to physicians who e studying or about to study ophthalmology as ay render them acceptable for examination and∙ cerication after they have fulfilled the necessary reirements. Any graduate or undergraduate of an proved medical school may make application for ∶mbership in this Group. Upon acceptance of the plication, information will be sent concerning the ˙iical and educational requirements, and advice to ∶mbers of the Group will be available through preptors who are members or associates of the Board. embers of the Group will be required to submit an-ially a summarized record of their activities.

The fee for∙ membership in the Preparatory Group ten dollars, but this amount will be deducted from e fifty dollars ultimately required of every candi-.te for examination and certification. For sufficient

reason, a member of the Preparatory Group may be dropped by vote of the Board.

ASSOCIATION OF INDUSTRIAL PHYSICIANS AND SURGEONS

The annual meeting of the Association of Industrial Physicians and Surgeons and Midwest Conference on Occupational Diseases will be held at the Palmer House, Chicago, June 6-9, 1938. The purposes of the organization are minimizing the morbidity and mortality in working people from industrial accidents and diseases, and all physicians and surgeons interested in this phase of preventive medicine are urged to attend. A. G. Park, 540 N. Michigan Avenue, Chicago, is Convention Manager, and is in charge of exhibits.

CITIZENS AID SOCIETY

The Cancer Institute Committee of the University of Minnesota Medical School has announced the 1938 Citizens Aid Society Lecture which will be presented at the Medical School on the evening of Tuesday, April 12. Dr. Edgar Allen of Yale University Medical School will present this Lecture, the title of which will be "Ovarian Hormones in Relation to Female Genital Cancer."

POSTGRADUATE COURSE FOR PHYSICIANS IN OBSTETRICS AND PEDIATRICS

Beginning in May the second state-wide Postgraduate Course for Physicians in Obstetrics and Pediatrics will be given in eight centers throughout the state. This is the course presented through the coöperated efforts of the Minnesota State Medical Association, the Medical School of the University, and the State Department of Health. It is financed by funds coming to the Division of Child Hygiene of the State Department of Health through Society Security appropriations.

The centers and dates for this year are, as follows:

May 4—Crookston
        Winona
May 11—Hibbing
        Willmar
May 18—Albert Lea
        Fergus Falls
May 25—Worthington
        Bemidji

The arrangements will be different this year from last. The sessions in each center will last all day, and the entire material will be presented in that one day. There will be four lectures in obstetrics and four in pediatrics given by two obstetricians and two pediatricians. This arrangement was decided upon after considerable discussion in order to meet some of the objections which∙ arose last year. Particularly, that the work extended over too long a period, making it difficult for the men to arrange for attendance. It was felt by most of those who discussed the question that in general the physician in practice could more readily arrange for one full day away from his office than he could for parts of a number of successive days.

Complete schedules for the course and an outline of the material to be presented will be mailed by Mr. R. R. Rosell, Executive Secretary of the Minnesota State Medical Association, to the physicians in and about the eight centers which have been selected.

RESERVATIONS, STATE MEETING

Hotel reservations for the 85th annual meeting of the Minnesota State Medical Association to be held in Duluth, June 29, 30 and July 1, should be made immediately according to the Committee on Local Arrangements of which Dr. R. J. Moe is chairman.

One of the best programs in the history of the organization has been arranged and an attendance of more than twelve hundred is expected from Minnesota and from surrounding states. Most of those who attend will plan, also, to take advantage of the dates and extend their trips, with their families, until after the Fourth of July holiday.

Several other organizations will be meeting in Duluth at the same time, according to the Committee, and will require accommodations.

Meeting headquarters are at the Hotel Duluth. A list of eight additional hotels has been selected by the committee, however, and excellent accommodations can be secured in any of them. The complete list with rates is printed below. Reservations should be made direct with the hotel chosen.

Hotel	Single	Double
Hotel Duluth, 231 E. Superior St.		
(With Bath)	$3.00 & up	$4.00 & up
Spalding Hotel, 5th Ave. W. & Superior St.		
(Without Bath)	1.50 & up	2.50 & up
(With Bath)	2.50 & up	3.25 & up
Lenox Hotel, 6th Ave. W. & Superior St.		
(Without Bath)	1.50 & up	2.50 & up
(With Bath)	2.25 & up	3.25 & up
Holland Hotel, 11 N. Fifth Ave. W.		
(Without Bath)	1.75 & up	2.75 & up
(With Bath)	2.50 & up	3.50 & up
Lincoln Hotel, 317 W. 2nd St.		
(Without Bath)	1.50 & up	2.50 & up
(With Bath)	1.75 & up	2.75 & up
McKay Hotel, 430 W. 1st St.		
(Without Bath)	1.25 & up	2.00 & up
(With Bath)	1.75 & up	2.75 & up
Cascade Hotel, 101 W. 3rd St.		
(Without Bath)	1.50 & up	2.00 & up
(With Bath)	2.00 & up	3.00 & up
Arrowhead Hotel, 225 N. 1st Ave. W.		
(Without Bath)	1.00 & up	2.00 & up
(With Bath)	2.00 & up	3.00 & up
Hamilton Hotel, 1418 E. Superior St.		
(Without Bath)	1.50 & up	2.00 & up
(With Bath)	2.50 & up	3.50 & up

WABASHA AND WINONA COUNTIES

The seventh annual joint meeting of the Wabasha and Winona County Medical Societies and the thirteenth annual dinner tendered by the Sanatorium Commission to the physicians of the counties served was held at Buena Vista Sanatorium, Wabasha, Minnesota, on Monday evening, March 14. There were thirty-four

in attendance, including doctors and four lay members of the Sanatorium Commission.

Dr. H. T. Sherman, president of the Wabasha County Society, officiated as toastmaster. Dr. James M. Hayes, president, and Mr. R. R. Rosell, executive secretary of the State Medical Association, gave talks on the aims and purposes of the State Association. Dr. I. W. Steiner, secretary of the Winona County Society, gave a report on the recent County Officers' Conference in Saint Paul.

The following papers were presented:

"Acute Abdominal Conditions," DR. JAMES M. HAYES, Minneapolis.

"Diagnosis and Treatment of Primary Carcinoma of the Lung," DR. THOMAS J. KINSELLA, Minneapolis.

"Intractable Nasal Hemorrhage, with Report of Case Requiring Ligation of the External Carotid Artery," DR. GEORGE L. LOOMIS, Winona. Discussion was opened by Dr. Eli E. Christensen, Winona.

WASHINGTON COUNTY

The regular meeting of the Washington County Medical Society was held March 8 with good attendance. The Secretary reported on the County Officers' Meeting and following that there was a discussion on the welfare board's activities.

There was also a report on the Mantoux tests showing that out of 305 pupils only twelve refused to take the test. There were forty-four pupils who were positive reactors, forty-three of whom were x-rayed. One pupil refused. There were also fourteen adults (teachers) tested, with three positives. Three children outside of the school were x-rayed. There was also a report on the vaccination questionnaire which disclosed the fact that quite a number of pupils throughout the grade schools had not been vaccinated.

Dr. E. V. Strand, of Bayport, spoke to the Society about his trip East. He visited the medical centers in Montreal, Boston, New York, Baltimore, and Washington. His experiences were well outlined and told in a manner which was enjoyable to listen to as well as instructive. He also mentioned the up-to-date equipment in the hospitals in these medical centers.

Dangers of Sodium Perborate in the Mouth

The most prominent ingredient used in recent years in dentifrices and mouthwashes for antiseptic purposes is sodium perborate. This has been inspired, no doubt, by its alleged efficiency in combating Vincent's infection. According to the clinical observations recorded in a recent questionnaire study by Isador Hirschfeld, chairman of the Committee on Scientific Investigation of the American Dental Association, perborate may cause (1) painful chemical burns of the oral mucosa (including the gingivæ); (2) less painful or entirely painless burns producing a milky-white discoloration, especially of the marginal gingivæ; (3) an inflamed condition of the oral mucosa, which predisposes the gingivæ and mouth generally to ready abrasion and infection through minimal traumatization, and (4) a form of "hairy tongue" which in some instances causes gagging or irritation of the soft palate and pharynx. Ample examples of the danger of this form of self medication have now been recorded and adequate proof offered. (J. A. M. A., Feb. 5, 1938, p. 445.)

WOMAN'S AUXILIARY

Mrs. J. F. Norman, Crookston, *President*
Mrs. A. A. Passer, Olivia, *Editor*

AN OPEN LETTER TO THE MEMBERS OF THE STATE MEDICAL AUXILIARY

Dear Auxiliary Members:

There are a number of matters which I want to bring to your attention, and I appreciate the privilege of communicating with you through the pages of MINNESOTA MEDICINE.

You will be interested to know that the Auxiliary will again show a nice gain in membership this year; at this writing, ten County Auxiliaries have reported a larger membership than in previous years. This is encouraging, for the reason that if the State Auxiliary wishes to continue as a vital reserve force for the Medical Association, it is necessary to grow numerically. The various groups are to be commended for the prompt attention given the payment of dues during March; as a result, the State, in turn, will be in a position to remit dues promptly to the National Auxiliary.

The mid-winter meeting of the Executive Board was held in Minneapolis on January 14 because it was possible for our National President, Mrs. Augustus Kech, to be with us on that day. Mrs. Kech recommended that the Minnesota Auxiliary assist the Medical Society by establishing a Clipping Bureau. Your president placed the matter in the hands of the Medical Advisory Board, and at a meeting of the Council which followed the County Officers' meeting on February 26, the idea was enthusiastically endorsed by the Council which went on record as stating that the Medical Association would accept this service with appreciation. You will have the privilege of deciding definitely about this as a project at the annual meeting; in the meantime, if you are interested, start clipping! Clip everything from your local newspapers which has any reference to medicine or local physicians; editorials are of especial interest. This service will be of great value to the Medical Association and we are hoping it will receive your active coöperation.

Another recommendation which was made by a special committee and adopted at the Board meeting, was to the effect that County Auxiliaries follow the State Constitution, Article X, with reference to delinquent members of said Auxiliaries. Other matters of interest to all the members were discussed at the Board meeting and will be included in the reports at the annual meeting.

The State Meeting will be held in Duluth June 29, 30 and July 1, and the annual business meeting of the Auxiliary will be held on Thursday, June 30. Plans are going forward to make this meeting one of lasting inspiration, and it is not too early for you to make your plans to attend. Duluth is famous as a hostess city and the women of the St. Louis County Auxiliary are busily engaged in making preparations for the

meeting. There is talk of a trip on Lake Superior on July 1, so try to have your plans include all three days of the convention. With your assistance and coöperation, the sixteenth annual meeting of the Minnesota State Medical Auxiliary will be a memorable one.

LORETTA M. NORMAN, *President.*

The Vitamin C Content of Commercially Canned Tomato Juice and Other Fruit Juices as Determined by Chemical Titration

The Council on Foods reports that many physicians have inquired about the vitamin C content of canned fruit juices. In order to obtain further information on this point, Dr. E. M. Bailey of the Connecticut Agricultural Experiment Station, New Haven, has supplied comparative data on the cevitamic acid content of Council accepted products by chemical titration. This survey covers all canned fruit juices which, at the time of the examination, were privileged to display the seal of the Council on Foods. The figures show that all brands of the canned fruit juices examined contained appreciable quantities of vitamin C. In terms of the average approximate number of international units of vitamin C per hundred cubic centimeters, the values are: pineapple juice 300, tomato juice 400, grapefruit juice 750, orange juice 900 and lemon juice 1,000. From the figures available, it would appear that canned orange juice is only slightly less potent in vitamin C than the fresh juice from which it is made. Approximately two and one-half volumes of canned tomato juice should be given in order to provide the vitamin C equivalent of one volume of fresh orange juice. If other juices are to be substituted, it is probable that the substitution could be made, other things being equal, on the basis of the vitamin C content. (J. A. M. A., Feb. 26, 1938, p. 650.)

Udga Tablets

The Bureau of Investigation reports that according to a Federal Trade Commission release for May 21, 1937, the Commission ordered Udga, Inc., to cease and desist from representing "through advertisements, circulars or testimonials, or in any other manner, that the product would cure stomach ulcers, gastritis, indigestion, dyspepsia and various other stomach ailments and diseases, including those caused or reputed to be caused by hyperacidity." William Fraser of St. Paul is president of Udga, Inc. Fraser is a voluminous advertiser and, among other advertising devices, publishes *Fraser's News*, a puff sheet devoted to the wonders of Udga Tablets. From Fraser's "Column of Health Comment" we learn: "Years ago, after I left the army . . . Back home in St. Paul, Minn., I learned first hand of a formula developed by a renowned physician for treatment of stomach acidity—that distressing condition so little understood by doctors generally . . ." Nowhere in the Fraser advertising available to the Bureau of Investigation is there any clue that Mr. Fraser has had any training in pharmacy, chemistry, physiology, pathology or therapeutics. According to the government chemists' analysis, each Udga Tablet contained about 9 grains of sodium bicarbonate, about 9 grains of bismuth subnitrate and about 8 grains of magnesium exide. The limited value of these common drugs is well known to every physician. Certainly they are not to be relied on in the indiscriminating and unsupervised treatment of gastric ulcer. (J. A. M. A., August 21, 1937, p. 605.)

PROCEEDINGS of the MINNESOTA ACADEMY of MEDICINE

Meeting of January 12, 1938

The regular monthly meeting of the Minnesota Academy of Medicine was held at the Town and Country Club on Wednesday evening, January 12, 1938. Dinner was served at 7 o'clock and the meeting was called to order at 8:15 by the president, Dr. R. T. LaVake. There were fifty-nine members and two guests present.

This being the annual meeting at which the President's address is read, no business was taken up.

DIAPHRAGMATIC HERNIA

E. M. JONES, M.D.
Saint Paul

Dr. E. M. Jones, retiring president, read his address on the above subject, illustrated with lantern slides. He requested that the paper be discussed. (Complete paper to appear later in MINNESOTA MEDICINE.)

Abstract

The diagnosis and treatment of diaphragmatic hernia has received increasing attention during the past few years. There is no reason to assume the condition to be more prevalent than heretofore, but rather that improvement in diagnostic methods has made its presence more easily and thus more frequently proven. Development in roentgenological technic, together with accurate clinical observation, has resulted in the placing of diaphragmatic hernia in the list of common conditions.

In 1853, Bowditch reviewed the subject of diaphragmatic hernia and reported a case seen at the Massachusetts General Hospital, observing that earlier writers believed that a wound of the diaphragm was always fatal.

Diaphragmatic herniæ are considered true or false depending on whether or not a sac is present. They are further divided into congenital and acquired, the latter possibly traumatic in origin.

These various types of herniæ are discussed from the standpoint of their occurrence and symptoms presented. Various points are emphasized that will aid in the diagnosis. There is also discussion of the congenital short esophagus and the surgical importance of differentiating it from a diaphragmatic hernia is emphasized.

Reduction of the hernia with repair of the hernial opening is the only means of definitely relieving the symptoms. As long as strangulation does not occur, the presence of abdominal viscera within the chest is not incompatible with life.

Many aspects of the treatment of diaphragmatic hernias are discussed.

Five cases of diaphragmatic hernia that have been operated upon are discussed and lantern slides were shown demonstrating the condition before and after

surgical repair. There are three cases of esophageal hiatus hernia and two that are traumatic. Two slides were shown of a congenital diaphragmatic hernia.

In this group of cases three were cured, there was one recurrence and one death.

Discussion

DR. J. F. CORBETT, Minneapolis: I want to congratulate Dr. Jones on his series of cases. It is master surgery and very few of us can point to so many cases. I saw one case that was a potential diaphragmatic hernia. This boy had been shot in the lower part of the left chest and when admitted to the hospital his condition was bad. The most marked symptoms were abdominal, but no fluid could be demonstrated in the abdomen. There was some blood in the chest and there was pain referred to the shoulder. For that reason, by means of an intratracheal positive pressure apparatus, I ventilated the lungs and opened the chest and found one of the most remarkable pictures I have ever seen. The bullet had cut the diaphragm and nothing had gotten into the abdominal cavity. We repaired the defect and, so far as we have been able to learn, he has been in good health since. The blood was what led me to go into the chest cavity. It was from the intercostal arteries. So, the manner of approach was correct but the main reason for selecting this route was fallacious.

DR. MARTIN NORDLAND, Minneapolis: Dr. Jones is to be complimented for his excellent discussion of this interesting subject. In this connection, I thought it might be of interest to report a case of congenital diaphragmatic hernia, recognized by the pediatrician three days after birth and which I operated upon five days after birth. The infant was delivered by the obstetrician by cesarean section.

From the time of birth the patient frequently became cyanotic when nursing and vomited after each feeding. Occasionally the vomitus contained a small amount of blood. The pediatrician noted bizarre sounds in the chest and an x-ray examination on the third day after birth revealed the presence of the entire stomach in the right side of the chest. A diagnosis of diaphragmatic hernia was established and an operation was advised. At operation on the fifth day, the stomach was replaced in the abdominal cavity and the diaphragm sutured. The suturing was accomplished with much more ease than in similar hernias in adults. The patient died on the twelfth day from pneumonia. The postmortem examination revealed the stomach had remained in good position in the abdominal cavity.

The case is of interest because of the early diagnosis, the predominating symptoms being cyanosis and vomiting and the positive diagnostic x-ray findings. I is of further interest because the hernia occurred on the right side of the diaphragm. Statistics reveal that only about 22 per cent of diaphragmatic hernias occur on this side. It has been frequently noted that infants with diaphragmatic hernias have other congenital deformities. This case had a large inguinal hernia, bilateral club-feet and a rather marked hypertrophic pyloric stenosis.

DR. O. H. WANGENSTEEN, University of Minnesota: Dr. Jones pointed out that internal hernias, of which diaphragmatic hernia is a type, become obstructed but do not strangulate as readily as do external hernia. This comes about because the structures about the apertures through which the intestine may herniate are not so unyielding as in external hernias, where ligaments like Poupart's or Gimbernat's cause obstruction and strangulation simultaneously. Strangulation, of course, does attend neglected obstructed diaphragmatic hernias. It is because of this lesser tendency to strangulation in diaphragmatic hernia that a short trial with suction applied to an inlying duodenal tube is in order before recourse is had to surgery. The gaseous distension and fluid retention in the stomach can be relieved usually by this means and reposition of the abdominal viscera herniated into the thorax can be then undertaken with less risk to the patient. A preliminary decompression of the colon as advocated by Truesdale is to be done only in those instances in which a "scout" x-ray film of the abdomen indicates that the colon is considerably distended. In diaphragmatic hernias of traumatic origin in which a portion of the colon becomes engaged and obstructed in the diaphragmatic aperture, Truesdale's suggestion of preliminary cecostomy is a good one. For, as has been repeatedly pointed out in recent years in the literature of bowel obstruction, the ileocecal valve and sphincter behave as a check-valve, permitting the entry of fluid and gas from the proximal reaches of the gut, but regurgitation of content from the obstructed colon into the ileum is precluded by the ileocecal valve. If such an obstruction goes unrelieved for long, perforation of the distended colon is bound to happen.

The para-esophageal hernias of which Dr. Jones spoke at length are, of course, not so likely to become obstructed. Occasionally, however, volvulus of the stomach may occur in an unusually large para-esophageal hernia. Such an occurrence has once come under my attention. In the main, however, obstruction or strangulation in para-esophageal hernias is decidedly unusual. It is difficult to escape the impression that surgeons have attacked these hernias with greater enthusiasm than they are justified in doing. In a few cases in which the roentgenologist made the diagnosis of para-esophageal hernia with confidence, I have been unable to demonstrate to my own satisfaction at operation that a hernia was actually present. After operation, the roentgenologist declares that the hernia is no longer present, and again re-examination after several months fails to disclose evidence of the hernia. Yet the patient continues to complain of the same symptoms as he did when the alleged hernia was discovered on roentgen examination. The large para-esophageal hernias, which Dr. Jones spoke of, should be repaired surgically when they cause symptoms and the physical status of the patient warrants undertaking operation. Many of you are undoubtedly familiar with the controversy which Prof. Cauerbruch and his erstwhile roentgenologist Berg, now of Hamburg, had over these so-called "Epiphrenische Glocken." Sauerbruch steadfastly maintained that these supra-diaphragmatic shadows of gastric mucosa which roentgenologists observed and described as para-esophageal hernias were often not hernias at all. My own experience with some of these is very much like that of Prof. Sauerbruch, and I would suggest that surgeons exercise some restraint in operating upon all para-esophageal hernias diagnosed as such by roentgenologists.

I had an interesting experience a short time ago with a congenital pleuro-peritoneal hiatus hernia in a man of twenty-seven (University Hospital No. 662347), which may interest you. Until he engaged in a wrestling bout in April, 1937, he had no symptoms referable to the hernia. The application of the "scissors-hold" to the abdomen caused him to become dyspneic and to have abdominal pain accompanied by vomiting. The seizure was soon over and he was again quite well until midsummer when a similar attack came on without apparent provocation. The spell for which he was finally hospitalized in October, 1937, came on during the night and he was brought to the hospital with the

picture of an acute intestinal obstruction. A scout film disclosed the presence of the stomach in the thorax. The left diaphragm could not be identified roentgenologically and it was suggested that the patient might have an eventration of the diaphragm—a suggestion which could not account adequately for the obstruction. Following employment of suction applied to a duodenal tube passed into the stomach, the dyspnea and cyanosis decreased and the abdomen softened. The stomach, however, could not be emptied completely, as indicated by subsequent films. The improvement attending employment of suction, however, was such that the needed operation could now be carried out with equanimity. At operation, the stomach, together with a good portion of the small intestine and colon as well as the spleen were found to have herniated through an hiatus in the left diaphragm. Employing a suggestion of Dr. C. H. Mayo (*Annals of Surgery*, 86:481, 1927), a catheter was introduced through the aperture into the left thorax; air was injected gently with a syringe and it was startling to observe how the small bowel and other viscera which could not be delivered by pulling, came back gradually into the abdomen spontaneously with the establishment of atmospheric pressure in the thorax. The edges of the diaphragmatic aperture were smooth and its location was typical for a congenital pleuro-peritoneal hiatus hernia. Dr. Weinberg, of Omaha, had told me of an excellent plan in the repair of such defects which he has since published (*Surgery*, 3:78, 1938), a plan which I found very helpful in closing the defect. After the placement of interrupted silk sutures, the peri-renal fascia—a very extensive sheet of strong tissue—was sutured over the site of repair. The patient has remained well. This suggestion of Weinberg should prove very helpful in the repair of large diaphragmatic defects.

In pleuro-peritoneal hernias of the right diaphragm, it is the liver which enters the thorax. The other intraperitoneal viscera can not enter the thorax because of the engagement of the liver in the diaphragmatic aperture.

I have had one operative experience with pleuro-peritoneal hiatus hernia in the newborn. Dr. Mayo's maneuver for the reduction of the herniated viscera was then not known to me. After return of the viscera to the peritoneal cavity and closure of the diaphragmatic defect, I found that I could not close the abdominal incision. The peritoneal cavity was too small to hold the returned viscera. I had to content myself with suture of the skin. At postmortem examination, the left kidney was still in the thorax.

DR. F. C. RODDA, Minneapolis: The diagnosis of congenital diaphragmatic hernia may present some difficulties. My own experience concerns two cases. In one child, diagnosis was made and the child operated upon, with excellent results. The other case was that of an infant four weeks of age with the prevailing symptoms of vomiting, cyanosis and collapse. The same roentgenologist who had confirmed our diagnosis in the first case made a similar diagnosis in this child. At operation, we found an enormously dilated stomach and much of the bowel in the left chest. The lung was collapsed and the diaphragm, which presented a very thin poorly-developed musculature, was crowded up to the apex, and, to our chagrin, we found a well-developed pyloric stenosis. Whether the findings were due to an injury of the phrenic nerve or a lack of development of the muscles of the diaphragm, we were unable to determine. There was no opening in the diaphragm and consequently no hernia; but the physical signs and x-ray findings were very similar to those found in a true hernia. The child died.

DR. KENNETH BULKLEY, Minneapolis: The discussion of diaphragmatic hernia is always instructive because none of us has seen many such cases. Little has been said here tonight regarding traumatic diaphragmatic hernia and for this reason I would like to report a diaphragmatic hernia, the result of a stab wound. This involves the case of a boy about ten years of age who was brought into Bellevue Hospital, New York, a good many years ago, just as I was making rounds. The history was that this boy immediately previously had been stabbed with a banana knife while attempting to steal bananas. The wound of entry lay in the left posterior chest, was about one inch in length, and through it protruded a tongue of fat which manifestly was omentum. At this time the boy had no abdominal symptoms whatsoever. The chest was opened through an intercostal incision, using a Lillienthal retractor, the omentum was pulled still further from the abdomen, amputated and reduced within the abdominal cavity, and a slit in the diaphragm about one inch in length was repaired without undue difficulty. The chest was closed without drainage; the pneumothorax cared for by aspiration, and the patient returned to his bed.

This case illustrates the necessity of bearing in mind the possibility of an intra-abdominal injury in cases of traumatic diaphragmatic hernia, particularly by stab wounds or gunshot wounds, inasmuch as on the following morning this boy showed very definite signs of an intra-abdominal hemorrhage of an extent sufficient to necessitate intervention. Following transfusion, the boy's abdomen was opened and there was found an exceptionally long cut of his spleen, bleeding profusely. This could be controlled only by a splenectomy, which was done. The boy went on to ultimate recovery.

DR. JONES, in closing: I wish to thank the members for their discussions. I have nothing particular to add, but wish to leave the thought that we should always bear in mind the possibility of the presence of a diaphragmatic hernia when making diagnoses referable to the chest and upper abdomen. It is not uncommon for an exhaustive examination to reveal nothing except a small diaphragmatic hernia. If circumstances permit the repair of the hernia, the patient is frequently cured.

The meeting adjourned.

ALBERT G. SCHULZE, M.D., *Secretary.*

Meeting of February 9, 1938

The regular monthly meeting of the Minnesota Academy of Medicine was held at the Town and Country Club on Wednesday evening, February 9, 1938. Dinner was served at 7 o'clock and the meeting was called to order at 8:15 o'clock by the president, Dr. R. T. LaVake.

There were forty-nine members and one guest present.

Minutes of the December and January meetings were read and approved as read.

Upon ballot the following men were elected as candidates for active membership in the Academy:

Dr. Lee W. Barry..........................St. Paul
Dr. Roy E. Swanson.................:....Minneapolis

The scientific program followed.

CLINICAL TETANUS: A SURVEY.

Report of Cases With Unusual Early Symptoms

E. A. REGNIER, M.D.
Minneapolis

Dr. Regnier read his inaugural thesis on the above subject.

Abstract

Twenty-nine clinical cases of tetanus are reviewed. Tetanus toxins are disseminated through the blood stream and not through motor nerve trunks as heretofore believed.

Trismus may be a late symptom of tetanus. Any regional muscle group may be primarily involved. Two cases are reported in which initial symptoms were all referable to the abdomen and simulated an acute abdominal catastrophe. A third case is reported in which the masseters were the last group of muscles to be affected.

A history of abdominal cramp followed by profuse perspiration, board-like rigidity and spasm of abdominal muscles, other findings of peritonitis being absent, should lead one to suspect tetanus.

Discussion

DR. CARL B. DRAKE, Saint Paul: There are some distinct disadvantages to the present prophylactic treatment of tetanus. There is a certain group of individuals who have a natural or acquired sensitivity to horse serum. There is a much larger group of individuals who, on account of their occupation, are very subject to injury in which infection to tetanus is quite likely. Considerable work has been done by some French investigators in developing an alum-precipitated tetanus toxoid. This toxoid contains no horse serum and two or three injections of 1 c.c. are given at two to three month intervals. In case of a suspicious injury an additional injection is given which raises the antitoxin in the blood sufficiently in most cases. I have not encountered any report of extensive use of the toxoid, which of course is necessary before its clinical value can be determined. It has been used sufficiently, however, to warrant its acceptance by the Council on Pharmacy and Chemistry.

DR. C. B. WRIGHT, Minneapolis: Are there any late sequelæ of tetanus such as neuritis or late cerebral symptoms? In looking through the literature I could not find any.

DR. J. A. JOHNSON, Minneapolis: I appreciate very much Dr. Regnier's thorough discussion of this subject, especially his description of the onset of muscular spasm in the abdomen, which is so apt to be mistaken for some intra-abdominal lesion.

My first introduction to tetanus was when I was ten years of age. One of my playmates received a firecracker injury on the 4th of July and died as a result of it. I still remember his terrible suffering.

It has been my misfortune during many years to see a large number of these cases. Over twenty years ago when I was house surgeon in a large hospital in Chicago, it was then our practice that all injury cases receive a prophylactic dose of antitetanic serum while still in the emergency room. During a period of five years I did not see a single case of tetanus develop in any of these cases. We saw, however, many cases that came to the hospital that had not had the prophylactic serum. This serum has been so well established as a preventative of tetanus that it must now be considered a criminal neglect not to administer it in cases that can be suspected of having been infected with tetanus.

At that time also we had considerable difficulty with some cases of post-operative tetanus developing in clean wounds. That was due to catgut. So much has been done in the sterilization of catgut that this condition is not now feared as it used to be. Years ago, after a case of tetanus had developed into advanced stages, the patient practically never recovered. As time has gone on, it has been my experience that more and more of these late cases have been cured; perhaps because now we are giving them larger doses, and I also believe the serum is more potent than it used to be. I believe avertin is one of the best methods of controlling the spasms, especially when they are continued and very severe.

DR. W. E. CAMP, Minneapolis: I would like to ask Dr. Regnier if he has any statistics on the number of cases that develop after head injury as compared to the number developing after injury to the extremities?

DR. REGNIER, in closing: In answer to Dr. Drake's remark about giving prophylactic serum, I wish to state that there has been developed a toxoid for prophylaxis of tetanus. There are very favorable reports, especially in foreign literature, about the use of alum-precipitated tetanus toxoid. This toxoid has been universally adopted in the French Army in the last few years. Some of our American biological houses now have tetanus toxoid on the market. There is no doubt but what there is danger in giving serum to an allergic individual, but these people can be desensitized. Unquestionably the use of toxoids would obviate this danger of serum reaction. Reports from the French Army, members of which have been using toxoid for a considerable length of time, state that once an individual has obtained immunity and is subsequently wounded, he is then given subsequent protective doses of toxoid.

My answer to Dr. Wright's question is that there are no permanent sequelæ of tetanus. Pathologically there are no typical lesions in fatal cases. These patients, when they survive the disease, become greatly emaciated and their muscles lose their tone and become exceedingly flabby, but there are no permanent structural changes.

Dr. Johnson stresses the use of prophylactic serum. I can think of no legitimate excuse for not using prophylactic serum in all puncture wounds, wounds harboring foreign bodies and wounds harboring secondary pyogenic organisms. As regards the amount, 1,500 units is considered standard but this dose must be repeated two or three times at weekly intervals in cases that have a great deal of suppuration and where the infections are prolonged. It is a well known fact that one prophylactic dose will not always be protective. One of our cases received prophylactic serum thirteen days after he was wounded and within forty-eight hours of the time tetanus developed. This case promptly died. Another case received prophylactic serum seven days after his injury and subsequently developed tetanus and survived the infection.

In reply to Dr. Camp's question about tetanus associated with head injuries, I am frank to state that there were only two cases in this series that might have had scalp wounds as the focus of infection. One of these cases had a hand injury, therefore the source of infection was not definitely determined. One other case had a neck wound and the incubation period in this case was only four days and terminated fatally. Infections following head injuries are rather infrequent but when they do occur are often very severe.

It is surprising, from a review of the literature, how few head injuries are complicated by tetanus infection.

I am very grateful to these gentlemen for their discussions.

RETROPERITONEAL DERMOID WITHIN THE PELVIS

MARTIN NORDLAND, M.D.

Minneapolis

This case is that of a patient who had an extraperitoneal tumor within the pelvis. It is of interest because of the difficulty experienced in its removal and because of complications caused by its presence during obstetrical delivery about five months previously.

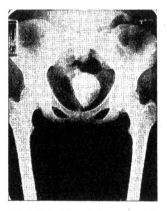

Fig. 1. Cyst anterior to the lower portion of the sacrum and coccyx.

The history of this case reveals that on September 2, 1937, the patient was brought into the hospital by her attending physician for the induction of labor because she was two weeks beyond the date of expected delivery. She had gained 65 pounds during pregnancy and seven pounds in the last week. Medication and bag induction failed to induce labor but a second attempt with castor oil and quinine caused the onset of pain on September 8, at about noon. Pains began slowly and continued with increasing severity without much progress all through the day of September 9. An obstetrical consultant was then called in by the attending physician, who had noted the presence of "a tumor in the vagina." Rectal examination had given this information. The consultant in his examination described the tumor as "antero-rectal." He stated that the tumor was tense and firm, contained fluid and was not tender and further that it extended in the direction of the left sacro-iliac joint. With the pains, the lower margin of the tumor extended down to about 1½ inches above the anal ring. The cervix was completely dilated above the protruding margin of the tumor.

They felt that aspiration was advisable and, with the

finger in the rectum, they inserted a large needle up to the left side of the rectum and punctured the tumor mass. Nothing was aspirated, but when they withdrew the needle it was filled with sebaceous looking material. A second attempt with a larger needle was also

since the delivery of her baby, it was thought best to postpone the surgical removal of the pelvic tumor for several weeks.

By the first of January, 1938, the patient returned to the hospital in very good condition. The two fistu-

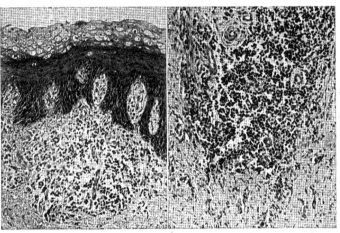

Fig. 2. Microscopic section of cyst wall showing characteristic lining with stratified squamous epithelium and chronic inflammation underneath.

Fig. 3. Microscopic section of cyst wall showing round cell infiltration, plasma cells and pus.

unsuccessful. The skin was then incised and a blunt scissors was directed upward in the same line and in this manner the tumor was widely opened. About one pint of heavy, cheesy, sebaceous material without odor was evacuated. The patient delivered about three hours later without difficulty.

They noted with interest that with each pain a long ribbon of the sebaceous material about 3 inches thick and 10 inches long would be evacuated. Most of the material was saved and by the time the baby's head was on the pelvic floor more than a liter of the material had been collected. Laboratory examination of the material showed it to contain much squamous epithelial and cholesterin substance. The patient promptly became infected and ran a temperature, the drainage became thinner and developed much offensive odor. It was necessary to reestablish drainage through the insertion of catheters into the cystic cavity on the ninth day. These catheters were inserted for a distance of about 10 inches, and as a result of the procedure the temperature dropped promptly. When the catheters were removed five days later, the temperature again became elevated and, with reinsertion and establishment of drainage, the temperature again receded. The patient left the hospital at the end of six weeks.

I was called to see the patient just before she was dismissed. She was still having recurrent elevations of temperature. Examination of the uterus revealed the fundus retroverted and pressed over to the right with the cervix behind the symphysis pubis. There were two fistulous openings high in the perineum near the lower left side of the vaginal outlet. Because her general condition was poor and because it was only five weeks

lous openings were still present and the patient stated that there had been varying amounts of discharge since she left the hospital in November.

Stereoscopic antero-posterior and lateral plates were made of the pelvis after the injection of the sinus tract with an opaque material. The tract was demonstrated from the region of the labia to a position anterior to the lower portion of the sacrum and coccyx, where there was a fairly large cyst (Fig. 1).

On January 12, 1938, the patient was taken to the operating room. Under general anesthesia a double elliptical incision 3 inches in length was made to the left of the vagina extending down to the perineum including both the fistulous openings. A No. 20 catheter was pushed up into the lower fistulous opening for a distance of about 12 inches. The contents were held in the sac by clamping the catheter. The fistulous tract was dissected out using the catheter as a guide and the lower end of the sac was exposed, dissected free from the ramus of the pubis and the hollow of the sacrum. With the assistant's finger in the rectum, it was possible to free the fistulous tract from the rectum without injury to that wall. The left vaginal wall was similarly protected by keeping a finger in the vagina during the dissection. Because it was impossible to get the highest portion of the sac from below, it was thought best to finish the operation through the abdomen. Two large cigarette drains were placed into the wound from below and the abdomen was opened in the midline below the umbilicus, the peritoneum over the left broad ligament split vertically so that the field of operation which was begun from below was exposed through this opening.

The remaining portion of the sac was dissected hrough this approach and a 3 inch pack was placed in he cavity so created. This was tied to one of the igarette drains introduced from below. The opening a the broad ligament was sutured and the abdomen losed. The mass removed with the fistulous tract as the size of a large fist. It was found in the pelvis etween the vault of the vagina and in front and lat-ral to the rectum. It was fastened to the ramus of he left pubis anteriorly and to the periosteum of the acrum near the left sacro-iliac joint. During the bdominal procedure, the left ureter and the femoral vessels were exposed. The sac contained sebaceous and suppurative material and had a smooth lining.

The laboratory submitted the following report: "Microscopic sections show .walls of cyst containing fibrous tissue some of which is elastic. It has a lin-ing, round cells, plasma cells and pus. Some points covered with stratified squamous epithelium with con-siderable chronic inflammation underneath" (Fig. 2 and Fig. 3).

Pathologically, dermoids are of interest even though they are quite commonly encountered by the surgeon of average experience. Dr. E. T. Bell has suggested that this tumor might be classified as an epidermoid. Bowles states that cystic teratoma must be distinguished from other dermoid tumors which are congenital ·se-questration tumors found at the lines of embryonic fusion and which arise by the development and inclu-sion of cells of ectodermal origin. It is possible for retroperitoneal teratomas to develop from the isolated blastomeres or germ cells of an accessory retroperi-toneal ovary. It is possible that this is what happened in this case. An ovarian dermoid is considered large when it reaches the. size of a grapefruit. Most der-moids range from the size of a heh's egg to an orange. As seen in the history above, this cyst contained more than a quart of sebaceous material at the time of de-livery and was as large as a good sized fist at the time of the operation. Koucky, in a recent analysis of a hun-dred cases of dermoids, states that a typical ovarian dermoid, cleansed of its fat and loose hair, reveals a projection into its cavity. This projection known as the plug, pseudomamma, or focus is covered with hairy skin and contains the parenchyma of the tumor. The rest of the cyst wall is smooth and glistening, reddish in color and wrinkled and 1 to 2 mm. in thickness. The plug or focus is the essential part of the dermoid. Its growth and secretory activity determines the size of the tumor. Forty-one per cent of Koucky's cases had a smooth interior and revealed only slight thickening of the lining to mark the site of the plug and focus. No focus·was demonstrated in this case. In his conclusion, Koucky states that dermoids usually occur in the 4th and 5th decades, seldom interfere with child-bearing and that the symptoms are usually due to pressure on the surrounding organs. Our patient was twenty-three years old, and the tumor was recognized because it did interfere with the delivery of the child. Roentgen ex-amination before delivery gave no information. The patient made an uneventful recovery following the removal of the cyst and is in good condition at the present time.

The meeting adjourned.

ALBERT G. SCHULZE, M.D., *Secretary.*

BOOK REVIEWS

Books listed here become the property of the Ramsey and Hennepin County Medical libraries when reviewed. Members, however, are urged to write reviews of any or every recent book which may be of interest to physicians.

BOOKS RECEIVED FOR REVIEW

THE COMPLEAT PEDIATRICIAN. Practical, Diagnostic, Therapeutic and Preventive Pediatrics. Revised Edi-tion. Wilburt C. Davison, M.A., D.Sc., M.D., Pro-fessor of Pediatrics, Duke University School of Medicine, and Pediatrician, Duke Hospital; formerly Acting Head of Department of Pediatrics, Johns Hopkins University School of Medicine, etc. 250 pages. Price, $3.75, flexible binding. Durham, N. C.: Duke University Press, 1938.

THE THOUSAND FORMS OF DISEASE. R. P. Byers, M.D. 29 pages. Price, $1.50, paper cover. Boston: Su-peruniversity Publications, 324 Newbury St., 1938.

OPERATIVE GYNECOLOGY. Fifth Edition.. Harry Stur-geon Crossen, M.D., Professor Emeritus of Clinical Gynecology, Washington University School of Medi-cine, etc., and Robert James Crossen, M.D., Assist-ant Professor of Clinical Gynecology and Obstetrics, Washington University School of Medicine, etc. 1076 pages. Illus. Price, cloth, $2.50. St. Louis: C. V. Mosby Co., 1938.

J. P. MURPHY—STORMY PETREL OF SUR-GERY. Loyal Davis. New York: G. P. Putnam's Sons, 1938. Price $3.00.

No American surgeon ever received more criticism at the hands of his fellow surgeons than did J. B. Murphy of Chicago. Few received more honors at the hands of the profession and public. This biography is beautifully written by a Chicago surgeon who knew J. B. and is as impartial as a biography could be. After reading the volume one can appreciate how this surgeon's dynamic personality, his inconceivable in-dustry and his unsuppressable ambition led him to the top of the ladder but not without his being the target for much mud slinging and some justifiable criticism. This biography reads like a novel and will prove in-teresting especially to one who ever had the privilege of attending one of J. B.'s clinics.   C. B. D.

HEART FAILURE. Arthur M. Fishberg. 788 pages. Illus. Philadelphia: Lea and Febiger, 1937.

Of the many volumes concerning heart disease which have appeared in recent years none has been of more value to the physician than the publication under re-view. The author has well succeeded in bringing to-gether the vast amount of work which has been done in recent years on problems concerning the circulation, and he has pointed out the reasonable deductions which can be drawn from this work. The work is essentially one on pathologic physiology of the circulation, a valuable contribution to our knowledge of the reasons for the various manifestations of circulatory disease.

The author's descriptions of and differentiations between cardiac failure and peripheral circulatory failure lead to an intelligent appreciation of the care of these conditions. They have been all too often regarded as simply heart failure.

The work may be divided into three major sections. The first describes the signs and symptoms which accompany heart disease, as well as the fundamental circulatory change which can be measured in quantitative terms. The methods of production of these changes are described. The second deals with the application of these fundamentals to the various types of circulatory failure, and the third part discusses the treatment which modern concepts indicate.

Any adverse criticism would be too insignificant to mention in discussing a work which has so much to offer the physician as does this volume.

JOSEPH F. BORG, M.D.

POISONING WITH CICUTA MACULATA OR WATER HEMLOCK

(Continued from Page 262)

in abundance. While one had eaten the roots, the other had partaken only of the flowers. It is interesting to note that the one who had eaten the root and stock was very sick and had convulsions, while the other who had eaten the flowers but no roots had no convulsions.

In the older boy, besides the violent convulsions, there was unconsciousness, protruding eyeballs, and frothing at the mouth. The froth was blood tinged. Cyanosis was extreme and the corneal reflexes absent. The jaws were set and there were severe twitchings of the muscles of the face. The abdomen was negative. The fingernails were cyanotic and the hands were tightly clinched.

During the convulsion it seemed as if the boy was about to die from suffocation. The convulsions lasted on the average of about ten minutes, being followed by a state of exhaustion. The patient remained cyanotic and unconscious. This patient had five convulsions. Following the last convulsion, the boy, exhausted, fell into a deep sleep.

The younger boy, who had eaten the blossoms, complained of general weakness, faintness and nausea. Slight cyanosis and nervous twitchings were also present. Dizziness was a prominent symptom. There was evidence of general collapse and the extremities were cold.

Treatment consisted of gastric lavage and enemas. In the other boy, it was necessary to use a metal mouth gag in order to pass the stomach tube. After his stomach was evacuated, it was necessary to administer morphine hypodermically. Stimulants such as strychnine, black coffee, strong tea, whisky, caffeine and sodium benzoate were administered. Artificial respiration was necessary. His urine showed a trace of albumin the first day. The second and third day the urine was increased in amount but it contained an abundance of blood and albumin. His condition remained the same until the seventh day when he appeared more rational and his appetite began to improve. There were still dark rings under his eyes. The urine had increased in amount and contained less blood and albumin. The kidney condition in general was treated by rest in bed, elimination, low protein and a salt-free diet. Iron, manganese and copper were given later to combat the anemia. Recovery followed.

The younger boy, who could swallow was given hot water containing tameric acid at thirty-minute intervals followed by lavage. This was followed by prompt recovery.

CLASSIFIED ADVERTISING

MINNESOTA MEDICINE

Journal of the Minnesota State Medical Association, Southern Minnesota Medical Association, Northern Minnesota Medical Association, Minnesota Academy of Medicine and Minneapolis Surgical Society.

| Volume 21 | MAY, 1938 | Number 5 |

ESTIMATION OF PERMANENT DISABILITY

GEORGE R. DUNN, M.D.
Minneapolis, Minnesota

THE Industrial Commission of Minnesota ultimately determines the amount of disability in a compensation case.

Members of the medical profession usually furnish an opinion or several opinions, as the case may be. This opinion is called an estimate of disability. The estimate of disability should be based on the permanent loss of general usefulness of the extremity or portion of the extremity involved. Occupation is not considered in making the estimate.

The estimate of permanent disability is expressed by the medical man as a certain percentage of loss of function of the extremity or portion of the extremity involved. For example:

10% loss of function of the right arm.
10% loss of function of the right hand and wrist.
10% loss of function of the right hand.
10% loss of function of the right thumb, index, middle, ring, or small finger, as the case may be.

Leg	200 weeks	
Foot and ankle	150 weeks	
Foot	125 weeks	
Great toe	30 weeks	
Second toe	10 weeks	
Third toe	10 weeks	70 weeks
Fourth toe	10 weeks	
Fifth toe	10 weeks	

A knowledge of these values is necessary for the medical man in furnishing an estimate of disability. For example, in a case involving the complete loss of the thumb with additional injury to the palm of the hand, the estimate would be based on a percentage of loss of function of the hand but would exceed a 40 per cent loss of function of the hand for the thumb alone (value 60 weeks) constitutes 40 per cent of the hand (value 150 weeks).

Certain losses by amputation are definitely fixed by law.

FINGER AMPUTATIONS

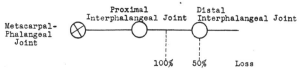

Amputation of distal phalanx 50 per cent and amputation of distal and half or more of middle phalanx 100 per cent of the finger.

Certain values in weeks have been fixed by law for extremities and component parts.

Arm	200 weeks	
Hand and wrist	175 weeks	
Hand	150 weeks	
Thumb	60 weeks	
Index finger	35 weeks	
Middle finger	30 weeks	160 weeks
Ring finger	20 weeks	
Small finger	15 weeks	

In case the terminal phalanx of a finger has been amputated (50 per cent of finger), and in addition there is limitation of movement at the proximal interphalangeal joint, due allowance must be made for the additional disability, i.e., 50 per cent (loss by amputation) plus additional disability due to the limitation of movement at the proximal joint.

If an amputation has been done below the

knee, leaving a satisfactory stump for a useful artificial limb, the disability constitutes the loss of a foot and ankle. Various other amputations of arms and legs as well as loss of hearing, loss of an eye, disfigurement, and certain combinations of these conditions are covered by law. Permanent partial disability and permanent total disability are also legally defined.†

However, in a large number of cases medical men must form an opinion of the percentage of disability by contrasting the injured member with the normal and, while no absolute rules or values can be set forth, certain principles may perhaps prove helpful, subject to proper correction.

In estimating disability of the arm, four important considerations are:

1. Range of movement.
2. Strength and stability
3. Pain.
4. Tactile sensation.

In estimating disability of the leg, five important considerations are:

1. Range of movement.
2. Strength and stability.
3. Pain.
4. Shortening.
5. Tactile sensation.

In evaluating pain, one is guided by complaints, muscle reaction, limitation of motion of joints, measured atrophy of the muscle and organic findings such as roughened joint surfaces, nerve lesions and other conditions. A fracture of the os calcis may cause little deformity of the foot but if the subastragaloid joint is rough and painful, there may be a considerable loss of function.

Tactile sensation can be fairly definitely tested and, especially in the hand, may cause a definite impairment of function.

Strength and stability of the various portions of the extremities are closely related and are of particular importance in the lower extremity. It must be remembered that full strength returns only with active prolonged use of an injured extremity. The injured member may be compared with the uninjured and the strength of the hands tested by a grip machine and fairly accurately measured.

Important nerve lesions may cause, through

†See Labor Laws of Minnesota.

muscular paralysis, loss of range of movement and loss of strength; and by the sensory nerve lesion, loss or impairment of sensation or pain.

Shortening, especially of the lower extremity, is of importance. The disability caused by shortening of the lower extremity, depending on the symptoms produced, frequently falls within this range:

Shortening of 1 inch................. 0-10% of leg
Shortening of 1-2 inches...............10-20% of leg
Shortening of 2-3 inches....:..........20-40% of leg

Range of movement, strength and stability usually reflect fairly well the disability present, for if movement is painful, the usual result is limitation of movement and diminished strength. Strength, as we have seen, can be fairly accurately determined by the grip machine or by actually comparing the strength of the injured and uninjured extremities in various movements against the resistance of the examiner's hands.

It consequently follows that in a large number of cases the estimate of disability is closely related to the loss of the normal range of movement. Certain portions of the normal range in certain joints, particularly the shoulder, are, undoubtedly, of greater value and more generally useful than other portions. This is a matter upon which any particular individual can but express an opinion and only roughly approximate.

To proceed in orderly manner, it would firs seem desirable to valuate the various norma joints with regard to the extremity as a whole Having fixed a value on the normal joint an knowing the normal range of movement of thi joint, it should be possible to fairly accuratel estimate the percentage of disability to the ex tremity occasioned by a certain loss of the nor mal range of movement at this particular joint

Finger

Let us first consider the finger. As dete mined by our Minnesota Law, the amputatic of the distal phalanx constitutes a 50 per ce loss of function of the finger and a phalanx ar a half or more constitutes 100 per cent loss.

If a finger amputated at the distal inte phalangeal joint constitutes a 50 per cent lo of the finger, then ankylosis of this joint aloi would seem to furnish a slightly more usef finger or perhaps a 40 per cent loss of functi of the finger. Obviously the loss of moveme of the two interphalangeal joints (proximal a distal) constitutes 100 per cent loss of the finger; therefore ankylosis of the proximal interphalangeal joint may be said to constitute 60 per cent of the finger.

Roughly, the middle finger can be flexed at the various joints from a straight line (180°)

DISTAL JOINT (40 PER CENT OF FINGER)
(RANGE 90°)

Roughly 10° loss of movement = 5% (loss of function of finger)
Roughly 30° loss of movement = 15% (loss of function of finger)
Exactly 45° loss of movement = 20% (loss of function of finger)

LOSS BY AMPUTATION (FINGER)

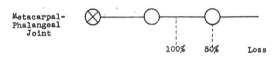

PERCENTAGE VALUE OF JOINTS OF FINGER

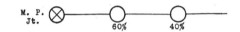

RANGE OF MOVEMENT OF JOINTS

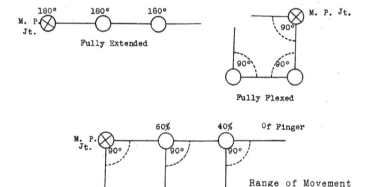

through 90° (to a right angle), each joint having a range of approximately 90°.

Having fixed the per cent of value of the normal joint with respect to the finger and the normal range of movement of this joint, one may then compute the percentage of loss to the finger of any certain number of degrees of loss of movement at this joint.

PROXIMAL JOINT (60 PER CENT OF FINGER)
(RANGE 90°)

Exactly 30° loss of movement = 20% (loss of function of finger)
60° loss of movement = 40% (loss of function of finger)
90° loss of movement = 60% (loss of function of finger)

If there is some loss of movement at both joints, compute the percentage loss to the finger at each joint and add the two to determine the total.

Loss of extension constitutes just as definite a loss of motion as loss of flexion and can be computed in the same manner.

Let us take a concrete example of disability to a finger which has a 30° loss of extension in

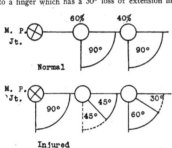

Normal

Injured

Flexion of Injured

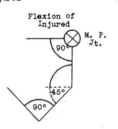

Extension of Injured

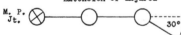

Dark lines represent range of movement at metacarpal phalangeal, proximal and distal interphalangeal joints, respectively. Dotted lines represent loss of normal range of movement.

the distal joint and a 45° loss of flexion in the proximal joint.

Thumb (60 Weeks)

The first metacarpal is relatively quite movable and in estimating disability to the thumb the metacarpal phalangeal joint may be valued at 60 per cent of the thumb and the interphalangeal joint at 40 per cent of the thumb. Comparison of range of movement should always be made between the normal and injured thumb as there is considerable variation in individuals but the average is probably 45° at the metacarpal phalangeal joint and 45° at the interphalangeal joint when the tip of the thumb is approximated to the palm of the hand at the base of the small finger.

LOSS BY AMPUTATION (THUMB)

NORMAL RANGE AND VALUATION OF JOINTS OF THUMB

Hand (150 Weeks)

In estimating disability of the hand, the function of the fingers is taken into consideration and, in addition to this, any disability to the palm or dorsum of the hand.

Wrist (Estimate Based on Hand and Wrist, 175 Weeks)

Complete ankylosis of the wrist in good position (30° dorsiflexion) probably constitutes approximately 30 per cent loss of the hand and wrist. One must consider that movement of the wrist, when lost, prevents the individual

	Metacarpal Phalangeal	Proximal	Distal Joints
		60%	40%
Value of Joint (% of finger)...........		90%	90%
Normal Range	90°	45°	60°
Range of Injured Finger...............	90°	45°	30°
Loss of Range....,.................	0°		

Loss (exactly) at Proximal Joint........ $\frac{45°}{90°}$ or ½ of 60% equals 30%

Loss (roughly) at Distal Joint.......... $\frac{30°}{90°}$ or ⅓ of 40% equals 15%*

Total Percentage Loss of Finger 45%

*Take closest 5 per cent.

making normal use of the hand by interfering with getting the hand into proper position. Any actual injury to the hand constitutes an additional disability. Wrist joint movements vary considerably but usually the normal and abnormal joint movements can be compared and a fairly definite estimate obtained.

WRIST (30 PER CENT OF HAND AND WRIST)

Average normal range as follows (but check with uninjured wrist):

Palmar Flexion	60°	Range 120°
Dorsiflexion	60°	
Radial Deviation	15°	Range 45°
Ulnar Deviation	30°	
Pronation	90°	Range 180°
Supination	90°	

Elbow (50 Per Cent of Arm)
Normal Range 145°

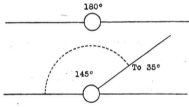

The normal range of the elbow is 145°. With these figures in mind, one can compute the portion of 50 per cent which a certain amount of the loss of the normal range occasions.

Shoulder (Including Scapular Movement)
(65 Per Cent of Arm)

Abduction	180°	
Forward Elevation	180°	
External Rotation	45°	135°*
Internal Rotation	90°	

*Judged by forearm with elbow at a right angle. Not important usually.

Shoulder and scapular movement need not be differentiated for this particular consideration.

External and internal rotation usually do not play a very important part as scapular fixation very rarely occurs.

Movement below the level of the shoulder would seem to be more valuable than movement above this level and value of movement would seem to decrease as the arm travels from the shoulder level to a straight overhead position. In the upper range (145° to 180°) a slight back-

ward or lateral bending of the body compensates and this range is infrequently used. A man 5 feet 6 inches in height with arm extended to 180° attains approximately the level of the hand that a man of 6 feet in height reaches with the hand when the arm is elevated to 145° at the shoulder.

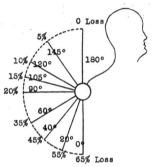

Toes

It is practically impossible to measure accurately individual joint movement in toes; consequently the arc of the tip of the toe describes

TOES (COMPARE WITH NORMAL)

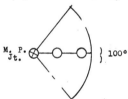

Range (Arc of Tip Approximately 100°)
Loss of 10° equals 10%
Loss of 50° equals 50%

in moving from full flexion to complete extension is a better index. Pain on movement is an important factor in disability of toes as a painful toe may easily be much more troublesome than an amputated toe.

Foot (125 Weeks)

Any injury to the foot involving more than disability to the toes but not affecting the ankle joint, should be estimated on the foot. This includes the toes, metatarsal and tarsal bones and the subastragaloid joint.

SUBASTRAGALOID JOINT (25 PER CENT OF FOOT)

Inversion ....35°⎫ Total 45°
Eversion ....10°⎭

Here again pain is an important factor. A painful subastragaloid joint may create more disability than an ankylosed joint; consequently subastragaloid arthrodesis may be indicated on occasions. Pain and stability are more important factors in the lower extremity than in the arm. On the contrary, loss of movement in the lower extremity is less important than in the arm.

ANKLE (25 PER CENT OF FOOT AND ANKLE)

Plantar flexion ....35°⎫ Range 45°
Dorsiflexion ....10°⎭

Knee (50 Per Cent of Leg) (Range 145°)

Ankylosis of the knee in a favorable position, 25° of flexion (155°) probably results in approximately a 50 per cent loss of function of the leg. In an unfavorable position the disability is higher.

ANKYLOSIS OF KNEE

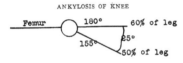

NORMAL RANGE OF KNEE MOVEMENT

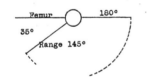

The most valuable range of movement of the knee probably lies between 155° and 85°. If the knee can not be flexed to 155°, it renders the leg very awkward. On the other hand, flexion beyond 85° probably becomes less important, relatively.

Stability of the knee is of great importance. An individual who has a good range of movement, but on account of lateral instability of the knee constantly requires a large knee cage, probably has approximately a 35 per cent loss of function of the leg.

Normal Range 145°
Value 50% of Leg

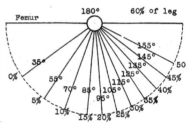

Hip Joint (60 Per Cent of Leg)

Abduction ....40°⎫ 70°
Adduction ....30°⎭

Internal Rotation .....30°⎫ 70°*
External Rotation ....40°⎭

*Judged by patella or foot with leg straight or by the leg (below the knee) with hip and knee flexed to a right angle.

Flexion ⎫ 135° (Important)
Extension ⎭

Abduction, adduction, internal and external rotation are usually not nearly as important as flexion and extension.

A fair degree of precision is desirable in determining these measurements. A grip machine, an instrument for measuring angles, and a tape measure are the only equipment necessary.

In expressing an estimate of permanent disability, one must bear in mind that one is estimating the amount of disability which will actually be permanent, that is, the amount of disability which will eventually be present after medical treatment and reasonable use of the extremity have largely accomplished all improvement possible.

The figures and percentages set forth are not based on any book or article but simply represent one opinion formed and gradually evolved over a period of years* and presented to the medical profession of Minnesota hoping that it may tend to clarify our opinions in this rather intricate matter.

*Somewhat similar but less comprehensive paper, withou diagrams, read at noonday session of Hennepin County Medica Society approximately ten years ago.

ENLARGEMENT OF THE HEART*
Its Recognition by the Radiologic Method

PHILLIP HALLOCK, M.D.

Minneapolis, Minnesota

TO determine the presence or absence of enlargement of the heart is obviously of great importance. Cardiac enlargement, i⁴ present, generally indicates myocardial disease. Furthermore, the extent of cardiac enlargement is a fair index of the severity of myocardial involvement and in a large measure provides the most satisfactory basis for prognosis.

For the establishment of a diagnosis of cardiac disease, the physician depends chiefly on the symptoms and physical findings. The time-honored symptoms associated with cardiac disease are of inestimable value and will continue to occupy a position of great importance in cardiac diagnosis. On the other hand, certain physical signs have met with reproach in the past and are continuing to be met with increasing disfavor because by their employment the range of precision afforded by such instruments as the electrocardiograph, the sphygmomanometer and the x-ray cannot be attained. The value and potentialities of the x-ray in modern cardiology is the subject I wish to discuss.

X-ray or radiologic visualization of the heart is now indispensable in cardiac diagnosis. It offers us an accurate and detailed knowledge of the heart as an anatomic structure, both in its normal and pathologic states, information which extends far beyond the reach and scope of percussion and palpation.

Gross enlargement of the heart can easily be detected in most cases by percussion and palpation. However, slight degrees of enlargement cannot be recognized with certainty by these methods. The difficulties encountered in the use of the percussion method in the obese, the emphysematous and in the female sex are well known. Furthermore, it is a highly subjective method in which the personal equation is far too great. Too often have we been disillusioned by the fantastic ideas that have been and still are held regarding the accuracy that can be obtained by percussion. It can give us only a rough estimate of the transverse diameter of

*From the Department of Medicine, University of Minnesota Hospital, Minneapolis. Read before the annual meeting of the Minnesota Heart Society, November 17, 1937.

the heart and tells, under favorable conditions, whether there is enlargement in the conus area.

While the percussion method should not be discarded in the routine bedside physical examination, its limitations and the inaccuracies that attend its use should be constantly kept in mind. Sir Thomas Lewis,⁸ in speaking of percussion, stated: "It is crucial in measuring to know the error of the method. To have an inaccurate measure may be regrettable, but to have it and not to know it is deplorable."

Because of the lack of faith in the percussion method, recourse has been made to the method of palpation in evaluating cardiac enlargement. This is a valuable bedside technic, but its scope is limited. It offers accurate information about the left ventricle. However, it can be misleading when there is displacement of the heart from any cause or when tachycardia is present.

The Radiologic Method

While the radiologic method for the visualization of the living heart has been employed for many years in Europe, it can be said that its use is still in its infancy in this country, particularly in this region. It is now a universally observed fact that the most experienced radiologists are skilled in the use of the fluoroscope and many will defer a final opinion until after the radioscopic examination has been completed. What information may one expect to gain by submitting the patient to routine radiological examination? Certainly no organ is so well placed for x-ray visualization as the heart. In the first place, it is almost completely surrounded by transparent lung tissue, and, by rotating the patient, it can be viewed from all aspects. An idea of its volume can be immediately obtained, as well as its position in the chest. In the act of turning the patient, each individual chamber can be identified and scrutinized as to size and shape. The great vessels of the heart as they emerge from their respective chambers and extend beyond their origins can be critically examined. In addition to the visualization of the component parts, the character and extent of pulsations of the heart and its pedicle can be recognized and evaluated. Calcification in the pericardium, aortic arch, and heart valves can be actually visualized. Lastly, in cardiac failure,

Fig. 1. Outline drawing of normal heart showing effect of changes in height of diaphragm on cardiac silhouette. Continuous line: the end of expiration. Dotted line: the end of deep inspiration. It will be noted that with the lowering of the diaphragm both cardiac borders moved toward the midline. The apparent increase in the size of the heart as a result of a high diaphragm often can give a false impression of cardiac enlargement.

secondary changes that occur in the lung fields and pleural spaces can be recognized.

To disregard this method of examination, Rösler[18] states, means to renounce much of what our best trained sense organ, the eye, can perceive. It has been rightly stated that the radioscopic method provides a means for performing a veritable biopsy of the living heart.[9]

The shape and position of the normal heart as seen by radioscopic examination is variable, depending on a number of factors. Indeed, the chief difficulty in the routine application of radiocardiology is not in the technic, which can be easily mastered, but lies in the interpretation of normal variability and in the recognition of slightly abnormal enlargement. The chief factors upon which alteration in shape and position of the normal heart depend are, for example, age, constitutional build, respiration and position of the diaphragm. It has been demonstrated on anatomical grounds that the contour of the chest cavity determines the form and position of all the organs contained therein. Hence, hearts contained in round chests have a more circular circumference, while those found in flatter chests are more oval in appearance. Individuals of the sthenic type, where the development of the trunk predominates, give the following picture: The mediastinal shadow is short and wide and the diaphragm is high in position. The heart shadow is decreased in height and tends to be boot-shaped—that is, it is tilted upward and to the left. On the other hand, those of the asthenic habitus,

in which development of the extremities and vertical dimensions prevail, give a different roentgenological picture. The mediastinal shadow is narrow and long, the diaphragm is low in position and the cardiac silhouette is centrally located, giving the so-called drop heart appearance. The high diaphragm resulting from increased abdominal obesity, meteorism or ascites may cause the heart to assume a transverse position, so that it looks larger than it actually is. Too often a diagnosis of cardiac enlargement is made in these cases, and occasionally healthy men are rejected for life insurance or positions involving physical strain because percussion or palpation suggests that the apex beat is outside the nipple line. The increase in transverse diameter of the heart with advancing age is often not due to an actual increase in heart size, but may be a result of two other factors. The diaphragm is situated higher and an arteriosclerotic and elongated aorta tends to push the heart down on the already elevated diaphragm, thus giving one the impression that there is an increased surface area of the cardiac silhouette. In children the diaphragm is high and the heart appears large in a relatively small chest. One has only to observe the large difference between the position, shape and apparent size of the heart in deep inspiration and expiration to be convinced of the marked variation in shape and apparent size that may occur (Fig. 1).

Parkinson[9] has emphasized the fact that slight scoliosis, particularly in children of school age, may displace the apex beat outward a trifle beyond the nipple line, and, in addition, may result in an exaggerated apex beat, which gives the examiner a false impression of cardiac enlargement. This source of error is present even in radiologic examination. However, by turning the patient slightly to the right, this distortion can be corrected and the cardiac shadow brought back into its normal position.

Cardiometry

Cardiometry, or the quantitative method of determining cardiac enlargement, consists of measuring the distance between certain landmarks on the cardiac silhouette and comparing these measurements with those of normal hearts. For many years investigators have elaborated methods for making cardiac measurements, and have compiled voluminous data upon which to establish normal standards for heart size. After

304

critically examining the literature, Rösler[18] states that the majority of publications on the subject reveal much evidence of vast waste both of energy and material with resulting confusion and contradictory conclusions. Probably the first method proposed, one which is still in vogue to-day, is the cardio-thoracic ratio, the relationship of the transverse diameter of the heart to the internal diameter of the chest at its base. In people of normal build, the diameter of the heart should not exceed 50 per cent that of the chest. However, variations are many and this method is too unreliable as a guide as to whether a heart is slightly enlarged.

The investigations of Hodges and Eyster[5] are worthy of note. They have shown that the cardiac transverse diameter could be best correlated with body size, providing height and weight were taken into consideration. As a result, they have developed a formula for predicting the transverse diameter of the heart. Their tables would appear to represent the most scientific attempt from which to estimate the mean physiologic heart size. Authors on the subject of cardiometry agree that the most accurate method to estimate heart size is by determining cardiac volume. Thus, Rohrer[14] attempted to determine heart volume by taking measurements in two planes, and succeeded in obtaining fairly accurate results. These results, confirmed by Kahlstorf,[6] have not yet been routinely introduced into clinical use. A method of determining surface area has been introduced with the hope that the cardiac area will afford a finer index of cardiac size than linear measurements. The difficulty of this method lies in the fact that the upper and lower borders of the heart cannot be sharply demarcated from the vascular shadow above and that of the liver below.

Cardiometry, complicated and bestrewn with imperfections, is, with few exceptions, hardly suitable for routine clinical use. I cannot recall in any instance that the numerical measurements of the heart have afforded me any information not gained by fluoroscopy and inspection of the six-foot film, except where measurements are utilized for comparative purposes in the same individual over a period of time.

Moreover, from an etiologic point of view, it is not so much the total size of the heart that concerns us, but rather the alterations that may occur in its shape. Enlargement of the heart rarely affects all chambers to an equal extent. It has its origin in a certain specified chamber or several chambers, depending on the location of the pathologic process. For example, the strain in hypertension is primarily on the left ventricle, which enlarges in its characteristic manner, in emphysema the strain is on the pulmonary artery and conus of the right ventricle, in mitral stenosis on the left auricle and the right ventricle. Enlargement, with rare exceptions, is therefore regional and in each instance a characteristic pattern of the heart shape is evolved, depending on the seat of the cardiac strain. It can be seen, therefore, why a change in the shape of the heart is of greater importance than the variation in heart size alone. By the recognition of the various patterns of the heart shape, we are thus able to obtain corroborative evidence of the cause of enlargement and to recognize localized changes in early stages. The successful application of the radiologic method in studying cardiac enlargement depends on the recognition of these various pathologic configurations in heart shape. Before this can be attempted, one must be thoroughly acquainted with the normal radiologic anatomy of the heart and great vessels as visualized in the chest from the standard three positions.

Radiologic Anatomy of the Heart

Anatomically the heart is a three-dimensional organ. Radioscopic examination permits study of the heart in three planes; namely, the anteroposterior, the right oblique, and the left oblique positions. In this routine method we inspect the contour of the cardiac chambers from three viewpoints.

In the anteroposterior view (Fig. 2) three borders are visible: the right, left and inferior. The right and left borders of the shadow are easily seen, the inferior border is for the most part lost in the shadow of the diaphragm. The right border beginning superiorly extends downward in an almost straight line for a short distance. This is the shadow of the superior vena cava which at its lower border forms a small notch where it blends into the convex shadow of the right auricle. Just medial to the notch is the origin of the ascending aorta. The right ventricle forms most of the shadow seen anteriorly.

The left border of the heart and great vessels is considerably longer than the right. The most superior shadow is semicircular in contour and constitutes the terminal portion of the aortic arch

hepatic angle in which is the shadow of the inferior vena cava. The latter is made visible when the patient takes a deep breath. Behind the contour of the posterior border of the heart is

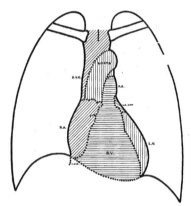

Fig. 2. Outline drawing from teleoradiogram to show normal relationships of cardiac chambers and great vessels in anterior position (after Parkinson and Bedford).

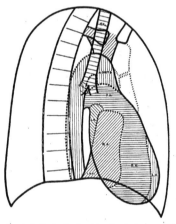

Fig. 3. Outline drawing from teleoradiogram showing normal relationships of cardiac chambers and great vessels in the right (d) oblique position. (After Parkinson and Bedford.)

and beginning of the descending aorta. It is often variable in prominence. This shadow is known as the aortic knuckle or knob. Just below this is a flat arch somewhat longer than the aortic shadow. This represents the beginning of the pulmonary artery and uppermost portion of the right ventricle (conus arteriosus). Inferior to this is a small arch, the left border of the left auricular appendage. The remaining and major portion of the silhouette is the left ventricle which forms an elliptical border extending into the left lung field and then turning back toward the midline.

The patient now makes a half turn to the left, bringing the right shoulder to the screen anteriorly so that he is examined through the right chest. This is the right oblique position (Fig. 3). This position affords an excellent view for studying enlargement of the left auricle, pulmonary artery and conus of the right ventricle. The shadow of the left auricle forms the upper two-thirds of the posterior border. Just inferior to this is the shadow of the posterior border of the right auricle. Below this is the cardio-

the clearly illuminated post-mediastinal space. To obtain maximum illumination through this space the patient should be rotated further to the left. (70°). Enlargement of the left auricle partly or completely obliterates the upper part of this space. Massive enlargement of the left ventricle obliterates the lower portion of this area. Anteriorly, if the rotation is only slight, the shadow of the lower portion of the left ventricle participates in the contour. If rotation is greater, the right ventricle becomes border forming. The greater portion of the anterior contour in the right oblique is formed by the conus region of the heart and the pulmonary artery and represents the so-called outflow tract of the right ventricle. This contour, like the one made by the left auricle, represents an important landmark in early pathologic lesions affecting the right side of the heart. Above this appears the shadow of the long aortic arch which sweeps posteriorly and superiorly to disappear in the shadow of the spine. The anterior mediastinal space, like the posterior one, should always re- remain clear. The aortic, pulmonary and left au- ricular impressions of the barium filled esophagus are best studied in the right oblique position.

of the aortic arch and inferiorly by the roof of the left auricle and posteriorly by the descending aorta. Under normal conditions it is fairly well illuminated. Crossing it is the left branch of

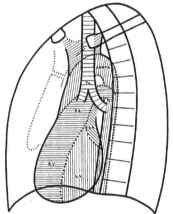

Fig. 4. Outline drawing from teleoradiogram showing nor- mal relationships of cardiac chambers and great vessels. In left (II) oblique position (after Parkinson and Bedford).

Continuing the routine fluoroscopic examina- tion, the patient is now turned half right and ex- amined through the left side of the chest (Fig. 4). It has been said that this radioscopic view will eventually prove to be most valuable in studying cardiac enlargement. Here, the cardiac shadow appears as if the heart were cut in sagittal section. In this view it is possible to closely estimate the position of the interventric- ular septum. The ventricles make up approx- imately two-thirds of the cardiac silhouette, the shadow of the right ventricle in front and the left ventricle posteriorly. Normally, the posterior border of the left ventricle stands well away from the spine. The stem of the pulmonary ar- tery is fairly well visualized in this view. The aortic arch is well seen sweeping up and poste- riorly. This is an excellent view in which to study pathologic changes that occur in the aorta; name- ly, those due to arteriosclerosis, hypertension, syphillis and congenital defects.

An important landmark in the left oblique position is the "aortic window" (Fig. 5). It is bounded superiorly by the inner concave border

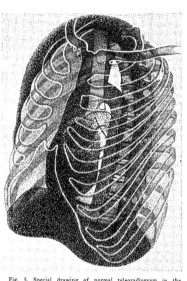

Fig. 5. Special drawing of normal teleoradiogram in the left (II) oblique position, to show the aortic window and super- aortic triangle (after Parkinson and Bedford).

the pulmonary artery and in it lies the left main bronchus. In pathologic states such as hyper- tension and arteriosclerosis of the aorta it en- larges. In massive enlargement of the pulmonary artery, especially its left branch, the window is obliterated. In enlargement of the left auricle it is made smaller and the left bronchus is ele- vated.

Recently, Parkinson and Bedford have de- scribed a new radiologic landmark in the left oblique position (Fig. 5). This is a translucent triangle seen surmounting the upper border of the aortic arch when the subject is rotated 45° or more. The anterior border is formed by the left subclavian artery, the posterior border by the spine, and the base by the roof of the aortic arch. The aortic triangle is diminished by elevation, elongation, or dilatation of the aortic arch. An intrathoracic goitre or aneurysm of the arch may encroach upon it. The triangle is enlarged by conditions which lower the aortic summit and by emphysema. By utilization of the base of the triangle as the upper point and the

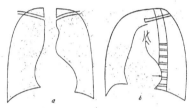

Fig. 6. Outline drawings from case of aortic stenosis in young male, aged twenty-two, blood pressure 108/87. Systolic thrill over aortic area. Harsh systolic murmur over aortic area transmitted to vessels of neck. (a) anterior view: aortic configuration with slight enlargement of left ventricle downward and to the left. The globular appearance suggests marked hypertrophy with slight dilatation. Fluoroscopic examination showed diminished pulsatory amplitude, tardus in character, of left ventricle and aortic shadow. (b) Left-oblique view: left ventricle border projecting into the vertebral shadow.

roof of the aortic window as the lower point of measurement, the measurement of the diameter of the arch of the aorta is often possible.

Left Ventricle.—The most vulnerable of all chambers of the heart to enlargement is the left ventricle. Fortunately, from a radiologic viewpoint, enlargement of this chamber is comparatively easy to recognize. The difficulty lies not so much in determining whether or not the left ventricle is enlarged but in deciding whether it is simply displaced to the left. As already stated, the apparent size of the left ventricle depends much upon the position of the diaphragm. Furthermore, considerable enlargement of the right ventricle, particularly from right-sided congenital lesions, can displace the left border outwards, giving one the impression that the left ventricle is enlarged. However, this point can be settled by turning the patient well into the left oblique position (left shoulder to the screen). When the left ventricle enlarges it does so posteriorly as well as laterally. If, in this view, the posterior border of the left ventricle extends beyond the anterior shadow of the spine it is to be considered enlarged. However, if it stands clear in front of the spine the apparent enlargement seen in the anterior position is in all probability a result of displacement rather than enlargement.

It is difficult, if not impossible, to recognize hypertrophy by radioscopic examination. It is only when dilatation has supervened upon the

hypertrophy that the increase in the size of the left ventricle can be recognized with certainty. The aortic valvular lesions which produce left ventricular enlargement are aortic stenosis, either

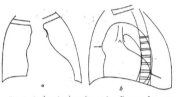

Fig. 7. Outline drawings from teleoradiograms from case of syphilitic aortitis and aortic incompetence. (a) Anterior view: large left ventricle, prominent ascending aorta which is irregular in outline and prominent aortic knuckle. (b) Left oblique view: Cardiac silhouette extends far into shadow of spine—left ventricular enlargement. Widened ascending aorta with localized outpouching.

arteriosclerotic or rheumatic in origin, and aortic incompetence which may be due either to rheumatism or syphilis. Isolated aortic stenosis alone, as a rule, causes only moderate enlargement the left ventricle (Fig. 6 a and b). Left ventricular enlargement due to arteriosclerotic stenosis of the aortic valves can at times be differentiated from that due to rheumatism by radioscopic examination. The differentiation lies in recognizing calcification of the aortic valve and calcification of the aortic arch in arteriosclerotic stenosis. Furthermore, in aortic stenosis due to arteriosclerosis, the aortic knob is quite prominent, and the arch of the aorta can be seen to appear as ectatic. Aortic incompetence can be differentiated from aortic stenosis without any difficulty by the character of the pulsations of both the aorta and left ventricle. In aortic stenosis the pulsations of the heart and aorta are small. In aortic incompetence as a result of a high pulse pressure, the amplitude is great. X-ray examination also can help in differentiating aortic insufficiency due to syphilis from that due to rheumatism. An aneurysm or out-pouching of the aortic arch speaks in favor of syphilis (Fig. 7 a and b). Syphilis of the aorta without involvement of the aortic valves is practically never a cause of cardiac enlargement.

Hypertension, whether primary or secondary, affects the left ventricle. The degree of enlargement depends on several factors; namely, the height of the diastolic pressure, age, constitutional type, and presence or absence of coronary disease. In the typical case the left ventricle enlarges in a boot-shaped manner and rather characteristic changes occur in the aortic arch. The aorta becomes uncoiled in that it diffusely dilates and elongates toward the root of the neck. This can be demonstrated in the left oblique view. The effect of this alteration is to increase the size of the aortic window.

Radiology is of invaluable aid in diagnosing congenital anomalies of the aortic arch. Persistent right-sided aortic arch can be diagnosed only by this method. The barium-filled esophagus can be seen to impress the arch on the left side instead of, as it normally does, on the right side, and the concavity of the aortic arch impression is directed to the right. Frequently, complete or partial coarctation of the aorta can be recognized by radioscopy. In this condition, a narrowing of the aortic arch just distal to the subclavian artery can sometimes be demonstrated (Fig. 8). The presence of hypertension in young adults should immediately suggest the possibility of coarctation of the aorta and the classical radioscopic findings which attend it should be sought.

Now that coronary thrombosis is so frequently recognized as a clinical entity, the complications that follow it can be determined with a fairly high degree of accuracy. Thus, formerly the diagnosis of cardiac aneurysm was relegated to the pathologist. It is now possible, by x-ray examination, to visualize the aneurysmal bulge in a fair proportion of cases. The common site for the development of the aneurysm is in the vicinity of the apical portion of the left ventricle for anterior infarction and along the posterior wall with posterior infarction. In both instances these aneurysms are radioscopically visible. We have recently observed an aneurysm of the lower posterior portion of the left ventricle when the patient was placed in the left oblique view. Roentgenological diagnosis of aneurysm of the heart is quite impossible when the lesion develops at the diaphragmatic surface or when it affects a septum. Calcification may occasionally be noted in the wall of the aneurysm.

Left Auricle.—Radiologic examination of the left auricle has contributed greatly not only to the recognition of mitral stenosis but also to a study of its effects on the enlargement of other cardiac chambers. Anatomically, the left auricle is situated entirely on the posterior aspect of the heart. For this reason it just rests against the

esophagus. It is not visible from the front, except a tiny portion of it which is known as the left auricular appendage. It is therefore beyond the reach of percussion.

Fig. 8. Coarctation of the aorta, partial, in female, aged thirty-two, who died of subacute bacterial endocarditis. Outline drawing from teleoradiogram in left oblique view, showing kink-like narrowing of aorta. Considerable dilatation of aorta proximal to site of stenosis. Postmortem control.

According to Assman,[1] the right oblique position (patient facing examiner with right shoulder to screen) with rotation about 70° is the most favorable position because then the retrocardiac space is well shown, being bounded above and below by clear spaces Parkinson has stated that next to the presystolic murmur, the posterior displacement of the barium filled esophagus is the best evidence for left auricular enlargement in mitral stenosis (Fig. 9a and b). The stages of left auricular enlargement from one of simple enlargement to where it has assumed aneurysmal size and extends into the right chest can be easily demonstrated by radioscopy.

It should be pointed out here, however, that displacement of the esophagus is not pathognomonic of mitral stenosis. Babey[2] has recently shown, in radioscopic studies confirmed by necropsy findings, that other conditions may displace the esophagus posteriorly. Long standing cases of auricular fibrillation without mitral stenosis eventually lead to left auricular enlargement. In complete heart block the left auricle sometimes becomes quite prominent. A greatly enlarged left ventricle not infrequently can push the left auricle posteriorly. In such cases the barium-filled esophagus convexity in the right oblique position is often long and gradual and not so abrupt or placed so high as in the left auricular enlargement found in mitral stenosis.

Right Auricle.—The right auricle forms the right lower border of the heart and is therefore clearly visible from the front. When enlargement appears on the right side of the heart, it should not be inferred that the right auricle is enlarged because lesions responsible for right auricular enlargement are rare. Enlargement in the region of the right auricle should rather in-

recognition of right-sided lesions. In the study of enlargement of the right ventricle it is important to recognize the fact that the outflow tract of the right ventricle represented by the

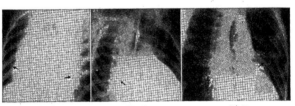

Fig. 9a   Fig. 9b   Fig. 10

Fig. 9. Mitral stenosis and aortic insufficiency, auricular fibrillation in male, aged forty-seven. (a) Left oblique view. Right ventricular enlargement shown anteriorly. Left ventricular enlargement indicated by cardiac shadow projecting into the shadow of the spine. The left bronchus is elevated by an enlarged left auricle. The aortic window is narrowed. (b) Right oblique view. The enlarged left auricle (balloon-like prominence) displaces the barium filled esophagus posteriorly and obliterates the retrocardiac space. Anteriorly, there is considerable prominence of the pulmonary conus. Just below this is noted a bulging of the mass of right ventricle which almost completely obliterates the lower portion of the anterior mediastinal space.
Fig. 10. Teleoradiogram, right oblique view, showing enlargement of the conus region of right ventricle. From case of emphysema. Postmortem control.

dicate displacement of the heart, dextrocardia, enlarged left auricle extending out from behind the right auricle, generalized enlargement of the heart, pericardial effusion or aneurysm of the ascending aorta. These conditions can all be differentiated by radioscopic examination. Lesions affecting the tricuspid valve are rare. However, when tricuspid stenosis does occur, enormous enlargement of the right auricle ensues. In organic tricuspid incompetence or more commonly in relative tricuspid insufficiency, some enlargement of the right auricle is expected. This condition can occasionally be seen in advanced stages of pulmonary disease in which the right heart alone is affected. In congenital defects of the auricular septum, the right auricle is often enlarged to a considerable extent, especially when there is a coexistent congenital mitral stenosis. Rarely, isolated enlargement of the right auricle may be seen in congenital auricular septal defects, in the absence of other congenital anomalies.

It should be further mentioned that long-standing cases of auricular fibrillation will, in time, cause enlargement of both auricles. By studying the radioscopic impressions of the barium-filled esophagus it is possible to differentiate left auricular enlargement from right auricular enlargement.

Right Ventricle.—Radiology has rendered a great service to cardiology in facilitating the

conus is the first to suffer enlargement from whatever may impose a strain on it. Fortunately, conus enlargement can be recognized in its early stages. First evidence of conus enlargement is best seen in the right oblique view with the patient well turned to the right (Fig. 10). In this position one sees a localized outpouching between the shadow of the pulmonary artery and the body of the right ventricle. When the enlargement becomes more pronounced, the conus becomes radioscopically visible on the left border of the heart in the anteroposterior view. With subsequent involvement, the body of the right ventricle becomes implicated and can be recognized best in the left oblique view (Fig. 9a). This is best demonstrated when the patient is turned well to the right (about 60°). Certain right-sided congenital lesions have fairly definite radiological appearances. By correlation of the shape of the heart with the auscultatory findings and the presence or absence of cyanosis it becomes possible to determine the location of the lesion with great accuracy.

Congenital heart lesions should no longer be looked upon as a matter of purely academic interest because, as Maude Abbott has shown, the prognoses in many types of congenital anomalies are extremely favorable. It is, therefore, important to recognize the type of congenital anomaly of the heart before venturing a poor prognosis. Radiology serves to distinguish congenital lesions from rheumatic valvular defects, occasionally a difficult task from purely clinical observations. The Tetralogy of Fallot, one of the common causes of cyanosis in congenital heart

looked if one expects to find an increase in the transverse diameter of the heart seen from the front. While the prominence of the conus is more common and exaggerated than enlargement

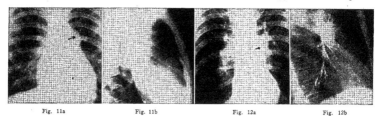

Fig. 11a   Fig. 11b   Fig. 12a   Fig. 12b

Fig. 11. Patent ductus arteriosus in female, aged twenty-two. Blood pressure 140/68. A machinery murmur and thrill in the second left interspace. Second pulmonic sound present. Telroradiogram: (a) Anterior view: moderate enlargement of entire cardiac silhouette chiefly right ventricular with marked prominence of shadow of pulmonary conus and artery. The aortic knob is small. Left oblique: (Illustration omitted). Aortic window obliterated by enlarged pulmonary artery. Marked enlargment anteriorly of body of right ventricle. Pulsations of Hilar vessels noted on radioscopic examination. (b) Right lateral: No left articular enlargement. Filling up of anterior mediastinal space by enlarged right ventricle and conus.
Fig. 12. Emphysema in male, aged forty-two. History of bronchial asthma for twelve years. Teleoradiogram: (a) Anterior view: prominence of pulmonary artery and of both of its branches (hilar vessels). (b) Right oblique view: oval shadow of enlarged pulmonary artery is well shown. Postmortem control.

disease, often gives a characteristic cardiac silhouette, namely a dextroposed aorta, small or normal sized pulmonary artery, and an enlarged right ventricle. Patent ductus arteriosus with a small aorta and dilated pulmonary artery and conus usually offers no difficulty (Fig. 11a and b).

Further contribution of the radioscopic method to the study of cardiac enlargement has recently been submitted by Parkinson and Hoyle[12] in their comprehensive treatise on the heart in emphysema. So convincing is their evidence that one need no longer doubt that the right heart is involved in this disease. In our studies on emphysema heart we have been able to confirm their findings. They have pointed out that cardiac measurements are invalidated because of the excessive width of the chest in emphysema. They further emphasize that the signs of right ventricular enlargement are different and elusive, being not nearly as easy to recognize as the signs of left ventricular enlargement to which physical signs are so largely directed.

Right ventricular enlargement in emphysema is most commonly recognized by the prominence of the conus which may be seen from the front but better yet in the right oblique view (Fig. 10). It has been shown by Kirch[7] that the far end of the outflow tract of the right ventricle, the conus, suffers first from increased pressure in the pulmonary circulation. The conus first lengthens rather than widens, and this is frequently over-

of the body of the right ventricle, nevertheless, enlargement of the right ventricle can best be seen with the subject rotated in the left oblique position to about 60°, where it forms the anterior border of the silhouette.

Another radiologic feature of emphysema heart is prominence of the pulmonary artery seen from the front (Fig. 12a). Here also, dilatation of its branches can be visualized. Prominence of the main pulmonary stem can be recognized roentgenologically in the two oblique positions (Fig. 12b). In the left oblique the stem and left main branch can be seen as one of the structures lying in the aortic window. Not infrequently the pulmonary artery may become enlarged to entirely obliterate the window. With barium paste, the so-called right pulmonic artery impression can be recognized on the esophagus. In enlargement the pulmonary artery impression becomes exaggerated.

A marked prominence of the pulmonary artery and conus or one of the main branches has often been erroneously interpreted as mediastinal tumor. Pulmonary artery enlargement is commonly observed in certain types of congenital defects: namely, in patent ductus arteriosus; auricular and ventricular septal defects; and in congenital aneurysm of the pulmonary artery or one of its branches. Among the acquired lesions that cause pulmonary artery enlargement are mitral stenosis, especially when associated with pulmonary valve incompetence, congestive failure, chiefly of the left ventricular type, and enlargement in the early stages of hyperthyroid heart (Fig. 13a and b). The pulmonary artery is likewise enlarged in pulmonary arteriosclerosis

ease was a rare association and that rheumatic fever was not an etiologic factor. The findings of mitral stenosis ruled out its presence. The cardiac shadow was normal in size in seven,

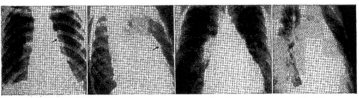

Fig. 13a   Fig. 13b   Fig. 14a   Fig. 14b

Fig. 13. Toxic adenoma in female, aged forty-eight. BMR + 68 per cent. Tachycardia, palpitation, and dyspnea on exertion. First sound at apex booming in character (pseudo-mitral stenosis). Harsh systolic murmur over pulmonic area. Teleoradiogram: (a) Anterior view: Prominence of pulmonic arch. No cardiac enlargement. Radioscopic examination showed hyperactive pulsations along all borders, particularly the pulmonary artery. (b) Right oblique view showing pulmonary artery prominence.
Fig. 14. Pulmonary arteriosclerosis in male, aged thirty-three. Only complaint is dyspnea on moderate exertion. Systolic murmur heard over pulmonic area. No diastolic murmur heard. Second pulmonic sound accentuated. Venous pressure normal. Circulation time: from arm to lung somewhat prolonged, twelve seconds. Circulation time: from lung to tongue normal. In the anterior view, the striking feature on radioscopic examination was the hilar dance (expansile pulsations of pulmonary stem and its branches). The smaller pulmonary vessels out further in the lung fields could be seen pulsating noticeably. Pulsations at the left lower border of cardiac silhouette is the right ventricle. These pulsations alternate in direction (see-saw movement), with prominence of pulmonary arc. Teleoradiogram: (a) Marked enlargement of cardiac silhouette. Chiefly right ventricular enlargement, with prominence of pulmonary arc. Aortic shadow not seen. Pulmonary arterial branches markedly enlarged. (b) Right oblique view: Mass of heart chiefly right ventricle. Left atrium not enlarged. The dense, bandlike shadow (indicated by arrows posteriorly) is the shadow of the dilated right main pulmonary artery. The left oblique illustration is omitted. It showed the aortic window filled out by the pulsating shadow of the pulmonary artery. There was very little, if any, enlargement of the left ventricle posteriorly. Anteriorly, enlargement of the body of the right ventricle was pronounced.

and rarely in syphilis of the pulmonary artery. The so-called hilar dance and pulsations of the pulmonary vessels are irrefutable evidence of pulmonary artery enlargement (Fig. 14). By radioscopy it is possible to distinguish cardiac enlargement from pathological conditions in the mediastinum or in the surrounding structures that may simulate cardiac enlargement, such as mediastinal masses, lung tumors, and spinal cord tumors. Differentiation is made possible by rotating the patient behind the fluoroscopic screen. In this manner extra-cardiac shadows can be separated from the silhouette of the heart.

Constrictive pericarditis.—There is one type of chronic heart disease in which surgery is unquestionably indicated and when carried out successfully leads to dramatic recovery. I am referring to chronic constrictive pericarditis, fifteen cases of which were reported by Paul White[15] in the St. Cyres lectures in 1936. He described the condition as one of a state of congestion without cardiac failure, which was brought about by a thick, rigid wall of pericardium surrounding the heart and the great vessels, in this manner embarrassing its action and mechanically obstructing the inflow of blood.

In discussion of his cases, he stated heart dis-

slightly enlarged in five, and moderately enlarged in three cases. In the case of constrictive pericarditis that we have recently studied the heart was normal in size. The clinical manifestations of chronic cardiac compression are distended cervical veins, cyanosis, ascites, enlargement of the liver, edema and hydrothorax, pulsus paradoxus, small pulse and low pulse pressure. However, before decortication of the heart is attempted, the clinician must make doubly sure that the constrictive phenomena exist. The opportunity to confirm the clinical findings is made possible by radioscopic examination. In this condition we usually see a normal sized heart which is fixed in position. The striking feature is that the heart is immobile. The act of respiration does not alter its size nor shape. Frequently, no pulsations of its borders can be discerned. If pulsations are present, they are markedly impaired and localized either to the right or left side of the heart. Occasionally, areas of calcification can be visualized in the thickened pericardium. The results reported by Churchill[4] and Beck[3] after performing pericardial resection are indeed striking and stand out among the great achievements of modern surgery of the heart.

Time will not permit me to discuss any further the usefulness of radioscopy to clinical cardiology. The clinician who has the radioscopic method at his disposal is equipped with a diagnostic facility equal to if not greater in importance than the electrocardiogram. Briefly, the radioscopic method gives us the following information. It replaces percussion and palpation because it gives the extent of cardiac enlargement with a much higher degree of accuracy. By the radioscopic method it is possible to determine slight changes in heart size and to distinguish whether, in doubtful cases, the heart is normal or enlarged. While it is possible that the cardiac silhouette is sometimes less informative than auscultation, as, for example, in early cases of mitral stenosis, aortic insufficiency and certain congenital defects, it gives us superior information regarding prognosis. Other things remaining equal, the smaller the cardiac silhouette, the better the prognosis. By the radioscopic method it is possible to recognize alterations in the shape of the heart. These alterations in shape inform us as to which chambers are involved, and to what extent, and give us a clue as to the etiologic basis for enlargement.

In conclusion, I would like to quote Dr. John Parkinson,[10] who comments about the present and future status of radiocardiology:

"Radiology can contribute to direct and exact knowledge in almost every variety of cardiac disease. . . . Though some will doubtless exaggerate its importance, it will steadily find its proper level among modern means of diagnosis. It is natural to regard with suspicion anything unfamiliar, and it is our duty to scrutinize any new method; but let not this defer our acquaintance with radiology of the heart—a novelty no longer. The modern physician will have his diagnostic powers extended and refined by adding radiology to his scheme of examination; he will supplement traditional methods by direct inspection of the internal organs. . . . Cardiology is now an important and integral branch of general medicine, nothing more and nothing less. It will advance and develop beyond a post-mortem pathology which is static. By radiocardiology we shall reach a more vital anatomy and physiology, and—earlier in disease—a dynamic pathology of the living heart."

References

1. Assman, H.: Die klinische Röentgendiagnostik der inneren Erkrankungen. 5th Ed., Berlin, 1934.
2. Babey, A.: Displacement of the esophagus by cardiac lesions other than mitral stenosis. Am. Heart Jour., 13: 228, 1937.
3. Beck, C. S., and Cushing, E. H.: Circulatory stasis of intrapericardial origin; the clinical and surgical aspects of the Pick syndrome. Jour. A.M.A., 102:1543, 1934.
4. Churchill, E. D.: Pericardial resection in chronic constrictive pericarditis. Ann. Surg., 104:516, (Oct.) 1936.
5. Hodges, F. J., and Eyster, J. A. E.: Estimation of transverse cardiac diameter in man. Arch. Int. Med., 37:707, 1926.
6. Kahlstorf, A.: Fortschr. a. d. Geb. d. Röntgenstrahlen, 45: 123, 1932.
7. Kirch, B.: Klin. Wchnschr., 9:769, 817, 1930.
8. Lewis, Thomas: Diseases of the Heart. The Macmillan Company, 1934.
9. Parkinson, J.: The radiology of heart disease. Brit. Med. Jour., 2:591, (Sept.) 1933.
10. Parkinson, J.: Enlargement of the heart. Lumleian Lectures, Lancet, 1:1391, (June) 1936.
11. Parkinson, J., and Bedford, D. E.: The aortic triangle. A radiological landmark in the left (or II) oblique position. Lancet, 2:909, 1936.
12. Parkinson, J., and Hoyle, C.: The heart of emphysema. Quart. Jour. Med., 6:59-86, (Jan.) 1937.
13. Rösler, H.: Clinical Roentgenology of the Cardiovascular System. Charles C. Thomas, 1937.
14. Rohrer, F.: Fortschr. a. d. Geb. d. Röntgenstrahlen, 24: 285, 1916-17.
15. White, P. D.: Chronic constrictive pericarditis (Pick's disease) treated by pericardial resection (St. Cyres Lecture). Lancet, 2:539, (Sept. 7) 1935; 597, (Sept. 14) 1935.

CONGENITAL SYPHILIS*
Analysis of the Problem in Minnesota

FRANCIS W. LYNCH, M.D.
Assistant Professor, University of Minnesota
Saint Paul, Minnesota

RECENT interest in the prevention and control of syphilis should be accompanied by increased attention to congenital syphilis, because it is a phase of the disease entirely controllable by prophylactic measures. Preventive therapy is almost uniformly successful after the early recognition of maternal syphilis by routine serologic studies of pregnant women. Since these preventive measures are not of recent development but have been recognized for twenty years, one may well inquire why additional cases of congenital syphilis are continually seen.

Although congenital syphilis is not a major public health problem in Minnesota it is interesting to note that over a ten-year period there is no appreciable change in the number of reported cases of this disease†

1927	125	1932	105
1928	67	1933	151
1929	103	1934	131
1930	163	1935	122
1931	134	1936	105
1927-1931—592		1932-1936—614	

The statistics for the two five-year periods are perhaps not comparable inasmuch as the profes-

---

*From the Division of Dermatology, University of Minnesota Medical School, Dr. H. E. Michelson, Director.

†Figures obtained by courtesy of Dr. O. McDaniel, Minnesota State Board of Health.

sion has been more alert in recognizing syphilis in recent years and much more prone to report new cases to the State Board of Health. It is possible that there has been an actual decrease in the incidence of congenital syphilis.

It was thought that analysis of the new cases recently observed at the University and Ancker Hospitals might disclose the reasons for the continued occurrence of congenital syphilis and point out a course to follow in future attempts to prevent this disease. During a period of two years a total of thirty-seven congenital syphilitics made their first visit to these two clinics. An additional fourteen patients were included in the study because they presented manifestations of active syphilitic infection during this period although the diagnosis had been made in previous years. In approximately one-third of the total cases, the physician or agency referring the patient to the clinic had already established the diagnosis.

	Univ. Ancker Hosp.	Total
Cases studied	26 25	51
New cases in two-year period....	21 16	37
Diagnosis known before admission	9 9	18 (35%)

Since the symptoms of congenital syphilis are well known the clinical investigation of this series was limited to a simple classification. The patients classed as suffering from early signs of congenital syphilis included examples of snuffles, rhagades, osteochondritis and cutaneous eruptions. It is unfortunate that in so many as twenty-two cases the disease was not recognized until the development of neurosyphilis or interstitial keratitis, conditions where treatment seldom returns the tissues to completely normal function.

	Univ. Ancker Hosp.	Total
Clinical manifestations		
Early	5 7	12 (24%)
Asymptomatic	12 5	17 (33%)
Interstitial keratitis	5 7	12 (24%)
Neurosyphilis	5 8	13 (26%)
(Three children had both keratitis and neurosyphilis)		

The relatively large number of children showing no clinical evidence of congenital syphilis is evidence of some progress toward lessening the damage resulting from this disease. Only a few of these children were referred to the clinic as a result of routine serologic studies. Most of them were members of families where the diagnosis of syphilis had been made on another in-

dividual a short time before. The entire family was then investigated and in the case of these children the disease was recognized before serious pathologic changes had taken place. It is unfortunate that a still larger number of cases could not have been recognized while the infection was still asymptomatic.

In the case of syphilis as with most other infections the chance for cure is much greater when the infection is recognized early. In an attempt to determine the amount of time lost before proper diagnosis, these patients were grouped according to their ages at the time of diagnosis. In nearly half the group the children were of school age before the disease was recognized.

	Univ. Ancker Hosp.	Total
Age at time of diagnosis		
Under 6 months..............	8 8	16 (32%)
6 months to 6 years...........	6 5	11 (22%)
6 years to 10 years...........	7 4	11 (22%)
Over 10 years.................	5 7	12 (24%)

Congenital syphilis presents a minor problem in Minnesota in comparison with many other communities, but in spite of the relatively favorable nature of the local situation thirty-seven new cases of this preventable disease have been observed at Ancker and University Hospitals within a two-year period. As it is unreasonable to expect complete eradication of congenital syphilis or any infectious disease, the question arises whether its incidence has reached an irreducible minimum in Minnesota. In the light of experience elsewhere, particularly in the Scandinavian countries, this question must be answered in the negative.

This state has been fortunate in the efforts of the State Board of Health in the control of syphilis and in the manner in which the public clinics have performed serologic tests on all pregnant women. The dermatologic and obstetric clinicians at the Medical School have taught for many years that every pregnant woman, whether in a clinic or under private care, should have a Wassermann test early in each pregnancy. The failure of many physicians to perform such tests is certainly not due to ignorance of their value but rather to discouragement after performing large numbers of such tests with only negative results. Nearly all physicians have known that intensive specific treatment is urgent after recognition of syphilis in pregnancy. Congenital syphilis is being observed in spite of this knowledge and must be regarded as a problem deserving further attention.

In the case of prevention of congenital syphilis, as in all medical advances, there has been a period of time, a lag, between the scientific discovery and its universal acceptance and application. To a certain extent such delay is inevitable, but every effort should be made to reduce it to a minimum. It was thought that study of the individual histories of these fifty cases of congenital syphilis might disclose information as to the cause of this "lag" and point out a course to follow in future efforts against the disease.

With reference to congenital syphilis the education of the medical profession has not been as successful as might be desired. It is evident that routine serologic study in pregnancy would result in almost entire prevention of the congenital infection but it is not clear in this group of cases how often the lack of this study was the fault of the attending physician. In one case, however, the presence of syphilis was demonstrated in the seventh month of pregnancy, yet the physician determined to "defer treatment until termination of the pregnancy" and a congenital syphilitic child was born. Another woman having neurosyphilis was admitted to a third hospital early in pregnancy. Although she was an inmate of this institution throughout her pregnancy, no specific therapy was given and a syphilitic child was born.

The physician has an added responsibility to avoid delay in diagnosis after the birth of the child. One infant suffered early from convulsions and at the same time presented a cutaneous eruption, yet the diagnosis was delayed until the child was seven months of age. A seven year old child gave a history of "sore eyes" since infancy but the cause was not recognized until after the development of neurosyphilis. A sixteen year old child had "always been sick" and the father was known to have syphilis but interstitial keratitis developed before the disease was recognized.

One woman had previously received inadequate treatment for syphilis yet no serologic study or antiluetic treatment was ordered during her pregnancy. Her child was sickly for the first few weeks and then failed to gain weight while the disease progressed until the child was admitted to the hospital at three months of age.

In this case treatment had been delayed too long and the child died a few days later.

These instances are all evidence of the need for further education of the profession in the available scientific knowledge. Another example of professional failure occurred in an institution which requires Wassermann studies on all women delivered. In this case, although the test was probably performed, no report was recorded, since the patient's laboratory sheet was misfiled. Several months later the child returned with congenital syphilis and the oversight was noted. An occasional error of this nature is probably to be expected though not to be excused.

A second reason for "lag" in the application of medical knowledge is the time required for education of the public. It is evident that continued effort is necessary to persuade women to report to their physicians in the first few months of pregnancy. If maternal syphilis is recognized this early, the proper treatment is almost always successful in preventing congenital syphilis. The present extensive publicity campaign against syphilis may overcome some of the objections of women to submitting themselves to routine Wassermann studies in private practice.

Every syphilitic woman when starting treatment should be told of the importance of regular therapy during pregnancy and should be made to realize the necessity of notifying her physician early in subsequent pregnancies. Her Wassermann test may then be negative due to previous treatment, yet further treatment is indicated for prevention of infection of the child although the mother herself might not otherwise require this treatment. In several instances in this series the mother knew of her infection yet received little or no treatment during pregnancy.

Since a certain element in the population will never accept responsibility in matters of health, whether individual, family or public, it is evident that education without control will not be sufficient. It is particularly in these cases that public health workers must be interested and active.

Recognition of this public responsibility leads to study of the third cause for "lag" in the attempts at control of congenital syphilis. In many cases in this series the available social service or public health facilities were inadequate. It is to the credit of these workers that many of the cases of congenital syphilis were brought to the clinics while the infection was asymptomatic or latent. Most of these asympto-matic patients represent brothers and sisters of previously recognized cases of congenital syphilis, or children of women in whom the disease was recognized long after pregnancy. The State Board of Control must also be credited with recognition of the disease before it was clinic-ally evident in four of these children who were submitted for examination as candidates for adoption.

The following cases from this series are cited as examples of failure of social workers or pub-lic health authorities. In one case of interstitial keratitis and another with neurosyphilis, the mothers had been under treatment for syphilis for one year before the children were brought to the clinic for examination. In another case there was a similar delay but the consequences were less serious as the child suffered only from iritis. In one case of interstitial keratitis, four years were allowed to elapse between recognition of the disease and institution of treatment. In the interim an extensive cutaneous gumma devel-oped. In the case of a very young infant, four months were lost after reference of the patient from the pediatric to the dermatology clinic be-fore he reported for treatment. One unfortu-nate youngster developed interstitial keratitis six weeks after admission to the clinic. He was awaiting the completion of arrangements for his treatment. A child referred from the Univer-sity Hospital to Ancker Hospital returned to the original clinic a year later without having re-ported at the Ancker Hospital. Neurosyphilis had been allowed to progress during this period of unnecessary delay.

The difficulty of placing on a single person or service the responsibility for the development and unrecognized progression of congenital syphilis is well indicated in the following his-tory. A woman first seen in the clinic in July, 1933, was treated for gonorrhea but no serologic tests for syphilis were performed. She returned to the obstetric clinic two years later, when rou-tine studies showed a positive Wassermann re-action but treatment was not instituted until seven weeks after her admission to a pre-natal clinic. The child was apparently normal at birth but was taken six weeks later to another hospital where clinical, serologic and roentgen studies

showed him to be syphilitic and he was referred back to the original clinic for treatment.

Summary

Though only thirty-seven new cases of con-genital syphilis have been observed in two years in the University and Ancker hospitals, it is evi-dent that many of these could have been pre-vented. The scientific background for such prophylaxis is well established.

In this study an attempt has been made to de-termine the reason for failure of these preven-tive measures and in many of these cases it has been possible to place the responsibility for this failure. The examples which have been cited serve to show that future attempts toward the control of congenital syphilis require greater in-terest on the part of the medical profession and the provision of more adequate social service and health department facilities. Education of the general public appears to be a minor factor in the prevention of congenital syphilis.

The following procedures are suggested as methods for the prevention of congenital syphilis and its serious effects on the child:

1. *Every woman with gonorrhea should have a Wassermann test in order to recognize early many cases of syphilis which are now passing unrecognized.*

2. *Every syphilitic woman should receive adequate treatment but should also be warned of the need to report to her physician early in any subsequent pregnancy and inform him of her syphilitic status.* (A woman who has once had syphilis usually requires treatment through-out each pregnancy. Patients whose disease is of more than eight years' duration and who have received "adequate" treatment previous to the pregnancy may be exceptions to this rule.)

3. *Every pregnant woman should have a Wassermann test early in pregnancy.*

4. *After the diagnosis of syphilis is made during pregnancy, treatment should be intensive.* (If it is started in the third or fourth month and at least ten arsenical and ten heavy metal injec-tions are given, a normal child may be expected. The dosage of the drugs and the division into courses are matters for individual arrangement.)

5. *At the time of delivery a Wassermann test should be performed on the maternal blood or the "cord" blood in every case.* (Collection of blood from the severed cord is a simple method

316

for determination of the serologic status of the mother only. Since the child's serologic identity is not established until several weeks after birth, a Wassermann test on cord blood does not prove the presence or absence of congenital syphilis. A positive Wassermann reaction on the cord blood, or the maternal blood, aids recognition of those cases in which syphilis has been acquired subsequent to the Wassermann tests performed earlier in pregnancy. Additional clinical, roent-genologic and serologic studies will establish the status of the child.)

If the medical profession were to follow these rules, even allowing for some lack of coöperation on the part of the patient, congenital syphilis could be practically eliminated in Minnesota. In the few cases where it might develop, the disease would be recognized and treated before irreparable damage was done.

PERSONAL SURGICAL OBSERVATIONS*

J. LAWRENCE McLEOD, M.D.

Grand Rapids, Minnesota

I WISH to present tonight a few observations on surgery in general as practiced by an average surgeon in a small hospital, and at the same time to report a few cases, each of which will, I hope, bring home some practical point.

It is my firm belief that those of us who practice in the smaller communities and institutions often give our patients closer individual service and attention and hence obtain better results than may be obtained in larger and better advertised surgical centers. In the larger centers the surgeon is likely to do less and less for the patient aside from the operation. Unless grave emergencies arise, the surgeon sometimes never sees the patient either before or after he meets him at the operating table, the operation often having been arranged for by the house staff alone. This is an additional wrong.

The closeness of personal contact between patient and surgeon so pleasant and profitable to both, which once prevailed even among busy surgeons in large centers has been largely disrupted, to the loss of both. The surgeon gains a little leisure and saves some wear and tear. The patient loses the solace and comfort he has a right to expect. *The two do not balance!!*

My personal opinon is that the operation itself is the least important to the patient's welfare, the preoperative and postoperative care far outweighing in benefit to the patient the actual technic.

*From the Itasca Clinic. Read before the Itasca Hospital Staff, Grand Rapids, Minnesota, September 2, 1937, and before the Range Medical Society, Virginia, Minnesota, October 19, 1937.

Preoperative Care

I shall dwell but a few moments upon this feature.

1. Patients who face any major surgical procedure are entitled to and should receive a full and careful physical check-up in the home or office before ever arriving at the hospital.

Any and every abnormality revealed or even suspected from the history or examination should be carefully checked into, and, if possible, remedied before the patient goes to the hospital.

I vividly recall a patient seen by two of us who suffered from recurrent attacks of angina pectoris. We had seen him in several attacks and had treated him and brought him out. The man was not satisfied and went away to a large Clinic. The Clinic got an indifferent history, gave the man a routine check, told him he had gallstones, and diagnosed his previous spells as gallstone colic. The man had his gallbladder removed (fortunately did not have an angina spell while in the hospital) and returned home only to have another angina spell in which he died. In my mind, the operation contributed to his untimely end. A thorough check-up with full history and coöperation between that Clinic and the home doctors would have been of considerable value.

2. The patient's chief resources on entering the operating room are his constitutional powers and his resistance, reinforced by cheery bravery; and all that can be done to increase these should be done. I have in mind two specific cases in which death postoperatively occurred partly, at least, because of lack of reserve.

One case was a woman who had been for some

time on a self-imposed restricted diet on which she lost twenty-five pounds from a normal weight of 160 pounds. She thought this would cure her gallbladder attacks and increase her beauty. Operation became imperative because of rapidly recurring attacks of colic and intractable vomiting, but the woman just faded out of the picture postoperatively because of lack of stamina.

A second patient, a strong, able-bodied and apparently robust young woman, was run down, however, from five pregnancies, the care of a large family and repeated gallbladder colic. Her examination revealed no really great physical handicap. After thirty-six hours in the hospital, during which time she rested well and was well checked, her gallbladder was removed. Thirty-six hours after the operation she developed a cardiac failure and died.

In both of these cases, a preliminary period of preparation with rest and general care might have spelled a different final result. It is unnecessary to go into great detail but there are a number of conditions such as anemia, jaundice, elevated blood pressure, obesity and alcoholism which require preliminary treatment prior to operative procedures.

3. Hospitalization for at least twenty-four hours prior to all major operations gives the patient a chance to become accustomed to new surroundings, nurses, attendants and hospital procedure. It further gives the sincere surgeon a chance to gain the patient's additional confidence and allay nervous misgivings. The preanesthetic preparation too can be performed in a more thorough and leisurely manner. This will all contribute to a better final result and it is our experience that a quiet day or two in the hospital before a major operation is *not* an additional expense because it will reduce the postoperative hospitalization a corresponding amount.

Let me say also that the old-time habit of giving laxatives preoperatively is a vicious practice. Unless the operation is for hemorrhoids or extensive perineal work, I can see no justification for causing the patient the fatigue of a day's diarrhea with its accompanying cramps, its tendency to produce gas pains and distress on succeeding days, and, above all, its dehydration, which is the very thing every surgeon should avoid. How utterly silly it is to give a purge which dehydrates and then intravenous fluid just

before or after operation to counteract dehydration. One has only to recall many appendectomies done without even a preliminary enema, which have resulted successfully, to understand the foolishness of this practice.

4. Every surgeon has his own pet theory about anesthetics and the preparation therefor. I shall not attempt to discuss any. Suffice it to say that once a regular routine has been tried and proven, it should be carried through in all cases and a surgeon in a small community has no right to attempt to make guinea pigs out of his patients with a lot of untried or half proven new drugs which some irresponsible agent tries to sell him.

So much for preoperative care.

Postoperative Complications and their Treatment

I quote:

"Many a well-fought surgical battle, won on the operating table, is needlessly lost in the convalescent room. The surgeon should personally attend to postoperative directions. There is too great a tendency to operate and get out—rather than operate and stay about.

"Many a cleverly performed operation has passed into death through faulty and inefficient after-treatment—while many a desperate and apparently hopeless operation has gone into brilliant recovery through after-treatment skill and efficiency. A patient may be put upon the road to recovery by operation—but unless he be wisely guided along that road, the operation may be unavailing. Even a bungled operation with a safe, speedy convalescence and satisfactory outcome, is more, far, to the patient than the cleverest operative technic followed by a long, painful, or hazardous, convalescence, and with an imperfect result.

"The surgeon's work and responsibility are only partly done when he has finished operating. Often much more judgment, and higher and broader surgical qualifications, are needed in the early recognition of conditions following operations, and in the after-guidance of those conditions to safety and full function, than was ever demanded in the mere operative technic. The surgeon who is an excellent operator but an indifferent postoperative fighter will probably lose more patients than the indifferent operator who is a hard and efficient postoperative fighter."[*]

The patient on return from the operating room and following recovery from the anesthetic should be allowed every possible freedom of position consistent with comfort. A pillow under the knees renders the abdomen less rigid and hence more comfortable. The postoperative nausea and vomiting are seldom prolonged and

_____
[*]Bickham, Warren S.: Operative Surgery, Philadelphia: W. B. Saunders Company, 1924. Volume I, page 289.

318

as a rule take care of themselves or the cause is apparent and the condition corrected by simple means. One very common postoperative error is wrapping the patient too warmly and causing excessive dehydration by sweating. Where possible, the patient should not be allowed to sweat excessively either on the operating table or after return to bed. What possible excuse can there be for proctoclysis, hypodermoclysis and intravenous therapy to restore the fluid balance if we at the same time permit dehydration by a hot pack of wool blankets and hot water bags?

I am happy to note also that, with the exception of operations on the stomach and duodenum, the patient is today allowed to have fluids practically *ad lib.* following operation. I feel that many cases of gas pains and general distress can be completely avoided if the patient is, encouraged to take nourishment in moderate amounts following almost all operations where the anesthetic has not caused unfavorable reaction.

Postoperative pain should be absolutely controlled for two or three days by large enough doses of an opiate to really do some good. Postoperative bleeding should always be investigated and the cause removed. Postoperative shock should not occur if the patient has been properly prepared and the operative procedure is within the physical strength of the patient. I believe no surgeon should plan to operate longer than two hours at any one stage. The patient just is not made to stand that prolonged shock to the nervous system under any type of anesthesia. If shock does occur, it must be combated with every device at the surgeon's command.

The major postoperative complications which I wish to discuss and illustrate with case reports are:

1. Pulmonary embolism.
2. Acute gastric dilatation (gastric paresis).
3. Obstruction.
4. Paresis and paralysis of the bowel.

Pulmonary Embolism.—This frightful specter rears its ugly head following surgical procedure every so often. There is no proven cause for it and no known prophylaxis or treatment. My single case is:

A woman, forty-six years of age, a hard-working farmer's wife, had for a good many years suffered from a large adenomatous goiter and recurrent gall-

bladder attacks. About three years before she had come to the hospital for cholecystectomy she had shown signs of marked hyperthyroidism. She refused treatment and allowed the toxins to do their damage for two years before she finally went to the University Hospital, where a successful thyroidectomy was done.

Her gallbladder symptoms had started to be more severe and frequent about the same time but we waited a year before suggesting gallbladder surgery. The gallbladder was readily removed and the patient convalesced satisfactorily although she was nervous and somewhat apprehensive. On the morning of the fourth day, the patient remarked to the nurse that she felt "better than she ever felt in her life." She requested a bed pan. The nurse got one, returned, helped her on the pan only to have the patient collapse and die in a few seconds.

Ingleby says of this condition:

"The patient who may be convalescing from an operation or apparently in good health suddenly becomes dyspneic and cyanosed. Death may be practically instantaneous. Survival is rarely as long as 10 minutes."

Inasmuch as we know of no prophylaxis and no treatment, the case is reported merely as one reason why a surgeon should always give a guarded prognosis and keep the back door open for a rapid run to cover in the face of such rare but always possible eventualities.

Postoperative Acute Gastric Dilatation.—This condition is also rare but its occurrence is frequent enough and serious enough to demand the most active measures for relief without which death usually occurs within twenty-four to forty-eight hours. It occurs in the second twenty-four hours following operation and it should be especially remembered that it may occur in connection with extra-abdominal as well as intra-abdominal operations. It has also been encountered in connection with various non-surgical conditions such as pneumonia and typhoid fever. Its cause is unfortunately not definitely known. but it appears that an atonic state of the stomach and overfilling of the organ with food or fluid play a part. Toxemia, an unusually long mesentery, duodenal obstruction and the like, have also been blamed.

A case in point was that of a young man of twenty-five years who, on August 4, 1937, at 5 a. m., left Nashwauk for the Twin Cities. On the way down, he became ill with considerable abdominal distress, nausea and protracted vomiting. In spite of his illness he completed his business in the Twin Cities and then drove home via Duluth and the trip home took fourteen hours, much of the time being spent vomiting by the roadside. He arrived home at 2 a. m. but did not see any physician till 4 p. m., August 5, when we admitted him to the hospital. He had a ruptured appendix. He was operated at once, the wound being closed with drainage.

The first twenty-four hours postoperative were very quiet and seemed normal. At 7 p. m., twenty-seven hours after the operation, he suddenly began to be distressed. His lips and fingernails became cyanotic, his pulse increased rapidly in rate and became irregular, his breath came in short apparently painful gasps. There was not much apparent distension but the epigastrium became markedly tympanitic. A rectal tube brought a little gas but no relief. He did not and could not vomit. He could not void. There was a small amount of purulent drainage from the wound. His lungs, because of heart failure, started to fill with mucus and secretions, and he had the so-called death rattle. His condition became alarming by 10:30 p. m. Many attempts to introduce the nasal suction tube were not successful. We then decided to try the large stomach tube. This failed to go down and so embarrassed the patient that he almost expired.

Because of our inability to get suction started in the orthodox manner, the patient was turned and placed in knee-chest position with several pillows under the hips, the face out over the edge of the bed. In this position, we got our tube down and got results. The patient showed considerable improvement. Nasal suction was continued for two days. Digitalis was given for the heart. Enemas and rectal tube produced results, proving that we had no intestinal paresis. Intravenous fluids were given repeatedly.

During the third postoperative day, the pulse fell rapidly and the boy proceeded to make an uneventful recovery.

Postoperative Obstruction.—I shall here consider only mechanical obstruction and consider paresis separately. Mechanical obstruction seldom occurs immediately after operation. Our cases have been seen months following operation.

One such case was that of a young man seen in June, 1933, with an appendix which had been ruptured several hours. He was very ill. Decision was made to operate and establish drainage. The appendix was not looked for but the drainage was established, the bowels mopped up and 300 c.c. of normal saline left in the abdomen. He had a stormy convalescence but left the hospital on the twelfth day.

Subsequently, he had several minor and one major spell with obstructive symptoms. The administration of mineral oils helped him, but on January 24, 1934, seven months after the operation, he came back to the hospital acutely ill, greatly distended, vomiting profusely and in great pain. Enemas and nasal suction were of no avail so an operation was performed. The ileocecal junction was found bound down tightly and the small bowel obstructed just where it emptied into the cecum. Adhesions in the entire area were dissected away and a search made for the appendix but none was

found. The lower end of the cecum seemed normal. The patient made a normal recovery and has had no trouble since.

In this case we know that the adhesions were the result of previous suppuration in the right lower quadrant. The resulting scar tissue finally closed off the small bowel. These postoperative obstructive cases ordinarily do well but it is important not to delay operation in the presence of an acute attack.

I believe that, where the patient's condition justifies it, it is good procedure to check for unnatural or unusual bowel adhesions at time of any operation in the lower right quadrant and to free such bands as may be found. Those patients who return after appendectomy and tell you that the operation did no good and in whom you can figure no definite pathology, are, I believe, cases in which the operation failed to release some of these obstructive bands.

Postoperative Paresis or Paralysis of the Bowel.—I turn now to consider this condition, which I regard as the most common serious postoperative abdominal complication. It occurs at times in individuals where there is neither excuse nor apparent cause for it. Simple abdominal surgery, with a minimum of handling of the bowel, may be followed by almost irreparable paresis, whereas a surgeon may check the viscera from one end to the other, perform an extensive operation and find the patient recovers without a gas pain.

The possible causes of accumulation of gas are: (1) excessive fermentation in bowel; (2) swallowed air; (3) arrested or modified intestinal peristalsis; (4) abdominal contraction; (5) relaxation of sphincters.

The distention from gas may become so great that a partial intestinal paresis may soon be converted into a total intestinal paralysis resulting in a distended inert tube. This may be further aggravated by mechanical obstruction occurring, in certain regions, through angulations due to its own overdistention.

No surgeon of any experience has failed to see this dreaded complication, and no surgeon who has seen it can fail to appreciate its serious possibilities. If there is any condition which calls for more patient, painstaking and prolonged effort on the part of the surgeon, I do not know what it is.

Until the last few years, the best weapon we

had to combat this complication was the colonic irrigation *properly carried out.* These last three words are important because the procedure requires anywhere from one-half to three hours, needs six to ten gallons of warm water and must be done patiently, gently, perseveringly, yet skillfully. The warm solution must play through the entire large gut persistently to help set up a normal peristalsis and often not till many gallons of water and much time has been consumed will the manipulator be rewarded by a gaseous return which spells success.

The above measure is as useful today as it ever was, but we now have a reliable ally in the Wangensteen nasal suction. When instituted early and run steadily over a period of many hours or days even, it can bring back normal function to a gut which otherwise would have remained completely paralyzed. I would recommend that both may well be used on any and every case which assumes serious proportions. The fact is that the surgeon might be better off if nasal suction was established as a routine procedure during the second and third day postoperatively in all extensive laparotomies. I confess that at present I am undecided whether forced feeding and plenty of agarmulsion will keep down gas formation and prevent distinion in a large percentage of cases or whether on the other hand the liquid diet may better be used along with nasal suction. In some cases, results have indicated that whichever method was used was not the best. At the present time, we are attempting to use the forced feeding agarmulsion plan in routine cases. However, when our best judgment gives reason to expect impending trouble because of the serious nature of a particular case we use the liquid diet and commence nasal suction early. Each procedure is of definite value in properly selected cases.

In extreme cases, the combined nasal suction and colonic irrigation cannot return peristaltic action to the distended and paralyzed bowel. If paralysis persists for some time, the last resource is an enterostomy. I wish to report such a case.

A man, aged forty-eight, was admitted to the hospital May 19, 1934, a few minutes after being first seen by me at my home. He had been ill three days. Pain had been severe on the first day, let up a while on the second, and then returned even worse on the third day. His abdomen was very distended and rigid, his temperature 102, pulse 100, respiration twenty-four. He was operated upon at once and a gangrenous ruptured appendix with abscess of the tip was removed and tubes

inserted without breaking down adhesions. The adjacent bowel was badly inflamed.

His recovery was stormy during the first six days. Enemas were very successful but little gas was obtained on nasal suction. Purulent drainage from the wound was considerable. The drainage tubes were removed on the seventh day and pus was pouring from the wound. Temperature and pulse had returned to normal. He began to become uncomfortable on the eighth postoperative day and on the ninth was much distended, vomited and his pulse rate was elevated. Nasal suction and enemas were both used with some success and both gave some relief. He was given two or more normal saline solutions with glucose intravenously each day to keep up his strength.

This routine was repeated for seven days and nights from the ninth to the sixteenth postoperative day without success. Then the abdomen was opened by a left rectus incision and a catheter was placed in a loop of the greatly distended jejunum.

We continued nasal suction and irrigations but now were able to drain out large amounts of liquid bowel content through the enterostomy opening. The battle continued until the twenty-first postoperative day, when fecal movement started per rectum, and on the twenty-second postoperative day suction was discontinued and the man took nourishment per os and held it. On the twenty-seventh postoperative day, we removed the enterostomy tube. Fecal drainage from the wound continued profusely, but on the thirty-fourth day, we strapped the wound with adhesive and the drainage lessened. He left the hospital on the forty-second day in good condition; the fecal fistula closed itself after he left the hospital. His recovery was rapid and he has had no abdominal trouble since.

This case is reported in order to demonstrate that no case should be regarded as too desperate. This man got to the cyanosis and death-rattle stage on different occasions. He was obviously about to die many times, but a dogged persistence for well over a month on the part of both surgeon and nurses was finally rewarded with success.

Let me repeat, therefore, that this type of abdominal complication is one which can today be handled successfully with the various mechanical measures at hand, but it requires the undivided attention of an interested and persistent surgeon who personally follows every symptom and treatment in detail.

Conclusions

I have attempted to bring out nothing spectacular or new, but merely to emphasize the importance of: (1) adequate preoperative examination and preparation; (2) postoperative vigilance, watching for symptoms of complications; (3) persistent treatment of all complications which may arise.

THE ETIOLOGY OF CHOREA*

CHARLES H. SCHRODER, M.D.

Duluth, Minnesota

SINCE we are to speak of Sydenham's chorea we should begin with Sydenham. His paper "On the Dance of St. Vitus" is really a very modest affair. Freely translated the opening paragraph would run about as follows:

"This is really a sort of convulsion. It affects boys and girls from the tenth year to puberty. It manifests itself with a lameness or weakness of one or the other leg so that the weaker member drags itself along behind in a semi-paralyzed manner. The hand of that side if applied to the breast or some other part is unable to remain in that same position even for a moment but is twisted around to another position by a convulsive movement—whichever way the weaker member is drawn. Before the cup can be placed to the mouth he exhibits a thousand gestures, circular in type; for he cannot move in a straight line to his mouth but his hand is turned aside by spasm and he twists it hither and yon until, at length, by mere chance placing the drink properly to his lips, he throws it suddenly into his mouth and eagerly drinks it,—accomplishing the act in such a way that all onlookers are moved to laughter."

The rest of the article is interesting, but I shall forego transcribing it. It is concerned mostly with therapy. Nowhere is there any suggestion of etiology unless we consider such, the reference to the age of the patients.

From the time of Bright, however, the close association of chorea with rheumatism was taken for granted. It is so taken today. Nevertheless Osler, in his masterly monograph on this subject, while not exactly challenging the assumption, showed that the connection was often difficult to demonstrate, stating that only 21 per cent in his series showed a close association. He did state, however, that there is no known disease which, at autopsy, shows such a large percentage of cardiac defects. Since that time there has been much discussion as to the relation of rheumatism and chorea.

Steiner stated that he could find only four cases of articular rheumatism in 252 cases of chorea. Coburn and Moore note that chorea frequently occurs without clinical or laboratory signs of rheumatic activity and that many patients develop no rheumatic stigmata even after repeated attacks of chorea. They state that the cases of so-called "pure chorea" will run from 30 to 50 per cent. Other writers express similar views.

Then, in 1935, J. R. Gerstley wrote a challenging paper in which he concluded that chorea should be looked upon not as a disease but as a syndrome developing in a child predisposed by heredity and constitution, after psychic exhaustion or infection. He draws attention to the importance of wretched home conditions, domestic crises and inadequate diets. He thinks that there is a distinct chorea temperament to be noted in certain intelligent, over-stimulated and markedly introverted children. He noted again the evident relation of the disease to puberty and suggests that the endocrine glands must be closely concerned. "Rheumatism is a concomitant, not a cause."

This is a pregnant sentence. Nevertheless, we shall ignore its implications for the present and ask ourselves what percentage of cases with chorea ultimately present clinical evidence of chronic valvular heart disease.

Pfaundler and Schlossman answer that ultimately one-half of all choreic cases will present such evidence. Abt says that 32 per cent of his cases showed "cardiac complications." Jones and Bland in their scholarly analysis of 482 cases of chorea state that with observation extending over an eight year period 54 per cent showed rheumatic heart disease. When rheumatism alone was present this percentage of endocarditis rose to 86 per cent and they make this striking statement: "Rheumatic heart disease is less likely to occur when chorea is part of the syndrome."

Of course, in the relatively few cases coming to autopsy, marked cardiac changes are uniformly found. I quoted Osler's striking statement in this connection. Fagge found cardiac disease in seventeen out of eighteen autopsies.

Now, practically all recent writers admit that there are cases of what we shall call "pure chorea." Jones and Bland place the percentage at 28 and say that in these cases, even over an eight year period, no frank evidence of rheumatic

*Read before St. Mary's Hospital Staff, Duluth, Minnesota, November 4, 1937.

ever could be found. However, Schwartz and eader studied carefully seventy-five cases of ure chorea and observed them from one to welve years. They state decisively that after even or eight years one hundred per cent eemed to show cardiac involvement. They ask: s it true of chorea, as of rheumatism, that the eart is always involved?

Of course, we are hampered by the fact that the etiological agent of rheumatism is still "sub judice." Only a few years ago Wilson made the statement that apparently identical organisms may be recovered from healthy children as well as from patients with rheumatism and related infections. It is also true that blood culture from typical clinical cases of rheumatism frequently may remain sterile. So we can hardly look to bacteriology to solve our problem.

As Swift has well pointed out, rheumatism, like tuberculosis, does not come on as a typical acute infection but often has a long latent period. Gerstley's remark then that chorea does not act like an acute infection would certainly not disprove its rheumatic origin.

As can readily be demonstrated, pathology, too, cannot solve the question. The Aschoff body, it is true, is pathognomonic of rheumatism as is the tubercle in tuberculosis and the gumma in syphilis. This peri-arteriolar inflammatory nodule has indeed been demonstrated by Poynton and Holmes and others, in the brains of patients dying with chorea, along with areas of encephalitis or with meningitis. The verruca on the valve is also indisputable as to origin. But over the cases that come to autopsy there is no dispute. If the patient with chorea dies he dies of rheumatism or its complications. The question still remains whether he can have chorea without rheumatism.

Now, we wish to put together a number of observations. Hassler and Moller show that heart disease not preceded by arthritis is more fatal than when so accompanied. It is likewise true that the gravest complications on the part of the heart occur in rheumatism that is not linked up with chorea. Likewise, the subcutaneous nodule, of bad omen, is much more common when chorea is out of the picture.

This can only mean that a higher degree of immunity or shall we say of allergy, using the word to define a reaction that restricts the virus to a narrow field, exists in some cases than in others.

It makes one wonder whether the allergic phenomenon in the brain itself is not the true cause of the chorea. Edema of the tissues is a marked feature in rheumatism. This edema is fairly well controlled by the salicylates and hence their clinical value, despite their lack of influence on the underlying pathology. If there was any evidence that one part of the brain more than another was affected in chorea, it would not be far fetched to conceive of a local tissue response here, similar to the reaction we picture in the joints or heart wall.

Heubner states that the peculiar character of the choreic movement cannot be referred to the motor centers or tracts (anterior central convolution and pyramidal tracts). The intended movement in chorea is exaggerated. Flexion, extension, rotation, supination are all irregular in time, character and degree. Cobb has shown in electro-myographic studies that one characteristic thing is the inability to sustain effort. Both voluntary and involuntary contractions are weakened. This may be confined to one side—the so-called hemi-chorea. Now it has been demonstrated that a lesion of the corpus luysii (subthalamic body) may produce a hemi-chorea and, as stated dogmatically by Martin and Alcock, "there is very little evidence that focal damage to any structure in the brain other than the corpus luysii or its emergent fibres results in hemichorea." This, of course, is organic, persistent chorea. We might mention in passing that the body of Luys lies in the mid-brain just below the optic thalamus and just internal to the fibres of the pyramidal tract as they pass down from the internal capsule to the cerebral peduncle. To the medial side is the nucleus ruber. Below is the substantia nigra. The corpus receives its main body of fibres from the lenticular nucleus of the corpus striatum.

That the lenticular nucleus and the corpus of Luys may be of prime interest in connection with choreic symptoms is evident from the beautiful work of S. A. K. Wilson on the anatomy and physiology of the corpus striatum and on the rare disease known as chronic lenticular degeneration.

These papers are much too elaborate to quote extensively. Suffice it to say here that he demonstrates that the nucleus lentiformis is practically independent of the cortex. It connects with the subthalamic body and nucleus ruber to form the so-called lenticulo-rubro-spinal tract. The function of this tract is to exert a steadying influence on the final common path (lower motor neuron) and to maintain the tone of skeletal muscle. In other words it has an inhibiting effect upon the cortico spinal or pyramidal tract and when this regulating function is in abeyance then appear involuntary movements, incoördinated movements and such symptoms as tremor and athetosis. The intended movement is exaggerated and incoördinate in time and degree, due to spasm and the attempt to anticipate spasm. And this is chorea.

In the disease known as chronic lenticular degeneration we have a toxic or infective factor acting selectively upon a basal nucleus. It is associated with marked liver pathology and certainly suggests the similar selective action that takes place in icterus gravis—the so-called "kern-icterus." In the disease first mentioned, classically described by Wilson, we have a selective action limited to the lenticular nucleus and corpus of Luys, and a wide train of symptoms embracing tremor, spasticity, dysarthria, dysphagia, paresis, et cetera.

It would seem to be reasonable to assume that the rheumatic virus also might exercise a selective action upon these nuclei and thus bring about this train of nervous symptoms that we have come to recognize as chorea. And if it be remembered that chorea occurs in those individuals presenting a high degree of resistance or allergic response, we might expect that localized edema would play a large part in the actual pathology. This might explain the rather dramatic response to certain lines of therapy, such as the injection of autogenous serum into the spinal canal or the induction of hyperpyrexia by diathermy or other means, or to such drugs as seem to have the power to induce a "reaction" accompanied by eosinophilia (sodium iodide, arsenic, nirvanol, foreign protein, et cetera).

This, of course, is mostly speculative and does not appear to include those cases unassociated with discernible infection—the cases of "pure chorea." It is possible of course that this is a misnomer and that the infection is there, although not clinically discoverable. It is really beside the point to refer to the sedimentation test as a distinguishing aid, because, admittedly, chorea only occurs in cases of low virulence. Possibly the test, after provocative therapy,

might prove of value. Nevertheless, unless all clinical observation is to be discredited, chorea does occur on a non-infectious basis and we have to face the question as to how this can be. What sort of mechanism is at work here?

Now, first of all is it possible that chorea can be caused on a purely psychic basis? What is the meaning of the seeming importance of the family's social set-up in Gerstley's experience?

Malamud calls attention to the fact that both the extra-pyramidal tract and the autonomic nervous system exert a marked influence on motor function. Also is it true that the vegetative nervous system is closely associated with the psyche? We have to reckon with the shadowy subject of conditioned reflexes and with the fact that abnormal motions may replace inhibited instinctive expression.

It is certainly possible to comprehend the possibility that under the influence of tremendous fright or excitement, with rapid breakdown of glycogen in the hepatic cells and production of excess of epinephrine, there might be augmentation of all nervous reactions and old pathways of conditioned reflexes and imitation arcs might be reopened. But could the expression in chorea-like movement be so close to chorea on an infectious basis as to defy differentiation? One is brought face to face with the fact here that Beattie and his confreres have been able to show that stimulation of certain hypothalamic centers can cause a widespread flow of impulses over the sympathetic system. The inference is plain, therefore, that these centers can and do act as a central depot for sympathetic reception. Thus a patho-physiological disturbance conceivably could be induced, by a different mechanism, in those very centers that would be concerned in a purely infectious process. In this connection we should mention that Obelli and others have shown that there is sympathetic innervation in skeletal muscle and a purely peripheral irritation might explain the mild twitchings often designated as "pre-choreic."

But what is back of this? Practically speaking, chorea may be said to be a pre-puberty disease. In other words the glandular activity and increased endocrine output of puberty changes the background in some way so that the choreic phenomenon ceases. The true explanation of this fact would go a long way to clarify our problem. One can hardly proceed further than

324

to restate the close connection between the endocrines and the normal functioning of the autonomic nervous system.

But perhaps we can proceed a step further. Widenbauer has brought forth some convincing evidence that the missing link in this whole discussion is the Vitamin B complex. On the basis of some very interesting case histories closely studied clinically and in the laboratory, he concludes that the "chorea constitution" (Gerstley also speaks of a typical chorea type) depends upon a long deprivation of Vitamin B. The neuropathic child and the young gravid woman are in similar stages of deprivation. The B complex is preeminently concerned in muscle, nerve and joint nutrition. Rheumatism and the various affections associated with chorea flourish when the supply is low. The very incidence of chorea, with a new year maximum and summer-fall minimum suggests the relationship. The complications of furunculosis and other staphylococcic skin lesions provide further evidence. He also points out the calcium deficit in chorea and the relationship of tetany and parathyroid deficiency with B avitaminosis.

Recalling that prominent symptoms of beri-beri are circulatory—to wit, enlargement of the heart, arrhythmia, exaggerated action, systolic murmur—this would seem to furnish an interesting parallel to those "mobile" heart symptoms that Trousseau called the distinguishing mark of rheumatism. That there is also a close parallelism of action between vitamin and hormone has often been suggested.

Nevertheless, this is not to get away from the whole question of infection. Beri-beri itself is more than an avitaminosis. The element of microbial action is by no means excluded. Matsumara and his colleagues claim that the principal etiologic element is a Gram-negative motile bacillus. However this may be, it does not seem possible in the present state of knowledge to make the dogmatic statement that chorea is dependent on an infectious process, or, on the other hand, that it is not related to infection.

The writer is not defending either view. His purpose is to arrange and digest the evidence.

MEDICAL BOOKS FOR THE LAITY

THOMAS E. KEYS, A.B., M.A.*
Rochester, Minnesota

M ANY people are reading and will read on medical subjects. The important immediate concern is that this material be authentic, well written, and on a subject of medical importance. Certainly the publishing field bears witness to the popular demand for medical knowledge. A glance at the Index Catalogue of the Library of the Surgeon-General's office (the largest medical library in the world) shows that members of the staff of the library have cataloged at least 1,500 manuals of popular medicine, 400 more extensive books on the subject and more than 140 popular medical journals. Most of the journals are extinct. Even syphilis, which until recently was whispered about over the radio as "the social disease," has been given wide publicity to help in its prevention and ultimate cure. Recent authoritative treatises published in 1937 on this subject have included: S. W. Becker's "Ten Million Americans Have It" (Lippincott), Morris Fish-

*Reference librarian, The Mayo Clinic, Rochester, Minnesota.

bein's "Syphilis, The Next Great Plague to Go" (McKay) and Thomas Parran's "Shadow on the land, Syphilis" (Reynal and Hitchcock).

An important medium for information on popular medicine and hygiene are the health journals. Such is *Hygeia*, the authority and reputation of which is above reproach.

The American Medical Association and the National Health Council also publish pamphlets on many subjects in the field of health and preventive medicine. The Department of Health and the Department of Labor of the United States contribute similarly to popular education on problems connected with good health. These pamphlets are published at cost and are available to all persons.

In establishing a basis for the selection of popular medical books the following criteria were used: (1) that they be written in words understandable to the average layman with a simple vocabulary and in well written, pleasing style; (2) that they be written on good authority on a subject of importance; (3) that they be published by a reputable house, and (4) that they do not attempt "cure-alls" or try to take the physician's place. The cure of disease we trust to our physicians and the progress of medical science bears witness that the ills of mankind are placed in safe hands.

For the rural communities there have always existed a few "family physicians" and home doctor books. One of the uses of these books, in days of poor transportation, was to suggest what to do before the doctor arrived. Today, they are worth while in cases of emergency. A recent book published on good authority is Dr. Morris Fishbein's "Modern Home Medical Advisor" (Doubleday, 1935). A book of the same type published primarily for social workers is Dr. R. C. Cabot's "Layman's Handbook of Medicine" (Houghton, 1937).

An interesting approach to the lay study of medicine lies in what may be termed "get acquainted books." These include books on medical history and biography. One of the most inspiriting books I have read is Gustav Eckstein's "Noguchi" (Harper, 1931). It not only introduces the reader to a remarkable personality but is a story of the fight against infectious diseases told in such a way that it is profitable to the laity. Hans Zinsser has written in a vivid manner the story of typhus fever in his "Rats, Lice, and History" (McClelland, 1935).

One cannot go very far in getting acquainted with medicine before coming into contact with the works of Sir William Osler. His essays, "Aequanimitas, with Other Addresses to Medical Students, Nurses and Practitioners of Medicine" (Blakistons, 1920, ed. 2) inspire in the reader great respect for the medical sciences. This is a type of book that will appeal especially to a first year medical student. Similarly, the excerpts from his writings in "Counsels and Ideals" (Houghton, 1921, ed. 2) make good reading. Perhaps the best written history of medicine from the standpoint of the laity is Osler's "The Evolution of Modern Medicine" (Yale, 1921). To become acquainted with the man one should read his life, "The Great Physician" (Oxford, 1934) by Edith Giltings Reid. A more scholarly biography is H. W. Cushing's "The Life of Sir William Osler" (Clarendon Press, 1925, 2 v.).

Other important medical biographies or autobiographies include Vallery-Radot's "Life of

Pasteur" (star edition), R. M. Wilson's "The Beloved Physician, Sir James MacKenzie" (Macmillan, 1926), Nathan C. Goodman's "Benjamin Rush" (University of Pennsylvania Press, 1934), Victor Heiser's "An American Doctor's Odyssey" (Norton, 1936).

In the field of medical history mention might also be made of Victor Robinson's "History of Medicine" (Froben reprint), H. W. Haggard's "The Lame, the Halt and the Blind" (Blue Ribbon, reprint, 1935) and Morris Fishbein's "Frontiers of Medicine" (Williams and Wilkins, 1933).

There is need for an authoritative popular book on human anatomy. Barnes and Noble have published an "Atlas of Human Anatomy" (1935) with colored illustrations by Franz Frohse and Max Brödel. This is good, but a more extensive book is needed.

In the field of physiology, the functional study of the human body, an excellent book is Dr. Logan Clendening's "The Human Body" (Knopf, ed. 3, 1937). Dr. Clendening included in his book, also, the body as it is related to disease and the development of medical science in the combat of disease. A recent book which promises to be of interest is A. J. Carlson's and Victor Johnson's "Machinery of the Body" (University of Chicago, 1937).

A large percentage of the patients who are being seen by physicians today are suffering from functional neuroses and chronic nervous exhaustion in general. Some of these patients, no doubt, have received from books not written for the laity information from which they have drawn faulty conclusions and they may have imagined their many ills. For the nervous patient himself, however, Dr. W. C. Alvarez has written his monograph, "Nervous Indigestion" (Hoeber, 1931). It makes enjoyable and profitable reading. Two books that deal with normal psychology are H. A. Overstreet's "About Ourselves" (Norton, 1927) and G. H. Dorsey's "Why We Behave Like Human Beings" (Blue Ribbon, reprint, 1930). Justification for neurotic personalities is expressed in L. E. Bisch's "Be Glad You're Neurotic" (McGraw-Hill, 1936). The history of insanity in America is well written in Albert Deutsch's "The Mentally Ill in America" (Doubleday-Doran, 1937). Books that share personal experiences in hospitals for the insane with the reader are the following: C. W. Beers' "A Mind that Found Itself" (Doubleday-Doran, reprint, 1932), M. M. Woodson's "Behind the Door of Delusion" (Macmillan, 1932) and W. B. Seabrook's "Asylum" (Harcourt, 1937). "Why Men Fail" (Century, 1928, edited by Morris Fishbein and W. A. White) is an analysis of the causes of failure, written for the average man or woman by the leading psychiatrists in the country. It also tells how failure may be turned into success.

An important bibliography on health books for the laity is that of Dr. Fishbein. This is published under the auspices of the American Library Association. A more up-to-date list may later be published by the Medical Library Association and also by the National Health Council. It is in this field that the intelligent layman must be directed if a national health program is to be realized.

It is through the efforts of both the laity and the medical profession that measures for preventive medicine and hygiene will be further adopted on a large scale. Authoritative books written for mature minds on this subject include the volume by W. E. Burkard and others: "Health and Human Welfare" (Ryerson Press, 1937), C. F. and N. W. Bolduan's "Public Health and Hygiene" (ed. 2, Saunders, 1936), and C. E. Turner's "Personal and Community Health" (ed. 4, Mosby, 1935).

While public hygiene deals with mass phenomena it is quite inseparable from personal hygiene. And it is important that the individual be schooled in how he can preserve his health and thus play his part in preventive medicine. C. W. Crampton's "The Boy's Book of Strength" (Mc-Graw-Hill, 1936) is written especially for the adolescent interested in athletics and is an outstanding book. Logan Clendening's "Health Chats" (McKay, 1936); W. W. Bauer's "Health Questions Answered" (Bobbs, 1937); C. E. Turner's "Personal Hygiene" (Mosby, 1937); and L. E. Hawkin's "Health in Youth and Age" (Hillman-Curl, 1937) are among the newer

books on this subject. M. J. Exner's "The Sexual Side of Marriage" (Norton, 1932) is a plain, frank, and practical book, and not poetically allusive like so many that have been written. The American Red Cross textbook on "First Aid" (revised edition, Blakiston's, 1937) is an excellent manual. It should be available in all homes in case of accident.

Books on diet should, I think, be recommended only on the advice of the physician. This should hold true for handbooks for patients suffering from such diseases as diabetes. In such diseases particularly, recovery depends on the intelligent coöperation of the patient. For patients suffering from arthritis, H. N. Margolis has written "Conquering Arthritis" (Macmillan, 1932).

To show up the quack and to help the laity to be on their guard against nostrums the American Medical Association has published "Nostrums and Quackery" (in three volumes, 1912-1936, volumes two and three edited by Arthur Cramp). Morris Fishbein has written "The Medical Follies" (Boni and Liveright, 1925) and "Fads and Quackery in Healing" (Blue Ribbon, 1935). An exposé of the drug racket is found in A. Rallet and F. J. Schlink's "One Hundred Million Guinea Pigs" (Vanguard Press, 1933). Of special interest to women is Mary Catherine Phillips' "Skin Deep; the Truth about Beauty Aids—Safe and Harmful" (Vanguard Press, 1934).

In conclusion, I might add that many books have not been included in this résumé. Some books have not met the requirements set up in the rules of selection, and of some books I have not had knowledge. If, however, I have suggested a few good books which may encourage others to read on a subject of vital importance and if I have shared with some of you my experiences in this field I shall have accomplished my aim.

LIVER EXTRACT IN GENERAL THERAPY

Case Report

J. J. HEIMARK, M.A., M.D.

Fairmont, Minnesota

FROM the time of my first impression of the efficacy of liver therapy in pernicious anemia, I have felt that it should be given a trial in other forms of debilitating diseases which were slow in recovery. Hence, during the several years in which liver has been on the market, I have used liver and liver extract in such cases. In using it on post-influenza cases routinely, I have felt that the therapy has shortened the period of exhaustion and general debility with which the patient has invariably contended for weeks and even months. Clinically, the same has held true for patients convalescing from pneumonia and empyema. I have also resorted to the use of liver extract in the treatment of those late winter and early spring patients from whom nothing tangible could be obtained except the histories of depletion and exhaustion so frequently attendant on long confining winters aggravated by minor ailments. It needed but trial to prove that liver extract had a decided restorative effect upon these patients far superior to that of other tonics and drugs.

It is an interesting thing to find that occasionally a case of essential hypertension will respond to liver. Again, others show no appreciable change. Since combining Rhodan with liver therapy in these cases, I have had more encouraging results than with any other form of treatment.

In piloting expectant mothers through to term with the usual pre-natal care I have found upon several occasions albumin in the urine and an increase in blood pressure towards the end of their pregnancies. After receiving 2 c.c. of liver extract two to three times a week for a couple of weeks, such patients have improved, their blood pressure has been lowered and the urine became albumin-free. I have considered these cases toxic types.

Recently I employed liver extract in the treatment of a patient with acute nephritis. Although to my knowledge it has not been recommended in the treatment of this disease, I am reporting the following cases with the suggestion that its use might merit further trial.

Case 1.—Mrs. J. H., aged thirty-nine, married and the mother of one child, consulted me February 23, 1936. She complained of headache, loss of appetite, swelling of the face, hands and legs. She had observed she was passing a decidedly small amount of urine during the day, and she stated that she had been getting progressively worse since she first noticed the onset of the trouble some one week previously. The scanty specimen of urine passed for examination revealed albumin 4 plus, casts and blood cells and cellular debris. The blood pressure was 178/118. There was marked edema of the entire body, especially of the extremities. I advised hospitalization, and upon refusal instructed that she be given complete bed rest and kept warm. Food was restricted to three glasses of skimmed milk or the same amount of home-made buttermilk per day—a Karell diet. Epsom salts were to be taken as needed. Before she left the office I gave her 2 c.c. of liver extract intramuscularly, and advised her to return in five days. On February 29, when she reported to the office

I gave her the second injection of 2 c.c. of liver extract. The urine showed no improvement, but she stated that she had been passing more urine, that the headache was leaving her, and that she felt better generally. On March 7, she received her third 2 c.c. of liver extract. The urine showed a definite decrease of albumin. The edema was practically gone. She stated she was feeling greatly improved, and the headache had left her. On March 15, the fourth 2 c.c. of liver extract was given. The albumin was one plus and the edema was gone. She stated she felt so well at this time that she hoped she would not have to report at the office for further treatment. On March 24 she was given her fifth and final injection of 2 c.c. of liver extract. The urine was negative for albumin. She stated she felt "just fine," and she looked well.

I did not see this patient again until April 15, 1936. The urine then was normal. The blood pressure was normal. She looked as well as at any time in the period that I had known her, and she stated that she had not felt so well for several years. I have seen her occasionally since that time, and she has remained well. On March 6, 1937, I examined the urine again and it was normal. The last time, January 26, 1938, the urine again was normal.

Case 2.—The use of liver extract in a case of orthostatic albuminuria was followed by the disappearance of the albumin. A boy of seventeen was seen in July, 1936. The diagnosis of orthostatic albuminuria had been made two years previously and he had been told that the condition was of no significance and that he would outgrow it as time went by. He had learned to test his urine and was able to demonstrate albumin most of the time. It appeared to be more abundant when he was tired or following strenuous exertion. The boy had become introspective and apprehensive about his condition.

The boy was a well built young man with splendid physique, and the picture of health. The urine contained albumin plus two, on a basis of four. He was given empirically 2 c.c. of liver extract intramuscularly at five-day intervals for five doses. Following the first liver extract injection, the albumin disappeared from the urine and has not recurred.

Case 3.—In another case of a boy of fourteen the injection of liver extract seemed to be of benefit. The boy's father told me that the boy had not complained of anything in particular but that he had observed throughout the summer a lack of energy and a marked diminution in his ability for sustained work. His appetite was poor, his skin pasty and pale, and he had gained no weight during the summer.

Physical examination was essentially negative, except that the boy did not look well. His tonsils were greatly enlarged but only moderately inflamed. The urine showed a strong plus albumin. Following two injections of 2 c.c. of liver extract at five-day intervals the albumin disappeared, and following tonsillectomy the urine remained albumin-free.

After having experimented with liver and liver extract in general disease, I have come to the conclusion that the clinical results have been so intriguing that I was finally prompted to make this report. It would, indeed, be interesting to follow this work under a purely scientific setting so that a more complete report could be made. I firmly believe that the full measure of the possibilities of liver extract in the treatment of disease other than pernicious anemia has not yet been taken.

328

◆ HISTORY OF MEDICINE IN MINNESOTA ◆

SURVEY OF PIONEER MEMBERS OF THE ST. LOUIS COUNTY MEDICAL SOCIETY

By RICHARD BARDON, M.D.

(Continued from April issue)

The Establishment of St. Luke's Hospital

The following article, written in 1921, was taken from the records of the hospital:

"In an old shack located on Third Ave. East, between Superior St. and the alley, St. Luke's Hospital opened for business. First steps for the organization of a hospital for Duluth were taken on October 18, 1882. One month later, the doors of the makeshift institution opened and members of the first board were hustling about to collect the $25, a month due for the structure. The town people being at that time more full of enthusiasm than cash, the first month's rent devolved upon the chairman of the board, Col. Charles H. Graves, and at the end of the first month's financial statement this contribution and a lone five dollar bill were all that glorified the treasury. For furnishings, the British Consul loaned the use of a range from the Government building, two beds had been begged from worthy citizens, as had one table, a few chairs and a blank book in which to register the rush of incoming patients. Mrs. Jessie Guion, an efficient matron, was engaged at $50 a month.

"At four o'clock on the afternoon of Nov. 18, a man on the Northern Pacific railroad broke his leg and by five o'clock the establishment of the hospital had been justified and has been ever since. This patient kept the hospital 'staff' busy for two months but added not a cent to the treasury until he was able to get back to work. A typhoid fever case caused temporary relief and excitement by paying $14 in advance only to have it efficiently counterbalanced by his remaining and requiring ten weeks care. One of the younger physicians, who had a very sick patient not long after, had him removed to the hospital, figuring that the man's death being only a matter of hours, an autopsy could be more conveniently performed with new equipment at hand. His plans went awry the following morning when he found his patient had recovered over night.

"It was a time of discouragement and stress to all concerned—a time when the water supply depended upon the strongest muscle and the largest pail; when the primitive means of sewage disposal and menace of typhoid necessitated most careful watching. Only the miraculous grit and determination of the board members carried this child of their brain to a sturdy maturity, though it was not long before 3,500 inhabitants of Duluth awoke to the needs the hospital was meeting and more and more opened their hearts and purses. Within two years the next step to a permanent building had been instituted and St. Luke's began climbing upward, this time to Second Avenue East and Fourth Street, where property had been purchased and a substantial building erected with a small indebtedness, some $1,700 being all that was assumed at that time.

"Rev. C. A. Cummings, the rector of St. Paul's Episcopal Church, was then the leading spirit in the organization of St. Luke's Hospital. He was aided by a board consisting of Col. Graves, G. V. I. Brown, Thomas B. Cullyford and Mrs. Ella B. Stone. The physicians of the town included Drs. Ritchie, Graff, Walbank, E. E. Collins, S. C. McCormick, C. F. McComb, George Davis and F. C. Sherwin.

"Upon the removal of the hospital to the new quarters on Second Avenue East, Mrs. Guion remained but a short time, to be followed by Miss Mary Scott as superintendent. The years following witnessed typhoid epidemics enough to try the staunchest heart and the new hospital was taxed far beyond its capacity and beyond the facilities it possessed to care for these patients.

"St. Luke's was also filling the rôle of a welfare institution, for at that time the Y.W.s and Y.M.s were not organized as they are now. The hospital seemed to be the center about which all charity and welfare work revolved and it was aided in many of these directions by the big-hearted men and women of the growing town who spent time, strength and energy to keep alive the sparks of helpfulness and assistance for those who blindly turned to this institution for help of all sorts. One father, mother and two children drove in forty miles to ask aid in locating an adventurous son who had set out unannounced to see the world. The hospital housed the parents and children for a week, while the means at hand were set in motion to find the young Columbus. Thanksgiving Day, 1884, according to the *Duluth Herald* of that date, found nineteen patients in the hospital enjoying a bounteous turkey dinner furnished by Thomas Cullyford, at that time proprietor of the St. Louis hotel. The account also notes but 'one female' amongst the patients, which at least was worthy of special mention.

"This hospital had one ward with fifteen beds, one private room, a sitting room on the second floor for the use of all patients and a small dispensary, used also for surgical emergencies. It was not many years before the limitations of the building were apparent and the present property at the corner of Ninth Avenue East and First Street was purchased. In 1900, the foundation was laid and on October 1, 1902, the present St. Luke's was opened, with a nominal capacity of seventy beds. The building cost in the neighborhood of $100,000, and at that time was considered one of the best equipped in this part of the country."

A later addition, greatly enlarging the hospital capacity, was opened in 1925.

St. Mary's Hospital

The following data concerning the organization of St. Mary's Hospital appeared in 1933, on the occasion of the forty-fifth anniversary of its foundation:

"In February, 1888, when Duluth was a pioneer city of a few thousand inhabitants, a small band of Sisters of St. Benedict—members of a religious community founded by St. Benedict for the purpose of caring for the sick and infirm —opened the City's second hospital in a small building at Twentieth avenue west and Third street." (Now St. Ann's Home.)

"Of that band, the last survivor, Sister Helen, died five years ago, but through the years younger members of the order took up the work and carried on under the direction of Mother Scholastica, the first president of the old St. Mary's Hospital Association.

"The first staff was composed of Mother Alexia Kerst and six other Sisters. The late Dr. W. H. Magie, one of the first members of the hospital staff, performed the first appendicitis operation at the hospital in 1891, and the first gastro-enterostomy operation in 1895.

"In those days, records still kept by the hospital disclose, patients came from miles around by carriage and sleigh. They were transported from floor to floor in a hand-operated pulley elevator, and their rooms and the wards were lighted by gas.

"In 1896, eight years after the first hospital was opened, the need for a larger building to accommodate the increasing number of patients resulted in the Benedictine Sisters purchasing the present hospital site at Fifth avenue east and Third street and constructing the first unit of the present hospital. In 1911, continued growth necessitated an additional wing having an increased bed capacity of sixty patients. In 1920, a new unit of six stories and a capacity almost equal to the then existing hospital building was added at a cost of $450,000.

"Other improvements included the out-patient department which was added in 1922; remodeling in 1924 to provide additional operating rooms, laboratory, supply room, an occupational therapy department, physical therapy department, a pediatrics department, x-ray offices, roentgenologist, orthopedic cast room and supply rooms.

"The hospital at present has a 290-bed capacity, forty Sisters on the administration and nursing staff, 104 student nurses, thirteen lay graduate nurses, three anesthetists, two physical therapists, an occupational therapist, a dietitian, eight laboratory technicians, and seven record room and office workers, eighty-eight physicians on the regular staff, seventy-three on the visiting staff and eight resident internes."

In the introduction to the medical history of St. Louis County, mention is made of the hospital ticket system. The Sisters of St. Benedict began to issue hospital tickets in the fall of 1898, and discontinued their sale on July 1, 1913, when the Working Men's Compensation Act was passed by the State Legislature. The tickets were sold to laboring men and lumberjacks, a ward ticket costing $9 and a double room ticket $12. Physicians and surgeons received as compensation $2 per week for each patient under their care while hospitalized. The hospital ticket system was not only of great benefit to the lumberjacks and laboring men in general, but also helped to build up the hospital.

PIONEER PHYSICIANS OF THE VERMILION AND MISSABE RANGES OF MINNESOTA

By OWEN W. PARKER, M.D.

I N a recent history of Minnesota, it is stated that Minnesota has furnished much of the testimony from which scholars have traced the history of the earth's crust. Here and there are rocks laid down in the early periods of geologic time, which tell of the conditions which existed here long before there were eyes to see or hands to record them.

Thus the records of the Vermilion and Missabe Ranges, which came to the white man's attention only about eighty years ago, have yielded scraps of information which, pieced together with other scraps, give us much of the story of the earth during its remote past. For instance, inasmuch as only the lowest forms of algæ have left their fossil imprints in these ores, geologists have concluded that the great iron ore depository era must have been contemporaneous with the beginning of life on the earth. Also, other evidence left in the rocks proves that since these huge bodies of iron rust were laid down, Minnesota's area has been elevated and depressed repeatedly. This northern area of Minnesota is said to be the backbone of the continent. It had thrust its nose above the waters long before the Appalachian System or the Rocky Mountains were formed. These systems are only infants in geologic age compared to our own section.

In this great drama, it is interesting and inspiring to contemplate that it fell to the lot of our present pioneers to discover this great body of iron ore, after it had been deposited in the earth's crust untold ages before, and to turn it to the use of mankind.

In this work of the pioneers, we find that the pioneer doctors did their part equally well.

The discovery of iron ore on the Vermilion Range in the neighborhood of Tower brought settlers and a rush of miners to this vicinity in 1883 and 1884. The first load of iron ore from the State of Minnesota was shipped to Two Harbors from Tower in 1884, and was hauled by the Duluth and Iron Range Railroad. Mr. Thomas Owens was the engineer. He afterwards become superintendent of the road and is still living at Two Harbors, and is widely known in this section.

On July 31, 1934, the fiftieth anniversary of this event was celebrated by the Old Settlers and Pioneers of the Vermilion and Missabe Ranges. A monument commemorating this momentous occasion was unveiled at Soudan, where it stands near State Highway No. 1.

It had been known for a number of years that there was iron ore in this vicinity, but no active operations had ever begun before. George Stuntz, who settled on Minnesota Point in 1852, was one of the active explorers. He interested George Stone, who in turn interested Charlemagne Tower of Philadelphia. Charlemagne Tower organized the Minnesota Iron Company and started developments in the vicinity of Tower at the Soudan Location. Tower, of course, was named after him and became the mother city of all the Range towns. The mining location of Soudan was kept separate from the business location which was at Tower from the very beginning and has ever remained separate so that at no time has there been any business of any kind in the way of stores in Soudan.

This community had experienced a gold rush following the Civil War, gold having been discovered on Gold Island, in Lake Vermilion, and other places, and as a result of these various rushes and trips the Vermilion Trail had been established through the efforts of George Stuntz. A monument to the memory of this great pioneer stands at the entrance of Hibbing, in Stuntz township.

With the rush of early settlers to Tower for the mining of iron ore, there came Dr. Isaac van Dusen. As far as can be ascertained, he was the first doctor. He remained there for about one year. It is stated that he was a homeopath.

In 1885, it is said, Dr. John Alden came to Tower and remained there about five years, until 1890. He was in private practice. During 1887 there were exploration camps at Ely, and Dr. Alden used to visit these camps at Ely, often riding on horseback to them, a distance of twenty to twenty-five miles.

I am told by old timers that for a few months in the summer of 1887 Dr. Alden had an assistant, a Dr. Anderson, stationed at Ely. He was a young man about twenty-five years of age. A little later Dr. Joseph B. Noble came to Tower and remained there for a number of years.

The first doctors for the mining company at the Soudan Mine, so far as can be learned, were Drs. Robert and William Hutchinson, who came originally from Capron, Illinois. One of them has a son living there at the present time who is a doctor. These men were the first doctors to take care of any iron mining company medical practice in Minnesota.

The Minnesota Iron Company erected the Soudan Hospital in the spring and summer of 1889. This hospital was the first on any of the iron ranges in Minnesota. It stands on its original site and is still owned by the mining company, having passed on to the Oliver Iron Mining Company when the U. S. Steel Corporation was organized in 1901.

The first doctor to come to this new hospital for the mining company was Dr. W. E. Harwood, of Joliet, Illinois, who took charge on May 1, 1889, and remained there until October 1, 1897. His health failed and he was forced to stop practice for a time and left for the west, living for a time at Denver, Colorado. After his health improved, he returned to the Range, locating at Eveleth to take care of the Minnesota Iron Mining Company's work at the Fayal Mine. In 1900, he established the Fabiola Hospital, and had associated with him Dr. Fred Barrett and Dr. Charles Lenont. Dr. Harwood later, after a number of years at Eveleth, gave up the work to specialize in his practice, and located in his former home in Joliet, Illinois, remaining there until the outbreak of the World War, when he joined the English Medical Service. He contracted pneumonia and died while in service at one of the surgical stations at the front in 1915 or 1916.

Dr. Harwood's first mining practice experience was at Ishpeming, Michigan, where he was an assistant to Dr. Bigelow, along with Dr. Shipman. He was a man of studious habits, fine character, and very conscientious in his work, always trying to improve himself, even through his last years. When he finally left the

Range, a testimonial dinner was given him, attended by a large number of his friends.

Associated early with Dr. Harwood at the Soudan Hospital was Dr. Wm. W. Richardson, a graduate of the Northwestern Medical College, who interned in Cook County Hospital. He came originally from Princeton, Illinois. This town happened to be the home at one time of a brother of William Cullen Bryant, the poet.

After Dr. Harwood left the Soudan Hospital on account of his health, Dr. Richardson became head of the hospital and continued so from October 1, 1897, to October 1, 1901.

After leaving Soudan, Dr. Richardson went to Alabama as surgeon for the Tennessee Coal and Iron Company, remaining until about 1905, when he located at Los Angeles, California, becoming a prominent surgeon and specializing there in bone and joint surgery. While operating in May, 1924, he was suddenly seized with a heart pain which compelled him to stop the operation and immediately go to bed. He lived only a few days. At autopsy, his death was found to be due to coronary thrombosis. He was a very capable man in medicine, well trained, and an excellent surgeon. He read German and took German medical publications even while at Soudan as a young physician. He held a teaching position in one of the medical schools at Los Angeles, and was in the World War, stationed somewhere in Europe. He was a great admirer of Christian Fenger, having worked with Fenger in Cook County Hospital. It was the privilege of the writer to be associated with him during his first few months on the Range. Dr. Wm. de La Barre of Minneapolis was also associated for a number of years with Dr. Harwood and Dr. Richardson of Soudan.

Dr. Charles Goodrich Shipman was the first physician to locate in Ely, Minnesota. As previously stated, there had been exploration camps in Ely during 1887 and Dr. Alden of Tower at times made visits to these Ely camps, but there had been no permanent physician until Dr. Shipman came.

Charles Shipman was born August 27, 1856, at Madison, Wisconsin. His father was a veteran of the Civil War and was commonly spoken of as Colonel Shipman. Dr. Shipman attended the Wisconsin University at Madison three years. His family moved to Chicago in 1874, and there he attended the old Chicago University for one year. He graduated from Rush Medical College in 1881 and was president of his class. He took special work in surgery under Dr. Moses Gunn, and during his final year was Dr. Gunn's clinical assistant. He practiced medicine in Chicago for one and a half years when in 1882 he received an appointment as assistant to Dr. Bigelow, chief surgeon of the mining companies at Ishpeming, Michigan. He remained four years at Ishpeming, when in 1886 he was appointed chief surgeon for the mining company at Bessemer, Michigan, on the Gogebic Range. He built a hospital and remained there about two years, but, his health failing, he sold the hospital and spent some months recuperating in California. Later he was appointed Chief Surgeon for the mining company at Ely, Minnesota. He left for that district in May, 1888, and walked into Ely the last five miles, carrying such medical equipment and instruments as possible. Among these were dentist's forceps, as the mining physicians in those days before dentists arrived had to do extractions. For many years in the attic of the Shipman Hospital at Ely there were some old amptuation knives about a foot or more long that Dr. Shipman had carried with him on this occasion, and there still remain some of his old dental forceps.

The railroad was built into Ely from Tower and the first passenger train was run on July 4, 1888, but when Dr. Shipman came in May, 1888, a portion of the track had sunk in a muskeg swamp about three miles out of Ely so that the track was impassable for trains.

Mrs. Shipman came on later in July, 1888. It took thirteen hours to make the trip from Duluth to Ely, Mrs. Shipman said, and the day coach left the track three times within the distance of 117 miles.

Dr. and Mrs. Shipman first had two rooms in Ely over a hardware store which was doing undertaking and there was a big sign, "Undertaking," in letters eighteen inches high. This was the source of many jokes at Dr. Shipman's expense. Before winter, Dr. Shipman had finished the building which was the first drug store in Ely, and which is still continued as a drug store. He lived in the store and had a front reception room and operating room and office.

During the spring of 1892 he started building the Shipman Hospital and finished it during 1893. When the panic of 1893 struck the whole country, it hit the iron ranges very hard, closing all mines. Someone said that during that year Dr. Shipman called the Shipman Hospital "Shipman's Monument"—it looked as though there would never be any use for it on the Range.

Dr. C. W. More of Eveleth, Minnesota, was Dr. Shipman's first assistant at Ely. Dr. More came to Minnesota in 1888, as assistant to Dr. S. C. Maxwell of Two Harbors, who had been appointed as physician to the employees of the Duluth and Iron Range Railroad Company at Two Harbors. About a year later, Dr. More accepted a position with Dr. Shipman at Ely and remained there over four years.

After Dr. More left Ely, Dr. H. E. Wunder came as assistant to Dr. Shipman, and remained until 1899. Later he was in charge of the Soudan Hospital, but left the Range about 1905, and now lives in Shakopee, Minnesota.

Of the many physicians associated at one time or another with Dr. Shipman, the pioneer physician, Dr. C. W. More, Dr. D. C. Rood, Dr. R. L. Burns,† Dr. George T. Ayres and the writer are still in this district—Duluth, Two Harbors and the Range.

Dr. Shipman left the Range in 1908 because of poor health. He went to Ocean Park, California, and for five years stopped the practice of medicine, then started in the practice of medicine again and practiced steadily five years until his death in 1918. He died suddenly in his own office, just after making a professional call on a patient.

Dr. Shipman was a man of magnetic personality, fine physique and handsome appearance. He was an excellent story teller and could tell innumerable stories in all the dialects, such as French, French-Canadian, Italian, Swedish, and especially the old Cornish miner dialects. He was an excellent entertainer and very hospitable, and was frequently visited by mining officials and other people of prominence who came through the Ely district. He was a sportsman and outdoor man, loved hunting, fishing, boating and baseball, having at one time been a player himself. He was also an excellent billiard player as well as an amateur boxer in his early life. He is still remembered by the old timers of the Range and is often spoken of in terms of affection and appreciation. He was an unusual character, and once one met him one never forgot him.

As a pioneer physician, he is entitled to great credit for the work he did in maintaining a high standard of medical practice on the Iron Range in the early days.

Dr. William H. Magie, one of the most prominent and able surgeons of Duluth and northern Minnesota, well remembered by all, built a small emergency hospital

---

†Since this was written, Dr. Burns has retired and gone to California to reside.

at Biwabik in 1892. Dr. Magie had been appointed surgeon of the Duluth, Missabe and Northern Railroad Company and for several of the mines operating in the Biwabik district.

The famous Merritt family of Duluth, Frank Hibbing and other explorers had done a great deal of work upon the Missabe Range, and it was commencing to open up at about this time. Dr. Magie placed in charge of the hospital Dr. Carroll Corson, who thus became the first physician to locate in Biwabik. In the same year, 1892, Dr. James R. Humphrey opened an office in Merritt, which was situated one mile east of Biwabik. He too was a surgeon for several of the mining companies operating in the district.

In 1893, the village of Merritt was almost destroyed by fire, and was never rebuilt. Dr. Humphrey moved his office to Biwabik where he built a small emergency hospital.

In 1894, Dr. Corson left Biwabik and Dr. Humphrey purchased the hospital owned by Dr. Magie. Dr. Humphrey operated the hospital and practiced in Biwabik until 1898, when he sold out to Dr. R. J. Sewall of Minneapolis. Dr. Sewall remained in Biwabik one year and removed to McKinley four miles west in 1899. Dr. Sewall sold the hospital in Biwabik to Dr. Charles W. Bray of Minneapolis, who moved to Biwabik in 1899. In 1906 the original building was destroyed by fire. A much larger hospital was built on the old site. This was operated by Dr. Bray, a greatly respected physician of Biwabik, until his death, July 8, 1937. Dr. Bray's wife, Mary B. Bray, is a graduate of the University of Minnesota Medical School, and assisted him very materially in the practice of medicine during their first few years in Biwabik. It is interesting to observe that of Dr. Bray's family of three sons and one daughter, all three sons are physicians, a truly medical family, and of the highest type.

Dr. H. L. Darms, with his wife, located at McKinley in 1892, very soon after the village had been organized. He served as mayor of the village in 1893. He left in 1894, going to Eveleth for Dr. More, who was sick. After this, McKinley was without a local physician until 1899, when Dr. R. J. Sewall moved there from Biwabik. In 1900 Dr. Sewall sold out to Dr. J. C. Farmer of White Bear, Minnesota, who practiced there until his death in 1921. Since that time, McKinley has had no resident physician.

The first doctor to settle in Virginia was Dr. James R. Humphrey, whom we have mentioned as having been early in Biwabik. This was in 1893. Dr. Humphrey was presumably in Virginia for only a short time, as he seems to have been in Biwabik until 1898. After him at Virginia came Dr. Stewart Bates, in 1893, and Dr. C. W. Miller. Dr. Bates built and operated the first hospital in Virginia.

Dr. Z. K. Brown came to Virginia in 1896 and died there from typhoid fever in 1899.

Dr. C. B. Eby was the first doctor to locate in Mountain Iron, about 1898. He was later associated with Dr. Avery and practiced in Virginia in 1901. He left the Range and later located in Spring Valley, Minnesota, where he lived until his death a few years ago. His death occurred while he was making a call to see a patient.

(To be continued in June issue)

EDITORIAL

MINNESOTA MEDICINE

OFFICIAL JOURNAL OF THE MINNESOTA STATE MEDICAL ASSOCIATION

Published by the Association under the direction of its Editing and Publishing Committee

EDITING AND PUBLISHING COMMITTEE

J. T. CHRISTISON, Saint Paul   C. B. WRIGHT, Minneapolis
E. M. HAMMES, Saint Paul   T. A. PEPPARD, Minneapolis
WALTMAN WALTERS, Rochester

EDITORIAL STAFF

CARL B. DRAKE, Saint Paul, Editor
W. F. BRAASCH, Rochester, Associate Editor
GILBERT COTTAM, Minneapolis, Associate Editor

Annual Subscription—$3.00.   Single Copies—$0.40
Foreign Subscriptions—$3.50.

The right is reserved to reject material submitted for editorial or advertising columns. The Editing and Publishing Committee does not hold itself responsible for views expressed either in editorials or other articles when signed by the author.

Classified advertising—five cents a word; minimum charge, $1.00. Remittance should accompany order.

Display advertising rates on request.

Address all communications to Minnesota Medicine, 2642 University Avenue, Saint Paul, or Suite 604, National Bldg., Minneapolis. Telephone: Nestor 2641.

BUSINESS MANAGER
J. R. BRUCE

Volume 21   MAY, 1938   Number 5

Surgical Relief of Adhesive Pericarditis

ADHESIONS between visceral and parietal layers of the pericardium may not be sufficient to cause symptoms. This condition is not infrequently first discovered at necropsy. When existing in conjunction with valvular heart disease, as is usually the case, thickened pericardium may aggravate the picture of valvular heart disease. When the pericarditis has been accompanied by extensive fibrosis of the parietal pericardium and has involved the surrounding structures of the mediastinum, the clinical picture may closely resemble cirrhosis of the liver, with enlargement of the liver, ascites with or without

dependent edema. These three clinical types were nicely described in an analysis of fifty-five proven cases by George Douglass Head* of Minneapolis in 1905.

Many a case of adhesive pericarditis has been erroneously diagnosed cirrhosis of the liver and its diagnosis is not easy. The history of a heart pain in conjunction with an attack of rheumatic fever is very important. A large heart not sufficiently accounted for by the valvular lesions present, an enlarged liver and ascites with little or no dependent edema should arouse the suspicion that adhesive pericarditis is causing cardiac hypertrophy through adhesion to the chest wall, diaphragm and mediastinal structures or perhaps by scar tissue interference with venous return to the right auricle. A fixed heart, systolic retraction at the apex and Broadbent's sign are all of some value, but fluoroscopic examination of the heart revealing a tugging of the diaphragm or hilus shadows is more likely to be of diagnostic value.

The idea of the possibility of surgical relief in certain selected cases was first proposed at the turn of the century. Delorme's suggestion of decortication was first considered too radical. Brauer's proposal, made in 1902, of removing the ribs overlying the heart was more conservative and more often employed, but proved inadequate in most cases as it relieved only the tug on the anterior chest wall and did nothing to relieve the constricting effect on the heart in diastole or the interference with venous return to the heart. Sauerbruch, in 1913, resected a portion of fibrosed pericardium in one case with relief of symptoms. Since that time numerous cases have been reported in which thickened adherent pericardium has been stripped off the heart muscle and removed, the adhesions having been separated even as far back as the vena cava. The experimental and clinical work of Claude S. Beck have been outstanding in this country and he has reported numerous successful results.

The operation of cardiolysis following the suggestions of Delorme is, needless to say, highly technical. Avoidance of the pleural spaces, strip-

---

*Head, G. D.: Chronic adherent pericarditis. St. Paul Med. Jour., 7:251-259, 1905.

ping off of thickened pericardium without injuring heart muscles and vessels, the use of negative pressure and the avoidance of postoperative "pneumocardiac tamponade" must all be considered.

However, close cooperation between cardiologist and surgeon in the selection of cases does afford some hope for surgical relief for a certain number of these chronic invalids. While clinical cases in which symptoms are produced largely by pericardial fibrosis amenable to surgical treatment are not common, some are doubtless overlooked. Since the results of operation in certain carefully chosen cases are so remarkably good, the development of the complicated technic by a limited number of surgeons is highly desirable.

John Shaw Billings (1838-1913)

ON April 12, 1938, occurred the hundredth anniversary of the birth of a man whom Sigerist has properly designated as one who "truly ranks among the great pioneers of American medicine." The occasion was fittingly commemorated by a joint meeting of the Johns Hopkins Medical Society and the Johns Hopkins Medical History Club and the proceedings are set forth in the April issue of the *Bulletin of the Institute of the History of Medicine*, of the Johns Hopkins University, named the John Shaw Billings Memorial Number, covering 163 pages.

The life of this remarkable man in detail has been written by Fielding H. Garrison and was published in 1915. It is a classic and deserves to be read by all who are in any degree interested in the upbuilding of scientific medicine. It is the story of the accomplishments of a man who did more to strengthen and elevate his profession than has anyone else in its history.

To attempt to cover the same ground, even in condensed form, within the limits of an editorial, is manifestly impossible. Only the highlights can be mentioned.

Billings' career began simultaneously with the outbreak of the Civil War. At twenty-three he received his commission, served with great distinction throughout the conflict and remained in the army for nearly thirty-four years. This experience resulted in the initiation of four of his great accomplishments: he was responsible for the production of the monumental Medical and

Surgical History of the War of the Rebellion; he developed the Army Medical Library, the Army Medical Museum and the Index Catalogue, all tremendous undertakings.

In 1876 he was approached by the Trustees of the Johns Hopkins Fund and induced to submit plans for the proposed Johns Hopkins Hospital, in competition with others. His plans were accepted and he was intrusted with the supervision of the construction, all, of course, with the consent of the army authorities. Notable as this service was, it was even less important than the part Billings played in the organization of the school and the selection of the personnel. The plans he proposed were radical to the point of being revolutionary at that time, but they were adopted, and the sanity of his ideas has been vindicated and proven by the subsequent developments. Seldom has so much responsibility rested on the shoulders of one man and never has it been more thoroughly justified.

He was called on to design other important hospitals, like Peter Bent Brigham, and made notable contributions to the literature of military medicine, the history of medicine, public hygiene, sanitary engineering and statistics. He was the author, according to Garrison, of "the most critical account of American medical literature (1876) and the best history of surgery that has been published in English (1895)." "He was," says the same authority, "a man of all-round ability . . . (who) did a giant's work for the advancement of American medicine."

Billings had a good heredity, but his people were poor and he secured his education at Miami with difficulty and personal privation. His training in the Medical College of Ohio was the usual two-year course of that period and he served an internship, an uncommon thing in to do in those days, in an obscure hospital. There must have been giant stature in his chromosomes, for he rose above these handicaps and left a heritage of almost unique accomplishment. Yet his name is scarcely known to the present generation. When Johns Hopkins is mentioned we think of Osler and Welch; the army suggests Beaumont, Sternberg, Reed and Gorgas; in medical history Sudhoff and Sigerist, all great and worthy men, but John Shaw Billings, quiet, self-effacing and competent, was the peer of them all, and without him some of them would not have had their great opportunity.

He retired from the army in 1896 at the age of fifty-eight, having served for thirty-four years. His plan was to spend the rest of his days in Philadelphia doing research, writing and teaching in the University of Pennsylvania but the Fates ruled otherwise. The Public Library system in New York was in a state of flux, with three disconnected organizations serving the public as best they could. The services of a trained and capable coördinator were needed and Billings was the man. Reluctantly he gave up his long cherished plans, put on the harness for more public work; and in this harness he died in 1913. But he had done one more big thing in a quiet way; those "seventeen years . . . saw dreams realized in a way given only to those who deserve success." To him it was just the day's work.

. G. C.

The College of Physicians and Medical Economics

THE program of the meeting of the American College of Physicians which was held in New York last month included at least two speeches which had nothing to do with scientific medicine. The presidential address by Dr. James H. Means took a slap at the attitude of the American Medical Association towards medical economic policies, and was widely heralded in the lay press as a revolt in the medical ranks of the country. The members of the College, to counteract any such impression, circulated a statement signed by 300 members, including President Means, denying that the College was in revolt against the organized medical profession. President Means' further remarks disparaging the importance of the present doctor-patient relationship suggest he has had little personal experience in the need of a doctor. His statement that "having a third party determine the size of, and even collect, the fee from the patient for the doctor is not only not an intrusion into the holy doctor-patient relationship but actually increases the likelihood of the patient's receiving from the doctor the best and wisest treatment the doctor is capable of giving" is hard to follow. If Dr. Means intends to convey the idea that collecting fees is distracting to the scientific practice of medicine, he is right. If, however, the majority of patients and practition-

ers prefer the present patient-doctor relationship to any other system so far offered, there is good reason to hold to our present system.

The other address by Dr. John P. Peters, professor of medicine at Yale University Medical School, was what one might expect from the secretary of the so-called "Committee of 430" doctors. The Committee having once declared itself in favor of more government influence in the practice of medicine, its secretary again makes a plea before the College for government subsidy for medical schools, hospitals and laboratories. He thinks the rich do not pay to support the institutions that care for the indigent, and yet enjoy medical advances' developed through the instrumentality of the indigent. He infers the rich do not pay taxes and that the indigent are used as guinea pigs for experimentation. He makes a plea for government subsidy for the productive phases of medicine developed by educational and research institutes and hospitals and distrusts the vagaries of philanthropists. Government direction, in his opinion, could be no worse. It is our impression that most of the advances in our country in medicine, as in other fields, have in the past been accomplished by private enterprise. Any advances that have been made in the Yale Medical School were made possible by the large endowment of Yale University, which was accumulated largely from gifts from the wealthy. On the whole, the speech resembles some we have recently heard from Washington, which have sounded like an attempt to accentuate class antagonism. Perhaps the speaker belongs in Washington.

Proposals for changes in policies regarding medical practice, education and research should properly be initiated within the ranks of our national organization. Activities of societies of specialists should be limited to scientific discussion. Our organization is a representative one and it is wiser to leave the disposition of medical problems to our chosen representatives.

Correction

The widespread report that Professor Moritz Oppenheim was one of several medical men of Vienna who had committed suicide was repeated in an editorial entitled "Nazi Persecution in Vienna" which appeared in our columns last month. This was an error which we take pains to correct. Professor Oppenheim is still alive, a fact which will be welcomed by many professional friends in this country.

MEDICAL ECONOMICS

Edited by the Committee on Medical Economics
of the
Minnesota State Medical Association

B. J. Branton, M. D.   W. F. Braasch, M. D., Chairman   J. C. Michael, M. D.
L. H. Rutledge, M. D.   A. N. Collins, M. D.

The State-Wide Survey

Has your county society started its survey of medical care and facilities in your own community? If not, the work should begin at once.

This survey, which means so much to the future of medicine in the United States, is being carried on in every county in the state. It is essentially a COUNTY SOCIETY SURVEY. Every member must do his part.

HAVE YOU DONE YOURS?

Study Under Way

Preliminary steps have now been taken for the state-wide survey of medical facilities by medical societies in Minnesota.

The first was an all-day meeting, Sunday, April 3, in Saint Paul, of the Committee on Medical Economics—chairman, W. F. Braasch, Rochester—where the following plans were formulated.

The Committee on Medical Economics, functioning through the Sub-Committee on Low Income and Indigent Problems, of which Dr. Coventry of Duluth is chairman, will have general supervision of the survey. It seemed best to group the county activities according to Councilor Districts, under the direct supervision of the respective councilors, who are familiar with the various local situations. In order to coordinate these state-wide activities the State Office of the Minnesota State Medical Association will assist county and district officers of the survey where it is needed and collect information required from state-wide health and welfare agencies.

It cannot be over-emphasized, however, that this survey is the individual problem of every county medical society, club, or district society in the State Medical Association. No one man

or group can be held responsible for the success of this campaign. It must be a coöperative movement—a share the work plan.

Help in Fact Gathering

Both state-wide and local welfare agencies will be asked to assist in gathering facts for the study. They will also be asked for their candid opinion concerning the adequacy of medical care in each locality and what suggestions they may have, if any, on practical means to improve it.

Dentists, pharmacists, social welfare workers, nurses, hospital executives, health officers, all will be asked to contribute to this study to the end that it may be authentic, accurate and comprehensive—and to the end, also, that no one can attack it, when the work is done, on the ground of prejudice or insincerity.

Preliminary Meetings

Preparations are now going forward in nearly all councilor districts for preparatory meetings of physicians to insure interest, information and enthusiasm for the work. Such meetings have already been held in district three under the direction of Councilor B. J. Branton of Willmar, in district five under the direction of Councilor George A. Earl of Saint Paul, in district two under the sponsorship of Councilor L. L. Sogge of Windom, and in district eight under the direction of Councilor W. L. Burnap of Fergus Falls.

Conferences have been arranged with the Governor, with Mr. Herman Aufderheide, director of the State Relief Agency, Mr. C. R. Carlgren, chairman of the State Board of Control, Mr. W. R. Sassaman, executive secretary of the State Planning Board. Arrangements have been made also for a general conference with state officials of the welfare and professional organizations whose interests involve care of the sick.

Forms to be Filled

Eight forms have been provided for the survey by the Bureau of Medical Economics of the American Medical Association to be filled out under the direction of the county societies and by individual members. A ninth form, not yet ready, is to be used to summarize the information secured on the others in each county. Copies of this summary will go to the State Office and to Chicago; one will remain with the county society, club or committee in charge of fact-gathering. A tenth form is to be supplied to state organizations for securing information of a state-wide character.

Work to be Pushed

The survey is to get under way at the earliest possible date and county officers are urged by the chairman in charge to make it their most important job until the work is finished.

Following are important talks on the subject given at the Sunday meeting by Dr. R. G. Leland, director, Bureau of Medical Economics, American Medical Association, and Dr. R. E. Scammon of the University of Minnesota, president of the State Planning Board:

DR. LELAND

You have no doubt heard it said that the survey of medical facilities initiated recently by the American Medical Association represents a change of front on the part of the association. You have heard, perhaps, that, confronted with criticism, with threats of legislative action, and with a demand for action on the part of the U. S. Public Health Service, the American Medical Association has at last been forced to form a positive policy and take action.

Nothing could be farther from the truth.

Policy Unchanged

It was sixteen years ago when the American Medical Association first announced its policy on health insurance. At that time the association went on record as officially opposed to health insurance except and unless it was organized and sponsored by local county medical societies. It has never deviated in any respect from that policy; but in 1935 the House of Delegates of the national body drew up the now famous Ten Points which definitely set out the principles that should be followed in any system for distribution of medical care, including health insurance. Later the American Medical Association specifically encouraged the formation of local community plans of various sorts, where they were needed and where they were under medical society sponsorship, for better distribu-

tion of medical care to low income groups. Many such plans were started in various parts of the United States with the advice and the assistance of the Bureau of Medical Economics of the association.

No Response

In 1937 after rejection of the proposal brought to the House of Delegates at Atlantic City by the New York State Medical Society for federal subsidy for care of the indigent, a resolution offering to confer with any qualified government agency on new plans for medical care in the United States was passed. Up to December, 1937, no agency had made any effort to take advantage of this offer.

In December, 1937, the United States Public Health Service and representatives of the American Public Health Association did approach the Board of Trustees for a conference on the matter and the plan for a survey of medical care by the practicing physician in his county society was formulated.

New Method

The American Medical Association has always been deeply interested in the public welfare. The survey represents, merely, a new method for attacking the problem of public welfare, not a new interest in the problem of care for the sick. It represents, also, the first time that medical men have ever been asked to make a study of medical problems.

A Medical Problem

Our survey should be regarded as the first step toward adjustment of our system of medical care to the changes of our times. I should like you to regard it, also, in the light of a medical problem.

The first step in the study of a medical problem is the collection of data; the second is a diagnosis based on the data collected; and the third is a recommendation for treatment.

This survey will be effective only if we handle it according to these three steps and in the light of a strictly impartial medical analysis.

Not "Just Another Study"

It cannot be too strongly emphasized that this is not a study to be made and forgotten. We medical men must work with public agencies to make whatever changes are necessary to keep in step with the changes of the times. The survey will provide us with the facts we need in order to make those changes effective.

The American Medical Association has been much criticized because "it had no plan." We have always had a plan. Our plan has consisted of an effort to make hundreds of plans, if need be, to fit every local community because no plan on earth could be made to fit every section of the United States. The object of this survey is to fit our plans, if they are needed, to the needs of the local community.

Is Obstacle Economic?

There is a wide-spread belief that an obstacle exists between physician and patient. We must find out just how real and how extensive this obstacle is and what is its cause. Is the obstacle wholly economic? Is it rooted partly in ignorance and lack of special health education? These are questions we must answer and problems that we must try to solve.

The effort need not be costly to the individual county society. It may require time and sacrifice on the part of some of you; but I hope you will carry it through to the conclusion, no matter what it costs. We must keep in mind that the medical profession is under fire of much criticism; we must keep in mind, also, our own objective, which is and always has been, the best possible medical care for all the people.

DR. SCAMMON

It has seemed to me as I have listened to the outline of your plans that this survey is going to be exceedingly valuable. Indeed, I'm not sure that I shouldn't go further and say that this survey is essential.

In the first place, the survey is tied up with the medical profession. And it is the doctors and the doctors, alone, who are in a position to evaluate the character and nature of the services needed.

In other countries where attempts have been made to reorganize medical care, the task has been done without the assistance of the medical profession. The results were almost invariably unfortunate until, after a period of time, the medical profession was called in to help. We have many examples of this sort of planning from above—and without the doctors—for medical care.

Wasted Years

In England, health insurance was worked out from above in a period of three months. It took twenty-five years of modification to get that original scheme down to a workable plan. If the medical profession had been called in in the first place a quarter of a century of effort would not have been wasted.

In the second place, this survey and resultant plans are to operate by taking small areas as units and working out problems individually there.

Here in Minnesota we have 87 counties. Some are growing, some are declining in population; some are urban, some are rural; some are prosperous and some are not. We are not faced with a simple problem when we undertake to study and adjust medical care in Minnesota.

We Must Have Patterns

It is therefore extremely important in my estimation to go at this problem in the manner suggested by this study. We must get a pattern for each state and for each locality of the state; and this is the only way to get it.

On some of the blanks provided for this survey you will, of course, not get a perfect return. This fact

should not constitute a cause for criticism. It is a fact that very few large surveys get a perfect return. Even insurance companies are unable to get them. It is possible on the basis of incomplete returns, however, to indicate "zones of confidence" in the returns. A process of cancelling out and evaluating will get at satisfactory answers in the end.

Choice: Data or Guessing

We never get anywhere at any constructive work without data. We must not expect that our results will be perfect; some variability is to be expected but this variability does not invalidate the usefulness of our attempt to collect facts.

The results of this survey may be merely a sampling. But we elect officers on a sampling process; not on the basis of a full vote. We have the choice of collecting data or of guessing. We can get the facts with a certain limit of error. And our best protection is certainly to work from information, even if it is not perfect, rather than from guessing. The public is best served where the medical profession takes the trouble to know where it stands.

DR. LELAND

Preliminary Preparations

The importance of preliminary organization for the survey cannot be over-estimated.

We must impress upon the individual medical man that this is "a medical analysis by medical men," that he, himself, is the only one who can push it through to a successful finish. We must not approach our task with a bias, either, or a preconceived notion that something must be done or that one plan or another is right or wrong, regardless. In some counties nothing needs to be done to improve distribution of medical care. We know that. But even in these counties we must have the information before we can safely come to such a conclusion.

By all means we should make use of findings of other organizations when we have reasonable assurance that the findings are accurate and honest.

For Accurate Sampling

I am very grateful to Doctor Scammon for his comments on the survey. Our findings will be samplings, only, as he told you. They will not be 100 per cent perfect nor will they lend themselves to mathematical statistical studies. But we must make an effort to have accurate sampling for all classes in a vertical rather than in horizonal lines. We must try to show the levels of service. Where osteopaths or chiropractors give a large amount of service, for instance, note should be made of the fact on the proper forms.

Community Project

We shall have failed seriously unless the confidence in the medical profession is in the crescendo as the study proceeds rather in the diminuendo in our communities. Our associates in the survey must be willing to go along with us, not only in getting information but in carrying out the recommendations that result.

In Michigan the survey is already underway. The governor gave his blessing, appropriated $10,000 to it and plans to use the results for purposes of his own.

In Pennsylvania where the study is also advancing rapidly, the work has been parcelled out by districts to members of the Committee on Medical Economics.

However you plan the details of the work in Minnesota, you must not fail to ask yourselves when it is completed: has every man had his day in court? If he has not, suspicion of prejudice and suppression of fact will defeat the purpose of the survey and render the work of no avail.

Forms Ready

The forms for this study were printed by the American Medical Association and all but two or three are ready for use. Of these last, one is for pharmacists; and one for state medical societies to record information from state agencies and state-wide health services. Summary forms for the county societies still remain to be supplied. On these summary forms each county society will be asked to summarize the information secured on the other eight forms. The county society will then keep the original forms from which the summary is made and make three copies of the summary, one for the state association, one for the American Medical Association and one for the county society.

The returns on Form 1 (on volume of free and paid for service of each physician, etc.) are to be anonymous; but a key method of some sort will doubtless be needed particularly in the large societies so as to know how many have sent in their returns.

To Every Man His Chance

Publicity will have to be carefully controlled. The first announcement that the medical profession of the state is going to make a survey of medical care in each county will be news. A brief statement of the purpose of the profession in making the survey will suffice for this story. Publicity thereafter should be confined to state journals and special bulletins and talks to the profession until the survey is completed and we are ready to tell the public what we propose to do about it.

Whether to go to non-members for information is a question to be determined by each society. You must always remember, however, that when the survey is over everybody must have had his say. We must not leave the door open to criticism by anyone, even non-members. Give everybody his chance in this survey, be he friend or foe.

Medicine in Charge

The power of a medical organization which acts as a unit to preserve essential values of medicine and to serve the public interest is well demonstrated in two spots in America today.

One is in British Columbia where a Health Insurance Act was drawn up with the aid of physicians several years ago and was so emasculated in passage that the physicians flatly refused to function under it. As a result of that refusal there is health insurance in name only in British Columbia, pending the passage of a new act which will meet with the approval of the medical men.

Washington Controversy

Illustration Number Two is to be seen today in the District of Columbia where the Group Health Association plan for employees of the Home Owners Loan Corporation has become focal point for conflict and newspaper attack.

As noted before in these columns, the Home Owners Loan Corporation received a grant of $40,000 from the government to enable it to start this group sickness insurance plan for employees of the corporation. The Comptroller General of the United States subsequently ruled that the grant was illegal; the House Appropriations Committee indicated its disapproval.

Declared Illegal

The United States district attorney of the District of Columbia ruled that the association is unlawful under the Healing Arts Act of the District of Columbia which declares that it is unlawful for any corporation to practice medicine. The corporation counsel also ruled that the Group Health Association is operating in violation of the insurance laws of the District of Columbia.

With tacit Administration approval the association persisted in its organization and operation in spite of these rulings. Six physicians were hired to take care of the 6,000 members of the association.

The complete history of the opposition of the District of Columbia Medical Society as it was outlined by Congressman Shafer of Michigan and published in the *Congressional Record* of Tuesday, March 29, is as follows:

When the scheme was first broached, the medical society offered its coöperation in good faith to help provide the medical care. There was only one proviso: that the program to be worked out should not violate the legal, ethical and professional standards of the society.

x for Six Thousand

It should be obvious to anyone that a plan whereby six physicians are hired to care for 6,000 people, the original grant for which was declared illegal by the Comptroller General and the plan of operation for which was also declared legal both under the Healing Arts law and the insurance laws of the District of Columbia, could not comply with the standard set by the District of Columbia Medical Society.

The Society accordingly ruled that its members could not participate in the plan because it involved the illegal practice of medicine. And when one of them accepted employment from the Group Health Association and refused to resign his job, the Society dropped him from membership.

Hospitals are naturally bound by the same standards as the medical society and they were also unable to maintain professional relationships with physicians who were engaged in medical practice that violated the law.

Test Cases

The physician dropped from membership is reported to have threatened suit against the Society, of course; also a test case involving a Group Health Association member and physician and one of the hospitals inevitably developed. This case was seized upon and touted for all it could be made to yield as a weapon against the Society.

The episode was shouted in the newspapers and a member of Congress from California hastened to introduce a resolution into Congress for an investigation, not only of the District of Columbia Medical Society, but of all constituent societies of the American Medical Association and the national association itself.

Resident Vindicated

The truth of the hospital episode was this: An appendicitis patient was sent to the hospital for operation by one of the Group Health Association physicians. The patient was informed that her association physician was not permitted to practice in the hospital but that she might call any other physician or surgeon whom she chose. She refused and left the hospital to be operated upon, two days later, in another hospital, and by another physician. Her appendix, at the time of operation, showed that her condition was not acute. As the resident at the

first hospital had originally declared, the case was not an emergency and he was not under obligation, therefore, to violate hospital rules to allow the operation.

The story told by the California congressman varied considerably from the facts and great capital was made of her dismissal from the hospital. In fact, it was noisily and erroneously reported that the appendix had ruptured after she left the first hospital and before operation.

Situation Precarious

As a result of the resolution and firmness of the Medical Society of the District of Columbia, the situation of the Group Health Association remains highly unsatisfactory and precarious. Only six physicians have so far been employed under it and these six physicians are not permitted to care for their patients in any reputable hospital in the District.

It is clear here, as in British Columbia, that the physicians themselves can control standards of medical care anywhere in the United States if they work together to maintain them.

In this connection it is important to make a note here of the fine address on the subject made in the House of Representatives by Congressman Shafer.

Champion in Congress

Said Mr. Schafer in the conclusion of a talk in which he reviewed the known facts of the Group Health Association controversy:

"In accusations of this kind (concerning the patient whose physician was refused permission to operate in the hospital) it is better to have the facts established immediately than to allow the medical profession to be exposed to loose charges. I have no doubt that an investigation would vindicate members of the District of Columbia Medical Society completely and for that reason I would support the resolution of the gentleman from California if it were not national in scope. . . . I am at all times ready to favor an investigation into charges against the medical profession or any of its reputable members because I believe that, except perhaps in isolated cases, such charges are idle gossip which would be disproved by an orderly investigation, and because I believe the medical profession is too important, its ideals are too fine, its service to humanity is too great and its necessity to human welfare too vital to allow it to be rendered suspect. I believe the members of the District of Columbia Medical Society whose conduct has been brought into question should be given full opportunity to establish in an orderly and convincing way the falsity of these charges."

Behind the Headlines

The American College of Physicians, a purely scientific association, was considerably startled, recently, to find its regular scientific meeting had been made the occasion for an entirely unsanctioned outburst of propaganda for the Committee of Physicians.

The first explosion was set off by Dr. John P. Peters of Yale, secretary of the now famous committee which released its proposals for Federal subsidy of medicine with considerable trumpeting in the lay press last November. Doctor Peters spoke before the College of Physicians at the personal invitation of Dr. James H. Means.

"Advantage of the Rich"

Said Doctor Peters:

"The practicing physicians offer solutions for health problems that overlook the production side (medical schools, hospitals and laboratories). Meanwhile the medically productive institutions are reduced more and more to philanthropy for their funds. . . .

"It is my impression that the government alone can assume the burden of providing, maintaining and correlating the necessary medical resources . . .

"It is rather amusing to reflect that, at the present time, most of the advances in medicine which the rich enjoy are developed in hospitals and institutions through the instrumentality of indigent patients. The fees which the rich pay, however, do not return to the support of those institutions but go to the practitioner who is exploiting new medical discoveries . . ."

Released in Advance

This interesting declaration received the sort of newspaper attention that such a paper always gets when it is given by a man who occupies a prominent place—and who hands his paper to the newspapers plenty of time in advance.

The second charge came from the retiring president, Dr. James H. Means of Harvard University, himself.

This time the American Medical Association was directly assailed as maintaining an attitude "close to standpatism."

"Like Jove on High Olympus"

"The behavior of the association is political," said Doctor Means. "It is partisan behavior; it champions a cause. At the present time the cause is something close to standpatism.

"But the policy can be changed at any time if the membership wills it. At the present time the membership of the American Medical Association is apathetic and inarticulate because it has no issues, no platforms set up to vote for.

"It is allowing the medical politicians to run things about as they please and official spokesmen, like Jove on high Olympus, hurl thunderbolts of wrath at all who differ in orthodox doctrine.

"As no democracy can be healthy without freedom of speech, real issues and an effective opposition party, it is desirable that those who believe in popular government bestir themselves to change this state of affairs."

Resentment Boiled

The effect of this well-timed challenge upon younger members of the College was electric, according to Minnesota representatives.

Resentment boiled up in all quarters. There was a general demand that the issue be thrashed out on the convention floor but wiser council prevailed.

Instead, a resolution was drawn up as follows and presented to the regents:

"Unfortunately an impression has been given to the press that the American College of Physicians is in revolt against organized medicine as represented by the American Medical Association.

"Inasmuch as the College has never taken any action, and inasmuch as we have reason to believe that this reported impression does not represent the opinion of the majority of the members of the College, we, the undersigned Fellows of the College, respectfully request the Board of Regents to correct this impression publicly."

Means, Signer

In the midst of a busy session, 400 signers to this petition were secured in the space of two hours. One of them, ironically, was said to be Doctor Means, himself.

An answer from organized medicine was immediately forthcoming. Said Dr. Morris Fishbein in a Chicago address the next night:

"Doctor Means has never taken any actual part in the affairs of the American Medical Association and his ignorance of what is going on is actually lamentable.

"If he had any real knowledge of the present activities of the association which include a nation-wide inventory of medical needs and a determination of means for satisfying them, he could not have spoken as he did . . .

"Dr. Means is, unfortunately, typical of a considerable number of physicians in laboratories or in full-time positions in medical schools who are unaware of medical practice outside of public hospitals or clinics.

Confiscatory Taxation is the Answer

"They have one chief objective . . . the securing of more and more government funds for the subsidizing of medical education, of hospitals and of the care of the sick.

"Their answer to the problem of medical care . . . is confiscatory taxation of industry and of the individual worker for the benefit of a bureaucracy."

To all of which Doctor Means issued the following meek statement in extenuation:

"I wish to correct a misunderstanding. It has been said that I am advocating a revolt against the American Medical Association. I am not advocating a revolt and nothing of the sort was mentioned in the speech which I made last night. What I did was to express the opinion that it would be wholesome if there should develop an enlightened opposition party within the democracy of the American Medical Association. This would be merely democracy functioning in a normal fashion."

Indignant Telegrams

It is reported, incidentally, that Doctor Means was promptly flooded with telegrams from all parts of the country—and that the prevailing tenor of these telegrams was indignation and a general demand for an explanation.

The real criticism of Doctor Means was not that he should hold opinions or that he should express them but rather that he should have expressed them when and where he did. The keenest resentment of all was expressed by College members who felt that they, a purely scientific body, had been placed in a false and unpleasant light before the country.

Silence Unfortunate

The whole episode gives rise to one obvious conclusion. The constituent state medical associations that make up the American Medical Association must hereafter vigorously express themselves on matters of economics, social welfare and the future of American medicine.

That the American Medical Association reflects the will of its constituent associations through their representatives in the House of Delegates is clear to anyone who is at all familiar with the sentiments and deliberations of this body. Under the Constitution the Board of Trustees must necessarily carry out the policies of the House of Delegates where such policies are clearly defined.

There is no doubt that a deliberate effort has been made by certain groups and agencies to promote a general impression that the American Medical Association does not truly represent organized medicine. These groups and agencies may be classified in a general way under the following headings: First, individual doctors who are not personally satisfied with the policies of the *Journal of the American Medical Association;* Second, politicians and others who want a complete change of method in the administration of medical care in the United States; Third, the patent medicine and proprietary medicine interests whose toes have been stepped on by the Council of Pharmacy and Chemistry; Fourth, the popular and ever growing number of throw-away medical publications supported by medical houses and exploiting uncensored medical advertising.

Knowledge—Judgment—Opinion

(Monthly Editorial Prepared by the Medical Advisory Committee)

Life to everyone is a contrast of emotions or thoughts.

To the child happiness, a smile, is easily changed into despair, a tear. The business man becomes a thinker in pessimistic or optimistic terms according to the stock market. The economists think in terms of supply and demand. They write volumes on their theories pro and con. The physician must make a diagnosis through scientific research before he can prescribe a treatment to cure or alleviate human suffering.

Your Medical Advisory Committee believes also that before a medical man endeavors to give an opinion about the results of others there are certain correlated facts that must be taken into consideration.

As a consultant or an expert he must have an extensive knowledge of the truths involved before he can pass sound judgment, which is the mental faculty of deciding correctly by the comparison of facts and ideas. His opinion then is worthy of consideration.

Too many of us in judging another man's work are inclined to do so hastily without study or reasoning. By giving erroneous opinions based on a lack of knowledge, and therefore faulty judgment, we start a large number of malpractice cases each year in Minnesota.

If without Knowledge, and hence lacking sound Judgment, we attempt to give correct Opinions and fail, the shame is ours and the results must be disastrous to the members of our profession.

Minnesota State Board of Medical Examiners

Self Styled Dutch Scientist Found Not Guilty by Duluth Jury

Re: State of Minnesota vs. Martin W. Pretorius.

Following a trial lasting three days in the District Court of St. Louis County, Martin W. Pretorius was found not guilty by a jury of eight women and four men. The defendant was charged, in an information filed by Thomas J. Naylor, County Attorney of St. Louis County, with practicing healing without a basic science certificate. The presiding judge was the Honorable Edwin J. Kenny.

Pretorius was arrested on July 14, 1937, at the Hotel Duluth where he was representing himself as an "Eminent South African Dutch Scientist—Hollywood Publisher—Newspaper Columnist and National Authority on Corrective Feeding and Body Culture." Pretorius represented himself as the founder and director of the Food Chemistry Educational Institute, Box 1857, Hollywood, California. Pretorius' method of operation was to give a number of free so-called health lectures during which people were solicited to take a so-called Martin Pretorius Home Study Course in Food Science and Rational Living. The cost of this course was represented as being $15.00. The pamphlet further stated that supplementary instructions would be given to "assist each student in solving their own health problem." * * * "Please indicate the conditions in which you and the immediate members of your family are particularly interested by placing an 'X' in the square provided." Then followed a list of eighty diseases and conditions including Bright's disease, cancer, epilepsy, tumors and tuberculosis.

According to the Clerk of the District Court of Atlantic City, New Jersey, one Martin J. Pretorius pleaded guilty on February 11, 1930, to practicing medicine without a license and was fined $200.00. Pretorius did not take the witness stand in his own defense, nor did he call any witnesses in his behalf. The defendant probably was aware that he would be questioned, in the event he took the witness stand, with respect to his educational qualifications, as well as his scientific attainments. It is interesting to note that when the State had completed the presentation of its evidence and a motion was made by the defendant for a dismissal of the charge on the grounds that "the evidence is insufficient to sustain the allegations of the complaint" and that "the facts proven are insufficient to constitute and show the commission of a public offense," the motion was denied after careful consideration by Judge Kenny. This shows that the Court was satisfied that the evidence was sufficient to sustain the allegations of the complaint and that the facts proven were sufficient to constitute and show the commission of a public offense.

The case was well tried for the State by Mr. Victor H. Johnson, Assistant County Attorney of St. Louis County. The defendant was represented by Mr. Jenswold of the law firm of Jenswold and Dahle.

Saint Paul Osteopath Removes Designation of "Aurist"

Re: Samuel M. Stern, D.O.

Following a complaint made to the Minnesota State Board of Medical Examiners that one Samuel M. Stern, a licensed osteopath with offices at 512 Hamm

Building, Saint Paul, was using the designation of "Aurist" on his door and stationery, an investigation was made of the matter by the Medical Board. A careful study of the osteopathic law of this state and other authorities, convinced the Board that an osteopath is not entitled to use that designation in Minnesota. The Minnesota osteopathic law specifically provides: "The practice of osteopathy is hereby declared distinct from that of medicine or surgery * * *." The Minnesota law also provides that an osteopath cannot furnish medicine for internal use, nor can he do major surgery. The accepted meaning of aurist undoubtedly is a physician who specializes in the treatment of diseases of the ear without any limitation as to the scope of the treatment. It seems logically to follow that the term osteopathy by the very nature of its statutory limitations, cannot, and does not harmonize with the accepted version of the term aurist.

The Minnesota State Board of Medical Examiners so notified Stern and after consulting with his lawyers, Stern removed the designation.

Wright County Optometrist Pleads Guilty to Practicing Medicine Without a License

Re: State of Minnesota vs. Benjamin E. Nelson.

On April 25, 1938, Benjamin E. Nelson, who maintains an office to practice optometry at Buffalo, Minnesota, entered a plea of guilty to an information charging him with practicing medicine without a license. Nelson entered this plea of guilty before the Honorable Leonard Keyes, Judge of the District Court for Wright County. After a presentation of the facts by Mr. Thomas P. Welch, County Attorney, and Mr. Brist on behalf of the State Board of Medical Examiners, Judge Keyes sentenced Nelson to a term of one year in the Minneapolis Workhouse. The execution of this sentence was stayed and Nelson was ordered to pay the costs of the prosecution, to refrain from practicing medicine and to report to the State Board of Parole. Nelson was arrested on March 8, 1938, following a complaint being filed against him by Mr. Brist, attorney for the State Board of Medical Examiners. The investigation conducted by the Medical Board disclosed that Nelson, despite a warning given him in 1935, was practicing medicine by prescribing diet, furnishing medicine to patients and examining specimens of urine. Prior to being warned in 1935, Nelson's method of operating was to give patients slips of paper which were to be taken to Beutner's Drug Store at Buffalo. These slips called for formula No. 1, No. 2, No. 3, et cetera. After he was warned, Nelson did his prescribing by word of mouth rather than in writing.

A most unusual incident occurred in the final disposition of the case, Nelson being represented by Mr. C. S. Hawker, a lawyer of Buffalo, who also was the Justice of the Peace before whom Nelson was arraigned. Mr. Hawker described Nelson as an outstanding citizen of Buffalo, while Nelson himself attributed his prosecution to the jealousy of the medical profession. It is a rather strange thing, but some persons who are prosecuted for practicing medicine without a license, never seem quite fully to understand that the question before the Court is their guilt or innocence, and that by entering a plea of guilty, the facts speak for themselves.

The State Board of Medical Examiners wishes to acknowledge the splendid coöperation of Mr. Welch, the County Attorney. Mr. Welch promptly instituted a prosecution when the evidence, consisting of numerous bottles of medicine and other exhibits, was presented to him.

OF GENERAL INTEREST

Scientific Exhibitors

The gold medal of the Southern Minnesota Medical Association will be presented to the physician presenting the best exhibit of his work at the Minnesota State Medical Association meeting in Duluth.

This medal is presented annually as an encouragement to individual research by Minnesota medical men.

Dr. Donald Lowell Paulson of Rochester was married to Margaret Willius of Saint Paul, early in March.

* * *

Dr. C. E. Anderson of Brainerd has been elected chief of staff of St. Joseph's Hospital in Brainerd.

* * *

Dr. Henry Silver, formerly of Sebeka, has moved to Belview, where he will engage in the practice of medicine.

* * *

Dr. and Mrs. M. M. Hursh of Cohasset have returned from the south after enjoying a vacation of several months.

* * *

Dr. and Mrs. F. M. Manson of Worthington have returned from a southern trip which included a Caribbean cruise.

* * *

Dr. Jerome Scanlan of Minneapolis has moved to Pine City to become associated with Dr. A. K. Stratte in the practice of medicine.

* * *

Dr. Arden L. Abraham of Minneapolis has become associated with Drs. Gage Clement and J. R. McNutt of Duluth, in the practice of radiology.

* * *

Dr. S. W. Harrington of Rochester presided at the meeting of the American Association for Thoracic Surgery, which met in Atlanta, Georgia, early in April.

* * *

Dr. and Mrs. E. J. Kaufman, formerly of Appleton, have located in Anoka. Mrs. Kaufman is also a physician, and both will engage in the practice of medicine.

* * *

Dr. William Elliott, formerly of Newark, Illinois, has become associated with the Lenont-Peterson Clinic of Virginia. Dr. Elliott specializes in urology and skin diseases.

* * *

Dr. Carl D. Kolset, who has practiced medicine in Sanborn for the past thirteen years, has announced his retirement from active practice. His practice will be continued by Dr. R. J. Cairns.

Dr. L. E. Claydon of Red Wing has returned from a trip to South America. After spending three weeks on the Amazon he visited Peru, Ecuador, Colombia and Venezuela, taking moving pictures of various places of interest.

* * *

Dr. H. E. Michelson of Minneapolis addressed the Stutzman County Medical Society in Jamestown, North Dakota, at their annual meeting on March 31. A banquet was served before the meeting, and members from the surrounding societies attended.

* * *

The New York Academy of Medicine will hold its Eleventh Annual Graduate Fortnight October 24 to November 4, 1938. This year's session will be devoted to Diseases of the Blood and Blood Forming Organs. Those interested may write Dr. Mahlon Ashford, care of the Academy at 2 East 103rd Street, New York City.

* * *

Dr. A. E. Henslin of Le Roy, treasurer of the Mower County Medical Society for more than fifteen years, was recently presented with a box of Nottingham cigars by the society members. Dr. Henslin has been incapacitated since January, due to a frost-bitten toe, but expects to have recovered in a few more weeks.

* * *

Dr. John L. McKelvey, at present a professor in the Peiping Union Medical College, China, has been appointed head of the department of obstetrics and gynecology at the University of Minnesota to take the position held for many years by Dr. Jennings C. Litzenberg, who will retire this spring. Dr. McKelvey was born in Kingston, Ontario, and is a graduate of Queens University.

The Board of Regents announces a gift of $10,000 from Mrs. John Dwan, the mother of Dr. Paul Dwan of the Department of Pediatrics, for the inauguration of a serum center at the University of Minnesota.

The Board of Regents also accepted a gift of $7,300 from the Citizens Aid Society of Minneapolis for the purchase of an additional Roentgen Therapy machine for the Cancer Institute.

* * *

Dr. R. M. Wilder of Rochester attended the meeting of the American Institute of Nutrition in Baltimore early in April, and conducted a round table discussion on diabetes at the meeting of the American College of Physicians in New York. He also addressed the meeting of the Postgraduate Assembly in Danville, Pa. Dr. Wilder will also attend the meeting of the Association of American Physicians in Atlantic City early in May, and will deliver the Mary Scott Newbold lecture before the College of Physicians in Philadelphia.

The Journal of Neurophysiology made its debut in January of this year. Its purpose is to concentrate in one periodical, experimental work on the functions of the nervous system, peripheral and central. Appearing bimonthly, contributions will be selected four weeks prior to publication, contributions not chosen to be returned to the author. This method will assure prompt publication of the important experimental work being done in this field. The editorial board consists of J. G. Dusser de Barenne and J. F. Fulton of Yale, and R. W. Gerard of Chicago. The publication is of particular interest to our readers in that Dr. Fulton, a former resident of Saint Paul, is a member of the editorial board. The publication doubtless fulfills a long present need and has our best wishes for its success.

* * *

Dr. Carl C. Chatterton last month was awarded the International Distinguished Service Medal for 1937 by the Cosmopolitan Club of Saint Paul. The medal is given each year to a resident of the city who during the past twelve months has rendered outstanding and unselfish civic service without remuneration. It is, of course, a recognition of Dr. Chatterton's services rendered crippled children at the Gillette State Hospital. For twenty-seven years he has been associated in this work and since Dr. Gillette's death has directed the policies of the State Hospital for Crippled Children. Dr. Chatterton has also shaped the policy for the Federal Social Security service in Minnesota in so far as it relates to crippled children and the set-up in this state is conceded to be the most efficient of any state.

* * *

Medical Department Reservists

The annual postgraduate course and clinical conference given by the Clinics in St. Louis for Reserves of the Medical Department of the United States Army will be held May 23 to 28, inclusive.

The regular enrollment fee of $10.00 is waived for Reserve Officers and the only expense will be a fee of $2.50 to cover the cost of the dinner honoring the Corps Area Commander and the cost of incidentals.

Appropriate military credits will be given for attendance.

* * *

Tenth Anniversary Medical Broadcast

Dr. William A. O'Brien gave his 520th weekly radio talk over WCCO, under the auspices of the Minnesota State Medical Association, Saturday, April 2.

The occasion marked a milestone in radio broadcasting in the Northwest, particularly in the use of radio for health education, and it was noted by a special tenth anniversary program at the regular program hour on Saturday, April 2, by Dr. J. M. Hayes of Minneapolis, president, and Dr. R. M. Burns, of Saint Paul, chairman of the radio committee of the Association, and by Max Karl, director of education for station WCCO.

A luncheon followed at which Doctor O'Brien was guest of honor and to which leaders in medical and health education and in radio activities in Minnesota

were invited. Among the speakers at this luncheon for which Doctor Burns acted as toastmaster were H. A. Bellows, station manager for WCCO at the time when the program began, Doctor Hayes, Dr. B. J. Branton of Willmar, R. R. Price, director of the extension division and chairman of the radio committee of the University of Minnesota, and many others.

Over the air and at the luncheon, physicians and experts in radio extended their congratulations to Doctor O'Brien and his sponsoring association and paid tribute to the unique radio gift of Doctor O'Brien which has enabled him to continue the program with continuously increasing popularity for this record period of years.

The Minnesota State Medical Association program, with Doctor O'Brien as speaker, was hailed as a model of its sort and acknowledged as one of the pioneers in educational broadcasting.

Radio officials pointed out, among other things, that Doctor O'Brien is accorded the unusual privilege of speaking only from notes rather than from a censored manuscript and that this faculty for talking spontaneously and directly to his listeners had much to do with his personal popularity as a speaker and teacher. Physicians pointed out that Doctor O'Brien, in all his years of regular broadcasting, had never veered from the standards of accuracy and medical ethics set for its public education program by the State Medical Association, that he had worked conscientiously with practicing physicians with whom his listeners discuss the broadcasts and that he had assisted materially in keeping medical men alert to new developments in practice.

The weekly program hour is now Saturday at 9:45 a. m.

Hospital Notes

Dr. C. I. Krantz of Duluth has been named chief of staff, and Dr. J. H. Peterson, secretary, of the Hearding Hospital, Duluth.

* * *

Minnesota Hospital Service Association

On the evening of April 18, the Minnesota Hospital Service Association held a dinner meeting to which were invited individuals from various Twin City activities to commemorate the occasion of the approval of the Association by the American Hospital Association. The Minnesota Association was one of thirty-eight throughout the country to receive this approval, and the only one in the state.

Mr. A. G. Stasel, Superintendent of Eitel Hospital in Minneapolis, and president of the Association, presided and paid tribute to the group of Saint Paulites who had the temerity and perseverance to initiate the Association which began its activities in June, 1933, as the Saint Paul Hospital Association, and in 1935 adopted its present name when the Minneapolis hospitals joined. Today

(Continued on Page 351)

◆ REPORTS and ANNOUNCEMENTS ◆

MEDICAL BROADCAST FOR MAY
The Minnesota State Medical Association Morning Health Service

The Minnesota State Medical Association broadcasts weekly at 9:45 o'clock every Saturday morning over Station WCCO, Minneapolis and Saint Paul (810 kilocycles or 370.2 meters).

Speaker: William A. O'Brien, M.D., Associate Professor of Pathology and Preventive Medicine, Medical School, University of Minnesota. The program for the month will be as follows:

May 7—Sun and Air
May 14—Research and the Hospital
May 21—Periodic Health Examination
May 28—Protective Foods and the Teeth

MEDICAL SEMINAR
ASSOCIATED HARVARD CLUBS

The Medical School Seminar at the 41st Annual Meeting of the Associated Harvard Clubs to be held at the Palmer House, Chicago, Illinois, on May 20, 21 and 22 next, promises to be an outstanding feature of the meeting. It will mark Dr. Burwell's first visit to Chicago in his official capacity as dean. The program is as follows:

The Harvard Medical School in 1938........ Dr. C. Sidney Burwell, Dean and Research Professor of Clinical Medicine.

Trends in Pre-clinical Teaching .... Dr. A. Baird Hastings, Hamilton Kuhn Professor of Biological Chemistry.

The Tutorial System in the Harvard Medical School.......... Dr. Walter Bauer, Associate Professor and Tutor in Medicine.

The Surgical Curriculum of Today....... Dr. Elliott C. Cutler, Moseley Professor of Surgery.

Discussion by......... Dr. Joseph T. Wearn, Professor and Head of the Dept. of Medicine, Western Reserve University, Cleveland, and Mr. Laird Bell, Chairman of the Educational Committee, Board of Trustees, University of Chicago.

The Seminar will begin about 2:30 p. m. on Saturday, May 21, immediately following a joint luncheon of all the schools beginning at 12:30 p. m., during which Frederick Roy Martin and William Allen White will speak briefly.

All graduates of the University are invited to attend. A limited number of admission cards are available for non-Harvard men who are particularly interested in medical education. These may be obtained by writing to Willard O. Thompson, M.D., Chairman of the Medical School Committee, 700 North Michigan Avenue, Chicago, Ill.

THE STATE MEETING

The 85th annual meeting of the Minnesota State Medical Association will be held in Duluth at the Hotel Duluth just before the Fourth of July holidays and therefore holds a special appeal this year, not only for those who are attracted by the distinguished scientific program but also for those who want to combine attendance at the meeting with a pleasant vacation in Northern Minnesota.

Unusual extra-meeting activities have been arranged for both the physicians and their wives so as to take full advantage of the place and time of meeting. One is the golf tournament to be held Saturday morning, July 2, following the close, Friday afternoon, of the scientific sessions. Another is the long boat trip on one of the big lake boats leaving the docks early in the morning and returning after luncheon in the afternoon.

The scientific session and exhibits, alike, are designed by the Committee on Scientific Assembly to be of value especially to the busy general practitioner. Emphasis is laid upon improved methods of treatment for conditions encountered in daily practice rather than upon the exceptional problems of medicine.

Among the interesting entries in the exhibit section is the prize-winning fracture exhibit of the Mayo Clinic, the exhibit on treatment of syphilis from the American Medical Association, the demonstration of pneumonia treatment by the Minnesota Department of Health and the demonstration of a simplified method of blood transfusion from the Department of Surgery of the University Medical School. In addition there will be daily lectures on diabetes at the exhibit and demonstration hours by the Committee on Diabetes and many other important exhibits by individuals and institutions, including an entire section devoted to scientific work of Duluth members and institutions.

Dr. Howard Haggard of Yale heads a distinguished list of guest speakers which includes Dr. Irvin Abell, president-elect of the American Medical Association; Dr. Roland Cron of Milwaukee; Dr. Hollis Potter of Chicago, who will give the annual Russell D. Carman lectureship; Dr. Edward Jackson of Denver; Dr. Philip Lewin of Chicago and Dr. Karl Meyer of Chicago; Dr. E. K. Marshall of Johns Hopkins and Dr. C. Anderson Aldrich of Winnetka, Ill.

For the medical economics section scheduled for Friday morning, July 1, from 11 a. m. to 12, the speakers will be Dr. J. M. Hayes, Minneapolis, president of the association, who will give his presidential address at that time; Chief Justice H. M. Gallagher of the Supreme Court of Minnesota and Mr. S. B. Houck of Minneapolis, representing the Minnesota Bar Association.

The first Herman M. Johnson memorial lecture will be given at a luncheon meeting to be held at the hotel Friday noon. Governor Elmer A. Benson, long a friend of Dr. Johnson and well acquainted with his work, will be the lecturer.

Dr. Haggard will give the principal address at a public health meeting to be held Wednesday night at the Lyceum theater. The public will be invited to this meeting, which is sponsored jointly with the State Association and the St. Louis County Medical Society by the St. Louis County Public Health Association.

The annual banquet of the association will be held Thursday night at the hotel, with Dr. Haggard and Dr. Abell as speakers. It will be followed by dancing.

Round table luncheons arranged for Monday and Tuesday represent a departure in state meeting programs. The subject for the Monday luncheon will be social hygiene, and Dr. W. A. O'Brien will be the principal speaker and discussion leader.

All of the speakers at the Tuesday morning session will be invited to attend the Tuesday luncheon to answer questions and lead the informal discussion of the morning's program.

The annual meeting of the Women's Auxiliary will be held Thursday morning, to be followed by the annual luncheon at the Northland Country Club. The usual Board meeting will take place Wednesday at the hotel to be followed in the late afternoon by a tea at the Woman's Club.

AMERICAN ASSOCIATION OF INDUSTRIAL PHYSICIANS

Preventive medicine will be the keynote of the 23rd annual meeting of the American Association of Industrial Physicians and Surgeons which will be held concurrently with the Midwest Conference on Occupational Diseases at the Palmer House in Chicago, June 6, 7, 8 and 9, 1938.

Dr. Edward C. Holmblad, 28 E. Jackson Blvd., Chicago, Chairman of the Program Committee, announces the most interesting program in the history of this organization.

Advance programs of the meeting are available to any doctor interested and will be sent without charge to any practicing physician interested in attending this meeting. The sessions will be open to any practicing physician in accordance with the educational program of the Association to spread the propaganda of preventive medicine, and absenteeism of employes.

For an advance copy of the program or for information on exhibits, address—Mr. A. G. Park, 540 No. Michigan Avenue, Chicago.

WASHINGTON COUNTY

The Washington County Medical Society met April 12. During dinner two representatives of the American Benefit Association spoke on the Association's hospital benefit insurance policy.

The survey of medical care to be conducted by the American Medical Association in coöperation with county societies throughout the country was explained.

The meeting was then addressed by Dr. Carl Larsen of Saint Paul on the subject of "Sinus Disease" with special emphasis on surgical treatment.

In Memoriam

John T. Gill
1858-1938

DR. JOHN T. GILL of Echo, Minnesota, died suddenly on February 28, 1938, while making a call. He was eighty years of age.

John T. Gill was born February 26, 1858, at Monroeville, Ohio, where he grew to manhood. He attended Western Reserve College at Cleveland, and in 1886 received his medical degree from the New York Medical College.

After practicing in Monroeville for four years, Dr. Gill went to Kansas City, Missouri, where he practiced two years in the Cherry Street Hospital. He than practiced two years in Chicago, moving in 1895, to Echo, Minnesota, where he had practiced for forty-three years. The esteem in which he was held by his many patients and friends in the locality in which he practiced so long was well expressed in local newspapers. He never refused to respond to a call even in the early days when long trips over the prairie in winter necessitated the use of cutter or bob sled.

Dr. Gill was married October 9, 1895, to Blanche McClure at Redwood Falls. He is survived by his widow and seven children. He was a member of the Masonic order and had served on the village council and school board and as health officer.

Clarence Moors Golden
1877-1938

DR. Clarence M. Golden, of Tyler, Minnesota, passed away on March 23, 1938. He had been in poor health for the past two years and confined to his bed since August.

Dr. Golden was born at Marston, Michigan, June 30, 1877. After attending local schools he was a student for two years at the University of Michigan and received his medical degree from the St. Louis College of Medicine in St. Louis, Missouri, in 1906.

On November 6, 1905, Dr. Golden was married to Helen Grant of Bemidji. Her untimely death occurred in 1935. Dr. Golden was a member of the Lenont Hospital Staff in Virginia, Minnesota, for some eight years before removing to Ruthton in 1914. In 1920 he became affiliated with the Tyler Clinic and Hospital, which has been established by Dr. A. L. Vadheim.

Dr. Golden served as county coroner of Lincoln County for four years and had been active in Red Cross work, especially at the time of the World War. He was an able surgeon and conscientious in the care of his patients. He is survived by his son Harold and a sister, Mrs. Ruth Simpson, both of whom helped care for him during his last illness. He is also survived by a half sister, Mrs. D. G. Knapp, and his stepmother, Mrs. O. J. Golden, both of Kalamazoo, Michigan.

Clarence R. Morss

1880-1938

DR. CLARENCE R. MORSS of Zumbrota passed away at the Colonial Hospital, Rochester, Minnesota, on March 23, 1938.

He was born in Ledgedale, Pennsylvania, May 1, 1880, and accompanied his family to Scranton, Pennsylvania, in 1893. He attended school in Lackawanna and Scranton and in 1904 graduated from Lehigh College with a B.A. degree. He received his M.D. degree from the University of Pennsylvania in 1908, having been a member of the H. C. Wood Medical Society during his internship at the Philadelphia Methodist Hospital the following year.

Dr. Morss arrived at Coleraine, Minnesota, in April, 1910, to become attached to the staff of the Coleraine Hospital, a United States Steel Corporation institution. Resigning from this work in 1913, he practiced in Duluth until February, 1914, when he moved to Zumbrota, Minnesota, remaining there until April, 1917, when he returned to Coleraine. In May, 1918, he joined the medical corps of the army and was stationed at Camp Greenleaf and later at Fort Oglethorpe before spending ten months overseas, principally in France. Upon leaving military service in September, 1919, he relocated in Zumbrota, where he has continuously practiced.

Dr. Morss was prominent in social and civic affairs at Zumbrota. He had been president of the Zumbrota Golf Club, president of the Commercial Club and president of the Board of Health. He was a member of the St. Louis County Medical Society, Minnesota State and American Medical Associations. He was also a Knight of Pythias and a member of the Presbyterian church.

Homer Francis Peirson

1867-1938

MARCH 24, 1938, marked the passing of one of Austin's oldest physicians, at least in years of service. Doctor Peirson had practiced in the community of Austin since 1896, when he went there from Minneapolis upon completion of his internship.

Homer Francis Peirson was born Stepember 11, 1867, on a farm near Stewartville, Minnesota, where his parents came from Wisconsin in 1854. In 1874 his parents moved to Grand Meadow and there he attended school. He then spent one year at Carleton College, Northfield, Minnesota. In 1891, he graduated from the University of Minnesota. He took up the study of medicine at the Rush Medical College in Chicago, where he graduated. He then spent one year in intern work at St. Mary's Hospital in Minneapolis.

Doctor Peirson took little part in local politics, but served as coroner for a number of years and as president of the old Mower County Medical Society the year he came to Austin. He was a member of the state and national medical societies for a number of years. He was a member of a number of fraternal

organizations, serving as medical examiner for them. Doctor Peirson had but two real interests in life—his profession and his family. He leaves a widow and two daughters. He was always kind and considerate in his home, a devoted father, and friendly to all.

Although he had been in failing health the past two years he refused to give up his life's work, his practice of medicine. He went each day to his office and it was there he suffered the cerebral hemorrhage from which he died a few hours later.

Ira M. Roadman

1865-1938

DR. Ira M. Roadman of Minneapolis died in February following an emergency operation performed during a vacation trip to Mexico.

Born in Stahlstown, Pennsylvania, he was educated in Cedar Falls, Iowa, and at Cornell College, Iowa, receiving his medical degree from Minnesota.

For several years Dr. Roadman was chief medical attendant for the Duluth, Missabe and Northern Railway at Duluth. He later practiced at Onamia, Minnesota, and during the World War was stationed at Fort Leavenworth in the Medical Corps. In 1919 he entered the United States medical service for Indians and was stationed at Ponsford, Minnesota. In 1931 he retired and had since lived in Minneapolis.

Dr. Roadman was a thirty-third degree Scottish Rite Mason and a member of the Methodist Church. He is survived by his widow, a son, Howard R., and a daughter, Bernice.

HOSPITAL NOTES

(Continued from Page 348)

the Association numbers 163,000, including dependents, in its membership, being surpassed by only one similar association, that in New York City.

After listening to selections rendered by a quartet of nurses from the Deaconess Hospital of Minneapolis, Mayor Gehan of Saint Paul presented the certificate of approval to the president of the Association and paid tribute to the officers and trustees of the Association.

Mr. E. A. Van Steenwyk, executive secretary of the Association, presented some interesting figures in connection with the Association. Since the beginning of the Association's activities a total of about $750,000 has been paid out to hospitals for service rendered; about 400 members are now daily provided hospital care with an overhead cost last month of 11.1 per cent; every fifth person one meets on the streets of the Twin Cities is a member or dependent of the organization; 46 per cent of the members have their hospital bills paid entirely by the Association; an additional 44 per cent pay less than $10.00 for their stay in the hospital, and the remaining 10 per cent pay over $10.00.

In concluding the program, Dr. W. A. O'Brien talked on the service hospitals supply, and mentioned the high standing of hospitals in Minnesota.

PERFORATING HEMORRHAGIC (ENDO-METRIAL) OVARIAN CYSTS.*

CHARLES A. HALLBERG, M.D.

In 1921 Sampson[1] published his first contribution dealing with a type of ovarian blood cyst heretofore variously designated as tarry, chocolate, perforating and hemorrhagic cyst. The term "ovarian cysts of endometrial origin" was suggested to distinguish this type of cyst from other ovarian hematomas.

As a result of the above and succeeding contributions by Sampson[2] dealing with this subject, the disorder was quickly accepted as a clinical and pathological entity and is now commonly designated as endometriosis or endometrioma of the ovary.

Endometrium within the ovary was first described by Russel[3] in 1899, which he believed represented an inclusion of the Müllerian duct. Pick[4] in 1905, in a notable study of ovarian hematomata, gave the first description of a typical chocolate cyst, and, furthermore, described the functional as well as morphological resemblance of the epithelial lining of the cyst wall to endometrium. The following quotation of his paper is from the translation by Graves[5]:

"As a result of the glandular development of the germinal epithelium, its invasion of the ovarian substance and the round cell proliferation of the surrounding stroma, there occurs in the ovary a form of adenoma which reflects a perfect likeness to the endometrium of the corpus uteri—adenoma ovarii endometroides; this tumor is especially likely to be associated with fibroids of the uterus.

"The ovary is in such cases either insignificant (pure adenoma) or cystic (cystadenoma) and may reach the size of a goose egg. The single or multiple cysts are distinguished by a syrupy chocolate colored or more reddish content; and a more or less pigmented mucus-like membrane of the type of endometrium of the corpus uteri. The pigment of the contents and the 'mucosa' is derived from hemorrhages which follow the participation of the endometrial-like tissue in the menstrual and other congestions of the internal genital organs."

The prevalent theories of origin of endometrial cysts of the ovary may be divided into two groups: (1) the serosal theory and (2) the implantation theory.

The serosal theory owes its development mainly to Robert Meyer.[6] He points out that the pelvic peritoneum has its origin in the cœlomic mesothelium. He demonstrated that stimulation or injury of the pelvic peritoneum by means of inflammation may produce, during the processes of healing, a metaplasia of serosal cells enabling them to develop endometrial-like glandular structures.

This theory may be applied to the germinal epithelium on the surface of the ovary. Pick, as noted in the above quotation, ascribed the endometrial structure within the ovary to metaplasia and invasion of the germinal epithelium.

Novak[7] suggests that disturbances in endocrine function may serve as a stimulant to the formation of aberrant endometrium.

Sampson's implantation theory arises from the observation of blood flowing from the fallopian tubes during a pelvic operation performed either immediately following a curettement of the uterus or, more commonly, at the time of menstruation. He proved that blood thus regurgitated through the fallopian tubes carried with it fragments of uterine or tubal mucosa. These fragments of endometrium, falling upon the ovary, possess the ability to invade its surface and, with continued growth, develop into glandular or adenomatous structures. The adenomata thus formed react to menstruation in a manner similar to that of the uterine mucosa. The accumulated and retained menstrual blood results in the formation of blood cysts.

On the surface of the ovary, these hematomata appear as single or multiple minute purple cysts. Deeper penetration into the ovary results in the formation of cysts varying in size, filled with menstrual blood. As the cysts gradually enlarge with each menstrual cycle, rupture eventually occurs, spilling the contents of the cyst into the pelvis. The escape of fragments of aberrant endometrium may result in the formation of new implants upon the various pelvic structures. Dense adhesions are formed between the site of perforation and adjacent pelvic structures.

King[8] believes that so-called endometrial cysts develop from structures within the ovary. He describes numerous instances of tarry corpus luteum cysts and tarry cysts of the atretic follicle identical in gross and histological structure with endometrial cysts. The origin of the epithelial lining of the cyst wall is not established but he states it arises probably by metaplasia from cells which are present in the ovary.

Pathology.—The diameter of endometrial cysts usually varies from 2 to 6 cm. They may be single or multiple. When multiple cysts exist, they frequently communicate with each other, suggesting the occurrence of rupture of the wall into neighboring cysts.

The outer surface of the cyst is bluish gray in color and usually presents a wrinkled appearance. There are two striking and characteristic features of the appearance of these cysts after their removal, namely the presence of one or more perforations of the cyst wall, with a thick roughened area of ovarian tissue around it, indicating the site of dense adhesions; the second, the exceptionally thick walls of the cyst which stand apart and do not collapse after the contents have escaped.

The lining of the cyst cavity is usually stained a deep brown, from the retained blood. The contents of the cyst resemble thick chocolate syrup.

*Inaugural thesis.

The diagnostic feature of endometrial cysts is the discovery of an epithelial lining. Sampson describes the epithelium as being low cuboidal or columnar resting on a vascular stroma, sometimes containing gland-like structures resembling uterine glands. The stroma shows evidence of recent or of old hemorrhage.

The extent of the epithelial lining is variable. It may be found only at the site of perforation; it may line the entire cyst or a part of it; or may occasionally be entirely absent.

According to Sampson's investigations, the epithelial lining may be more or less completely cast off in certain phases of its reaction to menstruation. As regeneration of the epithelial lining occurs, it may exist only in limited areas.

Portions of the cyst not lined by epithelium consist of ovarian stroma and usually some areas of luteal membrane.

The routine pathological examination in the hospital laboratory fails to discover epithelial structures in the majority of instances, and as luteal cells are commonly encountered, the pathological diagnosis is usually corpus luteum cyst. It, however, seems probable that if studies were made of the entire lining of the cyst, discovery of adenomatous structures would be materially increased.

Endothelial cysts are infrequent before the age of thirty and rare before the twenty-fifth year. Approximately 10 per cent occur in the second decade. Their number is about 25 per cent greater in the fourth decade than in the third. If pregnancy has occurred, it is commonly limited to a single instance.

Its incidence among single and married women is about equal. A history of a previous pelvic infection is notably infrequent.

The almost universal existence of dense adhesions to neighboring structures makes for a varied and extensive symptomatology. Additional complexities in diagnosis may be provided by associated endometrial implants disturbing the function of the urinary and intestinal tracts.

The leading symptom is pain, in the form of dysmenorrhea of the acquired type. Pelvic pain may be present or absent throughout the menstrual interval, but in any event it is almost certain to be increased a few days prior to and during the menstrual period. It is usually described as an aching in the lower abdomen and frequently as backache in the sacral region.

Some form of disturbance of the menstrual flow is the rule, usually causing prolonged or increased flow, or both. This group of symptoms are quite identical with those met with in a case of subacute or chronic pelvic infection.

The information obtained by pelvic examination is frequently misleading. The usual characteristic features of an ovarian cyst, namely, a rounded elastic tumor, movable and readily identified as being separate from the uterus, are physical signs entirely foreign to a typical adherent hemorrhagic cyst. Instead, one finds a mass of indefinite outline, almost invariably with more or less fixation, in most instances intimately attached to the uterus, often nodular in the lowermost portions and usually sensitive to pressure. They may particularly re-

semble uterine fibroids occurring near or in the cervix.

Not infrequently, a relatively small cyst with numerous perforations and extensive attachments to the uterus, broad ligament, small intestine, sigmoid and omentum will produce a mass filling one-half of the pelvis.

Surgical procedures in this disorder are necessarily governed by the age of the patient, the extent of involvement of the ovaries, the condition of the uterus, and the existence of endometrial implants in other organs. If the disorder is localized in one ovary, and implants elsewhere are absent, removal of the involved ovary has usually proved to be sufficient. With extensive bilateral involvement, removal of both ovaries, with or without hysterectomy, generally is indicated. In young women, excision of the cysts may be tried, though reports indicate that recurrence is likely.

Bibliography

1. Graves: Textbook of gynecology, p. 445. Philadelphia: W. B. Saunders Co. 1928.
2. King, E. S. J.: The origin of "endometriosis" of the ovary. Surg., Gyn. and Obst., 53:22, 1931.
3. Meyer, R., and Kitai: Endometrial adenomyosis and aberrant cells. Zentralbl. f. Gynak., 48:2449, 1924.
4. Novak, E.: Significance of uterine mucosa in fallopian tube with discussion of aberrant endometrium. Amer. Jour. Obst. and Gyn., 12:484, 1926.
5. Pick, L.: Tumor formation in the genitals in hermaphrodites. Arch. f. Gynak., 76:191, 1905.
6. Russel, W. W.: Aberrant portions of the Müllerian duct found in an ovary. Johns Hopkins Hospital Bull., 10:8, 1899.
7. Sampson, J. A.: Perforating hemorrhagic (chocolate) cysts of the ovary. Their importance and especially their relation to pelvic adenomas of endometrial type. Arch. Surg., 3:245, 1921.
8. Sampson, J. A.: Life history of ovarian hematomas. Amer. Jour. Obst. and Gyn., 4:451, 1922.

MEDIAN NERVE SUTURE, NEUROLYSIS OF ULNAR NERVE, PLASTIC REPAIR AND RESECTION OF ULNA FOR DEFORMITY OF HAND

ARTHUR F. BRATRUD, M.D.

This patient, Miss S. S., at present twenty-two years of age, was first seen in August, 1926. She gave the following history at that time. While living in Madagascar she accidentally fell out of a tree, landing on the right hand with the hand partially adducted and the hand flexed. This occurred about January 5, 1925. She received a compound fracture of the wrist, with one of the bones sticking out through the broken skin. She was attended by a physician on the island, who applied a cast after reduction of the fracture. An infection resulted and the cast was removed. This was followed by extension around the wrist by means of a bandage. This bandage cut into the skin and an infection resulted in the sides of the wrist as well as lower end of the forearm and wrist. She was up and out of bed by the first of February, 1925. The wounds were not entirely healed until August, 1925. Later she received massage treatments, during the time that she was in Madagascar. She stated that she could bend the hand at the wrist slightly, but had no motion in the fingers in any direction. She complained at that time that she had no feeling in the radial side of the palm of the hand or on the flexor surface of the thumb, first and second fingers, and very slight sensation on the ulnar side of the palm of the hand, and flexor side of the third and fourth fingers, as well as the corresponding area on the back of the hand. She also stated there was complete numbness on the back of the thumb, first and second fingers, and that she could turn the hand but very little.

When examined there was a dense, thick, heavy scar, about two and one-half inches in length, covering the entire flexor surface of the wrist and the lower part of the forearm. This seemed to be fixed to the bone. Pronation and supination at the wrist was very nearly nil. Fingers were held slightly separated, with no semblance of adduction, abduction, extension, or flexion. The hand was held in a position of abduction with the ulna pressing out into the skin and shoving the hand into that position. There was present very slight flexion and extension and slight abduction and adduction at the wrist.

This case presented a very poor outlook as far as ultimate good result was concerned. However, on August 23, 1926, she was operated upon at Fairview Hospital, at which time the following findings were present. There was complete severance of the median nerve at the wrist and a large amount of scar tissue around the ulnar nerve at this location. There was a mass of scar tissue between the profundus and sublimis digitorum muscles, and the ends of the tendons at the wrist. It appeared as though there were no tendons passing through this scar tissue. The mass of scar tissue, anterior to the radius, ulna and pronator quadratus muscle was completely dissected away. The median nerve was resected to a point when the fasciculi appeared normal. On account of the amount of the destruction of the median nerve it was extremely difficult to obtain apposition of the severed ends. A neurolysis of the ulnar nerve was performed. The hand had to be put up in an extreme degree of flexion in order to secure apposition of the severed ends of the median nerve, even after loosening this up into the middle third of the forearm. A predicle fat flap from the chest wall was then attached, splitting the fat fascia and replacing a layer between the scar tissue and the bones of the forearm, pronator quadratus and carpal bones. This left a good layer of fat anterior and posterior to the nerve and scar tissue. The pedicle flap wound was dressed with a parowax dressing as follows: Open sterile gauze is dipped in warm melted sterile parowax, and applied at once, before the parowax hardens to the skin and raw surfaces. This does not have to be removed before separation of the flap, and allows painless dressing. On September 7th, a resection of the pedicle flap from the chest to the right forearm was performed. A plastic closure of the raw areas of the chest was performed at this time. The flap was in very good condition. On January 5, 1927, a resection of the lower end of the ulna above the epiphysis was performed about one inch above the lower end of the bone, so as to allow the wrist to assume a normal position. In July, 1927, there was beginning return of sensation in the median nerve distribution of the hand.

This girl was advised to try to use the hand as much as possible, and to keep up massage as much as possible. Several years later a letter was received from her, stating that her hand was improving so much that she could bend and separate the fingers, and was beginning to play the piano. She was not seen again until December, 1937, at which time the following findings were present. There had been complete loss of growth of the radius on account of the destruction of the epiphysis which had resulted at the time of the original injury. This was present when first seen in 1926. The ulna had continued growth again after resection and was protruding downward so as to throw the wrist into the position of marked abduction. There was very slight pronation and supination present at the wrist. Flexion and extension at the wrist was present to a moderate degree. Abduction and adduction of the fingers was present and the fingers could be flexed, but not sufficient to close the hand completely. Intrinsic muscular action of the hand had returned completely. There was

complete return of sensation in both the median and ulnar nerve distribution. The pedicle flap which had been separated from the chest was extremely thick and heavy. When an attempt was made to move the fingers it appeared as though there was a large amount of scar tissue holding the tendons at about the level of the annular ligament.

On December 12 at New Asbury Hospital, the pedicle flap was loosened and a large amount of fat, with some skin, was removed. At that time the area which had practically nothing but scar tissue between the muscles and tendons, had a group of tendons completely down through the fatty tissues. The fat tissue posterior to the scar tissue and tendons was well preserved. There was a mass of scar tissue at the lower end of the pedicle flap. Adhesions were freed and a closure of the wound was performed. Incision was made laterally to the ulna and the distal end of the ulna resected. Since this time she has been making very nice improvement again. There was impairment of function for a few weeks after the last operation. Pronation and supination has increased since December 12. She can now flex the fingers so that the fingers almost touch the palm of the hand. Abduction and adduction of the fingers is not quite as good as previous to the last operation, but is improving constantly from week to week, so that ultimately it will probably be very nearly normal. On account of the contraction of the flexor tendons the fingers can be completely extended only when the hand is flexed. It is also noted that the hand is very much smaller than the normal hand.

The striking feature about this case was the fact that nerve suture was performed one year and eight months after the original injury. The opinion prevails that nerve suture after eighteen months gives practically no results. However, here is a case which shows practically complete restoration of function, with suture being performed one year and eight months after the original injury or severance. Whether the destroyed epiphysis of the radius in this case was caused by infection or the injury, is difficult to say. However, it impaired the growth of the bone in the radius. The other striking feature is the fact that tendons which were not present at the time of the first operation in August, 1926, had grown or regenerated down through the fat so that there was a mass of tendons extending down through the fatty tissues.

This girl is normally a right handed individual. Since her injury she has educated her left hand so that now she is practically a left handed individual.

Discussion

DR. KENNETH BULKLEY: It was with considerable pleasure that I had the opportunity of seeing this patient in consultation with Dr. Bratrud a short time before he operated upon her for the second time, and also to have again had the opportunity of examining her a few days ago. Dr. Bratrud is to be congratulated on obtaining so useful a hand for a patient who originally seemed to have a hand hopelessly crippled as far as any real use of it was concerned. This case should not only serve as a lesson in optimism to us, but can also be used as a text for a few remarks on four different problems which it illustrates.

The first relates to the viability of transplanted fat. There has long been a controversy, more or less, as to whether transplanted fat remains as such or gradually undergoes fibrosis. I believe this case illustrates the fact that it does maintain its identity and viability. The first full thickness transplant which Dr. Bratrud made and the remains of which you now see was infinitely thicker than it now is, since Dr. Bratrud at the second sitting dressed it down. The pad was characteristic, soft and pliable, and Dr. Bratrud informs me that at operation there was very little, if any, signs of fibrosis in it.

The second problem relates to tendon regrowth or which might possibly better be termed tendon refunction. Dr. Bratrud informs me that when he first operated upon this girl some 11 years ago at the point where the tendons emerged from the fleshy bellies of the flexor muscles they disappeared into a mass of what appeared to be fibrous scar tissue, and you will remember that he made no attempt to separate these, if they existed, one from the other, but simply undermined this mass of scar tissue, interposing fat beneath it and also superficial to it beneath his skin flap; and yet you have seen demonstrated tonight how a hand, practically useless in the form of a "claw," has re-educated or re-differentiated or possibly, to a certain extent, regrown its tendons so that at least to a very serviceable extent they now function.

The third point of interest in this case to me seems to be the lack of growth of the radial epiphysis, which is probably more common in fractures of the ends of the long bones in children than is generally recognized. Compere,* in a recent report from Chicago, has investigated the growth arrest in long bones after fractures including the epiphysis. About thirty-five per cent of all fractures that had been treated in his Clinic occurred in children fourteen years or younger and fourteen per cent of these fractures in children involved the growth epiphysis; and of these involved cases that were cared for and followed over a period of six months with x-rays, ninety-five per cent of them showed growth disturbances. The method used by Dr. Bratrud in each operative sitting for the correction of this radial deviation by resection of a portion of the ulna is the classical procedure commonly used.

To me the most astounding result obtained in this case was the regeneration of both the median and ulna nerves. You will remember that this girl suffered her primary injury south of the southernmost tip of Africa and was not operated upon here in Minneapolis by Dr. Bratrud until approximately twenty months later. If I understand the situation correctly the median nerve was found completely divided and an end-to-end anastomosis was necessary, with marked flexion of the wrist thereafter in order to bridge the defect which so commonly occurs in these nerve divisions; and yet nine months later this girl was already beginning to show signs of regeneration and today she has complete regeneration of her median nerve. This is an almost unheard of result as far as I know for nerve regeneration where the repair has been made later than the sixth or at most the ninth month following severance. The regeneration of the ulna nerve is possibly easier to understand inasmuch as I believe it was not completely severed but merely thoroughly embedded in scar tissue, requiring only a neurolysis.

In view of the fact that no one of us as individuals see any large number of nerve trunk injuries, possibly it would be of value to refresh our memories as to what goes on in the regeneration of a nerve trunk, and for that purpose I am going to close my discussion by quoting Campbell† on the subject:

"After complete or partial severance the ruptured nerve fibres separate; the distal segment loses its function and undergoes degeneration. The injury produces an effusion of blood, and migration of leukocytes takes place into and about the end of the proximal segment and throughout the entire distal segment. The axis-cyl-

*J.A.M.A., 105:2140-2146, Dec. 28, 1935.
†Campbell: A Textbook of Orthopedic Surgery, 1930.

inders perish, the myelin sheath is absorbed and the cells along the inner surface of the neurilemma cease to proliferate. The sheath shrinks and becomes empty except for scattered masses of nuclei and protoplasm. The degeneration occurs rapidly, beginning within twenty-four hours after the injury, and is complete in a few days. The leukocytes are replaced by connective tissue cells which absorb the fatty myelin and the axis-cylinders, and the degenerated nerve trunk becomes hard, fibrous and cirrhosed. In the proximal end of the divided nerve, an end-bulb is formed by curling up of the prolonged nerve fibres and fibrous tissue. While degeneration occurs in a few days, regeneration requires months. The exact method of regeneration is uncertain. Partial regeneration undoubtedly occurs in the distal segment, independently of the proximal, although complete regeneration is not possible unless the two segments are in apposition. The generally accepted theory is that the nerve is regenerated by the prolongation of the existing nerve fibrils in the proximal segment. The fiber, which is at first composed of myelin, pierces the granulation tissue between the nerve ends and enters into the empty sheath of the distal segment. It grows slowly along the scaffold of the degenerated trunk and function is re-established only when the new axis-cylinders have permeated the nerve."

Dr. S. T. MAXEINER: I realize that most reports of late nerve suture are not encouraging and nerve suture of long standing is often condemned. However, I would call your attention to the Clinic given by Dr. Kanavel before the American College of Surgeons in Chicago, at which time he reported a nerve suture in the case of a Seattle surgeon five years after the original injury. Regeneration was extremely slow but was progressive over the next five-year period and became so complete that the doctor is able to do his own surgery. This would suggest that nerve suture performed after the lapse of five years is not entirely hopeless.

Dr. G. R. DUNN: I certainly think that Dr. Bratrud is to be congratulated on this case. This case presented most unusual difficulties, the establishing of full thickness skin graft, freeing of the tendons, suturing of the nerves and correcting the growth disturbance. Each and every one of these procedures is difficult and that the four procedures should have given such an excellent functional result is quite remarkable. I think it is one of the best cases of this sort I have had the pleasure of seeing.

PRESENTATION OF A CASE WITH A LARGE CAVITY IN A POSTOPERATIVE LUNG ABSCESS WITH MULTIPLE LARGE BRONCHIAL FISTULÆ

W. A. HANSON, M.D.

Mr. E. N., thirty-seven years of age, married, was seen by us in February, 1934, with the following history. His past history and illnesses were irrelevant. He stated that while in the Orient at Java, on October 7, 1929, he was acutely ill and was operated upon for acute appendicitis. He was discharged from the hospital at the end of ten days feeling well. Four or five days later he began to have pains in the right chest followed by a persistent unproductive cough. The symptoms persisted more or less until January, 1930, when his cough became productive with a large amount of sputum, and "probably associated with a fever." At this time he was informed that he had "pleurisy." His weight had decreased from 145 to 115 pounds. During his travels from Hongkong, Shanghai, and Japan his cough became more persistent and at this time he raised considerable sputum

and "decayed lung tissue." His condition was diagnosed
as tuberculosis. Radiographs of his chest were interpreted as bronchiectasis. Following this he began to
raise blood and pus in his sputum. At Manila his right
chest was aspirated, obtaining "pus and water," and he
was informed that he had a lung abscess.

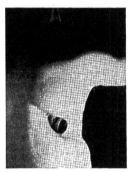

Fig. 1.

He returned to the United States in August, 1930. He
raised a pint of sputum in each twenty-four hours, consisting of blood, pus, and mucus, which had a foul odor.
Following bronchoscopy a diagnosis of bronchiectasis
was made. He had a continuation of his symptoms until
December, 1930, when he had a rather profuse hemorrhage from the lung. Following this he had aspirations
of the chest and a series of posterior rib resections
with beneficial results. Subsequently he developed a
large cavity with bronchial fistulæ, which we wish to
demonstrate this evening.

At this present time, his physical examination shows
a well developed male who weighs 142 pounds and is
5 feet 6 inches tall. His blood pressure registers 110
systolic and 70 diastolic in mm. of mercury. His pulse
is 72 beats per minute and his temperature is 98.6°. The
examination of the head, eyes, ears, nose and throat
reveals no abnormalities. The fingers reveal a moderate
clubbing, characteristic of chronic lung disease. The
right chest in the subscapular area shows a large
cavity about the size of two navel oranges with
many fibrous strands and bronchial fistulæ. One
fistula communicates with the main hilus bronchus. The
wound shows no evidence of infection. This is packed
daily. On removal of the packing he is very dyspneic
and is unable to talk above a whisper. The left chest is
free from abnormalities. Examination of the urine is
negative. His blood shows a hemoglobin of 78 per cent
(Dare) and 4,100,000 red blood cells per cubic millimeter of blood.

Radiographs taken of the chest show no abnormality
in the left lung field. The right chest shows resections
with partial regeneration of the fifth, sixth, seventh,
eighth and ninth ribs. There is a partial collapse of the
lower lobes and thickened basal pleura.

Comment.—This case is of interest first because of
the past and present disease and second from the standpoint of what method would be most efficacious in closing the large cavity and large fistulæ.

According to Dr. Carl Hedblom's collected series of

356

rainage of these abscesses is necessary and the Gracautery in the presence of an infected pleural ty or an empyema offers one method of obtaining nage and relieving the patient of his symptcms with the risk of dissemination of the infection. It does e a rather nasty condition in the chest, in that you have multiple pockets, communicating with your ‑ative wound, and all of the pus which originally ned up through the bronchus now comes out or ugh the wound. After a period of time, however, infection subsides, but the pockets still remain. The etion diminishes, leaving an epithelialized tract or ‑s of pockets which produce very little discharge. ou now surgically close up this wound, while there still abscess cavities present, even though they con no pus, you will probably induce a recurrence of trouble. This man now has multiple pockets which relatively clean and show little or no pus ordinarily, if they were closed up bv an external plastic collapse cedure he would undoubtedly develop cough and ectoration and have further difficulty.

his man, as he walks around, is not short of ith and can work, if he carries a tight pack in his ind. If he does not have a tight pack in his wound he scarcely speak above a whisper for most of his air es out through the external openings. He then loses wind and is not able to work. From a surgical stand it, there are two or three things which might be attempted. One is to convert all of these abscesses into single pocket and then do an external collapse procedure to bring the walls into contact to allow healing. muscle transplant might be turned into the pocket attempt to close the bronchial fistulæ, but this is her a difficult thing to do in this instance. Much of muscle on the back of his chest has been destroyed the previous surgical procedures, leaving very little a transplant into the fistulæ. Smaller fistulæ may closed by cauterization with silver nitrate, leaving a :an wound which will close by external plastic pro dure. If the fistulæ cannot be closed, and many of the ‑ge ones do not close readily, then you are confronted a very complicated proposition which may demand your ingenuity and maybe more than that to get l of it. In some instances it may prove wiser to let :ll enough alone and let the patient continue to work th his chest wall defect.

DR. OWEN WANGENSTEEN: There are two matters of eat interest in the case presented by Dr. Hanson: one the question of the etiology of the suppurative proc s in the lung which eventuated in the condition which ‑. Hanson has shown us; the other revolves about e more important consideration of treatment.

Both Drs. Hanson and Kinsella indicated that they lieved the process to have had its origin through an ibolic source—a thesis for which a plausible defense ay be prepared. Yet, I am inclined to believe that this is an ascending rather than a descending infection. ie patient, as Dr. Hanson stated, had an appendectomy r suppurative appendicitis: he left the hospital ten ys later while he was still ill; he continued ill and lost :ight from 145 to 115 pounds. My reaction would be at a subdiaphragmatic abscess developed, which subquently penetrated the diaphragm and lay outside the ng for a long time as an occult empyema. Only after lapse of about fifteen months did the abscess rup re into the lung, signalled by the spitting up of large iantities of sputum. Subsequently, the pulmonary ab ess ruptured into the pleural cavity at a site where ere was a free pleural space, for, as Dr. Hanson said, e patient became suddenly much worse and when the eural cavity was aspirated, considerable exudate was itained. There having been no evidence of pulmonary

suppuration earlier in life we can disregard primary bronchiectasis as a consideration—other than as an occurrence secondary to long continued pulmonary suppuration.

This interpretation of the story which Dr. Hanson related may appear a bit unusual. At this remote date, one can only speculate as to the probable sequence of events. But mindful of the long period of time intervening between the initial suppurative process in the appendix and the first suggestion of pulmonary suppuration, I do believe the facts as stated lend considerable weight to the ascending view which I have taken of the matter.

At the present moment, I have at the University Hospital a young woman who was operated upon for suppurative appendicitis three years ago. A subdiaphragmatic abscess developed and was drained. In the intervening years, she had continued to complain of pain near the spine at the level of the tenth to twelfth dorsal segments. A sinus had opened intermittently; it has been enlarged and explored but nothing has been found. On opening the tract widely, recently, I uncovered an occult empyema beneath the tenth and eleventh ribs. It had not yet ruptured through the lung to establish communication with a bronchus. More commonly, of course, the development of a pulmonary abscess follows closely upon the formation of the subdiaphragmatic abscess. Most of you, I am certain, are familiar, however, with the occurrence which I have described.

Drs. Hanson and Kinsella have considered the therapeutic agencies which one might invoke to close the bronchial fistulæ which the patient now has. In the light of the satisfactory condition of the patient and his relative freedom from discharge from the fistulæ, I would agree that an attempt should be made to close them. As Dr. Kinsella has pointed out there has been already considerable loss of available muscle tissue immediately adjacent to the fistulous openings. Whereas, implantation of a pedicled slip of muscle into a bronchial fistula or suturing a flap of muscle over the stomata is a very useful procedure and one to which I am quite partial (Journal of Thoracic Surgery, 1935:5: 27), I am inclined to believe that it would be difficult to make such a plan work here. Even though a suitable pedicled muscle flap might be mobilized to fill in the defect, it would be even more difficult to cover the defect and transplant muscle with skin satisfactorily—a very important consideration in the closure of these numerous and large bronchial stomata. The best plan of procedure, I believe, is the procedure of Lebsche (Deutsch Ztschr. f. Chir. 189, 279, 1925).

While Professor Sauerbruch was still at Munich, his assistant, Lebsche, described a very useful technic for dealing with numerous bronchial stomata, which condition he described as "Gitterlunge" or gridiron lung. The margins of the exposed lung are mobilized by freeing it from the adjacent skin and other structures. The margins of the mobilized lung are then sutured together, burying the stomata. It is wise, I believe, to insert a temporary drain (Surgery, 2:859, (Dec.) 1937, footnote) led off through sufficient thickness of the chest wall, such that a persistent fistula is not likely to form. The skin is then closed securely over the trough of inverted lung tissue.

In order to secure adequate relaxation of the structures of the chest wall to permit satisfactory skin closure over the plastic on the lung, it would be well, I believe, to perform here a preliminary resection of the third, fourth and fifth ribs anteriorly two or three weeks before. It is my impression that the Lebsche procedure for "Gitterlunge" would offer the most satisfactory solution in closing this unusual defect.

INTERNAL FIXATION IN INTRACAPSULAR FRACTURES OF THE NECK OF THE FEMUR

WILLARD D. WHITE, M.D.

Summary

The general problem of treatment of intracapsular fractures of the neck of the femur was discussed. Statistics were given on the mortality, which probably averaged about twenty per cent in patients over fifty years of age who were treated by the old Whitman method or other non-operative means. The mortality increased in direct proportion to the age. As to percentage of unions in the so-called conservative or non-operative treatment represented by the Whitman or Maxwell-Ruth methods, this was not over fifty per cent. In many series the percentage was less.

There have now been enough cases operated upon by internal fixation to give some idea of its success. The method is still comparatively new and it is difficult to establish accurate statistics but there is no question about the fact that the mortality has been decreased and the percentage of unions very markedly increased. There are further advantages in the economic saving and the increased comfort to the patient.

Lantern slides were shown to illustrate pre-operative and post-operative results and patients were presented, all of whom had been operated upon at least a year ago or more. It was demonstrated how these patients could walk, move their joints, et cetera. Some of the hazards or risks were discussed.

Twenty-four cases in which the author performed an operation were discussed. In the first eleven a reduction was accomplished, position checked with anteroposterior and lateral films, a Kirschner wire was inserted and a canulated short flange nail was inserted over the wire and driven into place. In one of these cases the wire bent, in another the wire broke and was driven in through the acetabulum into the pelvis and had to be removed from within the pelvis. Following this, twelve patients were operated upon and the joint opened, the fracture reduced under direct vision and the nail also driven in under direct vision. In the last case the nail was driven in directly through a lateral incision over the trochanter without the preliminary introduction of a wire. The position of the nail was perfect.

Many of the cases are too recent to warrant a report on final results but it was felt that the operative treatment of intracapsular fractures of the neck of the femur with internal fixation offered by far the best means we have to treat this lesion. In the main, a short flange nail of the Smith-Peterson type was used. It is admitted that other types of internal fixation would probably accomplish the same results. In two cases Austin Moore pins were used and were very satisfactory.

Discussion

DR. E. A. REGNIER: Dr. White has covered the field of internal fixation of fractures of the neck of the femur most thoroughly and I assure you he is not the only one who has made a mistake of judgment and of technic. One must appreciate that internal fixation does not assure a union but rather it insures union. Obviously, there are many methods by which this may be done. I believe, in the light of my short experience, that even though the end-results by internal fixation were no better than those from previous methods, I should still choose the former method because of the absolute relief from pain and the financial saving it affords the patient. When one recalls that these patients were formerly hospitalized twelve to sixteen weeks and in the best hands only 50 per cent of those who survived treatment had satisfactory results, an improved method of treatment is most welcome.

Dr. White mentioned the various methods that he had used in treating these fractures. I believe that the choice of method is optional. It has been my practice to do a closed reduction and subsequently to make a short incision laterally below the trochanter so as to drive the nail over the previously inserted Kirschner wire. I have always attempted to place the nail in a valgus position because this permits less strain on the line of fracture. I believe that the Austin Moore pins, flanged screws and Morrison pin will all maintain fixation but I do not believe that they are compatible with any degree of early unprotected walking. At the General Hospital our patients could not afford walking calipers, therefore we permitted them to walk with crutches two weeks after inserting Smith-Peterson nails. These people were permitted to go home any time after the third week and we soon learned that many of them discarded their crutches soon after leaving the hospital and walked on the nailed hip long before union could take place. I recently had an opportunity of seeing a follow-up x-ray of a man whose hip I nailed one year ago and who has been walking without protection ever since. I will show his film and I think you will agree that he has a perfect union in excellent position. I also had the privilege of nailing the hip in an eighty-six-year-old woman and she was permitted to walk without protection the week following her operation. She has now walked for seven months without any mishaps and is perfectly comfortable. However, I do not advocate unprotected walking short of four to six months. I believe it is perfectly safe to put a properly fitted walking caliper on these people as soon as their wounds are healed. I have done this on over thirty cases and have had no occasion to regret it. The youngest patient that I treated was thirty-eight years of age and the oldest eighty-six. There has been no mortality and up to date only one case has proven a failure. In this individual the head of the femur partly atrophied and rotated of the end of the nail, necessitating a reconstruction operation.

Internal fixation should maintain accurate anatomic reduction and relieve all pain. The relief of pain has been so immediate and so gratifying that it has been my practice to treat these immediately, as soon as the immediate shock of fracture has been relieved, usually a matter of twelve to twenty-four hours. Nothing can be gained by postponing operation. Many old people fail rapidly when confined to bed with Buck's extension and morphine to control their pain while awaiting operation. I believe that the small risk and minimal trauma from the operation more than offset the risk of postponement. They are less apt to develop pneumonia and have much more freedom and comfort after operation than before. I believe that this procedure will soon be recognized as a routine and practically an emergency operation. In other words, unless a patient is moribund or has some complicating disease such as severe diabetes, I can see no reason for postponing the insertion of a nail in a recent fracture. (Films were shown.)

Dr. V. Hart: There are a number of remarks I would like to make but the hour is late so I will just close by telling Dr. White that I have appreciated his instructive paper and that I heartily support his thesis.

Dr. E. T. Evans: I won't say anything about the methods of treatment, et cetera, because I think that in-

ternal fixation of the neck of the femur is here to stay. I think, however, that we have much to learn in cases such as this. In spite of the fact that Dr. White said he hesitated to give a report at such an early date this is probably worth much more than a series of cases with beautiful results, for it is by our mistakes that we are to learn. Dr. Cole and I have now done something over forty hip operations in the last year by the open method, not Watson Jones approach but Kocher's anterior fascial splitting approach, and with the exception of two or three cases we feel we have learned something on every hip we have done. We are becoming more and more convinced that in our open reductions we are obviating some of the difficulties we have seen tonight and that is said with the experience of two or three years of closed reductions in back of us. It doesn't mean that we won't switch back to the closed reduction because we are open to conviction that with some improvements in technic the closed reduction may offer the same results.

Harvey Nelson, *Secretary.*

BOOK REVIEWS

Books listed here become the property of the Ramsey and Hennepin County Medical libraries when reviewed. Members, however, are urged to write reviews of any or every recent book which may be of interest to physicians.

BOOKS RECEIVED FOR REVIEW

Workbook In Elementary Diagnosis for Teaching Clinical History Recording and Physical Diagnosis. Logan Clendening, Professor of Clinical Medicine, University of Kansas. 167 pages. Illus. Price, cloth, $1.50. St. Louis: C. V. Mosby Co., 1938.

Men Past Forty. A. F. Niemoeller, A.B., M.A., B.S. Author of American Encyclopedia of Sex, etc. Foreword by Winfield Scott Pugh, B.S., M.D. 154 pages. Price, cloth, $2.00. New York: Harvest House, 1938.

Management of the Sick Infant and Child. Fifth Edition. Langley Porter, B.S., M.D., M.R.C.S. (Eng.), L.R.C.P. (Lond.), Dean, University of California Medical School and Professor of Medicine, etc., and William E. Carter, M.D., Director University of California Hospital Out-Patient Department, etc. 875 pages. Illus. Price, cloth, $10.00. St. Louis: C. V. Mosby Co., 1938.

A Biological Approach to the Problem of Abnormal Behavior. Milton Harrington, M.D., Psychiatrist, Institution for Male Defective Delinquents, Napanoch, N. Y. Formerly Consultant in Mental Hygiene, Dartmouth College. 459 pages. Cloth. Lancaster, Pa.: Science Press Printing Co., 1938.

Pneumonia and Serum Therapy. Revised Edition. Frederick T. Lord, M.D., Clinical Professor of Medicine, Emeritus, Harvard Medical School; Member Board of Consultants Massachusetts General Hospital, etc., and Roderick Heffron, M.D., Field Director Pneumonia Study and Service, Massachusetts Department of Health. 148 pages. Price, cloth, $1.00. New York: The Commonwealth Fund, 1938.

THE 1937 YEARBOOK OF GENERAL MEDICINE. Chicago: Yearbook Publishers, 1937. $3.00.

The 1937 volume of the Yearbook of General Medicine is, as usual, an excellent piece of work. Most of the important developments in the field of internal medicine that have been brought forward in the past year have been reviewed. Of special interest to our own readers is the fact that among those authors mentioned we find the names of Drs. Lufkin, Mariette, Myers, Shapiro, Wangensteen, Cecil Watson and Ziskin.

The volume can, indeed, be recommended to all those interested in a general review of the important work of the past year.

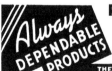

MINNESOTA STATE MEDICAL ASSOCIATION

Roster 1938

OFFICERS

J. M. Hayes, M.D. . . . . . *President* . . . . Minneapolis
W. R. McCarthy, M.D. . . . . *First Vice President* . . . . . . St. Paul
B. A. Smith, M.D. . . . . *Second Vice President* . . . . . . Crosby
E. A. Meyerding, M.D. . . . . *Secretary* . . . . St. Paul
W. H. Condit, M.D. . . . . . *Treasurer* . . . . . . Minneapolis
A. W. Adson, M.D. . . . . . . *Past President* . . . . Rochester
W. W. Will, M.D. . . . *Speaker, House of Delegates* . . . . . Bertha
J. C. Hultkrans, M.D. . . . *Vice Speaker, House of Delegates* . . . . Minneapolis
R. R. Rosell . . . . . *Executive Secretary* . . . . . . St. Paul

COUNCILORS*

First District
H. Z. Giffin, M.D. (1938).................Rochester
Second District
L. L. Sogge, M.D. (1938)....................Windom
Third District
B. J. Branton, M.D. (1940)................Willmar
Fourth District
J. S. Holbrook, M.D. (1939)................Mankato
Fifth District
G. A. Earl, M.D.(1940).....................St. Paul

Sixth District
C. A. Stewart, M.D. (1939).............Minneapolis
Seventh District
E. J. Simons, M.D. (1940).................Swanville
Eighth District
W. L. Burnap, M.D. (1939).............Fergus Falls
Ninth District
B. S. Adams, M.D. (1938)....................Hibbing

HOUSE OF DELEGATES, AMERICAN MEDICAL ASSOCIATION*

Members
W. A. Coventry, M.D. (1938).................Duluth
W. F. Braasch, M.D. (1938)...............Rochester
J. T. Christison, M.D. (1939)............St. Paul

Alternates
G. A. Earl, M.D. (1938)......................St. Paul
W. L. Burnap, M.D. (1938).............Fergus Falls
E. A. Meyerding, M.D. (1939)..............St. Paul

MINNESOTA STATE CERTIFICATION BOARD FOR PUBLIC HEALTH NURSING

E. J. Simons, M.D., ...Swanville

SCIENTIFIC COMMITTEES

(C.M.—Indicates Consulting Member)

COMMITTEE ON SCIENTIFIC ASSEMBLY
J. M. Hayes, M.D., *General Chairman*............Minneapolis
A. W. Adson, M.D................................Rochester
R. R. Rosell....................................St. Paul

SECTION ON MEDICINE
P. G. Boman, M.D................................Duluth
B. B. Souster, M.D..............................St. Paul
J. N. Libert, M.D...............................St. Cloud

SECTION ON SURGERY
Stanley Maxeiner, M.D.......................Minneapolis
V. S. Counseller, M.D..........................Rochester
R. C. Hunt, M.D.................................Fairmont

SECTION ON SPECIALTIES
W. A. O'Brien, M.D...........................Minneapolis

LOCAL ARRANGEMENTS
R. J. Moe, M.D...................................Duluth

COMMITTEE ON CANCER*
Martin Nordland, M.D. (1939)...............Minneapolis
W. A. O'Brien, M.D. (1938) (C.M.) *Vice Chairman* Minneapolis
Herbert Boysen, M.D. (1940).....................Welcome
A. G. Chadbourn, M.D. (1938)................Heron Lake
H. C. Cooney, M.D. (1940)......................Princeton
C. O. Estrem, M.D. (1938)..................Fergus Falls
O. J. Hagen, M.D. (1939)......................Moorhead
A. D. Haskell, M.D. (1938)...................Alexandria
R. S. Hegge, M.D. (1940).........................Austin
O. W. Holcomb, M.D. (1939)..................Minneapolis
F. A. Olson, M.D. (1939)....................Minneapolis

H. E. Robertson, M.D. (1938)...................Rochester
J. A. Slocumb, M.D. (1940).....................Plainview
A. E. Sohmer, M.D. (1939).......................Mankato
Waltman Walters, M.D. (1940)..................Rochester

COMMITTEES ON INDUSTRIAL HEALTH
1. Committee on Fractures
O. W. Yoerg, M.D...........................Minneapolis
B. J. Branton, M.D.............................Wilmar
H. D. Burns, M.D............................Albert Lea
B. J. Gallagher, M.D...........................Waseca
Carl Johnson, M.D..............................Dawson
D. F. Meyer, M.D..............................Faribault
R. S. Mitchell, M.D.......................Grand Meadow
Harvey Nelson, M.D..........................Minneapolis
C. I. Oliver, M.D.............................Graceville
E. N. Peterson, M.D............................Virginia
F. L. Savage, M.D..............................St. Paul
E. C. Webb, M.D.............................Minneapolis
W. F. Wilson, M.D............................Lake City

2. Committee on Asphyxia and Asphyxial Death
A. E. Cardle, M.D..........................Minneapolis
M. W. Alberts, M.D.............................St. Paul
A. J. Chesley, M.D.............................St. Paul
Clarence Jacobson, M.D.........................Chisholm
F. H. K. Schaaf, M.D.......................Minneapolis
S. M. White, M.D...........................Minneapolis
M. S. Nelson, M.D...........................Granite Falls

COMMITTEE ON DIABETES
H. B. Sweetser, Jr., M.D....................Minneapolis
Moses Barron, M.D..........................Minneapolis
A. H. Beard, M.D...........................Minneapolis
A. E. Cardle, M.D..........................Minneapolis
R. C. Hunt, M.D................................Fairmont

*Terms expire December 31, of year indicated.

360

E. H. RYNEARSON, M.D.........................Rochester
W. A. STAFNE, M.D.............................Moorhead
D. W. WHEELER, M.D..............................Duluth
R. M. WILDER, M.D.............................Rochester

HEART COMMITTEE

F. A. WILLIUS, M.D............................Rochester
J. W. GAMBLE, M.D............................Albert Lea
C. N. HENSEL, M.D..............................St. Paul
F. J. HIRSCHBOECK, M.D...........................Duluth
J. M. LAJOIE, M.D............................Minneapolis
F. H. K. SCHAAF, M.D.........................Minneapolis
B. R. KARN, M.D...............................Ortonville

COMMITTEE ON SYPHILIS AND SOCIAL DISEASES

S. E. SWEITZER, M.D..........................Minneapolis
C. D. FREEMAN, M.D.............................St. Paul
F. E. HARRINGTON, M.D........................Minneapolis
W. E. HATCH, M.D................................Duluth
H. G. IRVINE, M.D............................Minneapolis
F. W. LYNCH, M.D...............................St. Paul
J. F. MADDEN, M.D.............................St. Paul
H. E. MICHELSON, M.D.........................Minneapolis
P. A. O'LEARY, M.D............................Rochester

COMMITTEE ON DEAFNESS PREVENTION AND AMELIORATION

HORACE NEWHART, M.D.........................Minneapolis
W. L. BURNAP, M.D...........................Fergus Falls
C. E. CONNOR, M.D..............................St. Paul
F. E. HARRINGTON, M.D........................Minneapolis
J. T. SCHLESSELMAN, M.D.........................Mankato
D. L. TILDERQUIST, M.D...........................Duluth
G. H. WALKER, M.D................................Winona

COMMITTEE ON OPHTHALMOLOGY

W. E. CAMP, M.D..............................Minneapolis
W. L. BENEDICT, M.D............................Rochester
F. E. BURCH, M.D...............................St. Paul
V. I. MILLER, M.D................................Mankato
F. F. SLYFIELD, M.D..............................Duluth

COMMITTEE ON HOSPITALS AND MEDICAL EDUCATION

J. B. CAREY, M.D............................Minneapolis
J. K. ANDERSON, M.D..........................Minneapolis
W. C. CARROLL, M.D.............................St. Paul

W. McK. CRAIG, M.D............................Rochester
H. S. DIEHL, M.D............................Minneapolis
J. R. MANLEY, M.D...............................Duluth
J. A. MYERS, M.D............................Minneapolis
L. G. SMITH, M.D.............................Montevideo
A. H. ZACHMAN, M.D.............................Melrose
B. F. SMITH, M.D..............................Rochester

SUB-COMMITTEE ON PUBLIC HEALTH NURSING

H. F. BAYARD, M.D...........................Minneapolis
C. E. CAINE, M.D................................Morris
T. E. FLINN, M.D............................Redwood Falls
H. F. HELMHOLZ, M.D...........................Rochester
P. H. KELLY, M.D...............................St. Paul
A. G. LIEDLOFF, M.D.............................Mankato
A. A. PASSER, M.D................................Olivia
F. J. PLONDKE, M.D.............................St. Paul
C. L. SCOFIELD, M.D..............................Benson

COMMITTEE ON MATERNAL WELFARE

R. D. MUSSEY, M.D.............................Rochester
C. J. EHRENBERG, M.D.........................Minneapolis
E. C. HARTLEY, M.D.............................St. Paul
C. O. MALAND, M.D...........................Minneapolis
R. J. MOE, M.D..................................Duluth
O. J. SEIFERT, M.D.............................New Ulm
C. L. SHERMAN, M.D..............................Luverne
W. E. WILSON, M.D.............................Northfield

COMMITTEE ON MILITARY AFFAIRS

COL. F. L. SMITH............................Rochester
LIEUT. COL. J. J. CATLIN........................Buffalo
LIEUT. C. J. FRITSCHE..........................New Ulm
CAPTAIN RALPH CREIGHTON.....................Minneapolis
CAPTAIN D. P. HEAD..........................Minneapolis
LIEUT. COMM. DONALD McCARTHY................Minneapolis
MAJOR J. J. MORROW..............................Austin

HISTORICAL COMMITTEE

J. M. ARMSTRONG, M.D...........................St. Paul
H. B. ANNIS, M.D............................Minneapolis
RICHARD BARDON, M.D.............................Duluth
CHARLES BOLSTA, M.D..........................Ortonville
L. E. CLAYDON, M.D............................Red Wing
OLGA HANSEN, M.D............................Minneapolis
R. S. MITCHELL, M.D.........................Grand Meadow
M. C. PIPER, M.D..............................Rochester
G. E. SHERWOOD, M.D.............................Kimball

NON-SCIENTIFIC COMMITTEES

COMMITTEE ON PUBLIC POLICY

L. L. SOGGE, M.D................................Windom
G. I. BADEAUX, M.D............................Brainerd
L. A. BARNEY, M.D..............................Duluth
J. F. DuBOIS, M.D...........................Sauk Center
E. A. EBERLIN, M.D.............................Glenwood
R. C. GRAY, M.D.............................Minneapolis
W. A. FANSLER, M.D..........................Minneapolis
H. C. HABEIN, M.D.............................Rochester
J. M. HAYES, M.D............................Minneapolis
F. H. NEHER, M.D...............................St. Paul
M. O. OPPEGAARD, M.D..........................Crookston
W. C. RUTHERFORD, M.D..........................St. Paul
C. B. WRIGHT, M.D..........................Minneapolis

INTERPROFESSIONAL RELATIONSHIP COMMITTEE

F. J. SAVAGE, M.D..............................St. Paul
F. F. CALLAHAN, M.D............................Pokegama
C. W. DEL PLAINE, M.D.......................Minneapolis
GORDON KAMMAN, M.D.............................St. Paul
J. N. LIBERT, M.D..............................St. Cloud
C. W. MAYO, M.D...............................Rochester
E. M. McLAUGHLIN, M.D...........................Winona
M. O. OPPEGAARD, M.D..........................Crookston

COMMITTEE ON UNIVERSITY RELATIONS

A. W. ADSON, M.D.............................Rochester
W. A. COVENTRY, M.D.............................Duluth
J. M. HAYES, M.D............................Minneapolis
F. J. SAVAGE, M.D..............................St. Paul
W. W. WILL, M.D.................................Bertha

EDITING AND PUBLISHING COMMITTEE*

J. T. CHRISTISON, M.D. (1939)...................St. Paul
E. M. HAMMES, M.D. (1941).......................St. Paul
T. A. PEPPARD, M.D. (1942)...................Minneapolis
WALTMAN WALTERS, M.D. (1938).................Rochester
C. B. WRIGHT, M.D. (1940)...................Minneapolis

*Terms expire December 31, of year indicated.

COMMITTEE ON PUBLIC HEALTH EDUCATION

L. R. CRITCHFIELD, M.D., *General Chairman*.........St. Paul

Executive

L. R. CRITCHFIELD, M.D..........................St. Paul
R. M. BURNS, M.D...............................St. Paul
F. H. MAGNEY, M.D...............................Duluth
H. F. HELMHOLZ, M.D...........................Rochester
J. A. MYERS, M.D............................Minneapolis
A. B. STEWART, M.D.............................Owatonna

Child Welfare

L. R. CRITCHFIELD, M.D..........................St. Paul
E. C. BAYLEY, M.D.............................Lake City
L. V. BERGHS, M.D.............................Owatonna
A. J. CHESLEY, M.D.............................St. Paul
H. S. DIEHL, M.D............................Minneapolis
B. J. GALLAGHER, M.D............................Waseca
P. M. GAMBLE, M.D............................Albert Lea
J. S. GROGAN, M.D............................Minneapolis
H. F. HELMHOLZ, M.D...........................Rochester
A. J. HENDERSON, M.D.............................Kiester
C. D. LUFKIN, M.D.............................Northfield
F. J. NORMAN, M.D.............................Crookston
C. J. PLONDKE, M.D.............................Faribault
C. L. SCOFIELD, M.D..............................Benson
A. B. STEWART, M.D.............................Owatonna
A. K. STRATTE, M.D............................Pine City
T. H. SWEETSER, M.D.........................Minneapolis

Radio

R. M. BURNS, M.D...............................St. Paul
J. K. ANDERSON, M.D..........................Minneapolis
E. H. BOYER, JR., M.D...........................Duluth
E. A. HEBERG, M.D...........................Fergus Falls
R. A. JOHNSON, M.D..........................Minneapolis
J. A. MOGA, M.D................................St. Paul
M. C. PIPER, M.D..............................Rochester
J. T. PRIESTLEY, M.D..........................Rochester

E. D. Risser, M.D. .... Winona
E. T. Sanderson, M.D. .... Minneota
T. O. Young, M.D. .... Duluth

Speakers Bureau

F. H. Magney, M.D. .... Duluth
C. C. Allen, M.D. .... Austin
R. M. Burns, M.D. .... St. Paul
L. A. Hilger, M.D. .... St. Paul
C. P. Robbins, M.D. .... Winona
T. W. Weum, M.D. .... Minneapolis

Editorial

H. F. Helmholz, M.D. .... Rochester
B. J. Branton, M.D. .... Willmar
B. R. Karn, M.D. .... Ortonville
J. A. Myers, M.D. .... Minneapolis
Ivar Sivertsen, M.D. .... Minneapolis

First Aid

A. B. Stewart, M.D. .... Owatonna
D. H. Garlock, M.D. .... Bemidji
A. Gullixson, M.D. .... Albert Lea
B. A. Smith, M.D. .... Crosby

Red Cross

A. B. Stewart, M.D. .... Owatonna
D. H. Garlock, M.D. .... Bemidji
A. Gullixson, M.D. .... Albert Lea
B. A. Smith, M.D. .... Crosby

Tuberculosis

J. A. Myers, M.D. .... Minneapolis
E. S. Boleyn, M.D. .... Stillwater
C. F. Ewing, M.D. .... Wheaton
W. K. Foster, M.D. .... Minneapolis

COMMITTEE ON MEDICAL ECONOMICS

W. F. Braasch, M.D., *General Chairman* .... Rochester

Executive

W. F. Braasch, M.D. .... Rochester
B. J. Branton, M.D. .... Willmar
W. A. Coventry, M.D. .... Duluth
L. R. Critchfield, M.D. .... St. Paul
E. W. Hansen, M.D. .... Minneapolis
M. S. Henderson, M.D. .... Rochester
F. A. Olson, M.D. .... Minneapolis
L. L. Sogge, M.D. .... Windom
T. H. Sweetser, M.D. .... Minneapolis

Editorial

W. F. Braasch, M.D. .... Rochester
A. R. Barnes, M.D. .... Rochester
A. N. Collins, M.D. .... Duluth
Lennox Danielson, M.D. .... Litchfield
E. A. Meyerding, M.D. .... St. Paul
E. S. Platou, M.D. .... Minneapolis

Professional Education in Medical Ethics and Social and Economic Trends

E. W. Hansen, M.D. .... Minneapoli
L. A. Buie, M.D. .... Rochester
R. H. Creighton, M.D. .... Minneapoli
H. S. Diehl, M.D. .... Minneapoli
J. N. Libert, M.D. .... St. Cloud
I. L. Oliver, M.D. .... Gracevill
J. J. Swendson, M.D. .... St. Pau

Medical Advisory

B. J. Branton, M.D. .... Willma
W. L. Burnap, M.D. .... Fergus Fall
W. H. Hengstler, M.D. .... St. Pau

State Health Relations

T. H. Sweetser, M.D. .... Minneapoli
E. S. Boleyn, M.D. .... Stillwate
W. S. Broker, M.D. .... Waden
L. R. Critchfield, M.D. .... St. Pau
J. N. Dunn, M.D. .... St. Pau
C. L. Hanley, M.D. .... Duluth
W. E. Hart, M.D. .... Monticell
H. E. Hillboe, M.D. .... St. Pau
C. M. Johnson, M.D. .... Dawso
J. P. McDowell, M.D. .... St. Clou
J. L. McLeod, M.D. .... Grand Rapid
S. A. Slater, M.D. .... Worthingto

Low Income and Indigent Problems

W. A. Coventry, M.D. .... Dulut
V. S. Counseller, M.D. .... Rocheste
B. O. Mork, Jr., M.D. .... Worthingto
C. L. Oppegaard, M.D. .... Crooksto
L. I. Younger, M.D. .... Winon
A. H. Zachman, M.D. .... Melros

Industrial Relations

M. S. Henderson, M.D. .... Rocheste
S. H. Baxter, M.D., *Vice Chairman* .... Minneapoli
B. S. Adams, M.D. .... Hibbin
S. H. Boyer, Sr., M.D. .... Dulut
W. H. Cole, M.D. .... St. Pau
G. R. Dunn, M.D. .... Minneapoli
W. N. Graves, M.D. .... Dulut
R. C. Hunt, M.D. .... Fairmon
E. M. Jones, M.D. .... St. Pau

Contract Practice

F. A. Olson, M.D. .... Minneapoli
N. H. Baker, M.D. .... Fergus Fall
J. C. Hultkrans, M.D. .... Minneapoli
Paul Leck, M.D. .... Austi
R. F. McGandy, M.D. .... Minneapoli
E. N. Peterson, M.D. .... Virgin

Women's Auxiliary

to the

Minnesota State Medical Association

OFFICERS

RS. J. F. NORMAN.............................. *President* .... Crookston
RS. W. B. ROBERTS......................... *President-Elect* .... Minneapolis
RS. E. M. HAMMES...........................*Past President*..St. Paul
RS. J. J. RYAN.............................*First Vice President*...............................St. Paul
RS. JOHN DORDAL........................*Second Vice President*...................Sacred Heart
MRS. R. S. FORBES.........................*Third Vice President*................................. Duluth
MRS. J. M. HAYES........................*Fourth Vice President*.............................. Minneapolis
MRS. H. F. WAHLQUIST....................*Recording Secretary*............................... Minneapolis
MRS. G. A. MORLEY.....................*Corresponding Secretary*........................... Crookston
MRS. R. J. JOSEWSKI........................... *Treasurer* .... Stillwater
MRS. G. E. HERTEL............................. *Auditor* .... Austin
MRS. W. J. BYRNES........................... *Parliamentarian* .... Minneapolis
MRS. J. A. THABES, SR........................... *Historian* .... Brainerd

CHAIRMEN OF COMMITTEES

Advisory—MRS. W. J. MAYO.............. Rochester
Archives—MRS. S. S. HESSELGRAVE..........St. Paul
Editor—MRS. A. A. PASSER................... Olivia
Exhibits—MRS. B. F. DAVIS................. Duluth
Finance—MRS. MARTIN NORDLAND........ Minneapolis
Health Education—MRS. H. E. WUNDER.... Shakopee
Hygeia—MRS. W. W. WILL.................Bertha

Legislation—MRS. J. L. McLEOD........ Grand Rapids
Organization—MRS. W. B. ROBERTS........ Minneapolis
Printing—MRS. F. A. ERB............... Minneapolis
Public Relations—MRS. A. F. BRANTON...... Willmar
Resolutions—MRS. W. H. VALENTINE......... Tracy
Revisions—MRS. E. C. ESHELBY............ St. Paul
Social—MRS. F. J. ELIAS...................... Duluth

Councilor Districts

DISTRICT NO. 1

H. Z. GIFFIN, M.D..........................Rochester
Counties — Dodge, Fillmore, Freeborn, Goodhue, Houston, Mower, Olmsted, Rice, Steele, Wabasha, Winona

DISTRICT NO. 2

L. L. SOGGE, M.D...........................Windom
Counties—Cottonwood, Faribault, Jackson, Martin, Murray, Nobles, Pipestone, Rock, Watonwan

DISTRICT NO. 3

B. J. BRANTON, M.D........................Willmar
Counties—Big Stone, Brown, Chippewa, Kandiyohi, Lac Qui Parle, Lincoln, Lyon, Meeker, Pope, Redwood, Stevens, Swift, Traverse. Yellow Medicine

DISTRICT NO. 4

J. S. HOLBROOK, M.D.......................Mankato
Counties—Blue Earth, Carver, LeSueur, McLeod, Nicollet, Renville, Scott, Sibley, Waseca

DISTRICT NO. 5

G. A. EARL, M.D............................St. Paul
Counties—Anoka, Chisago, Dakota, Isanti, Kanabec, Mille Lacs, Pine, Ramsey, Sherburne, Washington

DISTRICT NO. 6

C. A. STEWART, M.D.....................Minneapolis
Counties—Hennepin, Wright

DISTRICT NO. 7

E. J. SIMONS, M.D........................Swanville
Counties—Aitkin, Beltrami, Benton, Cass, Clearwater, Crow Wing, Hubbard, Morrison, Koochiching, Stearns, Todd, Wadena

DISTRICT NO. 8

W. L. BURNAP, M.D.....................Fergus Falls
Counties—Becker, Clay, Douglas, Grant, Kittson, Lake of the Woods, Mahnomen, Marshall, Norman, Otter Tail, Pennington, Polk, Red Lake, Roseau, Wilkin

DISTRICT NO. 9

B. S. ADAMS, M.D............................Hibbing
Counties—Carlton, Cook, Itasca, Lake, St. Louis

MINNESOTA STATE MEDICAL ASSOCIATION

COUNTY SOCIETY ROSTER

BLUE EARTH COUNTY MEDICAL SOCIETY
Regular meetings, last Monday of each month
Annual meeting last Monday in December
Number of Members: 33

President
Koenigsberger, Charles.......Mankato

Secretary
Penn, G. E...................Mankato

Andrews, R. N...............Mankato
Benham, E. W...............Mankato
Black, William..............Mankato
Butzer, J. A................Mankato
Dahl, G. A..................Mankato
Denman, A. V...............Mankato
Edwards, R. T..............Elysian

Feldman, F. M.............Mankato
Franchere, F. W.........Lake Crystal
Fugina, G. R...............Mankato
Haes, J. E.............Vernon Center
Hankerson, R. G....Minnesota Lake
Hassett, R. G..............Mankato
Holbrook, J. S.............Mankato
Howard, M. I...............Mankato
Huffington, H. L..........Mankato
Jullar, R. O...............St. Clair
Kemp, A. F.................Mankato
Koenigsberger, Charles........Mankato
Liedloff, A. G.............Mankato

Lloyd, H. J................Mankato
Miller, V. I...............Mankato
Morgan, H. O., Jr............Amboy
Osborn, Lida...............Mankato
Penn, G. E.................Mankato
Schlesselman, J. T........Mankato
Schmidt, P. A........Good Thunder
Sohmer, A. E...............Mankato
Stillwell, W. C............Mankato
Troost, H. B...............Mankato
Vezina, J. C..............Mapleton
Wentworth, A. J............Mankato
Williams, H. O.........Lake Crystal

BLUE EARTH VALLEY MEDICAL SOCIETY
Faribault and Martin Counties
Regular meetings, first Thursday of February, May, August and November
Annual meeting, first Thursday in November
Number of Members: 36

President
Rowe, W. H...............Fairmont

Secretary
Chambers, W. C..........Blue Earth

Bailey, H. B...............Fairmont
Barr, W. H..................Wells
Blanchard, H. G............Fairmont
Boysen, Herbert............Welcome
Chambers, W. C..........Blue Earth
Cooper, M. D............Winnebago
Demp, P. W..................Wells
Farrish, R. C.............Sherburn

Folta, John...............Ceylon
Gardner, V. H............Fairmont
Hayel, T. E............Blue Earth
Helmark, J. J............Fairmont
Henderson, A. J..........Kiester
Holm, P. F..................Wells
Hunt, R. C................Fairmont
Hunte, A. F.......San Carlos, Ariz.
Jacobs, A. C...............Elmore
Johnson, D. W............Fairmont
Johnson, H. P............Fairmont
Krause, C. W.............Fairmont
Luedtke, G. H............Fairmont
Marken, M. H.............Fairmont

McGroarity, J. J...........Easton
Miller, H. A..............Fairmont
Mills, J. L..............Winnebago
Raymond, J. H...........Triumph
Rowe, W. H...............Fairmont
Russ, H. H..............Blue Earth
Sommer, A. W.............Elmore
Sybilrud, H. W...........Bricelyn
Thayer, E. A..............Truman
Vaughan, V. M...........Truman
Virnig, M. P...............Wells
Wilson, C. E...........Blue Earth
Youngman, R. A..........Fairmont
Zemke, E. E..............Fairmont

CAMP RELEASE DISTRICT MEDICAL SOCIETY
Chippewa, Lac Qui Parle and Yellow Medicine Counties
Regular meetings, every second Thursday in Fall and Spring
Annual meeting, March
Number of Members: 23

President
Johnson, C. M..............Dawson

Secretary
Westby, Nels..............Madison

Bacon, R. S.............Montevideo
Bergh, L. N.............Montevideo
Boody, G. J., Jr...........Dawson

Burns, F. M................Milan
Burns, M. A................Milan
Cress, E. E.................Boyd
Foshager, H. T........Clara City
Hauge, M. I.............Clarkfield
Hauge, M. M.............Clarkfield
Herbert, W. L........Granite Falls
Holmberg, L. J............Canby
Johnson, C. M.............Dawson
Jordan, L. S.........Granite Falls

Kath, R. H.............Wood Lake
Lee, W. N................Madison
Lima, Ludvig...........Montevideo
Nelson, K. G............Moorhead
Pertl, A. L................Canby
Roust, H. A............Montevideo
Smith, L. C............Montevideo
Tangen, G. M..............Canby
Westby, Magnus...........Madison
Westby, Nels..............Madison

CLAY-BECKER COUNTY MEDICAL SOCIETY
Regular meetings, three annually
Annual meeting, December
Number of Members: 24

President
Ingebrigtson, E. K........Moorhead

Secretary
Flancher, L. H..........Lake Park

Aborn, W. H................Hawley
Bergheim, M. C............Hawley
Bottolfson, B. T.........Moorhead
Carman, J. E.........Detroit Lakes

Duncan, J. W............Moorhead
Ellingson, A. R......Detroit Lakes
Flancher, L. H........Lake Park
Gosslee, G. L...........Moorhead
Gunderson, R. M........Lake Park
Hagen, O. J............Moorhead
Haight, G. G...........Audubon
Humphrey, E. W........Moorhead
Ingebrigtson, E. K....Moorhead
Larsen, O. O.........Detroit Lakes

Larson, Arnold........Detroit Lakes
Moberg, C. W..........Lake Park
Rice, H. G..............Moorhead
Rutledge, L. H....Detroit Lakes
Seitz, S. B............Barnesville
Simison, Carl ....Barnesville
Simison, C. W............Hawley
Stafne, W. A...........Moorhead
Thysell, F. A..........Moorhead
Thysell, V. D............Hawley

DAKOTA COUNTY MEDICAL SOCIETY
Regular meetings on call
Annual meeting December
Number of members: (Not yet reported)

President
Peck, L. D................Hastings

Secretary
Burns, L. S..........South St. Paul

ROSTER MINNESOTA STATE MEDICAL ASSOCIATION

EAST CENTRAL MINNESOTA MEDICAL SOCIETY
Anoka, Chisago, Isanti, Kanabec, Mille Lacs, Pine and Sherburne Counties
Regular meetings, three yearly
Annual meeting, November
Number of Members: 33

President

Schlesselman, George...........Anoka

Secretary

Ness, C. M................Cambridge

Arends, A. L...............Sandstone
Blomberg, W. R...........Princeton
Blumenthal, J. S...Columbia Heights
Bossert, C. S..................Mora

Brink, D. M...................Isle
Brownstone, Manuel.......Sandstone
Callahan, F. F.............Pokegama
Clothier, E. F.............Elk River
Cooney, H. C..............Princeton
Dedolph, T. H..............Braham
Dredge, H. P.............Sandstone
Halladay, G. J...........Rush City
Halpin, J. E...............Rush City
Hedenstrom, L. H........Cambridge
Holmes, A. E.............Rush City
Kelsey, C. G..............Hinckley
Kemp, M. W...............Anoka
McBroom, D. E..........Cambridge
Ness, C. M...............Cambridge

Nordman, W. F................Mora
Norrgard, H. T.............Milaca
Nygren, W. T.............Braham
Petersen, P. C............Braham
Peterson, A. A...............Mora
Richey, G. L.............Cambridge
Roehlke, A. B..........Elk River
Schlesselman, George...........Anoka
Spurzem, R. J................Anoka
Stephan, E. L............Hinckley
Stratte, A. K.............Pine City
Swensen, R. G...............Harris
Vik, Melvin................Onamia
Wasson, L. F..........Chisago City

FREEBORN COUNTY MEDICAL SOCIETY
Regular meetings, Quarterly
Annual meeting, December
Number of Members: 23

President

Barr, L. C...............Albert Lea

Secretary

Prins, L. R..............Albert Lea

Barr, L. C..............Albert Lea
Branham, D. S........Albert Lea
Burns, H. D.............Albert Lea

Butturff, C. R...............Freeborn
Calhoun, F. W..........Albert Lea
Donovan, D. I...........Albert Lea
Folken, F. G............Albert Lea
Freeman, J. P...........Albert Lea
Freligh, W. B...........Albert Lea
Gamble, J. W...........Albert Lea
Gamble, P. M...........Albert Lea
Gullixson, A.............Albert Lea
Jerome, Bourne......Philadelphia, Pa.

Kaasa, L. J..............Albert Lea
Kamp, B. A.............Albert Lea
Leopard, B. A..........Albert Lea
Manley, L. V....Northampton, Mass.
Palmer, C. J...........Albert Lea
Palmer, W. L...........Albert Lea
Prins, L. R.............Albert Lea
Schultz, J. A..........Albert Lea
Trombley, R. A............Emmons
Whitson, S. A................Alden

GOODHUE COUNTY MEDICAL SOCIETY
Regular meetings, none
Annual meeting, December
Number of Members: 21

President

Graves, R. B.........Red Wing

Secretary

Juers, E. H............Red Wing

Aanes, A. M.............Red Wing
Anderson, S. H...........Red Wing
Brusegard, J. F..........Red Wing

Claydon, D. R.............Red Wing
Claydon, H. F............Zumbrota
Claydon, L. E............Red Wing
Flom, M. G.............Zumbrota
Graves, R. B............Red Wing
Hartnagel, G. F..........Red Wing
Hedin, R. F..........Chicago, Ill.
Johnson, A. E............Red Wing
Jones, A. W.............Red Wing

Juers, E. H.............Red Wing
Liffrig, W. W..........Goodhue
Mack, J. J......Little Rock, Ark.
McGuigan, H. T.........Red Wing
Miller, F. J.......Spokane, Wash.
Smith, M. W............Red Wing
Steffens, H. A..........Red Wing
Vaaler, T...........Cannon Falls
Williams, M. R......Cannon Falls

HENNEPIN COUNTY MEDICAL SOCIETY
Regular meetings, first Monday each month excepting June, July, August and September
Annual meeting, October
Number of Members: 599

President

Ulrich, H. L........Minneapolis

Secretary

Campbell, O. J........Minneapolis

Abramson, Milton.......Minneapolis
Alexander, H. A........Minneapolis
Aling, C. A............Minneapolis
Allen, H. W............Minneapolis
Allison, R. G..........Minneapolis
Altnow, H. O...........Minneapolis
Andersen, A. G.........Minneapolis
Andersen, S. C.........Minneapolis
Anderson, D. D.........Minneapolis
Anderson, E. D.........Minneapolis
Anderson, E. R.........Minneapolis
Anderson, F. J.........Minneapolis
Anderson, J. K.........Minneapolis
Anderson, K. W.........Minneapolis
Anderson, P. A.........Minneapolis
Anderson, U. S.........Minneapolis
Andreassen, E. C.......Minneapolis
Andrews, R. S.........Minneapolis
Annis, H. B...........Minneapolis
Arey, S. L............Excelsior
Arlander, C. E........Minneapolis
Arling, L. S..........Minneapolis
Arnold, A. W..........Minneapolis
Arnold, D. C..........Minneapolis
Arvidson, C. G........Minneapolis
Aune, Martin..........Minneapolis
Aurand, W. H.........Minneapolis
Baken, M. P..........Minneapolis
Baker, A. T..........Minneapolis
Baker, E. L..........Minneapolis
Baker, Looe..........Minneapolis
Barber, J. P.........Minneapolis
Barron, Moses.........Minneapolis
Bass, G. W...........Minneapolis

Baxter, S. H..........Minneapolis
Bayard, H. F..........Minneapolis
Beard, A. H...........Minneapolis
Beckman, W. G.........Minneapolis
Bedford, E. W.........Minneapolis
Bell, E. T............Minneapolis
Belzer, M. S..........Minneapolis
Benjamin, A. E........Minneapolis
Benjamin, E. D........Minneapolis
Benjamin, H. G........Minneapolis
Benn, F. G............Minneapolis
Berger, A. G..........Minneapolis
Bergh, G. S..........Minneapolis
Berkwitz, N. J........Minneapolis
Berman, Reuben........Minneapolis
Bessesen, A. N., Jr...Minneapolis
Bessesen, W. A........Minneapolis
Blake, James............Hopkins
Blake, J. A.............Hopkins
Blaustone, H. M.......Minneapolis
Bloedel, T. F.........Minneapolis
Bockman, M. W. H......Minneapolis
Boehme, E. H..........Minneapolis
Boies, L. R...........Minneapolis
Booth, A. H...........Minneapolis
Boreen, C. A..........Minneapolis
Borgeson, E. J........Minneapolis
Borman, C. N..........Minneapolis
Bouman, H. A. H.......Minneapolis
Boynton, R. H.........Minneapolis
Bracken, H. M....Claremont, Calif.
Bratrud, A. F.........Minneapolis
Brooks, C. N..........Minneapolis
Brown, F. D..........Paynesville
Brown, E. H...........Minneapolis
Brutsch, G. C.........Minneapolis
Bryant, F. L..........Minneapolis
Bryant, O. R..........Minneapolis
Bulkley, Kenneth......Minneapolis

Bullard, M. J.........Minneapolis
Butler, John..........Minneapolis
Buxelle, L. K.........Minneapolis
Cable, M. L...........Minneapolis
Cabot, V. S...........Minneapolis
Cady, L. H...........Minneapolis
Callerstrom, G. W.....Minneapolis
Cameron, Isabell......Minneapolis
Camp, W. E...........Minneapolis
Campbell, L. M........Minneapolis
Campbell, O. J........Minneapolis
Cardle, A. E.........Minneapolis
Carey, J. B..........Minneapolis
Carlaw, C. M.........Minneapolis
Carlson, Lawrence.....Minneapolis
Carlson, L. T.........Minneapolis
Caron, R. P..........Minneapolis
Cavanor, F. T........Minneapolis
Chesley, A. J.........Minneapolis
Christenson, G. R.....Minneapolis
Christianson, H. W....Minneapolis
Clark, H. S..........Minneapolis
Clay, L. B...........Minneapolis
Cohen, B. A..........Minneapolis
Cohen, S. S........Oak Terrace
Condit, W. H.........Minneapolis
Cook, H. W...........Minneapolis
Corbett, J. F........Minneapolis
Corniea, A. D........Minneapolis
Cottam, Gilbert.......Minneapolis
Crafts, L. M.........Minneapolis
Cranmer, R. R........Minneapolis
Cranston, R. W.....St. Louis Park
Creevy, C. D.........Minneapolis
Creighton, R. H......Minneapolis
Curtin, J. F.........Minneapolis
Cutts, George........Minneapolis
Cutts, R. E..........Minneapolis
Dady, E. E...........Minneapolis

arks, A. H.............Minneapolis	Salt, C. G.................Minneapolis	Sweitzer, S. E...........Minneapolis
atterson, W. E...........Minneapolis	Samuelson, Samuel........Minneapolis	Swendseen, C. G..........Minneapolis
aulsen, E. L............Minneapolis	Sandt, K. E.............Minneapolis	Taylor, J. H............Minneapolis
ederson, R. M...........Minneapolis	Sawatzky, W. A..........Minneapolis	*Ternstrom, O. H........Minneapolis
ennington, Reuben.......Minneapolis	Schaaf, P. H. K.........Minneapolis	Thomas, G. E...........Minneapolis
eppard, T. A............Minneapolis	Schaefer, W. G..........Minneapolis	Thomas, G. H...........Minneapolis
etersen, J. R............Minneapolis	Scheldrup, N. H.........Minneapolis	Thomas, G. J...........Minneapolis
etersen, Thorvald.......Minneapolis	Scherer, L. R...........Minneapolis	Thompson, H. H.........Minneapolis
eterson, Henry..........Minneapolis	Schmidt, G. F...........Minneapolis	Tingdale, A. C..............Wayzata
eterson, H. O...........Minneapolis	Schmitt, A. F...........Minneapolis	Trueman, H. S...........Minneapolis
eterson, H. W...........Minneapolis	Schmitt, S. C....Los Angeles, Calif.	Tunstead, H. J..........Minneapolis
eterson, N. P...........Minneapolis	Schneider, J. P..........Minneapolis	Turnacliff, D. D........Minneapolis
eterson, O. H...........Minneapolis	Schottler, H. E..........Minneapolis	Tyrrell, C. C...........Minneapolis
eterson, P. E...........Minneapolis	Schultz, P. J...........Minneapolis	Ude, W. H.............Minneapolis
eterson, W. C...........Minneapolis	Schussler, O. F.........Minneapolis	Ulrich, H. L...........Minneapolis
etit, L. J..............Minneapolis	Schwartz, V. J..........Minneapolis	Undine, C. A...........Minneapolis
eyton, W. T............Minneapolis	Schwyzer, Gustav........Minneapolis	Wahlquist, H. F.........Minneapolis
funder, M. C............Minneapolis	Scott, F. H............Minneapolis	Walch, A. E...........Minneapolis
helps, K. A............Minneapolis	Scott, H. G............Minneapolis	Waldron, C. W..........Minneapolis
latou, E. S............Minneapolis	Seashore, Gilbert.......Minneapolis	Wall, C. E............Minneapolis
ollard, D. W...........Minneapolis	Seham, Max.............Minneapolis	Wangensteen, O. H......Minneapolis
ollock, D. K...........Minneapolis	Seifert, M. H............Excelsior	Wanous, E. Z..........Minneapolis
olzak, J. A............Minneapolis	Selleseth, I. F.........Minneapolis	Ward, A. W...........Minneapolis
oppe, F. H............Minneapolis	Shaperman, E. P.........Minneapolis	Ward, P. A...........Minneapolis
ratt, F. J.............Minneapolis	Shapiro, M. J...........Minneapolis	Warham, T. T..........Minneapolis
ratt, J. A.............Minneapolis	Sharp, D. V............Minneapolis	Watson, J. A..........Minneapolis
reine, I. A............Minneapolis	Slegmann, W. C..........Minneapolis	Webb, R. C...........Minneapolis
rim, J. A.............Minneapolis	Silver, J. D...........Minneapolis	Weisman, S. A.........Minneapolis
roshek, C. E...........Minneapolis	Simons, J. H...........Minneapolis	Westman, R. T.........Minneapolis
uello, R. O. B.........Minneapolis	Simpson, R. D..........Minneapolis	Wethall, A. G.........Minneapolis
uinby, T. F....Lake Wales, Florida	Siperstein, M. D........Minneapolis	Wetherby, Macnider.....Minneapolis
uist, H. W............Minneapolis	Sivertsen, Andrew.......Minneapolis	Weum, T. W...........Minneapolis
asmussen, R. C.........Minneapolis	Sivertsen, Ivar.........Minneapolis	White, A. A...........Minneapolis
eed, C. A.............Minneapolis	Skjold, A. C...........Minneapolis	White, S. M...........Minneapolis
egnier, E. A...........Minneapolis	Sloan, Julius...........Minneapolis	White, W. D...........Minneapolis
ewbridge, A. G.........Minneapolis	Smisek, P. M...........Minneapolis	Whitesell, L. A........Minneapolis
Reynolds, J. S..........Minneapolis	Smith, A. E............Minneapolis	Widen, W. P...........Minneapolis
Rice, C. O.............Minneapolis	Smith, A. M............Minneapolis	Wilcox, A. E..........Minneapolis
Richardson, F. S........Minneapolis	Smith, H. M............Minneapolis	Wilder, K. W..........Minneapolis
Richdorf, L. F..........Minneapolis	Smith, N. M............Minneapolis	Wilder, R. L..........Minneapolis
Rieke, W. W..............Wayzata	Soderlind, R. T.........Minneapolis	Wilken, P. A..........Minneapolis
Rigler, L. G...........Minneapolis	Solhaug, S. B...........Minneapolis	Willcutt, C. E.........Minneapolis
Rishmiller, J. H........Minneapolis	Spano, J. P............Minneapolis	Williams, Robert.......Minneapolis
Rizer, R. I............Minneapolis	Sperling, Louis.........Minneapolis	Wilner, L. H..........Minneapolis
Roan, C. M............Minneapolis	Spratt, C. N...........Minneapolis	Winther, Nora.........Minneapolis
Robb, E. F............Minneapolis	Stanford, C. E.........Minneapolis	Witham, C. A..........Minneapolis
Robbins, O. F..........Minneapolis	Stelter, L. A..........Minneapolis	Wittich, F. W.........Minneapolis
Roberts, S. W..........Minneapolis	Stenstrom, A. T.........Minneapolis	Wohlrabe, A. A........Minneapolis
Roberts, T. S..........Minneapolis	Stewart, C. A..........Minneapolis	Wohlrabe, C. T........Minneapolis
Roberts, W. B..........Minneapolis	Stewart, R. I..........Minneapolis	Woodworth, Elizabeth...Minneapolis
Robitshek, E. C........Minneapolis	Stomel, Joseph..........Minneapolis	Wright, C. B..........Minneapolis
Rochford, W. E.........Minneapolis	Strachauer, A. C........Minneapolis	Wright, C. D..........Minneapolis
Rodda, F. C............Minneapolis	Strout, B. S...........Minneapolis	Wright, F. R..........Minneapolis
Rodgers, C. L..........Minneapolis	Strout, G. E...........Minneapolis	Wright, S. G..........Minneapolis
Rosen, Samuel..........Minneapolis	Sturre, J. R...........Minneapolis	Wright, W. S..........Minneapolis
Rosenwald, R. M........Minneapolis	Sullivan, R. M.........Minneapolis	Wyatt, O. S...........Minneapolis
Rucker, W. H...........Minneapolis	Sullivan, R. R.........Minneapolis	Wynne, H. M. N........Minneapolis
Rud, N. E.............Minneapolis	Sundt, Mathias.........Minneapolis	Ylvisaker, R. S........Minneapolis
Rudell, G. L...........Minneapolis	Swanson, Cephas.........Minneapolis	Yoerg, O. W...........Minneapolis
Russeth, A. N..........Minneapolis	Swanson, R. E..........Minneapolis	Zaworski, E. A........Minneapolis
Rusten, E. M...........Minneapolis	Sweetser, H. B.........Minneapolis	Zierold, A. A.........Minneapolis
Sadler, W. P...........Minneapolis	Sweetser, H. B., Sr.....Minneapolis	Ziskin, Thomas.........Minneapolis
St. Cyr, K. J................Osseo	Sweetser, T. J.........Minneapolis	

KANDIYOHI-SWIFT-MEEKER COUNTY MEDICAL SOCIETY

Regular meetings, second Wednesday of month
Annual meeting, December
Number of Members: 35

President
Petersen, M. C............Willmar

Secretary
Scofield, C. L...............Benson

Anderson, L. W...........Atwater	Danielson, K. A...........Litchfield	Jensen, H. H.............Atwater
Anderson, R. E...........Willmar	Danielson, Lennox........Litchfield	Johnson, Hans...........Kerkhoven
Arnson, J. M............Benson	Dowswell, W. J..........Kerkhoven	Kaufman, E. J...........Appleton
Branton, A. F...........Willmar	Duluda, S. S............Dassel	Kaufman, W. C...........Appleton
Branton, B. J...........Willmar	Fredrickson, A. C....Lake Lillian	Lutz, E. H.............Willmar
Brigham, Frank..........Watkins	Fredrickson, G. U. Y....Lake Lillian	Macklin, W. E..........Litchfield
Daignault, Oscar.........Benson	Frisch, F. P.............Willmar	Nelson, K. L............Willmar
	Frost, E. M.............Willmar	O'Connor, D. C......Eden Valley
	Giere, S. W............Benson	Petersen, M. C..........Willmar
	Hedlund, C. J...........Atwater	Proeschel, R. K.........Willmar
	Hodapp, R. J...........Willmar	Scofield, C. L..........Benson
	Hutchinson, Henry.......Willmar	Telford, V. J...........Litchfield
	Jacobs, D. L...........Willmar	Wilmot, C. A..........Litchfield
	Jacobs, J. C...........Willmar	Wilmot, H. E..........Litchfield

LYON-LINCOLN COUNTY MEDICAL SOCIETY

Regular meetings, first Tuesday of month, Spring and Fall
Annual meeting, first Tuesday in November
Number of Members: 22

President
Helferty, J. K...............Tracy

Secretary
Workman, W. G...............Tracy

Akester, Ward ....Marshall	Ford, B. C.............Marshall	Potter, R. B............Hendricks
Bossingham, O. N....Lake Benton	Germo, Charles..........Balaton	Purves, G. H.........Lake Benton
Erickson, A. O............Ivanhoe	*Golden, C. M............Tyler	Robertson, J. B........Minneota
	Gray, F. D.............Marshall	Sanderson, E. T.........Minneota
	Helferty, J. K...........Tracy	Schmidt, P. G......Granite Falls
	Hermanson, P. E........Hendricks	Smith, L. A............Balaton
	Hoidale, A. D............Tracy	Thordarson, Theodore...Minneota
	Jacquot, C. L..........Marshall	Vadheim, A. J...........Tyler
	Johnson, P. C...........Tyler	Valentine, W. H.........Tracy
	Monson, L. J............Canby	Workman, W. G..........Tracy
	Persons, C. E..........Marshall	Yaeger, W. W..........Marshall

*Deceased.

McLEOD COUNTY MEDICAL SOCIETY
Regular meetings, first Thursday of month
Annual meeting, January
Number of Members: 19

President		
Goss, H. C..................Glencoe	Holm, H. H.................Glencoe	Sahr, W. G..............Hutchinso
	Jensen, A. H.............Hutchinson	Schmidt, W. R..............Glenco
Secretary	Jensen, A. M.............Brownton	Scholpp, O. W...........Hutchinso
Sahr, W. G..............Hutchinson	Klima, W. W...............Stewart	Sheppard, C. G........Hutchinso
	Langhoff, A. H............Glencoe	Sheppard, Fred ....Hutchinso
Clement, J. B........Lester Prairie	Lippmann, E. W.........Hutchinson	Sheppard, P. E..........Hutchinso
Fine, B. A................Winsted	McMahon, M. J..........Green Isle	Tinker, C. W..............Stewar
Goss, H. C................Glencoe	Ninneman, N. N.........Silver Lake	Trutna, T. J............Silver Lak

MOWER COUNTY MEDICAL SOCIETY
Regular meetings, last Thursday of month
Annual meeting, Tuesday before last Thursday in November
Number of Members: 26

President		
Leck, P. C....................Austin	Havens, J. G. W..............Austin	Melzer, G. R.................Lyl
	Hegge, O. H................Austin	Mitchell, R. S........Grand Meado
Secretary	Hegge, R. S................Austin	Morrow, J. J................Austi
Robertson, P. A..............Austin	Henslin, A. E.............Le Roy	Morse, M. P...............Le Rô
	Hertel, G. E................Austin	Robertson, P. A............Austi
Allen, A. W..................Austin	Johnson, O. J................Lyle	Rosenthal, F. H.......Grand Meado
Allen, C. C..................Austin	Kibler, F. E................Austin	Schneider, P. J.............Adar
Allen, H. B..................Austin	Leck, P. C.................Austin	Schottler, G. J.............Dexte
Cronwell, B. J................Austin	Lommen, P. A...............Austin	Sheedy, C. L...............Austi
Flanagan, L. G...............Austin	McKenna, J. K..............Austin	Thomson, J. M............Brownsdal
Grise, W. B..................Austin		

NICOLLET-LE SUEUR COUNTY MEDICAL SOCIETY
Regular meetings, first Tuesday, April, September, and December
Annual meeting, first Tuesday in December
Number of Members: 2

President		
Kerschbaumer, Louisa.......St. Peter	Ericson, Swan..............Le Sueur	Nilson, H. J.......North Mankat
	Freeman, G. H............St. Peter	Nissen, A. S.............St. Pete
Secretary	Grimes, B. P.............St. Peter	Olmanson, G. G...........St. Pete
Lenander, M. E.............St. Peter.	Gully, R. J...............St. Peter	Rossen, R. X.............St. Pete
	Hiniker, P. J.............Le Sueur	Sonnesyn, N. N...........Le Sueu
Aitkens, H. B............Le Center	Holtan, Theodore.........Waterville	Strathern, C. S..........St. Pete
Covell, W. W.............St. Peter	Kerschbaumer, Louisa......St. Peter	Strathern, F. P..........St. Pete
Curtis, R. A.............Le Center	Kolars, J. J..............Le Center	Traxler, F. J............Henderso
	Lenander, M. E...........St. Peter	Wolner, O. H.............St. Pete

OLMSTED-HOUSTON-FILLMORE-DODGE COUNTY MEDICAL SOCIETY
Regular meetings, first Wednesday every odd month
Annual meeting, November
Number of Members: 381

President		
Piper, M. C.................Rochester	Broders, A. C.............Rochester	Dickson, D. D............Rocheste
	Brown, A. E..............Rochester	Djx, C. R................Rocheste
Secretary	Brown, P. W..............Rochester	Dixon, C. F..............Rocheste
Anderson, M. J..............Rochester	Brown, R. W..............Rochester	Dockerty, M. B...........Rocheste
	Browne, H. C., Jr........Rochester	Dolder, F.C................Eyot
Adams, R. C.................Rochester	Brumm, H. J..............Rochester	Donath, D. H.............Rochest
Adson, A. W.................Rochester	Brunsting, L. A..........Rochester	Drips, D. G..............Rochest
Affeldt, D. E...............Kasson	Buchstein, H. F..........Rochester	Dry, T. J................Rochest
Ahlfs, J. J................Caledonia	Bule, L. A...............Rochester	Eaton, L. McK............Rochest
Allen, E. V.................Rochester	Burchell, H. B...........Rochester	Ecker, A. D..............Rochest
Alvarez, W. C...............Rochester	Bussey, C. D.............Rochester	Elkins, E. C.............Rochest
Amberg, Samuel ....Rochester	Butt, H. R...............Rochester	Emmett, J. L.............Rochest
Anderson, M. J..............Rochester	Cabell, C. L.............Rochester	Engle, D. H..............Rochest
Anderson, N. E..............Harmony	Cabot, Hugh ....Rochester	Erich, J. B..............Rochest
Annis, J. W.................Rochester	Cady, J. B...............Rochester	Erickson, C. W...........Rochest
Archer, G. F., Jr...........Rochester	Cameron, D. M............Rochester	Eusterman, G. B..........Roches
Arny, F. P..................Preston	Camp, J. D...............Rochester	Evarts, A. B.............Rochest
Baggenstoss, A. H...........Rochester	Campbell, S. J...........Rochester	Faber, J. E..............Rochest
Bajley, R. J........Spokane, Wash.	Canfield, W. W...........Houston	Fairchild, R. D..........Rochest
Bair, H. L..................Rochester	Carmichael, F. A., Jr....Rochester	Farthing, J. W...........Rochest
Baker, G. S.................Rochester	Chauncey, L. R...........Rochester	Fatherree, T. J., Jr.....Le Sueu
Baker, H. R.................Hayfield	Chew, E. M...............Rochester	Fawcett, C. E.........Stewartvi
Baker, R. L.................Hayfield	Clagett, O. T............Rochester	Figi, F. A...............Rochest
Balfour, D. C...............Rochester	Clark, L. W..........Spring Valley	Foley, M. P..............Rochest
Bannick, E. G........Seattle, Wash.	Clark, R. L., Jr.........Rochester	Foster, F. P.............Rochest
Bargen, J. A................Rochester	Cleveland, W. H..........Rochester	Fricke, R. E.............Rochest
Barker, N. W................Rochester	Clifton, T. A............Chatfield	Friedell, M. T...........Roches
Barnes, A. R................Rochester	Coffey, R. J.............Rochester	Furey, E. D..............Roches
Bedard, R. E................Rochester	Comfort, M. W............Rochester	Gaarde, F. W.............Roches
Beiswanger, R. H............Wykoff	Conner, M. P.............Rochester	Ghormley, R. K...........Roches
Belzer, L. H................Rochester	Conway, J. F.............Rochester	Gibson, W. R.............Roches
Belote, G. B................Caledonia	Cook, E. N...............Rochester	Giffin, H. Z.............Roches
Benedict, W. L..............Rochester	Corwin, W. C.............Rochester	Gober, O. B..............Roches
Bennett, R. L., Jr..........Rochester	Counseller, V. S.........Rochester	Goldstein, Moe ....Roches
Benson, K. W................Rochester	Cragg, R. W..............Rochester	Good, C. A., Jr..........Roches
Berkman, D. M...............Rochester	Craig, W. McK............Rochester	Goodson, W. H., Jr.......Roches
Berkman, J. M...............Rochester	Crandall, L. A...........Rochester	Graham, R. W.............Roches
Betlach, C. T...............Rochester	Crewe, J. E..............Rochester	Gray, H. K...............Roches
Bigelow, C..................Dodge Center	Crumpacker, L. K.........Rochester	Gregg, R. O..............Roches
Binger, M. W................Rochester	Cusick, P. L.............Rochester	Grindlay, J. H...........Roches
Birge, H. L.................Rochester	Cutler, H. H.............Rochester	Grinnell, W. B............Pres
Black, B. M.................Rochester	Davis, A. C..............Rochester	Groff, J. E..............Roches
Black, J. R.................Rochester	Davis, L. G..............Rushford	Guernsey, C. M...........Roches
Blake, T. W............Seattle, Wash.	Day, L. A................Rochester	Habein, H. C.............Roches
Blum, B. B..................Rochester	Dearing, W. H., Jr.......Rochester	Haines, D. J., Jr........Roches
Boland, M. F................Rochester	Deeds, C. D..............Rochester	Haines, S. F.............Roches
Boothby, W. M...............Rochester	Delmonjco, E. J..........Rochester	Hall, B. E...............Roches
Bowing, H. H................Rochester	Desjardins, A. U.........Rochester	Hallenbeck, D. F.........Roche
Braasch, W. F...............Rochester	Deuterman, J. L.........Elgin, Ill.	

Hammer, H. J.............Rochester	MacLean, A. R............Rochester	Rushton, J. G.............Rochester
Harrington, S. W.........Rochester	Madding, G. F............Rochester	Rutledge, D. I............Rochester
Hartman, H. R...........Rochester	Magath, T. B.............Rochester	Rynearson, E. H...........Rochester
Havens, F. Z.............Rochester	Maksim, George, Jr......Rochester	Sanford, A. H.............Rochester
Hawn, H. W..............Rochester	Mann, A. S., Jr..........Rochester	Sawyer, M. H.............Rochester
Heck, F. J...............Rochester	Mann, F. C..............Rochester	Schmidt, H. W............Rochester
Heilman, D. M. H.........Rochester	Mareley, D. M............Rochester	Schneider, H. H...........Rochester
Heilman, F. R............Rochester	Masson, D. M............Rochester	Searles, P. W.............Rochester
Helland, G. M..........Spring Grove	Masson, J. C.............Rochester	Secord, E. W.............Rochester
Helland, J. W..........Spring Grove	Matthews, M. W..........Rochester	Seedorf, E. E.............Rochester
Helm, Standiford ....Rochester	Mayo, C. H..............Rochester	Seldon, T. H.............Rochester
Helmbolz, H. F...........Rochester	Mayo, C. W..............Rochester	Sheedy, L. P..............Rochester
Hempstead, B. E..........Rochester	Mayo, W. J..............Rochester	Shelden, C. H.............Rochester
Hench, P. S..............Rochester	Maytum, C. K............Rochester	Sheldon, W. D.............Rochester
Henderson, M. S..........Rochester	McCarty, W. C...........Rochester	Shoemaker, Rosemary .....Rochester
Hendrick, J. A., Jr......Rochester	McDonald, J. R...........Rochester	Sibley, W. L..............Roanoke, Va.
Herrell, W. E............Rochester	McDonough, F. E.........Rochester	Sickler, J. R.............Rochester
Hertz, C. S..............Rochester	McKaig, C. B.............Pine Island	Simonton, K. M...........Rochester
Hewitt, E. S.............Rochester	McKinnon, D. A., Jr......Rochester	Simpson, W. C............Rochester
Hewitt, R. M.............Rochester	Mccray, P. M., Jr........Rochester	Skaug, H. M., Jr.........Chatfield
Heyerdale, O. C.........Rochester	Merritt, W. A...........Rochester	Skinner, I. C., Jr.......Rochester
Heyerdale, W. W.........Rochester	Meyerding, H. W..........Rochester	Slocumb, C. H............Rochester
Hildebrand, A. G........Rochester	Middleton, A. W.........Rochester	Smith, B. F..............Rochester
Hines, E. A., Jr........Rochester	Miller, J. M............Rochester	Smith, C. H..............Rochester
Hinshaw, H. C..........Rochester	Moersch, F. P...........Rochester	Smith, F. A..............Rochester
Hodgson, C. H..........Rochester	Moersch, H. J...........Rochester	Smith, F. D..............Rochester
Hollister, C. B., H......Rochester	Montgomery, Hamilton ...Rochester	Smith, F. L..............Rochester
Holman, J. C., Jr.......Rochester	Montgomery, T. R........Rochester	Smith, H. L..............Rochester
Horton, B. T...........Rochester	Morlock, C. G...........Rochester	Smith, L. A..............Rochester
Howell, L. P...........Rochester	Mousel, L. H............Rochester	Smith, N. D..............Rochester
Hubly, J. M............Rochester	Mulrooney, R. E.........Rochester	Snell, A. M..............Rochester
Hunt, A. B.............Rochester	Mundell, B. J...........Rochester	Snyder, J. M.............Rochester
Jackman, R. J..........Rochester	Mussey, R. D............Rochester	Soniat, T. L. L..........Rochester
Jensen, R. M...........Rochester	Nash, J. A..............Rochester	Sprague, R. G............Rochester
Jewett, R. E...........Rochester	Nass, H. A..............Mabel	Stalker, L. K............Rochester
Johnson, H. P..........Harmony	Neal, H. B..............Rochester	Steenrod, E. J...........Rochester
Johnson, R. B..........Lanesboro	Nehring, J. P...........Preston	Steffens, L. F...........Rochester
Joyce, G. L............Rochester	New, G. B...............Rochester	Stuhler, L. G............Rochester
Judd, E. S., Jr........Rochester	Norris, N. T............Caledonia	Sutherland, C. G.........Rochester
Jump, W. C............Kasson	Noth, P. H..............Rochester	Swartz, F. C.............Rochester
Kahler, J. E...........Rochester	Odel, H. M..............Rochester	Swift, E. V..............Rochester
Kearney, R. W.........Rochester	Olds, J. W..............Rochester	Swingle, H. F., Jr.......Rochester
Keith, N. M...........Rochester	O'Leary, P. A...........Rochester	Templin, D. B............Gary, Indiana
Kelly, M. H...........Rochester	Olsen, A. M.............Rochester	Tennison, W. J., III.....Rochester
Kemble, J. W.........Plattsburg, N. Y.	Olson, E. A.............Pine Island	Thompson, G. J...........Rochester
Kendrick, T. D. H.......Rochester	Olson, G. E.............West Concord	Tierney, C. M............Harmony
Kennedy, R. L. J.......Rochester	Onsgard, L. K., Jr.......Houston	Tillisch, J. H...........Rochester
Kepler, E. J...........Rochester	Onsgard, L. K., Sr.......Houston	Trueman, R. R............Rochester
Kermott, L. H., Jr......Rochester	Parker, R. L............Rochester	Tuohy, E. B..............Rochester
Kernohan, J. W.........Rochester	Parkhill, E. M..........Rochester	Vickers, P. M............Rochester
Kerr, J. G............Rochester	Patton, G. D............Rochester	Wagener, H. P............Rochester
Kierland, R. R.........Rochester	Paulson, D. L...........Rochester	Wasman, Morris...........Rochester
Kirklin, B. R..........Rochester	Paulson, J. A...........Rochester	Wakefield, E. G..........Rochester
Kirklin, O. L..........Rochester	Pearman, R. O. D........Rochester	Walsh, J. J..............Rochester
Koch, E. A. S..........Rochester	Pemberton, J. deJ.......Rochester	Walsh, M. N..............Rochester
Koch, F. L. P..........Rochester	Perozzi, Thelma ....Rochester	Walters, Waltman ....Rochester
Koelsche, G. A.........Rochester	Piper, M. C.............Rochester	Ward, C. E...............Rochester
Kowallis, G. F.........Rochester	Plummer, W. A...........Rochester	Washburn, R. N...........Rochester
Krusen, F. H...........Rochester	Pollock, L. W...........Rochester	Watkins, C. H............Rochester
Kvale, W. F............Rochester	Pool, T. L..............Rochester	Watterson, K. W..........Rochester
Laird, D. R............Rochester	Popp, W. C..............Rochester	Waugh, J. M..............Rochester
Lannin, J. C...........Mabel	Powers, H. F............Rochester	Weaver, D. F., Jr........Rochester
Leddy, E. T............Rochester	Prangen, A. D...........Rochester	Weber, H. M..............Rochester
Lemon, R. G...........Rochester	Prickman, L. E..........Rochester	Weir, J. F...............Rochester
Lemon, W. S...........Rochester	Priestley, J. T.........Rochester	Wilder, R. M.............Rochester
Lewis, E. B............Rochester	Pumphrey, R. E..........Rochester	Williams, H. L., Jr......Rochester
Lillie, H. I............Rochester	Ralph, R. D.............Rochester	Williams, R. V...........Rushford
Lipscomb, W. R.........Rochester	Randall, L. M...........Rochester	Willius, F. A............Rochester
Lloyd, S. J............Rochester	Rasmussen, T. B.........Rochester	Wilson, L. B.............Rochester
Lochead, D. C..........Rochester	Regan, J. F.............Rochester	Wilson, R. B.............Rochester
Logan, A. H...........Rochester	Rhorer, R. J............Rochester	Wilson, W. D.............Rochester
Logan, G. B...........Rochester	Risser, A. F............Stewartville	Wolff, L. W..............Rochester
Lord, G. A............Rochester	Rivers, A. B............Rochester	Wolfram, D. J............Rochester
Love, J. G............Rochester	Robertson, H. E.........Rochester	Woltman, H. W............Rochester
Lovelace, W. R.........Rochester	Rogne, W. G.............Spring Grove	Wood, H. C...............Rochester
Lovelady, S. B.........Rochester	Rosenberg, E. F.........Rochester	Woodruff, C. W...........Chatfield
Luden, Georgine..Victoria, B. C., Can.	Rosenow, E. C...........Rochester	Woodruff, Robert.........Rochester
Lundy, J. S............Rochester	Rosenow, E. C., Jr.......Rochester	Wrork, D. H..............Rochester
Macey, H. B...........Rochester	Rosenstiel, H. C........Rochester	Yeager, C. L.............Rochester
MacKay, A. R..........Rochester	Rucker, C. W............Rochester	Young, H. H..............Rochester

PARK REGION DISTRICT AND COUNTY MEDICAL SOCIETY
Douglas, Grant, Otter Tail and Wilkin Counties
Regular meetings, Second Wednesday every even month
Annual meeting, December
Number of Members: 60

President

Combacker, L. C.........Fergus Falls

Secretary

Boline, C. A............Battle Lake

Ahrens, R. S...........Fergus Falls	Baker, N. H.............Fergus Falls	Drought, W. W.........Fergus Falls
Arndt, D. W...........Frazee	Bergquist, K. E.........Battle Lake	Erickson, C. O.........Fergus Falls
Baker, A. C............Fergus Falls	Blakey, A. R............Osakis	Esser, John ....Perham
	Boline, C. A............Battle Lake	Estrem, C. O..........Fergus Falls
	Boyd, L. M.............Alexandria	Gardner, W. P.........Fergus Falls
	Boysen, J. E............Pelican Rapids	Griswold, F. E.........Hoffman
	Boysen, Peter ....Pelican Rapids	Hand, W. R...........Elbow Lake
	Broker, W. S............Wadena	Hanson, E. C..........New York Mills
	Burnap, W. L...........Fergus Falls	Haskell, A. D.........Alexandria
	Clifford, C. W..........Osakis	Heiberg, E. A.........Fergus Falls
	Combacker, L. C.........Fergus Falls	Jacobs, G. C..........Fergus Falls

Johnson, Q. V..........Fergus Falls
Katzberg, L. W..........Fergus Falls
Kierland, P. E..........Alexandria
Lee, W. A..........Fergus Falls
Leibold, H. H..........Parkers Prairie
Leland, J. T..........Herman
Lewis, A. J..........Henning
Love, F. A..........Carlos
Lund, C. J. T..........Underwood
McMahon, L. H..........Breckenridge
Miller, W. A..........New York Mills
Mouritsen, G. J..........Fergus Falls

Naegeli, Frank ....Fergus Falls
Nelson, W. I..........Minneapolis
Nelson, W. O. B..........Fergus Falls
Otto, H. C..................
Parson, L. R..........Elbow Lake
Patterson, W. I..........Fergus Falls
Paulson, T. S..........Fergus Falls
Powers, F. W..........Barrett
Randall, A. M., ...Ashby
Reeve, E. T..........Elbow Lake
Riley, J. B..........Fergus Falls
Rimer, E. W..........Breckenridge

Ross, W.' P.............Battle Lake
Satersmoen,' Theodore....Pelican Rapids
Sather, E. R..........Alexandria
Serkland, J. C..........Rothsay
Stemsrud, H. L..........Parkers Prairie
Steube, R. W..........Alexandria
Sutton, H. R..........Hoffman
Tanquist, E. J..........Alexandria
Vail, J. B..........Henning
Windsor, R. L..........Fergus Falls
Wray, W. E.................Campbell

RAMSEY COUNTY MEDICAL SOCIETY
Regular meetings, last Monday in every month excepting June, July, August
Annual meeting, last Monday in January
Number of Members: 336

President
Dunn, J. N..................St. Paul

Secretary
Wilson, J. A..................St. Paul

Abbott, J. S..................St. Paul
Ahrens, A. E..................St. Paul
Ahrens, A. H..................St. Paul
Alberts, M. W..................St. Paul
Alden, J. F..................St. Paul
Alexander, F. H..................St. Paul
Armstrong, J. M..................St. Paul
Arnquist, A. S..................St. Paul
Aurelius, J. R..................St. Paul
Ausman, C. F..................St. Paul
Backus, A. S..................St. Paul
Bacon, D. K..................St. Paul
Bacon, L. C..................St. Paul
Balcome, M. M..................St. Paul
Barry, L. W..................St. Paul
Barsness, Nellie..................St. Paul
Beadie, W. D..........Cannon Falls
Beals, Hugh ....St. Paul
Beck, H. O..................St. Paul
Bell, C. C..................St. Paul
Benepe, J. L..................St. Paul
Bennion, P. H..................St. Paul
Bentley, N. F..................St. Paul
Berrisford, P. D..................St. Paul
Bicek, J. F..................St. Paul
Binger, H. S..................St. Paul
Birnberg, T. L..................St. Paul
Bock, R. A..................St. Paul
Boeckmann, Egil ....St. Paul
Bohland, E. H..................St. Paul
Bolender, H. L..................St. Paul
Borg, J. F..................St. Paul
Bouma, L. R..................St. Paul
Brand, G. D..................St. Paul
Bray, E. R..................St. Paul
Briggs, J. F..................St. Paul
Broadie, T. E..................St. Paul
Brodie, W. D..................St. Paul
Brown, E. L..................St. Paul
Brown, J. C..................St. Paul
Bulinski, T. J..................St. Paul
Burch, F. E..................St. Paul
Burns, R. M..................St. Paul
Burton, C. G..................St. Paul
Busher, H. H..................St. Paul
Cain, C. L..................St. Paul
Caldwell, J. F..................St. Paul
Carroll, W. C..................St. Paul
Chatterton, C. C..................St. Paul
Christiansen, A. ....St. Paul
Christison, J. T..................St. Paul
Clark, H. B., Jr..................St. Paul
Clark, T. C..................Minneapolis
Colby, Woodard ....St. Paul
Cole, W. H...................St. Paul
Collie, H. G..................St. Paul
Colvin, A. R..................St. Paul
Connor, C. E..................St. Paul
Cook, C. K..................St. Paul
Countryman, R. S..................St. Paul
Cowern, E. W..........North St. Paul
Critchfield, L. R..................St. Paul
Culligan, J. M..................St. Paul
Dack, L. G..................St. Paul
Daugherty, E. B..................St. Paul
Daugherty, L. E..................St. Paul
Davis, Herbert ....St. Paul
Davis, William ....St. Paul
Dedolph, Karl ....St. Paul
Delavan, P. A..................St. Paul

*Deceased.

370

Derauf, B. I..................St. Paul
Dickson, T. H..................St. Paul
Dittman, G. C..................St. Paul
Donohue, P. F..................St. Paul
Dovre, G. M..................St. Paul
Drake, C. B..................St. Paul
Dunn, J. N..................St. Paul
Earl, G. A..................St. Paul
Earl, John ....St. Paul
Earl, Robert ....St. Paul
Edlund, G...................St. Paul
Edwards, J. W..................St. Paul
Edwards, T. J..................St. Paul
Ely, O. S.............South St. Paul
Emerson, E. C..................St. Paul
Endress, E. E..................St. Paul
Ernest, G. C..........South St. Paul
Eshelby, E. C..................St. Paul
Fahey, E. W..................St. Paul
Ferguson, J. C..................St. Paul
Fesler, H. H..................St. Paul
Flanagan, H. F..................St. Paul
Fogarty, C. W..................St. Paul
Fogelberg, E. J..................St. Paul
Foley, F. B..................St. Paul
Freeman, C. D..................St. Paul
Fritz, W. L..................St. Paul
Froats, C. H..................St. Paul
Gager, E. C..................St. Paul
Garbrecht, Arthur ....St. Paul
Gardiner, D. G..................St. Paul
Geer, E. K..................St. Paul
Gehlen, J. N..................St. Paul
Geist, G. A..................St. Paul
Ghent, C. H..................St. Paul
Gibbs, E. C..................St. Paul
Gilfillan, J. S..................St. Paul
Ginsberg, Wm. ....St. Paul
Goltz, E. V..................St. Paul
Grant, H. W..................St. Paul
Gratrek, Thomas ....St. Paul
Grau, R. K..................St. Paul
Greenberg, H. A..................St. Paul
Gruenhagen, A. P..................St. Paul
Hagaman, G. K..................St. Paul
Hall, A. R..................St. Paul
Hall, H. H..................St. Paul
Hammes, E. M..................St. Paul
Hammond, J. F..................St. Paul
Harmon, G. E..................St. Paul
Harthel, W. F..................St. Paul
Hartley, E. C..................St. Paul
Hassett, M. F..................St. Paul
Hauser, V. J..................St. Paul
Hawkins, V. J..................St. Paul
Heath, A. C..................Stillwater
Heck, W. H...................St. Paul
Hedenstrom, F. G..................St. Paul
Hengstler, W. H..................St. Paul
Hensel, C. N..................St. Paul
Heron, R. C..................St. Paul
Herrmann, E. T..................St. Paul
Hilger, A. W..................St. Paul
Hilger, D. D..................St. Paul
Hilger, L. A..................St. Paul
Hilleboe, H. E..................St. Paul
Hinkler, L. F..................St. Paul
Hochfilzer, J...................St. Paul
Hoff, Alfred ....St. Paul
Hoffman, M. H..................St. Paul
Holcomb, J. C..................St. Paul
Holcomb, O. W..................St. Paul
Holmen, R. W..................St. Paul
Holt, J. E..................St. Paul
Hopkins, G. W..................St. Paul
Howard, M. A..................St. Paul
Howard, W. S..................St. Paul
Hullsiek, R. B..................St. Paul
Ide, A. W..................St. Paul
Ikeda, Kano ....St. Paul
Ingerson, C. A..................St. Paul

Jesion, J. W..................St. Paul
Johanson, W. G..................St. Paul
Johnson, A. M..................St. Paul
Johnson, L. J..................St. Paul
Johnson, R. G..................St. Paul
Johnson, T. H....San Francisco, Calif.
Jones, E. M..................St. Paul
Kamman, G. R..................St. Paul
Kannary, E. L..................St. Paul
Kaplan, D. H..................St. Paul
Kasper, E. M..................St. Paul
Keefe, Rolland ....St. Paul
Kelly, J. V..................St. Paul
Kelly, P. R..................St. Paul
Kendrick, E. V..................St. Paul
Kennedy, W. A..................St. Paul
Kesting, Herman ....St. Paul
King, G. ....St. Paul
Klein, H. N..................St. Paul
Knauff, M. K..................St. Paul
Kugler, A. A..................St. Paul
Kvitrud, Gilbert ....St. Paul
Langenderfer, F. V..................St. Paul
Larsen, C. L..................St. Paul
Lax, M. H..................St. Paul
Leahy, Bartholomew..................St. Paul
Leavenworth, R. O..................St. Paul
Leitch, Archibald ....St. Paul
Leonard, G. J..................Hastings
Lepak, J. A..................St. Paul
Lerche, William ....Cable, Wis.
Leven, N. L..................St. Paul
Levin, Bert ....St. Paul
Levitt, G. X..................St. Paul
Lick, C. L..................St. Paul
Lippman, H. S..................St. Paul
Little, W. J..................St. Paul
Livingstone, J. W..........Hudson, Wis
Lowe, E. R..........South St. Paul
Lowe, T. A..........South St. Paul
Lundholm, A. M..................St. Paul
Lynch, F. W..................St. Paul
Madden, J. F..................St. Paul
Markoc, J. C..................St. Paul
Martineau, J. L..................St. Paul
McCarthy, J. J..................St. Paul
McCarthy, W. R..................St. Paul
McClanahan, J. H..........White Bear
McClanahan, T. S..........White Bear
McLaren, J. M..................Minnetonka
McNevin, C. F..................St. Paul
Meade, J. B..................St. Paul
Mears, R. J..................St. Paul
Medelman, J. P..................St. Paul
Meyerding, E. A..................St. Paul
Moga, J. A..................St. Paul
Mogilner, S. N..................St. Paul
Molander, H. A..................St. Paul
Moquin, M. A..................St. Paul
Moran, T. R..................Phoenix, Ar
Moriarty, Berenice ....St. Paul
Morrissey, F. B..................St. Paul
Mortenson, N. G..................St. Paul
Moss, M. N..................St. Paul
Moynihan, T. J..................St. Paul
Muller, R. T..................St. Paul
Myers, Thomas ....St. Paul
Naegeli, A. E..................St. Paul
Naslund, A. W..................St. Paul
Neher, F. H..................St. Paul
Nelson, L. A..................St. Paul
Nichols, A. E..................St. Paul
Noble, J. F..................St. Paul
Nye, K. A..................St. Paul
Nye, L. J..................St. Paul
O'Connor, L. J..................St. Paul
Oerting, Harry ....St. Paul
Ogden, Warner ....St. Paul
Ohage, Justus, Jr..................St. Paul
Olson, C. A..................St. Paul
O'Reilley, B. E..................St. Paul

Ostergren, E. W. ....St. Paul	Schons, Edward ....St. Paul	Thompson, F. A. ....St. Paul
Ouelette, A. J. ....St. Paul	Schuldt, F. C. ....St. Paul	Thoreson, M. O. ....St. Paul
Page, C. V. ....St. Paul	Schulze, A. G. ....St. Paul	Tifft, C. R. ....St. Paul
Pearson, F. R. ....St. Paul	Schwyzer, Arnold ....St. Paul	Tregilgas, H. R. ......South St. Paul
Pedersen, A. H. ....St. Paul	Scott, E. E. ....St. Paul	Van Slyke, C. A. ....St. Paul
Perry, C. G. ....St. Paul	Senkler, G. E. ....St. Paul	Veirs, Dean ....St. Paul
Peterson, D. B. ....St. Paul	Setzer, H. J. ....St. Paul	Veirs, R. S. ....St. Paul
Peterson, J. L. E. ....St. Paul	Shannon, W. R. ....St. Paul	Venables, A. E. ....St. Paul
Peterson, V. N. ....St. Paul	Shellman, J. L. ....St. Paul	Von der Weyer, William ...St. Paul
Plondke, F. J. ....St. Paul	Shillington, M. A. ....St. Paul	Waas, C. W. ....St. Paul
Prendergast, H. J. ....St. Paul	Shimonek, S. W. ....St. Paul	Walker, A. E. ....St. Paul
Prendergast, J. J. ...Carville, La.	Short, Jacob ....St. Paul	Walter, C. W. ....St. Paul
Radabaugh, R. C. ....Hastings	Simons, L. T. ....St. Paul	Warnock, R. W. ....St. Paul
Ramsey, W. R. ....St. Paul	Singer, B. J. ....St. Paul	Warren, C. A. ....St. Paul
Richards, E. T. F. ....St. Paul	Skinner, H. O. ....St. Paul	Warren, E. L. ....St. Paul
Richardson, H. E. ....St. Paul	Smisek, E. A. ....St. Paul	Watz, C. E. ....St. Paul
Ritchie, H. P. ....St. Paul	Smith, W. D. E. ....St. Paul	Webber, F. L. ....St. Paul
Ritchie, W. P. ....St. Paul	Snyder, G. W. ....St. Paul	Welch, M. C. ....St. Paul
Ritt, A. E. ....St. Paul	Sohlberg, O. I. ....St. Paul	Werner, O. S. ....Cambridge
Rogers, S. F. ....St. Paul	Souster, B. B. ....St. Paul	Wheeler, M. W. ....St. Paul
Rosenholtz, Burton ....St. Paul	Sprafka, J. M. ....St. Paul	Whitacre, J. C. ....St. Paul
Rosenthal, Robert ....St. Paul	Steinberg, C. L. ....St. Paul	Whitmore, Frank ....St. Paul
Rothrock, J. L. ....St. Paul	Sterner, E. G. ....St. Paul	Williams, C. K. ....St. Paul
Rothschild, H. J. ....St. Paul	Sterner, E. R. ....White Bear	Williamson, G. A. ....St. Paul
*Roy, Philemon ....St. Paul	Stewart, Alexander ....St. Paul	Wilson, J. A. ....St. Paul
Roy, P. C. ....St. Paul	Stinnette, S. E. ....St. Paul	Wilson, J. V. ....St. Paul
Runberg, G. N. ....St. Paul	Stoeckmann, A. E. ....St. Paul	Winnick, J. B. ....St. Paul
Rutherford, W. C. ....St. Paul	Stolpestad, A. H. ....St. Paul	Wold, K. C. ....St. Paul
Ryan, J. J. ....St. Paul	Stolpestad, H. L. ....St. Paul	Wolfe, H. H. ....St. Paul
Ryan, J. M. ....St. Paul	Strate, G. E. ....St. Paul	Wolff, H. J. ....St. Paul
Ryan, M. E. ....St. Paul	Strauss, M. L. ....St. Paul	Wolkoff, H. J. ....St. Paul
Sarrecki, M. M. ....St. Paul	Swanson, J. A. ....St. Paul	Youngren, E. R. ....St. Paul
Satterlund, V. L. ....St. Paul	Swendson, J. J. ....St. Paul	
Savage, F. J. ....St. Paul		Zander, C. H. ....St. Paul
Schoch, R. B. J. ....St. Paul	Teisberg, C. B. ....St. Paul	Zimmermann, H. B. ....St. Paul

RED RIVER VALLEY MEDICAL SOCIETY

Kittson, Mahnomen, Marshall, Norman, Pennington, Polk, Red Lake and Roseau Counties
Regular meetings, second Tuesday every quarter
Annual meeting, second Tuesday, December
Number of Members: 59

President
Borreson, Baldwin...Thief River Falls

Secretary
Oppegaard, C. L. ....Crookston

Adkins, C. M. ......Thief River Falls	Brown, L. L. ....Crookston	Morley, G. A. ....Crookston
Adkins, G. H. ....Grygla	Delmore, J. L., Jr. ....Roseau	Nelson, H. E. ....Crookston
Anderson, W. E....Thief River Falls	Delmore, J. L., Sr. ....Roseau	Norman, J. F. ....Crookston
Anderson, W. S. ....Minneapolis	Ederer, J. J. ....Mahnomen	Ohnstad, J. L. ....McIntosh
Behr, O. ....Crookston	Erickson, Eskil. ....Halstad	Oppegaard, C. L. ....Crookston
Berge, D. O. ....Roseau	Griffin, P. J. ....Fertile	Oppegaard, M. O. ....Crookston
Berlin, A. S. ....Hallock	Haugseth, Enoch. ....Twin Valley	Paradis, W. G. ....Crookston
Bertelson, O. L. ....Crookston	Hedemark, H. H...Thief River Falls	Parsons, J. G. ....Crookston
Biedermann, Jacob..Thief River Falls	Helseth, H. K....Thief River Falls	Pelletiere, E. V. ...Thief River Falls
Blegen, M. M. ....Warren	Henney, W. H. ....McIntosh	Reff, A. R. ....Crookston
Boardman, D. V. ....Twin Valley	Hodgson, H. H. ....Crookston	Rice, H. R. ....Roseau
Bohl, G. W. ....Ada	Hollands, W. H. ....Fisher	Roy, J. A. ......Red Lake Falls
Borreson, Baldwin..Thief River Falls	Holmstrom, C. H. ....Warren	Sather, R. O. ....Crookston
Bratrud, O. E....Thief River Falls	Johnson, H. C...Thief River Falls	Shaleen, A. W. ....Hallock
Brink, A. A. ....Baudette	Kahala, Arthur ....Crookston	Shedlov, Abraham ....Fosston
	Kirk, G. D. ......East Grand Forks	Stevens, John ....Gonvick
	Knutson, G. ....Greenbush	Stocking, F. P. ....Hallock
	Leitch, N. M. ....Warroad	Stuurmaans, S. H. ....Erskine
	Loken, Theodore ....Ada	Tanglin, W. G. L. ....Mahnomen
	Lynde, O. G. ......Thief River Falls	Torgerson, W. B. ....Oklee
	Mellby, O. E. .....Thief River Falls	Uhley, C. L. ....Crookston
	Mercil, W. F. ....Crookston	Wiltrout, I. G. ....Oslo

REDWOOD-BROWN COUNTY MEDICAL SOCIETY

Regular meetings, May, August, November, and February
Annual meeting, May
Number of Members: 31

President
Hovde, Rolf ....Winthrop

Secretary
Fritsche, C. J. ....New Ulm

Abbott, C. B. ....Springfield	Dysterheft, A. F. ....Gaylord	Nuessle, W. G. ....Springfield
Abraham, A. L. ....Minneapolis	Esser, O. J. ....Gibbon	Olson, K. L. ....Gibbon
Anderson, E. M. ....Lamberton	Fesenmaier, O. B. ....New Ulm	Peterson, R. A. ....Vesta
Brey, F. W. ....Wabasso	Fritsche, Albert ....New Ulm	Reineke, G. F. ....New Ulm
Cairns, R. J. ....Sanborn	Fritsche, C. J. ....New Ulm	Rothenburg, J. C. ....Springfield
Dubbe, F. H. ....New Ulm	Fritsche, T. R. ....New Ulm	Saffert, C. A. ....New Ulm
	Gibbons, F. C. ....Comfrey	Schroeppel, J. E. ....Winthrop
	Goblirsch, A. P. ....Sleepy Eye	Seifert, O. J. ....New Ulm
	Hammermeister, T. F. ......New Ulm	Vogel, H. A. L. ....New Ulm
	Hovde, Rolf. ....Winthrop	Vogel, J. H. ....New Ulm
	Kusske, A. E. ....New Ulm	Wahlberg, E. W. ....Morgan
	Mortensbak, H. E. ....Hanska	Weiser, G. B. ....New Ulm
		Wohlrabe, E. J. ....Springfield

RENVILLE COUNTY MEDICAL SOCIETY

Regular meeting, second Tuesday of each month
Annual meeting, November
Number of Members: 22

President
Dordal, John ....Sacred Heart

Secretary
Madland, R. S. ....Fairfax

Adams, R. C. ....Bird Island	Brand, W. A. ....Redwood Falls	Johnson, O. H. ....Redwood Falls
Billings, R. E. ....Franklin	Bushard, W. J. ....Bird Island	Lenz, J. R. ....Morton
	Cole, H. B. ....Redwood Falls	Loenholdt, E. H. ....Hector
	Cole, J. C. ....Redwood Falls	Madland, R. S. ....Fairfax
	Cosgriff, J. A. ....Olivia	Mesker, G. H. ....Olivia
	Dordal, J. ....Sacred Heart	Passer, A. A. ....Olivia
	Fawcett, A. M. ....Renville	Penhall, F. W. ....Morton
	Flinn, T. E. ....Redwood Falls	Potthoff, C. J. ....Morgan
	Gaines, E. C. ....Buffalo Lake	Preisinger, J. W. ....Renville
	Hartman, C. M. ....Fairfax	Sulsem, F. N. ....Sacred Heart

*Deceased.

RICE COUNTY MEDICAL SOCIETY

Regular meetings, at call
Annual meeting, December
Number of Members: 36

President
Huxley, F. R...............Faribault

Secretary
Plonske, C. J..............Faribault

Babcock, F. M.............Northfield
Beede, E. R...............Faribault

Dugan, L. F...............Faribault
Dungay, N. S..............Northfield

Engberg, E. J.............Faribault
Francis, D. W.............Morristown
Haessly, S. B.............Faribault

Hanson, A. M..............Faribault
Haynes, A. L..............Faribault
Huxley, F. R..............Faribault·
Kanne, C. W...............Faribault
Kucera, S. T..............Lonsdale
Lende, Norman.............Faribault
Lexa, F. J................Lonsdale
Lufkin, C. D..............Northfield
Lyght, C. E...............Northfield
McKeon, J. O..............Montgomery
Meyer, F. C...............Kenyon
Meyer, P. F...............Faribault
Moses, Joseph, Jr.........Northfield
Moses, R. R...............Kenyon
Nuetzman, A. W............Faribault

ST. LOUIS COUNTY MEDICAL SOCIETY

Carlton, Cook, Itasca, Lake and St. Louis Coun·
Regular meetings, second Thursday every month
Annual meeting, December

Number of Members: 215

President
Gillespie, M. G...............Duluth

Secretary
MacRae, G. C.................Duluth

Adams, B. S.................Hibbing
Addy, E. R..................Gilbert
Akins, W. M.................Eveleth
Anderson, H. R..........Deer River
Armstrong, E. L.............Duluth
Athens, A. G................Duluth
Ayres, G. T....................Ely
Bachnik, F. W...............Hibbing
Bagley, E. C................Duluth
Bagley, W. R................Duluth
Bakkila, Henry..............Duluth
Bardon, Richard.............Duluth
Barney, L. A................Duluth
Berdez, G. L................Duluth
Bianco, A. J................Duluth
Binet, H. E...........Grand Rapids
Birkland, O. N..............Hibbing
Blacklock, S. S.............Hibbing
Blakely, C. C...............Barnum
Boman, P. G.................Duluth
Bowen, R. L.................Hibbing
Boyer, S. H., Jr............Duluth
Boyer, S. H., Sr............Duluth
Braverman, N. J.............Duluth
Bray, P. N..................Duluth
Bray, R. B.................Biwabik
Buckley, B. P...............Duluth
Burton, J. L.................Buhl
Cantwell, W. F...International Falls
Carstens, C. F..............Hibbing
Chapman, T. L...............Duluth
Cheney, E. L................Duluth
Chermak, F. G...............Duluth
Chessen, James..............Duluth
Christensen, E. P......Two Harbors
Clark, F. F.................Duluth
Clement, T. G...............Duluth
Collins, A. M...............Duluth
Collins, H. C...............Duluth
Coventry, W. A..............Duluth
Coventry, W. D..............Duluth
Dahlin, I. T................Aurora
Davis, B. F.................Duluth
Doolittle, L. E.............Duluth
Doyle, G. C.................Duluth
Eckman, P. F................Duluth
Eckman, R. J................Duluth
Ekblad, J. W................Duluth
Elias, F. K.................Duluth
Emanuel, E. W...............Duluth
Engdahl, F. W.........Grand Rapids
Eppard, R. M................Cloquet
Estrem, T. A................Hibbing
Ewens, H. B................Virginia
Fankboner, A. V..............Buhl
Fawcett, K. R...............Duluth
Fellows, M. F...............Duluth
Fetterly, Warren...........Virginia
Feuling, J. C................Bovey
Fischer, M. McC.............Duluth
Fisher, Isadore.............Ceylon
Forbes, R. S................Duluth
Gendron, J. F........Grand Rapids
Gillespie, M. G.............Duluth
Gillespie, N. H.............Duluth
Goldish, D. R...............Duluth
Goodman, C. E..............Virginia

Gowan, L. R.................Duluth
Graham, Robert..............Duluth
Graves, W. N................Duluth
Hall, A. E.................Virginia
Haney, C. L.................Duluth
Hanson, E. O................Cloquet
Harlowe, H. D..............Virginia
Harris, C. N................Hibbing
Hatch, W. E.................Duluth
Hathaway, S. J..............Proctor
Hayes, M. F...............Nashwauk
Hedberg, G. A.............Nopeming
Hejam, W. C..................Cook
Heimark, O. E...............Duluth
Hilding, A. C...............Duluth
Hill, F. E..................Duluth
Hirschboeck, F. J...........Duluth
Hirschfield, M. S...........Duluth
Hoff, H. O..................Duluth
Hursh, M. M...............Cohasset
Jacobson, Clarence........Chisholm
Jensen, T. J................Duluth
Johnson, D. E...............Duluth
Jolin, F. M...........Grand Rapids
Jolin, R. V...........Grand Rapids
Junnila, B. O.........Grand Rapids
Keyes, C. R.................Duluth
Kiesling, I. H............Nashwauk
Klein, Harry................Duluth
Knapp, F. N.................Duluth
Kohlbry, C. O...............Duluth
Kotchevar, F. R............Eveleth
Kraft, Peter................Duluth
Krantz, C. I................Duluth
Kuth, J. R..................Duluth
Laird, A. T...............Nopeming
Lenont, C. B..............Virginia
Lepak, F. J.................Duluth
Litman, S. N................Duluth
Loofbourrow, E. H.........Keewatin
Lundquist, C. W............Hibbing
Macfarlane, P. H..........Chisholm
MacRae, G. C................Duluth
Magney, F. H................Duluth
Malmstrom, J. A...........Virginia
Manley, J. R................Duluth
Mareley, W. J............Nopeming
Martin, E. T................Duluth
Martin, W. C................Duluth
Mattson, C. H...............Duluth
Mayne, R. M.................Duluth
McCarty, P. D.................Ely
McComb, C. F................Duluth
McCoy, M. K.................Duluth
McDaniel, S. P............Virginia
McDonald, A. L..............Duluth
McHaffie, O. L..............Duluth
McKenna, M. J.........Grand Rapids
McLeod, L. L..........Grand Rapids
McNutt, J. R................Duluth
Mead, C. H..................Duluth
Merriman, L. L..............Duluth
Miners, G. A............Deer River
Mitby, I. L.................Hibbing
Moe, R. J...................Duluth
Moe, Thomas............Moose Lake
Monroe, P. B..........Two Harbors
More, C. W.................Eveleth
Morsman, L. W..............Hibbing
*Morss, C. R..............Zumbrota
Mueller, S. C...............Duluth
Nelson, E. H..............Chisholm
Nelson, R. L................Duluth
Nicholson, M. A.............Duluth

*Deceased.

372

SCOTT-CARVER COUNTY MEDICAL SOCIETY

Regular meetings, second Tuesday of the month
Annual meeting, June
Number of Members: 33

President
Cervenka, C. F..........New Prague

Secretary
Pearson, B. F..............Shakopee

Buck, F. H................Shakopee
Butler, J. K................Carlton
Cervenka, C. F..........New Prague
Crow, E. R...............Arlington
Dowidat, R. W............Cologne
Eklund, E. J...............Norwood
Emmerson, W. S............Mayer

Fischer, H. P.............Shakopee
Havel, H. W................Jordan
Hebeisen, M. B............Chaska
Henriksen, H. G..............Elko
Juergens, H. M........Belle Plaine
Klein, J. C................Shakopee
Kortsch, F. P...........Prior Lake
Maertz, W. F..........New Prague
Malerich, J. A.............Shakopee
Martin, T. P..............Arlington
Nagel, H. D................Waconia
Novak, E. E...........New Prague
Olson, C. J...........Belle Plaine

Ormond, D. T..............Waconia
Pearson, B. F.............Shakopee
Phillips, W. H..............Jordan
Pogue, R. E........Glendale, Calif.
Reiter, H. W.............Shakopee
Rick, P. F. W............Le Center
Schimelpfenig, G. T..........Chaska
Shrader, J. S...............Jordan
Simons, B. H...............Chaska
Westerman, A. E........Montgomery
Westerman, F. C........Montgomery
Woodworth, L. F........Le Center
Wunder, H. E.............Shakopee

SOUTHWESTERN MINNESOTA MEDICAL SOCIETY

Cottonwood, Jackson, Murray, Nobles, Pipestone and Rock Counties
Regular meetings, November and April or May
Annual meeting, November
Number of Members: 62

President
Sherman, C. L..............Luverne

Secretary
DeBoer, Hermanus..........Edgerton

Arnold, E. W...............Adrian
Basinger, H. P...........Windom
Basinger, H. R......Mountain Lake
Beckering, Gerrit...........Edgerton
Benjamin, W. G...........Pipestone
Bofenkamp, F. W..........Luverne
Brown, A. H............Pipestone
Carlson, J. V............Westbrook
Chadbourn, A. G........Heron Lake
Chunn, S. S...............Pipestone
Clark, H. H...............Edgerton
Cress, P. J..............Ellsworth
DeBoer, Hermanus..........Edgerton
Dolan, C. P.............Worthington
Doman, V. W.............Lakefield
Doms, H. C................Slayton
Engh, Sigfred.............Jackson

Halloran, W. H............Jackson
Halpern, D. J.............Brewster
Harrison, P. W.........Worthington
Hebbel, Robert.............Windom
Hitchings, W. S.........Lakefield
Johnson, R. E.........Worthington
Kelling, L. F............Lakefield
Kendahl, A. M..............Jasper
Kilbride, A. C........Worthington
Kilbride, J. S.........Worthington
Lohmann, J. G..............Jasper
Lowe, Thomas...........Pipestone
Maitland, D. P............Jackson
Maitland, E. T............Jackson
Manson, F. M.........Worthington
McCrea, J. M..............Fulda
McElmeel, E. F.........Pipestone
McLane, E. G.............Jackson
McLane, W. O.............Jackson
Mork, B. O., Jr......Worthington
Mork, B. O., Sr......Worthington
Nealy, D. E................Adrian
Pankratz, P. J......Mountain Lake

Patterson, W. E..........Westbrook
Piper, W. A......Mountain Lake
Priest, R. E.........Worthington
Rose, J. T..............Lakefield
Schade, F. L.........Worthington
Schutz, E. S......Mountain Lake
Sether, A. F...............Ruthton
Sherman, C. L.............Luverne
Sjostrom, L. E...........Storden
Slater, S. A.........Worthington
Sogge, L. L..............Windom
Stanley, C. R........Worthington
Stevenson, B. M..........Fulda
Stratte, H. C............Windom
Thorson, E. O...........Luverne
Tofte, Josephine......Minneapolis
Waller, J. D.............Wilmont
Wells, W. B..............Jackson
Williams, A. B............St. Paul
Williams, C. A..........Pipestone
Williams, L. A..........Slayton
Wright, C. O............Luverne

STEARNS-BENTON COUNTY MEDICAL SOCIETY

Regular meetings, third Thursday of the month
Annual meeting, third Thursday of December
Number of Members: 52

President
Clark, H. B................St. Cloud

Secretary
Libert, J. N...............St. Cloud

Adams, L. P...............St. Cloud
Barringer, P. E...........St. Cloud
Beuning, J. B..............Albany
Brigham, C. F............St. Cloud
Buscher, J. C............St. Cloud
Clark, H. B..............St. Cloud
Donaldson, C. S.............Foley
DuBois, J. F...........Sauk Center
Engstrom, G. F..........Belgrade
Evans, L. M...........Sauk Rapids
Fleming, T. N............St. Cloud
Freeman, W. L...........St. Cloud
Friesleben, William......Sauk Rapids
Gaida, J. B..............St. Cloud

Goehrs, H. W.............St. Cloud
Haberman, Emil............Osakis
Halenbeck, P. L.........St. Cloud
Hemstead, Werner........Brainerd
Henry, C. J................Milaca
Holdridge, George...........Foley
Johnson, Walfred........Sauk Center
Jones, R. N...............St. Cloud
Kern, M. J................St. Cloud
Kettlewell, R. B.......Sauk Center
Kingsbury, E. M.........Clearwater
Kohler, D. W...........St. Joseph
Koop, H. E............Cold Spring
Koop, S. H..............Richmond
Lewis, C. B..............St. Cloud
Mahowald, A.............Albany
McDowell, J. P...........St. Cloud
Meyer, A. A..............Melrose

Moynihan, A. F........Sauk Center
Myre, C. R.............Paynesville
Rathbun, C. A............St. Cloud
Richards, W. B..........St. Cloud
Rumpf, W. H.............St. Cloud
Sandven, N. O.........Paynesville
Schatz, F. J............St. Cloud
Sher, D. A...........Cold Spring
Sherwood, G. E...........Kimball
Stangl, Fred............St. Cloud
Stangl, P. E............St. Cloud
Stewart, N. E............St. Cloud
Sutton, C. S.............St. Cloud
Townsend, De Wayne.......Brooten
Walfred, K. A............St. Cloud
Watson, W. I.........Holdingford
Wenner, W. I...........St. Cloud
Wiechman, F. H..........St. Cloud
Zachman, A. H...........Melrose

STEELE COUNTY MEDICAL SOCIETY

Regular meetings, second Monday of month
Annual meeting, January
Number of Members: 18

President
Schaefer, J. F.............Owatonna

Secretary
McEnaney, C. T...........Owatonna

Berghs, L. V.............Owatonna

Carlson, V. W......Blooming Prairie
Dewey, D. H.............Owatonna
Ertel, E. O.............Ellendale
Farabaugh, C. L..........Owatonna
Flores, O. T.........Dodge Center
Hartung, E. H..........Claremont
Kreuzer, T. C...........Owatonna
McEnaney, C. T..........Owatonna

McIntyre, J. A..........Owatonna
Melby, Benedik......Blooming Prairie
Morehead, D. E.........Owatonna
Nelson, E. J............Owatonna
Roberts, O. W..........Owatonna
Schaefer, J. F..........Owatonna
Senn, E. W.............Owatonna
Smersh, J. F............Owatonna
Stewart, A. B..........Owatonna

UPPER MISSISSIPPI MEDICAL SOCIETY

Aitkin, Beltrami, Cass, Clearwater, Crow Wing, Hubbard, Koochiching, Lake of the Woods, Morrison,
Todd and Wadena Counties
Regular meetings, quarterly
Annual meeting, January
Number of Members: 95

President
Lamb, H. L.............Little Falls

Secretary
Badeaux, G. I...............Brainerd

Amundson, A. E.........Little Falls
Anderson, C. E..............Brainerd
Badeaux, G. I...............Brainerd
Beise, R. A................Brainerd
Benton, P. C................Staples
Borgerson, A. H.............Sebeka
Bosland, H. G.............Verndale
Bray, K. E..............Park Rapids
Burns, H. A.........Ah-Gwah-Ching
Campbell, R. W........Cass Lake
Cardle, G. E........Ah-Gwah-Ching
Carlson, C. E...............Aitkin
Carlson, H. A...............Walker
Christie, G. R.........Long Prairie
Christie, R. L.........Long Prairie
Cook, J. M................Staples
Davis, L. T................Wadena
Davis, R. D.............Clearbrook
Davis, T. C................Wadena
Dworak, A. F..............Walker
Eiler, John............Park Rapids
Ericsson, M. G.........Long Prairie
Fait, R. V.............Little Falls
Frost, H. T................Wadena
Garlock, A. V..............Bemidji
Garlock, D. H.............Bemidji
Gerber, M. P.............Brainerd
Ghostley, M. C.............Puposky

Gifford, B. L.............Long Prairie
Gorenflo, Leila..........Cass Lake
Grawn, F. A.............Northome
Grogan, J. S..............Wadena
Groschupf, T. P.............Bemidji
Grose, F. N...............Clarissa
Hanover, R. D.............Littlefork
Hanson, E. C.........Park Rapids
Hawkinson, J. P............Crosby
Hawkinson, L. F...........Brainerd
Healy, R. T.................Pierz
Hendrickson, R. R..........Wadena
Hesselgrave, S. S.........St. Paul
Higgs, W. W..........Park Rapids
Holst, C. F............Little Falls
Holst, J. B............Little Falls
House, Z. E.............Cass Lake
Houston, D. M.........Park Rapids
Hubbard, O. E.............Brainerd
Hubin, E. G...............Deerwood
Jacobson, D. J.............Blackduck
Jamieson, E. F.............Brainerd
Johnson, C. E............Pine River
Johnson, D. L.........Little Falls
Johnson, E. W.............Bemidji
Kelly, B. W.................Aitkin
Kerlan, Irvin.........Minneapolis
Kerlan, S. Z...............Aitkin
Lamb, H. L............Little Falls
Lee, H. W................Brainerd
Lenarz, A. J.........Browerville
Lund, W. J................Staples
Marcum, E. H.............Bemidji
Mark, Hilbert...........Minneapolis

Mason, J. A........International
McCann, D. F................Be
Mosby, M. E...........Long P
Moyer, R. E............Minnes
Mulligan, A. M............Bra
Nelson, N. P..............Bra
Petraborg, H. T..............A
Pierce, C. H................Wa
Potek, David.....International
Quanstrom, V. E............Bra
Ratcliffe, J. J...............A
Reichelderfer, C. F..........St
Ringle, O. F................W
Roberts, L. M...........Little
Rosenfield, A. B..............P
Shannon, S. S................C
Simons, E. J................Swa
Simons, S. J.................A
Smith, B. A..................C
Stafford, C. E................H
Stein, R. J.................
Swedenburg, P. A..........Swa
Thabes, J. A. Jr...........Bra
Thabes, J. A. Sr...........Bra
Vandersluis, C. W...........Be
Watson, A. M..............Roy
Watson, J. D...........Holdin
Watson, P. T...............Cass
Webster, L. J........Ah-Gwah-G
Whittemore, D. D............Be
Will, W. W...................B
Wilson, V. O..............Minne
Withrow, M. E....International

WABASHA COUNTY MEDICAL SOCIETY

Regular meetings, March, October
Annual meeting, first Thursday after first Monday in October
Number of Members: 14

President
Sherman, H. T............Plainview

Secretary
Wilson, W. F...........Lake City
Bayley, E. C...........Lake City
Bouquet, B. J..............Wabasha

Burlingame, D. A...........Mazeppa
Cochrane, W. J..........Lake City
Collins, J. S..............Wabasha
Ellis, E. W.................Elgin
Flesche, B. A...........Lake City
Frost, R. H..............Wabasha

Holt, G. W.................Wa
Mahle, D. G...............Plai
Ochsner, C. G..............Wa
Sherman, H. T.............Plai
Slocumb, J. A.............Plai
Wilson, W. F...............Lake

WASECA COUNTY MEDICAL SOCIETY

Regular meetings, at call
Annual meeting, December
Number of Members: 9

President
McIntire, H. M.............Waseca

Secretary
Olds, G. H.................Waseca

Bernstein, W. C.....New Richland
Chadbourn, C. R..........Janesville
Erickson, R. E.....New Richland
Gallagher, B. J............Waseca
Hottinger, R. C..........Janesville

McIntire, H. M.............
Oeljen, S. C. G............
Olds, G. H................
Swenson, O. J.............

WASHINGTON COUNTY MEDICAL SOCIETY

Regular meetings, second Tuesday in January, February, March, April, May, September, October,
November and December
Annual meeting second Tuesday in December
Number of Members: 16

President
Ewald, R. P...............Newport

Secretary
Boleyn, E. S............Stillwater
Boleyn, E. S............Stillwater
Brooks, G. F............Stillwater

Ewald, R. P..............Newport
Haines, J. H...........Stillwater
Humphrey, W. R.........Stillwater
Josewski, R. J.........Stillwater
Kalinoff, D............Stillwater
Linner, Gunnar.........Stillwater
McCarten, F. M.........Stillwater

Mingo, F. E................
Poirier, J. A..........Forest
Ruggles, G. McC.......Forest
Samson, E. R.............Sti
Strand, E. V................B
Stuhr, J. W...............Sti
Van Meier, Henry.........Sti

WATONWAN COUNTY MEDICAL SOCIETY

Regular meeting, at call
Annual meeting, December
Number of Members: 8

President
Bratrude, E. J.........St. James

Secretary
Grimes, H. B.............Madelia

Bergman, O. B...........St. James
Bratrude, E. J.........St. James
Bregel, F. L............St. James
Grimes, H. B...........Madelia

Hagen, O. E...............But
Hammar, L. M.............But
McCarthy, W. J............
Thompson, Albert.........St.

ROSTER MINNESOTA STATE MEDICAL ASSOCIATION

WEST CENTRAL MINNESOTA MEDICAL SOCIETY

Big Stone, Pope, Stevens, and Traverse Counties
Regular meetings, second Wednesday in January, April, July and October
Annual meeting, second Wednesday in October
Number of Members: 23

President
Shelver, H. J.............Ortonville

Secretary
Oliver, I. L.................Graceville

Arneson, A. I...................Morris
Bates, B. V...........Browns Valley
Behmler, F. W................Morris
Bergan, Otto................Clinton
Bolsta, Charles............Ortonville

Caine, C. E...................Morris
Cumming, J. F................Morris
Doleman, N. F................Tintah
Eberlin, E. A.............Glenwood
Elsey, E. McC.............Glenwood
Elsey, J. R...............Glenwood
Ewing, C. F.............Wheaton
Fitzgerald, E. T............Morris
Garrow, D. M..............St. Paul
Giesen, A. F...............Starbuck

Karn, B. R................Ortonville
Lindberg, A. L............Wheaton
Linde, Herman...............Cyrus
McIver, B. A..............Lowry
Mooney, L. P.............Graceville
O'Donnell, D. M.......Ortonville
Oliver, C. I.............Graceville
Oliver, I. L.............Graceville
Ransom, M. L.............Hancock
Shelver, H. J............Ortonville

WINONA COUNTY MEDICAL SOCIETY

Regular meetings, first Monday in January, April, July, October
Annual meeting, first Monday in January
Number of Members: 25

President
Tweedy, R. B..............Winona

Secretary
Steiner, I. W.................Winona

Benoit, F. T.................Winona
Christensen, E. E............Winona
Heise, W. F. C.............Winona
Keyes, J. D.................Winona

Lindsay, W. V.............Winona
Mattison, P. A............Winona
McLaughlin, E. M..........Winona
Meinert, A. E.............Winona
Nauth, W. W..............Winona
Neumann, C. A.............Winona
Nilles, L. J...........Rollingstone
Page, R. L...............St. Charles
Risser, E. D..............Winona
Robbins, C. P.............Winona
Roemer, J. E.............Winona

Roth, F. D................Lewiston
Satterlee, H. W..........Lewiston
Schaefer, Samuel...........Winona
Steiner, I. W.............Winona
Tweedy, G. J.............Winona
Tweedy, R. B.............Winona
Walker, G. H.............Winona
Whetstone, S. D..........Winona
Wilson, R. H.............Winona
Younger, L. I............Winona

WRIGHT COUNTY MEDICAL SOCIETY

Regular meetings, quarterly
Annual meeting, first Wednesday after first Monday in October
Number of Members: 18

President
Grundset, O. J............Montrose

Secretary
Catlin, J. J.................Buffalo

Anderson, W. P.............Buffalo
Bendix, L. H.............Annandale

Catlin, J. J..................Buffalo
Catlin, T. J..................Buffalo
Ellison, F. E...........Monticello
Greenfield, W. T..........Delano
Grundset, O. J...........Montrose
Harriman, L..........Howard Lake
Hart, W. E...............Monticello
Hoyer, L. J..........Howard Lake

Lee, J. L................Watertown
Peterson, O. L.............Cokato
Phillips, A. E.............Delano
Ridgway, A. M...........Annandale
Roholt, C. L.............Waverly
Rousseau, Victor.......Maple Lake
Thielen, R. D.........St. Michael
Thompson, Arthur............Cokato

Aanes, A. M.........Red Wing	Bailey, R. J.........Spokane, Wash.	Birkland, O. N.........Hibbing
Abbott, C. B.........Springfield	Bair, H. L.........Rochester	Birnberg, T. L.........St. Paul
Abbott, J. S.........St. Paul	Baken, M. P.........Minneapolis	Black, B. M.........Rochester
Aborn, W. H.........Hawley	Baker, A. G.........Fergus Falls	Black, E. R.........Rochester
Abraham, A. L.........Minneapolis	Baker, A. T.........Minneapolis	Black, William.........Mankato
Abramson, Milton.........Minneapolis	Baker, E. L.........Minneapolis	Blacklock, S. S.........Hibbing
Adams, B. S.........Hibbing	Baker, G. S.........Rochester	Blake, James.........Hopkins
Adams, L. P.........St. Cloud	Baker, H. R.........Hayfield	Blake, J. L.........Hopkins
Adams, R. C.........Bird Island	Baker, Looe.........Minneapolis	Blake, T. W.........Seattle, Wash.
Adams, R. C.........Rochester	Baker, N. H.........Fergus Falls	Blakely, C. C.........Barnum
Addy, E. R.........Gilbert	Baker, R. L.........Hayfield	Blakey, A. R.........Osakis
Adkins, C. M.........Thief River Falls	Bakkila, Henry.........Duluth	Blanchard, H. G.........Fairmont
Adkins, G. H.........Grygla	Balcome, M. M.........St. Paul	Blaustone, H. H.........Minneapolis
Adson, A. W.........Rochester	Balfour, D. C.........Rochester	Blegen, H. M.........Warren
Affeldt, D. E.........Kasson	Bannick, E. G.........Seattle, Wash.	Bloedel, T. J. G.........Minneapolis
Ahlfs, J. J.........Caledonia	Barber, J. P.........Minneapolis	Blomberg, W. R.........Princeton
Ahrens, A. E.........St. Paul	Bardon, Richard.........Duluth	Blum, B. B.........Rochester
Ahrens, A. H.........St. Paul	Bargen, J. A.........Rochester	Blumenthal, J. S.........Columbia Heights
Ahrens, R. S.........Fergus Falls	Barker, N. W.........Rochester	Boardman, D. V.........Twin Valley
Aitkens, H. B.........Le Center	Barnes, A. R.........Rochester	Bock, R. A.........St. Paul
Akester, Ward.........Marshall	Barney, L. A.........Duluth	Bockman, M. W. H.........Minneapolis
Akins, W. M.........Eveleth	Barr, L. C.........Albert Lea	Boeckmann, Egil.........St. Paul
Alberts, M. W.........St. Paul	Barr, W. R.........Wells	Boehme, E. J.........Minneapolis
Alden, J. F.........St. Paul	Barringer, F. E.........St. Cloud	Bofenkamp, F. W.........Luverne
Alexander, F. H.........St. Paul	Barron, Moses.........Minneapolis	Bohl, G. W.........Ada
Alexander, H. A.........Minneapolis	Barry, L. W.........St. Paul	Bohland, E. H.........St. Paul
Aling, C. A.........Minneapolis	Barsness, Nellie.........St. Paul	Boies, L. R.........Minneapolis
Allen, A. W.........Austin	Basinger, R. P.........Windom	Boland, E. W.........Rochester
Allen, C. C.........Austin	Basinger, H. R.........Mountain Lake	Bolender, H. L.........St. Paul
Allen, E. V.........Rochester	Bass, G. W.........Minneapolis	Boleyn, E. S.........Stillwater
Allen, H. B.........Austin	Bates, B. V.........Browns Valley	Boline, C. A.........Battle Lake
Allen, H. W.........Minneapolis	Baxter, S. H.........Minneapolis	Bolsta, Charles.........Ortonville
Allison, R. G.........Minneapolis	Bayard, H. F.........Minneapolis	Boman, P. G.........Duluth
Altnow, H. O.........Minneapolis	Bayley, E. C.........Lake City	Boody, G. J., Jr.........Dawson
Alvarez, W. C.........Rochester	Beadle, W. D.........Cannon Falls	Booth, A. E.........Minneapolis
Amberg, Samuel.........Rochester	Beals, Hugh.........St. Paul	Boothby, W. M.........Rochester
Amundson, A. E.........Little Falls	Beard, A. H.........Minneapolis	Boreen, C. A.........Minneapolis
Andersen, A. G.........Minneapolis	Beckering, Gerrit.........Edgerton	Borg, J. F.........St. Paul
Andersen, S. C.........Minneapolis	Beckman, W. G.........Minneapolis	Borgerson, A. H.........Seneka
Anderson, C. E.........Brainerd	Bedard, R. E.........Rochester	Borgeson, E. J.........Minneapolis
Anderson, D. D.........Minneapolis	Bedford, E. W.........Minneapolis	Borman, C. N.........Minneapolis
Anderson, E. D.........Minneapolis	Beede, E. R.........Faribault	Borreson, Baldwin.........Thief River Falls
Anderson, E. M.........Lamberton	Beek, H. O.........St. Paul	Bosland, H. G.........Verndale
Anderson, E. R.........Minneapolis	Behmler, F. W.........Morris	Bossert, C. S.........Mora
Anderson, F. J.........Minneapolis	Behr, O. K.........Crookston	Bossingham, O. N.........Lake Benton
Anderson, H. R.........Deer River	Bejse, R. A.........Brainerd	Bottolfson, B. T.........Moorhead
Anderson, J. K.........Minneapolis	Bejswanger, R. H.........Wykoff	Bouma, A. R.........St. Paul
Anderson, K. W.........Minneapolis	Beizer, L. H.........Rochester	Bouman, H. A. H.........Minneapolis
Anderson, L. W.........Atwater	Bell, C. P.........St. Paul	Bouquet, B. J.........Wabasha
Anderson, M. J.........Rochester	Bell, E. T.........Minneapolis	Bowen, R. L.........Hibbing
Anderson, N. E.........Harmony	Belote, G. B.........Caledonia	Bowing, H. H.........Rochester
Anderson, P. A.........Minneapolis	Belzer, M. S.........Minneapolis	Boyd, A. M.........Alexandria
Anderson, R. E.........Willmar	Bendix, L. H.........Annandale	Boyer, S. H., Jr.........Duluth
Anderson, S. H.........Red Wing	Benedict, W. L.........Rochester	Boyer, S. H., Sr.........Duluth
Anderson, U. S.........Minneapolis	Benepe, J. L.........St. Paul	Boynton, Ruth.........Minneapolis
Anderson, W. E.........Thief River Falls	Benham, E. W.........Mankato	Boysen, Herbert.........Welcome
Anderson, W. P.........Buffalo	Benjamin, A. E.........Minneapolis	Boysen, J. E.........Pelican Rapids
Anderson, W. S.........Minneapolis	Benjamin, E. G.........Minneapolis	Boysen, Peter.........Pelican Rapids
Andreassen, E. C.........Minneapolis	Benjamin, H. G.........Minneapolis	Braasch, W. F.........Rochester
Andrews, R. N.........Mankato	Benjamin, W. G.........Pipestone	Bracken, H. M.........Claremont, Calif.
Annis, H. B.........Minneapolis	Benn, F. G.........Minneapolis	Brand, G. D.........St. Paul
Annis, J. W.........Rochester	Bennett, R. L., Jr.........Rochester	Brand, W. A.........Redwood Falls
Archer, G. F., Jr.........Rochester	Bennion, P. H.........St. Paul	Branham, D. S.........Albert Lea
Arends, A. L.........Sandstone	Benoit, F. T.........Winona	Branton, A. F.........Willmar
Arey, S. L.........Excelsior	Benson, K. W.........Rochester	Branton, B. J.........Willmar
Arlander, C. E.........Minneapolis	Bentley, N. P.........St. Paul	Bratrud, A. F.........Thief River Falls
Arling, L. S.........Minneapolis	Benton, P. C.........Staples	Bratrude, E. J.........St. James
Armstrong, E. L.........Frazee	Berdes, G. L.........Duluth	Braverman, N. J.........Duluth
Armstrong, J. M.........St. Paul	Bergan, Otto.........Clinton	Bray, E. R.........Rochester
Arndt, H. W.........Frazee	Berge, D. O.........Roseau	Bray, K. E.........Park Rapids
Arneson, A. I.........Morris	Berger, A. G.........Minneapolis	Bray, P. N.........Duluth
Arnold, A. W.........Minneapolis	Bergh, G. S.........Minneapolis	Bray, R. B.........Biwabik
Arnold, D. C.........Minneapolis	Bergh, L. N.........Montevideo	Bregel, F. R.........St. James
Arnold, E. W.........Adrian	Bergheim, M. C.........Hawley	Brey, F. W.........Wabasso
Arnquist, A. S.........St. Paul	Berghs, L. V.........Owatonna	Briggs, J. F.........St. Paul
Arnson, J. M.........Benson	Bergman, O. B.........St. James	Brigham, C. F.........St. Cloud
Arny, F. P.........Preston	Bergquist, K. E.........Battle Lake	Brigham, Frank.........Watkins
Arvidson, C. G.........Minneapolis	Berkman, D. M.........Rochester	Brink, A. A.........Baudette
Athens, A. T.........Duluth	Berkman, J. M.........Rochester	Brink, D. M.........Isle
Aune, Martin.........Minneapolis	Berkwitz, N. J.........Minneapolis	Broadie, T. E.........St. Paul
Aurand, W. H.........Minneapolis	Berlin, A. S.........Hallock	Broders, A. C.........Rochester
Aurelius, J. R.........St. Paul	Berman, Reuben.........Minneapolis	Brodie, W. D.........St. Paul
Ausman, C. F.........St. Paul	Bernstein, W. C.........New Richland	Broker, W. S.........Wadena
Ayres, G. T.........Ely	Berrisford, P. D.........St. Paul	Brooks, C. N.........Minneapolis
	Bertelson, O. L.........Crookston	Brooks, G. F.........Stillwater
Babcock, F. M.........Northfield	Bessesen, A. N., Jr.........Minneapolis	Brown, A. E.........Rochester
Bachnik, F. W.........Hibbing	Bessesen, W. A.........Minneapolis	Brown, A. H.........Pipestone
Backus, A. S.........St. Paul	Betlach, C. J.........Rochester	Brown, E. D.........Paynesville
Bacon, D. K.........St. Paul	Beuning, J. B.........Albany	Brown, E. J.........St. Paul
Bacon, L. C.........St. Paul	Bianco, A. J.........St. Paul	Brown, E. J.........Minneapolis
Bacon, R. S.........Montevideo	Bicek, J. F.........St. Paul	Brown, J. C.........St. Paul
Badeaux, G. I.........Brainerd	Bjedermann, Jacob.........Thief River Falls	Brown, L. E.........Crookston
Baggenstoss, A. H.........Rochester	Bigelow, C. E.........Dodge Center	Brown, P. W.........Rochester
Bagley, E. C.........Duluth	Billings, R. E.........Franklin	Brown, R. W.........Rochester
Bagley, W. R.........Duluth	Binet, H. B.........Grand Rapids	Browne, H. C., Jr.........Rochester
Bailey, H. J.........Fairmont	Binger, H. E.........St. Paul	Brownstone, Manuel.........Sandstone
	Binger, M. W.........Rochester	Brumm, H.........Rochester
	Birge, H. L.........Rochester	

Brunsting, L. A.............Rochester
Brusegard, J. F............Red Wing
Brutsch, G. C............Minneapolis
Bryant, F. L.............Minneapolis
Bryant, O. R.............Minneapolis
Buchstein, H. F.............Rochester
Buck, F. H.............Shakopee
Buckley, R. P.............Duluth
Buie, L. A.............Rochester
Bulnaki, T. J.............St. Paul
Bulkley, Kenneth ....Minneapolis
Bullard, M. J.............Minneapolis
Burch, F. E.............St. Paul
Burchell, H. B.............Rochester
Burlingame, D. A.............Mazeppa
Burnap, W. L.............Fergus Falls
Burns, F. M.............Milan
Burns, H. A.............Ah-Gwah-Ching
Burns, H. D.............Albert Lea
Burns, M. A.............Milan
Burns, R. M.............St. Paul
Burton, C. G.............St. Paul
Burton, J. J.............Buhl
Buscher, J. C.............St. Cloud
Bushard, W. J.............Bird Island
Busher, H. H.............St. Paul
Bussey, C. D.............Rochester
Butler, J. K.............Carlton
Butler, John ....Minneapolis
Butt, H. R.............Rochester
Butturff, C. R.............Freeborn
Butzer, J. A.............Mankato
Buzzelle, L. K.............Minneapolis

Cabell, C. L.............Rochester
Cable, M. L.............Rochester
Cabot, Hugh ....Rochester
Cabot, V. S.............Minneapolis
Cady, J. B.............Rochester
Cady, J. H.............Minneapolis
Cain, C. L.............St. Paul
Caine, C. E.............Morris
Cairns, R. J.............Sanborn
Caldwell, J. P.............St. Paul
Calhoun, F. W.............Albert Lea
Callahan, F. F.............Pokegama
Callerstrom, G. W.............Minneapolis
Cameron, D. M.............Rochester
Cameron, Isabell ....Minneapolis
Camp, J. D.............Rochester
Camp, W. E.............Minneapolis
Campbell, A. M.............Minneapolis
Campbell, O. J.............Minneapolis
Campbell, R. W.............Cass Lake
Campbell, S. J.............Rochester
Canfield, W. W.............Houston
Cantwell, W. F.............International Falls
Cardle, A. E.............Minneapolis
Cardle, G. E.............Ah-Gwah-Ching
Carey, J. B.............Minneapolis
Carlaw, C. M.............Minneapolis
Carlson, C. E.............Aitkin
Carlson, H. A.............Walker
Carlson, J. V.............Westbrook
Carlson, Lawrence ....Minneapolis
Carlson, L. T.............Minneapolis
Carlson, V. W.............Blooming Prairie
Carman, J. E.............Detroit Lakes
Carmichael, F. A., Jr.............Rochester
Caron, R. P.............Minneapolis
Carroll, W. C.............St. Paul
Carstens, C. F.............Hibbing
Catlin, J. J.............Buffalo
Catlin, T. J.............Buffalo
Cavanor, R. T.............Minneapolis
Cervenka, C. F.............New Prague
Chadbourn, A. G.............Heron Lake
Chadbourn, C. R.............Janesville
Chambers, W. C.............Blue Earth
Chapman, T. L.............Rochester
Chatterton, C. C.............St. Paul
Chauncey, L. R.............Rochester
Cheney, E. L.............Duluth
Chernak, F. G.............Duluth
Chesley, A. J.............Minneapolis
Chessen, James ....Duluth
Chew, E. M.............Rochester
Christensen, A.............Winona
Christensen, E. P.............Two Harbors
Christenson, G. R.............Minneapolis
Christiansen, A.............St. Paul
Christianson, H. W.............Minneapolis
Christie, G. R.............Long Prairie
Christie, R. L.............Long Prairie
Christison, J. T.............St. Paul
Chunn, S. S.............Pipestone
Clagett, O. T.............Rochester
Clark, F. P.............Duluth
Clark, H. B.............St. Cloud
Clark, H. B., Jr.............St. Paul
Clark, H. H.............Edgerton

Clark, H. S.............Minneapolis
Clark, L. W.............Spring Valley
Clark, R. L., Jr.............Rochester
Clark, T. C.............Minneapolis
Clay, L. B.............Minneapolis
Claydon, D. R.............Red Wing
Claydon, H. F.............Zumbrota
Claydon, L. E.............Red Wing
Clement, J. B.............Lester Prairie
Clement, T. G.............Duluth
Cleveland, W. H.............Rochester
Clifford, G. W.............Osakis
Clifton, T. A.............Chatfield
Clothier, E. F.............Elk River
Cochrane, W. J.............Lake City
Coffey, R. J.............Rochester
Cohen, B. A.............Minneapolis
Cohen, S. S.............Oak Terrace
Colby, Woodard.............St. Paul
Cole, H. B.............Redwood Falls
Cole, J. G.............Redwood Falls
Cole, W. H.............St. Paul
Collie, H. G.............St. Paul
Collins, A. N.............Duluth
Collins, H. C.............Duluth
Collins, J. S.............Wabasha
Colvin, A. R.............St. Paul
Combacker, L. C.............Fergus Falls
Comfort, M. W.............Rochester
Condit, W. H.............Minneapolis
Conner, H. M.............Rochester
Connor, C. E.............St. Paul
Conway, J. F.............Rochester
Cook, C. K.............St. Paul
Cook, E. N.............Rochester
Cook, H. W.............Minneapolis
Cook, J. M.............Staples
Cooney, H. C.............Princeton
Cooper, M. D.............Winnebago
Corbett, J. F.............Minneapolis
Corniea, A. D.............Minneapolis
Corwin, W. C.............Rochester
Cosgriff, J. A.............Bird Island
Cottam, Gilbert ....Minneapolis
Counsellor, V. S.............Rochester
Countryman, R. S.............St. Paul
Covell, W. W.............St. Peter
Coventry, W. A.............Duluth
Coventry, W. D.............Duluth
Cowern, E. W.............North St. Paul
Crafts, L. M.............Minneapolis
Cragg, R. W.............Rochester
Craig, W. McK.............Rochester
Cranmer, R. R.............Minneapolis
Cranston, R. W.............Minneapolis
Creevy, C. D.............Minneapolis
Creighton, R. H.............Minneapolis
Crenshaw, J. L.............Rochester
Cress, E. E.............Boyd
Cress, P. J.............Ellsworth
Crewe, J. E.............Rochester
Critchfield, L. R.............St. Paul
Cronwell, D. J.............Austin
Crow, E. R.............Arlington
Crumpacker, L. K.............Rochester
Culligan, J. M.............St. Paul
Cumming, J. F.............Morris
Curtin, J. J.............Rochester
Curtis, R. A.............Le Center
Cusick, P. J.............Rochester
Cutler, H. H.............Rochester
Cutts, George ....Minneapolis
Cutts, R. E.............Minneapolis

Dack, L. G.............St. Paul
Dady, E. E.............Minneapolis
Dahl, E. O.............Minneapolis
Dahl, G. A.............Mankato
Dahl, J. A.............Minneapolis
Dahlin, J. T.............Aurora
Daignault, Oscar ....Benson
Daniel, D. H.............Minneapolis
Danjel, L. M.............Minneapolis
Danjelson, K. A.............Litchfield
Danielson, Lennox ....Litchfield
Daugherty, E. B.............St. Paul
Daugherty, L. E.............St. Paul
Davis, A. C.............Rochester
Davis, B. F.............Rochester
Davis, Herbert ....St. Paul
Davis, J. G.............Rushford
Davis, L. T.............Wadena
Davis, R. D.............Clearbrook
Davis, T. C.............Wadena
Davis, William ....St. Paul
Day, A. J.............Rochester
Dearing, W. H., Jr.............Rochester
DeBoer, Hermanus ....Edgerton
Dedolph, Karl.............St. Paul
Dedolph, T. H.............Braham
Deeds, G. D.............Rochester
Delavan, P. A.............St. Paul

Delmonico, E. J.............Rochester
Delmore, J. L.............Roseau
Delmore, J. L., Jr.............Roseau
del Plaine, C. W.............Minneapolis
Demo, P. W.............Wells
Denman, A. V.............Mankato
Derauf, B. I.............St. Paul
Desjardins, A. U.............Rochester
Deuterman, J. L.............Elgin, Ill.
Devereaux, T. J.............Wayzata
Dewey, D. H.............Owatonna
Dickson, D. D.............Rochester
Dickson, T. H.............St. Paul
Diehl, H. S.............Minneapolis
Diessner, H. D.............Minneapolis
Dittman, G. C.............St. Paul
Dix, C. R.............Rochester
Dixon, C. F.............Rochester
Dockerty, M. B.............Rochester
Doering, R. E.............Minneapolis
Dolan, C. P.............Worthington
Dolder, F. C.............Eyota
Doleman, N. H.............Tintah
Doman, V. W.............Lakefield
Doms, H. C.............Slayton
Donaldson, O. S.............Foley
Donath, D. H.............Rochester
Donohue, P. F.............St. Paul
Donovan, D. L.............Albert Lea
Doolittle, L. E.............Duluth
Dordal, J.............Sacred Heart
Dorge, R. I.............Minneapolis
Dornblaser, H. B.............Minneapolis
Dorsey, G. C.............Minneapolis
Dovre, C. M.............St. Paul
Dowidat, R. W.............Cologne
Dowswell, W. J.............Kerkhoven
Doxey, G. L.............Minneapolis
Doyle, G. C.............Duluth
Doyle, L. O.............Minneapolis
Drake, C. B.............St. Paul
Drake, R. B.............Minneapolis
Dredge, H. P.............Sandstone
Drill, H. R.............Hopkins
Drips, D. G.............Rochester
Drought, W. W.............Fergus Falls
Dry, I. J.............Rochester
Dubbe, F. H.............New Ulm
DuBois, J. F.............Sauk Center
Duff, E. R.............Minneapolis
Dugan, L. P.............Faribault
Dukelow, D. A.............Minneapolis
Duhde, S. S.............Dassel
Dumas, A. G.............Minneapolis
Duncan, J. W.............Moorhead
Dungay, N. S.............Northfield
Dunlap, E. H.............Minneapolis
Dunn, G. R.............Minneapolis
Dunn, J. N.............St. Paul
Duryea, W. M.............Minneapolis
Dutton, C. E.............Minneapolis
Dvorak, B. A.............Minneapolis
Dwan, P. F.............Minneapolis
Dvorak, A. F.............Walker
Dworsky, S. D.............Minneapolis
Dysterheft, A. T.............Gaylord

Earl, G. A.............St. Paul
Earl, John ....St. Paul
Earl, Robert ....St. Paul
Eaton, L. McK.............Rochester
Eberlin, E. A.............Glenwood
Ecker, A. D.............Rochester
Eckhardt, C. L.............Minneapolis
Eckman, P. F.............Duluth
Eckman, R. J.............Duluth
Ederer, J. F.............Mahtomen
Edlund, G.............St. Paul
Edwards, J. W.............St. Paul
Edwards, R. T.............Elysian
Edwards, T. J.............St. Paul
Ehrenberg, C. J.............Minneapolis
Ehrlich, S. P.............Minneapolis
Eich, Matthew ....Minneapolis
Eiler, John.............Park Rapids
Eisenstadt, D. H.............Minneapolis
Eitel, G. D.............Minneapolis
Ekblad, J. W.............Duluth
Eklund, E. J.............Norwood
Elias, P. J.............Duluth
Elkins, E. C.............Rochester
Ellingson, A. R.............Detroit Lakes
Ellis, E. W.............Elgin
Ellison, D. E.............Minneapolis
Ellison, F. E.............Monticello
Elsey, E. M.............Glenwood
Elsey, J. R.............Glenwood
Ely, O. S.............South St. Paul
Emanuel, K. W.............Duluth
Emerson, E. C.............St. Paul
Emmerson, W. S.............Mayer
Emmett, J. L.............Rochester

379

Kierland, P. E..............Alexandria
Kierland, R. R.............Rochester
Kiesling, I. H.............Nashwauk
Kilbride, E. A............Worthington
Kilbride, J. S.............Worthington
King, E. A................Minneapolis
King, G. L.................St. Paul
King, H. T................Minneapolis
Kingsbury, E. M...........Clearwater
Kinsella, T. J............Minneapolis
Kirk, G. P........East Grand Forks
Kirkhn, B. R..............Rochester
Kirklin, O. L..............Rochester
Kistler, A. J.............Minneapolis
Kistler, C. M.............Minneapolis
Klein, Harry...............Duluth
Klein, H. N................St. Paul
Klein, J. C................Shakopee
Klima, W. W................Stewart
Knapp, F. N.................Duluth
Knapp, M. E.............Minneapolis
Knauff, M. K...............St. Paul
Knight, R. R.............Minneapolis
Knight, R. T.............Minneapolis
Knutson, G. A.............Greenbush
Koch, E. A. S.............Rochester
Koch, F. L. P.............Rochester
Koelsche, G. A.............Rochester
Koenigsberger, Charles ....Mankato
Koepcke, G. M............Minneapolis
Kohlbry, C. O...............Duluth
Kohler, D. W..............St. Joseph
Kolars, J. J..............Le Center
Koller, H. M.............Minneapolis
Koller, L. R.............Minneapolis
Koop, H. E............Cold Spring
Koop, S. H.................Richmond
Korchik, J. P............Minneapolis
Kortsch, F. P...........Prior Lake
Kotchevar, F. R...........Eveleth
Kowallis, G. F............Rochester
Kraft, Peter................Duluth
Krantz, C. I................Duluth
Krause, C. W..............Fairmont
Kreuzer, T. C.............Owatonna
Krusen, F. H..............Rochester
Kucera, F. J..............Hopkins
Kucera, S. T..............Lonsdale
Kucera, W. J.............Minneapolis
Kugler, A. A...............St. Paul
Kuske, A. L...............New Ulm
Kuth, J. R..................Duluth
Kvale, W. F...............Rochester
Kvitrud, Gilbert............St. Paul

Lagersen, R. W..........Minneapolis
Laird, A. T..............Nopeming
Laird, D. R..............Rochester
Lajoie, J. M.............Minneapolis
Lamb, H. L..............Little Falls
Lang, L. A...............Minneapolis
Langenderfer, F. V..........St. Paul
Langhoff, A. H...........Glencoe
Lannin, J. C................Mabel
Lapierre, A. P...........Minneapolis
Lapierre, C. A...........Minneapolis
Lapierre, J. T...........Minneapolis
Larsen, C. L................St. Paul
Larsen, F. W.............Minneapolis
Larsen, O. O...........Detroit Lakes
Larson, Arnold.........Detroit Lakes
Larson, C. M.............Minneapolis
Larson, L. M.............Minneapolis
Larson, L. M...........Oak Terrace
Larson, P. N.............Minneapolis
LaVake, R. T.............Minneapolis
Lax, M. H..................St. Paul
Laymon, C. W............Minneapolis
Leahy, Bartholomew.........St. Paul
Leavenworth, R. O...........St. Paul
Leavitt, H. H............Minneapolis
Lebowske, J. A...........Minneapolis
Leck, P. C..................Austin
Leclercq, G. T. A........Minneapolis
Leddy, E. T...............Rochester
Lee, H. M................Minneapolis
Lee, H. W.................Brainerd
Lee, J. L................Watertown
Lee, W. A..............Fergus Falls
Lee, W. N..................Madison
Leibold, H. H........Parkers Prairie
Leitch, Archibald...........St. Paul
Leitch, N. M...............Warroad
Leland, H. R.............Minneapolis
Leland, J. T...............Herman
Lemon, R. G...............Rochester
Lemon, W. S..............Rochester
Lenander, M. E...........St. Peter
Lenárz, A. J.............Browerville
Lende, Norman.............Faribault

Lenont, C. B...............Virginia
Lenz, J. R.................Morton
Lenz, O. A...............Minneapolis
Leonard, G. J.............Hastings
Leonard, L. J............Minneapolis
Leonard, Sam.............Minneapolis
Leopard, B. A...........Albert Lea
Lepak, F. J.................Duluth
Lepak, J. A................St. Paul
Lerche, William....Cable, Wisconsin
Leven, N. L................St. Paul
Levin, Bert................St. Paul
Levitt, G. X...............St. Paul
Lewis, A. J................Henning
Lewis, C. B...............St. Cloud
Lewis, E. B...............Rochester
Lexa, F. J.................Lonsdale
Libert, J. N...............St. Cloud
Lick, C. L.................St. Paul
Liedloff, A. G...............Mankato
Liffrig, W. W...............Goodhue
Lillehei, E. J...........Robbinsdale
Lillie, H. I...............Rochester
Lima, Ludvig.............Montevideo
Lind, C. J..............Minneapolis
Lindberg, A. L............Wheaton
Linde, Herman................Cyrus
Lindgren, R. C...........Minneapolis
Lindquist, R. H..........Minneapolis
Lindsay, W. V................Winona
Linner, Gunnar............Stillwater
Linner, H. P.............Minneapolis
Linton, W. B.............Minneapolis
Lippman, E. S............Minneapolis
Lippman, H. S..............St. Paul
Lippmann, E. W...........Hutchinson
Lipschultz, Oscar........Minneapolis
Lipscomb, W. R............Rochester
Litman, B. A.............Minneapolis
Litman, S. N................Duluth
Little, W. J................St. Paul
Litzenberg, J. C.........Minneapolis
Livingstone, J. W......Hudson, Wis.
Lloyd, H. J................Mankato
Lloyd, S. J...............Rochester
Lochead, D. C.............Rochester
Loenholdt, E. H...........Hector
Logan, A. H...............Rochester
Logan, G. B...............Rochester
Logefeil, R. C...........Minneapolis
Lohmann, J. G...............Jasper
Loken, Theodore ....Ada
Lommen, P. A................Austin
Long, Jesse..............Minneapolis
Loofbourrow, E. H..........Keewatin
Loomis, E. A.............Minneapolis
Lord, G. A...............Rochester
Love, F. A..................Carlos
Love, J. C................Rochester
Lovelace, W. R............Rochester
Lovelady, S. B............Rochester
Lowe, E. R............South St. Paul
Lowe, Thomas..............Pipestone
Lowe, T. A...........South St. Paul
Luden, Georgine,
            Victoria, B. C., Canada
Luedtke, G. H............Fairmont
Lufkin, C. D.............Northfield
Lufkin, N. H.............Minneapolis
Lund, C. J. T...........Underwood
Lund, W. J.................Staples
Lundberg, R. I...........Minneapolis
Lundblad, R. A...........Minneapolis
Lundgren, A. C...........Minneapolis
Lundholm, J. A...........St. Paul
Lundquist, C. W............Hibbing
Lundquist, E. F..........Minneapolis
Lundy, J. S...............Rochester
Lutz, E. H................Willmar
Lyght, C. E..............Northfield
Lynch, F. W...............St. Paul
Lynch, M. J..............Minneapolis
Lynde, O. G........Thief River Falls
Lysne, Henry............Minneapolis
Lysne, Myron ....Minneapolis

MacDonald, A. E.........Minneapolis
MacDonald, D. A.........Minneapolis
MacDonald, I. C.........Minneapolis
Macey, H. B..............Rochester
Macfarlane, P. H..........Chisholm
Mach, F. B...............Minneapolis
Mack, J. J...........Little Rock, Ark.
Mac Kay, A. R.............Rochester
Macklin, W. E............Litchfield
MacLean, A. R............Rochester
Macnie, J. S.............Minneapolis
MacRae, G. C................Duluth
Madden, J. F...............St. Paul

McQuarrie, Irvine.........Minneapolis
Mead, C. H....................Duluth
Meade, J. R..................St. Paul
Mears, B. J..................St. Paul
Mecray, P. M., Jr..........Rochester
Medelman, J. P...............St. Paul
Meinert, A. E................Winona
Meland, E. L...............Minneapolis
Melby, Benedik......Blooming Prairie
Mellby, O. F........Thief River Falls
Melzer, G. R....................Lyle
Mercil, W. F................Crookston
Merkert, C. E..............Minneapolis
Merkert, G. L..............Minneapolis
Merrill, Elisabeth.........Minneapolis
Merriman, L. L................Duluth
Merrit, W. A...............Rochester
Mesker, G. H...................Olivia
Meyer, A. A..................Melrose
Meyer, E. L...............Minneapolis
Meyer, F. C...................Kenyon
Meyer, P. F.................Faribault
Meyerding, E. A..............St. Paul
Meyerding, H. W............Rochester
Michael, J. C.............Minneapolis
Michel, H. H..............Minneapolis
Michelson, H. E...........Minneapolis
Middleton, A. W............Rochester
Miller, F. J.......Spokane, Wash.
Miller, H. A................Fairmont
Miller, H. E..............Minneapolis
Miller, J. C..............Minneapolis
Miller, J. M...............Rochester
Miller, V. I..................Mankato
Miller, W. A........New York Mills
Mills, J. L................Winnebago
Milton, J. S..............Minneapolis
Miners, G. A...........Deer River
Mingo, F. E.....................Hugo
Mitby, I. J...................Hibbing
Mitchell, E. C..................Mound
Mitchell, R. S......Grand Meadow
Moberg, C. W...........Lake Park
Moe, J. H.................Minneapolis
Moe, R. J......................Duluth
Moe, Thomas...........Moose Lake
Moersch, F. P.............Rochester
Moersch, H. J.............Rochester
Moga, J. A.................St. Paul
Mogilner, S. N............St. Paul
Moir, W. W...............Minneapolis
Molander, H. A............St. Paul
Monroe, P. B.........Two Harbors
Monson, E. M.............Minneapolis
Monson, L. J....................Canby
Montgomery, Hamilton....Rochester
Montgomery, T. R..........Rochester
Mooney, L. P..............Graceville
Moorhead, M. B...........Minneapolis
Moquin, M. A..............St. Paul
Moran, T. R........Phoenix, Ariz.
More, C. W.................Eveleth
Morehead, D. E............Owatonna
Moren, Edward..........Minneapolis
Morgan, H. O., Jr..........Amboy
Morjarty, Berenice..........St. Paul
Moriarty, C. R..........Minneapolis
Mork, B. O..............Worthington
Mork, B. O., Jr........Worthington
Morley, G. A...............Crookston
Morlock, C. G..............Rochester
Morrison, A. W.........Minneapolis
Morrissey, F. B..............St. Paul
Morrow, J. J..................Austin
Morse, M. P..................Le Roy
Morse, R. W..............Minneapolis
Morsman, L. W.............Hibbing
Morss, C. R...............Zumbrota
Mortensbak, H. E............Hanska
Mortenson, N. G............St. Paul
Morton, H. McI...Vincentown, N. J.
Mosby, M. E..........Long Prairie
Moses, Joseph, Jr.........Northfield
Moses, R. R..................Kenyon
Moss, M. M..................St. Paul
Mouritsen, G. J.........Fergus Falls
Mousel, L. H...............Rochester
Moyer, R. E..............Minneapolis
Moynihan, A. F........Sauk Center
Moynihan, T. J............St. Paul
Mueller, S. C..................Duluth
Muller, R. T................St. Paul
Mulligan, A. M...............Brainerd
Mulrooney, R. E.............Rochester
Mundell, B. J...............Rochester
Murphy, E. F.............Minneapolis
Murphy, J. J..............Minneapolis
Mussey, R. D...............Rochester

*Deceased.

Myers, J. A..............Minneapolis
Myers, Thomas...............St. Paul
Myre, C. R...............Paynesville

Naegeli, A. E................St. Paul
Naegeli, Frank..........Fergus Falls
Nagel, H. D.................Waconia
Nash, L. A.................Rochester
Naslund, A. W..............St. Paul
Nass, H. A....................Mabel
Nauth, W. W................Winona
Neal, H. B.................Rochester
Neal, J. M................Minneapolis
Nealy, D. E...................Adrian
Neary, R. P..............Minneapolis
Neher, F. H.................St. Paul
Nehring, J. P................Preston
Neilson, H. F.............Minneapolis
Nelson, E. H...............Chisholm
Nelson, E. J...............Owatonna
Nelson, H. E...............Crookston
Nelson, Harvey..........Minneapolis
Nelson, H. S.............Minneapolis
Nelson, K. L.................Willmar
Nelson, L. A................St. Paul
Nelson, M. S...........Granite Falls
Nelson, N. P................Brainerd
Nelson, O. E..............Minneapolis
Nelson, O. L. N.........Minneapolis
Nelson, R. L..................Duluth
Nelson, W. E..............Minneapolis
Nelson, W. O. B.......Fergus Falls
Ness, C. M.................Cambridge
Neumann, C. A..............Winona
New, G. B.................Rochester
Newhart, Horace.........Minneapolis
Nichols, A. E...............St. Paul
Nicholson, M. A..............Duluth
Nilles, L. J............Rollingstone
Nilson, M. J.......North Mankato
Ninneman, N. N.........Silver Lake
Nissen, A. S...............St. Peter
Noble, J. F.................St. Paul
Noble, S. J.................St. Paul
Nordin, G. T.............Minneapolis
Nordland, Mattin........Minneapolis
Nordman, W. F.................Mora
Norman, J. A...............Crookston
*Norrgard, H. T............Milaca
Norris, R. H.............Minneapolis
Norris, N. T..............Caledonia
Noth, H. W...............Minneapolis
Noth, P. E.................Rochester
Novak, E. E.............New Prague
Nuessle, W. G..............Springfield
Nuetzman, A. W..............Faribault
Nutting, R. E...................Duluth
Nydahl, M. J.............Minneapolis
Nye, A. A...................St. Paul
Nye, L. L...................St. Paul
Nygren, W. T.................Braham
Nystrom, Ruth ....Minneapolis

Oberg, C. M.............Minneapolis
O'Brien, W. A...........Minneapolis
Ochsner, C. G..............Wabasha
O'Connor, D. C.......Eden Valley
O'Connor, L. J..............St. Paul
Odel, H. M.................Rochester
O'Donnell, D. M........Ortonville
O'Donnell, J. L.........Minneapolis
Oeljen, S. C. G...............Waseca
Oerting, Harry..............St. Paul
Ogden, Warner...............St. Paul
Ohage, Justus, Jr...........St. Paul
O'Hanlon, J. A...............Proctor
Ohnstad, J. L..............McIntosh
Olds, G. H...................Waseca
Olds, J. W.................Rochester
O'Leary, P. A.............Rochester
Oljver, C. I...............Graceville
Oliver, I. L...............Graceville
Olmanson, E. G.............St. Peter
Olsen, A. M................Rochester
Olsen, E. G..............Minneapolis
Olson, A. C..............Minneapolis
Olson, A. E..................Duluth
Olson, A. O..................Duluth
Olson, C. J..................St. Paul
Olson, C. J..............Belle Plaine
Olson, S. A.............Pine Island
Olson, F. A..............Minneapolis
Olson, G. E...........West Concord
Olson, K. L....................Gibbon
Olson, O. A..............Minneapolis
Olson, R. G..............Minneapolis
Onsgard, L. K., Jr.........Houston
Onsgard, L. K., Sr.........Houston
Oppegaard, C. L..........Crookston
Oppegaard, M. O.........Crookston

Oppen, E. G..............Minneapolis
O'Reilley, B. E..............St. Paul
Ormond, D. T................Waconia
Osborn, Lida................Mankato
Ostergren, E. W.............St. Paul
Otto, H. C.....................Frazee
Ouelette, A. J..............St. Paul
Owre, Oscar...............Minneapolis

Page, C. V..................St. Paul
Page, R. L..................St. Charles
Palmer, C. F...............Albert Lea
Palmer, H. A................Eveleth
Palmer, W. L..............Albert Lea
Pankratz, P. J........Mountain Lake
Paradis, W. G..............Crookston
Parker, D. M........Oakland, Calif.
Parker, O. W....................Ely
Parker, R. L................Rochester
Parkhill, E. M..............Rochester
Parks, A. H..............Minneapolis
Parson, L. R.............Elbow Lake
Parsons, J. G..............Crookston
Pasek, A. W.................Cloquet
Passer, A. A...................Olivia
Patterson, W. E..........Minneapolis
Patterson, W. E............Westbrook
Patterson, W. L........Fergus Falls
Patton, G. D................Rochester
Paulsen, E. L.............Minneapolis
Paulson, D. J..............Rochester
Paulson, J. A..............Rochester
Paulson, T. S...........Fergus Falls
Pearman, R. O. D.........Rochester
Pearsall, R. P.................Virginia
Pearson, B. F................Shakopee
Pearson, F. R................St. Paul
Pedersen, A. H.............St. Paul
Pederson, R. M...........Minneapolis
Pellettiere, E. V...Thief River Falls
Pemberton, J. deJ..........Rochester
Penhall, F. W................Morton
Penn, G. E...................Mankato
Pennie, D. F...................Duluth
Pennington, Reuben......Minneapolis
Peppard, T. A.............Minneapolis
Perozzi, Thelma...........Rochester
Perry, C. G..................St. Paul
Persons, C. E...............Marshall
Pertl, A. L....................Canby
Petersen, J. R............Minneapolis
Petersen, M. C..............Willmar
Petersen, P. C................Braham
Petersen, Thorvald.......Minneapolis
Peterson, A. A.................Mora
Peterson, D. B.............St. Paul
Peterson, E. N...............Virginia
Peterson, H. O...........Minneapolis
Peterson, Henry.........Minneapolis
Peterson, H. W..........Minneapolis
Peterson, J. L..................Duluth
Peterson, J. L. E............St. Paul
Peterson, N. P...........Minneapolis
Peterson, O. H..........Minneapolis
Peterson, O. L.................Cokato
Peterson, P. E...........Minneapolis
Peterson, R. A...................Vesta
Peterson, V. N...............St. Paul
Peterson, W. C...........Minneapolis
Petit, L. J.................Minneapolis
Petraborg, H. T...............Aitkin
Peyton, W. T............Minneapolis
Pfunder, M. C...........Minneapolis
Phelps, K. A.............Minneapolis
Phillips, A. E................Delano
Phillips, W. H................Jordan
Pierce, C. H..................Wadena
Piper, M. C.................Rochester
Piper, W. A..........Mountain Lake
Platon, E. S..............Minneapolis
Plondke, F. J.................St. Paul
Plonske, C. J..............Faribault
Plowman, E. T..............Marble
Plummer, W. A............Rochester
Pogue, R. E..........Glendale, Calif.
Pohl, J. F. M............Minneapolis
Poirier, J. A............Forest Lake
Pollard, D. W............Minneapolis
Pollock, D. W.............Minneapolis
Pollock, L. W..............Rochester
Polzak, J. A..............Minneapolis
Pool, T. L..................Rochester
Popp, W. C.................Rochester
Poppe, F. H..............Minneapolis
Potek, David......International Falls
Potter, R. B................Hendricks
Potthoff, C. J.................Morgan
Power, J. E...................Duluth
Powers, F. H................Rochester
Powers, F. W.................Barrett
Prangen, A. D..............Rochester

Pratt, F. J................Minneapolis
Pratt, J. A................Minneapolis
Preine, I. A..............Minneapolis
Preisinger, J. W............Renville
Prendergast, H. J...........St. Paul
Prendergast, P. J......Carville, La.
Prickman, L. E............Rochester
Priest, R. E..............Worthington
Priestley, J. T.............Rochester
Prim, J. A................Minneapolis
Prins, L. R...............Albert Lea
Proeschel, R. K.............Willmar
Proshek, C. E.............Minneapolis
Pumphrey, R. E..............Rochester
Purves, G. H.........Lake Benton
Puumala, R. H...............Cloquet

Quanstrom, V. E.............Brainerd
Quello, R. O. B..........Minneapolis
Quinby, T. F......Lake Wales, Fla.
Quist, H. W..............Minneapolis

Raadquist, C. S..............Hibbing
Radabaugh, R. C.............Hastings
Raihala, John..............Virginia
Raiter, F. W. S..............Cloquet
Raiter, R. F................Cloquet
Ralph, R. D................Rochester
Ramsey, W. R................St. Paul
Randall, A. M................Ashby
Randall, L. M..............Rochester
Ransom, M. L...............Hancock
Rasmussen, R. C..........Minneapolis
Rasmussen, T. B............Rochester
Ratcliffe, J. J..............Aitkin
Rathbun, C. A...............St. Cloud
Raymond, J. H..............Triumph
Reed, C. A..............Minneapolis
Reeve, E. T............Elbow Lake
Reff, A. R................Crookston
Regan, J. F................Rochester
Regnier, E. A.............Minneapolis
Reichelderfer, C. F...........Staples
Reineke, G. F...............New Ulm
Renier, H. H..............Shakopee
Rewbridge, A. G..........Minneapolis
Reynolds, J. S..........Minneapolis
Rhorer, R. J...............Rochester
Rice, C. O...............Minneapolis
Rice, H. G................Moorhead
Rice, H. R..................Roseau
Richards, E. T. F............St. Paul
Richards, W. B..............St. Cloud
Richardson, F. L............Coleraine
Richardson, F. S.........Minneapolis
Richardson, H. E.............St. Paul
Rickdorf, L. F...........Minneapolis
Richey, G. L..............Cambridge
Rick, P. F. W............Le Center
Ridgway, A. M.............Annandale
Rieke, W. O................Wayzata
Rigler, L. G.............Minneapolis
Riley, J. B..............Fergus Falls
Rimer, E. W.............Breckenridge
Ringle, O. F................Walker
Rishmiller, J. H.........Minneapolis
Risser, A. F............Stewartville
Risser, E. D................Winona
Ritchie, H. P...............St. Paul
Ritchie, W. P...............St. Paul
Ritt, A. E.................St. Paul
Rivers, A. B...............Rochester
Rizer, R. I..............Minneapolis
Roan, C. M..............Minneapolis
Robb, E. F..............Minneapolis
Robbins, C. P...............Winona
Robbins, O. F...........Minneapolis
Roberts, L. M............Little Falls
Roberts, O. W.............Owatonna
Roberts, S. W...........Minneapolis
Roberts, T. S...........Minneapolis
Roberts, W. B...........Minneapolis
Robertson, H. E............Rochester
Robertson, J. B..........Minneapolis
Robertson, P. A..............Austin
Robilliard, C. M...........Faribault
Robinson, J. M..............Duluth
Robitshek, E. C..........Minneapolis
Rochford, W. E...........Minneapolis
Rodda, F. C.............Minneapolis
Rodgers, C. L...........Minneapolis
Roehlke, A. B...............Elk River
Roemer, H. J................Winona
Rogers, S. F................St. Paul
Rogne, W. G...........Spring Grove
Roholt, C. L...............Waverly
Rohrer, C. A..............Waterville
Rokala, H. E................Biwabik

Rood, D. C.................Duluth
Rose, J. T.................Lakefield
Rosen, Samuel..........Minneapolis
Rosenberg, E. F............Rochester
Rosenfield, A. B.............Pequot
Rosenholtz, Burton..........St. Paul
Rosenow, E. C..............Rochester
Rosenow, E. C., Jr...........Rochester
Rosenstiel, H. C...........Rochester
Rosenthal, F. H........Grand Meadow
Rosenthal, Robert............St. Paul
Rosenwald, R. M..........Minneapolis
Roskilly, G. C. P..........Minneapolis
Ross, W. P.............Battle Lake
Rossen, R. X...............St. Peter
Roth, F. D................Lewiston
Rothenburg, J. C...........Springfield
Rothrock, J. L..............St. Paul
Rothschild, H. J............St. Paul
Rousseau, Victor........Maple Lake
Roust, H. A..............Montevideo
Rowe, O. W.................Duluth
Rowe, W. H................Fairmont
Rowles, E. K..............Coleraine
Roy, J. A............Red Lake Falls
Roy, P. C..................St. Paul
*Roy, Philemon..............St. Paul
Rucker, C. W...............Rochester
Rucker, W. H............Minneapolis
Rudd, R. F.............Minneapolis
Rudell, G. L...........Minneapolis
Rudje, C. N.................Kenyon
Rudie, P. S.................Duluth
Ruggles, G. McC........Forest Lake
Rulberg, G. N...............St. Paul
Rumpf, C. W...............Faribault
Rumpf, W. H..............Faribault
Rumpf, W. H..............St. Cloud
Rushton, J. G..............Rochester
Russ, H. H..............Blue Earth
Russeth, A. N...........Minneapolis
Rusten, E. M...........Minneapolis
Rutherford, W. C.............St. Paul
Rutledge, D. I.............Rochester
Rutledge, L. H.........Detroit Lakes
Ryan, J....................St. Paul
Ryan, J. M................St. Paul
Ryan, M. E................St. Paul
Ryan, W. J.................Duluth
Rynearson, E. H............Rochester

Sach-Rowitz, Alvin.......Moose Lake
Sadler, W. P.............Minneapolis
Saffert, C. A...............New Ulm
Sahr, W. G...............Hutchinson
St. Cyr, K. J...............Osseo
Salt, C. G..............Minneapolis
Salter, R. A................Virginia
Samson, E. R..............Stillwater
Samuelson, L. G.............Mankato
Samuelson, Samuel.......Minneapolis
Sanderson, E. T..........Minneapolis
Sandt, K. E.............Minneapolis
Sandven, N. O............Paynesville
Sanford, A. H..............Rochester
Sarff, O. E................Virginia
Sarnecki, M. M............St. Paul
Satersmoen, Theodore...Pelican Rapids
Satter, R. A..............Alexandria
Sather, R. O...............Crookston
Satterlee, H. W............Lewiston
Satterlund, V. L.............St. Paul
Savage, F. J................St. Paul
Sawatzky, W. A...........Minneapolis
Sawyer, M. H..............Rochester
Sax, S. G..................Duluth
Schaaf, F. H. K..........Minneapolis
Schade, F. L............Worthington
Schaefer, J. F.............Owatonna
Schaefer, Samuel.............Winona
Schaefer, W. G..........Minneapolis
Schatz, F. J...............St. Cloud
Scheldrup, N. H..........Minneapolis
Scherer, C. A...............Duluth
Scherer, L. R...........Minneapolis
Schimelpfenig, G. T.........Chaska
Schlesselman, George..........Anoka
Schlesselman, J. T.........Mankato
Schmidt, G. F...........Minneapolis
Schmidt, H. W.............Rochester
Schmidt, P. A.........Good Thunder
Schmidt, P. G........Granite Falls
Schmidt, W. R..............Glencoe
Schmitt, A. F...........Minneapolis
Schmitt, S. C....Los Angeles, Calif.
Schneider, H. H............Rochester
Schneider, P. J...........Minneapolis
Schneider, P. J..............Adams
Schoch, R. B. J............St. Paul
Scholpp, O. W............Hutchinson

Schons, Edward.............St. Paul
Schottler, G. J..............Dexter
Schottler, M. E..........Minneapolis
Schroder, C. H..............Duluth
Schroeppel, J. E...........Winthrop
Schuldt, F. C.............Minneapolis
Schultz, J. A.............Albert Lea
Schultz, P. J............Minneapolis
Schulze, A. G................St. Paul
Schussler, O. F..........Minneapolis
Schutz, E. S..........Mountain Lake
Schwartz, V. J...........Minneapolis
Schwelger, T. R.............Hibbing
Schwyzer, Arnold............St. Paul
Schwyzer, Gustav.........Minneapolis
Scofield, C. L...............Benson
Scott, E. E................St. Paul
Scott, F. H..............Minneapolis
Scott, H. G..............Minneapolis
Searles, P. W..............Rochester
Seashore, Gilbert.........Minneapolis
Seashore, R. T...............Duluth
Secord, R. W...............Rochester
Seedorf, E. E..............Rochester
Seham, Max.............Minneapolis
Seifert, M. H..............Excelsior
Seifert, O. J...............New Ulm
Seitz, S. B..............Barnesville
Seldon, T. H...............Rochester
Selleseth, E. F..........Minneapolis
Senkler, G. E...............St. Paul
Senn, E. W................Owatonna
Serkland, J. C..............Rothsay
Sether, A. F................Ruthton
Setzer, H. J................St. Paul
Shaleen, A. W..............Hallock
Shannon, S. S................Crosby
Shannon, W. R..............St. Paul
Shaperman, R. F.........Minneapolis
Shapiro, E. Z...............Duluth
Shapiro, M. J..........Minneapolis
Sharp, D. W.............Minneapolis
Shastid, T. H................Duluth
Shaw, A. W...................Buhl
Shedlov, Abraham...........Fosston
Sheedy, C. L................Austin
Sheedy, L. P...............Rochester
Shelden, C. H..............Rochester
Sheldon, W. D..............Rochester
Shellman, J. L...............St. Paul
Shelver, H. J..............Ortonville
Sheppard, C. G...........Hutchinson
Sheppard, Fred...........Hutchinson
Sheppard, P. E...........Hutchinson
Sher, D. A.............Cold Spring
Sherman, C. L...............Luverne
Sherman, H. T..............Plainview
Sherwood, G. E..............Kimball
Shillington, M. A............St. Paul
Shimonek, S. W.............St. Paul
Shoemaker, Rosemary.......Rochester
Short, Jacob................St. Paul
Shrader, J. S................Jordan
Sibley, W. L.........Roanoke, Va.
Sickler, J. R..............Rochester
Siegmann, W. C..........Minneapolis
Silver, J. D.............Minneapolis
Simjson, Carl............Barnesville
Simison, C. W...............Hawley
Simons, B. H................Chaska
Simons, E. J...............Swanville
Simons, J. H.............Minneapolis
Simons, L. T................St. Paul
Simons, S. J................Akeley
Simonton, K. M...........Rochester
Simpson, E. D...........Minneapolis
Simpson, W. C.............Rochester
Sinamark, Andrew...........Hibbing
Singer, B. J.............Minneapolis
Siperstein, D. M.........Minneapolis
Sisler, C. E..........Grand Rapids
Sivertsen, Andrew...Hollywood, Calif.
Sivertsen, Ivar.........Minneapolis
Sjostrom, L. E...............Storden
Skaug, H. M...............Chatfield
Skinner, H. O...............St. Paul
Skinner, I. C., Jr..........Rochester
Skjold, A. C..............Minneapolis
Slater, S. A..............Worthington
Sloan, Julius............Minneapolis
Slocumb, C. H.............Rochester
Slocumb, J. A..............Plainview
Slyfield, F. F................Duluth
Smesh, J. F................Owatonna
Smisek, E. A................St. Paul
Smisek, F. A.............Minneapolis
Smith, A. E.............Minneapolis
Smith, A. M.............Minneapolis
Smith, Archie M.........Minneapolis
Smith, B. A.................Crosby
Smith, B. F................Rochester

*Deceased.

Willius, F. A.	Rochester	Wohlrabe, C. F.	Minneapolis
Wilmot, C. A.	Litchfield	Wohlrabe, E. J.	Springfield
Wilmot, H. E.	Litchfield	Wold, K. C.	St. Paul
Wilson, C. E.	Blue Earth	Wolfe, H. H.	St. Paul
Wilson, J. A.	St. Paul	Wolff, H. J.	St. Paul
Wilson, J. V.	St. Paul	Wolff, L. H.	Rochester
Wilson, L. B.	Rochester	Wolfram, D. J.	Rochester
Wilson, R. B.	Rochester	Wolkoff, H. J.	St. Paul
Wilson, R. H.	Winona	Wolner, O. H.	St. Peter
Wilson, V. O.	Minneapolis	Woltman, H. W.	Rochester
Wilson, Warren	Northfield	Wood, H. G.	Rochester
Wilson, W. D.	Rochester	Woodruff, C. W.	Chatfield
Wilson, W. F.	Lake City	Woodruff, Robert	Rochester
Wiltrout, I. G.	Oslo	Woodworth, Elizabeth	Minneapolis
Windsor, R. L.	Fergus Falls	Woodworth, L. F.	Le Center
Winer, L. H.	Minneapolis	Workman, W. G.	Tracy
Wingquist, C. G.	Los Angeles, Calif.	Wray, W. E.	Campbell
Winnick, J. B.	St. Paul	Wright, C. B.	Minneapolis
Winter, J. A.	Duluth	Wright, C. D.	Minneapolis
Winther, Nora	Minneapolis	Wright, C. O.	Luverne
Witham, C. A.	Minneapolis	Wright, F. R.	Minneapolis
Withrow, M. E.	International Falls	Wright, S. G.	Minneapolis
Wittich, F. W.	Minneapolis	Wright, W. S.	Minneapolis
Wohlrabe, A. A.	Minneapolis	Wrork, D. H.	Rochester

MINNESOTA MEDICINE

Journal of the Minnesota State Medical Association, Southern Minnesota Medical Association, Northern Minnesota Medical Association, Minnesota Academy of Medicine and Minneapolis Surgical Society.

| Volume 21 | JUNE, 1938 | Number 6 |

PREVENTION OF SPONTANEOUS AND INDUCED ABORTION*

FRED J. TAUSSIG, M.D.

Saint Louis, Missouri

NOWADAYS we hear much talk about the conservation of our natural resources, reforestation, soil-preservation, and the control of damage by flood and famine. Not so much thought is given, however, to the even more important problem of conservation of our human resources. It is up to us as physicians to take the leadership in that direction. I know no more glaring example of the failure to practice conservation than in the wastage of human life associated with spontaneous and induced abortion. The avoidance of a pregnancy through contraception may limit production but it does no physical harm. Childbirth involves certain unavoidable risks to both mother and child, but there is the compensation of a new life added to our human resources. Abortion, on the other hand, has all these risks multiplied seven-fold without any of the compensations. With the exception of a small number of therapeutic abortions, it has nothing but liabilities as its sequel: the mother incapacitated, her health undermined at times, with death not an infrequent termination. The prevention of abortion therefore demands our most serious consideration.

Approximately six to seven hundred thousand abortions occur annually in the United States, and probably eight to ten thousand women lose their lives annually as a result of this condition. These estimates give one a conception of the magnitude of the problem. About one-third of these abortions are spontaneous and two-thirds are induced. Elsewhere[20] will be found the data, still rather meagre, upon which these figures are

based. I shall confine my remarks solely to the matter of causes and prevention.

Spontaneous Abortion

The more grateful portion of this study, because holding better promise for its relief, is that of spontaneous abortion. Here we have the eager coöperation of the patient and the measures employed are strictly medical, involving tests, examinations and procedures which are entirely within our own scope as physicians, as distinguished from the problem of induced abortion, in which the legislator, the economist and the social worker have an almost equal share of responsibility in preventive measures.

Since 1909 when I first ventured to write a brief monograph[21] on the "Prevention and Treatment of Abortion," there has been a definite advance in our knowledge of the causes and prevention of spontaneous abortion. At that time almost all abortions were attributed to some physical accident or trauma, and rest in bed together with the hypodermic administration of opiates were the only remedies used to combat the premature interruption of pregnancy. Habitual abortion was attributed to syphilis and patients were routinely placed on anti-luetic treatment. In the past three decades our increasing knowledge of the endocrine secretions and their modification during pregnancy has opened up a whole new field in the study of sterility and early abortion. Although we are far from having solved this problem, certain experimental data and clinical results point to the fact that we are at least on the right track and that the next decade should bring about a considerable reduction

---

*Read, by invitation, before the Hennepin County Medical Society, Minneapolis, January 3, 1938.

in the number of spontaneous abortions in those patients who can and will coöperate in carrying out the rather tedious and expensive method of treatment at present available.

Certain fundamental facts regarding the predisposing factors in spontaneous abortion have always been recognized. The general physical condition of the mother, more especially the condition of the uterus, in which the impregnated ovum was implanted, should be as near to normal as possible. Not infrequently pregnancy continues in spite of marked pelvic disease, but certainly the incidence of abortion in these cases is far in excess of the average. It has therefore been our aim to put the uterus in as normal a condition as possible.

Physical factors predisposing to abortion are: (1) retroversion; (2) fibroid tumors; (3) septate or infantile development; (4) deep lacerations of the cervix; (5) endometrial hyperplasia.

Since these causes have in the past been fully discussed, they will be considered only briefly in this paper. A considerable majority of retroverted uteri will rise out of the pelvis as pregnancy advances without complication. Nevertheless, gentle methods of bringing the uterus forward and holding it there with a pessary decrease uterine irritability and the chance of abortion. Gentleness is essential, however, since brusque manipulations predispose to interruption of the pregnancy. In the presence of fibroid tumors a decision will often be difficult, since pregnancy is ordinarily not interrupted. Where abortion has occurred without other apparent reason, it will usually be wise to do a myomectomy before allowing another pregnancy to take place. Septate and infantile uteri present physical conditions limiting the proper stretching of the uterine cavity. In the former, surgical excision of the septum is advisable. The infantile uterus may require no further treatment, since the pregnancy, even though terminating in abortion, has usually so dilated the cavity that a subsequent gestation is readily carried to term. Deep lacerations of the cervix may tend to abortion by predisposing to dislodgment of the lower pole of the ovisac, to decidual hemorrhage and decidual infection. They should in certain cases be repaired preceding a further conception. Endometrial hyperplasia, often a sequel of postabortive endometritis, may lead to renewed abortion if not corrected by a curettement. It can

result in faulty implantation of the ovum and so to fetal death.

Turning now from pelvic disorders to systemic infections as factors in abortion, two deserve special attention: (1) focal infections; (2) syphilis.

Curtis,[8] Reith[17] and others have demonstrated the occurrence of abortion in women who have a focus of infection, especially about the teeth or tonsils. Certain strains of streptococci, both in animals and humans, apparently predispose to decidual infection and abortion. Elimination of points of infection before the occurrence of the next pregnancy is therefore advisable. It would also be logical to give sulphanilamide in such cases, though I know of no reports in which this has been tried.

Syphilis is relatively simple of recognition and control, even though it is generally recognized that in the white race it rarely produces fetal death and interruption of pregnancy previous to the fifth month. In every case of abortion, however, it is wise to do a Wassermann test on husband and wife, and, if positive, institute specific treatment. McCord[9, 10] has shown that in the negro the virulence of syphilis may cause fetal death and abortion even in the first half of pregnancy.

It has been customary in the past to distinguish between maternal and ovular causes of abortion. In my recent book I still clung to this classification. The more we appreciate the close relationship between the endocrine secretions on the one hand, and the development of the ovum, its impregnation and implantation, and the associated irritability of the pregnant uterus on the other hand, the less does such a separation seem logical. The careful study of abortion ova, begun forty years ago by Mall[11] at the Carnegie Institute of Embryology at Baltimore and since then carried out in many other places, has brought convincing evidence of the importance of arrested development in the production of abortion. In fact I do not believe it an exaggeration to say that in two-thirds of spontaneous abortions such an abnormality of the hormonal secretions is the fundamental contributing cause. We have for a long time been skeptical about the stories of falls, strains, blows and other forms of trauma to which abortion has been attributed, since these injuries are relatively frequent during pregnancy and only in certain individuals seem to be attended by an expulsion of the ovisac. Sexual intercourse in the first trimester of pregnancy seems more definitely a contributing factor in abortion, but here it is plausible to assume that the physical contact may be less important than the associated stimulation of hormonal activities.

I shall consider the subject of endocrine pathology under three heads:

1. Preconceptional conditions influencing the development of the sex cells (ovum and sperm).
2. Developmental factors influencing the implantation and the nutrition of the ovum in the first trimester of pregnancy.
3. Hyperirritability of the uterine muscle, due directly or indirectly to an improper balance of endocrine secretions.

Preconceptional conditions.—It has long been noted by veterinarians and those engaged in animal experimentation that low fertility is usually attended by a high abortion rate. The bull with abnormal spermatozoa will produce a high percentage of abortions in his herd. The ovum is also frequently at fault, so that, if impregnated, its development will not progress beyond the stage of a primitive egg-mass. There is good reason to believe that many such abortions in women are not recognized but pass as an abnormal menstruation, since they do not materially disturb her physical condition. The more carefully we examine every extruded ovum in spontaneous abortions, the more we are impressed with the frequency of these so-called "blank cartridges," an unruptured amniotic sac in which no trace of embryo is longer visible. Occasionally a little nubbin of tissue will show a degenerated embryonal cell-mass. Such primarily blighted ova are frequently associated with relative sterility of the couple. Kane[6] found that of thirty-six children born to forty mothers who had previously habitually aborted, three showed malformations, and concludes: "It may be that preventing the expulsion of abnormal fetuses in the early months of pregnancy is combating nature's provision for the elimination of the unfit."

Unfortunately our knowledge of endocrine diagnosis and treatment is still in its infancy. We must grasp at straws in our preventive measures. The quantitative tests for estrogenic substance are not suitable for routine laboratory work. The basal metabolism test is our mainstay in

this work. If such a test indicates a hypothyroid condition in either husband or wife, it has been found that thyroid extract in moderate doses contributes both to increased fertility and to a more healthy ovum and sperm, so that the resulting impregnation is less apt to be followed by an abortion. Even with a relatively normal basal rate, it would seem that the pre-conceptional ingestion of small amounts of thyroid does no harm and may be of benefit.

Occasionally there have been observed mismated couples, who are sterile or have repeated abortions. In subsequent marriages both husband and wife may have healthy offspring. Tranquilli-Leali[22] has ascribed such a condition to incompatible blood groups. In thirty-eight of forty-one cases of habitual abortion he found husband and wife belonging to different blood groups. Further observations are required before we can definitely accept this hypothesis as true.

A routine careful examination of the spermatic fluid constitutes the most important point in pre-conceptional diagnosis and treatment. If this shows faulty morphology and motility, all possibly contributing causes, such as prostatic infection or endocrine disorders, should be corrected before allowing conception again to take place.

Developmental factors influencing the implantation and nutrition of the ovum, center largely around the proper functioning of the corpus luteum of pregnancy. Removal or destruction of this portion of the ovary shortly after conception invariably results in abortion, as proven by animal experimentation. Unfortunately we have as yet no quantitative physiologic test for the hormone produced by the corpus luteum, hence both our diagnosis and treatment are largely empiric. We know that the corpus luteum has a sedative effect on the uterine muscle just as anterior pituitary and estrogenic extracts have a stimulating effect. Consequently in cases of abortion not explainable on any other basis we assume a deficiency of corpus luteum or excess of estrogenic or anterior pituitary hormone. It seems fairly certain in any event both by animal experimentation and clinical experience that the injection of large amounts of progesterone (luteinizing hormone) in the early months of pregnancy does no harm and in a surprisingly large percentage definitely inhibits the tendency to abortion. Novak[13] rightly calls attention to the cases in which sedatives and rest without further medication prevent abortion, but in the forty-one cases of habitual abortion treated by Falls, Lachner and Krohn[5] the patients were up and around and received only progesterone with successful continuation of pregnancy to term in thirty-four cases. In Kane's series of forty cases of habitual abortion thirty-six were carried to term by the use of progesterone, but in this series thyroid extract was also given.

Whether this favorable effect of progesterone is primarily due to the prevention of an insufficient decidual reaction predisposing to faulty implantation or whether it is the countervalent in women who produce an excess of estrogenic or pituitary hormones remains at present unsolved.

In similar fashion we have abundant clinical evidence of the favorable effect of thyroid extract in preventing abortion, but we do not know in what way it acts. Many of these patients have a low basal metabolic rate. Werbatus,[25] treating twenty-four cases of habitual abortion with thyroid extract alone, reports only one failure. Aza[1] also speaks of good results with this treatment, and Litzenberg[8] stresses the value of thyroid extract in the treatment of sterility and abortion.

The interdependence of metabolic processes and the internal secretions is at no time more evident than during pregnancy and plays an important part in the etiology of abortion. E. C. P. Williams[26] has called attention to the frequency of low sugar tolerance in women who habitually aborted and found that by proper dietary control with or without insulin the incidence of abortion could be reduced. Vogt-Möller[23] and more recently Shute[19] have stressed the importance of a diet rich in Vitamin E. Vogt-Möller found a very low cholesterinemia present in habitual abortion and found that the administration of Vitamin E, in the form of wheat germ oil, corrected this condition and resulted in fifty-seven out of seventy-four cases being carried to term. Shute found that in many cases of spontaneous abortion the blood serum was resistant to tryptic proteolysis. This condition of the blood serum could be produced in rats by putting them on a diet devoid of Vitamin E. Hence he gives this vitamin in large amounts to patient having repeated abortions and found that the proteolyt-

ic reaction of the blood became normal and the pregnancy was carried to term. Shute believes that Vitamin E is one of the factors in the body that holds estrogenic substance in equilibrium during normal pregnancy.

The ingestion of large amounts of Vitamin C in the form of cantan has been advised by W. Schmidt,[18] since it has been claimed that this vitamin improves the function of the corpus luteum. He believes that in this way the tendency to abortion is reduced. Some writers stress the significance of calcium deficiency as a factor in abortion.

Hyperirritability of the uterine muscle, due directly or indirectly to improper balance of the endocrine secretions, has already been touched upon in the preceding paragraphs. Whether in these cases we are dealing with an excessive amount of estrogenic or pituitary hormones or an insufficient quantity of corpus luteum hormone it is difficult to say. In all events the hyperirritable uterine muscle under these circumstances, if subjected to any form of physical or psychic excitation, begins to undergo rythmic contractions that loosen and finally detach the placenta from its point of implantation, thus leading to an abortion. This cycle may occur at any time in the first two trimesters of pregnancy but is more apt to occur at the time of the expected menstrual period. At approximately four weeks intervals following the last menstruation there still persists a menstrual-like wave, at which time the uterus is more irritable and abortion more apt to occur. Exciting factors leading to abortion in such a hyperirritable uterus may be some physical strain or trauma, sexual intercourse, nervous exhaustion or mental shock. In some cases the period of greatest danger from abortion for some reason may be as late as the fourth or fifth month of gestation, hence it is advisable to continue the hormonal administration up to the period of viability of the child.

Summary of preventive treatment.—While for purposes of investigation it is better not to combine different therapeutic agents, since the specific effect of any one of them is thereby left in doubt, we are inclined in practice to recommend the use of all means that have any proven value.

As the first step, however, a careful review of all factors that may have led to previous abortions is desirable. Careful examination of the abortion products often point to the cause. The absence of an embryo, evidence of a missed abortion (one retained a month or more after fetal death), or an imperfectly developed decidual layer, point to endocrine factors. Basal metabolism tests, the determination of sugar tolerance, and Wassermann reactions on both husband and wife give additional information. Pelvic examination reveals the presence of fibroids, retroversion and deep cervical tears. A careful check of the husband's spermatic fluid must be made. All these are included under the head of preconceptional diagnosis and appropriate corrective treatment is instituted.

After conception we would still hold to a maximum of rest and sedative, particularly at the time of the expected menstrual wave. How far to go in this direction is a matter of individual choice, but certainly in the presence of bleeding or cramps, indicating a threatened abortion, absolute bedrest is essential. More debatable is the value of opiates under such circumstances. There is considerable evidence, as recently shown in the experiments of Falls, Lachner and Krohn,[5] that morphine in ordinary doses may stimulate rather than inhibit uterine contractions. If morphine is used at all, not less than one-third grain hypodermically should be given. Recently I have been more inclined to use barbiturates, since the combination of bedrest and opiates leads to constipation that in turn promotes intestinal, and hence uterine, peristalsis. Whenever possible, a case of threatened abortion should be handled in a hospital where absolute rest can be secured, away from the petty annoyances of the home.

And now a few words more about the technic of endocrine treatment. Unfortunately the manufacture and standardization of progesterone is an expensive process and we are faced by the practical problem of meeting the drug bills. If it is true, as claimed by Bishop Cook and Hampson,[2] that less than thirty rabbit units are probably insufficient, it means that the use of this product alone will cost not less than $30. Pratt[16] believes that the human female does not require as large an amount of progesterone as the rabbit to inhibit abortion. Kane[6] prescribes 1/25 rat unit of proluton every other day for ten doses, a series that is repeated every three weeks up to the end of the fourth month. Falls, Lachner and Krohn[5] give one rabbit unit twice daily in threatened abortion and prophylactically twice a week

up to the thirty-second week. My own experience would favor the use of the larger amounts.

There seems to be no contraindication to using thyroid extract in combination with some preparation of progesterone. The dosage employed by Werbatus[25] seems unduly high. He recommends one and a half grains three times daily up to four and a half months, and two grains three times daily thereafter up to the eighth month. I should feel it safer to use only one-half grain three times daily as suggested by Kane except in cases with persistent low basal rates. On the other hand some patients may require iodides to reduce thyroid activity. Thirty years ago habitual abortion was routinely treated by the administration of iodides and the occasional successes explained on the basis of a latent syphilis.

Vitamin therapy if carried out to the point recommended by Vogt-Möller, Shute and other enthusiasts is also very expensive. The wheat germ oil, used in Vitamin E treatment, must be given in large amounts. Shute uses 24 grains of such a preparation in the first twenty-four hours to produce the proper proteolytic reaction of the blood serum and four grains daily thereafter for the following months to keep it in that condition and so prevent abortion.

To summarize, then, in cases of spontaneous abortion, not due to lues, focal infection or gynecologic disease, I would employ a combination of progesterone, thyroid, Vitamin E, rest and sedatives. There is good reason to believe that such a combination, if carried out consistently for the first six months of gestation, will prevent almost every abortion except where there exists a primary defective germ-plasm.

Induced Abortion

We turn now to a consideration of the induced abortions and separate the legally from the illegally interrupted cases. In cases of hyperemesis, tuberculosis and certain forms of heart disease, therapeutic or legal abortion is resorted to less frequently than formerly, since our treatment of these conditions during pregnancy has shown material progress. The administration of intravenous glucose in hyperemesis has greatly reduced the number of serious toxemias that formerly required intervention. In tuberculosis the establishment of sanatorium treatment for pregnant women has lessened complications necessitating abortion. Fewer cases of heart disease are interrupted nowadays, since the prevention of decompensation is better understood. On the other hand we have realized during these decades that in an increasing number of cases of mental and nervous diseases, of moral irresponsibility and of marked physical depletion, a therapeutic abortion may be advisable to conserve the best interests of the family as a whole both from a health and eugenic standpoint. In most of these cases, while there may be argument as to the legal right to interrupt the pregnancy, there is no question as to the desirability of preventing conception. The incidence of therapeutically induced abortion can be reduced to a minimum by widespread carefully supervised instruction in contraception and by prompt sterilization of the individual where this is definitely indicated.

The illegally induced abortions, greatest in number, present our most difficult problem. Here again we must turn to a thorough study of underlying contributory factors to get some clew as to the best methods of prevention. In few countries outside of Russia has any attempt been made to analyze these causes, and Russian conditions are so different from our own that little assistance is gained from studying their reports. From a large series of thousands of women questioned in the abortion clinics of Russia as to the reason for desiring interruption of pregnancy the following report[20] may serve as a fair cross-section: poverty, 44 per cent; illegitimacy, 11 per cent; too many children, 22 per cent; unhappy married life, 9 per cent; fear of confinement, 4 per cent; medical reasons, 13 per cent; other reasons, 7 per cent. Poverty and large families, therefore, account for over half of the cases.

A clinical and social study of abortion was recently made by H. S. Pasmore[14] analyzing 117 criminal abortions that came to St. Mary Abbot's Hospital, London. Unfortunately methods of induction employed and the use of contraceptives in these cases are given more attention than analysis of the reasons for desiring the abortion. He found that religion apparently played no part, for the proportion of Catholics in this series was identical with the average for the population in that district. Abortion was relatively more frequent among illegitimate mothers. Another interesting study, published this year by R. Pearl,[18] deals with fertility and contraception among 7,500 white and negro

women in New York and Chicago. One out of eight of these women had at least one induced abortion. They were "deliberately causing from 1/6 to more than 1/5 of their aggregate reproductive wastage by the dangerous expedient of induced abortion." Pearl stresses the fact that these abortions occurred twice as frequently among those women who practiced contraception than among those that did not, and adds the comment: "The abortionist is called on to rectify the inadequacies of birth control." Her report does not, however, justify the assumption that the practice of birth control leads to the practice of induced abortion, since it is self-evident that women who were anxious at all costs to avoid having another child would almost without exception practice some form of birth control, and conversely that women who do not practice birth control usually accept with resignation the occurrence of a pregnancy and less frequently resort to abortion.

In Dr. Kopp's[7] analysis of 11,172 abortions in New York City, the number of induced cases increased directly with the number of children in the family. As evidence of increasing poverty in these larger families she noted that more of them were done by midwives, or were self-induced. The 1934 Children's Bureau report on maternal mortality[24] pointed out that although abortion was relatively more frequent among unmarried mothers (one in three as compared with one in five), 90 per cent of all who died from abortion were married women.

The causes of induced abortion may then be summarized as due to: Poverty; large families; domestic troubles; illegitimacy; and selfishness.

It would be a Utopian dream to attempt to eliminate all these evils. All we can hope for is to reduce their extent to some degree. Poverty will be with us for centuries to come, but even the poorest countries, such as Russia, have in recent years taken steps to provide free hospital care and medical service for expectant mothers so as to lessen the hardship of childbearing. Surely it is the function of the state to provid maternal and child welfare and when such program is carried out on a nation-wide scal it should materially reduce the temptation to re sort to abortion. In addition, when the famil gets beyond the three or four for whom th average parents can provide proper sustenance our efforts should be directed along the line o contraceptive education. We have only in the last two decades begun scientific research as to more certain and simpler methods of contraception and it seems not unlikely that these efforts will in the coming generation be rewarded by the discovery of measures that even the most dull-witted couple can employ with safety. When we have thus learned to limit the size of the family, the necessity for induced abortion should be reduced to a minimum.

Domestic troubles are largely dependent on poverty and too many children. When expectant mothers are deserted, the state should render financial and medical assistance if conditions require it. I do not wish to infer that the state should assume the full burden, but at any rate some help should be rendered to lessen the temptation to do away with the pregnancy.

The desire of the unmarried mother to induce an abortion is largely dependent upon our social code. How far this code should be modified to lessen the social ostracism now existing is for the coming generation to decide. If these foolish or unfortunate women were given a fair chance to earn a living for themselves and their child, more mothers would be inclined to carry on with their gestation and thus avoid the serious risks entailed upon instrumental interference.

Finally there is a large group of women who resort to induced abortions for no good reason except their personal convenience. Selfishness is an inherent trait in many of these women. The best corrective in these cases is to prove to them that for selfish reasons they would do better to carry their pregnancy to term. What these women do not appreciate is that every abortion carries with it a greater physical risk than a confinement, that the death-rate is seven times as great and that the resulting ill-health is probably ten to fifteen times as great. I am constantly impressed in private practice with the dense ignorance of intelligent women on this subject. Ten minutes of careful explanation will often make them change their plans and I know of no patients who are afterwards more grateful to their doctor for having saved them from taking such a false step.

I have left for the last the discussion of legal measures to control induced abortion. Since time immemorial the world has tried to limit this evil by punitive measures and utterly failed to ac-

complish anything except to increase the incidence of secret and more dangerous methods of interrupting pregnancy. I do not wish to infer that abortion should be legalized but I am convinced that punitive measures are a last resort and should be primarily directed against those individuals who make a profitable business out of its practice, those professional abortionists who through subterranean channels and paid agents induce women to resort to it as the easy way out. I notice that here in the State of Minnesota[12] you have recently caused the imprisonment of two midwife abortionists. As in other forms of crime, punishment of the criminal may be necessary but it is far less effective in producing results than a study of the cause of such crimes and their correction.

I am convinced therefore that the best results in reducing the incidence of criminal abortion can be obtained by:

1. More generous provision for the economic support and medical care of the expectant mothers among the poor.

2. Widespread information, especially among the poor, regarding the contraceptive methods that are at present available.

3. Intensive scientific investigation to discover safer and simpler methods of contraceptive practice.

4. An open discussion of this subject by both laity and profession so that the inherent dangers to life and health of the mother through induced abortion will be fully appreciated. Only in this way will the public appreciate the importance of preventing the decimating of the lives of expectant mothers and take the necessary steps for more effective control of the problem.

References

1. Aza, V.: Rev. Espana. Obst., 20:7-10, 1935.
2. Bishop, P. M. F., Cook, F., and Hampson, A. C.: Indications for clinical use of progestin; standardized corpus luteum extract. Lancet, 1:139, 1935.
3. Curtis, A. H.: Spontaneous recurrent abortion; inquiry into causes and preventive treatment. Jour. A.M.A., 84:1262, 1935.
4. Falls, F. H.: Cortical study of 500 cases of eclamptogenic toxemia. Am. Jour. Obst. and Gyn., 29:198, 1935.
5. Falls, F. H., Lachner, J. E., and Krohn, L.: Effect of progestin and estrogenic substance on human uterine contractions. Jour. A.M.A., 106:271, 1936.
6. Kane, H. F.: Use of progesterone in combating habitual abortion. Am. Jour. Obst. and Gyn., 32:110, 1936.
7. Kopp, M. E.: Birth Control in Practice. New York: Robert M. McBride Co., 1934.
8. Litzenberg, J. D.: The endocrines in relation to sterility and abortion. Jour. A.M.A., 109:1871, 1937.
9. McCord, J. R.: Syphilis of placenta. Am. J. Obst. and Gyn., 28:743, 1934.
10. McCord, J. R.: Syphilis and pregnancy. Jour. A.M.A., 105:89, 1935.
11. Mall, F. P.: Carnegie Inst., Wash., 12:56, 1921.
12. News Items. Jour. A.M.A., 108:564, 1937.
13. Novak, E.: Discussion. Jour. A.M.A., 106:273, 1936.
14. Pasmore, H. S.: A clinical and sociological study of

abortion. Jour. Obst. and Gyn., Brit. Emp., 44:455, 1937.
15. Pearl, R.: Fertility and contraception in New York and Chicago. Jour. A.M.A., 108:1385, 1937.
16. Pratt, J. F.: Discussion, Jour. A.M.A., 106:273, 1936.
17. Reith, A. F.: Streptococci as a cause of spontaneous abortion. Jour. Infect. Dis., 41:423, 1927.
18. Schmidt, W.: Behandlung des Schwangerschafts Erbrechen Muench. Med. Wchnschr., 1936, p. 358.
19. Shute, E.: Early diagnosis of abruptio placentæ and its treatment with germ oil. Am. Jour. Obst. and Gyn., 33:429, 1937.
20. Taussig, F. J.: Abortion, Spontaneous and Induced. St. Louis: C. V. Mosby Co., 1936, Chap. 26, pp. 24.37.

21. Taussig, F. J.: Prevention and Treatment of Abortion. St. Louis: C. V. Mosby Co., 1910.
22. Tranquilli-Leali, E.: Disaffinita del grippo sanguigno pa. terno-materno quale cause dostituzionale di aborto. Riv. Ital. di ginec., 13:490, 1932.
23. U. S. Children's Bureau: Maternal Mortality in fifteen states. U. S. Children's Bureau Reports, 1934.
24. Vogt-Möller, P.: Treatment of habitual abortion with wheat-germ oil (Vitamin E). Lancet, 2:182, 1931.
25. Werbatus, E.: Die Behandlung des habituellen Aborta mit Thyrecoidintabletten. Arch. f. Gynak., 160:589, 1936.
26. Williams, E. C. P.: Carbohydrate metabolism in cases of unexplained miscarriages. Lancet, 2:858, 1933.

POLIOMYELITIS IN MINNESOTA IN 1937*

JOHN F. POHL, M.D.

Minneapolis, Minnesota

ACCOUNTS of poliomyelitis occurring in Minnesota are available for many years. During the thirty-year period from 1908 to 1938 there have been 7,927 reported cases of the diseases in the State. The statistical history of poliomyelitis is punctuated by a considerable fluctuation in the year by year incidence of the disease, but, however variable, in no twelve-month period has the

abrupt increase over the thirty-seven cases reported for 1936, this number is not significantly above the average yearly expected level. It would appear (Table I) that the disease has not been very active in recent years.

Although the term is not well defined, there has been nothing in the nature of an epidemic in Minnesota since the year 1931. An aggregate of

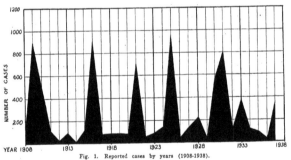

Fig. 1. Reported cases by years (1908-1938).

disease failed to make its appearance. An inspection of the charted course of poliomyelitis in Minnesota during the past thirty years (Fig. 1) indicates that there is a fairly sustained expected annual level of appearance of the disease, but that significant increases in incidence appear at fairly regular intervals.

The year 1937, with 354 reported cases, cannot be considered as unusual. Although a rather

the cases by ten-year periods (Table II), however, gives no indication that the disease shows any tendency toward spontaneous recession.

There have occurred 1,421 deaths attributable to poliomyelitis in Minnesota during this thirty-year period. This is an average mortality rate of 17.9 per cent. Although great advances have been made in medicine during this time, very littl has actually proven of benefit either in the pre vention or treatment of poliomyelitis. By ten year periods (Table II) there has apparently bee a significant decrease in the mortality rate of th

*The figures used were obtained from the Division of Preventable Diseases of the Minnesota Department of Health, through the courtesy of Dr. Orianna McDaniel, Director of the Division, and her staff. The paper does not represent any official report of the Department.

TABLE I. CASES AND MORTALITY BY YEARS

	Cases	Deaths	
1908	150	9	
1909	900	234	
1910	481	201	
1911	115	58	
1912	35	23	
1913	85	30	
1914	22	8	
1915	123	26	
1916	912	105	
1917	75	10	
1918	82	22	
1919	85	16	
1920	80	18	
1921	702	102	
1922	55	20	
1923	82	17	
1924	144	30	
1925	955	145	
1926	46	15	
1927	139	36	
1928	224	57	
1929	32	6	
1930	479	37	7.7%
1931	811	66	8.1%
1932	124	10	8.1%
1933	383	37	9.1%
1934	113	21	18.5%
1935	99	10	10.1%
1936	37	4	10.8%
1937	354	48	13.5%
Total	7927	1421	17.9%

disease. This might offer some hope that there is a tendency either toward a decreasing virulence of the causative agent or an increasing toleration by the host. It must be kept in mind, however, that these are only statistics. Considerable doubt must arise in regard to the diagnosis

of poliomyelitis made twenty-five or thirty years ago. It is only comparatively recently that the technic of examination of the spinal fluid has reached a stage of refinement where an unquestioned diagnosis can be ascertained. In 1937, there were forty-eight deaths, a mortality rate of 13.5 per cent. This is slightly above the average rate for the ten-year period which the year concludes.

TABLE II. MORTALITY BY TEN YEAR PERIODS

Year	Cases	Deaths	Mortality
1908-18	2898	704	24.3%
1918-28	2370	421	17.8%
1928-38	2659	296	11.1%
Total	7927	1421	17.9%

TABLE III. CASES BY MONTH BY ONSET OF SYMPTOMS, 1937

Month	Jan.	Feb.	Mar.	Apr.	May	June
Cases	3	1	1	1	0	1

Month	July	Aug.	Sept.	Oct.	Nov.	Dec.
Cases	13	64	173	71	18	8

The year 1937 demonstrated strikingly one of the typical features of the disease, marked seasonal variation of incidence (Fig. 2). Throughout the entire first half of the year only seven scattered cases were reported. In July there began an abrupt increase which mounted to almost epidemic proportions through August and reached its peak in mid-September. The four months of July, August, September and October accounted for 321, or approximately 91 per cent of the total 354 cases for the year. About half of the total number of cases for the year appeared in the single month of September.

The disease was proceeding with considerable acceleration in 1937 when the schools opened on September 7. This incident was attended by no noticeable increase in the rate of appearance of new cases which might be anticipated as a result of the segregation of large numbers of potentially infected children. On the contrary the apparent epidemic reached its peak within the week thereafter, and each succeeding week saw a progressive diminution in the number of new cases being reported. A few cases, however, continued to appear up to the close of the year (Table III).

peak of incidence appeared at approximately six years of age (Figure 3). By sex there was a preponderance of males, being 213 to 141 females.

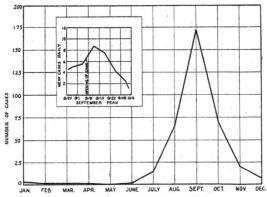

Fig. 2. Cases by month, by onset of symptoms (1937).

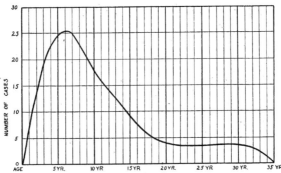

Fig. 3. Occurrence of poliomyelitis by ages (1937).

The majority of the individuals attacked in 1937 were between two and fifteen years of age, but there were victims in every year of life from birth to thirty-five. Three cases were reported in persons forty-four, forty-five and forty-eight years of age, respectively. The youngest child was six months of age, and there were three children under one year of age affected. The

Toleration of the infection varies considerabl at different age levels (Table IV). The genera mortality for 1937 was 13.5 per cent. Death di not claim any of the three infants under on year of age nor any of the three over thirty-five The period of life between the ages of twen and twenty-five appears to be the most vulner able, having had, in 1937, a mortality rate of 31.

er cent. No tabulation was made of the extent f paralysis at the different age levels.

Geographically, the cases in 1937 were fairly cattered in distribution, being reported from

seven were of the abortive type, compared with only ten cases of the abortive type appearing in the 165 cases occurring throughout the State at large. It is logical to assume that more suspected

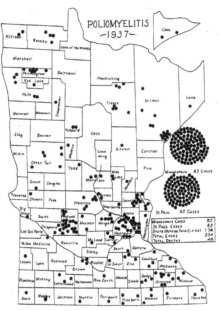

Fig. 4. Location of cases occurring in 1937.

fifty-six of the eighty-seven counties of the state (Fig. 4). The metropolitan districts of Minneapolis and Saint Paul, with a centralization of population, accounted for a good share of the cases. There were in addition minor centers of infection in other parts of the state, the principal one being in Kandiyohi County, from which twenty cases were reported.

The population of Minnesota (estimated 1934) is 2,602,000 people. The three largest cities, Minneapolis, Saint Paul and Duluth, comprise 32 per cent of the total population of the state. It appears that 189, or 56 per cent of the cases of poliomyelitis in 1937, were reported from these three centers of population. However, of the 189 cases occurring in these three cities, sixty-

cases of poliomyelitis are hospitalized in the larger cities, where hospital care is more readily available. The inference from this assumption, and from the figures regarding the abortive type of poliomyelitis, is that the diagnosis of poliomyelitis is facilitated in direct proportion to the accessibility of hospital and laboratory aid. If one considers only the cases showing demonstrable muscle weakness or paralysis, it appears that the three areas of condensation of population (32 per cent of state population) accounted for 46.6 per cent of the cases of poliomyelitis reported for the year 1937.

The classification of abortive and paralytic types of cases as applied to poliomyelitis depends on the demonstration of objective neurologic findings. The term paralytic is self-explanatory, indicating muscular weakness or paralysis. In addition, any patient showing depression of cutaneous or tendon reflexes, even though

TABLE IV. MORTALITY BY AGE GROUPS, 1937

Age	Cases	Deaths	Mortality
0- 5 yrs.	74	8	10.8%
5-10	101	11	10.9%
10-15	85	10	11.7%
15-20	40	7	17.5%
20-25	19	6	31.6%
25-30	16	3	18.8%
30-35	16	3	18.8%
Over 35	3	0	0.0%
Total	354	48	13.5%

no measurable muscular weakness can be demonstrated, is also classified as paralytic. The abortive case is one having suggestive symptoms, the diagnosis of which, in the absence of peripheral neurological changes, is made usually by examination of the cerebrospinal fluid. Considering that only ten cases were diagnosed as the abortive type outside of the large city districts in 1937, it is a fair premise that many cases of poliomyelitis are overlooked each year. In many cases this situation is admittedly unavoidable. Given even a suggestive set of symptoms, with hospital facilities distant or unavailable, the diagnosis of acute anterior poliomyelitis is not easily made with assurance. In the city of Saint Paul in 1937, with eighty-five reported cases of the disease, 51 per cent were abortive

in type. That is to say that an absolute diagnosis could be made in only half the cases without the aid of laboratory examination. For the three cities of Minneapolis, Saint Paul and Duluth, 36.4 per cent of the total cases were the abortive type.

With the greatest incidence of poliomyelitis occurring in the younger age groups it might be suspected that, as in the more common contagious diseases, there should be predictable increases in the occurrence of poliomyelitis at fairly regular intervals. The graphic record (Fig. 1) of the yearly incidence of the disease in Minnesota shows that this is borne out. Every five-year period from 1908 on has had one year with significant increase in the occurrence of the disease, except for the period just ended (Fig. 1). From these facts it would not be unexpected should there occur a considerable increase in the number of cases in the year or two immediately before us.

Summary

1. Statistics on acute anterior poliomyelitis in Minnesota are presented for the past thirty years.

2. During the past thirty years there has been no tendency for poliomyelitis to disappear in Minnesota.

3. There is a suggestion that the virulence of the causative agent is subsiding, or that man is developing a toleration for the disease. The difficulties in diagnosis, however, makes caution imperative in the interpretation of statistics.

4. The year 1937 showed only a moderate increase in the average annual level of incidence of the disease in Minnesota. There was a slight increase in the mortality rate above the level of preceding years.

Thiamin Chloride and Nicotinic Acid in Pellagra

Spies and Aring (J.A.M.A., April 2, 1938, p. 1081) report on the effect of the administration of vitamin B_1 in six cases of classic pellagra with peripheral neuritis. Irrespective of the cause of the pellagra, prompt relief of spontaneous neuritic pain resulted from the intravenous injection of thiamin chloride (crystalline vitamin B_1 hydrochloride). These observations suggest that vitamin B_1 deficiency plays a part in the development of clinical manifestations of peripheral neuritis associated with pellagra. The vitamin B_1 does not appear to cure the glossitis and stomatitis of pellagra but nicotinic acid, which has been referred to in *The Journal A.M.A.* (Jan. 22, 1938, p. 289; Feb. 26, 1938, p. 622), does relieve these symptoms. The Cincinnati investigators have demonstrated that all types of pellagra are benefited within twenty-four to forty-eight hours after the administration of nicotinic acid. Certainly both thiamin chloride and nicotinic acid deserve further intensive study in their relation to pellagra. (J.A.M.A., April 2, 1938, p. 1115.)

SACRAL BLOCK ANESTHESIA*

A Consideration of the Unusual Difficulties Encountered and a Report of Two Unusual Cases

R. CHARLES ADAMS, M.D., and EDWARD B. TUOHY, M.D., M.S. (Anes.)

Rochester, Minnesota

BY blocking the sacral nerves, anesthesia is produced which permits operations on the rectum, anus, urinary bladder, prostate, and perineum. Sacral block consists of a combination of caudal and transsacral block. By injecting only the caudal canal, complete anesthesia may be obtained in about 60 per cent of cases, using between 30 and 40 c.c. of a solution of 1 per cent procaine or metycaine. High caudal[1] block is a variation of caudal block in which larger quantities of the anesthetic solution are injected into the caudal canal and the resultant anesthesia obtained amounts to a peridural anesthesia from below upward. The extent of the anesthesia depends largely on the amount of the anesthetic solution injected which determines the height to which the solution rises. The amount of solution used varies from 40 to 90 c.c. and it is necessary to wait thirty minutes or more after injection to obtain complete anesthesia.

Ordinary caudal block must be supplemented in about 40 per cent of cases by transsacral block, in order to obtain complete anesthesia. This consists in blocking the second, third, and fourth sacral nerves bilaterally; occasionally it may be necessary to block the first sacral nerves as well. By combining caudal block with a bilateral block of the second sacral nerves, complete anesthesia may be obtained in about 80 per cent of cases. It is necessary, in all cases, to wait at least twenty minutes after injection to allow the oncoming anesthesia to become complete. For operations on the anus and on adjacent structures sacral block gives the following desirable features: (1) complete anesthesia, (2) complete relaxation, (3) anesthesia of the immediate field of operation only, (4) avoidance of certain systemic effects which frequently are associated with low spinal anesthesia, (5) systemic conditions which contraindicate both spinal and general anesthesia normally do not contraindicate use of sacral block, and (6) the anesthesia produced usually is of sufficient duration to permit the performance of the longest surgical procedures in the region.

The contraindications to the method are few: (1) infection in the region through which the needles must pass, such as infected pilonidal cysts and abscesses, owing to the danger of disseminating the infection, (2) idiosyncrasy to the anesthetic solution or to the vasoconstricting agent used in this solution, and (3) very nervous and hypersensitive patients.

Lundy's paper is a very detailed and complete treatise on the subject of the technic of sacral block. Only a few of the important steps of the method need be reviewed here. The skin over the sacrum is painted widely with an antiseptic solution, such as tincture of metaphen 1:200 or merthiolate 1:1000. The region is then draped. A solution of either 1 per cent procaine or 1 per cent metycaine[3] may be employed for the injection. The solution of metycaine produces a more rapidly oncoming anesthesia of a somewhat longer duration than procaine. Either solution gives satisfactory results. To 100 c.c. of the anesthetic solution, 1 c.c. of a solution of epinephrine (1:2600) is added. The addition of the epinephrine is essential if the anesthesia is to be of prolonged duration. At the time of injection, the solution should be warm, because a cold solution does not penetrate readily the nerve fibers. A solution which transmits a comfortably warm sensation to the volar surface of the forearm is of a correct temperature.

Before any wheals are raised or any injections are made, the position of the sacral hiatus and sacral foramina should be estimated and a drop of the anesthetic solution placed over the position of each. By so doing, the symmetry or asymmetry of the foramina in relation to the sacral hiatus becomes apparent. This preliminary step becomes very important when abnormalities of the bony sacrum exist. By its relation to the tip of the coccyx and to the sacral cornua, the position of the sacral hiatus is determined, the caudal needle is inserted and 20 c.c. of the anesthetic solution is injected very slowly. Before any solution is injected, frequent aspiration should be made with the bevel of the caudal

*From the Section on Anesthesia, The Mayo Clinic, Rochester, Minnesota.

needle in both anterior and posterior positions.

The dangers and effects caused by faulty position of the needles will be considered separately. The fluid should enter the caudal canal without resistance. The caudal needle is left in place until anesthesia has become complete. The transsacral portion of the block then is performed. Having identified the posterior superior spine, a point is taken one finger's breadth medial and inferior to it; this point is marked by a drop of solution. This corresponds on each side to the second sacral foramen. One finger's breadth below this point will be over the third sacral foramen and one finger's breadth below this, over the fourth. The position of the sacral hiatus will be found one finger's breadth below the fourth sacral foramen, medially. Should injection of the first sacral foramen be required, it will be found approximately one finger's breadth medial and superior to the posterior superior spine of the ilium. Wheals are raised over these points from below upward. The needles are inserted and the solution is injected. The amount required is usually 2 c.c. in the fourth, 3 c.c. in the third, and 10 c.c. in the second foramina. The foramina of the opposite side then are injected and, finally, in addition, 10 c.c. are deposited in the caudal canal. This brings the total amount of solution used to 60 c.c. If for any reason anesthesia is incomplete, a like amount may be used if required; this still will be within a safe limit of dosage.

Following completion of the block, the patient should not be tested for the presence of anesthesia for at least fifteen to twenty minutes. The testing should be done gently at first with the point of a needle on the skin posterior to the posterior margin of the anus. As the portion anterior to the margin of the anus is the last to become anesthetized, it should be tested last. If pressure with the needle occasions no discomfort, the same procedure is repeated with a tooth forceps. If the patient feels no pain, anesthesia may be considered complete. The presence of complete relaxation of the anal sphincter also should be noted. If an apprehensive patient is tested while the region is still sensitive, severe pain may be occasioned and this will lead the patient to interpret subsequent stimuli as painful, even after complete anesthesia has been obtained. The needles should not be removed until the anesthetist is assured that anes-

thesia is complete. The expected duration of t anesthesia is from one to two hours.

Conditions Affecting Sacral Block Anesthe

Sacral block is a procedure which requi considerable experience and skill in order to obtain uniformly good results, but with the aver case the experienced anesthetist encounters lit difficulty. On the other hand, cases are encou tered continually which vary from the avera normal case and these complications may owing to a variety of causes. In such cases, actual technic of performing the block becon more difficult and anesthesia is more difficult obtain. The latter section of this discussion v deal with the difficulties that may be encountei in abnormal cases and the various methods handling such cases.

Conditions giving rise to these difficulties n be classified as follows: (1) faulty position the patient during injection; (2) faulty positi of the various needles; (3) extremely nervc and apprehensive patients; (4) abnormalities the bony pelvis, such as differences between t male and female pelvis, previous injuries to t bones causing distortion of the landmarks a asymmetry, and osseous deposits in the fora ina; (5) abnormalities of the soft parts, such excessive subcutaneous fat, infection over region of injection, and formation of scars torting the soft parts, and (6) idiosyncrasies the solutions employed, such as sensitivity the anesthetic solution and sensitivity to vasoconstricting agent.

Faulty position of the patient.—The cor position of a patient for sacral block is the pr position with the arms extended, the elb semiflexed, the palms of the hands flat, and head turned to the side opposite the one b injected. Two small flat pillows are placed u the pelvis and the sacral rest is elevated mo ately. The patient is instructed to assum "pigeon-toed" position (toes together and t apart). This position makes the bony point the posterior part of the sacrum more promi and relaxes the muscles overlying them. patient also is instructed to relax the muscl that region as much as possible.

Faulty position of the needles.—The ca needle in place in the caudal canal of the will lie more nearly parallel with the horiz plane of the body (when the patient is in prone position) than when in the caudal canal of the female because of the greater degree of pelvic curvature of the latter. If this point is not remembered, it is easy to pass the caudal needle over the posterior wall of the sacrum. The bone always should be touched with the point of the needle, both anteriorly and posteriorly. When injecting the caudal canal, the palm of the hand should be placed over the sacrum so that any extravasation of fluid in that region will be appreciated. Frequent aspirations should be made before any solution is injected in order to make certain that the point of the needle is neither in a vein nor within the dura. If the point of the needle is kept below the level of the second lumbar vertebra there is little danger of this taking place. When there is any doubt regarding the aspiration of spinal fluid, the point of the needle should be withdrawn until no further aspiration can be made. In certain cases it is possible to aspirate a straw-colored cystic fluid on introduction of the caudal needle. In these cases, it is preferable to do a low spinal block, although the aspirated fluid obviously is not spinal fluid. When the bevel of the caudal needle has scraped the bony wall of the caudal canal, a hematoma may be formed and blood may be aspirated. This will also occur if the point of the needle has been introduced into a vein. In cases of carcinoma of the rectum particularly, the venous plexus within the canal seems to be very extensive. If aspiration of blood continues to occur with the point of the needle in various situations, this part of the injection should be delayed until the remainder of the block has been completed. This gives a chance for bleeding to cease. Even after bleeding has ceased, the injection into the caudal canal should be made with caution, because under such circumstances the solution may be absorbed more rapidly than normally into the circulation. When the aspiration of blood persists, the caudal injection should be withheld and the transsacral part of the block should be depended on for anesthesia.

The needles, when inserted correctly into the foramina, will be roughly at right angles to the caudal needle. In inserting these needles, no great amount of force should be used, especially if bone is encountered. The shaft of the needle should not be bent during the insertion. These errors easily may result in the breaking off of part of the needle under the skin. The wheals

should be raised slightly lateral to the foramen so that, before the needle is inserted, the skin may be pushed medially. This allows freedom of movement of the skin and subcutaneous tissue when inserting needles in the opposite side and prevents force being transmitted to those needles already in place. It is important that the point of the needle be inserted a distance of only a half finger's breadth into the foramen. If inserted too far the anesthetic solution will be extravasated anteriorly and will not reach the nerves.

Nervous patients.—Most patients tolerate the injection well if they are told what is about to happen and if injection of solution is made ahead of the needle, as the needle is being inserted through the tissues. A few patients are extremely intolerant. In many of these cases, if the injection can be made into the caudal canal and this injection allowed to take effect before the remainder of the block is attempted, the resultant anesthesia obtained may make the transsacral portion of the block bearable. Much apprehension may be combated by adequate premedication with morphine and pentobarbital sodium. Rarely is a patient so intolerant that his movements cause a needle to be broken. In such cases, it may be preferable to carry out the operation under intravenous anesthesia with pentothal sodium.

Abnormalities of the bony pelvis.—Differences between the male and female pelvis are the first consideration. The female pelvis is broader and the sacrum is more curved than that of the male. This results in some variation in the position of the needles both in the foramina and in the caudal canal. The fact that the male sacrum is more flat causes the caudal needle, when correctly inserted, to lie almost parallel with the horizontal plane of the body when the body is in the prone position. The curvature of the sacrum of the female results in the caudal needle pointing upward and more forward when in position, thus increasing the angle between the shaft of the needle and the horizontal plane of the body when the body is in the prone position. This feature must be borne in mind when inserting the caudal needle when treating women, for, if the plane of insertion of the needle is too flat, it may pass upward over the posterior surface of the sacrum instead of entering the canal itself.

The posterior superior spines of the female pelvis are farther from the midline than those of the male, because of the increased breadth of the former over the latter. As the second sacral foramen bears a constant relationship to the posterior superior spine, the imaginary lines passing through the two rows of needles inserted in the foramina of each side of a female pelvis will have a greater divergence from below upward than such lines passing through needles so placed in the male pelvis. In the latter, the two rows of needles will be more nearly parallel.

Injury and displacement of the bones are the second consideration. Old fractures involving the pelvis and the sacrum may result in varying degrees of displacement of the bones in whole or in part with accompanying distortion of the bony landmarks. Other factors leading to a similar condition may be congenital displacement or previous operations in the region. The coccyx itself may be displaced or absent. Although the sacral cornua usually can be palpated, among certain patients, particularly among the obese, definite prominences cannot be felt. Although the posterior superior spine on one side is usually symmetrical with that of the opposite side, some cases present wide discrepancies. However, even after injury to the sacrum there is usually a symmetrical relationship between the posterior superior spine and the second foramen of the same side and, also, between the foramina themselves. For these reasons, it is erroneous to use the needle inserted in the foramen on one side as a guide for inserting those on the other side.

Osseous deposits in the foramina are the third consideration. When inserting the needles in the foramina, only light pressure should be applied and, as the needle passes inward, this pressure should be decreased. Marked resistance usually indicates that the point of the needle is on bone and excessive pressure may result in breaking the tip of the needle or in hooking the point. Among some elderly patients, the foramina may be ossified partially or completely, leaving a small opening or none at all. In such cases, a cautious increase in pressure may be required to insert the needle. Undue movement of the patient's hips when the needles are in place also may result in breaking the shaft of a needle. During the injection of the anesthetic solution,

the shaft of the needles must be supported. If a large portion of a needle breaks beneath the surface of the skin and cannot be recovered, it will be preferable to incise the overlying skin and remove the needle at once. If only the point is missing, probably it will do little harm and will be better left alone.

Abnormalities of the soft parts.—Excessive subcutaneous fat is the first consideration. In the main, among obese patients there is greater difficulty in placing the needles correctly than among patients of average weight. In the latter, the bony landmarks usually may be seen as well as palpated. Increase in fat progressively masks these landmarks until none of them can be felt accurately. When such is the case, various digressions from the standard technic are necessary. The usual routine is to insert the caudal needle followed by those of the foramina. When none of the landmarks for inserting the caudal needle is palpable, the procedure should be reversed. Even among the most obese patients, a definite dimple in the skin will be evident overlying the region of the posterior superior spine. Using this as a landmark, one may locate the second, third, and fourth foramina on either side and insert the needles. The situation of those in the fourth foramen of either side then will serve as a guide to the location of the sacral hiatus. A needle 50 mm. in length may not be long enough to reach the foramina of such subjects and one 80 mm. in length should be used.

Infection in the region is the second consideration. One definite contraindication to sacral block is the presence of infection in the skin or subcutaneous tissue through which the needles must pass. Such conditions as infected pilonidal cysts, large abscesses or furunculosis of the skin, or infection from any cause make it advisable to perform a low spinal block or, possibly, to give an intravenous anesthetic. In the ordinary case, care must be taken to prevent introduction of infection, particularly from the region of the anus. The tip of the coccyx always should be palpated through a sterile towel. Multiple punctures by needles also increase the risk of infection. Occasionally, small pustules form at the site of the punctures because of careless technic.

Formation of scars is the third consideration. It is a frequent fault of beginners to be guided by the soft parts (gluteal cleft and midline) rather than by the bony landmarks. Such technic is certain to give rise to error, as the relation of the soft parts to the bones may possess any degree of variation, particularly following accident and injury. Accidents occur resulting in injury to the region in which the bones are not affected, but the overlying soft tissue may be so lacerated that, in healing, the resultant formation of scars with contraction may distort the normal contour of the skin grossly. Scarring from infection or from suppuration of long standing also may result in similar deformities. Two abnormal cases to be described subsequently will serve to bear out these conclusions.

Idiosyncrasies to the solutions used.—A patient may be sensitive to the anesthetic solution, to the vasoconstricting agent, or to both. Reactions to anesthetic solutions are frequent. Careful questioning of the patient before the injection is made may reveal this. The vasoconstricting agent is necessary to obtain duration of anesthesia but many patients are sensitive to epinephrine, and, in such cases, it should be omitted or cobefrin should be substituted. The preliminary injection should be made very slowly and should be discontinued if signs of hypersensitivity appear. Similar effects may result if the injection is made intravenously. Nausea and vomiting are complications which may occur. Inhalation of 90 per cent oxygen and 10 per cent carbon dioxide usually relieves these symptoms.

Case Reports

The following report of two abnormal cases is submitted in support of some of the previous statements.

Case 1.—A man, aged sixty-three years, weighed 140 pounds. Twenty years previous to his admission, he was run over by a wagon which weighed 4,300 pounds. One of the wheels passed over his pelvis. He was incapacitated for three weeks but was able to resume an active life about two months after the accident. Walking was not impaired. The reason for seeking medical attention at this time was because of increasing constipation and the passage of mucus and, recently, blood from the bowel. Examination revealed polypoid adenocarcinoma of the rectum, grade 1 (on the basis of 1 to 4), and hemorrhoids. The lesion was fulgurated under sacral anesthesia.

On examination of the sacral region at the time the sacral block was performed, gross bony abnormalities appeared to be present. The whole sacrum appeared to have been pushed to the right. However, the needles were inserted without difficulty and good anesthesia was obtained. Roentgenologic examination of the region did not reveal any distortion of the bones.

The accompanying photograph (Fig. 1) in which the landmarks are indicated by markings with a colored solution, will give the reader a clear picture of what had happened. The two upper dots are over the posterior superior spines, the next three are over the

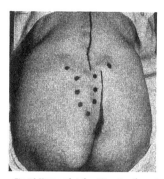

Fig. 1. Upper vertical line follows the alignment of the spines of the vertebræ; the lower line is a continuation upward from the gluteal cleft. The uppermost spot on each side overlies the right and left posterior superior spines, respectively; below them the pairs of three spots on each side overlie the second, third, and fourth sacral foramina, respectively. The lowest spot is the site of the sacral hiatus. Note how the skin overlying the sacrum has been pulled to the right by contracted fibrous tissue so that a continuation of the midline of the skin as extended upward from the gluteal cleft passes to the right of the sacral foramina on the right side.

second, third, and fourth sacral foramina of either side and the lower one represents the sacral hiatus. The midline of the skin has been extended upward from the gluteal cleft. The upper line marks the spinous processes of the lumbar vertebræ. The previous injury had torn the subcutaneous tissue so that the subsequent formation and contraction of scars which resulted had pulled the skin to the right, so that a line projected upward from the gluteal crest fell to the right of the right sacral foramina, giving the illusion that the bones had been distorted. This case shows the importance of relying solely on the bony landmarks.

Case 2.—A man, aged sixty-two years, had rectal trouble with an abscess near the rectum which began thirteen years previous to admission. Sinus tracts formed which periodically opened and closed, and at times new abscesses formed. Three operations had been performed in the past eleven years. In addition, his left leg had been run over thirty years previously. A stiff hip joint developed subsequently. On admission, the perirectal region contained many indurated masses, fistulous openings, and scars (Fig. 2). A sacral block was performed prior to operation and adequate anesthesia resulted. The prolonged suppuration and formation of sacral scars resulted in considerable distortion of the soft tissues as illustrated in Figures 3 and

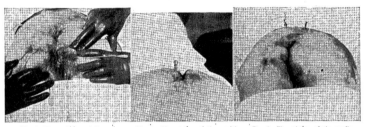

Fig. 2. The condition of the region of the anus previous to operation; probes have been placed in the multiple sinus tracts.

Fig. 3. The relation of the caudal needle, inserted in the caudal canal, to the gluteal cleft.

Fig. 4. The relation of the needle in the caudal canal and those in the various foramina to the gluteal cleft and anal region.

4. Figure 3 is an illustration of the caudal needle in place in the caudal canal. Note how the gluteal cleft has been displaced to the left. Figure 4 is an illustration of all the needles in place; a line projected upward from the gluteal cleft, passes through a line joining the foramina on the left side.

· Cases such as these are examples of the abnormalities which may occur in the region of the sacrum and how they may affect the performance of a successful sacral block. Sacral anesthesia has many advantages and few disadvantages. It supplies ideal operating conditions for the surgeon and involves a minimal risk to the patient.

References

1. Campbell, W. C.: Sacral block and high caudal block anesthesia. Proc. Staff. Meet. Mayo Clinic, 10:667-672, (Oct. 16) 1935.
2. Lundy, J. S.: A method for producing block anesthesia of the sacral nerves. Am. Jour. Surg., 4:262-270, (Mar.) 1928.
3. Tuohy, E. B.: The use of metycaine for producing block anesthesia of the sacral nerves. (In press.)

DIAPHRAGMATIC HERNIA*

E. MENDELSSOHN JONES, M.D.

Saint Paul, Minnesota

THE diagnosis and treatment of diaphragmatic hernia has received increasing attention during the past few years. There is no reason to assume the condition to be more prevalent than heretofore, but rather that improvement in diagnostic methods has made its presence more easily and thus more frequently proven. Development in roentgenological technic, together with accurate clinical observation, has resulted in the placing of diaphragmatic hernia in the list of commoner conditions. Too often in the past improper treatment has been due to failure in diagnosis. In obscure abdominal conditions the possibility of its existence must always be borne in mind.

In 1853 Bowditch reviewed the subject of diaphragmatic hernia and reported a case seen at the Massachusetts General Hospital, observing that earlier writers believed that a wound of the diaphragm was always fatal. He quotes Dr. Fothergell, whose letter to Dr. Mead about one

hundred years before gives a very interesting account of a case of diaphragmatic hernia. Dr. Fothergell says, "Everyone skilled in medicine, I think, will suppose from the history that the disease was a new one. But who would ever have conjectured that the diaphragm was divided asunder and that a large portion of the stomach and intestines had rushed through the opening into the breast." A century and a half before this letter was written, two cases were reported in the Opera Chirurgica by Ambrose Paré. One of these proved the fallacy of the older writers in believing a wound of the diaphragm was always fatal.

Bowditch collected eighty-eight cases and stated that he had carefully examined many works and journals from 1610 to 1846, believing that few more could be found.

Harrington points out that the clinical study of proven cases has established a fairly definite symptomatology, very helpful in making a diag-

*Presidential address before the Minnesota Academy of Medicine, January 12, 1938.

nosis or at least suspecting the presence of a diaphragmatic hernia.

At the Mayo Clinic between 1900 and 1925, thirty cases were recognized, of which nineteen patients were operated upon. From 1925 to 1935, one hundred and ninety-seven cases were recognized with one hundred and five patients operated upon. Harrington further points out that the condition is more common than believed at present, as he has made examinations of the diaphragm during other abdominal operations and has occasionally found a small hernia which had not been recognized clinically or roentgenologically before operation.

Diaphragmatic herniæ are considered true or false depending on whether or not a sac is present. They are further divided into congenital and acquired, the latter possibly traumatic in origin. In this classification a congenital hernia is understood to have been present at birth, the absence of a sac indicating that the hernial opening was due to the failure of the development or fusion of one or more of the anlagen of the diaphragm. Occasionally a congenital hernia has a sac and this is evidence of hernia formation after the complete separation of the pleural and peritoneal cavities.

The acquired hernia develops after birth and usually has a sac. This type generally occurs at the esophageal opening, the para-sternal foramen, or the lumbo-costal trigone.

A traumatic hernia may be caused by direct or indirect injury or by inflammatory necrosis of the diaphragm. In a direct injury such as a gun shot or stab wound, the hernia may occur at any point. When the injury is due to an indirect influence such as a crushing chest injury, the most frequent location of the rupture is the dome and posterior half of the left hemi-diaphragm. This type of hernia usually has no sac. When the hernia occurs at the esophageal opening there is a sac present. If the injury to the diaphragm is caused by inflammatory necrosis, the opening in the diaphragm is usually posterior and there is no hernial sac.

The symptoms in these cases depend on the structures involved in the hernia. When the stomach is the only organ involved, a very different picture is presented from that in which the intestines, as well, are herniated through the diaphragmatic defect. The diagnosis is not infrequently missed because the symptoms presented are referable to the chest; shadows may be present on the roentgenogram readily simulating a number of other conditions. It will be seen, therefore, that the possibility of a diaphragmatic hernia should always be borne in mind during routine chest x-ray examinations.

Herniations of the fundus of the stomach may result in typical cases of hour-glass deformity, and, because of the altered blood supply of the diaphragm and traumatism following its constant movement, ulceration may result. In some cases malignant changes have been found. With accurate observation loops of bowel or portions of the stomach may be seen in the chest without the administration of barium, if the possibility of hernia is borne in mind. The freedom of fluid or gas in the bowel, or the presence of some pleural thickening, may so mask the picture that an incorrect diagnosis is made. Truesdale cites a case in which such an error in diagnosis was made and a quantity of milk was removed by exploratory thoracentesis. Downs cites cases with death resulting from exploratory thoracentesis. Many patients with these conditions have been classed as neurotics because of the vagueness of their symptoms.

The manifestations of diaphragmatic hernia are frequently very complex and simulate those of various other organic conditions in the abdomen and thorax. Not infrequently one or more incorrect diagnoses have been made in these patients before the presence of a diaphragmatic hernia is discovered. It has often been confused with gall-bladder disease, gastric or duodenal ulcers, hyperacidity, secondary anemia, cardiac disease, carcinoma of the cardia, stricture of the esophagus, appendicitis, or intestinal obstruction.

In the congenital hernia the symptoms are usually present immediately after birth or at least in the early weeks or months of life. Many of these patients die a few hours after birth from respiratory and circulatory failure. Truesdale points out that diaphragmatic hernia may be more common than suspected from mortality statistics. He feels that autopsies are done less frequently in children than in adults and without a post mortem examination there is always a possibility of an error in diagnosis.

Should an infant with a diaphragmatic hernia survive a few weeks, the chief symptoms are cyanosis and dyspnea, but as the child grows older these symptoms become milder and those of a digestive disorder become more prominent. A patient with a congenital hernia living to adult life has an unusually fixed mediastinum. Such patients may be symptom-free, but when evidence of any disturbance does occur the picture is usually that of an intestinal obstruction.

Hiatus herniæ often cause considerable disturbance of respiration, circulation, and deglutition. In 1933, Junfer reported a case of an esophageal hiatus hernia in a man sixty-five years of age, the sac containing the stomach and most of the omentum. The esophagus measured only seventeen centimeters in length, and was believed to be a true esophageal hiatus hernia acquired early in life. The stomach had entered the chest early and since there was no traction on the esophagus, it remained short. It is readily understood that in this patient there had been no constriction of the stomach and the diaphragm maintained its normal rhythmic movements. In patients with a hiatus hernia with no other pathological complications the symptoms are fairly well understood, since more individuals of this type have been carefully studied. There is usually a sense of fullness in the substernal region and this is associated with substernal distress. Hiccough and heartburn are frequently present. If a large amount of food is taken just before retiring these symptoms are exaggerated. Relief is usually obtained by vomiting. Other cases may present epigastric fullness after meals. There is rarely a complaint of pain and the distress is substernal rather than epigastric.

The symptoms produced by traumatic hernia vary according to the viscera herniating through the diaphragmatic opening. As this type of hernia is without a sac there is usually a greater amount of abdominal contents passing into the thoracic cavity. When the opening is small, due to direct injury, such as a stab or gunshot wound, obviously only a small herniation can take place; in the indirect injury resulting from a severe blow or crushing chest injury, the hernial opening may be very large and the stomach, with most of the intestines, is frequently found in the chest. This is especially true if the diaphragmatic injury is on the left side. When it occurs on the right side the liver frequently is partially or wholly herniated through the opening and it is unusual to find any extensive herniation of the stomach and intestines.

In this type of a hernia the patient complains of abdominal cramps and considerable gastric distress, especially after eating. There may be respiratory distress evidenced by shortness of breath due to the pressure on the lung and mediastinum by the viscera in the pleural cavity. There may be constipation, and, when a laxative is taken, active peristalsis causes a gas rumbling in the chest which is audible to the patient. This is a very annoying symptom.

When one has this type of case under observation the possibility of an intestinal obstruction developing must be constantly borne in mind. Because of the general condition of cases that have had severe injury with resultant diaphragmatic hernia, it is frequently impossible to repair the hernia until the patient's condition improves.

The diagnosis of herniæ of the diaphragm has become much more frequent with the refined and exact roentgenological methods that are being used, and it is felt that x-ray demonstration is the only sure means of diagnosis. It has been pointed out that the x-ray is not infallible and not infrequently small herniæ are missed. Jenkinson and Roberts feel that less than five per cent of the small herniæ can be identified if the patient is examined only in the erect position. It is evident that close coöperation between the roentgenologist and the clinician is necessary as it is not uncommon to have these cases present a symptom-complex that is not understandable after the most searching examination, and as many of the conditions which cause symptoms referable particularly to the upper abdomen and chest simulate those presented by various types of diaphragmatic hernia, it is essential to keep this possibility in mind. This observation is applicable to the congenital, acquired, and traumatic types of hernia. In the traumatic cases the diagnosis should usually be rather simple, as the symptoms are more acute and the physical findings are much more definite. As pointed out, a good x-ray examination is most essential and this should be carried out in all cases that have had a direct or indirect injury of the chest. Any case that has had a crushing injury of the chest should have a complete gastro-intestinal examination, including a barium enema. If this routine is followed, most traumatic herniæ will be diagnosed. Pneumoperitoneum may be a helpful diagnostic aid in differentiating a diaphragmatic hernia from an eventration of the diaphragm.

Another condition that must be differentiated

from diaphragmatic hernia is the congenital short esophagus. In 1931, Findlay and Kelly discussed an anomaly that was characterized by congenital shortening of the esophagus and the presence of a portion of the stomach in the thoracic cavity. There was also a stenosis of the junction of the esophagus and thoracic portion of the stomach.

It is very important from a surgical standpoint to determine whether one is dealing with a shortening of the esophagus, with resulting partial or complete intrathoracic stomach, or whether there is a herniation of the stomach into the thoracic cavity.

One must also consider the possibility of the presence of a diaphragmatic hernia in cases of dextro-cardia.

Reduction of the hernia with repair of the hernial opening is the only means of definitely relieving the symptoms. There are undoubtedly many cases of diaphragmatic hernia that are symptom-free, and as long as strangulation does not occur the presence of abdominal viscera within the chest is not incompatible with life.

A most troublesome complication is that of intestinal obstruction, the mortality from intestinal obstruction being higher because of the necessity of the hernia repair. When the stomach is the only viscus involved, incarceration may occur and not strangulation, and the mortality is not as high. Truesdale advocates the employment of a two-stage operation to reduce the mortality occurring when dealing with cases complicated by intestinal obstruction. He advises first an appendicostomy or cecostomy to relieve the obstruction, the hernial repair being an operation of election.

In congenital hernia in infants the results of surgical repair have been disappointing, although some successful cases have been reported. The most favorable types are those passing through the left pleuroperitoneal canal, lateral defects in the septum, and small herniæ around the esophagus. The abdominal approach is preferred, as there are rarely any adhesions present. It is important to overcome the pneumothorax at the conclusion of the operation.

In discussion of the repair of the acquired type, the method of approach is dealt with in detail. Some surgeons prefer the thoracic operation while many prefer to use, when possible, the abdominal approach. If the hernia is on the right side, the thoracic approach is selected, since the

liver interferes with adequate exposure, making the repair difficult.

Harrington thinks there is less risk of thoracic complications when the abdominal approach is used, and he uses this approach in all cases of hernia through the left hemi-diaphragm. He feels it is of particular advantage in cases of hernia through the esophageal opening, as the herniated stomach is usually confined in a sac in the posterior mediastinum and does not enter the true pleural cavity.

It is sometimes necessary to do a combined thoracic and abdominal operation as the viscera may be involved by adhesions which can not be freed from either abdominal or thoracic exposure alone.

Crushing of the phrenic nerve is frequently done in the traumatic herniæ that have a large opening, since the repair of an inactive diaphragm is easier. Crushing does not cause permanent injury to the nerve, and the diaphragm resumes its activity again in six to nine months.

I wish to present five cases of diaphragmatic hernia emphasizing some of the clinical manifestations that have been discussed.

Case 1.—A woman thirty-five years of age was first seen on February 25, 1935. She stated that she had suffered more or less upper abdominal distress for nineteen years. At that time she fell, striking the handle bars of a bicycle so severely that the bar was broken. She subsequently had severe pain in the abdomen and was ill in bed a number of days. Since that time she has had occasional spells of nausea and vomiting after meals. The vomiting has been more frequent during the past three years, occurring almost daily. The attacks never came before meals and were always worse when lying down.

The clinical impression was that of gall-bladder disease. An x-ray examination showed a non-functioning gallbladder but all relevant physical findings at that time were negative. In March, 1935, a gastro-intestinal tract x-ray study showed a herniation of the cardiac end of the stomach through the esophageal opening.

She was kept under observation on medical management, but since the symptoms did not subside it was felt that the diaphragmatic hernia was the cause of her disability.

After reducing her weight 15 pounds, an operation was performed on May 18, 1936. The roentgenologic findings were substantiated. The hernia was reduced and the esophageal opening, which readily admitted three fingers, was sutured. She made an uncomplicated recovery. A radiograph taken June 4, 1936, showed the hernia reduced and a picture on October 17, 1937, shows no recurrence. At present she is in good health and has complete relief of her symptoms.

Case 2.—A woman thirty-three years of age was first seen on October 18, 1935. She had been well until one year before, when she developed attacks of heartburn followed by nausea and vomiting. Occasionally she noted sharp epigastric pain radiating from the umbilicus to the epigastrium and the right scapular region.

when her weight was found to have increased to 212 pounds. She stated that until June, 1937, she felt well and had had no return of the symptoms experienced before the operation in April, 1936. Since June, 1937, she has had attacks of smothering at night and at intervals

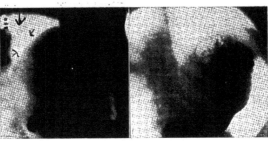

Fig. 1. Case 1. Esophageal hiatus hernia.

Fig. 2. Case 1. Radiograph taken one and a half years after repair. No recurrence.

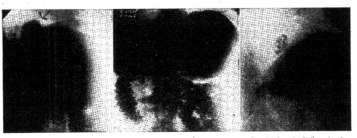

Fig. 3. Case 2. Shows esophageal hiatus hernia.

Fig. 4. Case 2. Radiograph taken three months after repair shows no recurrence.

Fig. 5. Case 2. Radiograph taken one and a half years after repair shows a recurrence.

The pain was relieved by vomiting and deep breathing. She had had nausea during the last six weeks and vomiting had become more frequent.

The patient was markedly overweight. Disease of the gallbladder or peptic ulcer was suspected, but x-ray examination showed a normally functioning gallbladder and there was no evidence of a lesion of the stomach or duodenum. There was found, however, a slight herniation of the cardiac end of the stomach through the esophageal opening. The diaphragmatic hernia was thought to be the cause of her symptoms and an operation advised.

She was put on medical management, reducing her weight from 210 pounds to 165 pounds.

On April 25, 1936, she was operated upon. The hernia was repaired and she made a good recovery. X-ray examination in June, 1936, showed no evidence of the hernia. This patient was last seen in October, 1937,

a gnawing sensation in the substernal region. The intervals between attacks ranged from a few days to three or four weeks. X-ray examination in October, 1937, showed a recurrence of the hernia. If this condition progresses her weight should again be reduced and another repair undertaken.

Case 3.—A woman sixty-one years of age was first seen in May, 1937. She dated the onset of her illness by an attack of whooping cough which she contracted when a child. Since that time she had noted heartburn, nausea, occasionally associated with vomiting, and pain in the back and under the left costal margin occurring one to three hours after meals. She could not eat large quantities of food without vomiting, and during the past year she had marked dyspnea after meals. The symptoms were aggravated when lying down.

She consulted several physicians because of stomach trouble, and had been on an ulcer diet several times.

Each time the symptoms were aggravated. There was nothing of note on general examination. On x-ray examination the gallbladder was reported as normal, but the gastro-intestinal examinations showed an extensive herniation, through the esophageal opening, of the cardiac end of the stomach.

very obvious finding of a loop of intestine in the thoracic cavity.

Case 5.—A man sixty-three years of age was first seen at home on November 10, 1935, by Dr. J. N. Gehlan of Saint Paul, Minnesota. The patient had been in

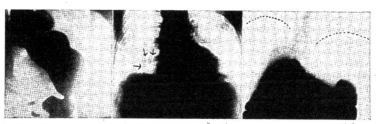

Fig. 6. Case 3. Large esophageal hiatus hernia.

Fig. 7. Case 4. Herniation of colon through opening in right diaphragm.

Fig. 8. Case 4. Barium enema one year after repair shows no recurrence.

On May 1, 1937, an operation was done for the repair of the hernia. The esophageal opening readily admitted three fingers. The immediate postoperative condition was satisfactory although her pulse rate was one hundred and forty. She was placed in an oxygen tent and stimulation was given. The day following the operation a blood transfusion was done and her condition improved. Forty-eight hours after the operation she had a sudden attack of dyspnea and cyanosis. A second transfusion was done but she continued to complain of dyspnea. Examination of the chest revealed no abnormalities. Later that day the patient appeared very alert and coöperating, but died suddenly following a short conversation with the nurse.

An autopsy revealed the cause of death to be multiple pulmonary emboli.

Case 4.—A man forty-three years of age was seen in June, 1935. He had been under treatment off and on since 1914 for duodenal ulcer. An x-ray study showed the presence of a duodenal ulcer with some pyloric obstruction. A gastro-enterostomy was advised and this was done in July, 1935. On opening the abdomen the liver and duodenal areas were obscured by the colon that ascended into the right thoracic cavity through an opening in the diaphragm. The opening was about 4 inches in length and there was a sac present. The colon was easily reduced as there were no adhesions between the colon and the hernial sac. The defect in the diaphragm was repaired. The duodenal ulcer was found and a posterior gastro-enterostomy was done. On further questioning of the patient it was learned that at the age of nine he had fallen from a horse, striking his right side. The probability is that the hernia dates back to this accident. He has gained weight since his operation and his gastric symptoms have disappeared. The interesting observation in this case is that the roentgenologist's attention was so focused on the stomach and duodenal examination that he did not observe the

an automobile accident on October 12, 1935. He stated that he fractured three ribs on the left side, that he had an injury to his left hip and back.

Immediately after the injury he was hospitalized and an adhesive dressing was applied to his chest. He developed bronchopneumonia and was in the hospital three weeks, after which he was moved to his home in Saint Paul. At the first examination at his home he said he felt fairly well but was bothered by a persistent cough and considerable expectoration. Examination of the chest showed dullness over the left side posteriorly. The breath sounds were suppressed and coarse râles were heard throughout the right chest. The right border of the heart was six centimeters to the right of the sternum. Abdominal examination showed no abnormalities. There was some tenderness in the lumbosacral region. On November 16, 1935, the cough had increased but the lung findings were unchanged. There was a slight temperature elevation and he complained of some abdominal distress. On November 21, 1935, he complained a great deal of abdominal cramps. The cough had improved but the dullness persisted in the left chest with bronchial breathing on the left side posteriorly. He was then sent to the hospital for x-ray study of his chest and his back, which showed a fracture through the first segment of the sacrum on the left side.

Stereoscopic studies of the chest showed impaired airation of the left lung with elevation and flattening of the diaphragm. There were numerous air-filled pockets with intervening areas of fibrosis. There was an area of consolidation in the base of the left lung, but this was somewhat obscured by a dense cloudiness. The right lung was clear. A diagnosis was made of thickened pleura with trabeculating adhesions in the lower left chest with the possibilities of a small amount of fluid and an area of consolidations in the left base. Because of this rather confusing report and the persistence of the symptoms, the clinician did a thoracen-tesis which proved negative.

A gastro-intestinal radiograph was made which showed that the entire stomach, all the jejunum, part of the ileum, and a loop of the colon had passed into the

mothorax was relieved. After the first week, however, his condition improved and he made a saisfactory re-covery. He developed an infection in the lower end of the operative wound and he now has a small incisional hernia. His general health at this time is exceptionally

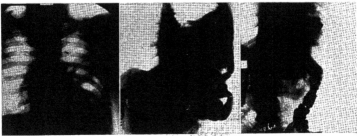

Fig. 9. Case 5. Chest plate showing numerous air-filled pockets with inter-vening fibrosis.

Fig. 10. Case 5. Entire stomach, the jejunum and part of the ileum seen in left thoracic cavity.

Fig. 11. Case 5. Barium filled colon seen in the left thoracic cavity.

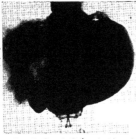

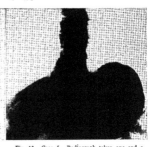

Fig. 12. Case 5. Radiograph taken three months after repair shows no recurrence.

Fig. 13. Case 5. Radiograph taken one and a half years after repair shows no recurrence.

left thoracic cavity through a rupture in the left hemi-diaphragm.

I was asked to see the patient November 30, 1935. He was still very nervous and weak, and was having considerable gastric distress and constipation, but as there was apparently no intestinal obstruction, I ad-vised close observation and postponement of the opera-tion until his general condition improved. On May 10, 1936, he was admitted to the hospital and the left phrenic nerve was crushed, and on May 16, 1936, the repair of the hernia was undertaken. A very large opening was found in the left hemi-diaphragm. For-tunately, no adhesions had formed between the abdomi-nal viscera and the pleura. The abdominal viscera was replaced in the abdomen and the defect in the dia-phragm was repaired.

The patient had a difficult time for a few days. He was placed in an oxygen tent immediately and the pneu-

good and roentgenograms taken in July, 1936, and Oc-tober, 1937, show no evidence of recurrence of the hernia.

Through the courtesy of Dr. Kano Ikeda, I am able to show a case of congenital diaphragmatic hernia:

Case 6.—One sees from the illustration that the de-fect is on the left side and the left thoracic cavity is crowded with abdominal viscera pushing the heart and lungs to the right thoracic wall. The radiograph shows the gas filled intestinal loops filling the entire left tho-racic cavity. It is readily understood that a hernia of this type is incompatible with life.

The abdominal approach was used in the sur-gical repair of the cases reported. Ethylene and

408

ether inhalation anesthesia was employed, and in the case of the large traumatic hernia the administration was by the intratracheal method. The defects in the diaphragm were sutured with silk

4. A thoracentesis is contraindicated until the possibility of a diaphragmatic hernia has been eliminated.

5. Operative repair of the diaphragmatic de-

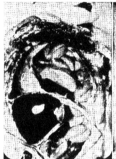 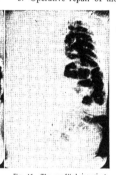

Fig. 14. Case 6. Congenital diaphragmatic hernia with the left thoracic cavity crowded with abdominal viscera.

Fig. 15. The gas-filled intestinal loops fitting the entire left thoracic cavity.

sutures together with living sutures of fascia lata which were taken from the patient's thigh.

In the first case of esophageal hiatus hernia, the hernial sac was removed, but in the second and third cases the stomach was freed from the hernia sac and the sac was allowed to retract into the posterior mediastinum.

It is very important to prepare these patients adequately for operation, as it is a severe operation that is frequently followed by considerable shock. It is therefore advisable to be prepared to use the oxygen tent for several days and blood transfusion will often be of great aid. The cases in which the viscera have been removed from the thoracic cavity frequently develop pleural effusion. This may be very slight but at times it is so extensive that it causes respiratory embarrassment and must be removed.

Summary

1. Improved roentgenologic methods have been a great aid in making a positive diagnosis of a diaphragmatic hernia.

2. A diaphragmatic hernia should always be considered when a confusing problem presents itself concerning the upper abdomen or chest.

3. In all severe chest injuries a careful x ray examination of the chest and gastro-intestinal tract including a barium enema should be carried out to determine the condition of the diaphragm.

fect after reduction of the hernia offers the only means of permanent relief.

6. Five cases of diaphragmatic hernia in which operation was performed are here reported. In this group three patients were cured, there is one recurrence and one death.

References

1. Ager, L. C.: Diaphragmatic hernia. U. S. Vet. Bur. Med. Bull., 6:971-973, (Nov.) 1930.
2. Barrett, N. R., and Wheaton, C. E. W.: The pathology, diagnosis, and treatment of congenital diaphragmatic hernia in infants. Brit. Jour. Surg., 21:420-433, (Jan.) 1934.
3. Bowditch, H. I.: Peculiar case of diaphragmatic hernia. Buffalo Med. Jour. and Mo. Rev., 9:1-39, (June) 1853.
4. Carman, R. D., and Fineman, S.: The roentgenologic diagnosis of diaphragmatic hernia, with a report of seventeen cases. Radiology, 3:26-45, (July), 1924.
5. Coley, B. L.: Hernia. Progressive Med., 2:30-37, (June) 1930.
6. Coley, B. L.: Hernia. Progressive Med., 2:43-52, (June) 1928.
7. Friedman, M., and Ehrlich, L. H.: Diaphragmatic hernia. Jour. Pediat., 8:38-40, (Jan.) 1936.
8. Gillespie, J. B.: Congenital shortening of the esophagus. Clin., ser. 25, 2:100-101, 1915.
9. Grulee, C. G.: Congenital diaphragmatic hernia. Internat. Clin., ser. 25, 2:100-101, 1915.
10. Harrington, S. W.: Surgical treatment of 105 cases of diaphragmatic hernia. Trans. West. Surg. Assn., 45:52-86, 1935.
11. Healy, T. R.: Symptoms observed in fifty-three cases of nontraumatic diaphragmatic hernia. Amer. Jour. Roent., 13:266-271, (March) 1925.
12. Hedblom, C. A.: Diaphragmatic hernia, In Lewis, Dean: Practice of Surgery. Hagerstown: Prior, 1930. Vol. 5, Chap. 7.
13. Jenkinson, E. L., and Roberts, E. W.: Lesions of the diaphragm. Amer. Jour. Roent., 38:584-591, (Oct.) 1937.
14. Truesdale, P. E.: Diaphragmatic hernia; its varieties and surgical treatment of hiatus type. Amer. Jour. Surg., 32: 204-216, (May) 1936.
15. Truesdale, P. E.: The thoraco-peritoneal operation for hernia of the diaphragm. Ann. Surg., 86:236-243, (Aug.) 1927.
16. Truesdale, P. E.: Hernia of the diaphragm; esophageal type in adults. New Eng. Jour. Med., 210:781-783, (April 12) 1934.

SYMPTOMATOLOGY OF THE VARIOUS LEUKEMIC STATES*

THOMAS A. PEPPARD, M.D.

Minneapolis, Minnesota

I DESIRE to present some observations concerning the symptoms and physical findings in leukemia, based upon a small group of thirty-four cases, and to present a brief clinical record of a few cases of special interest.

Ordinarily the diagnosis of leukemia may be made easily and with assurance. The clinical investigation at once indicates the necessity for an examination of the blood, and if, after this examination, for any reason we are still uncertain, the assistance of an expert blood cytologist in the great majority of instances will promptly and accurately establish the diagnosis. Not infrequently, however, atypical forms of the disease are encountered, and even though we include leukemia in our list of possibilities, we may find that we are unable to do more than this. A given case may at one time present evidence indicating one particular entity, and later give what appears just as good evidence for another. Again, a patient may at one time present the symptoms of a slowly progressive, chronic disease, and at another time show acute manifestations. It is necessary to keep in mind the essential dictum that the disease is one of the hemato-poietic tissues, and that the quantitative and qualitative changes found on blood examination are indicators of the changes going on in the blood forming centers.

The essential cause of the disease is, of course, unknown. At present, most observers class it with the tumors, though some argue for an infectious etiology. The preponderance of opinion and evidence seems to be in favor of the former.

Chart 1 represents Piney's ideas concerning hemato-poiesis.

In Chart 2, I have listed the presenting symptoms in a small series of thirty-four cases. I have grouped them merely as chronic, and acute or subacute. The symptoms are varied, quite as may be found in any text. Any of these individual symptoms alone means little, any of them occurring in a wide variety of conditions. Perhaps in presenting the clinical summaries, I may be able to group them in such a way as to make them mean more. At this point I merely want to comment on a few particular items. Weakness and fatigue were prominent complaints, even though the patient appeared quite robust and no anemia existed.

The frequency of the association of sore mouth, ulceration, necrosis, and bleeding, with the leukemic states (usually acute), recommends to the physician, laryngologist, and dentist, that he consider this relationship, even though a seemingly adequate cause may be present (Vincent's organisms). It is somewhat surprising perhaps that glandular enlargement does not appear with greater frequency; however, I ask you to compare it with the adenopathy in Chart 3 which illustrates the physical findings.

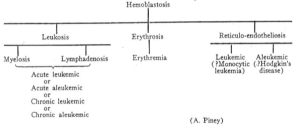

Hemoblastosis

Leukosis — Erythrosis — Reticulo-endotheliosis

Myelosis Lymphadenosis   Erythremia   Leukemic (?Monocytic leukemia)   Aleukemic (?Hodgkin's disease)

Acute leukemic or Acute aleukemic or Chronic leukemic or Chronic aleukemic

(A. Piney)

CHART 1

---

*Read before the Minnesota Academy of Medicine, November 10, 1937.

Jaundice was complained of in four cases; ough in six; itching in two; visual disturbance three; tender eyeball and pain on movement f the eyeball in one instance.

nodes may attain considerable size, though pressure symptoms are not the rule.

In addition to splenic and liver enlargement, these organs may also be tender, the spleen us-

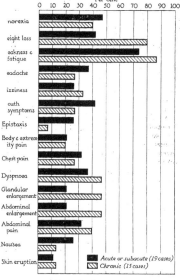

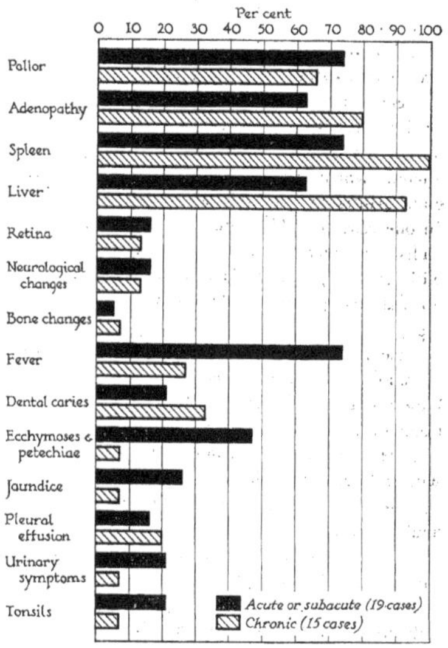

CHART 2. SYMPTOMS

CHART 3. PHYSICAL FINDINGS

It is highly important to pay attention to any skin lesion which may be present, for not infrequently a skin biopsy may be an important factor in determining the true diagnosis.

Priapism, though frequently mentioned, is a symptom which I have never encountered in this disease. Cabot failed to find it in a series of eighty-nine cases.

I have arranged the physical findings in the same general way in Chart 3. There is considerable difference in the degree of glandular enlargement in various parts of the body. The glands are usually discreet, moderately firm, freely moveable, and not attached to the skin or surrounding tissues. Usually the nodes are moderate in size, but not so large as those found in Hodgkin's disease or lympho-sarcoma. Occasionally the mesenteric, retro-peritoneal, and hilus

ually more often so than the liver.

The findings in the fundus oculi are principally engorged veins, with or without hemorrhages, with sometimes white streaks along the vessel walls, and increased tortuosity of the vessels. The peculiar color of the fundus is more often talked about than seen. Some authors estimate the incidence of retinal changes in as much as 65 per cent of cases.

Recent articles have commented upon the frequency of neurological findings. These have been carefully looked for, and not found in nearly the frequency reported by Weiss and Schwab (20 per cent).

Bone changes have not been found with any considerable frequency, although tenderness over the bones has been encountered when no lesion could be demonstrated. Sternal tenderness occurred more frequently in the myeloid types. In one patient symptoms were such as to suggest a possible osteomyelitis. One patient had infiltration of the fourth thoracic vertebra which resulted in a pathological fracture and this same person had areas of lessened density in the cranial tables.

The fever naturally more frequent in the acute group was variable and irregular.

Heart murmurs were frequent, sometimes readily explained by sufficient evidence of heart disease, sometimes explainable by the degree of anemia which was present. Subacute bacterial endocarditis may occur terminally as in sepsis. In one case, a child, a leukemic infiltrate had invaded the heart in such a way as to interfere with the coronary circulation and produce abnormal changes in the electrocardiographic tracing.

Case 1 illustrates the course of a patient with lymphoid leukemia whose course was rather longer than usual, with rather acute manifestations near the termination.

Case 2 illustrates rather typically a patient with reticuloendotheliosis.

Case 3 illustrates a hypocytic leukemia with acute symptoms.

Case 4 illustrates a myeloid leukemia which ran a short course.

It would appear that the greatest diagnostic difficulties consist in differentiation from pernicious anemia, Hodgkin's disease, cancer, benign lymph-adenosis, agranulocytosis, and aplastic anemia.

Conclusion.—A characteristic clinical picture together with typical blood findings readily establishes the diagnosis of leukemia. It is, of course, apparent that the qualitative blood changes are of more importance than the quantitative.

Even on encountering a low rather than a high total leukocyte count, leukemia must be considered, and when there is present adenopathy, enlargement of the spleen and liver, bleeding from the mouth or nose, a progressive downhill course, and a rapidly developing anemia, the chances are that leukemia is almost surely present.

Case Reports

Case 1.—A female, fifty-three years of age. Her father had died at the age of sixty-five of cancer of the stomach.

The patient had had no important illnesses. In

1914, she had a "nervous break-down," was in bed for eight months. Since 1923, she had gastrointestinal symptoms, consisting of pain and tenderness in the right upper quadrant, bloating, gaseous eructations, some nausea, and occasional vomiting. There was a tendency to constipation. There had been no jaundice. Menopause had occurred in 1925. She complained of weakness and fatigue, headache, some dizziness, slight dyspnea and palpitation on exertion. Patient had suffered from frequent upper respiratory tract infections.

Physical examination: The patient was well nourished, her color good. Some very small cervical nodes were palpable. Number of non-vital teeth were present. Heart and lungs were normal. The liver was not enlarged, the spleen not palpable. Fundus examination was negative. X-ray examination gave evidence of an abnormally functioning gallbladder.

The patient was seen and examined in 1927 by Dr. L. A. Nippert, who furnished the following findings: Hemoblogin, 77 per cent; erythrocytes, 4,540,000; leukocytes, 40,000, 17 per cent of which were polymorphoneuclears and 83 per cent lymphocytes, "all cells appearing mature and not those usually observed in leukemia."

I observed the patient during the years of 1929 and 1930, during which time her hemoglobin varied from 88 per cent to 83 per cent, the red blood cells from 3,870,000 to 4,480,000, and the total leukocytes from 22,000 to as high as 51,000. Most of the cells were lymphoid in character, but after much study the conclusion was reached that the condition was that of lymphatic leukemia. The Wassermann reaction was negative. The urine was always normal. The stomach contents showed normal findings, and the electrocardiographic tracing was normal. The basal metabolic rate was minus 21 per cent. During this time she was observed over a period of one month by Drs. Giffin and Roundtree, who satisfied themselves that the condition was leukemia, a skin biopsy showing changes characteristic of that condition. While the patient was not incapacitated, her weight diminished from 175 pounds to 157 pounds.

The patient was not observed from 1931-1933, but it was learned that she was receiving x-ray treatments. In August, 1933, she had some dental extractions and there was no excess bleeding.

In 1934, and up to March, 1935, she was observed by Dr. J. Davis of Minneapolis, who reported the findings as follows: Patient had lost in weight to 125 pounds by March, 1934. There was general lymph adenopathy, and the spleen was enlarged and palpable. Hemoglobin was 68 per cent, red blood cells 3,000,000, leukocytes 47,000. From the blood smears, the diagnosis was obvious, there being many immature forms. From this time the condition was progressive, the hemoglobin going down to 20 per cent, red blood cells 1,000,000, leukocytes 57,000 on February 28, 1935. There was considerable bleeding from the nose and mouth. Transfusions and the administration of liver did not modify the course, and the patient died March 1, 1935.

Diagnosis: Chronic lymphatic leukemia.

Comment.—Information is available concerning this patient over a period of approximately eight years. It is not uncommon to observe some of these patients with more or less characteristic blood changes, but with all relatively little impairment of the state of their general health. In the present instance the condition lasted longer than the average duration of about four years. Near the termination the symptoms become more acute.

Case 2.—R. L., a female, forty-nine years of age. Family history was unimportant.

The patient's general health had been good. Appendectomy had been performed in 1910. Radium had been applied to the pelvis in 1932, and she was said to have been anemic since 1932.

Following dental extraction, May 21, 1935, she bled profusely, was faint and weak, the face and jaw swelled, and there was a bad odor to the breath and a bad taste in the mouth. A chill occurred May 27, 1935, and the following day she entered the hospital.

Examination: The patient appeared well nourished; weight, 132 pounds. There was a marked pallor, swelling of the left lower jaw, but no fluctuation. Blood oozed from the gum margins, and there were large necrotic areas in the mouth. The regional lymph nodes were enlarged. Heart and lungs were normal. The abdomen was distended and the liver and spleen were not palpable. There was no general adenopathy.

Laboratory: hemoglobin at the time of admission was 37 per cent, red blood cells 1,500,000, leukocytes 1,000. Subsequently, the hemoglobin varied between 40 and 46 per cent. Three transfusions were given, and the red count was elevated to as high as 2,700,000. The leukocyte count varied from as low as 300 cells to as high as 2,400, the polymorphonuclear percentage generally about 20. There was variation in size and shape of the red cells and a few early forms were seen. There was some evidence of regeneration. The platelet count was 190,000 and on another occasion 250,000. The blood culture was negative. Smears from the mouth showed Vincent's organisms.

Culture: Fever ranged from 101 to 104.6 degrees, the pulse rate increasing in proportion to the temperature. There was much nausea, headache and weakness, and constant oozing from the mouth and gums. X-ray of the jaw showed infected area in the region of the tooth socket. There were ecchymoses and on June 5th frank hematuria. On June 9, hemiplegia, extensive retinal hemorrhage and coma supervened. Death occurred on this day.

Autopsy: Peritoneum, pleura, and pericardium were negative. The heart weighed 250 grams, and was entirely normal. The lungs were normal. The spleen weighed 250 gms., its cut surface appeared normal, and there was hyperplasia of the reticulum. The right kidney weighed 200 gms., the left was 175 gms., and they were normal except for blood in the pelvis. There was no general adenopathy. The rib marrow was not

gelatinous; the marrow of the middle of the femur was yellow but section shows hyperplasia, with mainly large round cells which showed no differentiation toward mature granulocytes or erythrocytes. There was no infiltration of the liver, lung, or kidneys.

Blood smears were reviewed by Dr. Downey who found the red blood cells and lymphocytes normal. A number of cells were found with rounded or indented nuclei with chromatin network resembling myeloblasts, the same as those found in the splenic sinuses and bone marrow which were termed differentiated reticulo-endothelial cells.

Diagnosis: Reticulo-endotheliosis (Monocytic leukemia).

Comment.—The extensive necrosis in the mouth is quite characteristic of this type of leukemia, the course of which is acute. The profound anemia serves to differentiate this condition from agranulocytosis. The head was not opened at autopsy, but quite likely there was a terminal cerebral hemorrhage.

Case 3—A. B., a male, thirty-one years of age. Family history unimportant.

History: This man had had childhood diseases without complications, influenza in 1918, gonorrhea in 1921, and fibrinous pleurisy in 1929. Syphilis was denied.

In October, 1935, he had an attack of abdominal pain, probably unaccompanied by fever, and constipation, and a surgeon considered the possibility of intestinal obstruction. After ten days he returned to work, was not up to par, but had no specific complaints.

On April 2, 1936, he experienced a moderately severe epigastric pain, dysphagia, a sense of pressure in the upper abdomen with tenderness, and loose bowel movements. There was a ten pound weight loss in two weeks. He complained of weakness, nocturia (1-3), dark urine, throat irritation, cough, and whitish sputum. On April 12, 1936, he entered the hospital.

Examination: Well nourished, weight 172 pounds, slight pallor, conjunctivæ icteric, ecchymoses, no general adenopathy. Lungs showed a shading at the left base, impaired resonance, over the lower third of the right base, diaphragmatic excursion, no pleural rubs. Heart normal, blood pressure 118/80. Liver extended 6.5 cm. below the tip of the ensiform, 5 cm. below the costal margin in the mid-clavicular line. Spleen extended half way from the costal margin to the umbilicus. A slight amount of peritoneal fluid was present. Rectal examination was negative.

Laboratory: Urine—the only significant finding was that of 4 plus urobilin and urobilinogen. The icterus index was 23. There was no increased fragility of the red cells. Bleeding time and clotting time were normal. One blood culture remained sterile. Blood Wassermann was negative. The hemoglobin, on admission, was 82 per cent, after two weeks 51 per cent, and thereafter varied between 55-48 per cent. Red blood count was 4,400,000, later reduced to 3,420,000. Leukocyte count varied from 2,900 to 3,400; differential: polymorphonuclears 7.7 per cent, lymphocytes 15 per cent, monocytes 8 per cent. One normoblast was observed, and no early leukocyte forms were seen at any time. Sputum was negative for tubercle bacilli. Twenty-five mgm. of urobilinogen was excreted in the urine in twenty-four hours; 350 mgm. urobilinogen in the stool. Cystoscopic examination and pyelograms were negative.

Autopsy: The heart weighed 250 gms. and there was a slight thickening of the edges of the mitral cusps, but no ulcerations nor fresh vegetations. The other valves were normal. The coronary vessels were normal. A minimal atheroma of the aorta was present.

The lungs were normal. At the hilum of the right lung was a mass of glands, 12 x 8 x 6 cm.

The spleen weighed 1,350 gms. The external and cut surfaces were studded with a large number of whitish firm nodules up to 5 cm. in diameter.

The liver weighed 4,050 gms., and was congested. There were numerous white nodules throughout, similar to those found in the spleen.

The right kidneys weighed 250 gms., the left 300 gms. They were pale and firm, and a 4 mm. nodule was present in the cortex of the right kidney.

Microscopic examination of nodules in the liver and spleen showed masses of cells resembling lymphocytes; much mitoses. The mediastinal lymph nodes showed leukemic metaplasia and also some necrosis. The kidney contained no leukemic infiltration in the parenchyma, but a subcapsular leukemic nodule. Imprint preparations from spleen and liver nodules showed large numbers of immature lymphocytes. Bone marrow of ribs and sternum appeared hyperplastic. On review of blood smears, no abnormal cells were found.

Course: There was irregular fever, with diurnal variations of from one to three degrees, gradually increasing from 100 degrees F. to 102. Pulse rate followed the temperature curve, increasing from a level of about 100 to 120. There was increasing weakness. There were attacks of abdominal pain with increasing distention of the abdomen. The liver and spleen enlarged. Ascites and dependent edema developed. There was sore mouth and nose bleed on occasion. The patient coughed and expectorated a clear mucoid material. The jaundice varied in intensity. He was given a transfusion of citrated blood on April 28, and on May 5, but became weaker and died on May 8.

Diagnosis: Aleukemic lymphoid leukemia.

Comment.—This patient died approximately thirty-six days after the development of his acute symptoms. The symptoms of cough and expectoration as well as difficulty in swallowing were undoubtedly related to the mediastinal glandular enlargement. Jaundice is not infrequently observed in the leukemias. It should scarcely be necessary to call attention to the fact that the term aleukemic refers to the absence of characteristic early leukocytic forms of cells in the circulating blood, and does not at all pertain to the total number of leukocytes. The not infre-

quent misapplication of the term has been one of the reasons for various attempts at altering the nomenclature, bringing forward such terms as hypocytic, hypercytic and normocytic to designate low, high, and normal total leukocyte counts. No especial need is seen for changing the terminology. Proper use of the present terms, with the necessary qualifications, very well suffices.

Case 4. (Courtesy of Dr. R. L. Sherer).—Male, sixty-two years of age. Family history was unimportant. Previous health had been good.

Acute onset occurred May 14, 1936, with nausea, vomiting, weakness and diarrhea. There were some body pains and chest pains, with increasing weakness and loss of weight.

Examination: A pallor, with slight icteric tinge was present. Fundus oculi were negative. There was moderate atherosclerosis. Blood pressure 140/90. Heart and lungs were normal. The spleen and liver were palpable and both moderately enlarged. Tendon reflexes were normal. Vibration sense was diminished over the lower extremities. The electrocardiographic tracing showed myocardial degeneration.

The patient entered the hospital June 2, 1936.

Laboratory findings: Hemoglobin was 45 per cent, red blood cells 1,980,000, white blood cells 5,800, 52 per cent of which were lymphocytes. There was considerable albuminuria with cylindruria. Test meal showed achlorhydria before and after histamine. Blood urea nitrogen on one occasion was 10 mgm., later as high as 29 mgm. Blood culture was negative. Subsequently, the hemoglobin varied between 40-35 per cent. There was little change in the number of red cells. After one week's time the total leukocyte count increased to 13,000; on June 16, it was 16,000, and on June 20, 20,000. There was gradual progressive increase in the immature forms of white cells, and although the anemia, the appearance of icterus, the achlorhydria, and the diminished vibration sense first suggested pernicious anemia, later study of the blood smears made the diagnosis apparent.

There was temperature variation from 98 to as high as 101 degrees. The patient expired June 24, 1936.

Partial autopsy only could be obtained. The spleen weighed 750 grams. The kidneys weighed 200 and 235 gms. The liver appeared to be of about normal size and weight. Sections of these organs showed leukemic infiltration. Diagnosis: Acute myeloid leukemia.

Comment.—In the present instance, as in not a few others, pernicious anemia was first suggested, not only by the general appearance of the patient, but by certain of the laboratory findings. While during the first week, treatment with liver extract produced a reticulocyte increase to 9 per cent, there was no improvement in the red blood cells, nor the hemoglobin.

414

A CASE OF WOHLFAHRTIA VIGIL CUTANEOUS MYIASIS IN MINNESOTA

CHARLES VANDERSLUIS, M.D., and D. D. WHITTEMORE, M.D.

Bemidji, Minnesota

"CUTANEOUS myiasis," as was so aptly stated by Walker,[10] "is an infestation of the skin and subcutaneous tissues by the larvæ of certain species of flies which feed upon these tissues during their period of growth, causing great suffering and often leading to secondary bacterial infection." With the invaluable assistance of Drs. William A. Riley and Reed O. Christenson of the Department of Entomology, University of Minnesota, we are able to present a proven case of cutaneous infestation of a young infant in Minnesota by maggots of the flesh fly *Wohlfahrtia vigil.*

M. B., a female infant of two and a half months, living in Crookston, Minnesota, presented a few small red pimples on her upper chest the morning of July 10, 1937. The mother observed that they became larger during the day, but she considered them due to the heat. Towards night the infant became irritable and began to cry. She cried all night in evident pain. She was brought to Bemidji on a visit the next morning, continuing to cry violently. The pimples on her chest became larger, were capped by yellowish white heads, and were surrounded by areas of redness and induration. The inflammatory bases of many closely grouped lesions on the right upper chest fused. That noon the mother suddenly noted lively crawling worms emerging from the pimples on the infant's chest, and she rushed the baby to us in great excitement. We noted about fifteen red macules, ten of them closely grouped on the upper right chest, and the rest scattered singly in the left axilla, left scapular region and left loin. The single lesions were like large, well developed acne pustules. The maggots were emerging from the confluent lesions on the upper chest, occupying an area about 6 x 8 cm. These lesions were the most advanced and seven or eight of them presented, at the apices, cleanly punched-out holes measuring about 3 mm. across. Each was surrounded by a small red area, and the deeper surrounding tissue was indurated. These holes contained the maggots. In most of the openings only one maggot was present but in several of them two and three were wriggling deep in the infant's hypoderm. In some areas the skin was undermined by tunnels between the holes, leaving but a fibrotic bloodless skeletal subcutaneous network. The maggots were actively feeding on the infant's tissues and when expressed or picked from an opening would rapidly crawl across the skin and enter another if possible. In some of the lesions not quite ruptured, maggots could be seen moving about under the inflamed necrotic epidermis. At least one maggot could be expressed from

each lesion, and such was the procedure followed in treatment.

On the anterior chest wall several free incisions were made to open up the tunneled hypoderm. The maggots

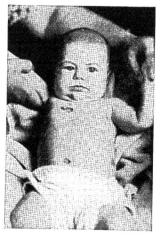

Fig. 1. Infant in authors' case.

were white, round, and segmented, measuring 4 to 8 mm. in length, and each had a black speck at the head. All of them, numbering about twenty, were removed from the baby and several placed in alcohol-formalin solution for study. It was noted that they lived several minutes in this preservative. The infant went to sleep immediately after all the larvæ had been removed. We placed azochloramid packs on the lesions and were forced to lose contact with the baby, due to the parents' anxiety to return to Crookston. Dr. W. F. Mercil saw the patient there and reported finding no more maggots. The child recovered uneventfully with treatment directed to clearing up the secondary inflammation from pus organisms (undoubtedly staphylococcus). The photograph represents the infant about one week following removal of the larvæ. Dr. Reed Christenson identified them as second stage larvæ of the Sarcophagid fly, *Wohlfahrtia vigil.*

Cutaneous myiasis is a medical curiosity in temperate parts of the United States, although it is not infrequent in the southern states. For many years it has been considered that the most common cause of human myiasis in the Western World is a Sarcophagid fly, *Cochliomyia macellaria*, which has been reported from Canada to the Argentine. It has been thought to have a "screw-worm" larva. It is somewhat larger than the housefly and deposits numerous eggs in open wounds, or in the nose or ear of individuals with a purulent discharge or odor which attracts the adult flies. Harris,[6] who reported a number of cases of screw-worm infestation, says that the larvæ may issue within a short time and begin at once to feed and burrow into all structures and cavities of the head, migrating into the eyes, middle ear, and brain, destroying tissues and causing infection and gangrene of soft parts and necrosis of bone. The larvæ then desert the host to pupate in five to fourteen days, leaving behind widespread devastation. Discharge of larvæ, and sero-sanguinous fluid, and the odor of wet gangrene are listed as the cardinal symptoms of infestation. The mortality is variously reported to run from 15 to 85 per cent.

In 1933, Cushing and Patton[2] made the astonishing discovery that the true "screw-worm" is the larva of a related but entirely distinct species, which they proposed to call *Cochliomyia americana.* It is this species which invades living tissue after entering through some wound. For a half century or more, *Cochliomyia macellaria,* a secondary invader, has been held responsible for invasions of living tissue which were really due to *C. americana.* The resultant confusion in medical and veterinary literature is such that case reports of the past must all be regarded with suspicion.[8]

Another family of flies, the Œstridæ, includes species whose larvæ are parasitic in animals and, occasionally, in man. Of these the bot-fly larvæ are commonly found in the stomach and intestine of horses. The eggs are laid on the hairs of the host and, when licked up, the larvæ enter the alimentary canal, where they remain until mature, when they are discharged in the manure and enter the ground to pupate. In the rare cases of human infection the larvæ are deposited on the skin, hatch, and penetrate the skin, moving about under the surface superficially and producing a characteristic creeping eruption, larva migrans, with narrow, slightly elevated, red, linear lesions. Its occasional resemblance

to scabies has been remarked. *Gastrophilus* is the most frequently cited causative genus.

Very different is the biology of the warble flies of cattle.[4] Here the eggs are likewise laid on hairs but the hatching larvæ bore into the skin of the animal host and migrate for months in the body tissues before they come to lie under the skin of the back in mid-winter. The rare human infections do not present the raised inflamed line of creeping eruption, but the larvæ migrate in the deeper tissues, occasionally manifesting their presence by tumor-like swellings and severe pain along the path of migration. Such a traveling lump may surpass the size of a pigeon egg, have the appearance of a furuncle, and, at the end of its migration, the warble stage, present a central opening on its surface in which the larva can be seen "appearing and disappearing after the manner of a jack-in-the-box."[1] This disease has been variously named as dermal myiasis, subcutaneous myiasis, and oxwarble disease. The larvæ of *Hypoderma lineata* and *H. bovis* have been identified as invaders in lesions of the above type. The so-called human bot *Dermatobia hominis* enters the unbroken skin (Dunn[3]) and produces similar painful tumors (non-migrating).

Wohfahrtia vigil as a human and animal parasite is little known about and has been found only in Canada and the northern part of the United States, due largely to the work of E. M. Walker[11] of the University of Toronto. Brauer and von Berganstamm in 1889 erected the genus Wohlfahrtia for certain flesh flies of the family Muscidæ formerly included in the genus Sarcophila. W. magnifica, the type species, is well known as a parasite of man and various domestic animals in Europe, particularly Russia, and has been considered the European analogue of our screw-worm fly. In all these cases the larvæ are noted to feed upon the mucous membrane and deeper tissues of the nose, gums, ear, and even the eye, but Walker finds no mention made of the larvæ ever penetrating the healthy skin, as must have occurred in the cases of infestation by W. vigil.

Nothing had been known of the larval habits of the North American species of Wohlfahrtia until the discovery of W. vigil as the cause of human cutaneous myiasis in Toronto in 1919 by Walker.[11] In 1931 he reported a total of sixteen cases having come to light since 1919, all in Canada and the northern United States. In 1934 there were four additional cases in Toronto besides 180 proven cases of Wohlfahrtia myiasis in dogs, cats, foxes, milk, ferrets, and rabbits. Dr. A. A. Kingscote of the Ontario Veterinary College, who reported the animal cases, says that "in very small animals from five to twenty larvæ will cause death usually within about ten days." There are isolated human cases reported in New York (Felt, 1925), New Hampshire (Sanders, 1928),⁹ Colorado (Knowles, 1925),⁷ and lately North Dakota (Gertson, 1933),⁵ the latter place only a few miles from Crookston. Dr. J. M. Aldrich, of the National Museum, writes: "The species ranges from Nova Scotia to North Dakota, or rarely further, but west of the Rocky Mountains it seems to be replaced by . . . Wohlfahrtia meigenii Shiner," a form which is not parasitic in the manner W. vigil is. Our case in Crookston appears to be the first reported in Minnesota, although a suspicious case was observed in the region of Duluth recently. Dr. Riley reports the death of many young mink, young foxes, and some cases of very young rabbits from the attacks of larvæ in this region, and he urged upon us the report of this human case.

All but one of the human cases of myiasis have occurred in infants less than one year of age, the average being two to five months. Felt reported the adult case of a conjunctival cyst filled with "living maggots provisionally identified as W. vigil." The small abscess-like lesions develop most commonly on the neck, chest, shoulders, and arms, showing our case typical in this respect. Lesions have also been observed on the palm, navel, cheek, and eyelids. In Walker's original words: "The small opening at the apex of the lesion is so strongly suggestive . . . of pus that on superficial examination a group of lesions might readily be considered impetigo; in fact, the diagnosis of impetigo was made erroneously in at least one of the cases reported. On closer examination it is readily seen that what appeared to be pus is, in reality, the posterior end of the larva. This may be seen to be moving . . . if pressure is exerted the larval body may be forced out. It can be seen to work its way by a wriggling movement along the skin surface. In most cases about twelve or fourteen of these lesions were present,

each with an external opening, and each containing one or more larvæ. In the earlier stages a slight macular rash may be present and at this time the young larvæ, 2 to 3 mm. long, may be found wandering over the surface of the skin. It thus appears that the larvæ may penetrate the skin at points distant from those where they were deposited by the parent fly. The development of the larvæ is very rapid, though variable. Scarcely more than 2 mm. long when born, they reach a length of about 20 mm. in from four to twelve days. In another day or two they emerge from the skin and drop to the ground and burrow into the earth and become puparia. After about eighteen days in this resting stage they emerge from the ground as adult flies. Most of the cases of myiasis due to this fly have occurred in June. The adult flies have been taken at various times during the summer months and have been found from the New England States to Alaska.

Norma Ford,⁴ through her studies of W. vigil in the field and in the laboratory, has learned much about the habits of the species. It is closely related to the house-fly and the blow-fly or "blue bottle," but unlike these diptera it does not breed in decomposing organic matter but rather is parasitic on living tissues. Experimentally it can be observed to prefer the eye of a living guinea pig to liver. Unlike the majority of common flies it deposits living larvæ or maggots instead of eggs, although rarely it has been observed to lay eggs when unduly excited or attracted to a favorable spot on a living animal. In feeding experiments it has been noted to pass up meat in favor of milk, sugar, and flowers. The flies are not attracted by the odors of decomposing substances. Ford found that all of the infested infants had been sleeping unprotected out-of-doors and that many had been living near a railroad track. She found that the flies were attracted by warmth and so stimulated to larviposition; thus she explains their greater activity near a warm railroad track in the summer. She also noted the greater activity of the females in the absence of direct sunlight, an interesting observation in view of the fact that a child is usually placed in a cool shady place when left outside. She remarked that in no case had the fly been known to enter houses. In our case · an exception may have occurred, since the mother states that at no time in the week preceding infection had the infant been left out-of-doors. The maggots were estimated to be about three days old. The nearest railroad track was three-fourths mile away.

If additional cases are encountered it is suggested that some of the living maggots be placed on raw meat and also some preserved in 70 per cent alcohol and sent to an entomologist. Again we wish to express our gratitude to Dr. W. A. Riley for his interest and many helpful notations.

References

1. Castellani and Chalmers: Manual of Tropical Medicine. 3rd ed., p. 1637, 1920.
2. Cushing, E. C., and Patton, W. S.: Ann. Trop. Med. and Parasitol., 27:539, 1933.
3. Dunn, Lawrence H.: Rearing the larvæ of dermatobia hominis in man. Psyche, 37:327, (Dec.) 1930.
4. Ford, Norma: Further observations on behavior of Wohlfahrtia vigil (Walker) with notes on collecting and rearing of flies. Jour. Parasitol., 22:309, (Aug.) 1936.
5. Gertson, G. D., et al.: Wohlfahrtia myiasis in North Dakota. Jour. A. M. A., 100:487, (Feb. 18) 1933.
6. Harris, S. T.: Human myiasis externa. U. S. Vet. Bur. Med. Bull., 5:412, (June) 1929.
7. Knowles, T. R.: Cutaneous myiasis. Colorado Med., 22:309, (Sept.) 1925.
8. Riley, W. A.: Personal communication.
9. Sanders, H. C.: Myiasis dermatosa. N. Eng. Jour. Med., 199:38, (July 5) 1928.
10. Walker, E. M.: Cutaneous myiasis in Canada. Can. Pub. Health Jour., (Oct.) 1931.
11. Walker, E. M.: Wohlfahrtia vigil as a human parasite. Jour. Parasitol., 7:1, (Sept.) 1920; Some cases of cutaneous myiasis with notes on the larvæ of Wohlfahrtia vigil (Walker). Jour. Parasitol., 9:1, (Sept.) 1922.

RELATIVE VALUE OF THE DIAGNOSTIC PROCEDURES IN THE ALLERGIC CHILD*

ALBERT V. STOESSER, M.D., and ROLLIN E. CUTTS, M.D.

Minneapolis, Minnesota

CUTANEOUS tests and trial or elimination diets play an important part in the diagnosis and treatment of allergic disorders of the child. Much has been written concerning the value of dermal testing in determining the causative agent in allergic disease. Early reports in the literature were chiefly concerned with the scratch method. The introduction of the intracutaneous method marked the onset of a controversy as to the relative merits of the two main methods of cutaneous testing. The pioneer investigators used extracts and solutions which had been crudely prepared and they differed greatly in their testing technic. It is not surprising, therefore, that these workers could come to no significant agreement on the matter.

Today the powdered and fluid extracts are definitely more potent than they were a decade ago and their quality will continue to improve. The powdered extracts need no longer be used for the scratch method. Glycerinized concentrated liquid extracts are now available. This material has led to the introduction of another technic. In place of the customary scratch through the upper layer of the epidermis, oblique and shallow punctures are made. This procedure is referred to as the pressure-puncture method of cutaneous testing. It is a relatively painless procedure when properly performed and

small children will tolerate it with little complaint.

The pressure-puncture method was adopted by the staff of the Pediatric Allergy Clinic of the University Hospital, the following technic being employed. The skin is cleansed with alcohol or ether or both and allowed to dry. The various glycerinized fluid extracts are then expelled from the glass capillary tubes upon the cleansed skin at intervals of about four centimeters. With a sterile sewing needle held nearly parallel with the skin, four to eight oblique pricks or shallow punctures are made into the epidermis by pressing the point of the needle through each drop of extract. A new needle is used for each test. The punctures are confined to an area not more than three millimeters in diameter.

Sufficient fluid extract to produce a positive reaction in susceptible children is carried into the epidermis by the multiple punctures and in a few minutes the excess fluid on the surface of the skin is gently wiped off. A similar test is carried out with a control glycerine solution and only those reactions in the test sites which are distinctly greater in intensity than that resulting from the control test are considered positive. The positive reactions (urticarial wheal surrounded by a zone of erythema) usually appear in sensitive patients in twenty to thirty minutes.

Three hundred consecutive cases of allergy in

*From the Allergy Clinic and Service of the Department of Pediatrics, University of Minnesota. Presented before the Fall meeting of the Southwestern Minnesota Medical Society at Fulda, Minnesota, October 7, 1937.

TABLE I. CLINICAL VALUE OF THE PRESSURE-PUNCTURE CUTANEOUS TESTS IN 300 ALLERGIC CHILDREN

| Allergic Disease | No. of Cases | Results of Treatment Based on Tests | | | |
| | | Good | | Poor | |
		No. Cases	Per Cent	No. Cases	Per Cent
Eczema	82	27	33	55	67
Allergic Rhinitis	36	6	17	30	83
Hay fever	44	35	80	9	20
Bronchial Asthma	120	74	62	46	38
Urticaria and Gastro-intestinal Allergy	18	2	1	16	89
Total	300	144	48	156	52

TABLE II. CLINICAL VALUE OF THE ELIMINATION DIETS IN THE 147 ALLERGIC CHILDREN FAILING TO RESPOND TO THE PRESSURE-PUNCTURE CUTANEOUS TESTS

| Allergic Disease | No. of Cases | Results Obtained from the Various Diets | | | |
| | | Good | | Poor | |
		No. Cases	Per Cent	No. Cases	Per Cent
Eczema	55	19	35	36	65
Allergic Rhinitis	30	8	27	22	73
Bronchial Asthma	46	2	4	44	96
Urticaria and Gastro-intestinal Allergy	16	10	63	6	37
Total	147	39	27	108	73

the child were tested by the method just described. The children ranged in age from six months to fifteen years. In 144 cases or 48 per cent the tests were of definite value in determining the exciting cause in the various allergic manifestations. The best results were obtained in hay fever and bronchial asthma. The causative agent was easily found in 80 per cent of the children with hay fever and in 62 per cent of those suffering with asthma. Only about 33 per cent of the cases of eczema gave positive skin tests which were found to be of clinical significance. Allergic rhinitis, urticaria and gastro-intestinal allergy made a poor showing. The results are summarized in Table I.

In 156 cases the pressure-puncture tests were of no value, and these children were not subjected at once to the intracutaneous testing. This method is painful and often rather difficult to

perform properly on the child. Therefore, the elimination diets were tried. The nine children with hay fever were omitted, leaving 147 cases. It was found that milk, cheese, egg, whole wheat, white potato, chocolate, tomato and orange were most frequently the offending foods. In thirty-nine cases the response to the trial diets was satisfactory. The best results were in urticaria, with eczema, and allergic rhinitis next. Those in bronchial asthma were the poorest, as may be observed in Table II.

The intracutaneous tests were next considered. The food allergens were placed in various groups in order to simplify testing but the inhalants were not mixed together. Pollens were excluded and therefore the nine cases of hay fever unsuccessfully treated were not tested. One hundred and eight children received the intradermal tests, the following technic being employed. The

TABLE III. CLINICAL VALUE OF INTRACUTANEOUS TESTS IN 108 CHILDREN FAILING
TO RESPOND TO THE PRESSURE-PUNCTURE TESTS AND ELIMINATION DIETS

| | | Results of Treatment Based on Tests | | | |
| | | Good | | Poor | |
Allergic Disease	No. of Cases	No. Cases	Per Cent	No. Cases	Per Cent
Eczema	36	2	6	34	94
Allergic Rhinitis	22	19	86	3	14
Bronchial Asthma	44	17	39	27	61
Urticaria	6	—		6	100
Total	108	38	35	70	65

TABLE IV. COMPARISON OF THE TESTS OBTAINED WITH THE PRESSURE-PUNCTURE
AND INTRACUTANEOUS TECHNICS IN THIRTY-EIGHT CHILDREN RESPONDING
FAVORABLY TO TREATMENT BASED ON THE LATTER METHOD

Case No.	Age in Years	Positive Pressure-puncture Tests	Positive Intra-dermal Tests	Allergens of Clinical Value
			Allergic Rhinitis	
1 S.J.	10	Vegetables	Cereals, vegetables	Cereals
2 R.D.	6	Cereals	Cereals, vegetables	Vegetables
3 J.B.	9	Dog dander, house dust	Feathers, house dust	Feathers
4 N.H.	9	Cereals	Feathers, orris root	Feathers
5 W.L.	7	Milk, cereals	Milk, cat and dog danders	Dog dander
6 T.B.	14	Feathers	Feathers, house dust, orris root	Feathers, house dust
7 L.E.	5	Cow dander, feathers	Banana, grape, pineapple	Banana, grape
8 S.S.	4	House dust	Orris root	Orris root
9 W.E.	11	Vegetables	Egg, cereals, vegetables	Cereals, vegetables
10 P.B.	9	Many weak reactions	House dust, orris root	Orris root
11 R.M.	13	,, ,, ,,	Milk, house dust	House dust
12 N.S.	13	,, ,, ,,	Cereals, vegetables	Cereals, vegetables
13 H.M.	13	,, ,, ,,	Cat and dog danders	Dog dander
14 L.N.	13	,, ,, ,,	Animal danders, orris root	Orris root
15 B.W.	11	,, ,, ,,	Milk, cereals, vegetables	Milk, cereals
16 I.A.	4	,, ,, ,,	Milk vegetables	Milk, vegetables
17 R.R.	10	,, ,, ,,	Wool, house dust	House dust
18 B.S.	10	,, ,, ,,	Wool, feathers	Feathers
19 W.B.	15	,, ,, ,,	Apple, feathers	Apple, feathers
			Bronchial Asthma	
1 B.S.	12	Cat dander, feathers	Milk, cat dander, feathers	Milk, feathers
2 R.F.	10	Silk	Animal danders, feathers	Feathers
3 L.B.	15	Wheat, peanut	Milk, cereals	Milk, peanut
4 U.L.	10	Cereals	Cereals, vegetables, house dust	House dust
5 L.R.	12	House dust, silk	House dust, orris root	Orris root
6 A.A.	12	Cereals, vegetables	Vegetables, mustard, chocolate	Chocolate, mustard
7 N.S.	8	Feathers, house dust	Egg, vegetables	Egg, feathers
8 E.B.	6	Egg	Animal danders, house dust	House dust
9 D.D.	9	Many weak reactions	Milk, feathers	Feathers
10 L.S.	4	,, ,, ,,	Cereals	Cereals
11 J.S.	11	,, ,, ,,	Vegetables, chocolate, house dust	Chocolate, house dust
12 R.F.	9	,, ,, ,,	Feathers, house dust	House dust
13 D.A.	7	,, ,, ,,	House dust	House dust
14 M.N.	11	,, ,, ,,	Chocolate, feathers	Chocolate, feathers
15 J.H.	6	,, ,, ,,	Animal danders	Dog dander
16 W.R.	8	,, ,, ,,	Cat dander, house dust	Cat dander
17 A.N.	4	,, ,, ,,	Milk, fruits, feathers	Feathers
			Eczema	
1 D.R.	2	Meats	Wool	Wool
2 H.J.	12	Many weak reactions	Vegetables, chocolate	Chocolate

outer aspect of the arm or the anterior aspect of the thigh is used. The skin is cleansed with alcohol and dried. A graduated 1 c.c. (tuberculin) syringe with a hypodermic needle of 27 gauge and a half inch in length is selected. After loading the syringe and ejecting all air bubbles, the needle is inserted into the corium through the integument. Not more than 0.01 c.c. of the sterile extract is injected. Control tests are similarly made with sterile extracting fluid. The tests are observed and read within ten to fifteen minutes.

In thirty-eight children good results were obtained by treatment based on the intracutaneous method of testing. Excellent results were obtained in the allergic rhinitis cases, the causative agent being found in 86 per cent of the children. Assistance was obtained in determining the underlying cause in 39 per cent of the children suffering with bronchial asthma. In eczema, however, the results were poor and the tests were of no value in the few remaining cases of urticaria. Table III present the results.

Interesting observations were made in the thirty-eight children responding favorable to the treatment based on the results of the intracutaneous technic when the positive reactions were compared with those previously obtained with the pressure-puncture method. The intradermal tests gave sets of positive reactions which often did not correspond very colsely with the positive tests of the pressure-puncture technic. Patients sensitive by skin testing to egg, milk or cereals by one method were found to give positive reactions to meats, vegetables or fruits by the other method. Food sensitivity by the pressure-puncture technic was found to be supplemented or replaced by inhalant sensitivity, by the intracutaneous technic, or the reverse might be true. For the sake of economy and clearness the data are summarized in Table IV. The children with definite positive tests by both methods are listed first and are followed by those in whom the pressure-puncture tests gave weak reactions to many allergens.

Incidentally the remaining seventy children in whom the intracutaneous tests were of no assistance in determining the cause of the allergic condition were subjected to less specific forms of treatment. In the cases of eczema, crude coal tar or its derivatives were used extensively. The orders concerning the application of the tar

were properly carried out in twenty-four children and fairly satisfactory relief was obtained, leaving ten children in whom the eczema was not controlled. The children with bronchial asthma were again examined and, in view of the poor response to the cutaneous tests, infection was now considered the most important cause of the asthmatic attacks. Tonsillectomy and adenoidectomy together with puncture and irrigation of the maxillary sinuses in some of the children was recommended. The operation was followed by prompt relief in eleven children, leaving sixteen cases in whom all forms of treatment were unsuccessful. The removal of the tonsils and adenoids gave relief to four of the six remaining children with urticaria and to the three with allergic rhinitis.

Summary and Conclusions

Three hundred cases of allergic disease in the child were subjected to a rather thorough investigation involving the various acceptable diagnostic procedures. This study yielded data of considerable value in determining the proper method of diagnosis and treatment for each allergic disorder.

First, the pressure-puncture cutaneous tests using glycerinized concentrated liquid extracts were applied to all the children. This technic was found to be tolerated by children of all ages from infancy through puberty.

1. The results of the treatment based on the positive reactions were satisfactory in 144, or 48 per cent, of the cases.
2. The procedure was of greatest value in hay fever and bronchial asthma, and of little value in allergic rhinitis, urticaria, and gastro-intestinal allergy.

Second, the elimination diets were tried. Excluding nine cases of hay fever, the diets were given to the remaining 147 children.

1. Thirty-nine of the cases, or 27 per cent, responded favorably.
2. The best results were obtained in urticaria and gastro-intestinal allergy. Only one-third of the cases of eczema and one-fourth of the cases of allergic rhinitis were helped by the diets. Little assistance was secured in bronchial asthma.

Third, the intracutaneous tests were applied to the 108 children who did not respond to the trial diets.

1. Treatment based ·on the results of this technic was satisfactory in thirty-eight, or 35 per cent of the cases.
2. The procedure was of greatest value in allergic rhinitis, and assistance was obtained in determining the causative agent or allergen in 39 per cent of the cases of asthma. Eczema made a poor showing.

These observations indicate that the allergic child could be treated with a minimum of time and effort if some attention was given to the fact that each allergic disease has a diagnostic procedure or procedures to which it responds best. In eczema the elimination diets and pressure-puncture tests are of greatest value; in allergic rhinitis, the intracutaneous tests; in hay fever, the pressure-puncture tests; in bronchial asthma, the pressure-puncture and intracutaneous tests; and in urticaria and gastro-intestinal allergy, the elimination diets.

◆ CASE REPORT ◆

ACUTE DISSEMINATED LUPUS ERYTHEMATOSUS ASSOCIATED WITH
MILIARY TUBERCULOSIS*

R. G. HINCKLEY, M.D., and C. A. McKINLAY, M.D.

Minneapolis, Minnesota

A PARTIAL review of the literature indicates that the association of acute disseminated lupus erythematosus with miliary tuberculosis has been of such relative rarity as to make this case of interest in that respect.

The patient, a male Hawaiian of Japanese extraction, twenty-five years of age, was admitted to the Students' Health Service on May 17, 1937. Prior to this illness, on admission to the University on September 27, 1932, the patient had been given a thorough routine physical examination. The findings at that time had been essentially negative, except for a positive Mantoux test (1-10,000 dilution), which was followed by a routine x-ray film of the chest, reported as negative on January 23, 1933.

History.—The illness began five days before admission, with chills, fever, and a dull ache between the shoulders, which became progressively worse. The patient stated that he had felt fairly comfortable when warm and in bed. Pain and chills had been simultaneous and frequent, but without regularity. Other complaints included occasional paroxysms of non-producive coughing and sensation of "heaviness in the chest."

Signs, Symptoms, and Clinical Course.—Examination on admission revealed a moderately inflamed pharynx, positive findings on the right side of the chest, temperature 104 degrees, pulse 118, and respiration 22. The positive chest findings were decreased motion on the right, dullness to percussion over the right base anteriorly and laterally, and massive showers of coarse, moist rales throughout the right lung above the area of dullness.

These signs and initial symptoms rapidly subsided. By the sixth day, the patient was apparently normal except for persistent constipation and minimal chest findings of a small area of decreased breath sounds and reinforced vocal resonance anteriorly at the right base and a few scattered sibilant rales posteriorly. The temperature began again to rise and leveled off at an approximate daily variation of 100 to 102 degrees; the constipation persisted; and a punctate erythematous rash appeared over the abdomen (May 27). Again the temperature mounted to an approximate level of daily variation from 102 to 105 degrees for one week (a peak of 105.6 degrees on June 1). The constipation was followed by diarrhea, and the abdominal rash altered to a generalized erythematous maculo-papular eruption—most marked on the trunk, but including the buccal mucosa. This rapidly became deeper in hue, morbilliform in character, and frankly coalescent. There was a moderate photophobia but no coryzal symptoms.

This rash faded in color, altered in character, and gradually localized primarily to the neck, face, knees, and elbows (June 3), but remained evident for the extent of the case. Cervical adenitis and mild bilateral palpebral conjunctivitis (similar to the general skin reaction) were noted. The face became edematous with brawny appearing skin, some grayish scaling and a V-line distribution over the neck and butterfly distribution over the nose and cheeks gradually becoming apparent. The temperature moderated but continued fairly constant throughout at an approximate daily variation of maximum peaks of 101 to 103 degrees. About the middle of this course (June 10) there was a very brief period of air hunger and rusty sputum which was probably an untoward therapeutic result. Gastro-intestinal upsets, with nausea and vomiting and an occasional period of diarrhea, were frequent in the latter period of illness. The patient was rational, and coöperative, except for brief periods of occasional delirium late in the afternoons of the last month. Bilateral chest signs were noted during the last month. The patient grew progressively moribund, and showed a profound terminal cachexia.

On August 3, the patient drank one and a half ounces of merthiolate solution—apparently with suicidal intent. When seen by the physician, he was nervous, sweating profusely, responsive and fully aware of the circumstances. The blood pressure was 70/0 and the pulse regular, extremely rapid, weak and

*From the Department of Preventive Medicine and the Students' Health Service of the University of Minnesota. Presented before the Minnesota Society of Internal Medicine, Nov. 8, 1937.

thready. Following emergency treatment and restorative attempts, signs of acute pulmonary edema developed, and on August 4 the patient expired.

Laboratory Studies.—Chest x-rays taken on May 18, May 25, June 1 and June 3 were all reported negative. One on June 25 showed broadening of the superior mediastinum probably due to motion. One on July 19 showed considerable distortion due to motion, but was reported as probably negative.

Urine analysis of eight specimens throughout the course of illness showed specific gravities of from 1.005 to 1.020, constant light traces of albumin, occasional pus cells, and on three occasions a few casts.

Complete blood counts were done on twenty-two specimens. These showed the white blood count most frequently at 2,400, gradually reaching 6-7000 during the latter days; high relative lymphocytosis, 50 to 75 per cent early, and shifting to a highly polymorphonuclear leukocytosis of 85 to 91 per cent in the later counts; red blood count of 4,000,000, dropping to 3,200,-000 before death, and hemoglobin starting at 89 per cent with 63 per cent finally. On one occasion (May 26) the platelets were 106,200.

Sputum was reported negative for pneumococci (types 1-8) on May 17 and June 8, and smears negative for acid-fast organisms on June 8. The urine and feces were reported negative for typhoid and related bacilli on May 28 and 29, and twenty-four hour urine specimen negative for acid-fast organisms, June 8. Blood was reported negative on agglutination tests for typhoid, paratyphoid, dysentery, and tularemia on May 26 and June 3; negative Wassermann, May 28; cultures and pour plates negative at 136 hour on June 1, June 5, and June 7; and guinea-pig inoculation with whole blood reported negative, June 8. Other miscellaneous reports were sedimentation rate on May 26, 1 hour –67 mm., 2 hour –96 mm.; NPN 26.2, June 10, BUN, 10.1, and spectroscopic blood showed evidence of metahemoglobin on June 8.

Therapy.—Other than general measures of dietary support, adequate nursing, etc., the case was subjected to few therapeutic measures. Two blood transfusions of citrated blood were given, one on June 3, of 400 c.c. and the other on June 10, of 300 c.c. Sulfanilamide was tried following the diagnosis of lupus erythematosus and while streptococcic septicemia was suspected. The patient received approximately thirty-two grams in divided dosage over a period of seventeen days. This treatment was initiated with equal quantities of soda bicarbonate, which had to be abandoned because of purgative results. On the sixth day of its administration after a maximum daily dose of grs. XV q.i.d., the patient developed air hunger and cyanosis, and blood spectroscopic analysis showed evidence of metahemoglobin. These symptoms rapidly disappeared upon the use of oxygen and temporary withdrawal of sulfanilamide followed by reduction in daily dosage. There were no noticeable or subjective symptoms of any beneficial effect. Emergency measures of the routine type were used terminally.

Autopsy.—The autopsy revealed: (1) Generalized miliary tuberculosis, involving the lungs, liver, spleen, kidneys, thymus, lymph nodes, and left seminal vesicle; (2) acute disseminated lupus erythematosus (regressing); (3) emaciation; (4) ingested merthiolate.

Discussion

Early in the course of the disease, attention was focused upon the physical findings in the chest, but there was no progression, and no x-ray changes were noted. The diagnostic study attempted to include elimination of bacteremia of any type, endocarditis, typhoid and related infections and pulmonary tuberculosis. Blood

cultures and common agglutination tests were negative and sputum examination did not reveal the causative organism. Serial x-ray films of the chest were interpreted as negative and a clinical diagnosis of miliary tuberculosis was not established. With the appearance of the skin lesion a diagnosis of acute disseminated lupus erythematosus was established by Dr. H. E. Michelson and Dr. F. M. Lynch, who studied the dermatological aspects of the case. The nature of the skin lesion, the fever, and the rather marked leukopenia were the basis of the diagnosis. Biopsy on June 4, 1937, offered confirmation in the nature of histopathologic changes. The finding of miliary tuberculosis at necropsy brings up the question of frequency of the association of lupus erythematosus and active tuberculosis. Keil[2] concluded from the study of 125 necropsy records in lupus erythematosus that only 20 per cent showed evidence of active or possibly active tuberculosis. In twenty postmortem examinations studied by Keil, one case of miliary tuberculosis was found in a case of sub-acute lupus erythematosus. Madden[3] reported nine cases at the University of Minnesota, and in three necropses no tuberculosis was found. O'Leary reported that five of ten cases of acute disseminated lupus erythematosus showed tuberculosis in some form, apparently not active. O'Leary[4] states the opinion from the evidence thus far that tuberculosis plays no significant rôle in lupus erythematosus, and that the syndrome is one of toxemia probably attributable to an infectious agent. Keil notes that the intensity of the cutaneous process cannot be correlated with the severity of the internal manifestations and looks on the visceral features and cutaneous lesions as due to a common cause. He feels that the patient with acute disseminated lupus erythematosus has a peculiar constitutional background, expressed in terms of an unstable vascular capillary system and that under stimulus of a variety of agents the vessels react to produce the unusual clinical picture. Goeckerman[1] emphasized the protean character of lupus erythematosus and the fact that the systemic manifestations with toxic or abdominal symptoms may predominate. He also noted that the sensitiveness of the patients to irritants in general and to removal of foci of infection was striking.

Summary

In the case of a young adult male, the clinical picture of acute disseminated lupus erythematosus developed with fatal termination, and the autopsy revealed in addition generalized miliary tuberculosis.

The rather unusual association of these diseases is reported.

References

1. Goeckerman, W. H.: Lupus erythematosis. Jour. A. M. A., 80:542-547, (Feb. 24) 1923.
2. Keil, H.: Conception of lupus erythematosis and its morphologic variants. Arch. Derm. and Syph., 36:729-757, (Oct.) 1937.
3. Madden, J. F.: Acute disseminated lupus erythematosis. Arch. Derm. and Syph., 25:854-875, (May) 1932.
4. O'Leary, P. A.: Disseminated lupus erythematosis. Minn. Med., 17:637-644, (Nov.) 1934.

PIONEER PHYSICIANS OF THE VERMILION AND MISSABE RANGES OF MINNESOTA

By OWEN W. PARKER, M.D.

(Continued from May issue)

Dr. Charles Lenont, whom we have spoken of as having first been associated with Dr. Harwood at the Fayal Mine and Fabiola Hospital, came to Virginia in January, 1901, and for one year maintained a small hospital and office in one of the store buildings on Chestnut Street. The present Lenont Hospital was built in 1903, and has been in continuous operation since that time, but has now been discontinued and remodeled, and houses the Lenont-Peterson Clinic.

The McIntyre General Hospital was built later in Virginia by E. H. McIntyre, who was there for a number of years and finally left, locating in the West.

Virginia has now just finished a fine new municipal hospital which is about ready for operation. Dr. Lenont is Chief of Staff.

Dr. James R. Humphrey, who has been mentioned as being one of the pioneer physicians of Biwabik and Virginia and was later associated with Dr. Shipman at Ely, was a Virginian by birth. He first entered the mining practice at Michigamme, Michigan, having succeeded his old preceptor, Dr. van Deventer, who had then left Michigamme to take a position in Ishpeming.

In January, 1881, he took postgraduate work in New York City, taking private instruction in physical diagnosis under Dr. Ed. J. Janeway, at Bellevue Hospital, and private instruction in operative surgery and surgical dressings under Dr. Joseph G. Bryant. He was in Butte, Montana, for a time and in other parts of Montana, and then came to the Iron Range of Minnesota early, as we have stated, about 1892. He left the Iron Range of Minnesota about 1902 and returned to his old home in Virginia and took over the management of a farm that he had become heir to, an old run-down southern estate of about 500 acres. The stone house on it had been burned during the Civil War. He began to improve the farm and bring it back to its pre-war beauty and fertility. He accomplished this with the same meticulous care and industry with which he did everything that he undertook. He died in his old home state of Virginia, January 10, 1922. He has a nephew practicing at Stillwater, Minnesota, Dr. Wade Humphrey, who at one time was associated with the Shipman Hospital staff at Ely.

Dr. Dana C. Rood was the pioneer physician of Hibbing. He came to Hibbing in 1893 and opened an office as physician for the iron ore mining companies around Hibbing. He was born in Windsor, Wisconsin, a small town near Madison, in 1864. His parents were natives of New York State. Soon after his birth, the family moved back to Watkins Glen, New York, in the beautiful Finger Lake country, where the doctor spent his early childhood and entered school. After finishing the public schools, he entered a preparatory school, or seminary, located at Dundee, New York. His family then moved to Wayne, Michigan. After his preparatory course he entered the University of Michigan, Medical Department, where he was graduated in 1886.

Following his graduation, he came on north and for part of 1886 and 1887 he was associated with Dr. Shipman at Bessemer, Michigan. He then left Dr. Shipman and opened an office in Duluth in 1888 and practiced medicine there. In 1890 he accepted a position in Zacatecas, Mexico, where he was located for about a year. Returning to Duluth from Mexico, he then, through the influence of Frank Hibbing, came to the Range and opened an office in Hibbing in 1892. Some of the doctors associated with Dr. Rood in his early days in Hibbing were Dr. John C. Rosser, Dr. G. N. Butchart, Dr. T. W. Stumm, and Dr. M. M. Ghent. The two latter located in Saint Paul and are now deceased. Dr. George F. Brooks, now located in Stillwater, Minnesota, was also an associate. In 1902, Dr. H. R. Weirick and Dr. S. S. Blacklock joined the staff and a year or so later Dr. W. F. Bullen, Dr. H. K. Reed, and Dr. E. E. Webber of Duluth.

As above stated, when operations began at Hibbing, Dr. Rood left Duluth and became the first physician of Hibbing. The Missabe Railroad reached Hibbing in the fall of 1893. The first train arrived in October or November of that year. After a trip by rail to Virginia, then to Mountain Iron, and from there on horseback, Dr. Rood first came to Hibbing in April, 1893, at which time there were a few tents and log cabins. In August, 1893, he returned to Hibbing to remain, sending in a few surgical and medical supplies, and established an office in the old Hibbing and Trimble building. At this time and for some months following, there was a severe epidemic of typhoid, and two months later Dr. Rood contracted the disease. It was not until the railroad reached there and he had partially recovered that he was able to get away from Hibbing.

About 1912 he left Hibbing and made his residence in Duluth, where he continues to live but still continues his association with the Rood Hospital at Hibbing. Hibbing has become one of the most famous and richest villages in the world. It is called the "Iron Ore Capital." Everything connected with this mining town has always assumed bigness. Along with its interesting history and growth has developed Dr. Rood's staff of physicians, which has become one of the largest medical organizations in the state.

When the north half of the village was moved to new Hibbing, the Rood Hospital was abandoned, and in its place the fine new Rood Hospital building was built at the new town of Hibbing.

The late Drs. Weirick and Bullen were pioneer members of this staff. Dr. S. S. Blacklock, contemporaneous with them, is now superintendent of the Rood Hospital.

Dr. Rood has seen all the amazing development of the great Hibbing district from its very beginning as a small rough mining camp where he went as its first doctor, practicing under difficult circumstances, to its present day greatness, truly a great drama of events to have lived through and have been associated with as first physician. The great village of Hibbing, among all its fortunate circumstances, was indeed fortunate in having a man of Dr. Rood's character and attainments as its pioneer physician.

Dr. Bertram Sage Adams, one of the early physicians on the Range, came to Hibbing in June, 1902, having been assistant to Dr. Bray at Biwabik in 1901.

He put a temporary shack up for an office, and started building a hospital at 426 Mahoning Street, moving into it in September, 1902. This was used for hospital and offices until 1915, when he built the hospital he is now using at 812 Third Avenue.

Dr. Adams has always been identified with all movements to improve medical practice on the Range. He is Councilor of the State Medical Association for this district, the only Range physician ever to hold this position.

Dr. Adams was born in Racine, Wisconsin, and graduated from the University of Minnesota Medical School in 1901. In June, 1902, he opened an office in

Hibbing, Minnesota, and at the same time opened the first medical office in the new mining town of Nashwauk, with Dr. James George in charge. During the first summer, a tent was used for office and living quarters by Dr. George while a new building was being erected. The following spring, Dr. George moved to Minneapolis, where he practiced until his sudden death about six years ago. His place was taken by Dr. John L. Shellman, who was associated with Dr. Adams for ten years, until he took postgraduate work in eye, ear, nose and throat work and then located in Saint Paul on the staff of Dr. Frank E. Burch, later with Dr. Ellwyn Bray establishing his own office in the Lowry Building in Saint Paul.

In the summer of 1903, Dr. Walter R. Schmidt became associated with Dr. Adams, and two years later opened an office in Chisholm. There he practiced until 1916, when he moved to Glencoe, Minnesota, where he is still practicing.

As previously stated, Dr. C. W. More of Eveleth came to Minnesota in the late eighties, was with Dr. Shipman at Ely for several years, then left and took a postgraduate course in New York, returning, as he says, broke financially. About this time, Mr. George St. Claire was opening a mine in Eveleth and upon the advice of friends, Mr. Joseph Sellwood and Mr. O. D. Kinney, Dr. More accepted a position as physician for the company at Eveleth. Dr. More states in his "Reminiscences of a Range Physician" that he came to Eveleth in June, 1894. The town had been started the year before, but hard times came on and it was partially deserted.

"When I arrived there was a saloon, a boarding house, three or four families, and a few shacks and tents where some of the miners lived. With borrowed money I bought a few drugs and dressings, a second-hand bed spring, a cheap mattress, moved into an unfinished and abandoned saloon shack, and took my meals in a large tent with the other mining employees. This dining tent was located near a small creek one could jump across. A hole had been dug near it by the proprietor of the tent, who was also the cook, to furnish water for washing clothes, dishes, et cetera. The summer was hot and dry. The inside top of the tent was black with flies. Typhoid fever resulted. The sick were cared for in tents, shacks, or wherever they lived. I was doctor and nurse, bathing the men, shaking out the dusty and dirty blankets and sheets if they had any. Most of the patients ran a temperature of 104 and 105. Some had complications. By September, the weather was getting colder. I had been running a low temperature for about three weeks, but kept going until one morning I did not have enough ambition to get up until someone came and wanted to know why I didn't go to see my patients. I was sent to St. Mary's Hospital in Duluth, where Dr. Sam H. Boyer, Sr., took care of me for two months. Drs. Bates and Miller of Virginia took care of the sick typhoid patients after I left. None of the patients in this epidemic of typhoid died. After leaving the hospital, I was laid up with phlebitis for three months. I returned to Eveleth in February, 1895. I went to work again considerably handicapped this time by being obliged to use a cane. I kept as an assistant the young physician who had been looking after my work during my absence, Dr. Darms. We had no hospital, but there was an empty one-story building boarded on the inside of the studding which we had made habitable by boarding up to the ceiling of the first floor on the outside and nailing some building paper on the inside and filling the space with sawdust. I put up two beds and heated the room by the box stove I had bought five or six months before. This makeshift camp served for a hospital for several months, when I had another one built, 25 x 40 feet, one story, but warmer and plastered, and filled with hospital beds. At one time we had nine patients with fractures, including a broken spine and a crushed pelvis."

This story of Dr. More's early experiences as a pioneer physician at Eveleth no doubt is illustrative of what most of the older pioneer physicians of the Range experienced. Dr. More is still on the Range at Eveleth. He probably has been in continuous practice for the mining companies on the Range longer than any other physician. He is Dean of Medicine on the Range. His long years of faithful service and devotion to his patients and to the practice of medicine, his fine character and unfailing integrity and absolute honesty entitle him to the greatest respect and honor. That his medical friends and lay friends are not unmindful of this is shown by the fact that they gave him a testimonial dinner in recent years as a token of their appreciation of him as a friend and physician.

Among Dr. More's early assistants were Dr. H. A. Darms, in 1894, previously mentioned, Dr. Wolner, Dr. E. B. Daugherty, now retired and living at Marine-on-St. Croix, and his brother Dr. L. E. Daugherty or Saint Paul, Dr. J. E. Arnold, now of Montana, Dr. F. J. Pratt, now of Minneapolis, Dr. W. A. Day, the late Dr. Fred Barrett, in 1898, and the late Dr. F. W. Bullen of Hibbing, in 1900. Dr. A. W. Shaw of Buhl became Dr. More's assistant in 1899, but left the More Hospital staff and moved to Buhl in September, 1901, and opened a temporary hospital in a store building. He was with Dr. More during the first smallpox epidemic in Eveleth, also during the time the town was moved from the Spruce Mine to its present site.

Buhl was organized in 1899, at the time of the opening of the Sharon Mine. The town was named after Frank Buhl of Sharon, Pennsylvania. Dr. Stuart Bates of Virginia, Minnesota, was the first physician in charge. Later, the Sharon Mine office was converted into a hospital.

Dr. Shaw was the pioneer physician of Buhl. His first assistant was Dr. R. R. Bailey, now of the Bailey Lumber Company. Dr. Shaw built a new hospital in 1918, and this was sold to the County in 1931, and is now used as a County Hospital. Dr. Shaw was at one time assistant in anatomy at the University of Minnesota under Prof. George A. Hendricks. Dr. Hendricks had previously been in the anatomy department at Ann Arbor, associated with the great anatomist, Corydon Ford.

The late Dr. Kirk of Los Angeles was one of the early physicians at Chisholm.

Associated early with the Rood Hospital was Dr. E. H. Nelson, who is still in Chisholm.

There have been many assistants or associates to these pioneer physicians of the Range, some of whom have become very prominent in medicine and surgery. Among them may be mentioned Dr. J. P. Sedgwick, Professor of Pediatrics at the University of Minnesota until his death, who was formerly with Dr. Harwood. Dr. George F. Dick, of Chicago, Department of Medicine, University of Chicago, who has done so much work in scarlet fever, was with Dr. Shaw about the years 1908-1909, leaving Dr. Shaw to study in Vienna. Dr. Frank Hirschboeck, prominent physician of Duluth, also was with Dr. Shaw a number of years. Dr. L. E. Daugherty, one of the prominent surgeons of Saint Paul, and his brother, Dr. E. B. Daugherty, were formerly associated with Dr. More at Eveleth. Dr. Robert Rizer, of Minneapolis, was formerly associated with Dr. Shipman at Ely, leaving Ely to become associated with Dr. Bertram Sippy of Chicago.

The late Dr. T. W. Stumm of Saint Paul was associated with Dr. Rood at the Rood Hospital at Hibbing. Dr. F. W. Schultz, Professor of Pediatrics at the University of Chicago, was on the Range for about one year, 1908-1909, at the Fabiola Hospital, Eveleth, associated with Dr. Harwood.

It may be said of the pioneer and early Range physicians that they were well-trained men and good doctors. Most of the men who came to the Range had had hospital internships and experience in hospital work before the medical schools of the country were requiring internships before graduation. The communities of the Range have been furnished with hospitals very early in their development and growth. Thus they have received a service which was not general over the State of Minnesota, at that time. These hospitals of the Range, that started almost with the beginning of the towns, have rendered a wide variety of service to almost every individual in the town, from the very minor things in surgery and medicine to the most complicated medical and surgical service, through their staff of physicians.

The Range Medical Society, organized a few years ago by the Range physicians as a subsidiary of the St. Louis County Medical Society, is a live, active organization, having had many excellent papers presented by men from Duluth, the Twin Cities, and Rochester, and having carried on postgraduate courses nearly every year in connection with the University Extension.

It is a far cry from the Iron Range of the day when Dr. Shipman walked through the muskeg swamp into Ely, when Dr. More settled in a saloon shack in Eveleth; when Dr. Rood first entered and saw the very beginnings of Hibbing, richest village in the world, and Dr. Shaw left Virginia on the "Old Wooden Shoe" at Gary, arriving at Buhl at 2 p. m., getting off at Buhl Station, a box car on a side track, and walking through a swamp on pole stringers, to find the Main Street of Buhl full of stumps. Yes, a far cry to the Range of today, with paved roads, white ways, wonderful school buildings, city halls and community centers, and hospitals, both general and contagious, a marvelous development to have occurred in the lifetime of a pioneer doctor. The frontiers of America have disappeared. The pioneers are fast disappearing, but when the last one has passed over the great divide, may the spirit of the Pioneer still live on, and may America never lose it.

(To be continued in July issue)

Western Electric 3-A Electrical Stethoscope

This portable electrical stethoscope is designed to aid the physician in hearing heart sounds and in diagnosing heart ailments. It has been developed particularly for physicians with impaired hearing, according to the firm. However, it is equally recommended to physicians with normal hearing in examining thick-chested individuals or detecting heart conditions during their early stages. It is claimed by the firm that other useful applications will be found in obstetric and lung fields. The Electrical Stethoscope essentially consists of a sensitive microphone, a vacuum tube amplifier and a receiver to reproduce the sounds. The two-stage amplifier, operated by dry batteries, will increase the loudness of the heart sounds about 20 decibels, or 100 times the intensity obtained with an ordinary acoustical stethoscope. The amplifier contains a filter which may be cut in or out of the circuit by means of a switch. The filter control diminishes the response at both the low and high frequencies; thus the intensity of normal heart sounds is lowered and the loudness of any existing murmurs is accentuated by the isolation. The Council reported that the instrument distorts in a measure the heart and breath sounds so that a certain amount of experience is necessary to learn the normal sounds as produced by it. Western Electric Company, New York. (J.A.M.A., April 2, 1938, p. 1111.)

MINNESOTA MEDICINE

OFFICIAL JOURNAL OF THE MINNESOTA STATE MEDICAL
ASSOCIATION

ublished by the Association under the direction of its Editing
and Publishing Committee

EDITING AND PUBLISHING COMMITTEE

. T. CHRISTISON, Saint Paul   C. B. WRIGHT, Minneapolis
. M. HAMMES, Saint Paul   T. A. PEPPARD, Minneapolis
WALTMAN WALTERS, Rochester

EDITORIAL STAFF
CARL B. DRAKE, Saint Paul, Editor
W. F. BRAASCH, Rochester, Associate Editor
GILBERT COTTAM, Minneapolis, Associate Editor

The right is reserved to reject material submitted for editorial
r advertising columns. The Editing and Publishing Committee
oes not hold itself responsible for views expressed either in
ditorials or other articles when signed by the author.

Classified advertising—five cents a word; minimum charge,
1.00. Remittance should accompany order.

Display advertising rates on request.

Address all communications to Minnesota Medicine, 2642 University Avenue, Saint Paul, or Suite 604, National Bldg., Minneapolis. Telephone: Nestor 2641.

BUSINESS MANAGER
J. R. BRUCE

Volume 21	JUNE, 1938	Number 6

State Meeting

THE stage is set for our annual meeting which is to be held this month in Duluth, almost two months later in the year than last year's meeting in Saint Paul. The time of meeting has been so planned that those attending can spend the week-end over the fourth of July in recreation in the north woods.

Perusal of the program, which appears in this number of the journal, shows that the main meetings of the Council and House of Delegates will be held in advance of the scientific sessions so as not to interfere with attendance at the general assemblies, which will this year replace sectional meetings. With clinics the third day, the program will occupy three instead of two days.

Nine outstanding specialists will appear as guest speakers on the program. Dr. Irvin Abell of Louisville, president of our national association and an outstanding surgeon, will address the Public Health meeting, open to the public, on the aims of the profession as they relate to the public. He will also give a talk to the profession on cancer. We all know of Dr. Howard W. Haggard of Yale, author of "Devils, Drugs and Doctors," who is equally famed as a public lecturer. He will address the Public Health meetings and will speak at the banquet Thursday evening.

Members of the Women's Auxiliary of the State Medical Association and the wives of state members who are not Auxiliary members are urged to attend the convention. In addition to the regular annual Auxiliary meetings, the St. Louis County Auxiliary members have arranged entertainment for visiting ladies, outstanding being a boat trip on Lake Superior on the Canadian liner Hamonic, on Friday.

The golf tournament for Association members is scheduled for Saturday following the meeting. For those who have never played the Northland course, there is the experience in store of watching a golf ball defy the laws of gravity by rolling up hill on the greens.

Some twelve hundred physicians are expected to attend the meeting. While most of those attending will be from Minnesota, an increasing number from neighboring states have been taking advantage of the scientific program in recent years and are again being invited to attend.

The Army Medical Library and Museum

THE present building of the Army Medical Library and Museum at Seventh Street and Independence Avenue in Washington was constructed by Congressional appropriation in 1887 and is now entirely obsolete and inadequate. Now pending in Congress is a bill providing for the appropriation of $3,750,000.00 to replace, in a better location, the present building with a modern fireproof structure of a type and style commensurate with the importance of this unique collection of books and specimens.

The Army Medical Library, now the largest

medical library in the world, was established in a small way by Surgeon General Lovell in 1836 and was known for many years afterwards as the Surgeon General's Library. It now contains approximately 300,000 books on medical subjects and, with the pamphlets, theses and other manuscripts, its collection numbers over a million separate items. By Acts of Congress of 1892 and 1901 the Library and Museum have been available to all scientific bodies and students. Thousands of readers and writers visit the Library yearly and by its inter-library loan system any reputable physician or scientist in this country may obtain any but the rarest books in its collection by making his request through the nearest library. It is the great central repository of medical literature, old and new, and contains many rare books, among them being about 460 of the existing 600 medical incunabula, or books published in the cradle age of printing, before 1500.

The oldest publication possessed by the library is Johannes Gerson's "De pollutione nocturna," printed in Cologne, in 1467, the only copy in the United States. Other rare old books are "Speculum humanæ vitæ" by Rodericus Zamorensis, printed in Rome in 1468, while among early writings on plague are "De epidemia" by Valescus de Taranta, Basel, 1470 and "Regimen pestilentiæ" by Alcanis Luis, printed in Valencia about 1490. The library has also a perfect copy of the first printed book on pediatrics, Bagellardo's "De infantium ægritudinibus," Padua, 1472, one of the two copies in the United States. Many of the incunabula are first editions. "De medicinis universalibus" by the Arabian physician Mesue the younger, printed in Venice in 1471, is the first purely medical book ever printed in the world.

The Library now receives two thousand medical journals and indexes every important article from every journal regardless of its country of origin or its language. The Index Catalogue of the Army Medical Library is world famous and has been in existence since 1879. It was characterized by the late Professor Welch of Johns Hopkins University, with the library itself, as "America's greatest gift to medicine."

The Army Medical Museum, now containing the largest number of pathologic preparations in America, was started in 1863 with specimens

from the hospitals and battlefields of the Civil War, and its enormous collection now covers the entire field of pathology. It maintains registries in seven important fields: eye, ear, nose and throat pathology, bladder tumors, lymphatic tumors, tumors in general, skin pathology and dental and oral pathology, all sponsored by national organizations interested in these various subjects, collecting and assembling the specimens with all available data in systematic fashion for ready consultation. With the Library, the Museum and the Index Catalogue, every resource for writing or research in any subject of any field of medicine is available under one roof. To the genius and industry of John Shaw Billings, whose career was epitomized in the editorial columns of MINNESOTA MEDICINE last month, is due the development of these three great activities, and the entire medical profession has been the gainer therefrom. It is little enough, it seems to us, that we lend our support to this movement to secure adequate housing for these priceless collections of books and specimens, where they may continue to give aid and support to the cause of scientific medicine.

G. C.

Insulin a Life Saver

SEVERAL years ago (1931) we called attention to the rise in the death rate from diabetes mellitus which had been unaffected by the discovery of insulin.* The death rate from diabetes had increased from 15.9 per 100,000 population in 1912 to 23.3 in 1928. In 1936 it had not receded and was 23.7. The explanation for such an unexpected increase was that either diabetes is more often diagnosed or is on the increase, or both.

How much of a boon insulin has been to diabetic individuals is well presented in a statistical analysis† of 2,271 deaths in diabetic patients seen by Joslin at the Baker Clinic in Boston between 1897 and 1928. The analysis of such statistics belongs to the sphere of the expert statistician and we are content to abide by the conclusions drawn by Dublin.

The patients are grouped according to the

*The Strange Case of Diabetes. Editorial. Minn. Med. 14:560, 1931.

†Joslin, E. P., Dublin, L. I., and Marks, H. H.: Studies, i Diabetes Mellitus, VI, Mortality and Longevity of Diabetics Am. Jour. Med. Sci., 195:596, 1938.

<table>
<tr><td>

In Memoriam

</td></tr>
</table>

F. Emerson Daigneau
1862-1937

DR. F. EMERSON DAIGNEAU was born at Hubbardton, Rutland, Vt., Ocober 1, 1862, and got his early education in the schools of that village. After attending Newton Academy at Shoreham, Vermont, he followed this with a course in the college at St. Hyacinthe, in the Province of Quebec. Later he went to New York and by his own resources worked his way through college there. He returned to Vermont and entered the medical department of the University of Vermont, graduating from there at the head of his class in 1886, with the degree of Doctor of Medicine. He received the highest honors of his class and the first prize established by the faculty for "general proficiency in examinations."

Dr. Daigneau practiced for a time at Somersworth, N. H., a year later came west to Saint Paul, and shortly thereafter came to the then growing city of Austin, where he remained until his death December 10, 1937. He was at one time a member of the Mower County Medical Society and the St. Olaf Hospital staff.

Dr. Daigneau was married March 31, 1888, to Miss Alice Merrick, of Somersworth, N. H., who survives him. He is also survived by six children: Donald V. and Ralph H. of Austin, Kenneth S. of New York, Maurice of Cleveland, Marcia L., now Mrs. P. H. Macfarlane of Chisholm, and Elizabeth A., now Mrs. T. E. Linnihan of Everly, Iowa.

Charles M. Storch
1870-1938

DR. CHARLES M. STORCH was born in Milan, Ohio, in 1870, and died March 13, 1938, at his home in Biloxi, Mississippi, after an illness of three years' duration.

Dr. Storch received his medical degree from the University of Michigan in 1891, after which he studied a year at the New York Polyclinic. He then became associated with his uncle, Dr. Charles Stewart, in Duluth. Moving to Grand Rapids, Minnesota, he devoted himself there to general practice for thirty-three years, until 1935, when he went to Minneapolis. Ill health prevented his carrying on active practice in Minneapolis.

Dr. Storch's father, Dr. August von Storch, was a graduate of Heidelberg University and for many years was a well known medical authority in Washington, D. C. He is survived by his widow, a half brother, Dr. Raymond Storch, a lieutenant commander in the United States Navy, and a step-son, Ralph E. Dawley, of Long Beach, California.

Dr. and Mrs. Storch moved to Biloxi about a year and a half ago, to occupy a home they had built there.

MEDICAL ECONOMICS

Edited by the Committee on Medical Economics
of the
Minnesota State Medical Association

W. F. Braasch, M. D., Chairman

SURVEY PROGRESS

Form No. 1 of the Survey on Medical Care was sent in May to all secretaries of county and district medical societies in Minnesota for distribution to members.

These forms should be filled in carefully and returned UNSIGNED to the county or district secretary.

The objective of this Survey is, fundamentally, to find out how many there are who are going without needed medical care and why.

This objective cannot be accomplished without the active interest and assistance of every physician.

HAVE YOU FILLED OUT AND RETURNED YOUR FORM?

If not, you should do so immediately. This is the most important task before American Medicine today.

The bulletin and instruction sheet which accompanied the Form is printed below in the hope that it will serve to re-emphasize in the minds of all physicians the importance of their part in this nation-wide effort.

Your Professional Future Is at Stake

Our whole system of medical practice in the United States has been challenged. There is criticism of the medical profession and of the adequacy of medical care on all sides.

ARE WE FAILING TO DELIVER ADEQUATE MEDICAL CARE TO ALL THE PEOPLE?

If we are, we must know the facts. Other groups who have attempted to study medical care have not presented a true picture of conditions because they have not had the active participation of the physician, who is the chief factor in the delivery of medical care in the United States.

NOW—THE AMERICAN MEDICAL ASSOCIATION, WITH THE ASSISTANCE OF HOSPITALS, NURSES, DENTISTS, PHARMACISTS, IS UNDERTAKING AN ACCURATE, HONEST, COUNTY-BY-COUNTY STUDY OF THE FACTS.

THIS IS YOUR STUDY—AND THE RESPONSIBILITY FOR MAKING NEEDED IMPROVEMENTS AS DISCLOSED IN THIS STUDY WILL BE YOUR RESPONSIBILITY. ABOVE ALL IT IS NOT TO BE JUST ANOTHER STATISTICAL EXERCISE TO BE FILED AWAY AND FORGOTTEN.

Following are the instructions for fill-out Form No. 1. They are numbered according to the question in each case. Forms are to be returned to me* unsigned.

1. If you have no exact figures, make a careful estimate.
2. Relief, Old Age Assistance, Farm Security patients, etc., included.
3. Make as accurate an estimate as possible.
4. Exact figures should be available here in most cases.
5. This refers to private practice as well as to public health services.
6. Make this reply as exact as possible.
7. This question should be answered frankly and fully.
8. Exact figures if available; otherwise give a careful estimate.
9. This is important. Answer in detail using extra sheet if needed.

*Secretary of Society.

Teachers Respond

Officers in charge of the Survey in Minnesota have been especially interested to note the enthusiasm and promptness with which other agencies have responded to the request for assistance in gathering pertinent information from their own records and experience.

Hospital, nursing and welfare organizations have taken an official hand in sending the appropriate forms to their member groups. The State Department of Education has sent forms to all superintendents of public schools in the state. Information is coming in rapidly from parochial and Catholic high schools all over the state and from the colleges, all of whom are communicating directly with the State Office.

Interest Is Keen

The speed and alertness exhibited by the principals of the Catholic secondary schools in responding to the request is an encouraging indication of the interest of these educators in the health of their charges and in the effort of the physicians to make accurate studies of their needs.

Below are comments selected at random from the large number of questionnaires already returned in spite of the fact that they reached the desks of the Sister Principals in the busiest month of the year.

It should be noted that a significant number attribute lack of proper care among their pupils to parental neglect.

It is obvious, also, in these comments that, while county medical societies are shouldering their responsibilities in many communities, in others not even a nurse has interested herself in the health of the school for years. It is the hope of the committee in charge of the Survey that this study will bring home to doctors everywhere the need to correct such situations as this wherever they are found. If the interest is great enough, some arrangement can always be made, and the best arrangements, as these answers indicate, are in the communities where the local doctors have taken a hand.

* * *

"We believe an annual dental examination would prove a great benefit. As there are several pupils in each classroom of our school who need glasses, a checkup on sight would be a great help."—Madison.

Parents Careless

"Arrangements for health supervision are made chiefly by the teachers and by the parents in our school. Nothing special is done in this line. The county nurse should do it but has not come around within five years or more. The fact is that even if the parents are told to take their child to a physician, it is not done. Many of our children lack needed medical care but it is due chiefly to carelessness on the part of the parents."—Collegeville.

* * *

"Every fall the physicians and a dentist from town come to examine our pupils but do not give free treatments. Last fall all our children were immunized against diphtheria and vaccinated for smallpox. The charge was 50 cents for each child. Our children are fairly well taken care of by their parents. We know of but one family that is in great need of medical care but has not the means to meet expenses. There ought to be a general fund to provide for this deficiency."—Loretto.

Legion, Lions Assist

"The local American Legion has sponsored a health program in the local schools the last two years. Previous to that we had a county nurse for a brief period of time. She visited the schools once during a term. Due to our doctors from both clinics who offered their services gratis and also to the coöperation of the able chairman of the American Legion Auxiliary, all the children whose parents consented were both vaccinated and immunized against diphtheria.

"Our pupils who suffered from poor eyesight and were too poor to pay for medical care of glasses were cared for by the local Lions' Club.

"The superintendents of the various schools here have agreed on engaging a nurse for the coming school term. Each school has been taxed for the purpose and our Reverend Pastor and his trustees will pay their apportionment."—Wadena.

"They Would Be Well Served"

"Arrangements with the county medical society were made for free vaccinations of whole families of indigent children. The people in this community would be well served if they took advantage of all services offered either free or at a small cost . . ."—Minneapolis.

* * *

"We as teachers feel that something should be done. We positively know that some pupils need medical attention for teeth, eyes, undernourishment, etc. Some children, for example, can read only when their eyes are at a certain angle. We have asked the parents to look after these children but we must have influential coöperation."—New Market.

* * *

"The need for medical care among the children of this particular school seems not great as the parents take exceptionally good care of them and willingly coöperate in any measures which are proposed to safeguard their health. From the standpoint of the teacher, however, it would be immeasurably valuable to us if through complete physical examinations we could become acquainted with the physical status of our children. Experience has taught us that often retardation is due to some unknown physical defect. If the health department is not able to appoint doctors to conduct these examinations periodically perhaps volunteers from the medical profession would give a day or a half-day to this work."—Minneapolis.

Need Nurse

"Common colds and coughs are greatly neglected. Skin diseases have gained some headway this year. A number of our pupils' eyes have been examined by oculists at our suggestion. We should deem it advisable to have the services of a nurse at least once a year."—Kimball.

* * *

"Some arrangements should be made for dental treatment or clinics for parochial schools. Ancker Hospital and Wilder Dispensary are overcrowded and do mostly extractions. Indigent pupils and those that could pay a little must neglect their teeth until decay progresses far enough for extraction."—Saint Paul.

* * *

"The county nurse visited our school once in four years. We have no doctor in this town."—Greenwald.

* * *

"No physician or nurse has called here since 1936. We have had good attendance at school this past school year and very little sickness. If any child living near by is sick we send him home immediately; if he lives at a great distance and has no telephone at home we give as much relief as we can by applying home remedies."—St. Leo.

* * *

"Three or four promises have been made to inspect our children; however, none was kept. We have received no attention this year."—Virginia.

Thanks to Doctors

"The medical care of the boys in this school is excellent—thanks to the splendid men of the Minnesota Medical Association who give generously of their time and service."—Minneapolis.

* * *

"Both medical and dental societies are willing to give treatment free of charge to pupils who are in need of such service."—Faribault.

BUTTER SUBSTITUTE CONTROVERSY

Did the A.M.A. discriminate against butter in favor of oleomargarine?

It did not.

Why did the A.M.A. refuse to standardize butter?

Because they found it impractical with their limited resources to inspect and standardize the innumerable brands and the constantly changing character of butter.

Their action was taken with no intent whatever to discriminate against butter in favor of any other product.

They took it for granted that everyone knew that natural butter fat was preferable to any substitute.

They also knew that Federal inspection was available to any producer of butter who wishes inspection and certification.

Why then did the A.M.A. continue to standardize and grade substitutes for butter fat?

Because there are many brands on the market which are being consumed by the public, some of which are of much higher nutritional value than others.

The public had no means of determining their comparative value.

The A.M.A. approved those brands which on analysis had the greatest food value. In this way the interests of the public were protected—not the manufacturers.

Such action in no way discriminated against butter or the farmer.

Iowa Protest

The Iowa State Medical Association passed a resolution on May 13 protesting the acceptance of substitutes for dairy products. The action was taken, without doubt, because of local agitation among Iowa dairy farmers and manufacturers of dairy products.

There has been similar agitation in Minnesota; but most physicians and others in Minnesota realize well the position of the American Medical Association. They know that everybody, including the "oleo" manufacturers, are aware of the superiority of butter as a food to any of its substitutes. They also know that there are millions of people in some sections of the United States who cannot afford to buy a sufficiency of dairy products for their families. People demand and use a cheap substitute and they are entitled to know, if possible, whether wholesome materials are used in the substitute and whether or not it is produced under wholesome conditions.

Public Duty

In investigating these substitutes as they apply and awarding the Seal of Acceptance to those whose materials, manufacture and advertising claims live up to the high standard

434

pital, or other vendor who is selected by client. This form will be presented to vendor, physician, dentist, hospital, or other, and will be authority for rendering the specified service. Responsibility for medical care is not accepted without his order except in emergencies."

Mr. Ervin richly deserves the thanks not only of those persons who are so unfortunate as to be out of work and on relief, but also the appreciation of each and every member of the medical profession, for his broad and fair-minded interpretation of this law. It seems only right and proper that when free choice is permitted as to the every-day commodities of life, such as food, clothing, etc., the principle of free choice of physician should be preserved.

MEDICAL CARE IN THE DOMINION

New plans for delivery of medical service are being worked out on an extensive scale these days by Canadian medical associations and the provinces and municipalities.

This development should be of great interest to physicians of the United States because conditions and people in various sections of Canada more nearly resemble those below the border than in any other country in the world.

Looking to England

It is quite natural, of course, that there should be a sympathetic feeling toward health insurance among a good many Canadian physicians since Canadians normally look to England to lead the way in many fields. It is interesting to note, however, that, where the mother country rushed headlong into health insurance and spent twenty-five years patching up discrepancies and undoing blunders, Canada is proceeding cautiously, gathering statistics, making local studies. If health insurance should ever become a reality there, on a national scale, it will be with full knowledge that the needs in the Western Provinces are quite different from those in the urban centers and that many little plans must be made to fit into the general pattern.

This was the gist of an address by Dr. F. W. Jackson, Deputy Minister of Health of the Province of Manitoba, before the Conference of State and Provincial Health Authorities of North America in Washington recently. Following are some of the types of service now

in operation in various parts of the Dominion as described by Dr. Jackson:

The Municipal Doctor System. By this system the municipality, local unit of government in Western Canada, covering an area of from 200 to 300 miles with a population of from 1,500 to 3,000 persons, hires the doctor on a salary basis. The salary varies from $3,000 to $4,000 yearly with certain perquisites and allowances for leaves to take post-graduate work, attend meetings. The municipal doctor is health officer and physician and he has the right to charge for a certain portion of his services.

System Is Spreading

This type of service has extended of late until it covers more than one-fifth of the rural municipalities of Saskatchewan already, with as many more preparing to institute similar plans. In Manitoba nine rural municipalities are receiving medical care under the plan with three or four others preparing to join them and two providing similar care for their urban residents on a *fee for services rendered basis.*

Lump sum basis with free choice of physician. In the Province of Ontario the Provincial government pays over to the medical profession a definite amount, varying from 35 to 50 cents per head, for medical care of the unemployed. The profession in return sees that care is provided. The doctors have divided the province into 11 districts with a local committee of physicians to supervise the service and distribution of funds for the district. The physicians send an account of services rendered at the end of each month, using the regular schedule of fees, and the physicians' committee prorates the total amount available. It appears to work out at about 40 per cent of regular fees paid to the physicians who do the work.

In the western provinces the same type of plan is operating in the cities.

Like Minnesota Plan

Fee basis with free choice of physicians. In Winnipeg a system of services upon a special fee basis has been set up with much the same type of regulation as governs medical care for the indigent in the majority of Minnesota counties. The city provides the funds but the administration is under complete control of the medical profession through a medical advisory committee which has authority to settle all disputes that may arise. The same plan is followed in most of the other cities in the Province of Manitoba.

It should be interesting to Minnesota physicians to note that in Manitoba wherever the service is in charge of the Manitoba Medical Association, a deduction of 5 per cent is made on all doctors' accounts. This 5 per cent is paid into the funds of the Association for defraying costs of supervision. It has resulted in the accumulation of a considerable sum of money above and beyond the amount needed to administer the service and this fund is to be held, according to Dr. Jackson, "in a trust fund to be used if and when consideration is given to some province-wide form of state medicine or health insurance."

Statistics for the Future

"The information obtained from the returns of the physicians under the plan in operation in Winnipeg," Dr. Jackson also remarked, "has been tabulated from year to year and we are now getting a fund of statistics which will be of real value in estimating the amount and type of illness and its requirement in terms of medical care in an urban community."

Health insurance acts have been passed in Alberta and in British Columbia. In Alberta, although the act was passed in 1934 setting forth all details, the plan has as yet not been put into operation. In British Columbia, as noted previously in these columns, the opposition of the organized medical profession has made it impossible to establish the plan. The opposition, according to Dr. Jackson, was due chiefly to the decision of the government not to include indigents in the scheme. A plebiscite on the question which took place in the summer of 1937 is said to have revealed public opinion in favor of some sort of Health Insurance.

"What the future may hold," said Dr. Jackson in conclusion, "remains to be seen; but one fact is apparent—as yet we have not the required information in Canada to allow us to set up in all its details, with any degree of actuarial accuracy, a scheme of adequate medical care for all groups of our population. We must get more information as to the amount and types of illnesses among the various groups of our population in the different sections of Canada and it would seem unwise for the Dominion or any province to embark on a wholesale scheme for the provi-

ECONOMICS SESSION

Chief Justice H. M. Gallagher will be principal guest speaker at the annual Medical Economics session to be held in connection with the State Meeting at Duluth, June 29, 30 and July 1.

Medical jurisprudence and our relations with the Bar have a place of particular prominence at this session. The second speaker is Mr. Stanley B. Houck of Minneapolis, Chairman, Standing Committee on Unauthorized Practice of the Law, American Bar Association.

Following these two talks scheduled for Friday morning, July 1, Dr. J. M. Hayes of Minneapolis will give the annual president's address. The subject, "Medical Problems in Minnesota," is timely and the active participation of President Hayes in medical, medical-economic and sociological affairs of the society assures a vigorous and individual paper.

"THE COMMUNITY PAYS"—Parran

"The community pays for preventable disease and disability. It pays in relief of the unemployables, in pensions and in institutional care. It would be cheaper for us as a nation to spend more for the prevention and care of disease than to continue to bear its money cost. It is, therefore, not only the humane but the practical consideration which brings to our attention the acute need for dealing courageously with unnecessary sickness in this country. Our efforts up to now have been sporadic, half-hearted, and frequently unscientific. The time seems opportune for the best minds in the medical profession to consider how medical knowledge can best be brought to fuller use by all of the people— how we may take up the lag between what we know and what we do. It should be possible for a national health program to be evolved which would be adapted to the varying needs of each state and community.

A practical program to utilize our scientific resources for life-saving would bring advantages to our profession almost as great as to the population which would be served."—Surgeon-General Thomas Parran, U. S. Public Health Service, before the Conference of State and Provincial Health Authorities of North America, April 9, 1938.

MINNESOTA STATE BOARD OF MEDICAL EXAMINERS

Cokato Chiropractor Pleads Guilty to Practicing Without a License

Re State of Minnesota vs. Harold A. Kirsch.

On May 2, 1938, the above defendant, Harold A. Kirsch, thirty-three years of age, entered a plea of guilty to an information charging him with practicing healing without a basic science certificate. Kirsch pleaded guilty at Buffalo, Minnesota, before the Honorable Leonard Keyes, Judge of the District Court for Wright County. After hearing the facts, Judge Keyes sentenced the defendant to pay a fine of $200.00 or serve sixty days in the Minneapolis Work House. The defendant is suffering from multiple sclerosis, and the Court, upon being advised of all the facts, suspended the sentence and placed the defendant on probation upon the condition that he refrain from practicing healing in any manner.

Kirsch, who stated that he was raised at St. Cloud, opened an office at Cokato, Minnesota, in the fall of 1937. He represented himself to the public as a chiropractor and an x-ray technician. He claims to be licensed to practice chiropractic in the State of Iowa, and that he formerly maintained an office at Mason City, Iowa. Following an investigation conducted by the Minnesota State Board of Medical Examiners, a complaint was filed against the defendant on February 1, 1938. Following his arrest Kirsch closed his office. The office has since been reopened by a licensed chiropractor. The defendant undoubtedly deserves considerable sympathy because of his physical condition; nevertheless, he was previously advised that he could not practice in Minnesota without a license, and consequently, when he opened up his office. the Board had no other alternative than to proceed with the case.

Austin Doctor Dies Following Arrest

Re State of Minnesota vs. Fannie Fiester.

On Wednesday, May 4, 1938, the Minnesota State Board of Medical Examiners received a telephone call from Mr. A. B. Anderson, County Attorney of Steele County, informing them that Mr. and Mrs. Anton Ruzek, R. F. D. No. 2, Blooming Prairie, were in his office to make a complaint that a lady doctor at Austin had performed a criminal abortion upon their eighteen year old daughter. The co-operation of the Medical Board was requested in making the investigation and Mr. Brist was assigned to this case.

Following the investigation, which was immediately made, and which included a long signed statement by the daughter, a complaint was filed on May 5, 1938, by the mother, and a warrant issued for the arrest of Dr. Fannie Fiester of Austin. Dr. Fiester was questioned by Mr. Edward T. Helgeson, Sheriff of Steele County, and Mr. Brist, and also by Mr. A. C. Richardson, County Attorney of Mower County. Dr. Fiester admitted having performed the criminal abortion and also admitted performing a number of other unlawful abortions. Dr. Fiester was very frank in her statements, and upon being arraigned in the Municipal Court at Austin, she was released on condition that she furnish a $500.00 bond. The matter was continued until Friday morning, May 6, at which time it was learned that Dr. Fiester was found in a serious condition and died that evening about 10 P.M. Mrs. Ruzek also filed a complaint against Mrs. Clara Cole of Blooming Prairie in connection with this case, and also a complaint against Lyle Cole, twenty-four-year-old son of Mrs. Cole. The complaint against Lyle Cole was filed in Steele County.

This statement is made by the Medical Board in fairness to everyone concerned, and particularly in view of the fact that the case ended in the manner that it did. The Board feels that Mr. Anderson and Mr. Stone, the Assistant County Attorney at Owatonna, Sheriff Helgeson, Mr. Richardson and Deputy Sheriff Enochson of Austin, were sincerely attempting to perform their duty in respect to this case, and that, while it had a tragic outcome, the entire matter should serve a worthwhile purpose.

Minnesota Physician's License Suspended for Two Years

In the Matter of the Revocation of the License of Harold Rees, M.D.

On May 13, 1938, the Minnesota State Board of Medical Examiners suspended for a period of two years the license to practice medicine held by Dr. Harold Rees of Minneapolis. Dr. Rees' license was suspended because of habitual indulgence in the use of narcotics. His case was called to the attention of the Board by a shortage in his supply of morphine and cocaine discovered by agents of the Bureau of Narcotics.

Dr. Rees is at the State Hospital at Willmar at the present time following his commitment from Hennepin County on April 13, 1938. Dr. Rees has been at Willmar on several previous occasions and the leniency shown him on those occasions accomplished nothing. If Dr. Rees leaves the hospital this time before he is discharged by competent authority his license will be revoked permanently.

Dr. Rees was born in Norway in 1869 and is a graduate of Rush Medical College in 1896. He was licensed in Minnesota by examination in 1900. Dr. Rees has practiced in the following towns in the past ten years: Saint Paul, Cambridge, New London, Ogilvie, Rose Creek, Rushmore and Minneapolis.

Medical Board Revokes Minnesota License of Indiana Physician

In the Matter of the Revocation of the License of George Henry Espenlaub, M.D.

At the regular meeting of the Minnesota State Board of Medical Examiners held on May 13, 1938, the Minnesota license to practice medicine held by Dr. George Henry Espenlaub now serving a one to ten year sentence in the Indiana State Prison at Michigan City, Indiana was revoked. Dr. Espenlaub, while practicing at Evansville, Indiana, was convicted of a felony, to-wit: assault and battery with intent to commit a felony, to-wit: Rape. Dr. Espenlaub was convicted by a jury and his conviction was upheld by the Supreme Court of Indiana. The record discloses that the crime was committed upon a patient in the office of Dr. Espenlaub.

Dr. Espenlaub was born in Evansville, Indiana, in 1898 and received his M.D. degree from Indiana University in 1922. He was licensed in Minnesota in 1923 by reciprocity with the State of Indiana. However, Dr. Espenlaub did not register with the Minnesota Board in 1928 under the Basic Science law nor has he registered since that date.

POTENCY OF LIVER PRODUCTS

As there is no satisfactory laboratory method which may be used for the standardization of anti-anemia preparations, the Committee of Revision of the Pharmacopeia has provided for an Anti-Anemia Preparations Advisory Board to pass on clinical data which manufacturers of these products might present, and if the data indicated a satisfactory degree of potency, the board would approve the product and it could be labeled under the U.S.P. title. Under the rules of the board the amount of liver supposed to be represented in the product may not be mentioned on the label, as it is likely to be misleading; a product derived from 100 Gm. of liver is not necessarily twice as potent as one made from 50 Gm. Products will now be labeled in units, and patients should receive for a maintenance dosage an average of about a unit each day. (J.A.M.A., March 19, 1938, p. 903.)

Dr. G. C. Edwards, formerly of Grove City, has opened an office in Cokato.
* * *
Dr. W. R. Kostick, formerly of Robbinsdale, has located in Fertile, where he will practice medicine.
* * *
Dr. and Mrs. E. O. Strassman have moved to Houston, Texas, where Dr. Strassman will practice medicine.
* * *
Dr. John S. Hamlon of Minneapolis has become associated with Dr. R. L. Page of St. Charles, in the practice of medicine.
* * *
Dr. William N. Freeman, Jr., of Perham, Minnesota, was married May 7, 1938, to Miss J'Austa White of Colfax, Washington.
* * *
Dr. A. W. Pasek, who has been practicing medicine at Lismore for the past year, has moved to Cloquet, where he will open offices.
* * *
Dr. E. M. Howg of Lennox, South Dakota, has located at Hills, for the practice of medicine. Dr. Howg was formerly a member of the Mayo Clinic staff.
* * *
Dr. Charlotte Miller of Fargo, North Dakota, is the first woman to finish a year's internship at St. Joseph's Hospital in Saint Paul. She received her diploma early in May.
* * *
Dr. Stella Wilkinson has located at Askov, where she will practice medicine. She is a graduate of the University of Minnesota and has recently been practicing medicine in Duluth.
* * *
Dr. Lyle Joseph Hay of Minneapolis was married on April 16 to Miriam Ilona Raihala, daughter of Dr. and Mrs. John Raihala of Virginia. Dr. Hay is at present an interne at General Hospital in Minneapolis.
* * *
Dr. W. C. Kaufman of Appleton has announced the addition of Dr. Frank E. Lipp on the staff of the Kaufman Hospital. Dr. Lipp was formerly resident physician at Neurological Hospital on Welfare Island, New York City.
* * *
Dr. D. C. Balfour and Dr. J. de J. Pemberton of Rochester attended the meeting of the Society of Clinical Surgery in Chicago, April 29 and 30. Dr. Balfour also attended the meeting of the American Surgical Association in Atlantic City early in May.
* * *
Dr. Ambrose Sprafka has opened an office in St Cloud for the practice of medicine. Dr. Sprafka is graduate of the University of Minnesota School of Medicine, and has just completed an internship at the Hospital St. Anthony De Padua in Chicago.

Dr. Dimitri Kalinoff of Stillwater was named to the Stillwater American Legion's Hall of Fame at a banquet held at the Lowell Inn early in May. Dr. Kalinoff was selected for his "unselfish service, without thought of gain" to the community within the past five years.

* * *

Dr. and Mrs. Owen W. Parker of Ely have returned from a recent automobile tour of the southern states, visiting all the Lincoln shrines and many other historic spots. One especially interesting to physicians was the home of Dr. Ephriam McDowell at Danville, Kentucky, where Dr. McDowell performed the first laparotomy in 1809.

* * *

Dr. and Mrs. John S. Lundy of Rochester returned from a three months' European trip, May 27. They toured Italy, Hungary, Germany, Holland, Belgium, France and England. Dr. Lundy was very favorably impressed with the work being done by European physicians as evidenced in the various clinics he attended while there.

* * *

Dr. H. L. Williams of Rochester attended the meeting of the American Laryngological, Rhinological and Otological Society, held in Atlantic City the last week in April, where he appeared on the program, and also attended the meetings of the American Laryngological Association and the American Otological Society, held the following week.

* * *

Dr. H. I. Lillie of Rochester attended the meeting of the American Laryngological, Rhinological and Otological Society held in Atlantic City the last week in April. Dr. Lillie was elected president of the Society at the last meeting. Dr. Lillie also took part in discussions at the meetings of the American Laryngological Association and the American Otological Society, held the first week in May.

* * *

The physicians in the Red Wing territory connected with St. John's Hospital were entertained at a banquet in St. James Hotel dining room on April 19, with members of the hospital board as hosts. The group included over fifty local physicians, and their wives. Dr. Branton of Willmar delivered the principal address of the evening. Dr. L. E. Claydon of Red Wing showed moving pictures taken on his recent trip to Mexico and South America.

* * *

Dr. Theodore Erickson of Montreal, son of Professor and Mrs. T. A. Erickson of Saint Paul, was married May 24 to Miss Mary Rachel Harrower, daughter of Mr. and Mrs. James Harrower of Cheam, Surrey, England. Dr. Erickson is a University of Minnesota graduate and at present is assistant neuro-surgeon at the Montreal Neurological Institute of McGill University. Miss Harrower is a graduate of the University of London and obtained her Ph.D. from Smith College. She has been a research fellow in the Neurological Institute.

HOSPITAL NOTES

The Nagel Hospital at Waconia has recently installed a new deep therapy x-ray unit.

* * *

Dr. Peter Ward, superintendent of the Miller Hospital, Saint Paul, was installed as president of the Minnesota Hospital Association at the close of the association's convention at the Nicollet Hotel, Minneapolis, May 21. Other officers elected were A. G. Stasel, Minneapolis, president-elect; Miss Amy Gunderson, Benson, first vice president; Dr. T. E. Broadie, Saint Paul, second vice president; Roy M. Amberg, Minneapolis, treasurer; and Arthur M. Calvin, Saint Paul, secretary.

New members of the board of directors are Miss Mabel Korsell, Grand Rapids; J. H. Mitchell, Rochester; Miss Esther Wolfe, Minneapolis; Dr. M. J. Hauge, Jr., Clarkfield; and Sister M. Patricia, Duluth.

Dr. A. F. Branton, of Willmar, was named delegate to the American Hospital Association for two years.

Eleven Deaths From a Cancer Treatment

In October, 1935, when the "Ensol" treatment was launched from Kingston, Ont., with what appeared to be carefully planned publicity in the newspapers, *The Journal* issued a warning to the effect that the product was being developed under uncontrolled conditions and that its exploitation would inevitably lead to grief for those concerned. Nevertheless a considerable number of doctors in various parts of the United States have used a product of this type in the treatment of cancer and it is obvious that at least has come to grief. It seems that the Biochemical Research Foundation of the Franklin Institute of Philadelphia prepared the product called B or Rex, which caused the deaths of 11 patients in Orlando, Fla. It seems likely that batch 152 was prepared on a Friday, some of it permitted to stand over Saturday and Sunday, and then sterilized on Monday. If the tetanus organism was present in the product it would have had two days in which to develop the toxin, so that when the product was sterilized on Monday a sufficient amount of tetanus toxin was present to cause death. These possibilities remain to be confirmed by more evidence—but certainly enough evidence is available to warrant the suggestion. At present there are being exploited to the American people a half dozen or more treatments of cancer that are in no way established as actually of value in the treatment of that condition. Enough is now known about the nature of cancer to indicate that the value of a cancer remedy cannot be established by sending it at random to physicians scattered all over the country, who use it in practice for a fee. The development, exploitation and promotion of "Ensol" and of its progeny "B" have been unscientific, unethical and unwarranted.—(J.A.M.A., April 9, 1938, p. 1194.)

MINNESOTA STATE MEDICAL ASSOCIATION
Eighty-Fifth Annual Session
June 29, 30 and July 1, 1938
Duluth, Minnesota

OFFICERS AND COMMITTEES

President—J. M. HAYES...................Minneapolis
Past-President—A. W. ADSON..............Rochester
First Vice President—W. R. McCARTHY.......St. Paul
Second Vice President—B. A. SMITH..........Crosby
Secretary—E. A. MEYERDING..................St. Paul
Treasurer—W. H. CONDIT................Minneapolis
Speaker, House of Delegates—W. W. WILL.....Bertha
Vice-Speaker,
House of Delegates—J. C. HULTKRANS....Minneapolis
Executive Secretary—Mr. R. R. ROSELL.......St. Paul

Committee On Scientific Assembly

J. M. HAYES, President ....Minneapolis
A. W. ADSON, Past-President ....Rochester
MR. R. R. ROSELL, Executive Secretary ....St. Paul

Section on Medicine

P. G. BOMAN ....Duluth
B. B. SOUSTER ....St. Paul
J. N. LIBERT ....St. Cloud

Section on Surgery

S. R. MAXEINER ....Minneapolis
V. S. COUNSELLER ....Rochester
R. C. HUNT ....Fairmont

Section on Specialties

W. A. O'BRIEN ....Minneapolis

Committees On Local Arrangements

General Chairman—R. J. MOE.
General Advisory—W. A. COVENTRY, F. H. MAGNEY, HARRY
  KLEIN, J. R. MANLEY, D. W. WHEELER.
House Arrangements—F. H. MAGNEY, C. M. SMITH, P. N.
  BRAY.
Public Relations—D. W. WHEELER, A. N. COLLINS, ELIZABETH
  BAGLEY, W. A. COVENTRY.
Scientific Exhibits—A. H. WELLS, S. G. SAX, A. G. ATHENS.
Commercial Exhibits—W. N. GRAVES, D. R. GOLDISH, M. F.
  FELLOWS.
Hotel Reservations—K. R. FAWCETT, N. J. BRAVERMAN.
Reunions—MARIO FISCHER, RALPH ECKMAN, S. MUELLER.
Golf—W. E. HATCH, W. D. COVENTRY.
Banquet—L. R. GOWAN, F. J. ELIAS, A. O. SWENSON.
Boat—W. C. MARTIN, C. H. MEAD, A. J. SPANG.
Clinical Programs—E. L. TUOHY, A. C. HILDING, M. H. TIB-
  BETTS, G. A. HEDBERG, W. E. HATCH, S. H. BOYER, JR.,
  F. J. HIRSCHBOECK, C. O. KOHLBRY, T. O. YOUNG, B. F.
  DAVIS, J. R. MANLEY.

ANNOUNCEMENTS

Luncheons.—Two Round Table Discussion Luncheons
have been arranged as a special feature of this meeting. The main dining room of the hotel has been reserved for these luncheon meetings. Tickets may be
purchased at the time of registration and at the door.

Wednesday.—The luncheon at 12:30 p.m. will be
devoted to discussion of Social Hygiene, particularly
to lay education on prevention and treatment of venereal disease. W. A. O'Brien, University of Minnesota,
will be principal speaker and discussion leader.

Thursday.—The luncheon at 12:30 p.m. will be
devoted to discussion of subjects introduced during
the Thursday morning session. The morning speakers, including the guest speaker, Dr. Lewin, will be
present to answer questions. Dr. O'Brien will be discussion leader.

440

Friday.—The luncheon period, beginning at 12:30,
will be devoted to the first Herman M. Johnson
Memorial Lectureship. First lecturer is the Honorable Elmer A. Benson, Governor of the State of
Minnesota, and long time friend of Dr. Johnson. J. M.
Hayes, president of the Minnesota State Medical Association, will preside and introduce the lecturer. Every
member is urged to attend.

* * *

Public Health Meeting.—The public will be invited
to attend the Public Health Meeting arranged for
Wednesday night at the Orpheum theater, next door
to hotel headquarters. Dr. Haggard, famous physiologist and radio speaker, author of the celebrated
series "Devils, Drugs and Doctors," and Irvin Abell,
Louisville, Ky., president-elect of the American Medical
Association, will be the principal speakers.

* * *

*The Minnesota Academy of Ophthalmology and Oto-
laryngology* will hold a special dinner meeting at the
Kitchi Gammi Club in Duluth on Friday, July 1, in
honor of Edward Jackson, of Denver. Dr. Jackson will
speak Wednesday at 4 p.m. before the Minnesota State
Medical Association and, under the sponsorship of the
Academy, he will also give a course of lectures Thursday, Friday and Saturday, June 30, July 1 and 2 on
"Practical Aspects of Physiological Optics in Refraction," at St. Mary's Hospital. Registration for this
course should be made with F. N. Knapp, 815 Medical
Arts Building, Duluth. The fee is $15.

* * *

The Southern Minnesota Medical Association, following its regular annual custom, will present a gold
medal to the individual physician who presents the
best scientific exhibit at this meeting. Judges will
be selected from among distinguished out-of-state visitors. The award will be made at the annual banquet
in the Ballroom, Thursday night.

* * *

Annual Banquet.—The annual dinner for members
and their wives, which was discontinued for a few
years owing to lack of proper facilities, will be resumed
again this year. It will be held Thursday at 6:30
p.m. in the Ballroom at the Hotel Duluth. Our celebrated guest speaker, Dr. Haggard of Yale, will be
the principal speaker. Dancing in the Ballroom will
follow dinner.

* * *

Golf Tournament.—The annual Golf Tournament will
begin Saturday morning, July 2, at the Northland
Country Club. Registrations for the tournament should
be made at the Registration Desk. Entrants will be
permitted to organize their own foursomes on a handicap basis. This is the first time the tournament has

SCIENTIFIC PROGRAM

Wednesday, June 29, 1938

Chairman: S. R. MAXEINER

Scientific Cinema:
Torek Operation for Cryptorchidism
WALTMAN WALTERS, Rochester

Obstetrical Hemorrhages
R. E. SWANSON, Minneapolis
Discussion: A. K. STRATTE, Pine City

Nutrition in Obstetrics
R. J. MOE, Duluth
Discussion: E. C. HARTLEY, St. Paul

Heart Disease in Pregnancy
J. F. BORG, St. Paul
Discussion: E. M. KASPER, St. Paul

Inflammatory Lesions of the Cervix and Vagina
L. W. BARRY, St. Paul
Discussion: W. F. MERCIL, Crookston

Scientific Cinema:
Congenital Absence of the Vagina—A New Surgical Treatment
V. S. COUNSELLER, Rochester

Carcinoma of the Colon and Rectum
IRVIN ABELL, Louisville, Ky.

Uterine Malignancy
ROLAND S. CRON, Milwaukee, Wis.

Round Table Luncheon:
Social Hygiene
Leader: W. A. O'BRIEN, University of Minnesota

Wednesday Afternoon

Chairman: B. B. SOUSTER

Scientific Cinema:
The Management of—Cancer of the Maxillary Sinus
                     Cancer of the Larynx
LAWRENCE R. BOIES, Minneapolis

Russell D. Carman Memorial Lecture:
The Diagnostic Roentgenology of Adult Pulmonary Tuberculosis with a New Suggestion as to Group Survey
HOLLIS E. POTTER, Chicago. Head, X-ray Departments Cook Co. and Presbyterian Hospitals

The Value of the X-ray in General Practice
C. G. SUTHERLAND, Rochester

Roentgen Therapy in Inflammatory Conditions
T. GAGE CLEMENT, Duluth

Scientific Cinema:
Eye Operations
CHARLES N. SPRATT, Minneapolis

Recognition and Treatment of Refractive Errors in Children
EDWARD JACKSON, Denver

Acute Mastoiditis
J. G. PARSONS, Crookston
Discussion: W. E. CAMP, Minneapolis

Eye Injuries
W. T. WENNER, St. Cloud
Discussion: E. P. BURCH, St. Paul

Wednesday Evening

PUBLIC HEALTH MEETING

Presiding Officer: M. G. GILLESPIE, Duluth
President St. Louis County Medical Society

Greetings
CARL SCHERER, Duluth. President, St. Louis County Tuberculosis and Health Society

Songs by the Normanna Male Chorus

441

Recent Advances in Medicine and Their Social Significance
HOWARD W. HAGGARD, New Haven, Conn.

Some Aims of the Profession as They Relate to the Public
IRVIN ABELL, Louisville, Ky.

Motion Picture: Emergency Treatment for Fractures

Thursday, June 30, 1938

Chairman: V. S. COUNSELLER

Scientific Cinema:
Os Calcis Fractures—An Improved Treatment
O. W. YOERG, Minneapolis

Fractures: General Principles
CLARENCE JACOBSON, Chisholm
Discussion: E. E. CHRISTENSEN, Winona

Emergency Treatment of Injuries
H. M. LEE, Minneapolis
Discussion: BENJAMIN F. DAVIS, Duluth

Abdominal Injuries
E. MENDELSSOHN JONES, St. Paul
Discussion: W. C. BERNSTEIN, New Richland

Intractable Low Back and Sciatic Pain Due to Protruded Intervertebral Disks: Diagnosis and Treatment
J. G. LOVE, Rochester
Discussion: HAROLD O. PETERSON, Minneapolis

Scientific Cinema:
Complete Rectal Prolapse—A Fascial Repair
C. W. MAYO, Rochester ·

Practical Pointers on Anesthesia
RALPH T. KNIGHT, Minneapolis
Discussion: E. B. TUOHY, Rochester

Rating of Disabilities
M. O. HENRY, Minneapolis
Discussion: R. M. BURNS, St. Paul

The Foot and Ankle—Their Discomforts, Deformities and Disabilities
PHILIP LEWIN, Chicago, Ill.

Round Table Luncheon:
Informal Discussion on Morning Program
.Leader: W. A. O'BRIEN, University of Minnesota

Thursday Afternoon

Chairman: P. G. BOMAN

Scientific Cinema:
The Transportation of the Patient with Fractured Spine
M. H. TIBBETTS, Duluth

Recent Advances in the Treatment of Burns
KARL A. MEYER, Chicago, Ill.

The Problem of Gastroduodenal Hemorrhage
A. M. SNELL, Rochester
Discussion: P. W. HARRISON, Worthington

Scientific Cinema:
Methods Used in Internal Fixations in Fractures of the Neck of the Femur
WILLARD D. WHITE, Minneapolis

Sulfanilamide in Bacterial Infections
E. K. MARSHALL, JR., Baltimore

A Type of Chronic Nervous Depression in Women with Response to Thyroid Medication
G. R. KAMMAN, St. Paul
Discussion: L. R. GOWAN, Duluth

What's New in the Treatment of Food Sensitiveness?
W. C. ALVAREZ, Rochester
Discussion: E. M. RUSTON, Minneapolis

Thursday Evening

ANNUAL BANQUET, BALLROOM

Toastmaster: J. M. HAYES

Introduction of Mrs. W. B. Roberts, Minneapolis, President Women's Auxiliary

Presentation of Southern Minnesota Medical Association medal

Greetings
IRVIN ABELL, Louisville, Ky.

Address
HOWARD W. HAGGARD, New Haven, Conn.

Dancing

Friday, July 1, 1938

Chairman: J. N. LIBERT

Scientific Cinema:
Ocular Aspects of Diabetes
WALTER H. FINK, Minneapolis

Clinics
Miller Memorial Hospital
St. Luke's Hospital
St. Mary's Hospital

Scientific Cinema:
Emergency Care of Traumatic Injuries to the Extremities
H. B. MACEY, Rochester

Installation of Officers
Presiding: J. M. HAYES, President

Report of the Secretary

Medical Economics
Presiding: W. R. McCARTHY, First Vice President

Address
HON. HENRY M. GALLAGHER, Waseca. Chief Justice, Supreme Court, State of Minnesota

Address
MR. S. B. HOUCK, Minneapolis. Chairman, Committee on Unauthorized Practice of the Law, American Bar Association

President's Address: Medical Problems in Minnesota
J. M. HAYES, Minneapolis

Luncheon:
Herman M. Johnson Memorial Lectureship
THE HONORABLE ELMER A. BENSON, Governor of the State of Minnesota

Friday Afternoon

Chairman: R. C. HUNT

Scientific Cinema:
Lumbar Ureterotomy for Stone—New Method and Technic
F. E. B. FOLEY, St. Paul

Some Practical Points in the Management of Nephritic Children
C. ANDERSON ALDRICH, Winnetka, Ill.

Acute Upper Respiratory Infections with Gastrointestinal Symptoms
E. D. ANDERSON, Minneapolis
Discussion: L. R. CRITCHFIELD, St. Paul

Peripheral Neuritis in Children
R. E. CUTTS, Minneapolis
Discussion: J. C. McKINLEY, Minneapolis

Congenital Heart Defects
T. J. DRY, Rochester
Discussion: R. N. ANDREWS, Mankato

Scientific Cinema:
Transplantation of the Ureters to the Sigmoid for Exstrophy of the Bladder
P. F. DONOHUE, St. Paul

Treatment of Upper Respiratory Infections
R. L. J. KENNEDY, Rochester
Discussion: ANDREW SINAMARK, Hibbing

The regular monthly meeting of the Minnesota Academy of Medicine was held at the Town and Country Club on Wednesday evening, March 9, 1938. Dinner was served at 7 o'clock and the meeting was called to order at 8:10 p. m. by the president, Dr. R. T. LaVake.

There were forty-six members present.

Minutes of the February meeting were read and approved.

The scientific program followed.

OPERATIVE DIVISION OF UNILATERAL FUSED KIDNEY*

With Case Report

·F. E. B. FOLEY, M.D.
Saint Paul

Abstract

The case to be reported is that of a unilateral fused kidney.

Brief lantern slide demonstration of the development of the upper urinary tract, at the same time pointing out the fault in normal development that gives rise to the anomaly of unilateral fused kidney, will add interest to description of the condition as clinically encountered. It should also make clear the features of the bilateral pyelo-ureterogram by which the condition is recognized. (Lantern slides.)

Unilateral fused kidney or "tandem kidney" or "crossed dystopia with fusion" is primarily an anomaly of the renal blastemata. It is one of the so-called fusion anomalies. Other anomalies of the same group are "horseshoe kidney" (fusion of lower poles usually, upper poles rarely) and "lump kidney" (conglomerate fusion). In unilateral fused kidney there is fusion between the lower pole of one kidney and the upper pole of the second kidney. The fused kidneys both lie to one side of the midline. Thus one kidney is ectopic across the midline. Almost regularly the lower kidney is the ectopic one and the fusion is at its upper pole. The ureter of the ectopic kidney crosses the midline to enter the bladder in normal position. Rarely the upper one of the two kidneys is the ectopic one. Only a few cases of this latter relationship have been reported.

The permanent kidney is formed from two elements. The ureteral bud arising from the Wolffian duct forms the excretory channels including almost the whole length of the tubules, papillary ducts, minor calyces, major calyces, pelvis and ureter. By branching growth the ureteral bud extends into and is covered by the renal blastema. The renal blastemata or nephrogenic cords are masses of mesodermal cells lying dorsal to the Wolffian ducts, one on each side, and entirely separate from the Wolffian ducts. From the renal blas-

*Dr. Foley gave a motion picture demonstration of the operation.

tema are developed the glomeruli and short connecting tubes that unite with the tubules formed from the ureteral bud.

At beginning formation of the permanent kidneys the two caudally placed renal blastemata lie close to each other but normally are completely separate. So far as I know it has not been determined just how and when fusion occurs, whether it is a primary fault in the formation of the blastemata, and present before the migration of the kidneys begins, or occurs during migration, particularly as the kidneys approach each other in passing through the narrow ring formed by the umbilical arteries.

Normally the migration of the kidney has three components of motion: ascent, rotation and axial deflection.

1. *Ascent.*—Normally the kidneys ascend to positions well up in the lumbar regions—the renal fossæ. When all possible ascent of the unilateral fused kidney has occurred its elongated form leaves its lower segment in abnormally low position. In addition the lower segment is drawn across the midline by the upper segment.

2. *Rotation.*—Normally the kidney rotates on its long axis so that the hilum, originally directed ventrally, is finally directed medially with the calyces extending laterally from the pelvis. Fusion of the two organs impairs this rotation particularly at the fused poles. In consequence some of the calyces of the unilateral fused kidney extend medially from the pelvis.

3. *Axial Deflection.*—Normally the long axis of the kidney, at first oblique toward the midline below, is deflected during migration to become oblique toward the midline above with the upper pole lying closer to the midline than the lower pole. Fusion of the two organs interferes with this normal axial deflection. In consequence, the long axis of the upper segment of the unilateral fused kidney remains oblique toward the midline below, the lateral movement of the lower pole being arrested by the fusion.

Because of these faults in development the "bilateral" pyelogram of a unilateral fused kidney with crossed ectopia of the lower segment representing the left kidney will show an upper (right) pelvis perhaps normally high in the renal fossa with its long axis oblique toward the midline below and its inferior calyces extending medially from the pelvis. The lower (left) pelvis will be abnormally low-lying, its axis extending obliquely downward from the lower pole of the upper (right) pelvis and even reaching somewhat across the midline while its ureter, crossing the midline, terminates in normal position in the left side of the bladder.

Case Report

The case to be reported is that of an unmarried woman, aged eighteen (Ancker Hospital record No. A-73402.)

The complaint was of left sided abdominal pain which had been present in variable degrees during the three years prior to her first admission to the hospital in August, 1936. At first the pain occurred in attacks. It was very severe, located in the left upper quadrant, appeared to be induced by exercise or other activity and to be relieved by lying down. At times the pain extended to the left lower thorax and to the left upper quadrant of the abdomen. Later constipation accompanying the attacks was noted. Weight loss of 15 pounds occurred.

Following almost complete relief of symptoms for a period of eight months the patient was admitted to the hospital for the third time, June 4, 1937. On this occasion there had been an attack of severe pain in the left lower quadrant followed by frequent periodic recurrences and finally by constant and persistent dull aching pain in this location. She was transferred to the urologic service.

The significant findings of the physical examination and laboratory investigations were: a rounded somewhat elongated mass lying below the umbilicus with its long axis extending longitudinally. The mass was slightly moveable in longitudinal direction and was tender to pressure. The mass transmitted the aortic pulsation but did not expand with it. On percussion, bowel tympany was present over the mass. The urine was normal, hemoglobin 57 per cent, leukocytes 3,600 per cu. mm., blood urea nitrogen 13.3 mgms. per 100 c.c. Excretion urogram: nearly normal function of each kidney; indefinite outlining of pelves and ureters with deformity typical of unilateral fused kidney with crossed ectopia of the left and lower segment. Cystoscopy: normal bladder mucosa and contour; ureteral orifices normal position and normal appearance. Indigo-carmine test of renal function: right—appearance time four minutes, deep concentration; left—appearance time seven minutes, moderate concentration. Bilateral pyelogram: clear outlining of deformity typical of unilateral fused kidney with crossed ectopia of the left and lower segment, no dilatation of the right pelvis or calyces, grade I dilatation of the left pelvis and calyces. Filling of the pelvis of the left segment produced pain identical with the pain complained of both as to character and location.

Diagnosis and summary of findings: Unilateral fused kidney with crossed ectopia of left and lower segment not accompanied by any significant pathologic change apart from the anomaly and responsible for painful symptoms.

Therapeutic indication: Operative division of the renal isthmus and correction of renal malposition.

A color motion picture film of the operation will now be shown. The malformed kidney was exposed through an extra-peritoneal right flank incision. The isthmus was divided between two rows of mattress sutures. The left kidney was displaced to the left and its upper pole was held medial to the vena cava by suturing the posterior parietal peritoneum to the posterior abdominal wall along the right border of the cava, the right kidney was fixed in normal position by the Foley nephropexy (Arch. Surg., 1929).

The result to date, ten months after operation, is excellent, there being complete relief of the pain complained of before operation. A bilateral pyelogram made two months following operation showed the right kidney and pelvis in normal position and of normal appearance and the position of the left pelvis somewhat improved.

At the time this operation was performed a cursory review of the literature disclosed no other case of division of the isthmus of the unilateral fused kidney without removal of one or the other half. Since

then further search has disclosed a total of fifty-one cases of operation on the unilateral fused kidney, most of them undertaken for concomitant pathologic change such as stone, hydronephrosis, etc. However, among the fifty-one cases, four cases of operation similar to that here reported were found.

In addition to this case of operative division of the isthmus of the unilateral fused kidney, we have performed the same operation in six cases of horseshoe kidney with equally satisfactory results in all save one case in which an unremoved stone and persisting infection made secondary nephrectomy necessary on one side.

It is submitted that unilateral fused kidney or horseshoe kidney causing only painful symptoms and not accompanied by pathologic change apart from the anomaly should be the object of surgical interference of the sort described here.

Discussion

Dr. W. F. Braasch, Rochester: I am compelled to say a few words of commendation and praise for the excellent presentation made by Dr. Foley and the unusual operation that he described. I remember that I discussed his paper on the separation of the isthmus with renal fusion four years ago and at that time I praised him for his originality; and now I again do so.

We urologists used to think that we were quite clever to make the clinical diagnosis of fused kidney prior to operation. Today it is getting to be an old story. Patients now come in frequently with the diagnosis already made by the local physician, by means of excretory urography. By employing this simple method of diagnosis it is no longer difficult to recognize renal fusion. On reviewing our records at the Clinic the other day, I found that during the past year a diagnosis of renal fusion was made in thirty-two cases. In a paper written by Judd, Scholl and myself some sixteen years ago, we described sixteen cases of renal fusion which had been operated on at the Mayo Clinic. One case among those reported (case No. 3) was operated on by Dr. C. H. Mayo in 1917, in which he made the first symphysiotomy for horseshoe kidney reported in this country. Rovsing first described this operation in 1910 and Papin later improved the operative technic. As far as I know, division of a unilateral fused kidney has not been done at the Clinic. We have operated on unilateral fused kidneys for such complications as stone and hydronephrosis, but have not bisected the kidney as Dr. Foley has described. Not all kidneys with unilateral renal fusion can be divided. In some cases the two renal pelves will be so closely related and the kidney assume such a shape that renal division will not be technically possible, or at least will offer considerable difficulty.

It should be remembered that there are difficulties in deciding whether a fused kidney should be operated. In many of our cases diagnosed clinically, we found no indication for operation. Apparent pyelectasis of moderate degree is often observed in the urogram with renal fusion, which has caused no symptoms. Although the pyelectasis in some cases is extensive, the patient has not complained of any pain. It may be difficult to determine whether actual stasis and obstruction are present. Patients also are observed who complain of pain but fail to show pyelectasis in the urogram. It can be very difficult to decide whether the apparent pyelectasis is the cause of the patient's symptoms. Of two cases in which the isthmus was

of two months, the vision cleared up and became quite satisfactory again. There has been no visual difficulty from that time until the present, when on examination the vision was: Right 20/200, Left 20/50. Fundus examination at this time showed some lens and vitreous haze, diffuse retinal edema with marked arteriolar spasm, thickening of the larger arterioles, arteriovenous compression and an edema of one diopter of each optic nerve. There were hemorrhages and cotton-wool patches in the right macular area.

General examination revealed marked arthritic changes in the hands and knees. Heart enlarged about 50 per cent with a widened base and marked sclerosis of the peripheral vessels. There was a slight trace of albumin, a few red blood cells and hyaline casts present in the urine.

After a period of rest in bed for two months there was a marked improvement in the vision of the left eye, although the blood pressure was still 180 systolic and 110 diastolic.

Comment.—Following a rather severe angiospastic retinitis with systolic pressure of 200, there was a complete remission for a period of fifteen years. Although such remissions are not uncommon, and sometimes occur even in cases of malignant hypertension, the picture now present is undoubtedly one of a more serious condition. The arterial and arteriolar thickening, visual disturbances, arteriolar spasm and some demonstrable swelling of the optic nerves are characteristic of the condition present. Marked improvement which resulted from rest in bed, sedatives, and some reduction in the pressure itself, are the indications of a fair prognosis of this condition.

Case 2.—Mr. J. J., aged forty-three, first came for examination on December 28, 1937, complaining of loss of vision in the left eye for the past few weeks. There had been some difficulty with vision since early in the Spring and it was becoming increasingly difficult to work. Hypertension had been present for the last five years and in June was associated with anorexia, fatigue, vomiting and diffuse abdominal pain. There was a weight loss of 15 pounds. He was in the hospital for a short period in June recovering from an attack of bronchitis.

On examination the vision was: Right 20/20, Left 20/200. Fundus examination revealed that the right optic nerve showed three diopters of swelling with marked arteriolar spasms and hemorrhages around the disk. The larger vessels showed a thickening and arteriovenous compression. In the left eye only a moderate swelling of the disk was present without hemorrhages or exudate. Visual fields showed a contraction of the right with nasal hemianopia of he left eye. The blood pressure was 250 systolic over 150 diastolic. The urine showed a trace of albumin and occasional red blood cells. Kidney function was 57 per cent. After a period of rest in the hospital with the usual sedatives and spinal puncture, there was a slow but steady rise in the pressure to 260 systolic, 160 diastolic. Headaches became more severe and cotton-wool exudates appeared in the right eye.

Comment.—Hypertension, which had existed for several years, was accompanied a few months before examination by definite symptoms of general weakness with evidences of arteriolar spasm. There was no improvement whatever following glucose and sucrose intravenously and a definite increase in blood pressure seemed to follow spinal fluid drainage. All of these measures are oftentimes sufficient to produce a remis-

sion of this condition, but at times the angiospastic
feature of the condition is so pronounced that there is
a sudden failure of the brain, heart or kidneys. It
is difficult to explain the field changes or the hypertensive or fundus findings.

Discussion

DR. W. E. CAMP, Minneapolis: Dr. Grant has very
thoroughly and very instructively presented these two
cases of malignant hypertension. With his permission,
I would like to show a few lantern slides completing
the ophthalmoscopic picture in these types of cases and
correlating these findings with the microscopic pathologic
change which is usually present. These slides were
made from serial sections of the eye of a case of
malignant hypertension, which died a renal death. According to Dr. E. T. Bell, about 5 per cent of all
cases of malignant hypertension die a renal death. The
slides show a marked edema of the optic nerve and
the surrounding retina with a small flat detachment
of the retina on either side of the optic nerve. The
marked sclerosis of the retinal and choroidal arterioles
is well demonstrated. The thickening is chiefly in the
intima and media and consists of fibrosis and hyaline
deposits. The cotton-wool exudate in the superficial
layers of the retina is found to be due to edema and
serum deposits containing a few large phagocytes or
macrophages. The "star-shaped" figure in the macular
region is due to lipoid exudate in the deeper layers
of the retina. These exudates with the ophthalmoscope
appear as small, yellowish-white, highly refractile bodies
and form an incomplete "star" in the macular region.
Fat stains show that they are lipoids in character and
when once formed are more permanent than the soft
cotton-wool patches described above. All of the above-
described features compose the picture of the retinitis
found in malignant hypertension.

DR. MOSES BARRON, Minneapolis: Dr. Grant's cases
are interesting both from the point of view of the
oculist and of the internist. It is rather unfortunate
that the terminology is often confusing. The oculist's
diagnosis of malignant hypertension usually applies to
those cases in which there is hypertension and which
develop retinal changes such as edema, narrowing of
the arterioles, hemorrhages, edema of the disc, as described by Dr. Grant. The internist, on the other hand,
generally uses the term to designate the type of case
represented by Dr. Grant's second case, and the one
illustrated by Dr. Camp; that is, malignant hypertension is meant to describe a case of essential hypertension which develops renal changes with renal insufficiency which usually results in death from uremia.
Very commonly the characteristic retinitis picture is
present. Dr. Camp mentioned that about 5 per cent
of these cases die of uremia. From our point of
view, about 95 per cent of these cases die of uremia.
The renal changes are often characteristic. In a paper
that was delivered before this Academy a year ago,
I tried to point out the characteristic changes in the
kidneys. The changes are degenerative; very pronounced are the changes in the arterioles with arteriolar necrosis. Dr. Grant's first case would be considered a case of essential hypertension with angiospastic involvement. Such cases often respond well
to spinal drainage. His second case, in which the
patient is progressively going down hill and in which
there developed symptoms of uremia, is a typical case
of malignant hypertension. Such cases do not respond
very well to spinal drainage. I wonder if Dr. Grant
would tell us on what basis he uses the term malignant
hypertension.

DR. GRANT (in closing): I think that, for the purpose
of differentiation, we have three types of hypertension:
(1) essential hypertension, with no signs except or-

446

MINNEAPOLIS SURGICAL SOCIETY

Stated Meeting, Thursday, April 7, 1938

MESENTERIC CYST

Case Report

W. C. Peterson, M.D.

· The first case of mesenteric cyst was observed in 1507 by Benevieni, a Florentine anatomist, who accidentally found such a cyst at autopsy and classified it as an anatomical curiosity. In 1880 Tillaux successfully operated on a cystic mesenteric tumor.

Mesenteric tumors are the rarest tumors in the abdomen but cystic tumors are four times as common as the solid neoplasms.

In a very complete article and bibliography by Dr. J. Ogle Warfield, Jr., from which I have very lavishly drawn my information, it is stated that probably 500 cases have been reported in the literature up to 1932. Briefly, mesenteric cysts may be classified according to origin as follows:

1. Embryonic retroperitoneal organs, such as germinal epithelium, ovary, wolffian or müllerian bodies.
2. Displaced embryonal intestinal tissue.
3. Dermal inclusions.
4. Angiomas of blood and lymph vessels.
5. Parasitic and bacterial infection.
6. Necrosis of lymph glands or solid tumors.
7. Trauma and foreign bodies.

Mesenteric cysts occur most commonly·in the fourth decade and women are affected twice·as often as men.

Diagnosis.—There are no pathognomonic signs or symptoms of mesentric cyst. However, an abdominal tumor which is rounded, cystic, mobile and not tender, should suggest such a cyst. The mobility is the outstanding sign. These cysts are located most commonly in the mesentery of the ileum and next most frequently in the jejunum, cecum, ascending and transverse colon.

Pathology.—These cysts may be so small as to be unrecognized, or so large they fill the entire abdomen. The cyst wall is usually composed of fibrous or elastic tissue with the lining so compressed that its cellular structure cannot be identified. Only occasionally is some tissue present which will identify the origin of the neoplasm. Malignancy is rare.

Complications.—Intestinal obstruction is the most common complication, occurs in one-third of the cases and of these the mortality is 50 per cent. Peritonitis, hemorrhage into the cyst, rupture into the bowel, torsion and impaction have all been reported.

Treatment.—1. Enucleation is the operation of. choice and has the lowest mortality, 9 per cent.

2. Enucleation with intestinal resection, 16.6 per cent.

3. Drainage or marsupialization has been done in some cases.

4. Aspiration.

Report of Case

A white spinster, seventy-five years of age, was seen October 4, 1937. Her past history was entirely irrelevant.

The patient ·had noticed a swelling in the abdomen for about three years. It was entirely painless and only troubled her by being in the way in adjusting her clothing.

Examination showed a very well preserved elderly woman, with normal findings except for a rounded protruding abdominal mass, not unlike a seven months pregnancy in a sparely nourished woman. The mass was not tender and was very freely movable.

Vaginal examination showed a small uterus.

Diagnosis: Large pedunculated ovarian cyst or fibroid.

Operation: A midline incision was made and on examination the tumor was readily seen to be in the transverse mesocolon. The posterior layer was incised and the cyst was dissected out quite readily except near the transverse colon. The thin areas in the colon were plicated, the rent in the mesentery closed and the abdomen sutured. The cyst was thin walled, weighed 2125 grams, was 15 cm. in diameter, and contained over 2 litres of bloody fluid. Recovery was uneventful.

References

1. Peterson, Edward W.: Ann. Surg., 96:340, 1932. ·
2. Warfield, J. Ogle, Jr.: Ann. Surg., 96:329, 1932.

Discussion

Dr. Martin Nordland showed slides demonstrating a case of mesenteric cyst. The case was previously reported before this Society.

Dr. J. F. Corbett: I have a case perhaps worth reporting from the standpoint of its unusual location. Like the essayist, I did not make a diagnosis beforehand. The tumor in this case I could feel but it did not seem to me at all movable. I expected to find something connected with either the tube or the ovary. When I opened the abdomen I found a cyst between the layers of the sigmoid at a very low level, practically where the mesentery comes down. I then recognized I was dealing with a cyst, thin-walled, and probably two or two and one-half inches in diameter.

In getting this out I found that because of the anatomical location the cyst had pushed its way somewhat into the bowel, leaving a paper thin mucosa only, so much so that I was afraid to close it without resecting the bowel. I therefore took out a complete segment of bowel and ·succeeded in making an end-to-end anastomosis. The pathologist reported a thin-walled cyst, undoubtedly embryonic in origin.

RECTO-URETHRO-VESICAL FISTULA, TRAUMATIC

Case Report

Robert F. McGandy, M.D.

The case I wish to report is that of a laborer, thirty-three years of age, whom I first saw in a rural hospital in Wisconsin, on September 26, 1932. He gave a history of slipping, falling backwards six feet, striking on a bolt which protruded eleven inches from a log. The bolt entered his perineum behind the rectum and went into the rectum in a somewhat sweeping fashion, penetrating the prostatic urethra and bladder. He bled considerably and was taken immediately to the hospital where he was seen by a doctor from a neighboring town. He was taken immediately

447

to the operating room where the doctor's examination revealed a large tear in the perineum, a three-inch tear in the posterior wall of the rectum and a six-inch tear in the anterior wall of the rectum. The doctor stated he could put his hand into the wound and noticed that the prostatic urethra had been torn for a distance of about one inch and a considerable amount of prostatic tissue had been torn away. The wound entered the bladder and urine could be seen coming out of it. The doctor attempted immediate repair of the rectum and let the rest of the wound fall together. That night, when the regular doctor at the hospital returned, the accident having happened at 8:40 in the morning, it was noticed that the patient was unable to void. The doctor was unable to pass a catheter and for this reason opened the bladder suprapubically and was able with difficulty to institute drainage through the urethra. He also left a drain in the suprapubic opening. The patient's temperature had been 102 for several days and his leukocyte count was 13,200. When I saw him, his temperature was between 99 and 100. The doctor had been irrigating the bladder daily. Urine was coming from the abdomen and urethra as well as the rectum. The patient was very restless, in extreme pain, markedly dehydrated and very toxic. An examination revealed a large three-inch long, foul smelling, pus discharging wound in the perineum and rectum. There was a tube inserted in the rectum and the stitches had sloughed away. As the patient could not be moved, I suggested more fluids, sedatives and hot packs to the perineum, in addition to what the doctor was already doing.

I saw the patient at the same hospital again on October 10, 1932. For the past five days the patient had had a high temperature and was suffering from a respiratory infection which proved to be pneumonia. He was still toxic and had a Vincent's infection in his mouth. Urine was coming from the abdomen and perineal wound. The urethra was not draining and the patient had a definite urethritis and epididymitis. Abscesses had formed in the shaft of the penis and drained pus. I felt the rectal wound had improved somewhat although the margins were angry. I could put my index finger in the rectal canal. I adjusted the catheter in the urethra and drainage was obtained through it. The blood chemistry was normal but the patient was becoming irrational at times. Definite suicidal tendencies had been noticed. The doctor stated that the patient had had voluntary stools. The urinary infection was apparently responding somewhat.

On November 17, 1932, this patient was transferred to the Northwestern Hospital in Minneapolis by ambulance. His temperature was 99 on admission and the patient presented the picture of exhaustion. He was discouraged and depressed. The nurse who came with him repeated the fact that he had many suicidal tendencies. He had a considerable amount of pain in his penis and perineum and he was poorly nourished. Urine drained suprapubically, through the catheter in the urethra as well as through the rectum. Urinalysis revealed a large amount of albumin with 50 to 75 pus cells per high powered field. There were two or three red blood cells per high powered field and many granular and hyaline casts. Wassermann reaction was reported to be negative. Hemoglobin was 74 per cent; red cells, 4,110,000; leukocytes, 16,500; non-protein nitrogen, 22.4 mgms. per 100 c.c.; creatinine, 1.2 mgms. per 100 c.c.

The patient was placed on regular bladder irrigations and urinary antiseptics. The urethral catheter was frequently changed and when out the fistula in the shaft of the penis drained. He was also given hot packs to his genitals and perineum. Fluids were forced and although sedatives were given, little success resulted from them. The patient had frequent suicidal tendencies in the hospital and had to be watched constantly. The condition of his perineum and bladder gradually improved. On November 28, with the

aid of a rectal speculum, I was able to pass a rubber catheter into the fistula opening in the rectum up to the bladder. I repeated this procedure on November 30 and injected some silver iodide emulsion obtaining an x-ray picture demonstrating a fistulous tract into the bladder.

Irrigation and urinary antiseptics were continued until December 8 when this patient was taken to the operating room, where under general anesthesia a perineal racket-shaped incision was made. As was to be expected, a considerable amount of scar tissue had formed both in front and behind the rectum. The rectum was dissected with difficulty from the surrounding structures after the method used in the old Whitehead operation for hemorrhoids. The dissection was carried upwards to a point about two centimeters above the entrance of the fistulous tract into the rectum. I could readily pass two fingers into the sinus opening, which led from the rectum up to the region of the posterior urethra and bladder. The fistulous tract was used to close the opening in the bladder and posterior urethra. This was reinforced with what remained of the prostatic capsule. It was thought best to sacrifice the rectum below the sinus opening. A new rectum was therefor pulled down in the manner used in the Whitehead operation. The sphincter musculature was markedly atrophied, retracted and composed of a considerable amount of scar tissue. However, what remained was approximated as best possible. The wound was drained. Fresh catheters were placed in the suprapubic and urethral channels.

The patient was placed on a low residue diet and sedatives. He was given subcutaneous fluids and definite steps were taken to prevent him from having a bowel movement. His temperature went up to 101 for the first three days. On December 10, two days after the operation, the patient became irrational and remained so until the 16th of December. He had to be placed in a straight jacket on December 12. Five days after the operation, he had a bowel movement consisting mainly of old blood. His thrashing around in restraints opened the perineal wound slightly. He was seen on December 15 by Dr. Hamilton, who felt we were dealing with an acute toxic delirium which apparently started originally after his pneumonia. I subsided with hallucinations and suicidal tendencies running along, only to become acute again following his present operation. The restraints were removed however, on the 17th of December, and the patient progressed quite well. I removed the suprapubic drain as soon as he became rational and on the 27th of December, I removed the catheter from his urethra. As I stated above he had several fistulæ in his penis, one being at the scroto-perineal angle. When the catheter was removed from the urethra, urine drained from these fistulous tracts, but many of the fistulæ in the shaft closed spontaneously. The rectal and suprapubic wounds closed normally and the patient was discharged from the hospital on January 18, 1933.

I did not see the patient again until February 2, 1933, when he returned from the country. He had gained ten pounds and his general condition, including his mental state, had improved remarkably. His complaints were that he noticed difficulty controlling his rectal sphincters during an attack of acute diarrhea from food poisoning. He also complained of dribbling of urine at the beginning and end of urination and the fact that he drained urine from a sinus opening at the junction of the perineum and scrotum. The suprapubic and perineal wounds had closed satisfactorily. I could put my index finger readily into his rectum. Because of the possibility of the opening tightening further I furnished him with some rectal dilators which he used regularly. I also began to dilate his urethra in the hopes that by so doing the fistula at the scroto-perineal angle would close spontaneously. Dilatation however, were usually followed by attacks of epididymitis, one of which necessitated surgical drainage

I, therefor, at a later date ligated the vas deferens on both sides and continued dilatation more vigorously. I was finally able to use a 28 French sound but the sinus persisted. For this reason, I placed the patient in the hospital again on November 15, 1933, repaired the sinus at the scroto-perineal angle. The tract was 1.5 inches long but was not difficult to repair. I used an indwelling catheter in the urethra for four days. The wound healed satisfactorily. I saw this patient a few months ago and he is doing very well and is working every day. He has no difficulty if he keeps his stools soft and does not allow his bladder to become over-distended before voiding.

IMPALEMENT OF THE RECTUM

With Report of Two Cases of Injury to the Bladder

GILBERT COTTAM, M.D.

Impalement of the rectum was used by the ancient as a form of punishment. The oldest collection of laws in the world, the Code Hammurabi (*circa* 2200 B.C.) contained specific allusion to it in the following words, as translated, in 1903, by C. W. Johns: "If a man's wife on account of another male has caused her husband to be killed, that woman upon a stake one shall set her." Pennington (A Treatise on the Diseases and Injuries of the Rectum, Anus and Pelvic Colon, 1923) mentions that in ancient Rome impalement was at first restricted to slaves who had been guilty of robbery and that later on, Nero resorted to it among other measures in his persecutions of the Christians. The Ottoman Turks used it soon after their irruption into Europe, for various offenses. In the Middle Ages it was used in Russia, Germany and Austria in cases of murder and witchcraft. It is said to have been used in the Inquisition. One of the English kings, Edward II, was murdered (A.D. 1327) in Berkeley Castle by having a red-hot skewer thrust up his rectum through a cow's horn used as an obturator. Pennington, on the authority of Fairlie, states that a form of impalement is in vogue today in the Malay Peninsula as punishment for female marital infidelity. A species of bamboo which grows with extraordinary rapidity, 24 inches in 24 hours, is used and the condemned woman is lashed to stakes over this bamboo, causing impalement in two days.

Accidental impalement of the rectum as it occurs in modern life is not a very uncommon injury. It happens in a wide variety of circumstances and with greatly differing vulnerating agents, but probably the most frequently encountered type is that which takes place in agricultural communities, in the manner about to be described. Those who are interested in the other types will find detailed information in the literature, of Weller Van Hook, of Chicago, whose article entitled "Rupture of the Rectum by Penetrating Bodies," with description of 58 cases collected from the literature, with one of his own included, published in *Medicine* for June, 1896, was the first contribution of the kind of any comprehensive importance to literature; of Herman Tillmans, who described 143 cases (including the vaginal type) in his article "Die Verletzungen u. Chir.

Krankheiten d. Beckens,' in *Deutsche Chirurgie*, 1905, Heft 62A; and finally in that of Otto W. Madelung, of Charlottenburg, entitled: "Die Pfählungsverletzungen des Afters un des Mastdarms" in *Arch. f. klin. Chir.*, 137:1-80, 1925, which contains an enormous bibliography covering eight and a half pages of closely printed references from all over the world. While, as the titles indicate, these two German articles just referred to deal with all kinds of wounds of the rectum and anus, a considerable number of impalements will be found to be described therein and some of these are of a nature to tax credulity, if it were not that they are fully authenticated by reliable observers.

Tonight our attention will be concentrated on the variety which occurs commonly in farming conditions and in a manner so uniformly similar that one description of the way in which it takes place will fit practically all cases. A farmer riding on top of a load of hay throws a pitchfork to the ground and slides down. The tines of the pitchfork have stuck in the ground and the handle stays up; the man straddles this handle and the point strikes his perineal region and is directed into the anus, in the manner described by Van Hook. One of five things is then obliged to happen: (1) The handle may merely enter the lumen of the lower bowel and do no more harm than cause contusions, abrasions and tears of the mucous membrane and sphincters; (2) it may penetrate the wall of the rectum anteriorly and damage the tissues of the recto-vesical septum, without injuring the bladder or entering the peritoneal cavity; (3) it may penetrate the anterior wall of the rectum and injure the bladder, without entering the peritoneal cavity, as in the first case I shall describe tonight; (4) it may penetrate the anterior wall of the rectum, traverse the recto-vesical septum, enter the bladder from behind and reach the peritoneal cavity through the top of the bladder, as in my own case, the second to be described tonight, or (5) it may penetrate the anterior wall of the rectum high enough to miss the bladder and reach the peritoneal cavity direct.

The immediate effects of an injury like this, no matter how extensively the parts involved are damaged, are often surprisingly slight. There is usually very little bleeding, no shock and a minimum of pain. In some of the cases reported the patient has removed the vulnerating agent himself and walked some distance afterwards. In a case reported by G. D. Whyte in the *Edinburgh Medical Journal* of March, 1911, page 255, a Chinaman had a piece of bamboo 8 inches long and 1.5 inches in diameter pushed up his rectum. He pursued his assailants for some distance, the piece of bamboo meanwhile working up into his lower bowel so that on admission the lower end could easily be felt in the iliac region, while the upper one passed under the rib margin where it could not be defined. This initial freedom from pain, shock, et cetera, is very misleading. Lay people do not appreciate the gravity of the situation and many doctors are slow to recommend intervention until peritonitis is well on the way and the chances of recovery even with operation are greatly diminished. Consequently, the super-

449

stition has arisen that these cases are better left alone and not operated upon.

This undoubtedly does apply to the non-penetrating cases, that is, those in which the vulnerating agent does not enter the peritoneal cavity, for most of these do

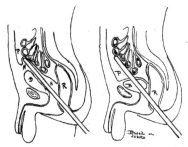

Fig. 1. *(left)* Dr. W. E. Morse's case. *P*, peritoneal cavity; *H*, hematoma; *B*, bladder; *X*, site of injury to bladder; *R*, rectum.

Fig. 2. *(right)* Author's case. *P*, peritoneal cavity; *B*, bladder; *R*, rectum.

recover under non-operative treatment, but where there is any doubt, we believe that it is safer to open the abdomen and take a look, for the odds are surely against the patient when fecal contamination of the peritoneum from the rectum occurs, or there is an open wound of the bladder into the peritoneum as well, if we sit back and do nothing but watch and wait. It is not always easy to estimate the depth of penetration in these cases. The distance of the fall before striking the vulnerating agent and the weight of the patient may afford some information, but the statement of a bystander who pulled it out is seldom reliable. The best evidence of deep penetration, if it be present, as it was in the two cases about to be described, is the ability to feel the end of the pitchfork handle, or whatever it is, through the anterior abdominal wall. In such cases we believe the indication for operation to be clear and undisputible, and as early as possible after the receipt of the injury.

I shall now describe as briefly as possible two illustrative cases with bladder involvement. Only the second is one of my own, the complete history of the first having come into my hands recently through the kindness of my friend Dr. W. E. Morse, of Rapid City, South Dakota, who handled it himself throughout.

Case 1.—Impalement of the rectum by pitchfork handle, with penetration of the anterior wall of the rectum, extraperitoneal injury of the bladder and massive retrocystic hematoma formation. Laparotomy, drainage and recovery (Dr. W. E. Morse's case).

C. W—, Bonita Spring, South Dakota, male, aged twenty-two, while hauling hay, on July 16, 1930, threw a pitchfork to the ground from the hayrack and immediately jumped from the load of hay, landing on the pitchfork handle, the fork having stuck in the

450

ground. The handle of the fork entered and penetrated the rectum for a distance of about 14 inches. The end of the handle could be felt a short distance above the pubes.

Examination showed the head, neck and chest free from evidence of disease or injury. The abdomen was acutely tender over the lower half, on both sides, with well defined rigidity of both recti. Rectal examination showed contusions in the anal area; the proctoscope revealed a perforation of the anterior wall.

Laparotomy under gas-ether anesthesia was performed within a few hours after the accident. It was found that the pitchfork handle had not penetrated into the peritoneal cavity but had stripped the peritoneum from the bladder to the anterior abdominal wall, with the formation of a huge hematoma in the traumatized area (Fig. 1).

The peritoneum was closed and the retrocystic traumatized area was drained by an extraperitoneal Penrose drain protruding anteriorly. A retention catheter of the mushroom type was left in the bladder and the patient returned to bed in good condition. Two days after the operation the patient was having a discharge of fecal material and gas through the retention catheter and a large amount of liquid which appeared to be urine was coming through the rectum. Eleven days after the operation, the intervening period having been quite uneventful, the temperature was normal, the patient feeling very well, there was less air coming through the bladder, less pain on urination and less fluid coming through the rectum. On the twentieth postoperative day the patient was sitting up and feeling very well; on the following day he was discharged from the hospital under observation, the rectal examination at that time showing that the channel of communication between the bladder and rectum was narrowed down to the size of a small lead pencil. Four days later he had to be readmitted on account of weakness, abdominal discomfort and pain in the rectum, due to fecal impaction in the rectum, relieved by enemas. Dr. Morse's records do not show the date of the final observation, but whenever it was the fistula had healed completely and the patient remained well.

Case 2.—Impalement of the rectum by pitchfork handle, with penetration of the rectum anteriorly, through-and-through penetration of the bladder into the peritoneal cavity and beginning peritonitis. Laparotomy, suture of the bladder, peritoneal drainage and tube drainage of the recto-vesical injury, recovery. (Author's case.)

R. P.—, Elkton, South Dakota, male, aged sixteen, was admitted on the morning of August 27, 1922, giving the following history: about 5:45 on the previous evening the patient jumped down from a wagon and struck a hay fork stuck in the ground, receiving the impact on his perineum. The fork handle entered the rectum and the end could be felt in front, just behind the anterior abdominal wall, a little below the umbilicus. Patient's father pulled out the fork handle. The immediate disability was slight; a physician who was called ordered hot applications and especially advised against any operation. During the night the father became alarmed by the boy's restlessness and complaint of increased pain, took him to a doctor in another town. This doctor catheterized the patient, obtaining only a small amount of fluid, although there had been no micturition since the accident, and also ordered him given an enema, which was found to contain some blood. This doctor realized the possibility of serious injury and brought the patient a distance of some sixty miles to me, early in the morning following the accident. I noted that the patient's facial expression appeared drawn and anxious, the pulse rapid and of none too good quality, the abdomen rigid throughout without localization and the lower abdomen tender to pressure. Rectal examination showed a longitudinal tear 1 inch long in the anterior wall, through which urine dribbled. Diagnosis: pitchfork handle injury of bladder through the rectum with possible intestinal injury; acute diffuse peritonitis.

Operation was begun exactly fifteen hours after the time the injury was received. Under ether the abdomen was opened through a right paramedian incision below the umbilicus. On opening the peritoneum a large amount of turbid fluid escaped and several coils of injected small intestine flaked with fibrin appeared. A transverse opening in the upper anterior wall of the bladder, in the median line, about 1 inch long, was soon found and repaired with two layers of catgut, the first of which included only the fibrous and muscular coats, the second closing and inverting the peritoneal coat (Fig. 2). A rapid exploration of the pelvis failed to disclose any intraperitoneal injury of the large or small intestines except a superficial abrasion of the small intestine at one point. A large black rubber fenestrated drainage tube was placed in the lower angle of the abdominal incision extending down into the pelvis. The rest of the abdomen was closed and the patient placed in the lithotomy position. The wound in the perineum was closed with a couple of interrupted sutures and a fairly large black rubber drainage tube placed in the wound in the rectum which was found to lead directly into the bladder and anchored externally. He recovered nicely and was discharged on the eighteenth postoperative day.

Conclusions

No one surgeon sees enough of these cases to be able to build up a series on which to form any conclusions. Most surgeons who report cases have seen only the one; so far, in a fairly extensive search of the literature I have found none who has reported more. Many surgeons of wide experience have seen none. Under these circumstances it is difficult to formulate a plan of action based on statistical study, applicable to the management of these cases. Van Hook and Tillmans, in their papers, estimate the mortality rate, by and large, at about 30 per cent. However; in Van Hook's collection of fifty-eight cases, the thirty in which penetration of the peritoneal cavity did not occur, all recovered, with or without abdominal exploration, while 71.4 of those in which such penetration did occur died. Many of these latter were cases of delayed operation or no operation, and so the figures are elusive in their significance.

I believe that the safest rule to follow is that postulated by Van Hook and other writers, that "operative measures suitable to the nature of the case should be undertaken with as much promptitude after these accidents as in cases of abdominal gunshot injury."

Discussion

Dr. Walter A. Fansler (by invitation): I very much appreciate the privilege of discussing the papers of Drs. Cottam and McGandy. I had the opportunity of examining the patient of Dr. McGandy, and consider the result quite remarkable. He complained of a little difficulty in controlling a liquid stool or his bladder if over-distended, but I felt that even this was quite largely a mental hazard. I have seen two other cases of this type which might be briefly mentioned. In the first instance the patient, a male, was backing down a ladder on the side of a railroad car. He dropped from the last rung and his anal region struck the end of a crowbar which was sticking upright in the ground. The crowbar entered the rectum through the anal canal do-

ing but slight injury to the anal canal. The rectum was pierced through the anterior wall at a point just above the prostate, the abdominal cavity being entered just posterior to the bladder. The abdomen was opened the following day by Dr. B. J. Branton of Willmar, who removed some pieces of overalls, and other extraneous matter. The rectum was repaired, and abdominal drains inserted. The patient left the hospital in two months with all wounds healed. I saw him sixteen months later. His complaint was a feeling of being unable to control his bowel. This, however, was a sensation, not a fact. He also stated that he had noted a little blood four days previously, and that he had pain during the act of defecation. A radiograph taken six weeks previously following a barium enema, was said to have shown some adhesions posterior to the rectum, but no interference with bowel function. The barium enema was retained without difficulty. Examination revealed that the anal canal could be dilated easily and painlessly to the diameter of one inch. The tone and contractile power of the sphincter was good. One and one-half inches from the anus on the midline of the anterior rectal wall, was a scar which extended upward and slightly to the left for 1.5 inches. It was well healed and not tender, and I felt the result was excellent. I saw the patient again six months later. At this time he complained of pain in the pelvis, particularly at night after a day of bending and stooping. He stated that the left lower portion of the abdomen swelled and that the scar of his abdominal incision was tender and painful. His appetite was poor and he had gas in his intestines. The findings upon examination were unchanged, and I could not but feel that the chief cause of symptoms was the threatened loss of compensation. I felt that operative procedure would be of no benefit and advised against it. However, his abdomen was explored at a later date by a local surgeon with the report of some adhesions about the sigmoid. My last report was that no benefit had been derived from the operation and my personal feeling was that no improvement would occur until the matter of compensation was settled.

The second patient was that of a young boy, sixteen years old, who was playing football on a vacant lot, from which the weeds had been cut, leaving some rather tall stumps. In the play he was pushed backward, sat on a weed-stump, which entered the rectum through the anal canal. The rectum was pierced on the anterior wall just above the prostate. I saw him in the General Hospital, sixty hours after injury. Rectal examination revealed the injury, but he had only a slight temperature and leukocytoses. He had slight distention and tenderness over the lowermost part of the abdomen. There was no abdominal rigidity, and we felt that, since sixty hours had elapsed with no graver symptoms than those present, we were justified in waiting further. In this case we were justified, as the boy's symptoms rapidly subsided and he was discharged from the hospital within a few days.

As has been pointed out, the occurrence of impalement or other similar rectal injuries, are so infrequent and the nature of the injuries so variable, that no predetermined or routine treatment has been determined. There are, however, certain facts which are of value when we are confronted with a patient suffering from this type of injury.

First it should be remembered that an elongated object entering the rectum will usually strike the anterior wall of the rectum, rather than the posterior wall which hugs the hollow of the sacrum. If the object be sharp, it will likely perforate at the first point of contact. If perforation does not occur here then it will almost surely take place near the site of the rectosigmoid juncture. At this point there is a distinct narrowing of the bowel, and just above there is a definite angulation. This angle is in some cases so acute that even

stition has arisen that these cases are better left alone and not operated upon.

This undoubtedly does apply to the non-penetrating cases, that is, those in which the vulnerating agent does not enter the peritoneal cavity, for most of these do

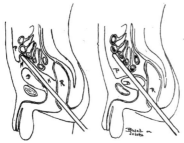

Fig. 1. *(left)* Dr. W. E. Morse's case. *P,* peritoneal cavity; *H,* hematoma; *B,* bladder; *X,* site of injury to bladder; *R,* rectum.

Fig. 2. *(right)* Author's case. *P,* peritoneal cavity; *B,* bladder; *R,* rectum.

recover under non-operative treatment, but where there is any doubt, we believe that it is safer to open the abdomen and take a look, for the odds are surely against the patient when fecal contamination of the peritoneum from the rectum occurs, or there is an open wound of the bladder into the peritoneum as well, if we sit back and do nothing but watch and wait. It is not always easy to estimate the depth of penetration in these cases. The distance of the fall before striking the vulnerating agent and the weight of the patient may afford some information, but the statement of a bystander who pulled it out is seldom reliable. The best evidence of deep penetration, if it be present, as it was in the two cases about to be described, is the ability to feel the end of the pitchfork handle, or whatever it is, through the anterior abdominal wall. In such cases we believe the indication for operation to be clear and undisputible, and as early as possible after the receipt of the injury.

I shall now describe as briefly as possible two illustrative cases with bladder involvement. Only the second is one of my own, the complete history of the first having come into my hands recently through the kindness of my friend Dr. W. E. Morse, of Rapid City, South Dakota, who handled it himself throughout.

Case 1.—Impalement of the rectum by pitchfork handle, with penetration of the anterior wall of the rectum, extraperitoneal injury of the bladder and massive retrocystic hematoma formation. Laparotomy, drainage and recovery (Dr. W. E. Morse's case).

C. W—, Bonita Spring, South Dakota, male, aged twenty-two, while hauling hay, on July 16, 1930, threw a pitchfork to the ground from the hayrack and immediately jumped from the load of hay, landing on the pitchfork handle, the fork having stuck in the

ground. The handle of the fork entered and penetrated the rectum for a distance of about 14 inches. The end of the handle could be felt a short distance above the pubes.

Examination showed the head, neck and chest free from evidence of disease or injury. The abdomen was acutely tender over the lower half, on both sides, with well defined rigidity of both recti. Rectal examination showed contusions in the anal area; the proctoscope revealed a perforation of the anterior wall.

Laparotomy under gas-ether anesthesia was performed within a few hours after the accident. It was found that the pitchfork handle had not penetrated into the peritoneal cavity but had stripped the peritoneum from the bladder to the anterior abdominal wall, with the formation of a huge hematoma in the traumatized area (Fig. 1).

The peritoneum was closed and the retrocystic traumatized area was drained by an extraperitoneal Penrose drain protruding anteriorly. A retention catheter of the mushroom type was left in the bladder and the patient returned to bed in good condition. Two days after the operation the patient was having a discharge of fecal material and gas through the retention catheter and a large amount of liquid which appeared to be urine was coming through the rectum. Eleven days after the operation, the intervening period having been quite uneventful, the temperature was normal, the patient feeling very well, there was less air coming through the bladder, less pain on urination and less fluid coming through the rectum. On the twentieth postoperative day the patient was sitting up and feeling very well; on the following day he was discharged from the hospital under observation, the rectal examination at that time showing that the channel of communication between the bladder and rectum was narrowed down to the size of a small lead pencil. Four days later he had to be readmitted on account of weakness, abdominal discomfort and pain in the rectum, due to fecal impaction in the rectum, relieved by enemies. Dr. Morse's records do not show the date of the final observation, but whenever it was the fistula had healed completely and the patient remained well.

Case 2.—Impalement of the rectum by pitchfork handle, with penetration of the rectum anteriorly, through-and-through penetration of the bladder into the peritoneal cavity and beginning peritonitis. Laparotomy, suture of the bladder, peritoneal drainage and tube drainage of the recto-vesical injury, recovery. (Author's case.)

R. P.—, Elkton, South Dakota, male, aged sixteen, was admitted on the morning of August 27, 1922, giving the following history: about 5:45 on the previous evening the patient jumped down from a wagon and struck a hay fork stuck in the ground, receiving the impact on his perineum. The fork handle entered the rectum and the end could be felt in front, just behind the anterior abdominal wall, a little below the umbilicus. Patient's father pulled out the fork handle. The immediate disability was slight; a physician who was called ordered hot applications and especially advised against any operation. During the night the father became alarmed by the boy's restlessness and complaint of increased pain, took him to a doctor in another town. This doctor catheterized the patient, obtaining only a small amount of fluid, although there had been no micturition since the accident, and also ordered him given an enema, which was found to contain some blood. This doctor realized the possibility of serious injury and brought the patient a distance of some sixty miles to me, early in the morning following the after-noon of the accident. I noted that the patient's facial expression appeared drawn and anxious, the pulse rapid and of none too good quality, the abdomen rigid throughout without localization and the lower abdomen tender to pressure. Rectal examination showed a longi-

ing but slight injury to the anal canal. The rectum was pierced through the anterior wall at a point just above the prostate, the abdominal cavity being entered just posterior to the bladder. The abdomen was opened the following day by Dr. B. J. Branton of Willmar, who removed some pieces of overalls, and other extraneous matter. The rectum was repaired, and abdominal drains inserted. The patient left the hospital in two months with all wounds healed. I saw him sixteen months later. His complaint was a feeling of being unable to control his bowel. This, however, was a sensation, not a fact. He also stated that he had noted a little blood four days previously, and that he had pain during the act of defecation. A radiograph taken six weeks previously following a barium enema, was said to have shown some adhesions posterior to the rectum, but no interference with bowel function. The barium enema was retained without difficulty. Examination revealed that the anal canal could be dilated easily and painlessly to the diameter of one inch. The tone and contractible power of the sphincter was good. One and one-half inches from the anus on the midline of the anterior rectal wall, was a scar which extended upward and slightly to the left for 1.5 inches. It was well healed and not tender, and I felt the result was excellent. I saw the patient again six months later. At this time he complained of pain in the pelvis, particularly at night after a day of bending and stooping. He stated that the left lower portion of the abdomen swelled and that the scar of his abdominal incision was tender and painful. His appetite was poor and he had gas in his intestines. The findings upon examination were unchanged, and I could not but feel that the chief cause of symptoms was the threatened loss of compensation. I felt that operative procedure would be of no benefit and advised against it. However, his abdomen was explored at a later date by a local surgeon with the report of some adhesions about the sigmoid. My last report was that no benefit had been derived from the operation and my personal feeling was that no improvement would occur until the matter of compensation was settled.

The second patient was that of a young boy, sixteen years old, who was playing football on a vacant lot, from which the weeds had been cut, leaving some rather tall stumps. In the play he was pushed backward, sat on a weed-stump, which entered the rectum through the anal canal. The rectum was pierced on the anterior wall just above the prostate. I saw him in the General Hospital, sixty hours after injury. Rectal examination revealed the injury, but he had only a slight temperature and leukocytoses. He had slight distention and tenderness over the lowermost part of the abdomen. There was no abdominal rigidity, and we felt that, since sixty hours had elapsed with no graver symptoms than those present, we were justified in waiting further. In this case we were justified, as the boy's symptoms rapidly subsided and he was discharged from the hospital within a few days.

As has been pointed out, the occurrence of impalement or other similar rectal injuries, are so infrequent and the nature of the injuries so variable, that no predetermined or routine treatment has been determined. There are, however, certain facts which are of value when we are confronted with a patient suffering from this type of injury.

First it should be remembered that an elongated object entering the rectum will usually strike the anterior wall of the rectum, rather than the posterior wall which hugs the hollow of the sacrum. If the object be sharp, it will likely perforate at the first point of contact. If perforation does not occur here then it will almost surely take place near the site of the rectosigmoid juncture. At this point there is a distinct narrowing of the bowel, and just above there is a definite angulation. This angle is in some cases so acute that even

451

with the greatest care a proctoscope cannot be advanced around it. Therefore this is a common site of perforation. In a few instances this narrowing and angulation does not occur, and the rectum and colon form a straight tube entering the abdominal cavity. This is undoubtedly the case in those rare instances where the end of the object causing impalement can be felt high in the abdominal cavity, and yet bowel perforation has not occurred. It is, I think, of some practical value to remember that in almost all cases of impalement the site of perforation will be not more than 6 inches from the anus and likely, less. The injury therefore should be easily visualized by the use of an anoscope or a short proctoscope. If no perforation can be found in this area the chances are that one does not exist.

In attempting to make a diagnosis the giving of enemas or the inflation of the bowel with air during proctoscopic examination should be avoided as foreign material may be forced into the peritoneal cavity. The walls of the rectum should be cleansed where necessary with moist gauze or applicators, and proctoscopic examination made without inflation.

An x-ray examination is a valuable adjunct in many of these cases for it may reveal the presence of gas in the peritoneal cavity, especially in those cases where some time has elapsed since the injury. It may also reveal the presence of foreign material.

Doctor Cottam commented upon the frequent lack of hemorrhage in these cases. This is because the majority of perforations occur on the anterior walls of the rectum in the relatively avascular area above the prostate. The blood supply of this portion of the rectum is derived almost entirely from the superior hemorrhoidal artery. This artery bifurcates upon the posterior aspect of the rectum, only its terminal branches extending anteriorly. He has also emphasized the unreliability of the statements of persons who witness the accident and the early lack of shock and other evidence of severe injury in these cases, even where perforation of the abdominal cavity has occurred.

To recapitulate all of the points brought out in these papers and their discussion, the following salient points may be kept in mind:

1. In the majority of cases the site of bowel perforation will be found on the anterior wall of the rectum, and seldom more than six inches cephalad to the anal orifice. It can therefore be easily visualized with a short anoscope or proctoscope, and if no perforation can be found in this area the chances are that one does not exist. If such an opening is found, careful probing is justifiable.

2. X-ray examination may reveal the presence of gas or foreign material in the abdominal cavity.

3. Enemas and inflation of the bowel with air are unnecessary and dangerous in cases of perforation. Proctoscopic examinations can be done without inflation and the walls of the bowel can be cleansed with moist gauze or applicators.

4. Statements of witnesses of the accident must be accepted with caution.

5. Hemorrhage, shock, severe pain, or other evidence of severe injury are frequently lacking immediately following the injury, even though perforation of the abdominal cavity has occurred. This must be kept in mind lest the surgeon be tempted to follow the policy of watchful waiting rather than making a thorough investigation.

6. Immediate exploratory laparotomy should be done in all doubtful cases. To wait for active signs of perforation is to court disaster. The exploration of a normal abdomen is not serious, but it is serious to allow a perforated bowel to go without early attention.

DR. C. D. CREEVY: I have never seen an impalement of the rectum in which the bladder was injured. I should like to congratulate both Dr. Cottam and Dr.

McGandy on the excellent results they have had in what must have been rather difficult situations.

My experience at the University Hospital includes one instance of impalement of the rectum with a pitchfork handle which entered neither the peritoneal cavity nor the bladder. The patient made an uneventful recovery without any operative therapy. I have seen one case of puncture of the sigmoid by a proctoscope which was repaired surgically within a few minutes of the accident but which caused death, indicating the virulence of the organisms that sometimes are present in the rectum. The rest of my experience has concerned lesions of a different type involving the rectum and bladder or urethra; included are a recto-urethral fistula which had followed a hemorrhoidectomy some thirteen years before. The communication was between the bulbous urethra and the anterior rectal wall just above the anal sphincter, so that the patient was able to void urine in a good stream through the anus, the urethra being shut off by a stricture just below it. The urine was clear. When the patient understood the nature of the operations that would be required he decided to continue his urination in the manner to which he had been accustomed for thirteen years. I still think this was a wise decision.

The second was a recto-urethral fistula following perineal prostatectomy done, of course, elsewhere, and which had already been repaired by Dr. Peyton, who did preliminary colostomy and cystostomy, followed by an operation similar to that which Dr. McGandy did in his patient.

The third was a case of a congenital communication between an imperforate anus and a prostatic urethra which was repaired by Dr. Wangensteen.

The only fistulous communication between the urinary tract and rectum which I have seen and treated personally was one which followed a series of operations for intestinal obstruction, also done elsewhere, beginning with an appendectomy, followed by drainage, followed by intestinal obstruction, followed by an operation for the relief of adhesions which, in turn, three or four days after the operation, was followed by the passage of feces and gas through the urethra. The condition had been present for about six months following the last operation when the patient was admitted to the University Hospital and the diagnosis, of course, was perfectly obvious from the symptoms. I was anxious to secure some films which could be made into a lantern slide for demonstration purposes and undertook to demonstrate the fistula by means of the x-ray. Barium given by mouth and by rectum failed to enter any fistulous communication. A cystogram was made and failed to show any communication between bladder and bowel. An opening could be seen high up on the posterior wall of the bladder with a cystoscope quite readily but nothing could be passed through it. When the abdomen was explored it was found that there was a perforation in the terminal ileum which communicated with the posterior wall of the bladder and which was very readily taken down and repaired, after which there was an uneventful recovery.

DR. T. H. SWEETSER: I wish to mention the case of a young man whom I saw at the General Hospital in 1933, in order especially to call attention to the possible value of intravenous pyelography and cystography in cases of the type under discussion this evening. This man, during a game of horseshoes, sat between turns on a tin can placed upside down on one of the iron stakes used in the game. The bottom of the tin can bulged farther each time he sat on it, and finally gave way and the stake entered the rectum. He developed abdominal pain in both lower quadrants, especially on the left; there was no nausea or vomiting and no external bleeding. He was given a hypodermic injection and sent to the hospital, where, on examination, only a tenderness and spasticity of the lower abdomen were found.

Exploratory laparotomy disclosed an intact peritoneum but marked edema of the tissues in the region of the rectum; no mention was made of the bladder. Four days later I was asked to see him because the urine at the time of admittance had showed blood, and later blood and pus cells. I suggested intravenous urography; I haven't heard that mentioned in the discussion thus far. There was noted thereby a mild bilateral hydronephrosis and hydro-ureter, and, more important in this case, a lack of concentration of the dye in the bladder, due apparently to leakage of urine into the surrounding tissues or into the rectum. Cystoscopy showed a wound in the base of the bladder and bits of clothing in the bladder cavity. The bladder was opened suprapubically, clothing, urine and feces removed, and the wound in the bladder base closed with a mattress suture of forty-day chromic catgut, avoiding the mucosa of bladder and rectum and pushing the knot down behind the bladder. A Freyer tube was placed for drainage. The urine, clear at first, showed some fecal contamination temporarily after three days, but cleared soon. The operative wound healed well and he voided easily and went home in excellent condition thirty-one days after his accident and twenty-six days after the cystotomy.

In this discussion, I wish mainly to call your attention to the safety and possible diagnostic value of intravenous urography in such cases.

DR. H. W. CHRISTIANSON (by invitation): I saw a case where a pitchfork tine had perforated through the rectum into the bladder. An indwelling catheter was placed in the bladder and a small drain was placed in the wound located in the rectal wall. This drain was removed in a few days and nothing further was done. The patient made a complete recovery.

One important fact might be brought out regarding the packing of these wounds. Drains or gauze packing should not be left in longer than is absolute necessary as they may produce a permanent sinus or fixed scar. This rule applies to any fistulous tract.

Accidents involving impalement of the rectum are very serious and it is, therefore, important to find out at once if the wounds are extra-peritoneal or intra-peritoneal.

DR. WILLARD WHITE: I would like to mention briefly a boy I saw at the General Hospital about 1925, as I remember. He had been playing ball and broke the bat. He put the blunt end of the bat on the ground and had a piece of board that he put across the upper or sharp end, and sat on this. Something happened so that he lost his balance, the board tipped up and the sharp end of the broken bat went into his rectum, penetrated the anterior wall of the rectum, through the posterior wall of the bladder and out through the fundus. I happened to be at the hospital on another emergency and I saw the boy about two hours after the accident, at which time there was very definite rigidity in the lower abdomen. We were satisfied that he had peritoneal irritation. We opened his abdomen and found urine and fecal material in the abdominal cavity and these perforations I mentioned.

These perforations, the two in the bladder and one in the rectum, were sutured. One point I would like to make now which I think you all know but may fail to remember and which is a very valuable thing in connection with extensive soiling such as you get in this type of thing. Pour in a great deal of normal salt solution and suck it out with the suction apparatus because it has been demonstrated with experimental animals that pathogenic organisms can be placed in the abdominal cavities of dogs and if the abdominal cavity is washed out thoroughly immediately and closed without drainage, about 80 per cent of these dogs will survive, whereas if they do the same thing except that they do not wash out the peritoneal cavities practically all of the dogs will die. It is a very good idea to irrigate the abdominal cavity and then use the suction apparatus.

An indwelling catheter was left in this boy and he got a bilateral epididymitis. There was some infection in the abdominal wound. However, he recovered. I followed him for a number of years. Since that time he has married and has at least two children. That was of interest to me because I wondered whether or not his bilateral epididymitis was going to sterilize him.

DR. H. F. BAYARD (by invitation): All of the cases reported here this evening have resulted in a favorable outcome, in spite of the fact that, as Dr. McGandy cites, the mortality rate reaches a level of something like 30 per cent. Two of the three cases within my experience have resulted fatally.

The first of these was a man who slipped off a runway while watching concrete being poured on a construction job. He impaled himself on one of the corrugated reinforcing rods protruding up above the concrete; this rod was somewhat over an inch in diameter. The injury was a complete denudation of the perianal skin, perforation of the lateral wall of the rectum as well as perforation of two loops of ileum. Peculiarly enough, this man made a recovery.

Another case, seen in consultation, resulted in a fatality. This case, as are many of the rectal traumatic lesions, was due to perforation of the lateral wall of the rectum by the handle of a pitchfork, the end of the perforation tract being at the base of the mesentery in one of the lower loops of bowel. A large postrectal abscess developed and was drained but an adynamic ileus and peritonitis developed and the boy died, as I recall the case, about one week after exploration of his abdomen.

These are usually very serious injuries and we should not be misled into thinking that the injury carries a low mortality rate.

The meeting adjourned.

HARVEY NELSON, M.D., *Secretary.*

The Prevention of Paralysis in Poliomyelitis

The seasonable outbreaks of infantile paralysis are not far distant. Last week a statement in the correspondence column of THE JOURNAL emphasized the necessity for complete rest for patients in the early stages of this disease. Complete rest is so important that it is usually far better to leave the child in bed at home when the disease is first suspected than to move the patient any appreciable distance to a hospital. When these patients are disturbed or moved as little as possible a majority in whom the disease has not progressed beyond the early stages escape paralysis entirely. Should the patient have paralysis, especially of the extremities, the affected part should be immobilized properly at the earliest moment. Early rest of a weakened muscle under these circumstances will help prevent permanent crippling. Infantile paralysis can be suspected when there is fever, headache, irritability, possibly vomiting, perhaps a tremor in the hands, and especially a tender rigid spine, which makes it impossible for the child to touch his chin to his knee. When such manifestations are present, the spinal fluid may be examined to confirm the diagnosis. Thus far there is no specific effective remedy in the acute stages of infantile paralysis nor any generally accepted preventive.—(Jour. A.M.A., May 14, 1938.)

◆ REPORTS and ANNOUNCEMENTS ◆

MEDICAL BROADCAST

The Minnesota State Medical Association Morning Health Service

The Minnesota State Medical Association broadcasts weekly at 9:45 o'clock every Saturday morning over Station WCCO, Minneapolis and Saint Paul (810 kilocycles or 370.2 meters).

Speaker: William A. O'Brien, Associate Professor of Pathology and Preventive Medicine, Medical School, University of Minnesota. The program for the month will be as follows:

June 4—Chronic Illness.
June 11—Burns.
June 18—Arthritis.
June 25—Orthodontia.

HENNEPIN COUNTY MEDICAL SOCIETY

Dr. J. S. Reynolds was elected president at the annual meeting of the Hennepin County Medical Society, held May 2, 1938. Other officers elected were: Dr. W. E. Patterson, first vice president; Dr. F. J. Pratt, second vice president; Dr. L. M. Daniel, secretary-treasurer, and Dr. T. A. Peppard, librarian.

Dr. F. A. Willius, of Rochester, addressed the members on "A Less Common Manifestation of Rheumatic Heart Disease."

NORTHERN MINNESOTA MEDICAL ASSOCIATION

Announcement has been made by the program committee that the fall meeting of the Northern Minnesota Medical Association will be held at Crookston, Minnesota, on Monday and Tuesday, August 29 and 30. Further announcement as to the program will follow in a subsequent issue.

REDWOOD-BROWN COUNTY

The Redwood-Brown County Medical Society held its annual meeting at the Turner Hall in New Ulm on Wednesday, May 4. The meeting was preceded by a banquet with the Ladies Auxiliary, following which Dr. J. G. Love and Dr. Bayard Horton of the Mayo Clinic gave talks respectively on "Diagnosis and Treatment of Head Injuries," and "Histamine Treatment of Migraine Headaches."

Election of officers resulted as follows: President, Dr. Walter G. Nuessle, Springfield; vice president, Dr.

Howard Vogel, New Ulm; secretary-treasurer, Carl J. Fritsche, New Ulm; censor for three years, Dr. Francis C. Gibbons, Comfrey; delegate to 1939 convention, Dr. Cornelius A. Saffert, New Ulm; alternate, Dr. Kenneth L. Olson, Gibbon.

The Medical Economics or "Contact Committee" was unanimously re-elected: Dr. Albert Fritsche, New Ulm, Chairman; Dr. T. F. Hammermeister, New Ulm; Dr. O. J. Seifert, New Ulm; Dr. E. J. Wohlrabe, Springfield; Dr. A. P. Goblirsch, Sleepy Eye.

SOUTHWESTERN MINNESOTA SOCIETY

A highly successful interprofessional dinner meeting was sponsored by the Southwestern Minnesota Medical Society on April 28 at the Hotel Thompson in Worthington.

Eighty-five men, representing dentists, lawyers, physicians and others, were present.

District Judge Charles A. Flinn introduced the first speaker, who was Mr. James H. Hall, president of the Minnesota State Bar Association. Dr. L. M. Cruttenden of Saint Paul, secretary of the Minnesota State Dental Association, followed him. Dr. Cruttenden was introduced by Dr. C. L. Perrizo, also a dentist, of Jasper. Dr. Cruttenden reviewed the history of dentistry since the establishment, one hundred years ago, of the first dental college.

Dr. B. J. Branton of Willmar, councilor of the third district, represented the physicians on the program. Dr. C. L. Sherman of Luverne, president of the Southwestern Society and of the Southwestern Sanatorium Board and member of the State Board of Medical Examiners, introduced Dr. Branton. Dr. Branton's theme was application of the Golden Rule in the relations between physicians and all of their professional associates.

WRIGHT COUNTY MEDICAL SOCIETY

The Wright County Medical Society met at Delano on Wednesday, April 20, twenty-two doctors being present. Dr. H. M. N. Wynne and Dr. R. I. Rizer of Minneapolis spoke on "Endocrines."

The home economics class of the high school served a four course dinner for the doctors and their wives at 6:30. During the afternoon the ladies were entertained by Mrs. A. E. Phillips and Mrs. Theodore Greenfield at Mrs. Phillips' home.

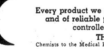

MINNESOTA MEDICINE

Journal of the Minnesota State Medical Association, Southern Minnesota Medical Association, Northern Minnesota Medical Association, Minnesota Academy of Medicine and Minneapolis Surgical Society

| Volume 21 | JULY, 1938 | No. 7 |

POLIOMYELITIS WITH SPECIAL REFERENCE TO THE DRINKER RESPIRATOR THERAPY*

ALBERT V. STOESSER, M.D., and WALLACE S. SAKO, M.D.

Minneapolis, Minnesota

E ACH year, more and more information concerning acute anterior poliomyelitis is placed on record. Some reports deal with the etiology of the disease, others with the diagnosis and many suggest new forms of therapy.

In the last six months of the year 1937, a fairly large number of cases of poliomyelitis were admitted to the University and Minneapolis General Hospitals. These patients were closely followed and interesting observations were made. The majority of the patients were admitted during the months of August and September. Three-fourths of these were between the ages of one and fourteen and the lowest mortality was found in the years from five to nine. There was an equal distribution as to sex. The size of the family did not seem to influence the incidence of the disease. There were no cases of second attacks.

In this series, the average maximum temperature was 103.9 F. and the white blood cell count averaged 8,900. The leukocyte count showed no definite relation to the temperature, indicating the blood response and presumably the antibody response to be slow or absent. The majority of the spinal fluid cell counts were between 50 and 100. The cell count generally fell gradually from the level found at the onset of the disease until the period just preceding the most extensive paralysis. At this time it rose again, falling slowly thereafter. The polymorphonuclear cells in the spinal fluid slowly decreased as the disease progressed and the mononuclears corresponding-

ly gradually rose until about the fourteenth day, when they were practically one hundred per cent. The course of the disease could not be predicted by the temperature, the white blood cell count or the spinal fluid findings.

The distribution of the paralysis was of interest. There were fourteen cases with paralysis of the muscles of the trunk and abdomen. This was a higher number than was expected. Most outstanding, however, was the incidence of cases having respiratory difficulty. Minnesota has experienced during the past ten years three periods during which there have been an unusual number of cases of poliomyelitis. Each time there has been a corresponding increase in the number of patients admitted to the hospitals. Among the hospital cases the incidence of patients with difficulty in breathing has increased until during the latter half of the past year it reached a rather alarming figure. Seventy-nine cases of poliomyelitis were admitted to the University and Minneapolis General Hospitals from July 1, 1937, to December 31, 1937, and of this number twenty-nine patients had some respiratory distress. Tables I and II summarize these observations.

Thunberg, in 1926, first used the barospirometer for artificial respiration. The patient was entirely enclosed in an air-tight cylinder. Drinker, Shaw and McKhann[4, 5] reported, in 1929, a modification of the barospirometer so that the patient's head could be outside the air-tight cylinder. Since then the Drinker respirator has been widely used for the treatment of respiratory failure in poliomyelitis. In Minnesota, however, where respirators are scarce, physicians must

*From the Department of Pediatrics of the University of Minnesota.

Year	University and General Hospitals	City of Minneapolis	State of Minnesota
1928	14	34	223
1929	14	4	30
1930	13	46	475
1931	65	143	810
1932	8	10	122
1933	47	94	382
1934	9	9	109
1935	6	13	98
1936	6	8	31
1937	83	95	358

TABLE II. TYPES OF POLIOMYELITIS DURING YEARS
OF HIGHEST INCIDENCE

University and Minneapolis General Hospitals

TYPE	1931	1933	1937*
Abortive	1	0	6
Non-paralytic	31	17	18
Encephalitic	1	0	1
Paralytic			
Spinal	26	17	25
Spinal respiratory	1	2	8
Bulbar	4	7	15
Bulbo-Spinal	1	4	6

*Six months period (July 1, 1937, to Dec. 31, 1937).

know the indications for this form of therapy especially in view of the fact that the recent small epidemics of poliomyelitis have been accompanied by a high incidence of cases with respiratory embarrassment. Some patients respond very well to the Drinker respirator; others do not respond and are even made worse. Physicians tend to place all their cases with respiratory difficulty into the machine. The authors feel that this is a poor procedure and offer, therefore, in this brief communication, the newer knowledge of the Drinker respirator therapy.

The most important problem is the careful selection of the patients for treatment. The following classification has been found to be of great assistance.

Spinal Cases

Spinal cases in which there is a direct paralysis of the muscles of respiration innervated by the nerves from the dorsal and cervical spinal cord. The intercostal muscles, the diaphragm, or both, are involved. Paralysis of the intercostal muscles is determined by watching the expansion of the chest during inspiration. The magnitude of expansion is more readily estimated by

pressing firmly on the upper abdomen, thus diminishing the excursion of the diaphragm. Paralysis of the diaphragm is determined by observing the movement of the abdominal wall during inspiration. If there is no abdominal movement, or if the abdomen is drawn inward during inspiration, it indicates weakness or paralysis of the diaphragm.

The individual with spinal respiratory paralysis usually advances to the stage where he lies in bed motionless, the eyes having a fearful stare. The face is dusky and the lips are cyanotic. The alæ nasi dilate with every inspiration and the accessory muscles of respiration, especially the sternocleidomastoid, are visible with every inspiration. The chest and the abdomen become practically vibrationless. The patient cannot sleep, but when he is placed in the Drinker respirator the response is usually dramatic. The cyanosis disappears and the face assumes its natural color. The facial expression is that of satisfaction. After the patient's breathing and the respirator become synchronous, the individual falls into a deep sleep which may last many hours.

The early respirators had three speeds: 15, 30 and 45 per minute. Later models had two speeds: 15 and 30 per minute. The latest type is so constructed that all degrees of speed can be obtained and the machine can be tilted as desired. Eight of our patients with respiratory difficulty were of the spinal type and all were placed in the Drinker machine. None of these died in the respirator although one died after removal from the machine, of peritonitis which followed a recto-vaginal fistula. The initial rate of 30 per minute was used in the majority of our cases, and then the rate was adjusted to correspond as nearly as possible to the normal respiratory rate of the patient—faster in children and slower in adults. Children were started at about 10 cm. of negative water pressure, which was gradually increased with age to 15 cm. or 20 cm. for adults. In each case the machine was operated at the lowest negative water pressure at which the patient had complete relief of symptoms.

The patients placed in the respirator remained in it undisturbed except for rotation from side to side several times daily. The efficiency of the respiratory muscles was observed when the machine was opened to give nursing care. I

improvement began, the respirator was opened for longer intervals and then, following the suggestions of Emil Smith,[12] the patients were asked to cough. If they could, they were removed from the machine and watched carefully for cyanosis. However, when the patients were able to breathe without effort but could not cough, they were kept a part of each day in the machine until such time as they were able to cough.

There was some mechanical difficulty in giving adequate nursing care to the patients in the respirator. The disadvantages of the machine were as follows:

1. The temperature was difficult to regulate.
2. The frequent incontinence of urine and sometimes of feces increased the tendency to skin irritation.
3. The rubber collar was uncomfortable and irritated the neck.
4. Early orthopedic treatment could not be carried out as desired.

Bulbar Cases

Bulbar cases in which there is involvement of the nuclei of the cranial nerves with apparent injury of the respiratory center. The damage to the bulbar nerves supplying the muscles of the pharnyx and the larynx is often ushered in by a nasal quality of the voice, by choking attack or by regurgitation of fluids through the nose. Various grades of aphonia and impaired ability to cough or swallow are present. Advanced cases may be heard breathing with an ominous gurgling in the throat. Attempting to swallow causes a choking attack. Secretions around the glottis which seem to prevent deep inspirations, cause the breathing to simulate paralysis of the respiratory muscles. Deep inspirations tend to aspirate fluid into the larynx and are frequently interrupted by a forced expiration. However, extreme irregularity of breathing, both as to depth and rhythm, is an indication of damage to the respiratory center.

Nine of our patients had pharyngeal paralysis with some interference in proper breathing. None was treated with the Drinker respirator and all recovered. Two patients also had facial paralysis, and this cleared up satisfactorily. There were, however, six bulbar cases with definite respiratory difficulty. Two patients were placed in the Drinker respirator but they did poorly and expired in a short time. It was apparent

that the machine caused aspiration of material from the throat and at the same time overcame the reflex choking and coughing by which this material could be ejected. The next case, therefore, did not receive the respirator therapy, the following measures being substituted:

1. The foot of the patient's bed was elevated to facilitate drainage of secretions away from the larynx and into the posterior pharynx, where they were removed by suction.
2. Postural drainage was used during the choking spells when the condition of the patient permitted.
3. Nothing was given by mouth and vomiting was almost eliminated. Plenty of parenteral fluid was administered and large whole blood transfusions were also given.

In spite of these procedures, the patient rapidly became worse. Choking attacks occurred with temporary severe anoxemia resulting in deep cyanosis. Aspiration of mucus and vomitus into the bronchial tree took place, producing evidence of bronchial obstruction leading to a complete cessation of breathing at times. Excessive fatigue due to the continual interference with inspiration by the unswallowed material in the pharynx or the actual inspiration of this material was the cause of death. However, the three remaining patients did not have such an extensive involvement of the bulbar nerves as was present in the previous case. All were treated without the Drinker respirator by the method outlined above. At first, it was difficult to refuse the use of the respirator to these cases, but as they progressed favorably the thought of using the machine vanished.

Bulbo-spinal Cases

Bulbo-spinal cases have, as the term indicates, both spinal and bulbar involvement. This is manifested by paralysis of intercostal muscles, the diaphragm, or both, and some paralysis of the pharynx. If the paralysis of the pharynx is unilateral, as indicated by difficulty in swallowing, the respirator may be effective. If the paralysis of the pharynx is bilateral, as indicated by a total inability to swallow, the machine is ineffective. This was easily demonstrated by the fact that five of our six bulbo-spinal patients were placed in the Drinker respirator, and none survived. They all had a bilateral paralysis of

TABLE III. REPORTS IN THE LITERATURE OF POLIOMYELITIS CASES TREATED WITH THE DRINKER
RESPIRATOR AND THE RESULTS OBTAINED

Year Author	Spinal Respiratory Treated	Died	Pure Bulbar Treated	Died	Bulbo Spinal Treated	Died
1929—Drinker & McKhann[4]	1	1				
1930—Shambough, Harrison & Farrell[10]	1	0			2	2
1931—Shaw, Thelander & Limper[11]	10	1	5	5		
1932—Wilson[14,15]	23	3	20	13		
1932—Wesselhoeft & Smith[13]	9	0	5	4	16	13
1933—Harper & Tennant[7]	7	0	17	17		
1934—Crone[3]	9	5	5	3		
1934—Landon[8]	56	29	2	2	30	22
1935—Fischer & Stillerman[6]	8	0	10	7		
1936—Brahdy & Lenarsky[1,2]	51	24	12	12		
1937—Stoesser & Sako	8	0	2	2	5	5
Grand Total of Cases	183	63	78	65	53	42
Mortality Per Cent		34		83		80

the pharynx. The one patient who did not receive the Drinker respirator therapy was not very ill. He was frightened by the machine and fought it. There was only a partial involvement of the muscles of respiration and a unilateral pharyngeal paralysis. This patient recovered.

The pathological lung changes in patients who have expired in the respirator have always been of great interest to those taking care of poliomyelitis patients. The following changes are commonly reported in the literature:[9] (1) rupture of the alveoli due to emphysema; (2) pneumothorax; (3) pulmonary atelectasis; (4) pulmonary congestion; (5) pneumonia.

Most of these conditions can be eliminated in the spinal respiratory cases if the machine is used properly and the patients are systematically turned and carefully nursed. However, those with the more severe bulbar involvement die and at necropsy reveal changes such as were found in our group, namely: pulmonary edema, bloody fluid in the pleural cavities, subpleural petechial hemorrhages, and hemorrhagic bronchopneumonia.

The experience gained from our small series of cases has confirmed the observations of other writers who state that those unfamiliar with respiratory failure in poliomyelitis are apt to

TABLE IV. SUMMARY OF TREATMENT OF POLIOMYELITIS CASES WITH RESPIRATORY
DIFFICULTY

University and Minneapolis General Hospitals,
July 1, 1937–Dec. 31, 1937

Type of Case	Treat-ment
Spinal respiratory with paralysis of intercostal muscles and diaphragm	A
	B
Bulbar with pharyngeal and/or laryngeal paralysis	A
	B
Bulbo-spinal with paralysis of respiratory muscles and pharyngeal paralysis	A
	B

A—Cases treated with the Drinker respirator.
B—Cases in which the Drinker respirator was not used any time.

overestimate the value of the respirator in th[is] disease because they fail to differentiate the typ[e] of respiratory failure. The spinal respirato[ry] case has a very good chance of being saved [by] the machine. On the other hand, in the bulb[ar] type with glosso-pharyngeal and vagus involv[e]ment the respirator often offers little hel[p]. Tables III and IV emphasize still more the i[m]portance of the foregoing statements.

Summary and Conclusions

Recent small epidemics of acute anterior poliomyelitis in Minnesota appear to reveal an increasing incidence of cases with respiratory difficulty. The respirator devised by Drinker and McKhann has been found to be of great help to the patients with difficult breathing. However, all patients are not benefited to the same extent.

Proper selection of the patients is essential. This is especially important in epidemic periods when the number of Drinker respirators available is less than the demand. Our experience with a small number of cases has shown the respirator to be of unquestionable value in the treatment of those patients with high spinal involvement. The machine gives them the rest so essential for recovery.

The Drinker respirator is of little or no value in the care of patients whose respiratory difficulty is bulbar in origin. The machine may overpower the choking and cough reflexes and in some cases even cause forcible aspiration through the larynx of secretions from the throat.

The bulbo-spinal cases may respond to the Drinker respirator provided the pharyngeal paralysis is unilateral. If the paralysis is bilateral and the patient cannot swallow, the machine is ineffective.

Bibliography

1. Brahdy, M. B., and Lenarsky, M.: The treatment of respiratory failure in acute epidemic poliomyelitis. Am. Jour. Dis. Child., 46:705, 1933.
2. Brahdy, M. B., and Lenarsky, M.: Respiratory failure in acute epidemic poliomyelitis. Jour. Pediat., 8:420, 1936.
3. Crone, N. L.: The treatment of acute poliomyelitis with the respirator. New Eng. Jour. Med., 210:621, 1934.
4. Drinker, P., and McKhann, C. F.: The use of a new apparatus for the prolonged administration of artificial respiration; a fatal case of poliomyelitis. Jour. A.M.A., 92:1658, 1929.
5. Drinker, P., and Shaw, L. A.: An apparatus for the prolonged administration of artificial respiration: a design for adults and children. Jour. Clin. Investigation, 7:229, 1929.
6. Fischer, E., and Stillerman, M.: Acute anterior poliomyelitis in New York in 1935. A review of 686 cases. Am. Jour. Dis. Child., 54:984, 1937.
7. Harper, P., and Tennant, R.: Treatment of respiratory failure in poliomyelitis. Yale Jour. Biol. and Med., 6:31, 1933.
8. Landon, J. F.: An analysis of 88 cases of poliomyelitis treated in the Drinker respirator with a control series of 68 cases. Jour. Pediat., 5:1, 1934.
9. Murphy, M. D., and Bauer, J. T.: Lungs after treatment of asphyxia neonatorum in the Drinker respirator. Report of thirty necropsies. Am. Jour. Dis. Child., 45:1196, 1933.
10. Shambough, G. E., Jr., Harrison, W. G., Jr., and Farrell, J. L.: Treatment of the respiratory paralysis of poliomyelitis in a respiratory chamber. Report of 3 cases, with one recovery. Jour. A.M.A., 94:1371, 1930.
11. Shaw, E. B., Thelander, H. E., and Limper, M. A.: Respiratory failure in poliomyelitis. Its treatment with the Drinker respirator. Calif. and West. Med., 35:5, 1931.
12. Smith, Emil: Respiratory failure and the Drinker respirator in poliomyelitis. Jour. A.M.A., 100:1666, 1933.
13. Wesselhoeft, C., and Smith, Edward C.: Results of the use of the Drinker respirator in thirty cases of respiratory failure in poliomyelitis. New Eng. Jour. Med., 207:559, 1932.
14. Wilson, J. L.: Acute anterior poliomyelitis: Treatment of bulbar and high spinal types. New Eng. Jour. Med., 206:887, 1932.
15. Wilson, J. L.: Respiratory failure in poliomyelitis; treatment with the Drinker respirator. Am. Jour. Dis. Child., 43:1433, 1932.

SYPHILIS IN THE TRANSIENT*

PAUL A. O'LEARY, M.D.

Rochester, Minnesota

DURING the past few months you have noticed in the press or have heard over the radio considerable discussion about syphilis and gonorrhea. A campaign has been launched for the dissemination of knowledge in regard to syphilis, similar to the educational program regarding tuberculosis which has been actively carried on for many years. There are many reasons why the time seems appropriate for the carrying out of such a program, and I shall discuss this shortly. It is worthy of comment, however, that in the years gone by the editors of newspapers believed that their readers were not ready for such a campaign and that they could not use the words "syphilis" and "gonorrhea" in the public press. This attitude has gradually changed, and newspapers and magazines now contain information in regard to the venereal diseases. Surgeon General Parran of the United States Public Health Service precipitated the idea of such a campaign and has enthusiastically established it as a nation-wide enterprise. That the people of this country are in the mood to receive information about venereal diseases is evidenced by the fact that the momentum of the campaign has carried it from the hands of the Surgeon General to become a problem managed by the individual states.

There are numerous reasons why syphilis should be discussed in public rather than behind closed doors, as has been the case heretofore. We now have data based on extensive research which permits us to say without reservation that early

*From the Department of Dermatology and Syphilology, The Mayo Clinic, Rochester, Minnesota. Read at the Midwest Conference on Transiency and Settlement Laws, Saint Paul, Minnesota, March, 1937.

syphilis is definitely curable. I should like to emphasize the fact that cure applies to early syphilis. When we speak of late syphilis, that is, when the disease has passed the early stage, we are compelled to speak of an arrest of the disease rather than cure. By "arrest" we mean checking the progress of the disease in the heart or other internal organs. We know, now, that we can cure 85 per cent of the patients who come to us with a fresh infection and follow out the course of treatment which is recommended. It is by proper treatment of early syphilis that the late complications of the disease can be avoided.

Another reason why we are ready for a program of publicity is the success of such undertakings in Europe. The campaign in Denmark has been highly successful. There were less than 200 new cases of syphilis last year in Denmark, and I believe that in about thirty of these cases the patients were sailors who apparently had acquired the disease in some foreign country. In England, likewise, the campaign has been effective and has materially reduced the number of new cases of syphilis in that country. This decrease in the number of new infections is due not only to the fact that the treatments are furnished free but rather to the more important stipulation that the patient *must* remain under treatment until released by his physician.

A significant point for consideration is that in most cases of syphilis and gonorrhea the disease is acquired between the ages of seventeen and thirty-two years. Youths at this age are not impressed with the seriousness of the disease and, in most instances, are unable financially to arrange for proper treatment; this fact is, no doubt, a not infrequent cause of transiency. These boys are afraid of transmitting the disease to some of the relatives and because of their embarrassment and shame start out "on the road," spreading the disease as they go. Not only is it necessary that treatment be made available to these patients, but it must be made compulsory so that they will be forced to remain under treatment until they are no longer infectious, or able to transmit the disease.

Syphilis is infectious only during the early phase of the disease and is seldom infectious after the fourth year of its existence, regardless of whether the patient has received treatment or not. In other words, if an individual has had syphilis for more than five years and has been

treated, there is practically no danger of his spreading the disease. In a man who has acquired syphilis and has had some treatment and has married five years after he acquired the disease, the likelihood is that his wife will not be infected and accordingly his children will not have the disease. However, if he marries within the first five years after he acquired the disease, the chances are that he will infect his wife, who in turn will infect the children, since the disease is transmitted to the children by the mother. This limitation of the infectiousness of the disease makes it an ideal disease for a public health program. We can absolutely eliminate the problem of infectiousness in cases of early syphilis by the adequate treatment of the patient. Treatment for two weeks will so heal the acute lesions that the infected individuals cannot spread the disease even though they will not be cured during this short time. We cannot do this with tuberculosis or other diseases of an infectious nature. Syphilis, therefore, lends itself to a universal health program because it is an ideal disease for the application of successful public health measures.

When I was first asked to discuss my impressions of the medical needs of transients, I was rather chagrined because I had had no contacts with transients. I did, however, have access to some reports on the incidence of venereal diseases among transients. It is unfortunate that no definite or concrete program was established in regard to venereal diseases early in the plans for the care of transients. The statistics which I was able to gather were from scattered sources and their interpretation was influenced by the enthusiasm of the medical officers who happened to be in control of the various areas. The United States Public Health Service at their Venereal Disease Clinic at Little Rock, Arkansas, took care of 1,125 patients with syphilis in 1934. Eight hundred forty-nine of these were on relief and 276 were self-supporting. Of these patients 65 per cent were between the ages of sixteen and thirty years; 24 per cent had acute syphilis, 63 per cent had latent syphilis, and 13 per cent had late syphilis. The 63 per cent who had latent or dormant syphilis may or may not have been in need of treatment. They were not, however, in an infectious state and hence were not a menace to the community. They may have been in need of care and perhaps room and board, but they were not of particular danger to anyone. Thirteen per cent had late syphilis, that is, syphilis of the heart or liver or nervous system. These patients were in need of treatment, perhaps in need of hospital care, to keep them from becoming state or county charges.

I have emphasized this particular group of figures because they represent incidence of damage from syphilis as it affects the populace as a whole. We know that less than a third of patients who have syphilis are going to have serious trouble from the disease, while two-thirds of those infected will have little if any trouble from the infection.

In Baltimore, there were 55,000 transients, of whom slightly less than 10 per cent had syphilis. Among the colored males, however, the incidence of syphilis was 23 per cent.

The Emergency Relief Bureau of New York City examined 40,000 men, of whom 3,100, or 8 per cent, had syphilis.

The report from Minnesota was obtained from two sources: Camp Independence and the Medical Health Center in Minneapolis. Camp Independence, during the three years of its existence, reported to the State Board of Health, 1,023 patients who had venereal diseases—702 had syphilis and 321 had gonorrhea. Of the 702 syphilitics, 176 had acute syphilis and hence were in danger of transmitting the disease. I have not been able to obtain statistics on the incidence of gonorrhea that are worthy of discussion. At the Minneapolis center, a group of 2,783 men received special examinations for evidence of syphilis. Of this number, 308 had syphilis and 107 had a history of syphilis; in other words, 11 per cent had syphilis. The reports on gonorrhea revealed fifty cases of acute gonorrhea and 700 men who gave a history of having had gonorrhea in the years gone by. The incidence of syphilis among colored men was 35 per cent.

Thus far I have been endeavoring to establish the fact that syphilis among transients is not a new problem. Syphilis among transients has always been a problem to those of us who have been interested in the disease. We will be able to do more, however, with more money available. I say this, having in mind the greatest appreciation for what has been done by the medical profession and charitable groups who for many years have given of their time, effort, and even material things for these patients, all

of which has been contributed without thought or hope of compensation.

From these reports we find that the incidence of syphilis among transients is only slightly higher than is the estimated incidence among the populace as a whole. The United States Public Health Service estimated that 10 per cent of adults in this country have syphilis. The reports indicate that in the transient groups in the large cities, in the South, and in the Northwest, the incidence of syphilis varies from 10 to 21 per cent among the white population and up to 37 per cent among Negroes. The incidence of gonorrhea could not be estimated.

Under the provisions of the Social Security Act, the United States Public Health Service has available money which may be used for a venereal disease campaign. The law specifies that this money be allotted to the various states according to population, special health problems, and financial needs, at the request of the state health officials supported by the governing state authorities. The tentative plan of the campaign against venereal disease, as outlined by Surgeon General Parran, has as its general theme the elimination of syphilis and gonorrhea by making proper treatment available to all who need it. Some of the features of this campaign are worthy of emphasis.

For example, we have no accurate statistics as to the incidence of syphilis, so one of the first features of the program will be to require that all patients who have syphilitic disease be reported to the state boards of health. The reporting of these patients is a requisite in many states at the present time. A second feature is that treatment for syphilis is to be available, free of charge, to anyone who seeks it. In some states the Health Department will furnish to physicians the necessary remedies, such as salvarsan, bismuth, and mercury, on request. The number of venereal disease clinics is sufficient to give adequate care to patients in the majority of the urban centers, but in the rural districts such provisions are lacking and it will be necessary to create some method whereby the patients in these communities will be treated and the doctor who cares for them will be paid for his efforts. A fourth important point in the venereal disease campaign will be the organization of a group of field workers by the state health departments. It will be the duty of these workers to trace all contacts, to arrange for the care of pregnant women who have syphilis and for the care of children who have congenital syphilis, and to locate and return for treatment patients who have had acute syphilis but who have discontinued treatment. When a diagnosis of gonorrhea or syphilis is made by a physician and treatment instituted, his problem does not end there but must include an effort to examine the individuals exposed to this patient. The success of this campaign will, in a great measure, depend not only on the efficiency of this "contact corps" but also on the creation of laws that will require these patients to remain under treatment until they are no longer a menace to their neighbors.

A fifth important item is provision of hospital beds for these patients. Patients who have acute syphilis should be isolated until they have been rendered noninfectious. The patient who has syphilis of the heart or liver, or late syphilis of the nervous system, may also be in need of a hospital bed, and just as much so as any other patient in the hospital.

I wish to emphasize also the effort to standardize the state laboratories where the diagnostic tests for venereal diseases are carried out. This is a technical detail which is already being worked out.

Finally, we must disseminate by the press, in pamphlet and in magazine, and by radio, knowledge regarding these diseases. A program for the postgraduate training of physicians in this field, under the combined direction of the state medical society, the public health service, and the American Medical Association, is also essential to the success of this plan.

What, then, are the medical needs of the transient who has a venereal disease? May I call attention again to the fact that venereal disease among transients is not a new problem to those of us who have been concerned with venereal diseases for these many years. True, we may have a different name for these patients, but the problem is no more acute. The evidence clearly indicates that the incidence of venereal disease among the unemployed is lower than it is among a low wage earning group. In the State of Minnesota, the patient who has venereal disease and is in need of treatment has not been neglected if he has sought aid. True, if neglect was evident, it occurred particularly in the rural areas, or if it occurred in the cities it resulted

from the refusal of the patient to continue the treatment recommended by the clinics. I do not believe that anyone in the State of Minnesota who was in need of treatment for syphilis and applied for it was ever refused such treatment. In other words, I am endeavoring to establish the fact that there is no need for undue excitement or extreme measures to combat a problem that has been with us for a long time and that has in this state been rather well taken care of by the medical profession and the health department, in accordance with the funds granted them and abetted by the generosity of those who have given of their time and efforts gratuitously. The granting of additional funds to the State Health Department, which has been in direct contact with the problem, and has handled it very satisfactorily for the last twenty years, will permit of the early and rapid establishment of additional personnel trained in the epidemiology and the treatment of these venereal diseases.

I have made mention of the fact that this is not a problem involving only the transient; it involves indirectly or otherwise the entire populace of this commonwealth. The evidence indicates that the incidence of venereal diseases among transients in the Northwest is lower than it is in the South, due no doubt to the fact that venereal diseases are more common among the colored race. It is shown from the statistics gathered in this state that about 10 per cent of the transients will have syphilis, and that of this number a third will be in need of active treatment and two-thirds will have the disease in mild form. This last group is not infectious and consequently not a menace to the community. Treatment is given in the early cases with the idea of cure and of preventing the patient from spreading the disease. In the late cases it is given for the purpose of arresting the disease, extending life expectancy, and maintaining the individual's capacity as a wage earner. I have been informed that there will be some 6,000 or 7,000 unemployed men in this state during the coming summer months, of whom approximately 700 will have syphilis. Of this number approximately 250 will be in dire need of treatment. If this treatment is to be effective and if the patient is to derive benefit of a worth-while nature, regulations must be enacted to compel him to remain under treatment until dismissed or at least released as noninfectious. The experience of the

United States Public Health Service has shown that patients who have early syphilis have continued treatment on an average of six weeks, whereas cure in early syphilis is not possible before six months of continuous treatment, as an absolute minimum, has been given. The entire campaign will fail if measures are not at hand to compel these patients to remain under treatment until they are cured. The transient who has venereal disease must be cared for either in a transient camp or in an institution already provided with equipment and personnel for the care of these diseases, or by the local physicians. The granting of additional funds to these already established agencies will readily provide for care of the transient in the urban areas. The occasional case encountered in the rural communities can best be treated by the local health officer or physicians.

The medical profession of this state has,

through a duly appointed committee,* agreed to encourage and work wholeheartedly in the campaign against venereal diseases. The Minnesota State Board of Health has played an active part in combating the disease by the treatment of these patients. With additional financial help they could reëstablish and maintain treatment facilities adequate not only for the transient but for the people of the state who need such medical care. In closing, may I emphasize that the transient who has a venereal disease is, after all, as he has been for many years, the problem of the health department. He is merely one part of the entire venereal disease problem in the state, which, if it is to be cared for efficiently, should be handled by a unit of the health department which is organized, experienced, and ready to cope with the entire problem in this commonwealth.

*S. E. Sweitzer, M.D., Chairman; F. E. Harrington, M.D.; W. E. Hatch, M.D.; J. F. Madden, M.D., and Paul A. O'Leary, M.D.

CHORIONEPITHELIOMA WITH REPORT OF A CASE*

Survey of Incidence in Saint Paul Hospitals

CHARLES W. FROATS, M.D., F.A.C.S.

Saint Paul, Minnesota

CHORIONEPITHELIOMA is a rare malignant tumor arising from the chorionic epithelium of the fetal villi following hydatidiform mole, abortion, and term pregnancy. The tumor may develop before the products of gestation have been expelled and has been described as occurring in the tube and ovary. Sänger, in 1889, first recognized the disease and applied the term "deciduoma malignum." Marchand, in 1895, correctly identified the tumor cells as derivatives of both layers of the chorionic epithelium and his views gradually became accepted. In 1898, he proposed the name chorionepithelioma.

Individual reports differ as to the incidence of chorionepithelioma. In a period of eighteen months, seven cases were found in 2,700 autopsies in Vienna. According to Curtis,[3] Symmers at Bellevue found none in 12,000 autopsies. Curtis,[4] in a coördinated clinical experience with Watkins covering sixteen years, found none, al-

though constantly on the lookout. As noted by Gough,[8] Kimbrough (1934) observed two in 8,375 confinements; Winter (1934), three in 8,000 confinements; St. Sommer (1934), one in ten years among 18,000 confinements; and Joravieff (1933), one in 26,000 confinements. Sherman[17] (1935) in a thirty-four year study of hydatidiform mole at the New York Lying-in Hospital found one in 182,119 obstetrical and 14,280 gynecological patients. Schumann[16] (1937), in an analysis of its frequency in Philadelphia over a five-year period covering 207,707 pregnancies, found fifteen, or one in 13,850 pregnancies. Cosgrove[2] (1938) reported three developing in 20,450 confinements at the Margaret Hague Maternity Hospital.

The true etiology of this disease is unknown. In all but rare exceptions pregnancy has preceded the growth. Teacher[18] reported a series in which the age incidence ran from seventeen to fifty-five years, averaging thirty-three. The majority occur in multipara. It is a disease of the child-bearing years and of fertile women, with

*Presented at the annual meeting of the Minnesota Society of Obstetrics and Gynecology, Saint Paul, Minnesota, April 23, 1948.

the incidence paralleling the degree of fertility. In Teacher's[18] monograph he found 8 per cent with the first pregnancy, 15 per cent with the second, and 28 per cent with the second and the third. Lynch and Maxwell[11] report the statistics of Briquel as 21 per cent occurring in the second pregnancy, 20 per cent with the third, and 47 per cent with the fourth or more.

Antedating so many chorionepitheliomas, hydatidiform mole has been considered as a predisposing condition. From Polloson and Violet's series of 455 cases, as reported by Curtis,[3] 45 per cent were found occurring after hydatidiform mole; 30 per cent after abortion; 21 per cent after labor at term; and 2.5 per cent followed ectopic gestation. In a series of 500 cases of hydatidiform mole, Findley[7] stated 31.4 per cent were followed by chorionepithelioma. Bell[1] gives the statistics of Sunde as 44 per cent occurring after hydatidiform mole; 30 per cent after abortions; and 22 per cent after labor at term. In 1922, Novak[14] estimated one per cent of moles became malignant and Teacher[18] believes five per cent too high. Polak[15] (1931), in discussing a paper on choriomas by Schmitz, stated that in ten years he had seen forty or fifty cases of moles and none became malignant and in the same interval ten chorionepitheliomas were not preceded by moles. In Schumann's[16] report, eight of the fifteen chorionepitheliomas were preceded by moles, while in Cosgrove's[2] analysis all three cases developed after molar pregnancies. With the incidence of malignancy following mole as 5 per cent or more, this in itself must be considered a grave condition.

The location of the tumor is most commonly in the area of the placental site. Grossly it invades the uterus as a soft, vascular mass, usually differentiated from the mucosal layer. It may be located on the endometrium, in the myometrium, or may grow through the wall and protrude into the peritoneal cavity or broad ligaments. The tumor, microscopically, is composed of masses of syncytium and nests of Langhans cells independent of villi with penetration into the wall of the uterus. There is invasion of blood vessels, mitosis of Langhans cells, very little stroma and intravillus vessels or lacking entirely. Hemorrhage and necrosis is common. The two types of cells vary in proportion in different tumors. Attempts have been made to classify these tumors. Mathieu and Palmer[12] and Gough[8] pre-

fer Ewing's classification into: chorioadenoma, choriocarcinoma and syncytial endometritis. It is considered one of the most malignant and destructive neoplasms known. The reported mortality rate varies from 10 to 60 and 70 per cent. Findley[7] states there is a higher recovery rate from chorionepithelioma following mole than from that following abortions and full term pregnancies.

The period of latency varies from a coexistent appearance with the pregnancy to months and years. Usually it follows in weeks or months but may occur any time thereafter during the life of the patient. Metastases occur by way of the blood stream. Lesions in the lungs and vaginal walls are usually the first to appear.

Lutein cysts of the ovaries are regularly observed as in hydatidiform mole. They are usually bilateral and vary from small multiple cystomata to large tumors. These are probably due to excessive hormonal influence with stimulation of follicle growth and luteinization. Several investigators have shown that they are the result of excessive pituitary stimulation.

The usual clinical symptom is persistent bleeding following abortion, molar pregnancy or fullterm pregnancy. The greatest difficulties are encountered in early abortions, where the bleeding may be thought to be due to placental remnants, and after labor wherein the physiologic bleeding may obscure the development of the growth.

The clinical value of the Aschheim-Zondek (1928) reaction for the study of normal and abnormal pregnancies has been well demonstrated. This biological test for anterior pituitary-like hormone is now an established aid in the diagnosis of chorionepithelioma. A number of authorities have shown that in hydatidiform mole and chorionepithelioma the amount of gonadotropic substance is much greater than that excreted during normal pregnancy. Due to the abnormal activity of the chorionic elements in these conditions the hormone secretion is increased to such an extent that even high dilutions result in positive reactions. On the basis of a quantitative reaction both the Aschheim-Zondek test or the Friedman modification may be used as a diagnostic aid. Ehrhardt[6] obtained a positive reaction in a case with 1/520 c.c. of urine and in another with 1/260 c.c. Levanthal and Saphir[10] reported 330,000 mouse units per liter of urine in an early case and Kurzrok[9] observed a reaction as high as one million mouse units.

As recorded by Mazer and Edeiken,[13] in 1929 Fels and Roessler made several observations, namely: that with hydatidiform mole and chorionepithelioma much higher quantities of prolan are secreted than in normal pregnancy; the quantitative estimation of the hormone is an accurate guide in differentiating both of these conditions from uterine bleeding in the course of pregnancy due to other causes; presence of increased hormone for longer than two weeks after normal pregnancy or more than eight weeks after a mole pregnancy is pathognomonic of chorionepithelioma; continued presence of the hormone after the complete removal of the growth is indicative of metastasis.

Only living chorionic tissue causes positive reaction and the reaction becomes positive before clinical diagnosis of metastasis can be made. Mathieu and Palmer[12] diagnosed two early cases with the history of a mole and the persistence of anterior pituitary-like hormone in the urine. If a positive reaction should recur after having been reported negative following the expulsion of a mole, care should be exercised in differentiating between a new pregnancy and chorionepithelioma. With the advance of pregnancy, prolan concentration increases and twin pregnancies show a higher titer than single. Herein the quantitative biologic test lends a most definite aid, but should not be the determining factor to the exclusion of the history and clinical findings. In the opinion of a number of investigators the biological test is more dependable than the findings from examination of uterine scrapings. Histological diagnosis from curettings is not always easy and may be inconclusive or even misleading. To establish the diagnosis by this method the operator must obtain a portion of the growth invading the wall of the uterus. Mistaken diagnoses have resulted in delay of proper treatment or the unnecessary removal of pelvic organs. Curettage is unreliable in that the growth may be located away from the uterine cavity in the myometrium. Levanthal and Saphir[10] (1934) and Cosgrove[2] (1938) each reported a case in which curettage would have been of no value. Moreover curettage carries the danger of perforation, infection, and possible dissemination.

Two reports have been made on a negative

Aschheim-Zondek in the presence of chorionepithelioma: one by Fahlbusch in 1930, related by Mathieu and Palmer,[12] and another in 1937 by Schumann.[16] Schumann[16] believes radical operation is indicated whenever persistent fetal elements are found, especially if bleeding occurs, in spite of negative Aschheim-Zondek reaction.

The degree of malignancy cannot be predicted, and the prognosis depends on early recognition. The hope of curing any malignant disease depends on recognition in its early stage of proliferation. It is therefore advisable to have repeated Aschheim-Zondek or Friedman tests made in all women who continue to bleed after the expulsion of a mole, or in those with abnormal bleeding of an undetermined cause following pregnancy. Titus[19] suggests performing the test every two weeks until negative, and thereafter every four weeks for six months. Mathieu and Palmer[12] recommend monthly tests for one year.

Upon the diagnosis of this disease the early removal of all tissue containing malignant elements would be the ideal treatment. The clinician is then confronted with the question as to which type of operation offers the best hope of cure. The usual procedure has been to perform an abdominal panhysterectomy with removal of both tubes and ovaries. The abdominal operation permits better exposure and there is less trauma to the tissues. Lynch and Maxwell[11] advised the most extensive removal that the individual case will stand. Mathieu and Palmer[12] believe that in chorionepithelioma diagnosed early and the growth confined to the uterus it is unnecessary to remove the ovaries if they appear normal. They report an early case with only supravaginal hysterectomy and no recurrence after two years. Gough[8] maintains the lutein cysts are due to the disease and of no causative significance, and that the removal or conservation of the ovaries is optimal. He recommends the removal of the cervix. Total hysterectomy was the method of choice in Cosgrove's[2] three cases and no recurrences had appeared after 26, 23 and 11 months.

Few reports have been made of treatment by irradiation, its use having been limited chiefly to inoperable cases and metastatic growths. Davis[5] (1936) reports its successful use following supravaginal hysterectomy in a case complicating a placenta previa. In his opinion operable cases should be preceded or followed by thorough radiation. Titus[19] recommends preliminary radiation with radium, followed by hysterectomy and a subsequent course of deep x-ray therapy. Irradiation should be effective as the growth is of fetal origin and such tumors are particularly susceptible to this kind of therapy.

The records of six representative hospitals in the city of Saint Paul were reviewed to determine the local incidence of chorionepithelioma.

Hospital A, 1928 to 1937 inclusive, reported 430 abortions, 6,310 confinements, one mole—no chorionepithelioma.

Hospital B, 1927 to 1937 inclusive, reported 589 abortions, 4,941 confinements, one mole—no chorionepithelioma.

Hospital C, 1928 to 1937 inclusive, reported 270 abortions, 2,995 confinements, one mole—no chorionepithelioma.

Hospital D, 1932 to April, 1938, inclusive, reported 1,279 abortions, 8,150 confinements, seven moles—no chorionepithelioma.

Hospital E, 1932 to April, 1938, inclusive, reported 365 abortions, 3,705 confinements, three moles—no chorionepithelioma.

Hospital F, December, 1920, to April 7, 1938, inclusive, reported 330 abortions, 7,282 confinements, four moles—no chorionepithelioma.

In a total of 3,263 abortions, 33,383 confinements and 17 moles (36,646 pregnancies in all), there was no record of a chorionepithelioma.

It should be stated that one of the hospitals reported one mole and four chorionepitheliomas. However, upon investigating two of these charts and the pathological reports, they were omitted as entirely inconclusive. Of the remaining two, prepared sections of the surgical specimens were submitted to Dr. E. T. Bell for examination. Dr. Bell reported no chorionepithelioma present.

Report of Case

The following constitutes the report of a chorionepithelioma of the uterus antedated by the expulsion of an hydatidiform mole.

Mrs. J. S., thirty-four years of age, married at twenty-two, had five children living and well. There was a history of a spontaneous miscarriage at four or five months in March, 1934, unattended by a physician. Menses were regular until mid-summer, the last menstrual date not being definitely known. She first consulted her physician August 16, 1934, complaining of a tired, worn-out feeling and nervousness. His examination showed her weight to be 142 pounds, blood pressure 128/75, and hemoglobin 70 per cent. She was again seen August 30, 1934, and under medication her hemoglobin had risen to 80 per cent and she felt some better. On September 24 she reported again with the complaint of slight uterine bleeding, but no associated cramps. Examination revealed a uterus about two and

a half months pregnant. The patient was put to bed for one month, including one week of hospitalization. The bleeding recurred upon being upon her feet. On November 7 abortion was induced by the bougie method after consultation with another physician. The induction was successful and a mass the size of a fist was expelled, described as meaty in appearance. The specimen was examined by Dr. E. T. Bell and reported as hydatidiform mole. Moderate bleeding continued for three weeks and several particles of tissue were passed. On November 30, 1934, the physician performed a dilatation and curettement with the removal of particles of vesicular tissue. This tissue was not examined. December 19, 1934, the uterus was of normal size and no bleeding had occurred. January 2, 1935, the patient reported to her physician that bleeding had recurred that day.

The patient was first seen by me in consultation January 4, 1935, with the complaint of uterine bleeding of two days' duration, and slight lower abdominal cramps. The amount was described as slightly in excess of the usual menstrual flow. There had been no evidence of bleeding for thirty-three days following the dilatation and curettement.

The family history was essentially negative.

Examination showed a well developed woman of 138 pounds weight, temperature 97.2, pulse 80, blood pressure 118/72, chest and abdomen normal. Pelvic examination: vulva, urethra, and glands negative; perineum somewhat relaxed; vaginal walls normal in appearance; old healed lacerations of cervix with chronic cervicitis present; fundus retrodisplaced, uniform in outline with the suggestion of being slightly enlarged; nothing palpable in either adnexal region. Laboratory findings: urine normal; hemoglobin 75 per cent; red blood count 4,000,000; white blood count 10,500.

Bearing in mind the history of the mole, it was, nevertheless, assumed that this was her first menstrual period following the dilatation and curettage, and retrodisplacement and slight subinvolution of the uterus was determined. It was suggested to the patient's physician that hormone tests for the presence of persistent hydatid reaction be made and that she be observed for the possible development of malignancy. On January 26, 1935, a Friedman test was positive. This was an undiluted specimen. The physician reported that she was continuing to have a slight bloody discharge off and on. February 27, 1935, a Friedman test was again positive. Through a misunderstanding the request to the laboratory for dilution of the urine was omitted. Her physician reported that irregular bleeding continued and the uterus was enlarged.

The patient was again seen by me March 12, 1935. Bloody vaginal discharge had continued at intervals. General examination was much the same as on previous visit. Her weight remained the same and the temperature was normal. Pelvic examination: inspection of vulva and vaginal walls showed no implants; thin bloody discharge from cervix; uterus definitely enlarged to the size of a 3 to 3½ months pregnancy, quite uniform in outline and slightly tender; adnexa

466

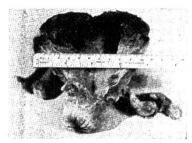

Figure 1. Photograph of gross specimen showing the entire uterus and its appendages with the anterior surface incised to expose the tumor in the fundus.

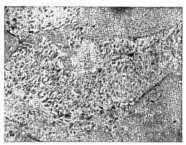

Fig. 2. Photomicrograph showing masses of chorionic epithelium in the uterine muscle independent of villi. The tumor cells are largely the Langhans type, but there are a few syncytial cells at the periphery of the section.

not palpable. Laboratory findings: hemoglobin 72; red blood count, 3,870,000; white blood count, 11,200; differential—lymphocytes, 33, large mononuclear 1, neutrophiles 65, eosinophils 1 per cent. Sedimentation rate moderately rapid, Wassermann negative, blood grouping 11. X-ray of chest negative for metastases. A clinical diagnosis of chorionepithelioma was made and operation advised.

On March 15, under spinal anesthesia, the abdomen was opened. The uterus was enlarged to the size of a three and one-half months' pregnancy. The growth, confined to the fundus and slightly nodular on the serous surface, presented a striking multicolored appearance. The ovaries were only slightly enlarged and cystic. A panhysterectomy was carried out, with the removal of both tubes and ovaries.

The uterus and its appendages weighed 320 grams. The inside diameters of the tumor measured roughly 5 by 7 cm. The pathologic report made by Dr. E. T. Bell of Minneapolis was chorionepithelioma of the uterus; numerous follicular and luteal cysts of the ovaries.

The patient made a good recovery and was discharged from the hospital March 29, 1935, on her fourteenth postoperative day. Deep x-ray therapy consisted of a total of 143 per cent skin erythema dose to the pelvis in ten treatments over a period of eighteen days, through four portals.

No immediate biological tests were made on this patient following surgery and radiation. The follow-up of this patient has been restricted to personal communications. The first one of these was received in July, 1936, in which the patient stated she had gained 17 pounds in weight, and, except for being a little nervous, felt well and worked hard every day. Recent communications in the last few weeks from both the patient and her physician were to the effect that she remains in good health and there is no evidence of recurrence. I believe that she may be considered cured.

Subsequently, on May 12, 1938, a Friedman test was negative.

Summary

1. The subject of chorionepithelioma has been reviewed.

2. The incidence of chorionepithelioma among 36,646 pregnancies and abortions in six Saint Paul hospitals has been given, substantiating the reported rarity of the condition.

3. A case report has been presented.

References

1. Bell, E. T.: Textbook of Pathology. Philadelphia: Lea and Febiger, 1938, p. 363.
2. Cosgrove, S. A.: The value of hormonal findings in hydatidiform mole and chorionepithelioma. Am. Jour. Obst. and Gyn., 35:581, (April) 1938.
3. Curtis, A. H.: Obstetrics and Gynecology. Philadelphia: W. B. Saunders Co., 2:969, 1933.
4. Curtis, A. H.: Chorionepithelioma of the uterus. Surg., Gyn. and Obst., 54:861, (June) 1932.
5. Davis, M., Edward, and Brunschwig, Alex.: The roentgenotherapy of chorionepithelioma. Am. Jour. Obst. and Gyn., 31:987, (June) 1936.
6. Ehrhardt, K.: Aschheim-Zondek pregnancy reaction. Surg., Gyn. and Obst., 53:486, (Oct.) 1931.
7. Findley, P.: Hydatidiform mole. Am. Jour. Obst., 75:968, (June) 1917.
8. Gough, James A.: A study of five patients with chorionepithelioma. Am. Jour. Obst. and Gyn., 34:267, (August) 1937.
9. Kurzrok, Raphael: The Endocrines in Obstetrics and Gynecology. Baltimore: The Williams and Wilkins Co., 1937, p. 247.
10. Leventhal, M. L., and Saphir, Wm.: Chorionepithelioma: early diagnosis by quantitative determination of anterior pituitary-like principle. Jour. A.M.A., 103:668, 1934.
11. Lynch, F. W., and Maxwell, A. F.: Pelvic Neoplasms. New York: D. Appleton and Co., 10:300, 1931.
12. Mathieu, A., and Palmer, A.: Early diagnosis of chorionepithelioma. Surg., Gyn. and Obst., 61:336-343, 1935.
13. Mazer, Charles, and Edeiken, L.: The value of the Aschheim-Zondek reaction in the diagnosis and prognosis of chorionepithelioma. Am. Jour. Obst. and Gyn., 26:195, 1933.
14. Novak, Emil: Hydatidiform mole and chorionepithelioma. Jour. A.M.A., 78:1771, (June) 1922.
15. Polak, J. O.: Discussion. Am. Jour. Obst. and Gyn., 21:593, 1931.
16. Schumann, E. A., and Voegelin, A. W.: Chorionepithelioma, with especial reference to its frequency. Am. Jour. Obst. and Gyn., 33:473, 1937.
17. Sherman, J. T.: Study of seventy-eight patients with hydatidiform mole. Am. Jour. Surg., 27:237, 1935.
18. Teacher, John H.: On chorionepithelioma. Jour. Obst. and Gyn. British Empire, 4: (July and August) 1903.
19. Titus, Paul: The Management of Obstetric Difficulties. St. Louis: C. V. Mosby Co., 1937, p. 221.

SPINA BIFIDA CYSTICA OF THE PELVIS: DIAGNOSIS AND SURGICAL TREATMENT*

ALFRED W. ADSON, M.D.

Rochester, Minnesota

A PATIENT who recently came to The Mayo Clinic because of spina bifida cystica of the pelvis presented an unusual problem for diagnosis because of the location and rarity of the lesion and also because a new operative procedure was required. This experience I believe justifies a report of the findings and the surgical technic employed. Since there still remains some confusion about the types of operations to employ for spina bifida, and some uncertainty about the proper time to operate, I shall review our experiences in the general discussion of the subject.

Spina bifida is one of the common deformities of the newborn; it occurs once in 1,000 to 2,000 births. There are two varieties. One is known as spina bifida cystica and the other as spina bifida occulta. The spina bifida cystica has three subdivisions. The first is simple meningocele, which represents a herniation of the meninges through a defect in the spinal canal. The cystic wall is composed of arachnoid and dura, which are covered with thinned fascia and skin. The meningocele contains no nerve elements. The second variety is known as myelomeningocele. This is similar to a meningocele except that nerve roots enter the wall of the cystic mass. The third variety is known as a syringomyelocele. It resembles the first variety in that it is composed of a sac but differs from the first and second varieties in that it contains a dilated portion of the conus medullaris, and nerve fibers end blindly in the wall of the sac. The first variety is rarely associated with any form of paralysis; the second variety is associated with a varying degree of sensory or motor disturbance; the third variety usually is associated with very marked paralysis. At this point, I should like to emphasize that a plastic repair on the cystic mass rarely improves the paralysis. Therefore, the parents of the patient should be informed of this fact before operation is performed.

An associated hydrocephalus of the communicative type may accompany any one of the three

varieties. However, it is most frequently associated with the third variety. If the two coexist, each requires separate surgical consideration. It has been observed that a repair of a large cystic spina bifida in cases in which there is no obvious evidence of hydrocephalus may result in a hydrocephalus as the spina bifida has served as a reservoir during the early weeks of life. Spina bifida may occur in any portion of the spinal canal. It occurs more frequently in the lumbosacral region than in other parts of the spinal column. However, it does occur in the craniocervical and in the cervical region, but it is rarely seen in the upper thoracic region. The spinal defect may include from one to ten vertebræ.

Spina bifida occulta is characterized roentgenographically by a bifid spinal column and by the appearance of a small dimple covered by a tuft of hair. It rarely produces clinical symptoms in early life, but the progressive myelodysplasia may cause symptoms later in life. This manifests itself by increasing sensory and motor disturbances and impairment of the rectal and vesical sphincters.

Analogous to the developmental defects of the spinal cord observed in the later stages of spina bifida occulta is a condition that is known as myelodysplasia, except that it occurs without a demonstrable bony defect.

Etiology

One of the oldest theories, strongly championed by Morgagni in 1779, rejected by most writers since von Recklinghausen's[12] comprehensive dissertation on spina bifida, in 1886, and recently rediscovered and espoused by numerous writers, is the theory of hydromyelia. According to this theory the choroid plexus, activated perhaps by a hormone, secretes such a large quantity of spinal fluid that it either prevents union of the medullary folds or ruptures them after union has taken place. Interference with the absorption of spinal fluid is advanced as the alternative mechanism. The rapid accumulation of fluid then is given as the primary cause; the resulting cyst is

*From the Section on Neurologic Surgery, The Mayo Clinic, Rochester, Minnesota. Thesis presented before the Minnesota Academy of Medicine, April 13, 1938.

interposed as a bulging mass between the lateral mesodermal structures, preventing the approximation and fusion of the lips of the medullary groove. One of the main supports of this theory lies in the fact that spina bifida is often associated with hydrocephalus, which is rapidly made worse or, if not already present, may rapidly be produced by operative closure of the spinal defect. The assumption of an excessive amount of spinal fluid obviously depends on the further assumption that the choroid plexus is secreting fluid at this early embryonic period. This hypothesis seems inadequate when the whole problem is considered; one of its most serious objections is the fact that the choroid plexus does not begin secreting fluid until about the tenth week, 2.4 mm. embryo (von Monakow),[9] whereas all writers agree that the spina bifidous deformity is produced no later than the third week. Further, the cases in which there is a failure of the entire neural canal to close certainly represent a more serious type of the same fundamental defect and must accordingly be explained on the same basis; it seems highly improbable that the amount of spinal fluid secreted is so immense that the entire canal, from its cephalic to its caudal ends, would be torn open or union prevented throughout by the flow of the choroidal secretion. Complete absence of the cord, or amyelia, which accompanies many of these severe types (Schmaus and Sacki)[13] must also be explained by a more comprehensive theory. Mention of micromyelia, diastomyelia, and diplomyelia, which occur with spina bifida and without it, would still further embarrass the theory. It is also irreconcilably at variance with the observation that the portion of the spinal cord involved lacks all evidence of pressure myelitis, with its disintegrating nervous tissue; on the contrary, it is seen to have remained at a standstill in its embryonic development, with embryonic nerve cells and embryonic blood vessels, as the area medullovasculosa (von Recklinghausen).[12] Associated defects, such as harelip, cleft palate, and club feet, are considered by recondite inference to be the results of pressure on the nerve centers. While it must be admitted that the added area of absorption supplied by the cyst often prevents the occurrence of hydrocephalus, it would seem more reasonable to suppose that the faulty absorption of spinal fluid may also be based on some developmental defect.

An associated cardiovascular defect has been suggested as a possibility.

von Recklinghausen[12] believed that spina bifida is primarily due to a failure of the mesodermal envelope of bone and dura to approximate; he looked on the ectodermal dysontogenesis as secondary. The fact that a myelodysplasia of this type may occur without defects in the bone controverts this theory; it suggests that the defect may be primary in the medullary plate. The types of spina bifida cystica and spina bifida occulta not accompanied by defects in the nervous system argue for the reverse. The necessity for making one primary and the other secondary is not apparent. Whatever the exact mechanism may be, it does not complete our search for the more fundamental process in which we are primarily interested.

There is much evidence against assuming that the basis is germinal, or developmental, and such cause has been generally discarded. I do not believe that this is altogether justified. Thus, the presence of developmental defects in one case, in which the closely related defect of enuresis and sacral dimple were transmitted to six persons on the male side, through three generations, is clearly an instance of heredity. Two other cases, in which the same defect appeared in siblings, do not furnish conclusive evidence, since maternal environmental factors might have been just as potent and quite as likely as developmental factors. On the whole, the hereditary element hangs on a very tenuous thread; it must be assumed for occasional cases, but these are not numerous enough to argue for its acceptance as the sole cause.

Experimental Production of Spina Bifida and Other Anomalies

Recent work[17] among biologists cannot be disregarded as some writers are disregarding it simply because it has been carried out on lower forms of life. The experimental production of spina bifida by modification of the environmental medium has taught us a great deal. A brief review of this evidence is profitable. Probably the most striking demonstration of the importance of environment in the production of spina bifida was that produced by Hertwig,[5] in 1896, who subjected the axolotl, a salamander, to different concentrations of sodium chlorid solution. He found that a 0.5 per cent solution had no effect, a 0.6 per cent solution produced monsters in 50 per cent, while 0.7 per cent solution resulted in development of spina bifidous monsters in every case. Stockard, using *Fundulus heteroclitus*, the common minnow, produced spina bifida by using magnesium chlorid. Cyclops could be produced in at least 50 per cent of cases, which was somewhat more frequent than spina bifida. It was also demonstrated that alcohol, ether, and the alkaloids could be used with similar results.

In order to demonstrate the applicability to man of these factors of monster production, Werber used substances produced in the human metabolism, namely butyric acid and acetone. He exposed *Fundulus heteroclitus* in the two, four, eight, and sixteen cell stages, to the action of 1-12/1-14 gm. molecular solution of butyric acid in sea water, from fifteen to twenty hours; he produced a great variety of monstrosities, the extreme defect being the development of only an eye or an ear, the rest of the embryo failing to appear. Higher percentages of acetone killed the embryos, while lower concentrations resulted in the development of monsters. Werber[15,16] concluded that faulty maternal metabolism might well be the underlying cause of dysontogenesis. Disastrous maternal effects of diabetic patients are well known. Keibel and Mall[6] found that the chorion of nearly all monsters had been the seat of inflammatory processes which in time might well have interfered with normal metabolism. The frequent association of hydramnios makes this all the more probable.

Chemical methods are not the only ones by which monsters have been produced artificially. One of the other simplest devices is a modification of gravitational forces on frogs' eggs. Simply turning upside down (Conklin)[4] frogs' eggs in the two-cell stage may cause the development of double-headed or double-bodied monsters. A redistribution, by centrifugalization, of the heavier elements of the eggs constitutes another method. In the ascidian (sea squirt) eggs, in which different kinds of protoplasm give rise to different organs and tissues, this rearrangement may result in marked dislocation of organs. That the problem is complex is shown by the fact that some varieties develop normally in spite of this artificial rearrangement (Morgan).[10]

Lewis[8] adopted the remarkably simple method of destroying different portions of the eggs of *Fundulus heteroclitus* by operation-needling, and

so forth, and demonstrated that the organs predetermined in the portion of the egg destroyed did not develop. He could thus produce a developmental defect in any portion of the body he desired. Kellicott found that subjecting the eggs of *Fundulus heteroclitus* to a temperature of the average household refrigerator, for a few hours or days, sufficed to produce every variety of defect.

That physicochemical action may produce developmental mental defects was demonstrated by Bardeen,[3] who exposed both male and female frogs to the x-ray for one hour, prior to fertilization. He learned that exposure to the x-ray of the ovum or the sperm sufficed to influence the subsequent development of the eggs in such a manner that marked abnormalities, including spina bifida, resulted. Baldwin[2] produced spina bifida in frogs by exposing a given part of the egg to the action of the ultra-violet ray.

The mechanism by which various factors influence the developing organism is also disputed. I can only refer to these briefly. Mall assumed that nutritional factors *in utero* resulting from diseased fetal members underlie monster production. Werber postulated the theory of blastolysis, according to which a part or wedge of the germ substance is destroyed, resulting in anomalous fusion or dispersion of the part split off. Stockard[14] believes that he has proved, by the use of magnesium with its well-known anesthetic or inhibitory action, that an inhibitory action is responsible. Kellicott,[7] espousing the hypothesis of disorganization, believes that this must take place before differentiation by gastrolysis, through interference with the organization of the fertilized ovum. The discovery of the deleterious action of the x-ray and radium on the sperm, prior to fertilization, added another complication, since it proved that an abnormal character of the gametes may in some instances suffice to produce the defect.

von Recklinghausen's demonstration that the area medullovasculosa contains elements retaining early embryonic characteristics is of fundamental importance and prohibits the acceptance of the current theories, in the strictest sense, as an explanation of the large group of cases not dependent on hereditary factors; or is it possible that lack of abnormality of function and metabolism, secondary to the apparent isolation of

470

these elements, in the area medullovasculosa suffices to explain their embryonic appearance.

In view of the foregoing clinical observations and the facts adduced through experimental methods, it seems that spina bifida cannot be explained on the basis of any single factor, but by one or more of the following causes: abnormal character of the gametes or mechanical, chemical or physico-chemical factors influencing the embryonic rudiments, either before or after differentiation; the mechanistic action of accumulated cerebrospinal fluid could act only as a secondary cause. A conception as broad as this seems to destroy all semblance of a theory; indeed, any precise formulation of a theory which does not take all these factors into account would be dogmatic, premature, and untenable at the present stage of knowledge.[17]

Symptoms

The physical deformity of a spina bifida cystica is obvious. The cystic masses vary in size from those which are similar to an English walnut to those which are larger than a grapefruit. The roentgenogram reveals the extent of the bony malformation. The neurologic examination reveals findings according to location and extent of the involvement of the nerves or spinal cord. It does not disclose any change in the presence of a meningocele, it shows but few nerves missing when a myelomeningocele is present and gives evidence of marked anomalies of the nerves and spinal cord if a syringomyelocele is present. Hydrocephalus[11] frequently accompanies the third variety but rarely is associated with the other two, and never is associated with a spina bifida occulta.

Surgical Considerations

Oftentimes surgeons are called upon to repair spina bifida cystica as soon as it is observed after birth. Occasionally, this can be done with success, but, judging from our own experience, it is evident that operations on babies carry a much higher mortality than do operations that are performed at a later date, let us say, at a period from six to nine months following birth. There are other advantages in waiting. First, an apparent hydrocephalus may not be evident at the time of birth but will be evident in six to nine months following birth. Second, neurologic findings are often difficult to demonstrate in a small child. Therefore, by waiting for six to nine

months it becomes much easier to demonstrate neurologic findings. A third reason for delaying the operation is that the parents can observe for themselves whether or not an accompanying hydrocephalus exists and whether or not any paralysis is caused by the anomalous condition. They should be thoroughly informed of these findings and should also be instructed concerning the results of the operation. They should be told frankly that the operation consists of a plastic closure and that the operation will not alter the hydrocephalus nor will it restore any function to the paralyzed extremity. It is well to go into detail concerning the object of the operation. The parents should be told what to expect in the way of results. The two first varieties, namely, meningocele and myelomeningocele, lend themselves to surgical treatment, but the syringomyelocele rarely presents a true indication for surgical treatment. Occasionally, one finds it advantageous to repair the cystic mass, but little is accomplished by attempting to free the conus medullaris from the scar tissue. Occasionally, one is able to free nerve filaments in order that they may fall back into the lumbosacral canal. When this is possible there may be some subsequent improvement in that particular nerve.

If an accompanying hydrocephalus exists, it is usually of the communicative type. Occasionally, repeated spinal punctures and limitation of the fluid intake may control the situation. If the child is a particularly healthy one, the surgeon may be justified in performing a Tracy-Putnam operation. This operation includes two separate openings of the lateral ventricles, through which the choroid plexus is coagulated for the specific purpose of decreasing the amount of cerebrospinal fluid secreted. Unfortunately, neither procedure guarantees that the hydrocephalus will be controlled. Since it is impossible to guarantee a control of the hydrocephalus, there is danger that the plastic repair may not hold and that leakage of cerebrospinal fluid may follow; when this does occur, there is always the danger that meningitis may develop.

If the obstetrician, as well as the parents, have been convinced that the plastic repair of the spina bifida cystica should be deferred until the child is six to nine months of age, they both ask two questions: (1) "How shall the spina bifida be cared for?" (2) "In the event that it leaks, how shall the leakage be controlled?" In our experience we have observed that the spina bifida can be protected nicely by the application of a doughtnut-like ring that is made of cotton and held in place with roller bandage. The ring can be fastened to the back with adhesive plaster. It serves as a wall about the cystic mass and thus prevents undue pressure on the mass if the patient is lifted or allowed to roll on his back. With this protection, the child can be handled just as any other child is handled during the early months of life. Frequently, abrasions or ulcerations are present on the thinned-out skin in the dorsal portion of the sac. When these occur, the macerated area can be treated with sterile petrolatum, or preferably sterile borated petrolatum. The crusts can be removed from time to time with pledgets of cotton soaked in liquid petrolatum which has also been sterilized. After the abrasion has healed, the cystic tumor should be washed daily with soap and water, and powdered with any good antiseptic powder. If a rupture has taken place, so that the cerebrospinal fluid leaks from the cystic mass, we find that a similar treatment may be employed, except that the child should be kept more or less in the prone position on a pillow, with the head slightly lower than the cystic mass, which prevents any hydrodynamic pressure on the sac itself. Occasionally, one is justified in aspirating the sac; this is done by sterilizing the skin at the base of the sac and introducing a needle through normal skin, directing the needle superficially into the mid-portion of the sac. Following aspiration of the sac, it is well to apply gentle pressure with a binder over a sterile cotton dressing. The cotton dressing never should be applied directly on a macerated area. It is much wiser to cover the macerated area with a strip of vaseline gauze before applying sterile cotton dressings.

The reason for waiting from six to nine months is that it allows one to evaluate the situation, to determine the degree of paralysis, if any exists, and to determine whether or not there is a coexisting hydrocephalus. It also allows the child to develop so that additional feedings of gruel and semisolid food can be given. The reason for not waiting longer than nine months is that the operation, if it is to be performed, should be performed before the child attempts to stand, for at this time he is very likely to fall onto the sac and thus press it unduly.

In selecting an operation, one should choose an operation that will permit a thorough exploration of the contents of the spina bifida before a plastic closure is made. It is unwise to employ the older technic, which consists of freeing the sac along its base, tying and transfixing it without an observation from within, as it may include a knuckle of roots or cord when in reality they have not become a part of the sac. There is no need to worry about a recurrence of the spina bifida cystica if there is no hydrocephalus. We have learned that it is unnecessary to employ any sort of bone graft, since a good plastic closure suffices to protect the nerves or cord in the spinal canal. This argument is substantiated by the fact that one never sees a spina bifida cystica result following a laminectomy for fracture of the spine or for the removal of an intraspinal tumor.

Spina Bifida Occulta

The symptoms that result from the associated myelodysplasia make their appearance in early adult life. They are characterized by deformity of the feet, disturbance in the reflexes, the appearance of sensory changes and the loss of control of the bladder and rectum. The symptoms increase as the age of the patient increases. Exploratory operation has been performed in a number of these cases. Some investigators have reported lipomatous masses which they believe have been responsible for the symptoms. Others have found hypertrophy of the ligamentum flavum, but unfortunately the surgical results have been rather disappointing, since the degeneration takes place in the conus medullaris whenever the lesion involves the lumbar or sacral region. Spina bifida occulta is not confined to the lumbosacral region and fortunately may exist without producing clinical symptoms.

Surgical Technic.—The patient is anesthetized while on his side.[1] Ether, administered by the drop method, is the anesthetic most commonly used. After the patient has been anesthetized, he is placed on his abdomen over a pillow with the head lower than the spina bifida cystica, in order that the cerebrospinal fluid will not drain from the ventricles when the sac has been opened. The skin is thoroughly cleansed with green soap, washed with ether or alcohol, and a solution of merthiolate is applied as an antiseptic. Following adjustment of the sterile linen, the sac is opened longitudinally in order to permit an internal exploration of the sac. If no nerve elements are present, a circular incision is made in the meninges peripheral to the defect in the spinal column, in such a manner as to permit an apposition of the meningeal flaps over the defect. Occasionally, it is advisable to reflect a flap of lumbar fascia across and suture to the opposite side in order to reinforce the closure of the meninges. After removing the redundant tissue the wound is then closed. It is preferable to use number 0 chromic catgut for the subdermal sutures. The skin is closed with interrupted silk sutures and the wound is covered with collodion dressings. Collodion dressings have the advantage of protecting the wound from contaminations of urine and feces. In the event that nerve elements have been found to enter the walls of the sac, it may be necessary to resect these along with the redundant tissue, but whenever it is possible to free nerve filaments or a portion of the cord and permit it to fall into the spinal canal, this should always be done. The freeing of adhesions oftentimes does permit a number of nerve elements and occasionally the cord to seek their former position, but even though this has been accomplished, too much credit should not be given to the operative procedure in the hope that additional recovery will take place in the paralysis. I have seen improvement in sphincteric control.

In the event that paralysis does exist as a result of the anomalous condition of the nerve and spinal cord, the relatives should be told that the situation might later be improved by orthopedic measures. In some instances, braces may be made. In other instances, fixation of flail joints may assist in the use of the extremity. The most serious sequela is the difficulty that is associated with incontinence of the bladder and rectum. The patient should be instructed to eat food that will regulate the bowels, and thus, by the aid of an enema, manage the daily evacuation. The patient should be instructed to develop automatic control of the bladder. Evacuation often can be initiated by a massage of the lower part of the abdomen. Urinals may need to be worn continuously. Catheterization should be avoided whenever possible. In a few instances, presacral neurectomy has proved of value in regulating evacuation of the bowels and bladder. In still fewer instances, lumbar sympathectomy has proved of value in relieving the vasomotor changes of the lower extremities, by improving the circulation and preventing ulceration.

Report of Case

A single woman, aged twenty-two years, whose father was a physician, first came to the clinic on September 4, 1935. Her chief complaint was pain situated in the region of the sacrum. The pain had first been noted when the patient was thirteen years of age. The appearance of the pain had been intermittent. At times it had been so severe that it had compelled her to go to bed for two or three days. She did not complain of a true sciatica, but said that the pain

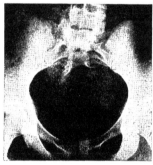

Fig. 1. Malformation of the sacrum caused by a spina bifida cystica that originated in the sacral region and extended into the pelvis.

did extend to the left knee. The pain had no relation to the time of day. The patient had been told that she had some abnormality of the sacrum and that she had a tumor in the pelvis. She had not had any other symptoms and the previous history was not significant. Examination disclosed tenderness in the left lower quadrant of the abdomen and a cystic mass that was situated in the hollow of the sacrum. Orthopedic examination revealed a marked lumbar lordosis, in addition to some tenderness over the lumbosacral region and over both sacro-iliac joints. Pelvic examination disclosed no abnormality except for the palpable mass previously mentioned. Examination of the blood and urine did not disclose any abnormality. Flocculation tests were negative. The roentgenograms revealed an absence of the lower half of the sacrum (Fig. 1). This was explained as a probable congenital aplasia. A neurologic examination failed to reveal any abnormality. The cystic tumor was found on rectal examination. A tentative diagnosis of a dermoid was made, but inasmuch as the patient was not urged to undergo operation at her initial visit to the clinic, she returned home without any surgical treatment.

The patient returned on July 21, 1936, with instructions to consult me in view of my interest in the treatment of sacral tumors. She then informed us that after she had left the clinic in September, 1935, she had continued to have sacral pain. This had been so severe that an exploratory laparotomy had been performed elsewhere in October, 1935. A retroperitoneal cystic mass had been found in the hollow of the sacrum, pos-

and was less firm than a dermoid or a chordoma. However, both of these tumors had to be considered in the differential diagnosis. I ventured the opinion that we were probably dealing with a spina bifida cystica which had resulted from an anomalous development

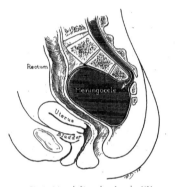

Fig. 2. Schematic illustration of a spina bifida cystica which was situated in the pelvis posterior to the rectum and in the retroperitoneal space.

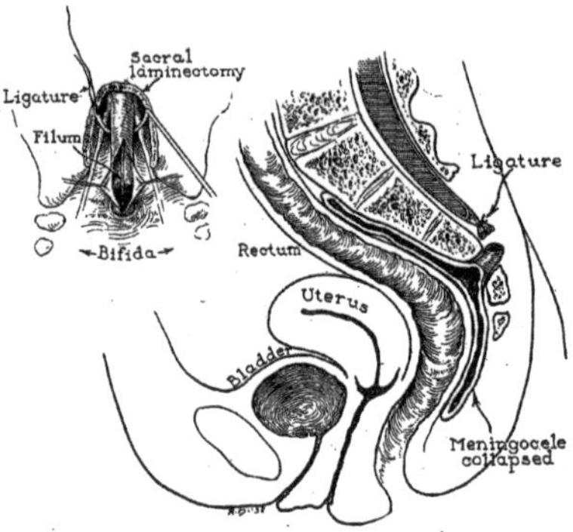

Fig. 3. Exposure of the caudal end of the sac through a small laminectomy wound, the resection and closure of the sac; this procedure permits the pelvic spina bifida cystica to drain into the soft tissues and collapse.

terior to the rectum. The mass had not been opened or removed. The abdominal wound had been closed, without any surgical intervention. In May, 1936, the patient had spent six weeks in bed because of a persistent fever. For a few months previous to her second admission to the clinic, she complained of persistent paresthesias which had involved the left foot and leg. At times, the pain had extended upward along her left side, but had not involved the face. She did not complain of any objective loss of sensation. Her menstrual history did not indicate any abnormality. She was free from all other symptoms except constipation, which had been troublesome at times. She had not noted any dysuria or urinary frequency. At times, she thought that her abdomen had swelled, at least it had appeared to be tender in the left lower quadrant. Urinalysis did not reveal any abnormality. Additional roentgenologic examination of the spinal column revealed the same finding that previously had been observed. The proctoscopic examination revealed nothing abnormal in the rectum or sigmoid colon. The proctologist observed a large, soft cystic mass which was situated posterior to the rectum. The results of neurologic examination again were negative. The ophthalmologic examination likewise did not reveal any abnormality. At this time, it became my good fortune to be the patient in consultation. I reviewed the history and the findings and proceeded to carry out a digital examination of the rectum. I could palpate a soft fluctuant mass, about the size of a kittenball, situated posterior to the rectum in the hollow of the sacrum. The mass was definitely cystic

of the sacrum, and I advised an exploration of the sacrum through a laminectomy performed over the third and fourth sacral vertebral segments.

The laminectomy was performed opposite the third and fourth sacral segments of the vertebral column, through a dorsal midline incision. Upon exposing the dural sac, it was found to communicate with the pelvic mass. I opened this at the lower end of the incision and found that the cerebrospinal fluid in the subarachnoid space communicated with the fluid within the pelvic mass (Fig. 2). I then had to determine whether or not it contained nerve elements and found that the only structure that passed down through the dural sac into the pelvis was the filum terminale, which measured about 2 mm. in diameter. There were no nerve elements in the sac at this location. The nerve fibers had left the dural sac at a higher level.

The problem that confronted me was how to remove this sac, but it soon became apparent that it was impractical to attempt to remove the pelvic mass. Therefore, I decided to divide and ligate the dural tube, in the sacral canal, thus closing the caudad end (Fig. 3). This was accomplished by a purse-string suture and additional reinforcing ligatures. Upon exploring the pelvic mass I found that I could introduce a catheter for a distance of 5 inches. Subsequent exploration with the lighted retractor showed that the arachnoid lining of the dural sac was rather gray in appearance and free from any unusual masses. This convinced me that I was not dealing with a dermoid and that I was dealing with a spina bifida cystica which had extended an-

474

teriorly into the pelvis in the retroperitoneal space posterior to the rectum. After aspirating the cerebrospinal fluid in the pelvic portion of this sac, the walls were seen to collapse as a result of the increased intra-abdominal pressure. Thus, it occurred to me that if I left the distal portion of this sac open, it would automatically close itself and become adherent. Therefore, I proceeded to treat it in this manner. The wound was closed and the patient cared for very much as we care for other patients who have spina bifida. The patient remained under observation in the hospital for sixteen days and was dismissed from the clinic twenty-one days after the operation, which was on July 22, 1936. During her postoperative convalescence, it was necessary to catheterize her for the first five days. A postoperative neurologic examination did not furnish any additional information. The patient said that the pain was less severe than it had been but that she was still conscious of some paresthesia on the outer aspect of the left foot and around the saddle area of her buttock. A rectal examination on the day of her dismissal did not reveal any pelvic mass. It was impossible to palpate any sort of fullness; therefore, it was apparent that the mass had been thoroughly collapsed and had remained collapsed. It perhaps was held in place by the pelvic organs. In a letter dated April 3, 1937, the patient said that she had returned to work and was feeling normal.

Comment

Spina bifida usually appears through defects in the lamina but it has been known to appear laterally through the spinal canal and in a few instances has appeared anterior to the vertebral column. I have had occasion to observe a previous case in which the spina bifida was situated anterior to the sacral vertebræ. There had been a projection of a diverticulum of the spina bifida through the rectum. The patient was operated on for a rectal polyp and death resulted. The case reported is unique in that the mass was situated anterior to the sacrum as a result of a congenital anomaly in the anterior portion of the sacrum. The tumor and the bony erosion resembled a dermoid situated in this position. The tumor also resembled a chordoma which had extended into

the pelvis, except that a chordoma is much firmer to palpation than was the mass in this case. The digital examination of this particular mass gave one the impression of a distended bladder except that the mass was situated on the opposite wall of the pelvis. The case is also unique because a cure was effected without removing the pelvic sac. This further confirms my opinion that a spina bifida cystica is a herniation of membranes through a spinal defect and that a cure can be effected without bone graft and without a folding in of the membranes; all that was necessary in this particular case was a division and a ligation of the dural-arachnoid tube at a place where the caudal sac normally would end.

References

1. Adson, A. W., and Beckman, E. H.: Spina bifida, its operative treatment. St. Paul Med. Jour., 19:357-363, 1917.
2. Baldwin, W. M.: The action of ultraviolet rays upon the frog's eggs. 1. The artificial production of spina bifida. Anat. Rec., 9:365-381, 1915.
3. Bardeen, C. R.: Variations in susceptibility of amphibian ova to the x-rays at different stages of development. Anat. Rec., 3:153-165, 1919.
4. Conklin, E. B.: Heredity and environment in the development of men. Princeton, Princeton University Press, 1916, pp. 309-360.
5. Hertwig: Quoted by Keibel, Frank, and Mall, Franklin.
6. Keibel, Frank, and Mall, Franklin: Manual of Human Embryology. Philadelphia: J. B. Lippincott Co., 1910, vol. 1, pp. 231-240.
7. Kellicott, W. E.: The effects of low temperature upon the development of Fundulus. A contribution to the theory of teratogeny. Am. Jour. Anat., 20:449-482, 1916.
8. Lewis, W. H.: The experimental production of cyclopia in the fish embryo (Fundulus heteroclitus). Anat. Rec., 3:175-181, 1909.
9. von Monakow, C.: Zur Entwickelung und pathologischen Anatomie der Rautenplexus. Schweiz. Arch. f. Neurol. u. Psychiat., 5:378-392, 1919.
10. Morgan, T. H.: The effects produced by centrifuging eggs before and during development. Anat. Rec., 3:155-161, 1909.
11. Penfield, Wilder: Hydrocephalus and spina bifida. Surg., Gynec. and Obst., 60:363-369, (Feb.) 1935.
12. von Recklinghausen, F.: Untersuchungen über die Spina bifida. Virchow's Arch. f. path. Anat., 105:243-330; 373-455, 1886.
13. Schmaus, H., and Sacki, S.: Pathologische Anatomie des Rückenmarks. Wiesbaden: J. F. Bergmann, 1901, pp. 490-496.
14. Stockard, C. R.: The artificial production of one-eyed monsters and other defects which occur in nature, by the use of chemicals. Anat. Rec., 3:167-173, 1909.
15. Werber, E. I.: Is pathologic metabolism in the parental organism responsible for defective and monstrous development of offspring? Bull. Johns Hopkins Hosp., 26:226-229, 1915.
16. Werber, E. I.: Experimental studies on the origin of monsters. Jour. Exper. Zool., 21:285-574, 1916.
17. Woltman, H. W.: Spina bifida; a review of 187 cases, including three associated cases of myelodysplasia without demonstrable bony defect. Minnesota Med., 4:244-259, 1921.

CARCINOMA OF THE GALLBLADDER*

W. C. CARROLL, B.S., M.D., F.A.C.S.

Saint Paul, Minnesota

IT is not with the idea of offering anything new that this paper is written, but to call attention to a condition which I think has not been given enough thought and consideration in the care of cases with gallbladder disease.

"As the pendulum of surgical opinion swings from conservatism to radicalism, and back again, it is often difficult to establish the accepted course to pursue. In April, 1911, W. J. Mayo wrote, "Ten years ago, we heard a great deal about "innocent gallstones," which means that gallstones existed without symptoms and that their presence was not suspected until postmortem examination brought them to light. We can not now escape the conviction that gallstones did cause symptoms and that we, as diagnosticians, and not the gallstones, were innocent." Andrews would take serious exception to the above quotation, for he recently said, "I think the operation on silent stones is a scandal." The question I would raise at this time is, how often do we see "silent stones"? A careful history taken after we know that a certain patient has stones will usually elicit the fact that symptoms were present even though they were mild and entirely disregarded by the patient. It certainly is not necessary to have colics to have symptoms of gallbladder disease. As we have hypersensitive patients, we also have hyposensitive ones. The latter will uncomplainingly carry their troubles, and conceal symptoms which will be uncovered only by the most searching questioning.

Carcinoma of the gallbladder is of sufficient frequency to make it a factor of serious consideration when we must pass judgment on a case of gallstones. The exact percentage of malignancy is difficult to evaluate as many cases both of gallstones and malignancy go undiagnosed. It is usually ranked sixth in frequency of malignancy of the digestive organs. Surgical experience in various large clinics in this country place the percentage from 1 to 2.5 per cent of all operations on the gallbladder. Collected statistics from cases reported by Wilkie, Deaver, Smith, Judd and Gray, Miller, French, Sherrill and McCarty

show that there were 393 carcinomas in 35,054 operations, an incidence of 1.12 per cent. Boyce and McFetridge[2] in the *International Surgical Digest*, Critique Section, state, "Looking at the facts from another angle a certain proportion of patients with gallstones develop cancer. Leutz, in 557 cases of cholelithiasis, found that malignancy developed in 5.1 per cent of women over thirty-nine years of age, and in 4.3 per cent of both sexes. Rolleston found the incidence of malignancy following cholelithiasis to be 4.5 per cent; Moynihan 5 per cent; Ridel 7 to 8 per cent; Graham 8.6 per cent and Schroeder 14 per cent. In five of the eighty-four cases reported by Magonn and Renshaw from the Mayo Clinic in 1921, the malignancy had developed at the site of a previous cholecystostomy for stones, and similar cases have been put on record by F. K. Smith, Mayo Robson, Knapp, Lett and others."[3] Judd has stated that those who develop malignancy of the gallbladder have had stones. Clinicians who will not accept this statement in its entirety must admit that cancer will not develop in a healthy gallbladder. An argument against this theory is the fact that experimentors have been unable to produce cancer in animals by the introduction of gallstones or other foreign bodies into the gallbladder. Barlow made the suggestion that calculi taken from malignant gallbladders are radio-active. Petrac and Krotkina used nineteen guinea pigs and inserted small radium tubes in twelve, and produced malignancy in two, after 136 and 158 weeks, respectively. However, two of the controls, in which only sterile glass capsules were inserted, also developed malignancy with metastasis at the end of sixty-six and 166 weeks. Other observers feel that a chemical factor either independent or in association with stones is responsible for the new growths. However, if we recognize the chronic irritation theory, there seems to be a causal relationship between stones and malignancy. As regards sex distribution, almost three-fourths of the reported cases have been in women, somewhat higher than the average distribution of benign lesions. There are records of carcinoma of the gallbladder in all decades, over the age of

*Read before the Saint Paul Surgical Society, February 10, 1938.

twenty, but the majority fall between the ages of fifty to sixty-five.

Papillomata are of such frequent occurrence that one would hardly believe that there is a relationship between them and malignancy. Nevertheless, cases have been observed where there are areas of epithelial proliferation extending through the muscle wall and some specimens show a close resemblance to papillary carcinoma. If there is at least a possible relation between these apparently benign looking, wart-like growths and the development of cancer, we then must look upon such a gallbladder as being better out, and not just regard it as many would, along with the strawberry type, as a metabolic disturbance incapable of causing any damage.

Pathology.—There are four generally recognized types of carcinoma of the gallbladder, and they can usually be differentiated by the naked eye: (1) scirrhous; (2) papillary; (3) mucoid-colloid; (4) squamous cell (epithelioma).

1. The scirrhous type is the most common, starting as a small infiltrating tumor, or thickening, which is at times overlooked in its early stage, but in its later development involves the whole gallbladder, contracting down on the stones so as to make it difficult at times to identify the organ itself. Microscopically, it is that of an adenocarcinoma It extends very early into the liver and the glands along the common duct.

2. The papillary type originates at the fundus or neck of the bladder and grows out into the lumen as a coarse villous or solid fungating mass. It is often associated with empyema as it early obliterates the cystic duct. Microscopically, it is that of a columnar cell adenocarcinoma.

3. The mucoid, or colloid type, is bulky and soft, and can be recognized by its jelly-like appearance. Microscopically, there are trabaculæ of fibrous tissue with large spaces of pseudomucin. Tumor cells are few and are found singly or in small groups. These cells contain small drops of mucin which enlarge, bursting and discharging their contents into the connective tissue.

4. The squamous type is the least common, and can as a rule only be differentiated microscopically. It is seen as an epithelioma made up of cells of squamous type with prickle cells, and only occasionally do epithelial pearls occur. The usual explanation of a squamous cell type in the gallbladder is that it arises from a previous leu-

koplacia which has been caused by irritation from pre-existing gallbladder disease.

Dissemination of any type is usually by local excision, distant metastases being encountered at post mortem. The lungs are involved in 10 per cent of the cases. The liver, on account of its intimate association and direct blood and lymphatic supply, is involved very early. In the right lobe, there frequently forms a large hard mass, while, at times, multiple nodules are found throughout the entire organ, which becomes greatly enlarged. The regional lymph nodes also are the seat of early metastases. The node by the cystic duct enlarges, blocking both the duct and artery, resulting at times in hydrops or more frequently empyema. The carcinomatous bladder is more subject to empyema than others. From this first gland, the others along the common duct and retroperitoneally become invaded.

Clinical Features.—Apparently, as yet, we have no signs by which an exact diagnosis of carcinoma of the gallbladder can be made in its early stage. The usual symptoms of gallbladder disease are present in the well taken history, varying in degree from those of a severe colic to the mildest indigestion. In two recently observed cases, there was a distinct change in the character and degree of the distress, the discomfort becoming more continuous and unrelated to food intake. The colic present earlier in the course of the disease in these cases had given way to more constant pain, which was the one symptom that finally made the patients consent to operation. Nausea, vomiting, anorexia, weight loss and jaundice, and finally cachexia, with or without signs of empyema of the gallbladder, are symptoms which appear as the disease advances. Jaundice may be an early symptom if the glands become involved and cause pressure on the common duct. The earlier the jaundice occurs, the sooner death will follow. Diarrhea and extreme weight loss have been noted in certain cases before any symptoms of biliary disease have attracted attention.

Various authors have tried to classify the disease according to symptoms but the overlapping and bizarre complaints make this extremely difficult. If we wait until a tumor mass is felt before advising operation, we will find that the patient is well beyond any surgical relief. This is the stage in which most of the patients are seen.

Cholecystography might be of possible value in early diagnosis, as Kirklin has suggested that a filling defect more than 2 cm. in diameter with an irregular border should arouse suspicion of malignancy. The necessity of well taken films and proper interpretation, of course, is very obvious. Boyce and McFetridge further observed in this review: "The only solution of the problem seems to be the constant recollection that malignancy of the gallbladder is a definite possibility in all cases of persistent retention of bile and the consideration of malignancy as a possible diagnosis of all cases of cholecystitis or cholelithiasis in individuals over forty, or even younger. If the possibility of its occurrence is not constantly borne in mind, the diagnosis will always be missed."

Treatment.—At the present time, the majority of patients with carcinoma of the gallbladder are seen too late for radical removal. Any operation, except in the very early cases, usually renders the patient more uncomfortable than before. If a cholecystectomy is at all feasible, it should be done and the lymph nodes along the cystic duct removed. The electrosurgical unit is of value for this operation as a portion of the liver about the gallbladder fossa where direct extension takes place should be removed. Gastroenterostomy may, at times, be indicated to relieve the pyloric obstruction. The immediate mortality, especially in the jaundiced cases, is usually very high, and those that survive operation, succumb in a few months. Every series on record has the same discouraging picture. Webber, at the Mayo Clinic, studied thirty cases according to Broders index, correlating the clinical findings with the microscopic picture. He found that in the groups graded I and II, palpable tumors were present in two cases, while there were twelve in Grades III and IV. Furthermore, the duration of life in Grades I and II was thirty-four months against 4.8 months for those of Groups III and IV.

Early operation in gall bladder disease will, undoubtedly, prevent the occurrence of carcinoma, as well as ward off many of the other possible complications. Heyd, former president of the American Medical Association, writes editorially, "Preventative medical thought and wise judicious surgery would suggest the early removal of chronically infected gallbladder and not delay until the accident of infection initiates a fulminating acute cholecystitis," and further he states, "Teachers of surgery who lend their prestige and give support to a policy of waiting, provide authority for timid surgeons, inexperienced operators and procrastinating practitioners."

Having personally observed patients with gallstones go through long periods of watchful waiting, hoping that nothing very serious will develop except an occasional colic, and then later seeing them with the more serious complications of damage to liver and pancreas, empyema, and, in a few, malignancy, I can wholeheartedly subscribe to Dr. Mayo's saying: "Innocent gallstones —a myth!" I believe the mortality in gallbladder operations performed before the development of complications should, in competent hands, be less than the incidence of malignancy alone. Individual case reports are of very little value as the usual picture is well known, but upon seeing a small but increasing number of these cases, which might have been avoided but for procrastination on the part of either patients or their physicians, I feel that too little attention has been called to this usually avoidable tragedy.

References

1. Andrews, Edmund: Pathogenesis of gallbladder disease. Minn. Med., 19:131-141, (Mar.) 1936.
2. Boyce, Frederick F., and McFetridge, E. M.: Carcinoma of Gallbladder. Intl. Surg. Digest, 21:67-79, (Feb.) 1936.
3. Broders, A. B.: Personal communication.
4. Erdman, J. F.: Malignancy of gallbladder. Ann. Surg., 101: 1139-1143, (May) 1935.
5. Heyd, Chas. Gordon: Acute cholecystitis, why delay? Surg., Gyn. and Obst., 65:550-551, (Oct.) 1937.
6. Illingworth, C. F. W.: Carcinoma of gallbladder. Brit. Jour. Surg., 23:4-18, (July) 1935.
7. Mayo, William J.: Innocent gallstones, a myth. Jour. A.M.A., 56:1021-1024, (April 8) 1911.
8. Rhodes, R. L., and Greenblatt, R. B.: Carcinoma of gallbladder. South. Med. Jour., 30:315-318, (March) 1937.
9. Windbigler, Chauncy: Personal communication.

RECURRENT "TROPICAL" LYMPHANGITIS*

With Report of a Case

RUDOLPH C. LOGEFEIL, M.S., M.D., and ROY A. HOFFMAN, M.D.

Minneapolis, Minnesota

SIMPLE acute lymphangitis is a rather common affection accompanying infected wounds of the hands and feet, and is usually due to infection from streptococci, less often to staphylococci, gonococci, or pneumococci. The bacteria may enter the lymph vessel directly from the infected wound, or pass through the wall of the vessel from without. However, inflammation of the lymphatics may occur without a primary focus of infection. It may occur during the course of acute infectious diseases, herpes, and especially erysipelas. Such chronic infectious diseases as gonorrhea, syphilis, tuberculosis and bubonic plague may show lymphangitis. Other forms occur after roentgen irradiation, sunburn, poison ivy and insect bites.

Osler[5] offers a pathologic classification of acute lymphangitis as follows: simple, purulent, and proliferative. The chief features of the simple form are hyperemia, edema and infiltration of the vessel walls and perilymphatic tissue with a resulting thickening which may become necrotic or proliferative. The condition returns to normal if the existing cause is removed. Otherwise, it may lead to a chronic process.

The purulent form shows more thickening of the wall, the lumen becomes filled with pus or a fibrino-purulent mass which, between the valves, gives a beaded appearance. Abscesses may form along the course of the lymph vessel or in the regional lymph nodes, and septicopyemia may result.

The acute proliferative type occurs chiefly in gonorrhea, the principal feature being a marked perilymphangitis.

Chronic or recurrent lymphangitis results in a partial or complete obliteration of the lymph vessel due to hypertrophic changes resulting from a proliferation and induration of the connective tissue of the vessel wall and surrounding tissues. When affecting an extremity, chronic edema or elephantiasis are the most important clinicial features.

Goeckerman,[1] in discussing recurrent lymphangitis, distinguishes between lymph-edema and solid edema, applying the former term to stasis of lymph resulting from mechanical obstruction like that following radical amputation of the breast without infection, while restricting the term solid edema to the end-process of recurrent lymphangitis.

Recurrent lymphangitis may be defined as repeated attacks of simple acute lymphangitis, due to an inflammatory process in the cutaneous lymphatic vessels caused by the streptococcus hemolyticus. The involved part shows a well defined area of redness, swelling and local pain, which spreads by direct continuity and is associated with general febrile symptoms. Suppuration may occur when the subcutaneous tissues are involved, and the whole process turns into the suppurative form. It occurs in temperate climates during the hot months, but is much more common in the tropics or sub-tropics, where it is called recurrent tropical lymphangitis. This is probably due to the fact that profuse sweating, dehydration and irritation of the skin predisposes it to infection. Although erysipelas affects the skin somewhat similarly it is more frequent during the colder months of the year, probably due to the increased frequency of upper respiratory infections. Also meteorological studies have shown that the frequency of erysipelas corresponds with an increase of humidity in the air. Other streptococcic infections, such as scarlet fever and rheumatic heart diseases, are common in temperate and cold climates, but scarce in California, and almost unknown in Puerto Rico.

My case is that of a white male, thirty-one years of age, single, who for the past eleven years has had recurrent attacks of inflammation of the lymphatics in the lower extremities, followed by edema.

He was born in Kentucky in 1906 and lived there for four years, before moving to Ohio. During early childhood he suffered no other illnesses than an attack of typhoid fever at the age of two and a second attack at the age

---

*Read before the meeting of the Minnesota Society of Internal Medicine, May, 1937.

of eleven. At twelve he was seriously ill with an acute bronchitis and an associated jaundice which persisted for a period of five weeks. A tonsillectomy was performed at the age of sixteen. There was no history of venereal diseases. His father and mother are living and well. His grandmother, mother, and brother have had acute rheumatic attacks, accompanied by high fever, and a moderate amount of swelling and pain in the hands and feet, lasting about a week.

The patient was apparently in good health until August of 1925, at which time he had a blister on his left heel which became secondarily infected. This condition cleared up in about a week under treatment, but recurred a month later and necessitated hospitalization for a ten day period. At the end of that time there was no further evidence of infection and he remained in good health until August, 1926, when he sustained an abrasion to the skin of the lower left leg. Within twelve hours he had a severe chill followed by a high fever and the typical clinical picture of an acute lymphangitis and lymphadenitis of the left leg and groin. The treatment consisted chiefly of rest, elevation of the limb, and application of local wet packs. The infection gradually subsided and within five weeks he was able to return to work.

In July, 1927, during a spell of very hot weather, without any evidence of external injury, he developed pain in both groins with tender, swollen glands, and evidence of lymphangitis of both legs, accompanied by high fever and the same constitutional symptoms as before. This attack subsided in ten days, after which he resumed his work.

Similar attacks occurred the next three summers, always during spells of hot weather, with complete recovery from each attack, except that there was a persistent gradual increase in the edema of both lower legs. He had no recurrence during the summer of 1931, all of which time he spent in Duluth, Minnesota. From 1931 to 1936 he had somewhat milder recurrences each summer, the most severe attack occurring in August, 1936, at which time he first came under my observation. About two weeks before this attack he came to my office complaining of edema of both lower legs below the knees.

Physical examination at that time was entirely

negative except for edema of the lower extremities and an epidermophytosis infection between the toes, commonly known as "athlete's foot." Tests for patency of the internal veins of both legs proved them to be normal. Urinalysis showed an occasional cast; P.S.P. 77 per cent in two hours; hemoglobin 83 per cent; rbc. 4,-170,000, wbc. 8600, P.M.N. Neut. 69 per cent, P.M.N. Eos. 4 per cent, large mono. 1 per cent, large and small lympho. 26 per cent; blood urea 15.6 mg. per 100 c.c. blood; Wassermann negative; basal metabolic rate minus 3.

A sedimentation rate of 55 mm. in 45 minutes was the only finding of consequence in any of the blood tests.

Six days later, during a spell of very hot weather, he suddenly had a severe chill, followed by a temperature of 105, and became acutely ill. Both lower legs were swollen, rather tender, with glandular enlargement of both inguinal regions. These glands were acutely inflamed, tender to touch, and they were more numerous and larger on the left side. He was sent to the Swedish Hospital, where laboratory tests revealed the usual febrile urinary findings, white blood count 30,500; differential count of 91 per cent P.M.N.; 5 per cent large Mono., 3 per cent small Mono., and 1 per cent transitional cells. The blood culture, Wassermann and tests for tularemia mellitensis and typhoid were negative.

The patient's temperature was 104.2 degrees on admission to the hospital and increased to 105.6 shortly afterward. He was irrational at this time. A septic temperature curve persisted for the next five days, fluctuating between 100 and 103 degrees, and gradually descending to normal on the sixth day.

The most interesting finding was the appearance of the extremities. There was an area of redness and a rash beginning at the ankle and spreading upward. The skin became hot, swollen and glistening; the margin of the rash was sharply demarcated but not palpably raised. As the rash advanced, the center of the affected area became somewhat pale and edematous. It spread from below upward by direct extension and extended to the knee joints or slightly above. However, a red streak extended up along the cords of the lymphatics to the regional lymphatic glands in the groins. As the temperature began to fall and the general con dition of the patient improved, the rash concurrently began to fade and practically disappeared when the temperature was normal. However, the limbs remained swollen and painful for many days afterward, and there was slight desquamation of the skin on the affected parts. The edema persisted and continued to remain increased over that present before the attack.

The above description is typical of all his attacks, but some, however, were not as severe as this one. Except for the persistent edema the patient remained well until August, 1937, when, during a spell of very hot weather, he had a similar but milder attack while working in North Dakota. This attack lasted about eight days and then left him again with a slight increase in the edema of the extremities. On close quizzing I found he had noted peeling between the toes practically every summer, and had treated this during one previous summer, following an attack. Altogether the patient has had fifteen attacks. Several summers he has had two attacks, and in 1930 had three attacks. The only summer he was free from it was in 1931 when he spent the entire summer in cool Duluth, Minnesota. In 1929 he received vaccine from a gland removed from the groin by Dr. Duff, but apparently this was of no help. The microscopic examination of this gland showed only chronic inflammation. He suffered no complications in any of the attacks except a persistent pachyderma.

I feel that my case is similar to those reported by Janero Suarez[7] under the title "Recurrent Tropical Lymphangitis." This disease occurs quite frequently in the southern part of the United States and is endemic in Puerto Rico and other sub-tropical countries. It attacks chiefly young people, more commonly females, who are most susceptible during menstruation and the puerperium. Over 90 per cent of Suarez's series occurred in the lower extremities, 81 per cent being limited to one leg. When present in both legs, one is usually more affected than the other. It gives no immunity to the patient; on the contrary, one attack predisposes to another. Recurrences may take place frequently or may be months or years apart, and are most common between the ages of twenty and forty. However, it has been noted that a severe attack is usually followed by a long re-

mission. Patients have been known to have sustained fifty or sixty attacks, often occurring regularly, every four to six weeks. Chronic edema or pachyderma results in a majority of the cases. Suarez believes the mechanical lymphatic obstruction or bacterial infection is in itself capable of producing elephantiasis. Mates[4] and Grace[2] believe that bacterial infection plays an essential etiological role in the pathology of elephantiasis. Drinker[3] and his associates have demonstrated in remarkable experiments on large police dogs that spontaneous attacks of lymphangitis occurred where lymphedema or experimental elephantiasis was produced by total destruction of the lymphatics in the hind legs. Hemolytic streptococci were cultured from the tissues of the affected leg, which could be transferred to other dogs, but only in limbs previously operated upon. In view of the fact that humans are more susceptible to streptococcal disease than canines, previous obstruction of the lymphatics is not essential for the production of acute lymphangitis, but, when present, predisposes to future attacks.

In Suarez's[7] series of 139 cases, ninety-one showed a definite focus of infection, 72 per cent of which were epidermophytosis interdigitalis. Removal of this infection was usually followed by cessation of attacks. One can usually get a history of focal infection or injury preceding the first attack. Occasionally cases occur in which no local lesion can be found. Suarez had two cases of this kind. They were classified as allergic. The redness, heat, edema and fibrosis probably represent "an allergic phenomenon to a protein fraction of the streptococcus or its toxin."

The symptoms and physical findings during a typical attack in my case correspond well with those described in Suarez's series. Incubation period was two to three days, while relapses occurred in 4 per cent of his cases. Chronic lymphedema and subcutaneous abscesses are the most common complications.

Otero and Lebron[6] demonstrated the presence of agglutinins against streptococci in practically every case of recurrent tropical lymphangitis. They give a positive allergic reaction to streptococcus filtrate, which disappears during the febrile stage. However, they found a definite increase in the antistreptolysin content of the blood, during an attack. They also believe that acute attacks are preceded by hemolytic streptococcus infections.

The presence of an area of redness with a well-defined margin, spread by direct continuity, pain and the accompaniment of constitutional symptoms, distinguishes recurrent lymphangitis from other erythematous lesions. Abscesses, cellulitis and thrombophlebitis may at times be confused.

Prognosis is very favorable, no deaths having been reported. Morbidity is great, however, due to recurring attacks. Disability produced by the elephantiasis is of considerable importance. Treatment consists of the following:

1. Removal of any possible focus of infection.
2. Proper care of the feet, especially during hot weather, with elimination of any possible epidermophyton infection.
3. Goeckerman[2] has had gratifying results in the early stages in seventeen cases from the use of foreign protein given intravenously and filtered roentgen rays applied locally.
4. Moving to a cool climate during the hot summer months is good prophylactic treatment.
5. The treatment of the elephantiasis is a difficult and lengthy problem.

Conclusions

1. I believe this case represents a definite clinical entity, occurring sporadically in this country, more commonly in the south, but which is endemic in tropical countries and described under the title of recurrent tropical lymphangitis.
2. It occurs only in hot weather.
3. An infective lesion or abrasion can usually be found, especially in the initial or early attacks. The initial attack predisposes the patient to further attacks. Severe attacks may produce some temporary immunity.
4. Injury to the lymphatics of the extremity with resulting chronic obstruction and an acquired allergy to hemolytic streptococcus, plus hot weather, may cause recurrences without infection or injury to the skin. This has been borne out by clinical and experimental observations.
5. Treatment, except prophylactic, has been unsatisfactory.

Bibliography

1. Goeckerman, Wm. H.: Recurrent lymphangitis. Minn. Med., Dec. 13:902, (Dec.) 1930.
2. Grace, A. W.: Filarial lymphangitis, considered as a mild erysipelas resulting from hypersensitiveness to a B. hemolytic steptococcus of a particular type. Roy. Soc. Trop. Med. and Hyg., 28:259-276, (Nov.) 1934.
3. Homans, John, Drinker, C, K., and Field, M. E.; Elephantiasis and the clinical implications of its experimental reproduction in animals. Ann. Surg., 100:812-832, (Oct.) 1934.
4. Matas, R.: The surgical treatment of elephantiasis and elephantoid states, dependent upon chronic obstruction of the lymphatic and venous channels. Am. Jour. Trop. Dis. and Prev. Med., 1:60, 1913.
5. Osler, Wm.: Modern Medicine, Philadelphia: Lee, 4: 583, 1908.
6. Otero and Lebron: Quoted by Suarez.
7. Suarez, Jenoro: Clinical findings in 139 cases of recurrent tropical lymphangitis. Puerto Rico Jour. Pub. Health and Trop. Med., 12:81, (Sept.) 1936.

INTESTINAL OBSTRUCTION DUE TO CALCIFIED MESENTERIC GLANDS

JOHN M. CULLIGAN, M.D.

Saint Paul, Minnesota

IN ROUTINE roentgenograms of the abdomen shadows of calcified mesenteric glands are a rather common finding. In the large majority of cases they are more or less of academic interest and surgical interference is not indicated. It is interesting to speculate upon their etiology and pathogenesis.

The primary causative agent is of course the tubercle bacillus. The human and the bovine types have been isolated from the glands. The human type is isolated from the glands of patients with tuberculosis elsewhere in the body whereas the bovine type is isolated usually from the glands of children who have ingested milk from tuberculous cows. Approximately 60 per cent of the cases are of the latter type.

The clinical course of the disease is variable. In the majority of patients no definite history of symptoms which might lead one to suspect the disease can be elicited. The disease is discovered late when a roentgenogram of the abdomen is made. The roentgenographic findings, when the diagnosis is made this way, are typical shadows of calcified glands usually having characteristic features. They present moth-eaten shadows of different density varying in diameter

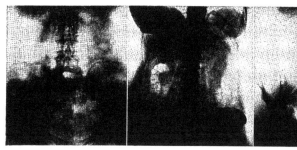

Fig. 1. Roentgenogram showing a large mesenteric gland in the right lower quadrant of the abdomen, measuring 8 x 5 centimeters. Gaseous distention of the small bowel can also be seen.

Fig. 2. Roentgenogram showing a small mesenteric gland in the right lower quadrant of the abdomen measuring 2 x 2 centimeters. The degree of obstruction may be demonstrated by the dilated loops of small bowel.

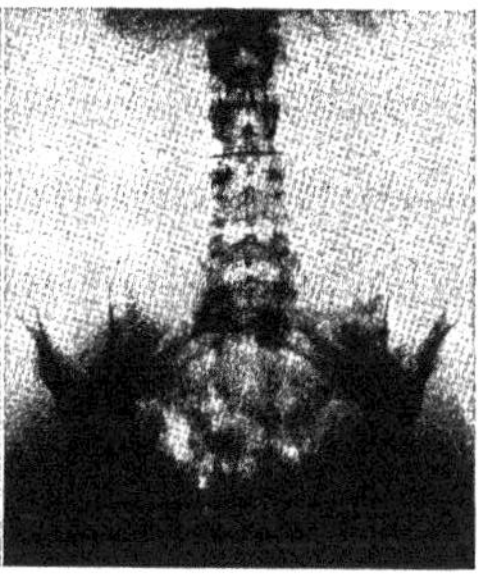

Fig. 3. Roentgenogram showing two large and multiple small shadows of calcified mesenteric glands. The largest measures 4 x 3 centimeters. No dilatation of the bowel is evident.

from one to five or six centimeters or more. They may be found any place in the abdomen but are usually located in the region of the umbilicus, probably a little more often on the right side.

Early in the disease an entirely different picture may be seen. The so-called acute type may give rise to definite clinical symptoms and signs. These are usually pain, colicky in character, associated with nausea and vomiting and abdominal tenderness in the region of the umbilicus or over the right lower quadrant of the abdomen. Exploration at this time will reveal enlarged caseating nodes in the mesentery.

Subacute types may be characterized by indefinite and vague abdominal complaints associated with pallor, weakness, and occasional attacks of slight fever. At times, the glands may be palpated.

Recently, we have observed three cases which were of the asymptomatic chronic type until obstruction of the bowel developed. From the size of the glands found at operation and because of their hard calcified nature, it was apparent that they had been present for many years, but the patients had had no symptoms referable to them. In two of the three patients, complete obstruction of the bowel was produced in the first attack, and in one chronic recurring partial obstruction was produced. The diagnoses were made from the findings of obstruction and the presence of shadows in the roentgenograms suggestive of calcified mesenteric glands.

Case 1.—A seventy-one-year-old woman was seized by severe abdominal cramps and abdominal distention. Within twelve hours vomiting occurred. This persisted. The patient was unable to defecate or pass flatus even with enemata. A roentgenogram (Fig. 1) revealed a large calcified shadow suggestive of a mesenteric gland. At operation through a right rectus incision, the entire small bowel was found injected and distended. The point of obstruction was in the right lower quadrant involving the ileum about twelve inches above the ileocecal valve. A large calcified gland was present in the mesentery close to the bowel. Cicatrization formed adjacent to it completely obstructed the bowel. The gland was excised, a few adhesions cut, and the collapsed bowel distended as the gas passed on. The patient made an uneventful recovery.

Three months later, she again presented herself with obstruction of the bowel. This time, it was due to a strangulated right inguinal hernia. This was freed and the hernia repaired. She again had had an uneventful convalescence.

Case 2.—A forty-six-year-old married woman was awakened at two o'clock in the morning by severe abdominal cramps. She slept very little during the remainder of the night. A hypodermic injection of morphine was administered at nine a. m. The patient was first seen at eight p. m. Paroxysms of pain were present and visible peristalsis could be seen. She obtained slight relief from enemata. A roentgenogram of the abdomen (Fig. 2) showed distention of the bowel and a shadow suggestive of a calcified mesenteric gland. Exploration, through a right rectus incision, revealed a greatly distended upper ileum. An obstructing band at the site of a calcified mesenteric gland encircled the bowel. This was cut and gas escaped into the collapsed bowel beyond the obstruction. The gland was excised. The patient made an uneventful convalescence.

Case 3.—A twenty-five-year-old single woman had had an appendectomy five years previous to the time I saw her. She complained of intermittent attacks of abdominal pain associated with abdominal distention. This pain could be relieved by enemata. Roentgenograms of the abdomen revealed two shadows of calcified mesenteric glands (Fig. 3). At operation, a constricting band bound the bowel to one of the glands. This was cut and the glands excised. Convalescence was uneventful and there has been no return of pain.

BROMIDES, THEIR USE AND ABUSE*

GORDON R. KAMMAN, M.D., F.A.C.P.

Instructor in Nervous and Mental Diseases, University of Minnesota,
Saint Paul, Minnesota

WITH the gradual elimination of industrial hazards, with increased efficiency in the control of epidemic diseases, and with the speeding up of modern living conditions, there has been in recent years a great increase in the number of functional nervous diseases afflicting the general population of our country. Man formerly used his skeletal muscles to subdue his natural enemies and to convert natural resources into the essentials of life. In modern times the burden has been lifted from our physical bodies and a great load thrown upon our psychological and emotional mechanisms. As a result of this change, the administration of hypnotics and sedatives which act upon the nervous system represents one of the most common procedures in modern medical practice. Millions of dollars are spent annually for the purchase of these drugs, and as a result of carelessness on the part of the medical profession they are frequently used by the laity without medical supervision. These drugs effect no cure. Their function is merely to mitigate; to intercede between man and his environment; to serve as a buffer which absorbs part of the constant and unrelenting barrage of stimuli to which man is subjected. There is scarcely any group of drugs more freely employed than sedatives and hypnotics, and prominent in this group are the salts of bromine. Inasmuch as the functional conditions in which these drugs are given are usually prolonged states, cumulation often occurs; but because of their extreme diversity, the symptoms of bromide intoxication are frequently missed. The complex of the busy doctor, plus the neurotic patient, plus the "salty medicine," is a common one; and the oft-repeated statement, usually delivered over the telephone; "keep taking that salty medicine," many times does much more harm than good. There are times when I suspect that a physician's skill as a psychotherapist stands in inverse proportion to the amount of bromide that he prescribes.

True, the salts of bromine are too valuable as therapeutic agents for us to decry their use, and it would be no more logical merely on account

of a few cases of bromide poisoning to condemn them as a whole than it would be to condemn digitalis because of the occasional occurrence of digitalis poisoning. In my experience, however, bromide intoxication seems to be occurring with such increasing frequency that, in spite of numerous contributions already made to the literature on the subject, it seems justifiable again to call the attention of physicians to certain dangers inherent in the use of bromides, and to point out specific methods for the diagnosis and treatment of bromide intoxication. Credit should be given to Wuth[17] for awakening interest in bromide intoxication and for publishing in 1927 a simple laboratory method for the quantitative estimation of the bromide content of blood serum.

The purpose of this paper is to call attention to the fact that bromides even in therapeutic doses may produce mental symptoms in susceptible individuals. These symptoms range from a mild clouding of consciousness to an active delirium, and from mental depression to stupor and coma. In recent years, I have observed a number of patients who have manifested symptoms of bromide intoxication which have slowly cleared up after withdrawal of the drug. These have usually been elderly individuals with varying degrees of arteriosclerosis, or cardiac and renal insufficiency; or younger persons who could not or would not take sufficient food, or were anemic and undernourished. It is probable that some of the exacerbations of mental symptoms and of the psychoses which occur from time to time in patients under our care are due to drug intoxication from our therapeutic effort rather than to the underlying conditions which we are trying to treat. One has frequently seen acutely disturbed psychotics in full restraints and requiring feeding by nasal tube become quiet and coöperative within forty-eight hours after discontinuance of a bromide ration of 45 g (3.0 gm.) a day.

Incidence

The first case of bromide intoxication was reported by Huette[3] in 1850, and for many years following this, reports of the condition were very infrequent. With the shift in preponderance

---

*Thesis presented before the Minnesota Academy of Medicine, October 13, 1937.

from infectious and physical diseases to neuropsychiatric disorders, the use of the salts of bromine as therapeutic agents has increased and more and more cases have been reported in recent medical literature. Apparently, the incidence of bromide intoxication and bromide delirium is higher than one ordinarily suspects. Among 505 admissions to the state hospital at Harrisburg, Pa., during the two years beginning June 1, 1931,[6] there were fifteen unquestionable cases of bromide psychosis. Among 238 admissions to Johns Hopkins hospital over a six month period[17] there were twenty cases of bromide intoxication, an incidence of 8.4 per cent. Among 1,000 consecutive patients admitted to the Colorado psychopathic hospital, forty-four showed an excess of bromide in the blood, and in seventeen (1.7 per cent) the mental symptoms were due solely to bromism.[13] During 1935, 2.7 per cent of the patients admitted to the Psychiatric Clinic at the New Haven Hospital in Connecticut showed definite signs of bromide intoxication.[7]

Pharmacology[14]

The effects of the bromine ion are largely confined to the central nervous system. Whatever other effects it produces are relatively insignificant and may be considered as secondary to those on the central nervous system. The slowing of respiration, the reduction of body temperature, and the slowing of all the physical processes may be attributed to lessened movement and consequent decreased heat production incident to the depressing action upon the central nervous system. All parts of the nervous system are affected, but the higher cortical centers seem to be most susceptible to the drug. Thomas[11] working with rabbits found that the amount of bromide absorbed by various portions of the central nervous system depends, in part, upon the water content of its various tissues. By feeding different rabbits known quantities of bromide, Thomas was able to show that the bromide content of the gray matter of the central nervous system was about 150 per cent that of the white matter when the content was calculated in milli-equivalents of bromide per gram of dry weight. Bastido[1] has shown that in bromidized dogs stimulation of the motor areas does not produce convulsions. In humans under the influence of bromide, the higher intellectual centers are retarded and the reaction time is pro-

longed. There also is a depressing effect on the spinal cord and the spinal reflexes are inhibited. Ordinary doses of bromide have no effect on the circulation, but larger doses depress the heart and vasoconstrictor centers, lessening arterial tension.[9]

When ingested, bromides are readily absorbed from the stomach and appear in the urine a few minutes later. However, elimination takes place very slowly, and after a single does of bromide by mouth, although the drug may be detected in the urine in a few minutes, it also may still be found in the urine as long as twenty days afterward. Bearing this in mind one should not have any difficulty in appreciating the cumulative effect of oft repeated doses of bromide over a long period of time.

Landheimer, in 1901, was the first to recognize the important influence of the intake of chlorides upon the retention of bromides. Bromides are not excreted by the kidneys as rapidly as chlorides but they tend to displace the latter in the blood and other body fluids. The displaced chlorides are excreted by the kidneys in preference to the bromides. This permits an accumulation of the bromides with consequent lowering of the chloride content of the body. A diminished chloride intake (insufficient food, or a nasal feeding formula containing insufficient chloride, *vide infra*) increases the risk of bromide intoxication. Conversely, an increased chloride intake facilitates the elimination of bromide. When 25 to 30 per cent of the blood chloride is replaced by bromide, symptoms of intoxication usually appear. Bennoulli states that a replacement of more than 40 per cent of the chlorides in the blood by bromide is fatal. It can be seen, therefore, that when a patient is receiving bromide medication, his chloride intake is of paramount importance. In order to maintain the chloride-bromide equilibrium, according to Rylan,[8] the chloride intake should be four times the bromide intake. If the bromide intake equals the chloride intake, intoxication will occur in about three weeks. According to Wuth[17] the average hospital patient takes about 7.4 gm. chloride in twenty-four hours. At Mounds Park Sanitarium, in St. Paul, the average daily diet contains 12 gm. of chloride exclusive of what the patient adds to his food after it is served to him. This amount of chloride is enough to balance 3 gm. (45 grains) of bromide per twenty-four hours, provided the patient eats all of his food. However, the standard nasal feedings, for which there are several formulæ, contain an average of 3 gm. of chloride per twenty-four-hour ration.[18] The average twenty-four-hour bromide dose for a neuro-psychiatric patient being 3 gm. (15 gr. three times a day) it can readily be seen that if Rylan's computations are correct, patients on nasal feeding and regular bromide medication should show signs of bromide intoxication in about three weeks. In my experience this has frequently been the case.

The question has frequently been raised as to whether the effect of bromide is dependent primarily upon the excess of bromide itself or upon consequent diminution of the chlorides. The effect of a single dose of bromide is too rapid for chloride diminution to be a factor. Furthermore, it is possible to narcotize dogs with bromide before diminution of chlorides has had time to play any conspicuous part.[14]

Symptoms of Bromide Intoxication

The clinical picture of bromide intoxication is extremely variable, and according to Katzenelbogen[14] and his associates, the only accurate method of establishing the diagnosis is the determination of an excess amount of bromide in the blood. While it is true that there are no pathognomonic symptoms of bromide delirium, and while it is also true that one encounters many cases in which the cutaneous manifestations of brominism are absent, I believe that it is possible to separate the types of brominism into two large clinical groups: simple bromide intoxication or depression, and bromide delirium or psychosis.

Simple bromide intoxication or depression consists of a state of mental sluggishness in which the patient thinks and acts with great difficulty, but is oriented and doesn't exhibit delusions or hallucinations. He is dull/stupid, and indifferent. His face is pale, expressionless, and may or may not show a rash. The eyes are heavy lidded, the expression staring, and the patient complains of headache. All the mental and physical reactions are retarded, memory may be impaired for recent events, and the gait is ataxic. There is anorexia, flatulence, nausea, and constipation. All tendon reflexes, as well as the corneal and pharyngeal reflexes, are reduced or absent. The pulse may be rapid and the temperature somewhat elevated.

Bromide delirium or psychosis, as has been stated before, is not an independent nosological entity. It is like any other toxic delirium and belongs to what Adolph Meyer calls the dysergasic state. The dysergasic state embraces all the exogenous psychoses, acute delirious manias, toxic-infectious psychoses, infective-exhaustive psychoses, deliria of fever, and drug deliria described by other authors. In addition to disintegration of function at the biological level (ataxia, tremor, slurring speech, et cetera) there is always dysfunction at the psycho-biologic level. Consciousness is clouded to a degree varying from patient to patient, and often from one minute to the next in the same person. There almost always is disorientation to some degree in all spheres, and the outstanding feature is great distractability. Thinking is incoherent, and there may be delusions and hallucinations which run a rapid course. The hallucinated objects are usually moving and multiple. Sometimes there are illusions in which the patient's bed becomes a boat or a train and his conversation indicates that he has a sensation of being in motion (vestibular irritation?). Some patients have transient manifestations of the Korsakow phenomena. Restlessness may become extreme and the patient may call out loudly, shout or scream, and become very disturbing to others. Restraints usually are necessary because patients react to hallucinatory experiences and delusional ideas. They try to join relatives whom they fancy are in an adjacent room, they may run away, jump out the window, et cetera. There sometimes is miming of familiar or occupational activities, and the miming may be of varying degrees of elaboration such as sewing, smoking or going through the complicated movements of dressing or undressing. Wolff and Curran[16] cite a bromide patient who had a police record and fancied that he was in a bootlegging drama. He thought that he was about to be "put on the spot" and enacted a scene rich in activities of fear and defense. Another patient built a bathing platform and jumped from the top of the table to the floor which he believed to be a lake.

One frequently must answer the question: "In a given patient, for what part of the psychotic picture are the bromides responsible?" Levin[5] states that if in an attempt to control the symptoms of a psychosis a patient is given bromide and there is no subsequent change in the psychotic picture, the case cannot be regarded as one of bromide psychosis. On the other hand, if following the administration of bromide the psychotic picture changes, the possibility of a bromide delirium must be considered. Bromide deliria usually clear up in from two to six weeks following discontinuance of the offending drug. However, either the underlying psychosis may persist after termination of the delirium and cause the psychiatrist mistakenly to dismiss from his mind the possibility that a bromide delirium ever existed, or a bromide intoxication theoretically may give rise to a chronic psychosis so that a patient who is not psychotic before the delirium fails to return to his normal health many months after the bromides have been discontinued.

Harding and Harding[2] believe that there exists a rough correlation between the amount of bromide in the blood and the type of mental reaction resulting therefrom. Patients with simple bromide intoxication or depression usually show a serum bromide of 100-150 mg. per 100 c.c. while a serum bromide of 150-300 mg. produces bromide delirium or psychosis. Serum bromides above 300 mg. c.c. often cause the patient to become more or less stuporous. On the other hand, Katzenelbogen, et al,[4] studied a number of cases and concluded that there was no distinct correlation between toxic symptoms and the bromide level in the blood. Patients with serum bromide as high as 385 mg. did not show any clinical symptoms of bromide intoxication; in other cases, acne, loss of pharyngeal reflexes, vertigo, ataxia and weakness were observed in patients with serum bromide as low as 147 mg. These workers conclude, therefore, that in following patients under bromide treatment it is the clinical picture and not the laboratory findings which should be primarily reckoned with in regard to the menace of bromide intoxication. According to Wuth,[17] however, any serum bromide in excess of 150 mg. should be considered as being in the "toxic zone." Max Levin[8] agrees that a serum bromide over 150 mg. will tend to produce symptoms. Moreover, when the serum bromide is high, the psychosis may begin to clear up before the content gets back to 150 mg., or it may persist after it has fallen below the level. The underlying psychiatric makeup of the patient has a great deal to do with this. Walter[15] suggests that it might be due to altered permeability of the meninges.

Course

The duration of symptoms of bromidism following discontinuance of the drug is from two to six weeks. According to Levin[8] this duration is determined by the following factors:

1. Organic brain disease which undoubtedly retards recovery.
2. Pre-existing psychoses which probably have the same effect.
3. Even in the absence of 1 and 2, there probably are constitutional differences in the speed with which delirium clears up.
4. The duration after discontinuance may vary according to the duration of symptoms before discontinuance of the drug. For example, a delirium which had been present for several weeks before the bromide was discontinued probably will take longer to clear than one which has lasted for only a few days.
5. The administration of sodium chloride probably hastens the clearing up of the delirium.

Treatment

Naturally, the first thing to be mentioned under the treatment of bromide intoxication is prevention. Bromide dosage should be kept down to the minimum and should not be continued over a long period of time. A patient receiving bromides must receive chlorides. One must be especially careful in dealing with old people, arteriosclerotics, and patients suffering from cardiac decompensation or renal insufficiency.

When bromide intoxication does occur, the first thing to do is to discontinue administration of the drug in spite of intense restlessness and a disturbed mental condition. Bromides, as well as all other sedatives, must be withheld. Some writers believed that there was a "withdrawal delirium" probably analogous to the psychotic manifestations accompanying the withdrawal symptoms of chronic morphinism. However, in the case of bromides, the delirium depends upon a certain concentration of bromide in the blood, together with the/resistance of the patient. As far as is known, following the abrupt withdrawal of bromides, there are no secondary reactions unless something intervenes to reduce the resistance of the patient. For this reason, the first procedure in the treatment of brominism should be to discontinue the drug. Next, the chloride content of the blood must be increased and this is best done by the intravenous administration of normal salt solution: and the giving of Na Cl by mouth. I usually give a capsule of 15 gr. (1.0 gm.) Na Cl four times daily. Patients who are very restless usually respond to hydrotherapy in the form of continuous baths or neutral body packs. When giving packs, care should be exercised that the pack is not warm enough to cause the patient to perspire excessively, for in that manner more chloride will be lost from the body. Elimination through the intestinal tract may be accomplished by a course of calomel followed by a saline cathartic. Sometimes spinal drainage helps to overcome restlessness and to eliminate bromide from the central nervous system.

With patients who are extremely disturbed and who are approaching a state of exhaustion and in whom the need for immediate rest is imperative, either paraldehyde by mouth or sodium amytal intravenously is usually adequate. I have used retention enemas of paraldehyde in olive oil, but with this form of administration there is some danger of producing gangrenous proctitis. Additional treatment of bromide intoxication or delirium is purely symptomatic and not complicated.

Toenhart[12] states that with bromides in the blood serum, hydrobromic acid is secreted by the stomach, neutralized, absorbed by the intestine, and later re-excreted into the stomach, thus producing a vicious circle. If in bromide intoxication the ratio of bromides to chloride is anywhere near the ratio of these ions to each other in the blood stream, then gastric aspiration should offer a rational and effective method of relief. Toenhart advocates gastric aspiration repeated several times daily over a period of several days. This removes as much of the bromide as possible, but chloride is necessarily removed also, so must be replaced either intravenously or orally. With Toenhart's method it is possible to remove as high as 1,240 mg. (20 gr.) of bromide in eight hours using continuous gastric aspiration with a negative pressure apparatus.

Many cases diagnosed as bromide delirium or psychosis were seen in hospitals not equipped to run serum bromide determinations, so we cannot consider these as proven cases. However, the history, clinical picture and subsequent course in every one of the unproven cases is so characteristic that we seem justified in assuming that they were cases of true bromide psychosis. Some of these were superimposed upon pre-

existing psychoneurotic conditions. Only a few typical ones will be cited, and then we will go on to proven cases. For the sake of brevity irrelevant features of the histories, physical findings, and clinical courses will be omitted.

Case Histories

Case 1.—A white man, aged fifty-four, was taken to a hospital with fractures of the right femur and tibia suffered in an automobile accident. There was a history of preceding chronic alcoholism. The fractures were reduced under ether anesthesia and a spica cast applied. The immediate post-traumatic course was uneventful, but on the third day the patient developed signs of delirium tremens. He was given 20 gr. of sodium bromide five times a day and occasional hypodermics of morphine. He became semi-stuporous, progressively more noisy and disturbed and developed hallucinations of sight and hearing. He was disinclined to eat and his feeding was neglected. The more disturbed he became, the more bromide he was given. After ten days, his condition had become serious and I was asked to see him. The patient was semi-stuporous, noisy, incoherent, restless and in full restraint. The lids were heavy, eyes glassy, breath fetid, and tongue furred. Speech was slurring, and when the patient attempted to reach for anything (restraints had been removed during the examination) it could be seen that his arms were very ataxic. All tendon reflexes were abolished but there were no pathological reflexes. The temperature ranged between 100 and 102° F. and the pulse varied around 104. A tentative diagnosis of bromide poisoning was made. All sedatives were discontinued, a spinal drainage was done, and the patient was given saline solution intravenously and NaCl by mouth. The serology on the spinal fluid was normal. On the third day the patient was much more quiet, and from then on there was a gradual amelioration of all psychotic symptoms. On the tenth day after treatment was instituted the patient was discharged from the hospital.

Case 2.—An unmarried white woman, twenty-four years old, developed symptoms of a mild anxiety neurosis, following the unsatisfactory termination of a love affair. She was mildly depressed and disinterested, had occasional crying spells, was unable to sleep at night, and wished that she were dead. Her attending physician sent her to a hospital and prescribed 20 gr. of a bromide mixture three times a day and at bedtime. On the sixteenth day of treatment the patient became confused and hallucinated. She thought that the trees outside her window were waving at her and that voices were coming from the light socket on the wall. She was restless, resistive and could be heard occasionally to call out loudly for various members of her family who she imagined were in an adjoining room. I was asked to see her on the twenty-third day after she entered the hospital and found her in an active delirium. She was somnolent and restless, it was impossible to secure her attention, most of her answers were irrelevant and she was completely disoriented for time and place. She spoke frequently of small aeroplanes she saw flying around her room. The neurological examination showed the pupils to be small but active to light. The patient was unable to accommodate. There was a fine bilateral nystagmus and the speech was slurring. All tendon reflexes in the arms and legs were brisk but no pathological reflexes were elicited. Coördination could not be tested. A diagnosis was made of bromide intoxication superimposed upon an anxiety neurosis and eliminative and supportive treatment was instituted. All sedatives were discontinued, NaCl was given parenterally and by mouth, and the patient was fed by nasal tube. I did not see her again but her physician reported that three weeks after treatment had begun all signs of delirium had disappeared and the clinical picture had returned to the original one of an anxiety neurosis. From then on, this patient's illness ran a course typical of this disease and she eventually made a complete adjustment.

Case 3.—A thirty-five-year-old white man was taken to a hospital in a distant town, suffering from chronic alcoholism. He had been drinking on an average of a quart of cheap whiskey every day for three months. For two weeks prior to his admission to the hospital he had been mildly confused and in the habit of taking long walks alone in the country. One day he was picked up in a neighboring town in a dazed condition, not knowing how he got there. He was taken to the hospital and placed on bromides and chloral by mouth. On the eleventh day his mental condition had become much worse and I was asked to see him. I found a powerfully built man lying in bed secured by restraints on all four extremities. He was yelling, cursing and shouting. Distractability was extreme and the patient was completely disoriented. Any examination was practically impossible but the patient's chart showed that his temperature was varying between 100° and 102° F. rectally and the pulse around 120-140. Very little / food had been taken. The chart also showed that during the eleven days the patient had been in the hospital he had received 2,200 gr. (14.6 gm.) of bromide, 1,100 gr. (7.3 gm.) of chloral, 45 gr. (3.0 gm.) of phenobarbital and several hypodermics of hyocin. Immediate discontinuation of all sedatives was advised, and NaCl was given intravenously and by nasal tube. Restlessness was controlled by warm, moist body packs, and on two occasions it was necessary to administer ½ ounce (7.5 c.c.) of paraldehyde in an oil retention enema to control the restlessness. I did not see the patient again but the attending physician reported that he made gradual but steady improvement, and in three weeks was discharged from the hospital in good condition.

It must be admitted that in none of the above cases was the existence of bromide intoxication proven by laboratory methods. However, the fact that the patients were steadily growing worse under bromide medication, developed an acute delirious psychosis, and improved promptly and consistently upon withdrawal of the drug and replacement by chlorides, is significant. In the following three cases definite laboratory evidence of elevated serum bromide was obtained at the height of the psychoses. Blood bromide determinations were made by Miss M. Seltz, laboratory technician at Mounds Park Sanitarium in St. Paul. The LaMotte comparator was used. As a colorimetric method, this is fairly accurate.

Case 4.—A white man, sixty-nine years old, was admitted to a hospital on February 25, 1937, complaining of intense vertigo associated with attacks of nausea and vomiting. From the description of the symptoms, I believe that he was suffering from a labyrinthitis. The physical, neurological and psychiatric examinations were negative throughout. Because of a mild hypertension and some signs of renal insufficiency, the patient was placed on a salt-free, meatless diet, and was given 15 gr. (1.0 gm.) sodium bromide six times a day. To offset this amount of bromide, he should have taken 360 gr. (20 gm.) NaCl every twenty-four hours but he was on a salt-free diet. After a few days the patient's vertigo and vomiting ceased and he was in good spirits and progressing satisfactorily. By March 10 he was up and walking around but still receiving bromide and no salt. On March 12, he began to have thickness of speech and anorexia (nurse's notes). He developed fever and pain in the chest and x-ray films showed a bilateral basal bronchopneumonia. A medical consultant was called by the attending physician and his notes state that the patient was too confused to permit a satisfactory examination. Mental confusion and restlessness continued and the patient was given frequent hypodermics of dilaudid. The febrile condition lasted for about ten days and during that time the patient did not take anything by mouth, so received no bromides. After his fever subsided his mental condition persisted and I was asked to see him on March 27, 1937. He had not received any bromide for fifteen days, but he was confused, restless, disoriented and hallucinated. He expressed delusions of infidelity and many of his formulations had a marked persecutory trend. The speech was slurring and the eyes staring but the skin was clear. The patient's mental condition was such that commitment to a state hospital had been advised. In reviewing his chart, I found that the patient had received 1,350 gr. (90 gm.) of sodium bromide in fifteen days, but no NaCl. Fifteen days after the last dose of bromide, his serum bromide still was 160 mg. per 100 c.c. This is in the toxic zone. NaCl by mouth and parenterally was advised and paraldehyde was used to control the restlessness. On the fourth day the patient was eating well, but was still confused and disoriented. On April 8, eleven days after treatment was started, the patient was walking out of doors, and on April 11, two weeks after institution of NaCl and supportive treatment, the patient was discharged from the hospital perfectly clear and rational mentally.

In this case it might be argued that the patient was suffering from a toxic delirium secondary to his pneumonia. I am inclined to doubt this, first, because the pneumonia was not a very toxic one, and the delirium was present to some degree before the temperature rose. Furthermore, the delirium continued for some time after the pneumonia had subsided, it was accountable for by an excess of serum bromide and it subsided when treatment for bromide delirium was instituted.

Case 5.—A white man, aged forty-two, with a history of occasional alcoholic excesses, was greatly upset by the death of his wife on March 1, 1937. He began to drink excessively and on March 10 consulted his family physician, who made a diagnosis of chronic alcoholism and melancholia. The patient was advised to stop drinking, which he did, and was placed on 20 gr. NaBr four times a day. On March 24 his gait became ataxic and his speech slurring. By March 28, his arms also were ataxic and it was impossible for him to feed himself. He was mildly confused and, because of the mental state and the ataxia, syphilis of the central nervous system was suspected and the patient was sent to the hospital for study. I saw him on March 28 and found him to be well oriented, but very sluggish mentally. There was profound emotional depression with a strong tendency to cry at the slightest provocation. The speech was slurring, there was a fine bilateral nystagmus, and all tendon jerks were reduced. There was marked bilateral ataxia of the arms and legs. The blood Wassermann was negative and the cerebrospinal fluid gave normal serology and cytology. The blood serum bromide was 310 mg. per 100 c.c. Under NaCl treatment, moist body packs, massage, and withholding all sedatives, the patient improved gradually and was discharged from the hospital on April 20 completely recovered from his ataxia, slurring speech, and mental sluggishness, but still emotionally depressed to a modest degree.

This was a case of simple bromide intoxication and had not yet gone on to the stage of delirium or psychosis. The clinical picture was very similar to that of tabo-paresis.

Case 6.—M.P., a white woman, aged fifty-two, was first seen by me in consultation on March 3, 1937. She was suffering from a moderately severe anxiety neurosis with numerous gastro-intestinal preoccupations. The neurological and physical examinations gave normal findings. A plan of treatment was outlined and the patient made satisfactory progress, being discharged from the hospital by her physician on April 9, 1937. On April 23, I was asked to see her again because she had returned to another hospital in a state of acute delirium. She had gone home taking 20 gr. of bromide mixture four times a day. We learned from relatives that she had had a return of her gastro-intestinal symptoms and since going home had eaten very little. When I saw her the second time she was confused, totally disoriented, and noisy enough to disturb other patients in the hospital. She was extremely restless, her speech was slurring, the lids were heavy, and the eyes had a dull staring expression. The tongue was dry and furred and the breath was foul. The neurological examination, as far as could be carried out, was normal. Blood serum bromide was 275 mg. per 100 c.c. The usual treatment was instituted and at the time of this report, May 2, 1937, the patient is more clear mentally, quiet, but still restless.

Comment

It will be noted in the above cases that the patients were taking moderately heavy doses of bromide over relatively short periods of time. However, none of them was eating a sufficient amount of food and, consequently, not getting enough chloride. This probably accounts for the early appearance of toxic symptoms in these cases. The fact that toxic symptoms were present for only a short time before treatment was instituted accounts for their rapid disappearance after treatment was begun.

The question naturally arises — why, with thousands upon thousands of people receiving bromide medication, do we not encounter more cases of intoxication? That is a difficult question to answer but I believe that it can be explained, in part, on the basis of individual susceptibility. Some people have a lower "delirium threshold" than others. We all know individuals who become delirious with relatively slight rises in temperature regardless of the cause. On the fever up to 105° to 106° F. without showing any signs of delirium. Then there is the question of individual susceptibility. Some people get sick on as little as 15 gr. (1.0 gm.) of potassium iodide a day, and then there are others who can take 200-300 gr. daily without the slightest difficulty. The individual variations in susceptibility to alcohol are too well known to merit discussion here. Decreased powers of elimination due to arteriosclerosis and renal insufficiency also favor intoxication in some cases, and in others the presence of another toxic factor such as alcohol or toxemia due to infection tends to aggravate the clinical picture. I feel, therefore, that one or more of several factors are necessary to produce bromide intoxication. These are: the administration of moderately large doses of bromide, decreased chloride intake, low delirium threshold, heightened individual susceptibility and impaired elimination or the presence of another toxic factor such as alcohol or infection

490

Summary and Conclusions

1. Due to the increase in functional nervous diseases more bromides are being prescribed than formerly.

2. In susceptible individuals bromides may produce mental symptoms even where given in usual therapeutic doses.

3. The effects of bromide are largely confined to the central nervous system. Bromide tends to displace chloride in the blood stream.

4. With the administration of bromide an adequate chloride intake is necessary to prevent bromide intoxication.

5. The toxic effects of bromide may be described as simple bromide intoxication or depression, and bromide delirium or psychosis.

6. Blood serum bromide in excess of 150 mg. per 100 c.c. is in the "toxic zone."

7. The duration of symptoms of brominism following discontinuance of the drug is two to six weeks.

8. Treatment of bromide intoxication consists of discontinuing the drug and all other sedatives, the administration of NaCl orally and parenterally, hydrotherapy, and, in urgent cases, quick acting and rapidly eliminated sedatives. Spinal

drainage sometimes helps, and gastric aspiration has been recommended to help eliminate the bromide.

9. Three probable cases and three proven cases are briefly reported.

References

1. Bastido: Quoted by Wainwright.
2. Harding, G. T., Jr., and Harding, G. T., III: Bromide intoxication. Ohio State Med. Jour., 30:310-313, 1934.
3. Huette: Quoted by Sharpe.
4. Katzenelbogen, S., Goldsmith, H., and White, P.: Bromide intoxication, its relation to the amount of bromide in the blood and the barrier permeability to bromide. Am. Jour. Psych., 13:637-644, 1933.
5. Levin, Max.: Bromide delirium and other bromide psychoses. Am. Jour. Psych., 12:1125-1158, 1933.
6. Levin, Max: Bromide psychosis: Diagnosis, treatment and prevention. Ann. Int. Med., 7:709-714, 1933.
7. Preu, P. W., Romano, J., and Brown, W. T.: Psychosis with bromide intoxication. New Eng. Jour. Med., 214:56-62, 1936.
8. Rylan, Chas. J., Jr.: Bromide intoxication or bromide psychosis, Virginia Med. Month., 61:292-296, 1934.
9. Sharpe, J. C.: Bromide intoxication. Jour. A.M.A., 102: 1462-1465, 1934.
10. Swanson, Ethel: Personal communication.
11. Thomas, Alice M.: The distribution of halides in animal tissue following bromide administration. (To be published.)
12. Toenhart, O. A.: Treatment of bromide intoxication. Wis. Med. Jour., 34:901-903, 1935.
13. Wagner, C. P., and Blumberg, D.: Incidence of bromide intoxication among psychotic patients. Jour. A.M.A., 95: 1725-1728, 1930.
14. Wainwright, Chas. W.: Bromide intoxication. Int. Clin., 1:78-95, 1933.
15. Walter, F. K.: Theorie und Praxis der Permiabilitats prufung mittels der Brommethode. Arch. f. Psych., 79:363, 1927.
16. Wolff, H. G., and Curran, D.: Nature of delirium and allied states. Arch. Neurol. and Psychiat., 33:1173-1215, 1935.
17. Wuth, Otto: Rational bromide therapy—New methods for its control. Jour. A.M.A., 88:2013-2017, 1927.

ACUTE PULMONARY EDEMA OCCURRING DURING PREGNANCY OR LABOR*

F. J. SCHATZ, M.D.

Saint Cloud, Minnesota

ACUTE pulmonary edema as a terminal complication of pregnancy or labor is a most serious one and a rather frequent complication of eclampsia, occurring in almost one-third of the eclamptic cases. Its incidence in eclampsia without convulsions is even higher.

Acute pulmonary edema occurs late in the course of pre-eclamptic and many fatal cases of eclampsia, and during labor in cases with cardiac decompensation without audible valve lesions. It has been suggested that it may develop in the fatal cases of eclampsia as an end-result of the failure of the pulmonary circulation. On the other hand, the fact that not all cases of pulmonary edema end fatally seems to exclude this explanation.

Slemons[4] found acute pulmonary edema in six of seven cases of eclampsia without convulsions which came to autopsy.

King, et al,[3] report a series of thirty cases of ante- and intrapartum eclampsia with four cases of edema of the lungs with three recoveries. The fatal case was a colored woman, who had marked pulmonary edema on admission. The edema was relieved by appropriate treatment. She was delivered by a very easy low forceps operation seventeen hours after admission. Through a misunderstanding, ether was used as the anesthetic with a recurrence of the edema, broncho-pneumonia and death. The edema has been reported in all stages of pregnancy from the second month[1] through to term, during delivery[6] and in the puerperium. However, its greatest incidence is after the fifth month of pregnancy. It is more frequent in multiparas than in primiparas[5] and

*From the Obstetrical Department, St. Cloud Hospital. Read before the joint meeting of the Stearns-Benton and Upper Mississippi medical societies at Little Falls, Minnesota, October 21, 1937.

rarely seen in non-pregnant subjects. While it may complicate many types of cardiac lesions, in most cases it follows mitral disease, and many patients with mitral lesions have no disturbance during pregnancy or labor. In some reported cases, however, there has been no history of cardiac symptoms before pregnancy.

Pathogenesis

Bustos Moron[1] summarizes the old theories of pathogenetic mechanism of this conditions as follows: (1) a mechanical disturbance, pulmonary hypertension and acute weakness of the right ventricle; (2) a reflex disturbance originating in aortitis and peri-aortitis; and (3) a toxic element which is always present. These are all elements which collaborate in the production of the syndrome. On the other hand, today the mechanism of the attack is considered due to a severe left ventricular insufficiency. Bustos Moron believes, along with Waldorp, that within a few seconds after the occurrence of the left ventricular defect, a sudden pulmonary flux is produced, the whole parenchyma becomes congested from vertex to base, and the serous transudate causes edema of the lung. According to my observation, the edema comes on in a few minutes after the initial cough. There is a marked bronchorrhea, fine sub-crepitant and bubbling râles with some impaired resonance. This confirms the diagnosis made on the basis of the facies and the repeated cough, with an abundant or scanty yield. The pulse is lost, there is an increase in frequency and sudden hypertension, dyspnea increases to orthopnea, consciousness may be lost, and death may follow unless proper therapeutic measures are instituted.

Symptoms

The onset is sudden, the cough persistent, and there is a sense of thoracic constriction soon followed by increasing dyspnea and precordial pain. There is marked cyanosis and spumous, salmon-colored expectoration containing blood. Fine râles may be heard at the lung bases and later throughout the lungs of the bubbling type.[2] The increased respiratory sounds obscure the heart tones, but a systolic murmur or a diastolic rumble may be heard at the apex. The pulse is rapid and thready or may be hard and tense, especially in the eclamptic type. The blood pressure is variable, the differential pressure tending to diminish. The temperature is normal or even subnormal. Albuminuria will be present at the end of the attack even in the absence of a pre-existing nephritis.

Types

Szer[5] distinguishes three clinical types of acute pulmonary edema in pregnancy. In the acute type, suffocation is intense and the patient may die within a few minutes with a pink froth on her lips. In the bronchoplegic type, expectoration is absent but the patient has severe dyspnea with thoracic pain. Signs of cardiac weakness appear rapidly. The patient does not cough and fluid accumulates in the bronchi and lungs. Cyanosis is marked; the blood pressure decreases and death may follow quickly in spite of treatment. The subacute forms are most frequently encountered. These are characterized by a nocturnal pseudo-asthma, described as a cardiac asthma by some authors, which awakens the patient. There is dyspnea with pink, foamy expectoration. Examination will reveal localized areas of edema. These attacks may be repeated frequently at night until the acute form appears.

Diagnosis

The typical forms are readily diagnosed. Diagnosis is based on the sudden onset of cough, the intensity of the edema, the characteristic edema and the auscultatory signs.

The condition may be confused with asthma, but in the latter there is a history of a previous attack and the dyspnea is of the expiratory type. Expectoration appears only at the end of the attack. The sputum is thick and contains eosinophiles. Pulmonary embolism and suffocating pneumothorax must be excluded in the diagnosis of the bronchoplegic type and this is affected by the pain in the side and the absence of expectoration.[5]

Pathology

In an autopsy reported by Teel, et al,[6] the gross and microscopic findings were interpreted as indicating that the patient suffered from a true acute toxemia of pregnancy. The pathologic lesions in the liver, kidney and lungs were similar to those found in fatal cases of eclampsia, except that they were less marked. The findings in the heart and lungs were interpreted as indicative of "acute left ventricular failure, resulting in marked pulmonary congestion and edema with slight emphysema." The heart weight (335 grams) and the subendocardial fibrosis of the myocardium and the mitral leaflets were insufficient to justify a diagnosis of chronic heart disease. No organism could be demonstrated in the myocardium or grown from a spleen culture.

Prognosis

The immediate prognosis is based primarily upon the amount of expectoration and the condition of the blood pressure but also depends largely on the promptness with which treatment is instituted. A large amount of expectoration is a favorable prognostic sign. Gallop rhythm, alternating pulse and a decrease in the differential blood pressure indicate insufficiency of the left ventricle and, consequently, offer a poor prognosis. In the presence of persistent râles at the bases, high diastolic pressure and arrhythmia, a guarded prognosis is indicated.

If the patient survives delivery and the early puerperium, the ultimate outlook as regards chronic cardiovascular and renal disease is good. Teel, et al, reported six cases, with two deaths. Three of the surviving patients were alive and well without cardiac, vascular or renal sequelæ, eight, six and two years after the attacks. King, et al, report four cases with one immediate maternal death.

Treatment

The basis of the treatment of acute pulmonary edema is heroic doses of morphine with atropine and heart stimulants, with venesection to reduce the venous hypertension and relieve the pulmonary circulation. Immediate relief follows the removal of 500 to 700 c.c. of blood. Peripheral venostasis has been recommended as an alternate to venesection.

Cardiac weakness indicates a cardiac tonic, ouabain, which acts rapidly when given intravenously. Assuming that the attacks are similar in mechanism to classical cardiac asthma, Teel, et al, feel that digitalization is indicated. These same authors also believe that the prophylactic use of digitalis in all eclamptics and patients with severe non-convulsive toxemia in and above the fourth decade of life should be considered. The results obtained by digitalization in the severe decompensated hearts at times are not what one would expect even with larger doses than that usually given.

From the obstetrical viewpoint, Szer believes that, while there is no fixed rule, early interruption of the pregnancy is indicated in those cases in which signs of grave cardiac insufficiency are present at the onset of pregnancy. Cesarean section should be considered when serious attacks occur repeatedly in spite of medical treatment. From a limited experience, Teel, et al, concluded that significant clinical improvement was not to be expected until the uterus was emptied. The optimum time for interference appears to be between twelve and forty-eight hours after the attack. This delay gives sufficient time for digitalization before the interruption of the pregnancy is undertaken.

Delay, as suggested by Teel, et al, may be tried in patients with a favorable cardiac condition and a mild lung involvement. The edema, however, may become suddenly severe and terminate fatally. In the more severe cases, the treatment must be instituted promptly and the uterus emptied as soon as possible. The bleeding after delivery is profuse and appropriate treatment must be instituted to control same.

When acute edema of the lungs occurs towards the end of pregnancy, it is often followed by labor. If necessary, dilatation may be completed manually and delivery effected by means of forceps or version.

Case Reports

Case 1.—Mrs. J. T. L., gravida 1, aged twenty-seven, had had the diseases of childhood, smallpox, tonsillitis, influenza, tonsillectomy, dyspepsia with urticaria of one week duration in 1932, Schoenlein's disease with a kidney complication and mitral insufficiency following an upper respiratory infection in 1923. Her last menstrual period was December 25, 1926, and the date of expectancy was calculated for October 1, 1927. The family history was negative. Edema of the lower extremities appeared when she was six months pregnant. Because of financial difficulty, she continued with her professional work as a nurse, which necessitated being on her feet a great deal. She was advised to discontinue working but refused. October 1, 1937, she was admitted to the hospital with a generalized edema and a mild respiratory embarrassment, temperature 98.2, pulse 80, respirations 28, blood pressure 160/120. Urinalysis of a catheterized specimen showed sp. gr. 1.014, acid, albumin, 2 mm. ring, acetone, diacetic acid, R. and W. B. C. Other physical findings were negative including examination of the heart.

She was given castor oil and a hot pack to stimulate elimination; spontaneous rupture of the membranes occurred four hours later. Her progress was slow and the patient was in labor forty hours. Morphine and scopolamine with ether in oil per rectum and magnesium sulphate intramuscularly were used during the first stage of labor. The head remained high in the right transverse position; the cervix was about two-thirds dilated. Suddenly the patient developed a cough with râles in both lungs, temperature 98.3, pulse 114, respirations 48. Appropriate medication was given and the patient prepared for delivery. Labor was terminated by manual dilatation of the vagina and cervix, with a difficult high forceps operation. The baby was in fair condition. A severe postpartum hemorrhage occurred after the expulsion of the placenta. The uterus was packed and 1 c.c. each of pituitrin and ergot were given by hypo. The estimated blood lost was 750 c.c., pulse 118, respirations 50. The patient's condition was poor. There was considerable bleeding the first postpartum day partially controlled with ergot. The labored breathing continued for twenty-four hours. The lungs were free of râles by the fifth postpartum day. The patient was able to leave the hospital on the thirteenth postpartum day. A subsequent pregnancy fifteen months later was normal throughout.

Case 2.—Mrs. J. L., gravida 4, aged forty, had her last menstruation August 4, 1928. She had had rheumatism in 1923, spontaneous full-term delivery in 1927, and rheumatism in 1928 when two months pregnant. Urinalysis at this time showed albumin, hyaline and granular casts, R. and W. B. C. No blood pressure readings were recorded at this time by the attending physician. There was no prenatal care.

The patient was first examined by me April 11, 1929. She was in labor and she was coughing, breathing, laboriously, cyanosed, and sitting up and stooped forward. Crepitant râles were heard in both lungs, and a systolic heart murmur heard at the apex and transmitted to the axilla. Morphine 0.01 (gr. 1/6) with atropine 0.0004 (gr. 1/150) was given with relief in one-half hour. The patient was prepared for delivery, anesthetized, catheterized, the cervix dilated manually, and forceps applied to the head in L. O. A. position. Delivery was easily accomplished. The baby was thin but in good condition. The lungs were clear after forty-eight hours. The patient made an uneventful recovery following her delivery. The heart and kidney condition remained unchanged. The patient was up and about the tenth postpartum day.

On May 9, 1929, while sitting at the table after supper, she was suddenly seized with a severe attack of coughing with labored breathing, cyanosis, expectoration of a serous, frothy, blood-tinged fluid (about 500 c.c.). Bubbling râles were heard in both lungs, the heart was rapid and a systolic murmur was heard over the aortic area which was transmitted into the neck, and a systolic murmur over the heart apex transmitted into the axilla. Morphine 0.01 (gr. 1/6), atropine 0.0004 (gr. 1/150), were given by hypodermic and the atropine had to be repeated in a half hour before the patient got any relief from the edema of the lungs. The heart was digitalized, and the morphine and atropine had to be given daily for a week before the lungs remained

clear. The swelling gradually became generalized with accumulation of fluid in the peritoneal cavity. The urinary output diminished until there was complete suppression. The patient expired February 19, 1930, from cardio-renal dropsy. Necropsy was not obtainable.

Case 3.—Mrs. J. W., gravida 2, aged thirty-three.

The patient was seen in consultation and referred by Dr. A. Mahowald. At the age of thirteen, she had had pain during and after urination for three or four days. She had had many of these attacks up to the time of her marriage seven years ago. She had had measles at the age of twenty-one, and edema of the lower extremities during the last month of her first pregnancy. She went to term and was delivered by an easy forceps operation. She had her last menstrual period March 25, 1930. The date of expectancy was January 2, 1931.

About one month prior to the development of the complication, she was examined by her physician for swelling of the lower extremities. On the afternoon of January 1, 1931, she developed a mild cough with free expectoration of fluid which gradually increased in amount. At about eleven P. M., the patient was awakened, smothering, with fluid escaping from her nose and mouth, coughing severely and breathing with difficulty. The family physician was called and he immediately took her to the hospital. She did not remember anything other than riding fast in a car. She was admitted to the hospital at 12:55 A. M.. Her physician ordered a hot pack and an enema, and magnesium sulphate was given by mouth, but was not retained. At 3:10 A. M., she was given 0.03 (gr. ½) codeine with some relief for one hour. At 4:30 A. M., he took her to the delivery room and packed the cervix with sterile gauze to induce labor, but was unsuccessful. The patient was seen by me at 7:30 A. M. She was sitting up in bed supported by a back rest. Serous blood-tinged fluid was escaping from the mouth and nose; she was coughing and vomiting simultaneously and struggling for air. The patient was cyanotic, cold and clammy, and there were bubbling râles in both lungs. The heart tones were regular, rapid, and difficult to detect; the pulse 120, respirations 42. Urinalysis: Albumin 2 mm. ring; hyaline and granular casts, R. and W. B. C. Morphine 0.01 (gr. 1/6), atropine 0.0004 (gr. 1/150) was given by hypo, and the atropine was repeated in ten minutes. The lung condition cleared sufficiently to allow the patient to be moved to the delivery room and prepared for delivery. The patient was placed in a semi-Fowler position; oxygen was given for the cyanosis; she was anesthetized with N₂O. After catheterization, the cervix was dilated manually, forceps were applied to head in R. O. P. position and the head was so delivered. The baby was in good condition. The patient was given ergot 1 c.c. per hypo to stimulate uterine contraction. Oxygen was given for the cyanosis. The placenta was expressed. Some 500 c.c. of blood was lost after the placenta was expelled. The tendency to bleed was marked and ergot had to be repeated in an hour. Two hours after delivery atropine was given for recurrence of the edema. The patient coughed a great deal the day of delivery, with free expectoration of bloody mucus. The blood pressure after delivery was 140/100, the temperature 101, pulse 100, and respirations 40. The progress was uneventful after the second day and the patient was discharged on the eleventh postpartum day. The blood pressure on the day of discharge was 110/70.

Her third pregnancy was without complication. She had her last period on December 25, 1931, and delivered spontaneously on August 28, 1932, one month earlier than the date of expectancy. A trace of albumin with moderate swelling occurred at the end of the seventh month with a blood pressure of 150/110. The blood pressure returned to normal and the urine was free of albumin following rest, diet, and the limitation of the fluid intake. Her weight the day of her first visit, February 28, 1932, was 182 pounds and the blood pressure 110/70. The day of her delivery her weight was 189.5 pounds and B. P. 130/88.

Her fourth pregnancy in 1936 was normal throughout.

Case 4.—Mrs. H. L., gravida 6, aged thirty-six, had had five full-term pregnancies, of which four were normal. During her fifth pregnancy, on the day of delivery, she developed a severe headache, vomiting, and numbness in the lower extremities. Her blood pressure was 160/100. The urinalysis of a catheterized specimen showed albumin 2 mm. ring; sp. gr. 1.020, hyaline and granular casts, R. and W. B. C.

She had had her last period September 16, 1930. The date of expectancy was June 23, 1931. The heart, kidney, and blood pressure were normal throughout the gestation. During the week prior to entering the hospital, she had respiratory difficulty which would occur from one to two hours after lying down at night. She was examined about midnight, June 7, 1931, in her home. The patient was delirious and did not recognize her family. She was sitting up and struggling for air. There were many râles in both lungs; no heart murmurs could be heard. Her temperature was 98, pulse 128, and respirations 30. She was taken to the hospital and admitted at 12:10 A. M. A noncatheterized specimen of urine showed a trace of albumin. Blood examination: R. B. C. 4,250,000; W. B. C. 9,400; Hbg. 76%. Codeine sulph. 0.03 (gr. ½) was given for the relief of the edema of lungs and restlessness. The patient was relieved by the medication and was in fair condition in the morning. At ten o'clock A. M., the membranes were ruptured artificially. Castor oil and quinine were given. Contractions started three hours later, and she was in labor one hour and ten minutes before the baby was born. Fifteen minutes prior to delivery she suddenly developed cyanosis, a severe cough, labored breathing, and râles in both lungs. Her pulse was 160, and respirations 32. The patient was placed in a semi-Fowler position. Atropine 0.0006 (gr. 1/100) with whiskey 15.0 (oz. ½), pituitrin 0.3 (Mv.) were given to hasten delivery. The baby was delivered spontaneously in good condition. The placenta was expelled by the Credé method. The patient's condition was fair when she was taken to her

room. She was placed in Fowler's position. Digitalis was given for the heart, oxygen for the labored breathing and cyanosis, morphine sulphate 0.01 (gr. 1/6) for restlessness and cough and ergot 1 c.c. to check the severe bleeding. After the fifth day the lungs were clear. The patient left the hospital on the eleventh postpartum day. The pulse was 96 and respirations 28. The patient's progress was slow and stormy. The heart was digitalized but never responded well to treatment. She died suddenly August 17, 1933, when she left her bed for elimination purposes.

Case 5.—Mrs. L. R. B., gravida 1, aged twenty-four, had had her last menstruation May 31, 1936. The estimated date of delivery was March 6, 1937; the date of delivery February 27, 1937. She was in labor sixteen hours.

This patient had had scarlet fever, measles, pertussis, diphtheria, chorea and rheumatism. She had had two attacks of rheumatism at the age of nine and sixteen years, her second attack lasting sixteen weeks. An appendectomy had been performed at the age of nineteen.

Physical examination on October 14, 1936, showed a well-nourished female sixty-seven inches tall, weighing 199.5 pounds. Her blood pressure was 170/70. All other physical findings were normal except that the heart was enlarged and a systolic murmur could be heard over all of the valve areas. She was about five months pregnant and her pelvis was large. The kidneys remained normal throughout the gestation and she gained 17.5 pounds from the time she presented herself for observation to the time of delivery February 27, 1937. The blood pressure dropped to 150/70 and gradually rose to 190/60 the day of delivery. The first pains came on about 3 A. M. and she entered the hospital at 7:15 A. M. Castor oil was given to stimulate contractions. On rectal examination, the head was mid-pelvic, the cervix thinned out and dilated about 2 cm. The fetal heart tones were heard to the right and below the umbilicus, 150 per minute.

The patient's heart condition was satisfactory and she was given her first dose of morphine and scopolamine at 2:05 P. M. At 3:15 P. M. she developed a slight cough which came at frequent intervals and fine subcrepitant râles were heard in both lungs; pulse 118, respirations 24. She was given atropine sulphate 0.0006 (gr. 1/100) with improvement. At 7 P. M., she had a recurrence of the lung symptoms and digitalin 0.0013 (gr. 1/50), strychnine 0.0016 (gr. 1/40) atropine 0.001 (gr. 1/75), were given by hypo. The atropine was repeated in twenty minutes. By this time the patient was cyanotic, the skin clammy, breathing labored, pulse 140 and there was free expectoration of blood-stained serum. She was taken to the delivery room and oxygen was given while being prepared for delivery. Under nitrous oxide anesthesia the perineum was dilated. The head in R. O. A. position was delivered by an easy forceps operation, the shoulders and body were delivered by the Christeller maneuver, the cord was clamped and cut, and the placenta expressed. One c.c. each of ergot and pituitrin were given per hypo to control the uterus. Some 400 c.c. of blood were lost. The oxygen was started as soon as the child was delivered and kept up for fourteen hours before the cyanosis and lung edema began to subside. The heart stimulation had to be repeated at regular intervals, with morphine for restlessness and ergot to control the uterus. The labored breathing, edema and cyanosis gradually cleared and after forty-eight hours the patient was symptom-free, with the pulse returning to normal. The heart stimulation was continued and the patient was discharged the tenth postpartum day. The digitalis was kept up for two months and her final check April 15, 1937, showed the B. P. 150/60 with the heart condition improved so that the patient was able to resume her household duties.

Case 6.—Mrs. J. M. A., gravida 3, aged thirty-three, had had edema with her two previous pregnancies. Her complaint at this time was difficulty in breathing, especially when she was lying down. This condition, which she attributed to the varnishing of her home, had been of two weeks duration. When moving about she had less difficulty in breathing.

The patient was seen in the home by Dr. C. B. Lewis and taken to the hospital. The edema and cyanosis were generalized and there was morbid dyspnea, with many moist bubbling râles and expectoration of frothy, blood-stained, serous fluid. Her B. P. was 160/90, pulse 100, and respirations 30. Labor was induced and the baby was delivered with forceps. The patient's condition was poor. Cardiac stimulation and oxygen were given but she expired one and one-half

hours after delivery. Bedside notes show that so postpartum bleeding continued up to the time of d

This case is reported with the permission of Dr B. Lewis and W. L. Freeman of St. Cloud, Min ta.

Conclusions

1. The strain of labor added to a weak heart musculature with or without the pres of a valvular lesion is a definite factor in cau acute pulmonary edema.

2. With appropriate treatment before, du and after delivery, maternal mortality from monary edema should be reduced to a minin

3. Severe bleeding occurred in five of th cases and was responsible for one maternal d

4. With proper antenatal care in subseq pregnancies, a recurrence of the pulmo edema may be prevented.

References

1. Bustos Moron, R.: Cardiac insufficiency in the month of pregnancy. Presna med. argent., 15 1099, 1929.
2. Bustos Moron, R.: Acute pulmonary edema during nancy; pathogenetic study. Ber. û d. ges. Gyn Geburtsh., 16:574, 1929.
3. King, E. L., Mayer, George A., and Ayo, T. B.: The sodium isoamylethyl barbiturate in the treatme eclampsia. Am. Jour. Obst. and Gyn., 23:867-871,
4. Slemons, J. M.: Eclampsia without convulsions. Hopkins Hospital Bulletin, 18:448-455, 1907.
6. Teel, H. M., Reid, D. E., and Hertig, A. T.: C asthma and acute pulmonary edema. Surg., and Obst., 64:39-50, 1937.

HYPERPYREXIA IN THE NEWBORN

Report of Infant With 107° F. by Rectum at Age of Fifty-three Hours

LARRY F. RICHDORF, M.D., Ph.D., and W. H. FORD, M.D.

Minneapolis, Minnesota

HYPERPYREXIA of 107° (rectal) in a newborn is unusual enough to warrant detailed analysis. In the case to be reported, this temperature was observed at the age of fifty-three hours. In the newborn a temperature as high as 104° (rectal) on the third day, or thereabout, is not necessarily associated with an unfavorable prognosis. In fact, in many a newborn moderate fever is transitory and recovery occurs without special treatment. The causative factors of transitory fever have been the subject of a great deal of controversy. Infection, inanition, dehydration, and birth trauma have been considered.

Salmi summarized the literature in 1935 and reported his observations in a series of infants delivered normally, by cesarean section, and by

forceps. Transient fever of 100° to 104° onset from the second to fifth day occurr 20 per cent of the 225 infants of n delivery. Long labors (over twenty-five h were three times as frequent in the infants festing fever as in the fever-free group. birth weight was above 3,500 grams i per cent of the cases showing fever, wl only 30 per cent were above this weight fever-free group. The incidence of tran fever in the newborn was increased whe membranes had been ruptured early (ten before delivery), when meconium was p in the amniotic fluid, or when vaginal exa tions had been done.

Twenty-five per cent of infants deliver cesarean section and 50 per cent of tho livered by forceps showed this phenomenon of fever. Salmi calls our attention to the fact that labor had been in progress a long time in many of the cases delivered by these two methods. Thus, long, hard, complicated labors *predispose* to temperatures ranging from 100° to 104° in the newborn.

Case Report

Baby boy F., weighing eight pounds, four ounces, was born March 26, 1936, at 5:15 p. m., the first baby (first pregnancy) of a mother nineteen years of age. Both mother and father were in good health. Labor was of fifteen hours' duration and normal except for an episiotomy. Nembutal (4½ grains) and scopolamine (1/200 grain) analgesia was used during labor and nitrous-oxide gas anesthesia during delivery. The amniotic sac ruptured one hour before the birth of the child. The amniotic fluid was definitely stained with meconium.

Mucus was removed from the nose and throat by suction with a soft rubber bulb before the infant made perceptible respiratory movements, and later, in the nursery, mucus was removed again in the same manner. During the first twenty-four hours after birth the weight loss was 4½ ounces and the temperature went from normal at birth to 102.2° rectal. During the second twenty-four hours the baby received 12 ounces of complement and water by mouth and 3 ounces of 5 per cent glucose in normal saline by rectum. During this twenty-four hours the rectal temperature ranged from 100.2° to 102.2° and the weight loss was 9½ ounces. This occurred without diarrhea or vomiting being present. At the age of 53 hours the baby's rectal temperature went up to 107°.

Examination at this time showed a somewhat spastic child, very hot to touch, with respirations 90 per minute. The thighs were flexed on the abdomen. The abdomen was slightly distended but no abnormal findings were noted on palpation. There was a slight areola of redness around the umbilical cord. The fontanelle was boggy but was not bulging, and it did not move with respiration. The mucous membranes of the nose, tongue and mouth were dry. The lungs were negative to percussion and auscultation. The heart was very rapid, estimated 200 beats per minute. Dehydration was obvious, and serious respiratory disease or cord infection was suspected.

Treatment: Whole blood (10 c.c.) and normal saline (100 c.c.) were given subcutaneously. One or both of

these fluids were given in like manner every three or four hours. One ounce of 5 per cent glucose in water was given by gavage every three hours. During the first twenty-four hours of this treatment, the baby received 40 c.c. of whole blood from the mother and the father, and 550 c.c. of normal saline subcutaneously and 240 c.c. of 5 per cent glucose by gavage. The whole blood and normal saline were absorbed very rapidly. The respirations and heart rate came down to normal and the temperature dropped to 101.4° rectal within twenty-four hours after the beginning of this treatment. The weight curve was interesting. In spite of the fact that 15 ounces of fluid had been forced by mouth and rectum, the baby lost 14 ounces in weight in the fifty-three hours from birth until the time the temperature went up to 107°. The baby was not disturbed during the succeeding twenty-four hours, but forty-eight hours after subcutaneous fluid was started the baby had gained 17 ounces.

Breast milk was started twenty-four hours after the beginning of the subcutaneous fluids. The milk was expressed from the mother and given by bottle every four hours. The baby nursed well when it was put to breast forty-eight hours later. Both baby and mother were discharged from the hospital on the tenth day in good condition, the baby weighing 8 pounds 7½ ounces, or 3½ ounces over birth weight.

The areola about the cord disappeared but the cord remained attached for several days after leaving the hospital. An umbilical secretion was obvious for four months, during which time a slight hernia developed. This healed by strapping with adhesive tape. Examination at six months showed a perfectly normal child.

Summary

1. A large first-born baby developed a temperature of 107° rectal at the age of fifty-three hours.

2. There was marked dehydration, possibly respiratory or cord infection.

3. Rapid and complete recovery followed treatment with whole blood and normal saline subcutaneously, and water and glucose by gavage.

References

1. Abt: Transitory fever in the newborn. Pediatrics. Philadelphia: W. B. Saunders Co,, 1923.
2. Brennerman: Transitory fever in newborn. Practice of Pediatrics, Hagerstown, Md.: W. F. Prior, 1937. Vol. I, Chap. 42, p. 108.
3. Salmi, T.: Ueber den Einfluss der protrahierten resp. komplisierten Gekurt auf die "transitorischen" Fiefererscheinungen bei Neugeborenen. Acta Pediatrica, 17:469-497, 1935.

CASE REPORTS ◆

ABDOMINAL PREGNANCY AT EIGHT MONTHS*

PHILIP N. BRAY. M.D.. M.S.
Duluth, Minnesota

THE literature on abdominal pregnancy was carefully reviewed by Cornell and Lash† (1933). In their series of 236 cases taken from the literature, their private cases, and the records of the Cook County Hospital, they reported that only 35 per cent were diagnosed correctly before operation. It is felt, therefore, that the presentation of another of these unusual cases is warranted, inasmuch as considerable diagnos-

-attached to a vital organ. Also, they advised, when necessary, to combine marsupialization with drainage.

H. O., a white female, aged twenty-eight years, was admitted to the Minneapolis General Hospital September 8, 1933. The patient had had no prenatal care. She was a gravida ii, para i. Last normal menstruation was December 16, 1932, of four days duration. January 16, 1933, she flowed one day. February 22,

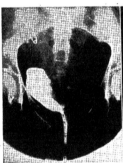 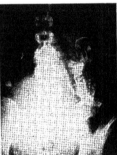 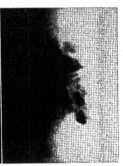

Fig. 1. Cystogram, taken after 50 c.c. of 12 per cent sodium iodide were injected in the bladder. The bladder is distorted, its mid and left portions are flattened out.

Fig. 2. Anterior posterior radiograph, showing the fetus in the left lateral portion of the abdomen.

Fig. 3. Lateral radiograph of the abdomen, showing the breech presenting.

tic help may be obtained by use of the cystogram and the other usual x-ray studies.

In the cases reported by Cornell and Lash, the condition was found most frequently in the first and second pregnancies. They found that in the eighty-six cases in which the baby was born after six months, the infant mortality was 22 per cent, whereas in the sixty cases in which the baby was born alive in the eighth and ninth months, the infant mortality was about 35 per cent. They found a maternal mortality of 14.3 per cent (thirty-four cases) in the total of 236 cases. Cornell and Lash concluded that removal of the placenta in toto is best when the placental blood supply can be ligated and when the site of the placenta is not

1933, she passed two small blood clots, then had no bleeding at all until four days before admission to the hospital.

The patient felt life June 1, 1933, and, she thought, until the day of hospital admission. She had never had any severe rupture-like pain, nor shoulder discomfort. Starting four days before admission at about 9:00 A. M., she had had moderate abdominal cramps coming about every two hours, bleeding a little less than that of a normal period, and frequency without pain or burning, to the extent of voiding about every forty-five minutes. Her bowels had moved that day, the stool being a little constipated, but not more so than usual.

Examination showed blood pressure 116/68, temperature 98.8°, pulse 78 and respiration 20. There was secretion from the nipples. A symmetrical pelvic mass was present on the right side extending within 3 cm. of the navel. The abdomen was soft, showed no peritoneal irritation, no fluid, no shifting dullness. On the left side of the abdomen there was a mass extending up to the costal arch. The upper pole felt

*From the Department of Obstetrics, Minneapolis General Hospital, University of Minnesota School of Medicine.

†Cornell, Edward L., and Lash, A. F.: Surg., Gynec. and Obst., 57:98, 1933.

like a fetal head, and could be palpated distinctly. The lower pole lay just above the pubic bone and could not be palpated distinctly. No fetal movements were felt nor heart beats heard. Pelvic examination showed a little sanguinous discharge from the vulva, floor was competent, and there was no evidence of

Dr. J. H. Simons and the writer. A lower midline suprapubic incision was made. Examination of the abdominal cavity showed the omentum to be attached to the mass in the right lower abdomen. The mass was the encapsulated placenta. The omental blood supply to the placenta was ligated in dissecting out

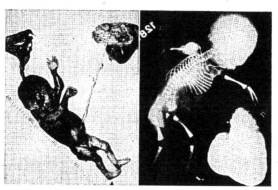

Fig. 4 *(left).* Photograph of baby and placenta, showing the baby's length and maceration.
Fig. 5 *(right).* Radiograph of baby, showing no evidence of syphilis in the long bones.

infection. Vaginal walls and cervix were only slightly blue, and the cervix was a little soft. There was a little bleeding from the cervix, about like that of a normal period. A symmetrical uterine-like mass, about the size of a three months pregnancy, occupied the right pelvic fossa. The breech, which lay to the left of the inlet, displaced this uterine-like mass to the right. Nothing abnormal was palpable in the cul-de-sac or either adnexa, but the left adnexa was a little tender.

A cystogram was taken after injection of 50 c.c. of 12 per cent sodium iodide in the bladder. The picture showed the bladder to be distorted, its mid and left portions being flattened out, apparently by the breech.

Anterior posterior and lateral radiographs were made, which demonstrated a single fetus lying anterior posterior and slightly transverse in the left lateral portion of the abdomen with the head to the left of the midline anteriorly opposite the first, second, and third lumbar vertebræ, and with the back posterior. There was a marked over-riding of the cranial bones, apparent collapse of the calvarium, and accentuation of the curves, indicating that the fetus was dead. The position of the fetus was one of extreme abnormality. Its density coincided with the continuation of the curves of the uterine mass, and its appearance definitely indicated that it was outside of the uterus.

The laboratory analysis showed hemoglobin 73 per cent; white blood count 10,500; polymorphonuclears 73 per cent; lymphocytes 25 per cent; and monocytes 2 per cent. Urine was entirely normal.

A preoperative diagnosis was made of:

1. Probable left extrauterine pregnancy with myomatous uterus or

2. Incarcerated dead fetus in a myomatous uterus.

Operative Record.—The patient was operated on by

the placenta from its capsule. Further examination showed the uterus to be the size of a three months pregnancy lying in the true pelvis. The placenta was a trilobed mass adherent to the posterior abdominal wall, intestinal coils, and omentum. The placenta rested just above the uterus, but distinctly separate from it, and a little to the right of the midline. The lower portion extended over the brim of the pelvis posteriorly. Examination of the adnexa showed both ovaries to be normal. Both tubes appeared slightly thickened, but otherwise they also were normal. The appendix was not observed. Examination showed a dead female fetus in the left abdomen. The fetus had probably been dead only a short time, as there was very little maceration. The baby lay anterior posterior with head anterior, back posterior, and breech presenting. The amniotic sac had not ruptured. There were many adhesions between the amniotic membranes and viscera. The sac was firmly attached to the baby's head. Almost the entire area of the amniotic sac was adherent to intestines and abdominal wall, but these adhesions were easily released. The omentum, containing large blood vessels, was attached to the anterior surface of the placenta, to the ascending colon, descending colon, and small intestine. The cord extended from the opening on the left side of the placental sac over intestinal coils to the fetus. The placenta obtained most of its blood supply through the large omental vessels, and lay in a capsule of two portions, a rather thin amnion and an outer thick membrane.

The fetus and membranes surrounding it were liberated and the baby extracted with the cord. There was no line of cleavage to the outer thick placental sac, so this was opened and the placenta peeled out. There was considerable bleeding which was easily controlled by temporary packing. This thick sac remaining after the placenta was removed was cut down to its mesenteric attachments, leaving enough to approximate the edges together with a running suture. A Penrose drain was inserted to take care of any oozing that might occur. After ascertaining that there was no free bleeding, the abdomen was closed.

During the operation the patient's blood pressure went down. to 70/30. 1,000 c.c. of 10 per cent glucose solution and 600 c.c. of citrated blood were given in the right cubital vein. The pressure went up to 110/70, and the patient was returned to the ward in good condition.

The fetus measured 41 cm. crown heel, 28 cm. crown rump, and weighed 1,355 grams. The cord was 35 cm. long. The placenta weighed 735 grams, was the size of a grapefruit, and was composed of three equally large lobes.

Microscopic section of the placenta showed chorionic villi and trophoblasts with blood clots. Rather large areas were hyalinized and necrotic. The surface at one point was infiltrated with lymphocytes and eosinophiles. The microscopic diagnosis was placental tissue with infarcts.

The maternal blood came back Wassermann-positive, Kahn 4 plus. This was repeated with similar findings. The patient gave no history of syphilis, and had had no treatment. The baby had been dead long enough so that no blood was obtainable for the Wassermann test. Radiograph of the baby's long bones showed no evidence of syphilis.

The patient made an uneventful recovery, running a low grade postoperative temperature for five days, the highest reading being 100.4° on the day following operation. The Penrose drain was removed on the third day, and the patient was discharged on the fifteenth day.

ACUTE LYMPHATIC LEUKEMIA WITH REMISSION

H. G. BOSLAND, M.D.

Verndale, Minnesota

J. P., a white female, aged three, was first seen December 25, 1936, for what seemed to be an attack of upper respiratory infection with inflamed manifestations. She was obviously quite ill with high fever, rapid pulse and chills. Onset had occurred two days previously with the usual symptoms of a "head and chest" cold. The other members of the family were just recovering from the "flu."

Physical findings were acute tonsillitis and pharyngitis, a moderate bilateral cervical adenitis entirely commensurate with the throat pathology, a few rather coarse râles in either lung, temperature 103 by axilla, and a general appearance of pallor combined with what seemed to be a state of excellent nutrition but which also gave the appearance of being abnormal as a kind of generalized tissue swelling of a resilient type. The mother stated that all of her children and particularly this one had been large, heavy, and well-nourished as infants. The urine was normal.

The father, mother, one sister and two brothers are all living and well. There had been no deaths in the family. The mother had gone to full term with all of her pregnancies and had had normal deliveries. There had been no miscarriages nor stillborn infants.

Treatment was symptomatic for fever and restlessness, ice packs to cervical glands, mustard plasters to chest, swabbing of throat, and hot drinks. The following day the temperature was down to normal, the patient had rested well and appeared much improved clinically. No thought of leukemia at this time entered my mind, my diagnosis being acute tonsillitis and an upper respiratory infection.

The patient was not seen again until January 30, thirty-five days later, at which time the father called me because the child's "cold" had become worse again. The interval history revealed that she had not seemed to recover her usual strength and vigor and was often irritable and peevish. She had continued to have a watery rhinorrhea and an occasional slight fever but otherwise seemed well in that her appetite was fairly good and she played. Two days previous, she had

become definitely worse. After a short examination, it was decided to take her to the hospital. Her temperature was 104.2 (r). An acute pharyngo-tonsillitis was present with a red angry looking patch on the right anterior pillar covered by a whitish exudate. The cervical nodes had increased in size, especially in the sub-mandibular region on the left, where the mass was very firm, somewhat tender, fixed, and seemed to represent a coalescence of several nodes. The ears were normal. The chest was normal on physical examination and x-ray. The urine was normal. Examination of the blood revealed a white count of 1,300, red count 2,450,000, Hgb. 30 per cent. In the differential, no pmns. could be identified with certainty. The predominating white cells were young lymphocytes. A blood smear was submitted to the pathology department of the University of Minnesota, the report returning with a diagnosis of acute lymphatic leukemia.

Symptomatic therapy was instituted: liquid diet, ice collar, sedatives. Liver extract was given parenterally in the hope that it might combat the neutropenia and anemia. Iron was given by mouth. Liver extract injections were made January 30, 31, February 4, 7, and 8. The temperature descended to normal in two days and remained within normal limits for five days. During this time, she consumed small amounts of liquids and a few soft foods, played with toys, noted her surroundings and in general seemed contented. Her face, however, was pasty, pallid, and puffy, the eyelids swollen. On February 5, the white count was 3,350, the red count and Hgb. unchanged. February 6, her temperature suddenly shot up to 104.4 (r) and the patient appeared extremely toxic. The swelling of the face and bloated appearance of the body increased. The sub-mandibular mass increased to the size of a lemon, was very tender, firm, and fixed. A mass in the left temporo-parietal region of the scalp which seemed fixed to the underlying periosteum and bone became more pronounced. A point of interest in this connection is that not only was this enlargement present at the very onset of illness in December but it had resulted from a blow sustained in falling about three weeks before and had not subsided in the interval. In retrospect, after the diagnosis of acute leukemia by blood study was unmistakable, this incident had a significance which at the beginning I failed to appreciate.

The patient continued to lose ground rapidly. She was listless, apathetic, and evinced no interest in her surroundings. She did not play and took only sips of fluid when urged. Her temperature remained high and the pulse ran at 140 to 150, fair in quality at times but most often poor. February 8, because of an obstructive edema of the throat, she could swallow nothing. The floor of the mouth was swollen to such an extent that the mucous membrane, pale, watery, and distended, protruded over the lower incisors between them and the tongue. There was no bleeding from mucous membranes nor had there been at any time previously during her illness. February 9, a transfusion of 200 c.c. of citrated blood was given into a right antecubital vein. About eighteen hours after the transfusion, she was able to swallow liquids again. The temperature slowly fell to 101 by February 11, and the patient improved somewhat clinically. She was more contented, less distressed and irritable. The prognosis was of course as hopeless as ever and the child was discharged from the hospital when the father decided that if she must die she might just as well die at home.

February 13, two days after discharge from the hospital, her axillary temperature was 105 and the white count 6,000. Swelling of left cervical nodes rapidly increased. Inguinal and axillary nodes were palpable but small. At no time did these nodes become larger. Blood smears were submitted on this day and the report showed no more immature leukocytes but the polymorphonuclears showed severe toxic changes. The differential count was: polymorphonuclears 68 per cent, lymphocytes 30 per cent, monocytes 2 per cent. By February 19, the mass under the left jaw was fluctuating. It was incised and thick pus was freely evacuated. By February 22, her general appearance and condition were good. The patient was rapidly recovering strength, appetite, and normal activity. On February 25, the white count was 6,000, the blood smear report showed great improvement: no immature leukocytes and polymorphonuclears no longer appeared toxic. In the differential the polymorphonuclears were 58 per cent, lymphocytes 36 per cent, monocytes 6 per cent. Thus, during the following month, the patient was to all appearances and from all evidence a normal, healthy child.

On March 30, the father informed me that the patient had been worse again for the past week because of a "cold." On examination the child presented an appearance of marked toxemia and prostration. The temperature was high, the pulse weak and rapid, and the skin was literally covered by firm gray-blue nodules varying in size from that of a match head to that of a walnut, the largest infiltrated area being in the left temporo-parietal region. This mass, although less discolored than the remainder, had begun to assume a cyanotic hue. On close questioning the parents recalled that during the first week in March several of these

nodules had been noted below the left clavicle, but inasmuch as they were small and painless and no more of them developed I was not advised of the circumstance. Furthermore, the child seemed well and happy. Shortly after her "cold" began, however, many more nodules rapidly appeared. The white count was 160,000; Hgb. 60 per cent. Examination of the chest revealed a large area of dullness suggesting pneumonic consolidation in the anterior portion of the left lower lobe. Because of abdominal distention, enlargement of the liver and spleen could not be definitely determined. There was no ulceration in the throat nor was there any evidence of bleeding from mucous membranes. A blood smear was submitted to the Department of Pathology, University of Minnesota, and again showed a typical acute lymphatic leukemia, nearly all of the white cells being immature lymphocytes. The child appeared moribund and the parents were so advised. General symptomatic measures of therapy were instituted and for the lack of anything better to do an injection of liver extract was given into the buttocks.

Due to the severity of the weather conditions and the comparative inaccessibility of the farmhouse, the child was not seen again until five days later, at which time examination revealed that the cutaneous nodules had all, to a marked extent, faded in color and diminished in size. The large temporo-parietal mass had decreased to one-third of its previous size. The other scalp nodules were scarcely palpable, whereas five days before they had been very obvious to sight and touch. The area of dulness in the chest had diminished. Clinically, she had definitely improved. Her eyes were brighter, she took an interest in her surroundings, and talked a little for the first time in a week. The temperature and pulse, however, remained rather high and the white count was 140,000. The possibility of liver extract playing a rôle in the child's improvement seems too remote for consideration for, of course, in all probability its use was coincidental with an attempted reversion to normal on the part of the hematopoietic mechanism. Yet, it is conceivable that some factor or factors in the body may be essential to prevent an uncontrolled over-production of certain blood cells just as the factor which is known to be present in liver extract is essential to initiate and sustain a state of normality in red cells where, one might say, under-production exists. The premise of a system of checks and balances in a blood cell controlling mechanism or mechanisms, which, in the normally functioning human body, prevents a shift toward abnormality in either direction is not without logic. There being at hand no other preparation which might conceivably provide whatever it was, if anything, that was lacking in this instance, liver extract was selected. Thus, I tried to justify submitting this already unhappy child to the additional discomfort of liver extract injections.

From about April 1 to April 9, clinical improvement was steady, being most marked the first five days following March 30. The nodules continued to disappear, although more slowly. Nodules known to exist one day would have disappeared entirely the next. The large temporo-parietal mass became hardly palpable. The

(Continued on Page 527)

MEDICINE IN WASHINGTON AND CHISAGO COUNTIES

ONE of the upper tributaries of the Mississippi is the St. Croix River, which forms part of the boundary between Wisconsin and Minnesota. It is also the eastern boundary of Washington and Chisago Counties. In the past it was the only approach to this region. Explorers, voyagers, and missionaries traveled its waters as it was one of the routes between the Mississippi and Lake Superior.

Until the treaties of 1837 with the Sioux and Ojibway Indians, there were few, if any, white settlers along its banks. White men knew the valley as a place of danger and the Indians referred to it by the ominous name of the "Valley of Bones," due, no doubt, to the frequent encounters then between the two hostile tribes.

With the signing of the treaty, the St. Croix valley was open for settlement. Lumber was the incentive which attracted the white man, and with the coming of the lumberman, medical history of the region begins. Among the first to arrive was a Dr. Fitch. In 1837 he and a group of others, including Franklin Steele, Jeremiah Russell, and a Mr. Maginnis, came from Fort Snelling and built a rough cabin near the falls. They then separated to search for pine, Dr. Fitch exploring the Sunrise River. A year later Dr. Fitch returned in association with the St. Croix Lumber Company. No other information about him is available except that he is said to have come from Galena, Illinois. Scarcely more is known about a Dr. Green, who came up the river in the fall of 1838, also looking for lumber. Green and his companions returned the following spring with complete materials for a mill, and on April 27, 1839, they drove in their stakes and formed at Marine the first permanent settlement in Minnesota. The mill was completed and at work by fall. Green remained at least two years, cutting timber near Kettle River. It is doubtful whether either Fitch or Green practiced; if they did it was probably incidental, for it was evident that their prime interest was lumber. This doubt is verified by the fact that all the early records speak of Dr. Christopher Carli, who came in 1841, as the first practicing physician north of Prairie du Chien. Dr. Carli's history is more complete than that of his predecessors.

Dr. Carli was born at Frankfort-on-the-Main December 7, 1811. He was educated at Heidelberg University, where he studied medicine. In 1832 he came to this country and practiced for three years in Buffalo, New York, before returning to Germany. However, after two years he again came to America, this time spending a year in Chicago, then a year in New Orleans, then going back to Chicago again. On May 24, 1841, he settled in Dakotah, St. Croix valley, on the site that is now Stillwater. His practice extended from Lake Pepin to Lake Superior, and from Menominee, Wisconsin, westward. He was always ready to visit a patient, on foot, skates or snowshoes, by horse or birchbark canoe. He was a member of the first city council of Stillwater and officiated as city and county physician, and coroner. He opened the first bank in Stillwater, and started the first drug store, which he afterwards sold to Dr. Henry Murdock. He also opened a stone quarry, dealt in real estate, and had many other avocations, for, like most of the pioneer physicians, he was obliged to rely on something besides his profession for his support. He lived in Stillwater until his death in 1887.

As more settlers came to the valley another physician, Philip Aldrich, arrived. He was born in 1792. There is no record of his early life or education. He came in the early forties and was mail carrier for the entire valley. At different times he brought mail from Prairie du Chien and Fort Snelling, going as far as the falls and treating patients along the route on every bimonthly visit. Whether he had ever earned the title of Doctor or not, he performed the duties of physician wherever he was able. He was a prominent citizen and occupied many public offices, including judge of probate and justice of the peace. He donated land for the town of Buena Vista. Although a Wisconsin man, he was well known and active on the Minnesota side of the river.

The next newcomer, Dr. J. M. Covey, also settled at Stillwater in 1844. He was a regular physician, having received a medical education in his native state of New York. He is described as being a sociable but eccentric man, and slightly deaf. He died in 1851 supposedly from the effects of sleeping in a newly plastered room. In 1846 and 1847 two more physicians arrived about whom practically nothing is known. The first was a Dr. De Witt, who located at St. Croix Falls, and the other a Mrs. Page, a practitioner of the Thompsonian school at Hudson. At the close of the Mexican war came Dr. Otis Hoyt, who stayed at St. Croix Falls until 1851, practicing medicine and "delivering pleasing lectures on the Mexican war," in which he had served. He also practiced a year in Stillwater, then moved to Hudson, where he remained until his death in 1885. He was the most prominent physician in Western Wisconsin for many years.

One other physician arrived in the forties, a Dr. Wright, who settled at Marine in 1849. Nothing is known about him except that he died there in 1851. It is interesting to know that he was reported to have died of cholera. Since Asiatic cholera occurred at Stillwater about that time, it is possible that it also reached Marine, brought by the river boats. Dr. Wright is referred to as the first physician at Marine, which adds to the belief that Dr. Green never practiced there.

During the next decade a tremendous number of immigrants poured into the valley, and with them the necessity for more medical care increased. Epidemic and other diseases, new babies, the treacherous current of the river, the knives that were freely drawn in the saloons, and the frequent accidents with the dangerous circular saws of the lumber mills conspired to provide a steady stream of patients, and doctors arrived in rapid succession to fill the need. Drs. Pugsley and Ahl came to Stillwater in 1850, and in the years from 1854 to 1857 they were joined by Drs. Murdock, Noyes, Muller and Rhodes. Marine became the home of Drs. Cooley, Reiner and Gaskill, and in 1854 Dr. L. B. Smith, the first resident physician of Chisago County, settled at Taylors Falls. Smith had spent a year in St. Croix Falls (the town directly across the river, in Wisconsin), where even on the day of his arrival he found a patient waiting for him, a man who had been caught in a running saw, and whose arm was badly mangled. Amputation was necessary, but unfortunately the baggage which contained the doctor's larger instruments had not arrived, having been sent on a slower steamer. The operation was, therefore, performed as well as possible with a few small pocket instruments and a crude joiner's saw, and it is recorded that the patient recovered quickly. Smith was followed in 1855 by Dr. E. D. Whiting, who many years later married the widow of Dr. Smith.

Also in 1855 came Dr. E. W. Johnson of Lakeland, and Dr. J. W. Comfort of Wyoming. All of these physicians remained for many years and were prominent in their profession as well as in other activities.

Dr. H. W. Murdock's drug store, which he purchased in 1854 from Dr. Carli, appears to have been a busy place at this time, for many advertisements appear in the *St. Croix Union*, the only newspaper published in Stillwater at that time. For example, the following appeared first on February 13, 1855:

PILLS, PILLS

Pills old and young, of all qualities, kinds
and descriptions. Enough to physic the territory at

Murdock's City Drug Store

Later, the doctor added a full line of perfumery, patent medicines, pure wines and liquors "for med. or mech. purposes," cigars, a soda fountain, paper hangings, oil paints and dye stuffs. He took as his partner Dr. O. G. Babcock, who came in 1855. Babcock moved to Afton in 1858, remaining there until his death in the fall of 1870. Carli's many activities are suggested by advertisements in the *Union*. On August 25, 1855, he advertised a hotel for rent, and offered for sale hardwood, 50 wheelbarrows, a two-horse wagon, 250 barrels of lime, 1,000 bushels of corn, 250 bushels of oats and 50 barrels of flour. Hoyt advertised land for sale. Crandall and Babcock also had a drug store, as did Pugsley and Reiner. These latter two were partners in practice at that time, as were Carli and Noyes. Later both partnerships were dissolved. In 1858 Pugsley formed a partnership with a newcomer, a Dr. Harlow. This partnership also was discontinued after several months. Apparently it was the custom for a newcomer to associate himself with a physician already established until he became known to the community.

In politics, in the forming of towns, and in the civic activities of their communities, many of the physicians played a prominent rôle. Reiner was a state senator; Gaskill a member of the first legislature. Reiner and several others served on the school board. Carli and Murdock helped organize the Stillwater fire department. Gaskill served three years as supervisor of the town of Marine. Later he was elected councilman, then elected and re-elected president of the council, and when Marine became a village he helped draft the charter. He was also a trustee of the state prison. Whiting was a representative in the legislature, and Carli was chosen president of the Old Settlers Association. Nearly all the doctors served as county, city or prison physician.

There is little information about diseases and epidemics in the earlier years of the settlements. The usual troubles were all present: tuberculosis, typhoid, scarlet fever and diphtheria. Asiatic cholera also reached Stillwater, carried there by the river steamers. Two interesting interviews with oldtimers are worth quoting in this connection. The first, Captain Stephen Hanks, of Albany, Illinois, remembered the cholera quite well:

"In 1851 or 1853," he said, "when I was rafting logs from the St. Croix to St. Louis, four of my men died of cholera on the way down. Two were taken ill in the evening and were dead in the morning. We stopped at the sand point between Willow River and Catfish Bar and I furnished the wood for coffins and Bowles made them. We buried them about a mile and a half above Catfish Bar on the top of the bluff. The rest of my crew deserted at Willow River. . . ."

The other interview, with E. W. Durant of Stillwater, included the following information:

"When the cholera first appeared on the river we were much afraid of it, but later, although it became very common, we paid little attention to it. The cholera came in 1849 to 1851, and spread from New Orleans up the river. All boats carried cheap board coffins and buried those who died when they stopped to take on wood, at night, if possible. . . . Another time, on the steamer "Cora" on the way up we buried several and at Stillwater landed a family of whom several died. Again, I attended two men on a log raft at Stillwater. I saw them in the evening and called again in the morning; one man at that time had lost half his weight and was very filthy, lying in a pool of mucus and bowel discharge. He died shortly after sunrise. I think four or five of that family died on the same trip up. We landed a cholera patient at Prescott, but I saved him; I used to give them Perry Davis' Pain Killer internally and rub it on externally as well."

There is no way of estimating the extent of communicable diseases, because if any records were kept, they have since been lost. While the newspapers carried some death notices they rarely mentioned the cause of the death, and even when they did it was often such a vague term as "inflammation" or "complication" or merely "fever." Not all deaths were reported. This may have been due to the lack of news value in most cases, but it was evidently also due, in part, to a sense of civic pride which led the editors of the papers to deny any lack of health in their own communities. Epidemics were often reported by the papers of another town, but denied by the citizens of the town in which the epidemic was reported. It is hard to tell which was correct. However, deaths of a more sensational nature—fights and accidents—were often recorded. The latter were amazingly frequent, especially in the sawmills. Probably the mills had no safety devices then such as they have now, or possibly the men were careless; certainly the fast-running saws made an appreciable cut in the life and health of the community. One physician alone, in later years, reported five such injuries in three weeks.

The close of the decade of the fifties found the following physicians practicing in Washington and Chisago Counties: in Stillwater, Ahl, Carli, Dyson (a homeopath who came in 1858), Harlow, Muller, Noyes, Pugsley and Rhodes; in Marine, Cooley, Gaskill and Reiner, although the latter had spent two years in Stillwater; in Taylors Falls, Smith and Whiting, and at Lakeland, Dr. E. Johnson.

The next few years of medical history were much concerned with the Civil War, for many practitioners left to accept military positions. Some were killed; some settled elsewhere when the war ended; some stayed in the army. In 1861 Dr. Muller took an appointment as surgeon at Fort Ridgley. In April, 1862, Dr. Reiner was sent to Kentucky by Governor Ramsey to help care for the wounded. Dr. Reiner returned in May with "encouraging accounts."

The *Stillwater Messenger* for September 2, 1862, published the announcement that Dr. E. G. Pugsley was to leave, having been appointed assistant surgeon of the First Minnesota. On May 5, 1863, Dr. C. P. Garlick was appointed assistant surgeon of the Fourteenth Wisconsin Regiment, and in July, Dr. L. B. Smith was appointed an assistant surgeon, and left in April, 1864. Dr. Rhodes, in July of that year, obtained a situation in the Post Hospital at Memphis. He later became surgeon in a Minnesota regiment.

In the *Stillwater Messenger* for October 11, 1864, a note appeared that E. G. Pugsley, who had returned honorably discharged in February, 1864, had become assistant suregon in the Ninth Regiment. Pugsley built up an extensive practice in Glasgow, Missouri, though he never went back there after the war. Dr. L. B. Smith of Taylors Falls was killed the day before the battle of Tupelo, the division to which he belonged having been ambushed by Forest's troops. Smith "was a tall man of fine personal appearance, with the air of an officer, for which reason, doubtless, some sharpshooter singled him out for destruction.'

A Dr. H. M. Patterson died, although the war was only indirectly the cause of his death. The *Stillwater Messenger* for February 12, 1868, carried the following announcement:

"Dr. H. M. Patterson died on Sunday morning, a victim of a disease contracted during the late 'cruel war.' A boy in appearance, he was a man in soul. We knew him for years in the military, and during the past eighteen months we have met him almost daily in the civil walks of life. He was a promising young man of twenty-six years, proficient in his profession and the soul of honor and generous impulses."

There is practically no other information about Patterson—when he came or where he practiced.

Dr. Muller apparently never returned to practice in Stillwater, though he visited the town occasionally. Most of the other physicians did return, however, to the valley.

Besides serving in the army at this time, the physicians took an active part in both local and state affairs. At a meeting of the board of county commissioners in September, 1862, Gaskill was appointed county examiner of school teachers in the first district. In February, 1863, Noyes was appointed prison physician. Drs. J. B. Phillips and E. D. Whiting were mentioned as being at a legislative district convention at Marine in September, 1866. In April, 1868, there was a notice in the Stillwater paper by J. R. M. Gaskill, district clerk, and in August and October the *Taylors Falls Reporter* announced that Drs. Marshall and Griswold had been appointed examining surgeons for pensions. The next year some mention is made of "Senator Dr. Noyes." Whiting served in two sessions of the Minnesota state legislature (1860-1861) as a representative. Rhodes was also very prominent in civic affairs at this time.

Political activities were not the only ones in which the doctors took part. Christopher Carli advertised himself as a banker and broker. Ahl ran a hotel. Whiting made an extensive trip through Europe in 1867, visiting the Paris exposition and stopping at all the principal cities of the continent. In 1869 Rhodes invented and patented a very useful "spark-catcher" for the draft of parlor stoves. The same year a young men's course of lectures was planned, among which was one by Dr. A. J. Stone on "The Physical Education of the Coming Man,' and one by Dr. Reiner on education. Dr. Kinkle was to have spoken, but was too busy at the last moment. Dr. Stone at this time issued a prospectus for a medical and surgical journal which appeared in Saint Paul a year later, in June, 1870. It was a monthly magazine called *The Northwestern Medical and Surgical Journal.* Stone was both editor and proprietor. Three Stillwater physicians were among those who, in 1869, formed the State Medical Society; they were Rhodes, Noyes, and Stone.

Among the newcomers of this decade were several very reputable practitioners as well as many disreputable ones. In 1860 came Dr. Hiram Murdock, the father of Dr. H. M. Murdock, who had been practicing in the valley for several years, and of Dr. G. W. Murdock who came to Taylors Falls in 1865. Hiram Murdock originally practised at Stillwater, but moved to the Falls in 1862, and stayed there until his death four years later. In 1861 Dr. G. M. Lambert came to Stillwater and in 1862 Dr. George Taylor to Point Douglas. In 1862 we find the following newspaper item:

EYES, EYES, EYES!

Dr. J. A. Gilison, operator on the eye,
will make a short stay in Stillwater at
the Sawyer House . . .

Gilison highly recommended himself, offered to cure any ailment presented, and advertised "no charge for examination or opinion." He returned frequently to Stillwater and was typical of a large group of doctors who traveled from town to town, leaving behind a trail of useless medicines and valueless advice. In 1865 came Dr. C. A. Brooks, formerly an army surgeon, and the above mentioned Dr. G. W. Murdock. A peculiar and unfortunate event marked the arrival of Dr. Brooks. His first call, the day after his arrival in Stillwater, was to return to Minneapolis to attend his brother, who had been accidentally and fatally shot. In 1866 several physicians arrived. Drs. Marshall, Griswold and Spicer all came to Taylors Falls and settled there; also, the papers mentioned Dr. J. B. Phillips of Marine. In 1867 and 1868 a Dr. Carrington practised at Taylors Falls, and Dr. N. W. Beckwith, an eclectic, and Dr. H. Runge came to settle in Stillwater. Runge had a rather varied career. Born in Germany in 1817, he went to school in Russia, and graduated after a six-year course in the University of Berlin. He then studied to become a veterinary surgeon in Copenhagen for two years. After that he returned to Moscow and practised until 1863. Then he went to South America and later to Iowa, where he stayed until 1867, when he came to Stillwater. Later he spent eight years in Minneapolis, returned to Stillwater, and in 1880 settled permanently at Osceola. In 1868 Dr. Garnet spent the summer in Taylors Falls; and Dr. W. H. Cavin, formerly of Hudson, moved to Stillwater. In 1869 Drs. A. J. Stone, G. W. Hart, and J. C. Kinkle settled in Stillwater, and in 1870 Drs. Jordan, Morrow and A. J. Murdock began to practise in the valley, the latter at Taylors Falls. Some of these newcomers formed temporary partnerships with other physicians. Among these partnerships were Gaskill and Brooks (at Osceola), Kinkle and Noyes, Stone and Jordan, Spicer and Griswold.

With the coming of more physicians to the St. Croix valley, it was natural that some sort of a medical society be formed. There is no record of when the first one was formed, but in the *Stillwater Messenger* of May 27, 1862, the following brief announcement appeared:

"The next quarterly meeting of the St. Croix Valley Medical Association will be held at Hudson on the 27th day of May, 1862, at 10 o'clock A.M. Surgical operations will be performed and advice given gratuitously for those who choose to present themselves before the association."

Evidently, then, there was some sort of medical society at the time, although there is no other record of its activities. It must have broken up later, probably due to the comings and goings of the physicians during the war, because in 1871 there were attempts to form a new organization.

The general health of the people in the counties during these years was poor, and epidemics were constantly being reported. Diphtheria was an ever present cause of worry; a large percentage of deaths reported in the papers were attributed to it. In March, 1863, the *Messenger* reported that "the dreadful disease prevails to a considerable extent in Hudson, having caused several deaths there." The same item recommended the use of ice, broken into small pieces and swallowed by the patient at intervals "until relief is experienced." Among others, one of Dr. Carli's daughters died of the disease in January of the following year. The Taylors Falls papers, in February, 1860, reported the disease prevalent, and stated that several children there had died of it. As to smallpox, in May, 1864, the Stillwater paper reported as follows:

"We are reliably informed that this dreaded disease has made its appearance at Marine, having been brought to that place by a young man from Fort Snelling. When he was first taken down, it was not known to be smallpox, and many of the friends and neighbors called in to see him, thus spreading the contagion in an alarming manner. We have no further particulars. Our people would do well to take every precaution to guard against the disease as we can hardly hope to escape a visitation of the dreadful scourge."

Apparently it did not immediately spread to Stillwater, although early in 1870 it was said to be "all around." Ten or twelve cases were reported at the Falls, thirty or more in the vicinity of Prescott, and one light one, the first in eight or ten years, in Stillwater. The Taylors Falls papers reported seven cases in Osceola (on the Wisconsin side of the river), most of them mild, but one fatal. The schools there were closed because of it. The paper also quoted Dr. Carli as saying that it could be checked in a short time by vaccination, diet and quarantine. Apparently there was some attempt to isolate cases at this time, although it was not strict enough to stop any epidemic. Among other diseases, the chief ones mentioned were lung fever and hydrophobia. The *Messenger* of January, 1867, remarks: "Our physicians say that there is more sickness in this place and vicinity at this time than ever before known. The prevailing disease, which has assumed an epidemical type, is lung fever." Curiously enough there were actually no cases of hydrophobia reported, although there were constant complaints and much fear of unmuzzled dogs. One death from cholera was reported in August, 1863, a few miles from Stillwater, and measles and other less serious epidemics made their appearance.

Statistics concerning the diseases in the state prison at Stillwater at this time are available, and show fairly well the frequency of illness in that institution. In 1866 there were nearly two cases of sickness to every prisoner; in 1867 over five; in 1868 over six; and in 1870 over four. The number of convicts at the beginning of the year 1867 was only thirty-five; at the beginning of 1868, forty-five, and at the beginning of 1869, forty-two. Conditions in the prison gradually became better after 1868, there being fewer illnesses per prisoner, although of course more prisoners. On reading reports of the prison at this time one's greatest surprise will probably be that there was not more illness and a much higher mortality rate. While the food was generally agreed to be excellent, and some sanitary regulations were strictly enforced by the warden, nevertheless the ventilation, heating, toilet facilities and especially the drainage were very poor. Even several years later, when the Board of Health made its first report, the site was described as unfavorable; the soil about the prison was saturated by springs; stagnant water covered the prison yards at all times, making the lower walls damp. The lower tier of cells was untenable, having two inches of water standing on the floors, and the walls bulged noticeably and "might fall at any moment." The well in the yard was muddy from surface drainage. The privy was described as being in a filthy condition, and refuse from the kitchen was simply thrown out in the yard. The air was damp and musty, and the cells were ventilated only by four-inch openings into an air shaft, which most prisoners closed up in the winter because of the inadequacy of heating. The cells were only five by seven feet. Of course, the prisoners worked from six to six, with only a half hour for lunch, or, in winter, from five to seven, but they spent the rest of their time in these cells, eating and sleeping in them. The dark cells, for refractory prisoners, were "offensive and not properly ventilated," and the custom of chaining misbehaving convicts to the doors, in a standing position, pre-vailed. Besides these, later reports by prison physicians and inspectors reported bathing facilities most primitive, laundry arrangements poor, and the kitchen very poor, though the food was good. The hospital was inadequate and in many cases sick prisoners had to be treated in their cells. In 1876 the prison physician was still urging that a sewer be built, as there had never been even the most primitive one. He urged also that a competent medical graduate be employed as hospital steward, as the position was then filled by an incompetent convict. In 1877 the prison was so crowded that some of the five by seven cells held two convicts. It would be highly unfair, however, to blame prison officials for the poor conditions, as they were simply an echo of conditions in most of the towns at that time. Stillwater itself was far from modern in sanitary ideals. The average person at that time was quite ignorant, and new ideas were probably hard to introduce. For example, in the *Taylors Falls Reporter* in the spring of 1866, there appeared an excellent article on trichina, with illustrations, by a Chicago physician. In the following issue of the *Reporter* appeared a long comment on "the atrocious trichina story," saying what a hoax and fraud the former article was, that trichinosis existed only in a certain small part of Germany, where pork was eaten raw and uncured, and it was caused by the diet of the hogs, which ate snakes and vermin. The article assured its readers that trichinosis was never found in the corn-fed hogs of the surrounding territory.

When the decade closed, the following physicians were in the two counties: Ahl, Brooks, Carli, Gaskill, Griswold, Kinkle, Lambert, Marshall, Morrow, A. J. Murdock, Noyes, Reiner, Rhodes, Runge, Spicer, Stone and Whiting. Probably Drs. Beckwith, Cavin and Dyson should be included, although there is no further record of either their presence or their departures. Babcock and Jordan had both died in 1870; Johnson left in 1864, Geo. W. Murdock in 1868, and Hart in 1870. Muller and Pugsley both settled elsewhere after the war; Smith was killed, and Taylor of Point Douglas left after a year. The *Reporter* of February, 1870, said that there were only eleven licensed physicians in the district, which included Washington, Chisago, Pine and Kanabec Counties. In Washington County, in 1869, according to the report of the committee of credentials in the State Medical Society, there were four regular and five irregular practitioners.

(To be continued in August issue)

EDITORIAL

MINNESOTA MEDICINE

OFFICIAL JOURNAL OF THE MINNESOTA STATE MEDICAL
ASSOCIATION

Published by the Association under the direction of its Editing
and Publishing Committee

EDITING AND PUBLISHING COMMITTEE

J. T. CHRISTISON, Saint Paul   C. B. WRIGHT, Minneapolis
E. M. HAMMES, Saint Paul   T. A. PEPPARD, Minneapolis
WALTMAN WALTERS, Rochester

EDITORIAL STAFF

CARL B. DRAKE, Saint Paul, Editor
W. F. BRAASCH, Rochester, Associate Editor
GILBERT COTTAM, Minneapolis, Associate Editor

Annual Subscription—$3.00   Single Copies—$0.40

Foreign Subscriptions—$3.50

The right is reserved to reject material submitted for editorial
or advertising columns. The Editing and Publishing Committee
does not hold itself responsible for views expressed either in
editorials or other articles when signed by the author.

Classified advertising—five cents a word; minimum charge,
$1.00. Remittance should accompany order.

Display advertising rates on request.

Address all communications to Minnesota Medicine, 2642 University Avenue, Saint Paul, or Suite 604, National Bldg., Minneapolis. Telephone: Nestor 2641.

BUSINESS MANAGER
J. R. BRUCE

Volume 21   JULY, 1938   Number 7

Clinico-Pathological Conferences in Hospitals

THE Council on Medical Education and Hospitals of the American Medical Association is
charged with the duty of the certification of hospitals for the training of interns and resident
physicians. This is what it says about one feature of its requirements:

"Necropsy performance in hospitals has rightly become a criterion of the scientific attitude of the staff.
It reflects a desire to elevate the practice of medicine,
an eagerness for scientific accuracy and a recognition
of pathology as a sound basis on which to build clinical knowledge. To interns and older physicians alike
there is a steady accrual of knowledge through repeated postmortem studies *in which pathologic and
clinical manifestations are carefully correlated.*"

"To comply with the requirements of the Council
a hospital approved for intern training must maintain
a necropsy rate of at least 15 per cent of its deaths
in order to supply an adequate amount of teaching material for the instruction of the house staff. *Surgical
as well as necropsy specimens can be used to advantage in clinical pathological conferences, which should
be conducted weekly or biweekly in accordance with the
amount of material available.*" (The italics are ours.)
(J.A.M.A. 110:974, March 26, 1938.)

Again, the American College of Surgeons is
responsible for the accrediting of hospitals for
standardization and here is clause (b), section
3 of its Minimum Standard for Hospitals:

"That the medical staff review and analyze at regular intervals their clinical experience in the various
departments of the hospital, such as medicine, surgery,
obstetrics and the other specialties; the medical records of patients, free and pay, to be the basis for such
review and analysis."

(Am. Coll. of Surg. 1938 Year Book, p. 57.)

So much for what may be called the letter
of the law. There are additional reasons why
clinico-pathological conferences have become
necessitous. In private or voluntary hospitals,
for instance, the opportunities for teaching interns and giving them a chance to put what
knowledge they have acquired into practical
application are very much less than in the larger
public institutions, consequently positions in the
latter type of hospital are much more sought
after and the private hospitals have difficulty in
securing their interns. Having done so, however, are these private hospitals not obligated
morally to make up, as far as they possibly can,
the deficiencies in their teaching and clinical
opportunities for their interns? Certainly they
are, and in no better way can they do it than
by carrying on well planned conferences. Every
hospital has an abundance of material, in both
the living and the necropsy fields, and it is the
duty of every staff, we believe, to see that such
material is made available and presented properly each week. If the hospital has a full-time
pathologist who is capable of taking charge of
it, so much the better, but sometimes the hospital's internal arrangements point to the wisdom of a different plan, with a well informed

return. It is this that builds up and maintains the spirit of these undertakings and makes them indispensible.

G. C.

Vitamin K

IN 1935 Henrik Dam reported the isolation of a material, deficiency of which in the diets of chicks resulted in fatal hemorrhage. He found this fat-soluble material in pig liver fat and designated it vitamin K. Subsequently, this compound was prepared in concentrated form and recently has been crystallized by Almquist. Thus, in a short time, another apparently essential animal nutritive product has been recognized and some of its basic chemical properties determined.

So-called vitamin K apparently is distributed widely in nature. In the plant kingdom its distribution appears to be confined almost entirely to the photosynthetic portion of the plant and in this its distribution is radically different from that of provitamin A. Considerable amounts of vitamin K have been found in alfalfa, kale, spinach, dried carrot tops, chestnut leaves, tomatoes, oat sprouts, and many other plants. In addition, it is found in soy bean oil and in the unsaponifiable portion of dog liver fat and pig liver fat.

The vitamin can be prepared from fish meal, rice bran or casein after the ether extracted material has been allowed to putrify and then subsequently extracted with petroleum ether. Under these conditions it appears that bacteria may cause the synthesis of this material but just what organisms can accomplish this synthesis are not as yet definitely known. However, Almquist and his associates recently have isolated a "fish meal organism" which closely resembles Bacillus cereus and which contains, and is capable of producing in fish meal, considerable amounts of vitamin K. The vitamin also is present in the droppings of chicks, in dried normal acholic feces of man, in dried colon bacilli, Bacillus subtilis, Staphylococcus aureus and many other microörganisms. Presumably the vitamin is present in the lipoid fraction of these bacteria but further data will be necessary before it can be assumed that the vitamin K found in alfalfa is the same substance as that present in microörganisms.

The exact physical and chemical properties of vitamin K are at present incompletely known but some properties seem to be definitely established. Physically it is a colorless, crystalline, fat-soluble material which is stable in air at 120° C. but is rapidly destroyed by alkali or sunlight. The substance apparently has a high molecular weight and contains a small amount of nitrogen but no sulfur or phosphorus.

Among young chicks which are given diets deficient in vitamin K there develops a tendency to bleed which is somewhat in proportion to the deficiency of prothrombin in the circulating blood. The syndrome in chicks is characterized by bleeding from the pin feathers and hemorrhages into muscles under the skin and in the abdomen, together with dark erosions on the lining of the gizzard. Frequently, low levels of hemoglobin are present and not infrequently fatal hemorrhages may develop very suddenly. Administration to these chicks of materials which contain vitamin K results in cessation of bleeding and an accompanying rise in the level of prothrombin. These phenomena are the basis for all known biologic assays of vitamin K.

The available experimental data are too meager to justify offering an explanation of the mechanism by which vitamin K affects prothrombin. Although prothrombin, so far as is known, does not contain a lipoid component, the possibility is not excluded that vitamin K, or a derivative thereof, might be present as a prosthetic group which is held in firm combination with the rest of the prothrombin molecule.

The recent demonstration that in the circulating blood of individuals who have jaundice there is a deficiency of prothrombin, has led to the clinical use of vitamin K as a therapeutic aid in the prevention and control of this abnormal bleeding. Independently, several groups of investigators have reported the successful elevation of the prothrombin level and in some instances inhibitory effects on actual bleeding of individuals with jaundice.

These results give some hope for control of the hemorrhagic diathesis in jaundice. However, simpler methods for estimation of the level of prothrombin in the blood and a more easily available and at the same time nearly chemically pure source of vitamin K are much needed at present. The recent successful use of injectable concentrates of vitamin K gives hope of standard dosage and of a standard method of administration.

H. R. B.

The A.M.A. Meeting

THE eighty-ninth annual session of the American Medical Association at San Francisco was outstanding in many respects. The attendance was large considering the location, approximately 6,000 registrants. As usual in recent years, much time was spent by the House of Delegates on economic questions. The president, Dr. J. H. J. Upham, in his address referred to the multiplicity of medical meetings and to the increasing growth in many localities of postgraduate courses, the demand for which appeared to be growing. He depreciated the lay control of scientific medicine and favored the campaigns on cancer, tuberculosis, and syphilis.

Dr. Irvin Abell, president-elect, was most enthusiastic over the excellent type of medical service now rendered to the American people, comparing the low morbidity and mortality here with that of other countries. He estimated that medical service rendered to the poor by American physicians amounted to over a million dollars a day. He said there should be no compromise between the profession and lay groups in the manner in which that service should be rendered. He also favored graduate extension.

President Wilbur of Stanford niversity stressed the need for more and better instruction for graduate and undergraduate students and suggested a three year pre-medical preparation for prospective students of medicine, adding that the quality of the applicant was of more importance than anything else.

Dr. Rudolph Matas of New Orleans was awarded the distinguished service medal of the Association. This is bestowed for outstanding achievement in Medicine and Surgery each year. Dr. Rock Sleyster of Wisconsin is the new president-elect.

Dr. H. H. Shoulders of Tennessee was elected Speaker of the House of Delegates succeeding Dr. Nathan B. Van Etten of New York.

Dr. Austin Hayden of Chicago and Dr. C. B. Wright of Minneapolis were each elected to succeed themselves as trustees for the ensuing five years.

The technical exhibits were many and varied. The scientific exhibits were generally considered very good but hardly the equal of the past few years.

Meeting places for the next three years were selected as follows: St Louis, Missouri—1939; New York City—1940; Cleveland, Ohio—1941.

The Duluth Meeting

THE annual meeting of the Minnesota State Medical Association held at Duluth, June 28 to July 1, was one of the most successful in the history of the Association. The program throughout was exceptionally interesting. Those in charge of the program were fortunate in obtaining a number of noted men from outside the state, among them being Dr. Howard W. Haggard of Yale University, and Dr. Irwin Abell, president of the American Medical Association.

Dr. George A. Earl of Saint Paul, the president-elect, will succeed Dr. J. M. Hayes at the end of the calendar year. Dr. J. C. Jacobs of Willmar was chosen first vice president, and Dr. A. M. Hanson of Faribault, second vice president. Dr. B. B. Souster of Saint Paul was elected secretary, succeeding Dr. E. A. Meyerding. Dr. W. H. Condit was re-elected treasurer.

Dr. H. Z. Giffin of Rochester was elected chairman of the Council. Dr. L. L. Sogge of Windom was re-elected to the Council from the Second District; Dr. B. S. Adams of Hibbing was re-elected from the Ninth District, and Dr. E. Mendelssohn Jones of Saint Paul was elected from the Fifth District, succeeding Dr. George A. Earl. Dr. W. A. Coventry of Duluth and Dr. W. F. Braasch of Rochester were re-elected delegates to the American Medical Association.

Dr. W. W. Will of Bertha was re-elected speaker of the House of Delegates. Dr. E. A. Meyerding, who has retired as secretary, was elected vice-speaker of the House of Delegates, and was presented with a gold medal for distinguished service to the Association over a period of many years.

The next annual meeting will be held in Minneapolis.

In Memoriam

Henning F. B. Wiese
1889-1938

DR. HENNING F. B. WIESE was born June 17, 1889 at Nordfjord, Norway, the son of Christian and Johanna Wiese. He was the youngest of seven children. His paternal great grandfather and grandfather were physicians in Norway. His maternal grandfather and one uncle also practiced medicine in Norway. His father was an expert accountant. One of his brothers is a physician in Norway and a sister is married to an English physician who resides in Paris, France.

Dr. Wiese attended the Gymnasium at Oslo, Norway, from 1904 to 1907, after which he entered the University of Oslo, graduating in 1915 with the highest honors of his class. He served his internship in the Rikshospitalet in Oslo, at the end of which time Dr. Mathiesen of Eau Claire, Wisconsin, who was Dr. Wiese's godfather, invited him to spend some time with him and Dr. Midelfart in their clinic, which he did, staying one and one-half years. From there he entered the Mayo Foundation at Rochester, Minnesota, where he spent three years. He was called by Dr. Schilling, the chief surgeon, to the Ullevaal Sykehuse in Oslo, Norway, at which hospital he served as surgeon for two and one-half years.

He received the degree of Master of Science in Surgery in 1922 from the University of Minnesota. He was a Fellow of the American College of Surgeons and the American Medical Association and a member of the Minneapolis Surgical Society. He was a member of the Kristiania Surgical Society and the Norwegian Medical Society; also a member of the Alumni Association of the Mayo Foundation.

During the World War Dr. Wiese held the commission of First Lieutenant in the Medical Reserve Corps and the heavy artillery of the Norwegian Army.

He gave his services for many years to the Wells Memorial Clinic and the Ebenezer Home and he was a member of the Surgical Staffs of Asbury, Swedish, Fairview and Deaconess Hospitals.

Dr. Wiese was married on December 16, 1922, to Juanita Wood, daughter of Frederick and Fanny Wood of Eau Claire, Wisconsin. They have two children, Karin, age 14, and Stetson, age 11.

Above all else Dr. Wiese loved his family and his home, and it was his desire to remain there throughout his final illness, which lasted seven months. It was my privilege in association with Dr. Charles Hallberg to see him a great deal in the final weeks of his illness and to note the faithfulness with which his beautiful and talented wife cared for him. He was brave, patient and considerate of others to the end, which came at noon, Friday, April 29, 1938.

Dr. Wiese was one of the most ethical surgeons

(Continued on Page 528)

MEDICAL ECONOMICS

Edited by the Committee on Medical Economics
of the
Minnesota State Medical Association
W. F. Braasch, M.D., Chairman

State Meeting

The Minnesota State Medical Association was holding its 85th Annual Meeting at the Hotel Duluth in Duluth as this issue of MINNESOTA MEDICINE went to press.
See the August issue for a complete résumé of events of this meeting.

AT SAN FRANCISCO

It is probable that there were more interested lay spectators in all parts of the country than ever before when the House of Delegates of the American Medical Association met in San Francisco in June, 1938.

Since the eventful session of 1937 in Atlantic City, the celebrated controversy, so-called, between the American Medical Association and the Committee of Physicians with their 430 signers broke into the headlines. Medical policies and plans—once "caviar to the general"—abruptly became front page news, along with strikes, mobbings, elections.

The floodlight of publicity seldom reflects facts with anything like a scientific accuracy. The rank and file of physicians saw themselves aligned there with that quaint survival of another day, the "stand patter," and were naturally astonished and resentful.

It was natural too, perhaps, that the proposal made some time ago by which the physicians should organize and go into the propaganda business for themselves should gather momentum as a result.

Better Counsel

Fortunately, better counsel prevailed at San Francisco. The American Medical Association will not organize a bureau after the pattern of meat packing interests, the soap interests, the patent medicine interests, the liquor interests.

The spectacle of a publicity bureau financed by

doctors, complete with slogans, contact men, expense accounts and high powered advertising experts is unappetizing, still, to the majority of doctors. They have no skeleton to hide, no pork barrel to roll over. They want to take care of sick men to the best of their ability and they want to help well men to stay well. In the process, they wish to earn a sufficient income to provide for their families. Of the two objectives they are probably just a little more interested in taking care of the sick than they are in providing a livelihood—and that is a special distinction they hold over many other professional and business men.

Unnecessary Luxury

There seems to be very small reason for such men to indulge themselves in the modern luxury of a gigantic publicity bureau and advertising campaign.

The advantage to be gained, even in modern America, which operates to some extent through a nice balance, made up of horse trading and manipulation between pressure groups, would probably not be worth the effort. It might, in fact, produce a grave and unfortunate reaction and the expense involved would be terrific. In fact, the demand for funds for the new venture might well eat into the great services to the public for which doctors are justly proud—their machinery for protecting medical education, their great Councils, their public health education.

The resolution which rejected the proposal of three states was definite, though it suggested; by way of gesture, to those who clamored for a new relation to the public and press, that all spokesmen for organized medicine conduct themselves in the Latin phrase, with "suaviter in modo"; the same time, they maintained the absolute essential "fortitur in re." It passed without dissenting vote.

No Split in the Ranks

Thus, the American Medical Association emerged from the storm and stress of another year without the split predicted in the headlines by the 430 episode; and it is still firmly established, as to public policy, upon the foundation of the famous ten principles.

One of the ten points was modified, it is interesting to note, to disapprove the inclusion of the special medical services such as pathological examinations, x-ray work and anesthesia in group hospitalization contracts and providing for removal of hospitals from the association's approved list where either the public or the profession is exploited.

The large number of hospital insurance proposals now being promoted publicly and privately made a specific clarification on these points essential and desirable.

For a Department of Health

The Federal Department of Public Welfare included in the recent government reorganization bill was condemned from the start by the House of Delegates. In its place, the delegates at San Francisco again approved a cabinet department of health which should be directed by a medical man as secretary.

It was appropriate and essential that the delegates should point out specifically that they—and not the special societies or individuals anywhere —are the truly qualified representatives of medical practitioners in America and that their actions in San Francisco reflect the policies and beliefs of organized medicine in the United States. Members of the house who are affiliated with other special societies were urged to work toward a closer coöperation between all medical groups in the country.

Survey

Dr. W. F. Braasch of Rochester, chairman of the Minnesota State Medical Association's Committee on Medical Economics and also chairman of the American Medical Association's advisory committee on the current nationwide survey of medical facilities, presented an encouraging report to the delegates. This survey will lay the first sound foundation for changes where they may be found necessary in the current system of handling medical care for the indigent or the low income groups, and will be complete within the year, it is hoped. It will constitute a

great contribution on the part of American medicine to the social readjustments necessary to our time.

Members who visited the American Medical Association exhibit at Duluth found a complete progress report to date from Dr. R. G. Leland, director of the Bureau of Medical Economics of the American Medical Association, and in direct charge of the national survey.

Reëlection for another five years of Dr. C. B. Wright of Minneapolis to the Board of Trustees, of course, is gratifying to Minnesota.

ECONOMICALLY SPEAKING

[Monthly Editorial Prepared by The Medical Advisory Committee]

A survey of the present economic situation finds the business man generally viewing it with distrust. Everywhere dissatisfaction with today's set-up is apparent.

Many educators and parents are becoming resentful of the rather radical departure from the old fashioned teaching of the 4 R's and fundamental ABC's.

Ministers find a new alarm in the wandering away from the old time religion of our forefathers and a tendency in some nations to scoff at the teachings of the Church.

Lawyers view the promulgation of the totalitarian state with concern knowing that if the new tendency in thought is carried out, the law of the land may be that of the dictator.

Men of medicine see in the future possible abandonment of the patient-doctor relationship with all that it means, complete state controlled health service and its many possible dire results.

But your Medical Advisory Committee has noted with marked satisfaction during the last year a tendency for the approximate 2,500 members of our State Association to think more as a group than as individuals knowing that that which effects one effects all; that the malpractice cases are lessening in Minnesota, smaller verdicts are being obtained in courts, there are fewer professional testifiers in evidence. Our medical work is becoming more effective in the state, and we are better united with each other; therefore, the public is served better. Rural and urban lines are being eliminated.

Not Utopia as yet, but we are thankful for the few miles we have gained on the road to a better understanding. Your neighbor's trouble or success reflects on you and should be your concern. A good neighborly spirit makes for contentment.

MINNESOTA STATE BOARD OF MEDICAL EXAMINERS

Non-medical "Interne" Pleads Guilty to Practicing Medicine without a License

Re: State of Minnesota vs. Halsted.

(Photo courtesy of Minneapolis Star)

On June 1, 1938, Hugh David Halsted, twenty-six years of age, entered a plea of guilty in the District Court at Minneapolis, to an information charging him with practicing medicine without a license. Following a statement of facts to the Court, Judge Edward A. Montgomery, sentenced Halsted to one year in the Minneapolis Work House and placed him on probation for one year. On April 19, 1938, Halsted was tried before a military court at Fort Snelling on a charge of misrepresenting his rank as an officer and misrepresenting his qualifications as a physician. He pleaded guilty to both charges and was given a dismissal from the military service of the United States.

The investigation conducted by the Minnesota State Board of Medical Examiners, which resulted in the filing of a complaint against Halsted by Mr. Brist on behalf of the Board, disclosed that Halsted was born September 29, 1911, at Milwaukee, Wisconsin. Before moving to Minneapolis, in the summer of 1929, Halsted resided in Chicago, and Chattanooga, Tennessee, graduating from high school in the latter place. From 1930 to 1933, inclusive, Halsted was a truck driver for the Harriet Laundry in Minneapolis. For a short period in 1934, Halsted worked as a shoe salesman for Dayton's Department Store. Along in the late summer and early fall of 1934, he spent some spare time at the Minneapolis General Hospital. Halsted stated that he always had a desire to be a physician and this prompted him to "hang around" the Minneapolis General Hospital. From October 10, 1934 to January 1, 1935, Halsted acted as an interne at Minneapolis General Hospital, according to a letter written by Dr. C. E. Remy then superintendent. From January 1, 1935, to June 25, 1935, Halsted was an interne at $50.00 per month at the Deaconess Hospital in Minneapolis. When inquiry was made at Deaconess as to why no investigation had been made of Halsted's credentials as a physician, the explanation was given that Halsted had previously been at Minneapolis General, and they assumed his credentials were in order. On July 5, 1935, after fraudulently representing himself as a physician and a graduate of the medical school at Northwestern University, and that he was licensed to practice medicine in Illinois. Halsted signed a contract to act as contract surgeon for the CCC Camps in Minnesota. No investigation was made at that time by those in charge to ascertain Halsted's qualifications. He was assigned to Camp No. 703 at Schroeder, Minnesota. In October of that year he was transferred to Allen, Minnesota. During the winter of 1935 and 1936 he was at Camp No. 724 at Bay, Minnesota. In the spring of 1936 he was transferred to Two Harbors, and subsequently to Rochester and Fort Snelling. In September, 1935, Halsted received a commission as a first lieutenant in the Medical

Reserve Corps of the United States Army. This commission was obtained upon his fraudulent representations with respect to his medical training.

In September, 1937, Halsted "promoted" himself to a Captaincy in the Medical Reserve Corps. Following his marriage in 1936, Halsted was paid $262.00 per month by the Government. In February, 1938, inquiry was made concerning Halsted's qualifications as a physician which led to his court martial on April 19th. The only medical education that Halsted ever received was in the Extension Division of the University of Minnesota in the year 1930-1931, at which time he was enrolled in a class in General Inorganic Chemistry. In the school year 1931-1932, he was enrolled again in a similar extension course and the records indicate that he failed.

This case again emphasizes the necessity of more care being exercised by hospitals in Minnesota in the selection of their internes. Halsted violated the Medical Practice Act of Minnesota while he was at Minneapolis General, at the Deaconess Hospital and in the CCC Camps. At no time, during his career, did he have any right to represent himself as a physician and surgeon, nor to assume to act in that capacity. Judge Montgomery, in passing sentence, remarked that he did not understand how Halsted got by as long as he did. While he was at Fort Snelling, Halsted resided at 2284 Highland Parkway, St. Paul; at the time of his arrest he resided at 4039 Pillsbury Avenue, Minneapolis.

Minneapolis Drug Addict Sentenced to Ten-year Term for Obtaining Morphine by Misrepresentation

Re: State of Minnesota vs. Kathrine Burkhardt.

On June 8, 1938, Kathrine Burkhardt, 36 years of age, entered a plea of guilty to an information charging her with obtaining morphine by fraud, deceit, misrepresentation and subterfuge. She was sentenced by the Honorable Edward A. Montgomery, Judge of the District Court at Minneapolis, for a term of not to exceed 10 years in the Women's Reformatory at Shakopee.

The defendant, a drug addict, is the first person to be prosecuted under the Minnesota Uniform Narcotic Drug Act for obtaining morphine by fraud or misrepresentation. This law was passed in 1937 by the Minnesota Legislature and provides, among other things, as follows:

"Sec. 18. Restrictions on obtaining drugs.

(1) No person shall obtain or attempt to obtain a narcotic drug, or procure or attempt to procure the administration of a narcotic drug, (a) by fraud, deceit, misrepresentation, or subterfuge; or (b) by the forgery or alteration of a prescription or of any written order; or (c) by the concealment of a material fact; or (d) by the use of a false name or the giving of a false address.

(2) Information communicated to a physician in an effort unlawfully to procure a narcotic drug, or unlawfully to procure the administration of any such drug, shall not be deemed a privileged communication."

The maximum penalty for a violation of the Act is 5 years imprisonment in a state penal institution. The defendant in this case received a 10-year sentence because she had two prior convictions for felonies in the United States District Court.

The Minnesota State Board of Medical Examiners was asked to coöperate with the Federal Bureau of Narcotics at Minneapolis in the prosecution of this case. The facts indicated that the defendant was a addict and between March 26, 1938, and May 30, 1938, had obtained 19 prescriptions for a total of 233¼ grain morphine sulphate tablets from six Minneapolis physicians. She obtained these prescriptions by misrepresenting her physical condition and falsifying her name and her address. On being questioned by Judge Montgomery, the defendant stated that she was raised at Wabasha, Minnesota, and that her true maiden name was Katherine Mahoney; that her married name was Burkhardt and that she was divorced in 1926. She stated that she had been addicted to the use of morphine for the past 16 years. On being questioned by Judge Montgomery with respect to her physical condition she stated that she suffered from chronic asthma: that she had a tumor on her spine and that she suffered from adhesions following an operation. The defendant gave her true address as 1155-15th Avenue S. E., Minneapolis, where she resided with a sister.

The defendant used many aliases in obtaining these prescriptions, among them being the names of Barnes, Berg, Varnes, Fairchilds, Johnson and Peschkie. In 1933, the defendant was sentenced by Judge Nordbye in the Federal Court in Minneapolis, to a three year term in the Federal Industrial Institution for Women at Alderson, West Virginia. This sentence was imposed for a violation of the Harrison Narcotic Act. In 1936, the defendant was sentenced by Judge Joyce in the Federal Court at St. Paul for a 10 months term in the Minneapolis Work House for a similar offense. The defendant also was in the Minneapolis Work House on four different occasions for vagrancy and once for the unlawful possession of morphine, in addition to the foregoing sentences in Federal Court.

The Minnesota State Board of Medical Examiners wishes to express its appreciation of the fine coöperation displayed in this case by the Federal Bureau of Narcotics in Minneapolis under the supervision of Mr. Harry D. Smith, and also the fine coöperation shown by Mr. Ed J. Goff, County Attorney, and his assistants Mr. Peter S. Neilson and Mr. Allen T. Rorem. The Medical Board believes that the enforcement of this particular provision of the Minnesota Uniform Narcotic Drug Law will greatly reduce the number of addicts who go about this state and attempt to procure morphine from one physician after another for the sole purpose of satisfying their craving for narcotics. The Medical Board wishes again to particularly caution the medical profession against furnishing or prescribing narcotics for these addicts. Most of them will not submit to a physical examination nor do they want to be hospitalized. The Medical Board feels that the imposition of a few more sentences like the one in this case, will go a long way toward solving this problem. There can be no question but what these persons need medical treatment and hospitalization, but it goes without saying that their addiction cannot be removed in a period of a few months.

ORALSULIN

No oral insulin preparation has been accepted by the Council on Pharmacy and Chemistry. Over eleven years ago *The Journal*, in discussing "Enterocap Oralsulin," (Dec. 4, 1926, p. 1935), pointed out the lack of evidence for the efficiency of orally administered preparations of insulin and pancreas. No new evidence has been found to necessitate a revision of the statement published at that time. Recently the federal authorities charged with the enforcement of the Food and Drug Act seized a shipment of Enterocap Oralsulin and declared the product adulterated and misbranded. According to the government report, examination showed that the preparation contained no insulin and that the labeling bore false and fraudulent representations regarding the curative or therapeutic effects of the product (Notice of Judgment 27373). No products of Lafayette Pharmacal, Inc., stand accepted by the Council on Pharmacy and Chemistry. (J.A.M.A., May 28, 1938, p. 1858.)

OF GENERAL INTEREST

Dr. Floyd F. Clark, who has practiced in Duluth for more than thirty years, is a candidate for county coroner.

* * *

Dr. Hamilton Montgomery of Rochester recently addressed the Chicago Dermatological Society, of which he is president.

* * *

Dr. C. B. Wright of Minneapolis was reëlected a member of the Board of Trustees of the American Medical Association at the convention in San Francisco.

* * *

Dr. Jere W. Annis (Minn. '35), for the past three years a fellow in medicine at the Mayo Foundation, has located in Lakeland, Florida, where he will practice internal medicine.

* * *

Dr. William Musfelt of San Diego, California, has finished his graduate course at the U. S. Veterans facility of Minneapolis, and has been transferred to Camp Custer, Mich.

* * *

Dr. W. R. Kostick is now located in Fertile, with offices over the Fox Theatre. Dr. and Mrs. Kostick and baby daughter moved to Fertile from Robbinsdale, where the doctor had formerly practiced.

* * *

The bill which was pending before Congress providing for a new building for the Army Medical Library and Museum, of which editorial mention was made in the June number of MINNESOTA MEDICINE, was passed by Congress and the building provided for.

* * *

Dr. L. J. Leonard of Minneapolis, who recently filed as candidate for Hennepin County coroner, is one of the few men in the United States who is both a practicing attorney and physician, and the only one in the Northwest licensed to practice both medicine and law.

* * *

Dr. Robert Leighton, Jr., a graduate of the University of Minnesota, who served his internship at Minneapolis General Hospital, on June 1 became associated in the practice of medicine and surgery with Dr. W. F. Cantwell of International Falls.

* * *

Dr. G. B. Cross and family have left Hills, where they have lived for seven years, and moved to Lakeville, where Dr. Cross will be affiliated with the hospital at Farmington, as well as taking care of the practice at Lakeville.

* * *

The marriage of Miss Rose Jessen of Saint Paul and Dr. Maurice C. Rousseau, son of Dr. and Mrs. Victor Rousseau of Maple Lake, took place on June 18. Dr. Rousseau is a graduate of the medical school of the University of Minnesota, and his bride is a graduate of the St. Joseph's School of Nursing.

Dr. R. A. Murray of Hibbing took over the practice of Dr. S. Z. Kerlan of Aitkin, the latter part of June. Dr. Murray has been associated with Dr. J. R. Manley of Duluth. Dr. and Mrs. Kerlan have left for California, where their son, Robert, will enter the University of California this fall.

*

Dr. F. J. Hirschboeck of Duluth, program chairman; Dr. Charles N. Hensel of Saint Paul, president; and Dr. M. H. Hoffman of Saint Paul, secretary-treasurer, were in charge of the program for the semi-annual meeting of the Minnesota Society of Internal Medicine held in Duluth on June 4. The meeting was attended by fifty medical men from all sections of the state.

* * *

Dr. Archie Nissen has been appointed Assistant Superintendent of the St. Peter Hospital, succeeding Dr. Ralph Rossen, who was recently named Superintendent of the Hastings State Hospital. Dr. Nissen is a graduate of the University of Minnesota School of Medicine, where he specialized in psychiatry, and later did graduate work. He has served for the past two years on the medical staff of the St. Peter Hospital.

Among other similar courses offered at various centers in the state during May, an all-day postgraduate course in the care of mothers and babies was given at Worthington. The course was arranged under the auspices of the State Department of Health, the University of Minnesota, and the Minnesota State Medical Association with Dr. A. J. Chesley, secretary of the department of health, and Dr. E. C. Hartley, director of the division of child hygiene, in charge. The faculty for the course included Dr. Rae T. LaVake, Dr. Samuel B. Solhaug, Dr. Edgar J. Huenekens and Dr. Irvine McQuarrie of Minneapolis. Such gatherings are financed by the social security funds granted for the purpose to the state department of health.

* * *

Attendants at the American Medical Association convention in San Francisco in June were Drs. W. F. Braasch, H. H. Bowing, J. F. Wier, B. E. Hempstead and F. J. Heck, C. F. Dixon, and Waltman Walters, all of Rochester, Minnesota.

Dr. Braasch is a member of the House of Delegates of the Association and took part in the program of the American Board of Urology. Dr. Bowing addressed the meeting of the Los Angeles Cancer Society, and spoke both before the meeting of the A.M.A. and the meeting of the American Radium Society. Dr. Heck spoke before the A.M.A. meeting and also at the meeting of the American Society of Clinical Pathologists. After speaking before the section on surgery of the A.M.A., Dr. Walters went on to Vancouver, B. C., to deliver a series of talks at the summer school of the Vancouver Medical Association.

REPORTS and
ANNOUNCEMENTS

MEDICAL BROADCAST FOR JULY

The Minnesota State Medical Association Morning Health Service.

The Minnesota State Medical Association broadcasts weekly at 9:45 o'clock every Saturday morning over Station WCCO, Minneapolis and Saint Paul (810 kilocycles or 370.2 meters).

Speaker: William A. O'Brien, Associate Professor of Pathology and Preventive Medicine, Medical School, University of Minnesota. The program for the month will be as follows:

July 2—Artificial Respiration.
July 9—Body Temperature Regulations.
July 16—Summer Complaint.
July 23—Art of Relaxation.
July 30—Teething.

AMERICAN CONGRESS OF PHYSICAL THERAPY

An intensive course in physical therapy will be held September 7-10, 1938, at the Palmer House, Chicago, just preceding the 17th annual convention of the Congress of Physical Therapy. The course will consist of lectures, conferences, clinics and demonstrations arranged primarily for physicians but open to a limited number of technicians properly sponsored. Applications should be sent to the Congress headquarters, 30 N. Michigan Avenue, Chicago. Upon acceptance, a fee of $25.00 will be required.

EAST CENTRAL MINNESOTA SOCIETY

The East Central Minnesota Medical Society met at Pokegama Sanatorium at Pine City on May 27, 1938. Dr. Walter P. Gardner, Anoka, and Dr. Edward J. Coffman, Anoka, were accepted as transfers into this society.

Dinner was served and in the evening a scientific program was presented by guest speakers. Dr. O. H. Wangensteen discussed thoracic surgery and a discussion of his subject was presented by Dr. D. Greth Gardiner. Dr. R. E. Hultkrans spoke on "Chronic Low Back Pain" and Dr. Stewart Shimonek followed with a short discussion of this subject.

SCOTT-CARVER SOCIETY

At the annual meeting of the Scott-Carver Medical Society held at Mudbaden, June 14, Dr. C. A. Stewart, of Minneapolis, spoke on "Dietary and Nutritional Problems in Pediatrics."

The following officers were elected for the coming year:

President—Dr. Earl Crow, Arlington
Vice President—Dr. Harold Havel, Jordan
Secretary-Treasurer—Dr. B. F. Pearson, Shakopee
Delegate—Dr. C. F. Cervenka, New Prague
Alternate—Dr. J. C. Klein, Shakopee
Censor—Dr. Alvin Westerman, Montgomery

PROCEEDINGS of the MINNESOTA ACADEMY OF MEDICINE

Meeting of April 13, 1938

The regular monthly meeting of the Minnesota Academy of Medicine was held at the Town and Country Club on Wednesday evening, April 13, 1938. Dinner was served at 7 o'clock and the meeting was called to order at 8:15 by the president, Dr. R. T. LaVake.

There were fifty-seven members and two guests present.

Minutes of the March meeting were read and approved.

Dr. H. E. Hullsiek read the Necrology Committee's Memorial to Dr. John T. Rogers, and a motion was carried that it be spread upon the records of the Academy and a copy sent to the family.

JOHN THOMAS ROGERS*
1867-1938

The Civil War was in every sense a social revolution. Through the sweep of the conflict the planting aristocracy of the South was as completely ruined as were the clergy and the nobility during the French Revolution. The very economic foundations of the planting system, including slavery itself, were destroyed.

Even before the unrest associated with the freeing of the slaves, the South had at no time a static population, and to the migrating groups Kentucky had ever added her share. Beginning with the settlement by Daniel Boone in 1775, through its admission to statehood in 1792, and up to 1890, it had been first an outpost, and finally a point of departure for those seeking fortune elsewhere. By 1880 it was no longer frontier, but a great commonwealth with thousands of prosperous citizens. Still the blue-grass state annually sent out many who could not resist the beckoning will-o-the-wisp of fortune. The last great migration occurred between 1880 and 1890. This exodus was the result of the moral and material disintegration incident to the great war. In this decade 50,000 souls left the state which, during its history, furnished the rest of the Union with some twenty governors, many senators, attorney-generals, justices, and other high officials. It was at this time that the Rogers family left Kentucky for Minnesota.

William Edward Rogers was born at Cane Ridge, Bourbon County, Kentucky, on August 12, 1835. On June 10, 1857, he married Margaret Vernon, descendant of Jacob Spears, revolutionary soldier. The fifth of their eight children was John Thomas Rogers, born July 18, 1867, at Versailles, Kentucky.

There is nothing to indicate that John Rogers' childhood was in any way different from that of any son of a comfortably landed proprietor of the South. However, before he was far on his way to manhood, the aftermath of the great civil strife descended with a

vengeance and, like so many others, William Rogers sought fortune elsewhere. It is not strange that in 1886 he chose Minnesota.

St. Paul was in its first exuberant flush of youth. The population was 110,000; it claimed 864 manufacturing establishments, while 18,000 persons and 142 trains passed through the union station daily. The Robert Street bridge and that to Dayton's Bluff were being built; 3,573 buildings of various types had been completed that year; and the city was served by thirty-five newspapers and periodicals. As a further mark of progress, it was noted that already some of the horsecars had been powered with cables.

The Rogers settled in St. Paul after a brief sojourn in the Dakotas. Young John was left in Louisville to complete his studies at Transylvania University, after which he joined them. The first note of him in this hustling and rather awe-inspiring city of French, Germans, and Irish from down river, is a listing in the St. Paul directory for 1887. Rogers, John—clerk for W. E. Rogers, real estate, 42 Globe Building—boards with W. E. Rogers, Chatsworth & Owasco.* How long he was employed by his father is not definitely known, and for some time he clerked in a haberdashery on Robert Street. Both of these positions were temporary and it apparently was not until he met Dr. Charles A. Wheaton that plans for his future were crystallized. Neither is it known in what manner he met Dr. Wheaton, but it probably was as a patient since he was sent to Brainerd at the instigation of Dr. Wheaton, with a note to a friend of the doctor's, remaining in the north woods six weeks. It might easily have been otherwise, since his father's office and the doctor's were but a block apart.

In 1888 he is living with his family in St. Anthony Park, and is a student with the firm of Wheaton and MacLaren. Dr. Wheaton at this time lived at 351 Washington Avenue, facing Rice Park, some three blocks from his office. Coming to St. Paul in 1877, he was well established in practice and was one of the northwest's surgical leaders. Young John helped about the office, read in the doctor's extensive library, and made himself generally useful. He assisted at operations, slept in the office and, in the absence of telephones, answered the night-bell, notifying Dr. Wheaton and driving him on calls.

In 1881 the St. Paul Medical College had taken into its faculty certain Minneapolis men, had moved to Minneapolis, and became the Minnesota College Hospital. In 1885 the St. Paul members resigned and again started the St. Paul Medical School, while the Minnesota College Hospital reorganized and became the Minnesota Hospital College. In 1888 the St. Paul Medical School and the Minneapolis institution surrendered their charters and became the College of Medicine and Surgery of the University of Minnesota,

---

*Memorial to Dr. John T. Rogers, read at the regular meeting of the Minnesota Academy of Medicine, on April 13, 1938

*Now Fairmount Avenue.

with a faculty of twenty-nine and Perry Millard as dean. The course of lectures consisted of three years of six months each, and it was here that John Rogers began his medical education in the fall of 1888. Living in St. Anthony Park, he took the Great Northern train at Merriam Park each morning and rode to the 10th street bridge. Here he got off and crossed the river to the medical school which was on 6th street, across the street from the old St. Barnabas' hospital.

. Now for the first time were felt the tremors of the impending social and economic upheavals that were to mark the end of an epoch, that of the end of the period of free land—the last of the frontier. The post-war deflation had set in and the Rogers family had not been long enough in the new surroundings to have become well-established in business. John's father and brother, Nat, were in the stock business at South St. Paul, but with little surplus money left for medical studies. His arrangement with Dr. Wheaton not only was an opportunity to observe the practice of medicine and surgery first-hand, but was important from an economic standpoint as well. The financial status of the young aristocrat from the south was at times a sore burden.

One of the many stories he told to the writer dealt with the time when, because of well-worn shoes, he found himself wellnigh walking on the ground. His chief, affluent and a smart dresser, had noted this and caused a pair to be made, ostensibly for himself, but actually to John's measure. He brought them to the youth apologetically, saying that they did not fit him, and wondered if the young man might wear them, since it seemed a shame to allow them to be wasted. To quote Dr. Rogers, "Doctor, I was a proud young fool, I was extremely humiliated. That night when I walked across the bridge on the way to dissect I dropped the shoes into the river. I borrowed two dollars from a classmate and bought a pair of very fine shoes with paper soles." He told Dr. Wheaton the others had been stolen. I have heard Dr. Rogers repeat this story many times, with considerable amusement. It is an evidence of the fierce pride which, tempered by experience and maturity, was so great an asset in later years, and which so often enabled him to hold fast to what he felt was right.

Assisting at operations both in and out of the city —these were the days of weekend excursions to smaller cities with hospital facilities, and included turkey-shoots, banquets, poker-games, and Sunday morning surgical field-days—answering the office night-bell, driving Dr. Wheaton, dissecting evenings, spending the summer of the final year at the City Hospital, thus went the three years of from 1888 to 1891.

In 1891 President Harrison's difficulties with restless labor were beginning. The populist party was organized, great talk went on of gold and silver, the slogan "16 to 1" was mouthed about, falling wheat prices brought ruin of thousands, and on the streets of Chicago a curious crowd watched a vehicle which rolled along with no horse attached to it. In the realm of medicine, Witzel was performing his first gastrostomy, Quincke introduced spinal puncture, Bier brought out

his hyperemia, a general aseptic ritual for surgery was standardized, and for the first time Halsted announced the use of rubber gloves. With this year came the end of John Rogers' first struggle for a foothold in the practice of medicine. His hardest days were behind him. Licensed to practice on April 10, 1891, and graduated in June of the same year, he is now a full-fledged physician associated with two of the best known men in the city, Dr. Charles Wheaton and Dr. Archibald MacLaren. He has left the family home; probably to be nearer his work, and is living at the Seville Flats.

Those who know him are acquainted with his meticulous methods in the matter of records and correspondence. It is questionable whether John Rogers ever ended a day's work without having completed his records and attended to his correspondence. Thus it is not surprising to find in a small pocket diary (an advertisement by the Maltine Company), careful notes of his first patients. He graduated in June, 1891, and what is probably the record of his first private patient appears on the page for June 12th, as follows: Wm. Swab—bartender—incised wound of forearm made by dirty knife—treatment: wound scrubbed with 1/2000 bichloride—iodoform dusted on—wound sutured with catgut—no inflammation.

. On July 16th occurs the following: Dutchman—porter in saloon—got in row with waitress who stabbed him in buttock with butcher-knife. Wound three inches deep, very painful, bleeding profusely. Treatment: irrigation with 1/1000 bichloride, one silkworm suture, iodoform gauze. Union by first intention.

Apparently his first operation was a tonsillectomy. On September 20th this appears: Morris J.—Tonsillectomy. Enlarged and frequently inflamed tonsils—both removed under cocaine—no pain—little hemorrhage—no attack several months afterwards. On January 5, 1892, a cervical repair, and in February a breast abscess. In April a fractured clavicle and in June a mastoid abscess, described as follows: Baby T., 6 months old. History unsatisfactory. Had been scarlet fever in home but baby had not taken it. Did well for two weeks when it began to bleed after a dressing. Local doctor called but it didn't succeed with acid—I saw child 48 hours afterward almost in collapse—still bleeding—applied compress—administered whiskey—hot applications to body—recovered.

And so the record goes, with careful notes, comments, his own explanations of failure to get desired results—on through 1892—an abscess of the femur, another mastoid, in October of that year the first of a remarkable—for that time—series of ectopic pregnancies, described with great detail and occupying two pages of small script, a repair of a cervix and perineum. On February 29th of this year, John Rogers joined the Ramsey County Medical Society.

At the age of 26 years, on April 4, 1894, he read his inaugural thesis before the Minnesota Academy of Medicine, entitled, "The Use of Wet Dressings and Poultices in Surgery." In this paper he cites his success with 1/3000 hot bichloride of mercury solution used as a wet dressing, as a substitute for the still-popular flaxseed poultice, which he condemns. He states that a recent communication from one of the men at Johns Hopkins says that flaxseed poultices are still used in that institution in cases of stitch abscess. He ends by saying, "I believe the day is not far distant when adequate incisions will be small ones, large drainage tubes will be entirely dispensed with, and irrigations unnecessary." A bold statement for 1894!

By this time his case-book includes such operations as excision of the superior maxilla, extra-uterine gestation, repair of crushed foot, mastoid abscess, suture of tendons, amputation of leg, varicocele, pyosalpinx, curettage, appendicitis, hemorrhoids, pelvic abscess, varicose veins, hysterectomies, anal fistula, Dupuytran's contraction, compound fractures, hernia, amputation at the thigh, osteomyelitis, and others. A widely varied surgical practice for a young man four years after graduation.

In June, 1895, he was appointed Clinical Instructor in Diseases of Children at the University of Minnesota. On June 20th of that year he read before the Gynecological Section of the Minnesota State Medical Society the first of his papers on ectopic gestation, with a report of sixteen surgically-treated cases.

Considering that it was but six years since Tait had published his work on extra-uterine gestation, it is again an evidence of the young doctor's progressive spirit when he says he believes that this condition "could and should be diagnosed before rupture in a large majority of cases." He states that if the operation be in the hands of experts and the patient operated upon before rupture, the mortality should not be greater than 2 per cent. This number of cases was unusual for the time, and called forth a rebuke from a surgeon in an eastern clinic attended by Dr. Rogers. The young surgeon had taken part in the discussion following an operation for ectopic pregnancy, mentioning his experience and that of his colleagues in St. Paul. The eastern surgeon apparently felt that the young man from the raw middlewest was overstepping the bounds and remarked witheringly that if these doctors had sixteen such cases there must be very uncommon women in St. Paul. Dr. Rogers had the better of it. He took great glee in his reply, which was to the effect that the women in St. Paul were in no way unusual, but it was possible that the doctors were.

In 1897 he published a paper on the operative treatment of tumors of the upper jaw, and in May of that year was appointed Clinical Instructor in Surgery at the University of Minnesota. It was also in this year that he and Dr. A. B. Stewart of Owatonna were sent as delegates to the meeting of the American Medical Association in Philadelphia, one being certified to attend the International Medical Congress in Moscow. They left St. Paul in May, sailed on the City of Rome, arriving in Edinburgh on June 16th, after two or three days in Glasgow.

Here they took courses in practical pathology, morbid anatomy with Alexander Bruce, and had the run of the Surgeon's hall and the Royal Infirmary. In July they left Edinburgh on bicycles for Vienna by way of Dublin, London, Paris, Lausanne, Berlin and Prague, arriving after a six-week's trip. In Vienna

they settled down for several months of study. They took courses in pathology, special dissection, general medicine, gynecology, and a course in blood disease with technic of staining specimens. Dr. Stewart says in a recent letter, "John was a diligent student and a delightful traveling companion. I learned much with him and from him."

Changes have occurred in the firm in the past three years. In 1897 it became Wheaton, Wheaton and Dennis, John Rogers having left January 1, 1897, to practice alone at 145 Lowry Building. Bob Wheaton having died suddenly in 1898, the firm became Wheaton, Rogers and Dennis.

In June of that year Dr. Rogers presented before the State Society a paper on contused wounds of the abdomen and their surgical treatment. Here he makes a plea for early recognition of intra-abdominal injuries resulting from contusions, emphasizing the point that this condition had not been adequately dealt with in the literature, which he says is "incomplete and unsatisfactory in its treatment of this condition." He hopes to create more interest in this type of serious injury, leading to further study and more frequent reports of cases, since, as he says, ". . . the advances in modern surgery have made it possible to explore the abdomen with impunity and almost with safety." In the year 1901 Dr. Rogers was elected President of the Minnesota Academy of Medicine.

It is now 1902. The Spanish-American war has come and gone with its scandals and profiteering, the beginning of the Roosevelt ascendency, and the beginning and end of the United States' short-lived fervor for foreign expansion. John Rogers is now associated with Dr. Wheaton, the firm name being Wheaton and Rogers. Reading papers at meetings, giving talks in and out of the city, participating in both development of the education and economic side of medicine as well as the purely scientific, he was adding rapidly, through ability as well as personality, to what had already become a large following. Two more papers on ectopic gestation, one reporting twenty cases, both plead for earlier diagnosis and proper treatment, showed that when John Rogers believed himself to be right the chips might fall where they would. He handled without gloves those who, he felt, through failure to grow with medical science were failing in their duty. A paper written on cancer of the breast, one read at the Academy on surgical cases, immobilization of the lower jaw, and one on tumors of the upper jaw and their operative treatment had appeared. The last mentioned was written six years after graduation, and reported several personal cases.

In 1903 the firm became Wheaton, Rogers and Gilfillan, with offices at 170 Lowry Arcade, and in 1905 Wheaton, Rogers and Colvin. During these years we find Dr. Rogers appearing before assemblies with papers on such subjects as tuberculosis of the kidney, differential diagnosis of gallstones, surgery of the bileducts, surgical treatment of the gallbladder, gunshot injuries of the brain, gastric ulcer, intussusception. One article, entitled, "The Health Instinct," appeared in *Popular Science Monthly.*

During this, the gilded age in American scientific,

economic and social development, with revolution occurring with disturbing frequency in all branches of thought, John Rogers was not only an interested onlooker but an enthusiastic participant. The progress in science, the frequency of innovation in medical and surgical circles, the swiftness with which yesterday's beliefs were cast aside for today's, were staggering, and taxed one to keep abreast. Dr. Rogers' writings through these years show not only an attempt to do so, but a reasonable success.

The volume of surgery done in those days by any one or a group of surgeons is worth noting. At the time under discussion more of the work of this group was done at St. Luke's Hospital than at other institutions. We know that it was not all confined to one institution, and also that there were the above-mentioned weekend excursions to smaller towns, with operations on Sundays. Yet, in one of these years, over a hundred patients were operated upon by this firm at St. Joseph's Hospital. During the years from 1880 to the early 1900's much of the surgery from Minnesota to the West coast was done in the Twin Cities, as is shown in the variety of the cases. No one city could have furnished certain rather uncommon types of cases in such numbers as the records show.

Dr. Wheaton, having retired by 1912, the firm became Rogers and Colvin. At this time the City Hospital staff was reorganized with Dr. Rogers as chief. When the American College of Surgeons was founded in 1913 he was one of the founders. In January of this year he became Assistant Professor of Surgery at the University of Minnesota; and, in 1914, he married Lillian Hallam Cooley, making a European trip as his honeymoon. In 1914 he was president of the Minnesota State Medical Association. In his presidential address he dealt with such subjects as the liquor question, medical licensure, legislation, medical defense and expert testimony, ending with a discussion of the then burning question of medical education and the Medical School. Here again, his remarks show a refusal to compromise with what he believed to be wrong. In 1915 the Rogers-Colvin partnership was dissolved and Harry Zimmermann entered Dr. Rogers' office as surgical assistant, the firm becoming Rogers and Zimmermann. In 1916 he was made Associate Professor of Surgery.

Through all these years, the seed of an idea was growing in the mind of one of St. Paul's pioneer business men, the development of which was to be of untold benefit to those less favored than himself. This man was Charles T. Miller, erstwhile clerk for J. J. Hill and one-time partner of W. F. Davidson in the steamboat business. It had long been Mr. Miller's wish that a hospital be built and named for the one whom he held in such high regard and esteem—John Rogers. Dr. Rogers refused to accede to this wish, insisting that the hospital be named for its donor. Mr. Miller died without having carried out his plan, but it was periodically discussed by his widow and Dr. Rogers. When she died several years later, she made a bequest of $1,400,000 for the building and equipping of a hospital, a board of trustees being named at the

522

same time. The sole stipulation was that there were to be fifty free beds, with no distinction as to color, race or creed. Dr. Rogers was named chairman of the board.

In 1917 a site was purchased and plans drawn for a hospital of 150 beds. According to the estimates made at the time, this could be built for $400,000, leaving $1,000,000 for a maintenance endowment. In the months intervening between the planning and the actual time of construction, the war had forced building costs so high that it was seen that the building as planned could not be erected and equipped and the endowment left intact. It was thus decided to postpone the building to a more favorable time, and allow the fund to grow.

Meanwhile, we had entered the war. In the summer of 1918, Surgeon General Gorgas arrived in St. Paul on a tour of the country in search of hospital facilities for American soldiers soon to return from France. After examining the Miller Hospital plans he advised the Board that if they would increase the number of beds to 250 and complete the structure, the government would take it over for a term of years. Patriotism and expediency finally caused the Board to accept this offer. The contract was let, construction rushed, and by the fall of 1918 the building was well under way.

In November 1918 came the armistice. With neither warning nor explanation, a telegram arrived unqualifiedly cancelling the afore-mentioned offer. The Board now found itself in a difficult position. It was obvious that the increased size of the hospital, together with still high construction costs, would leave little of the endowment fund for maintenance. After months of effort and after finally believing their troubles to be over, the Board suddenly found themselves, through a combination of circumstances, in a worse situation than before. Insurance, fire-protection, interest, heating, and other costs were mounting alarmingly. Permission was finally obtained from the court to use the endowment fund for the completion of the building, which was finished in November, 1920.

In order that the hospital might open, it was necessary to borrow, for the purpose of equipment, approximately $150,000. This was accordingly done, and the hospital opened its doors to the first patient on December 1, 1920.

The Charles T. Miller Hospital was not named for John Rogers, but those of us who know him realize that it is as much a monument to the dogged persistence, untiring effort, and almost fanatic devotion to an ideal, of one who was carrying out the wishes of a friend, as though the institution were named for him. It is safe to say that the only time in his life that John Rogers incurred the displeasure of anyone, was during the planning and building of this hospital, and then only because he held out against any and all influences which in his mind might in any way obstruct the furtherance of a great project. Fortunately, it was but a short time before all ill-feeling toward Dr. Rogers and the Miller Hospital was dissipated. From the time of its inception to the time of his death, John Rogers made the Miller Hospital his one thought. His complete success is shown, I believe, in the fact that in no year since its opening has the hospital cared for less than 1,000 free patients, reaching a high mark of 1,775 in 1937.

From the several months of conferences with his confrères who were eventually to be financially responsible for the hospital's opening, came the idea of an association to practice medicine in a group. From this grew the Miller Hospital Clinic which was organized in 1922 and continued for the practice of medicine and the training of younger men until it was dissolved in 1934.

In looking back over my years of association with Dr. Rogers, I should say there were, of his many good qualities, three that were outstanding. The one obvious to all was, of course, his great personal charm, which instilled in those meeting him for the first time a feeling of respect and trust. The second, and not so obvious, was his tremendous capacity for work, with apparently little effort. John Rogers had a powerful physique, one which most of his life enabled him to outdo physically not only his contemporaries, but often younger men. As a woodsman he was indefatigable. His hunting partners for thirty years will testify to this. It was well known to his associates that he could do twice as much work as most, see an astonishing number of patients, and at the same time give the impression of being quite at leisure. At any time he was ready and willing to help with another's problem, be he intern, nurse, doctor, or friend—for John Rogers was interested in people. And, lastly, he was honest.

Had Dr. Rogers neither prescription-pad nor scalpel, I believe he could still have accomplished more for ailing humanity than many physicians. He had the very rare and precious quality which enabled him to do for a patient the one thing that a patient wants done when he consults a doctor—that of being made to feel better. Meeting and talking to John Rogers had that effect. Samuel Bard said one hundred years ago—"The physician who confines his attention to the body knows not the extent of his art. If he knows not how to soothe the irritation of a troubled and enfeebled mind, to calm the fretfulness of impatience, to rouse the courage of the timid, and even to quiet the compunction of an over-tender conscience, it will very much confine the efficacy of his prescriptions; and these he cannot do, without he gain the confidence, esteem, and even the love of his patients." I know of no one having incorporated in his makeup to a greater extent these qualities than had John Rogers.

The last three years of his life he was far from well. Following the death of his wife he was beset with evils of body as well as spirit. He had the misfortune to break his leg and was confined for some time. A year ago he had a rather severe gastric hemorrhage, which he feared might be of malignant origin, but which was later proven not to be. He refused to cease entirely seeing patients although he spent increasingly more time away from his office. But a year ago he made a world tour with his daughter. He had been about as usual and the news of his sudden death from heart failure came as a surprise on January 2, 1938.

In the year 1755 a little girl walked with her mother

along a London street. Jostled to one side and being too tiny to see, she complained to her mother. The occasion was the passing of Samuel Johnson and some friends along the narrow sidewalks of Temple Bar. "Hush, child," said the mother to the little one, "a great man has passed by."

———

Upon ballot the following men were elected as candidates for membership in the Academy:

Dr. Albert Snell, Rochester, Associate Member.

Dr. Gilbert Thomas, Minneapolis, Active Member.

It was decided to have a non-scientific summer meeting at the country home of Dr. Archa Wilcox, and that Dr. Wilcox and a selected committee should decide just when the meeting is to be held.

The scientific program followed.

———

SPINA BIFIDA CYSTICA OF THE PELVIS

Diagnosis and Surgical Treatment

ALFRED W. ADSON, M.D.

Rochester, Minnesota

(See page 468, this issue)

Discussion

DR. F. C. RODDA, Minneapolis: We have had the following experience. Operation for the repair of spina bifida in infants two to four months of age, in which the hydrocephalus seemed to be quiescent, has been followed by a very sharp and rapid increase in the size of the head. On the other hand, where the operation has been delayed until the child has reached the age of ten or twelve months, we have not had this difficulty. It would appear as though the sac acted as a sort of safety valve in the early months of life. I should like to ask Dr. Adson if that is a factor in his selection of a nine months' age limit.

DR. F. R. WRIGHT, Minneapolis: What is the general outlook as to prognosis of these cases? Do they recover and make physiologically healthy individuals, or do they recover just sufficiently to be taken care of by somebody else?

DR. ARNOLD SCHWYZER, Saint Paul: I rise to discuss this paper because Dr. Wright has asked the question as to whether these patients are any good afterward. I saw, a few weeks ago, a man who came in with his mother who was sick. She said, "You know, I think some twenty-three or twenty-four years ago you operated on our baby. This fellow here is that baby." In this case there was a large meningocele in the upper cervical region, and this young man was a regular giant in size and strength. His neck showed a somewhat irregular scar. The worst forms are the myeloceles where the whole medullary canal is open. Inside of the edge of skin there is the zona serosa and, in the center a granular looking surface, the medullary tissue. In the median line above and below, one can see a little dimple which represents the entrance to the medullary canal. I have operated on two such cases, but there is not great opportunity to do much for the condition. Both babies lived, but the paralysis of the lower extremities persisted. The cord lies open in the center. For a couple of days before operation we try to get the area clean by using saline irrigations and a salicylic acid solution. Then the myelocele is closed. Both of these patients were paralyzed and stayed paralyzed, so far as we know, except that one of them, the child of a doctor, has shown considerable im-

523

provement in the feet. They are not entirely paralyzed.

(Note: Inquiry after the meeting from the father of this child with myelocele and an open central medullary canal reveals that the child can move the thighs and stretch and bend the knees. The feet are being treated orthopedically, and there is a grave sensory deficiency.)

Of tumors of the anterior area of the sacrum, Dr. Adson mentioned chordomas and teratomas. The first surgical case I had in my practice was a man sent to me by another doctor. The lesion was congenital. At birth it had apparently fluctuated, was incised by the attending physician, and never healed. The man was a poor farmer's helper and had always slept in the hay out in the barn because there was such a terrific odor about him. He was 18 years old when he came to see me. His was a presacral teratoma, between the sacrum and rectum.

A case of chordoma which I had in this area was brought before this Academy some time ago. [Meeting of October 7, 1936. Published in MINNESOTA MEDICINE, 20:15, (January) 1937.]

I should like to ask Dr. Adson if the sac in his case was injected with an obliterating fluid like alcohol.

DR. F. E. B. FOLEY, Saint Paul: This is one of the most interesting papers I have heard presented before the Academy. Dr. Adson has presented the subject of meningocele in a way most instructive and helpful to those concerned with the clinical surgical problem. My own interest is more in the physiology and pathologic physiology of the condition. This interest carries over from experimental work on the physiology of the cerebrospinal fluid done in association with Dr. Harvey Cushing in 1920. I would like to ask some questions bearing on this phase of the matter.

Is not the hydrocephalus developed following removal of a large meningocele always of the communicating type? Obstructive hydrocephalus due to occlusion of the aqueduct or the foramina entering the subarachnoid space should exist independently of the meningocele and not be influenced by its removal. Does occurrence of a communicating hydrocephalus in response to removing a meningocele indicate that the lining of the cyst had been a pathway for absorption of fluid and had protected the individual from hydrocephalus? Is removal of this absorbing surface directly responsible for the hydrocephalus?

In commenting on hydrocephalus secondary to removal of a meningocele, Dr. Adson mentioned the theory of Morgagni. This theory presupposes that the choroid plexus behaves as a secreting gland and that the cerebrospinal fluid is a true secretion. The experiments which I devised and carried out in Dr. Cushing's laboratory disprove this. They showed conclusively that the choroid plexus is not a secreting gland and that the fluid is a product of purely physical factors—filtration, osmosis and diffusion. A mixture of solutions of iron ammonium citrate and potassium ferrocyanid was supplied to the subarachnoid space from a manometer. The animal was then given a hypertonic salt solution intravenously. Incident to the increased absorption of cerebrospinal fluid and fall of fluid pressure thus induced, a considerable volume of the citrate-ferrocyanid mixture was displaced from the manometer into the subarachnoid space. On perfusing the animal with formalin containing hydrochloric acid, insoluble granules of Prussian blue were precipitated from the mixture at the sites to which it had reached. It was found that a reversal of flow in the aqueduct had occurred and that fluid now moved from the subarachnoid space up the aqueduct into the ventricles. There was a heavy deposit of Prussian Blue over the ependymal cells of the choroid, between these cells and in the choroidal vessels. The experiment proved that the increased osmotic value of the blood had reversed the flow of fluid through the choroid plexus which now ceased production of fluid and became a pathway of fluid absorption. Some years later these experiments were re-

peated and verified by Freemont-Smith: They show conclusively that the fluid is a product of purely physical factors and is not a true secretion. May it not be possible to put this fact to good purpose in the surgical treatment of meningocele?

DR. ADSON, in closing: In reply to Dr. Rodda's question as to whether or not a balance develops between the secretion and absorption of cerebrospinal fluid in communicating hydrocephalus, I wish to say that it is my opinion that a balance does develop when there is not too large a difference between the factors involved; that is, when the absorption mechanism is capable of absorbing most of the fluid secreted.

In reply to Dr. Wright's questions as to whether or not surgery is worth while, I wish to emphasize the point that I made in the paper. This was that the surgical treatment of spina bifida cystica is not indicated in the presence of an extensive hydrocephalus, nor is it indicated in the presence of a syringomyelocele when extensive paralysis is manifest. In the remaining group of cases it is definitely indicated and worth while.

I doubt if surgery is of material value in the treatment of spina bifida occulta. Occasionally, adhesions may be relieved and a fatty tumor found which, when removed, may give some relief; more often than not, however, nothing can be done from the surgical point of view. The symptoms most usually are the result of a myelodysplasia.

In reply to Dr. Foley's question as to whether or not the choroid plexus is a secreting gland, I wish to state that I am familiar with his experimental work and agree with him that the cerebrospinal fluid is not a secretory product of the choroid plexus but is a transudate as a result of various physical phenomena. However, the point that I wished to make was that the cerebrospinal fluid was eliminated by the choroid plexus into the lateral ventricles and had to find its way into the subarachnoid spaces. Otherwise a hydrocephalus would result.

CASE REPORT

FREDERIC E. B. FOLEY, M.D., and
JOHN E. DEES, M.D. (by invitation)
Saint Paul

The case to be reported is that of a married woman, aged fifty-five (Ancker Hospital record No. A6941). The patient had been treated for three years in the cardiac clinic of the Ancker Hospital for auricular fibrillation. She was admitted to the hospital on January 8, 1938, complaining of severe pain in the left flank and back for the preceding thirty-six hours. The onset had been sudden. The pain was severe and constant, being localized in the left costo-vertebral region and flank. There was no downward radiation. On three occasions since the onset of the attack she had noted gross blood in the urine. There had been no other urinary symptoms, no chills or vomiting.

On admission significant findings on physical examination were a temperature of 100° F, marked obesity and extreme tenderness to palpation over the left flank and costo-vertebral region. No mass was palpable. There was a rapid auricular fibrillation with an apical heart rate of 160 per minute, the blood pressure being 120/90. Except for a few râles in the bases of the lungs, there were no signs of decompensation.

Laboratory examinations showed the hemoglobin to be 78 per cent, leukocyte count 25,800, sedimentation rate 55 mm./hour, urea nitrogen 28 mmg. per cent.

The urine showed an occasional leukocyte and granular cast, no erythrocytes, 1-albumin, no sugar and it was sterile on culture.

On January 10 x-ray of the abdomen was negative for a rather large left renal shadow. Intravenous urography showed a well functioning, apparently normal right kidney with no excretion of dye from the left kidney in thirty minutes. Cystoscopy was then carried out. The bladder was negative. A No. 6 catheter was easily passed to the left kidney. There was no drainage of urine from the catheter but irrigation of the left renal pelvis with normal saline solution reproduced the patient's pain. The catheter was left in place for five hours at the end of which time it was removed as there had been no drainage of urine through it. Retrograde pyelography was not carried out at this time as the patient's temperature was 102° F.

The temperature subsided slowly from a maximum of 102 on January 10, reaching normal on January 18, the tenth day of hospitalization. Spontaneous pain in the kidney disappeared by the fifth day of hospitalization and tenderness to pressure by the seventh day.

On January 18 the left ureter was again catheterized. There was no drainage of urine nor could any be aspirated from the renal pelvis. The ureteral catheter was removed and a bulb catheter wedged into the left ureteral orifice. A pyelo-ureterogram was made after the injection of 11 c.c. of 20 per cent hippuran solution, which amount reproduced the patient's pain. The resulting picture showed an essentially normal, unobstructed ureter and kidney pelvis. A diagnosis of massive embolism of the left renal artery was made at this time.

Two days later cystoscopy was again carried out. Indigo-carmine appeared in good concentration in three minutes from the right ureter but none during ten minutes observation was seen to come from the left side. A No. 14 bulb catheter was wedged into the left intramural ureter and left in place for thirty-five minutes during which time there was no drainage of dye or urine through it.

The patient left the hospital on January 23. At this time there were no symptoms referable to the urinary tract. The urine contained many erythrocytes and leukocytes. The tachycardia had disappeared under digitalis.

The patient has been re-admitted for study on three occasions since discharge, two, three and four and one-half months respectively after the onset of her illness. Intravenous urography and cystoscopy after the injection of indigo-carmine intravenously as well as ureteral catheterizations have consistently showed an absence of excretion of dye or urine by the left kidney. Bulb pyelo-ureterograms have shown a progressive decrease in the capacity of the left renal pelvis and ureter from 11 c.c. on January 18 to 4 c.c. on May 16. The size of the pelvis and renal shadow have decreased markedly, the general configuration of the pelvis being preserved in miniature. There have been no urinary symptoms or evidence of other embolic episodes.

Cursory review of the literature in connection with this case report discloses publications on the subject beginning in 1856 when Traube first reported the condi-

tion. Schultz, five years previously, had ligated the artery in an experimental animal and observed atrophy of the kidney. Blessig, in 1859, in a similar experiment concluded that the renal artery was necessary, not only for the function, but for the nourishment of the kidney. He found that its ligation was followed in the first few days by venous engorgement and that this might cause actual hemorrhage if thrombosis of the vein also occurred. This latter observation is difficult or impossible to explain reasonably. With total occlusion of the artery, hematuria should be expected only in the presence of a patent vein. In such event venous pressure in the cava being higher than in the venules of the kidney, there should be engorgement of the kidney with diapedesis and blood in the urine the result. Why bleeding should occur in the presence of occlusion of both artery and vein is hard to understand and would seem to indicate fault in the experiment.

Buchwalden and Littin, in 1876, ligated the renal vein and found initial enlargement of the kidney with shrinkage of the kidney beginning by the sixth day and finally with establishment of collateral venous circulation through capsular renal vessels and lumbar veins with some preservation of function. This was corroborated in 1913 by Morrell and associates. These investigators found that following ligation of the artery rapid necrosis, atrophy and death of the kidney invariably resulted.

Westerborn, in 1937, reported careful observations and operation in a case very similar to the one here described. He also made some animal experiments. He found that one and one-third hours is the longest period of arterial occlusion that will be followed by total recovery of the kidney. He reports that occlusion of an hour and a half invariably results in impaired function. He concludes that embolectomy if done at all should be done in the first hour and certainly not later than two hours.

Eisendrath, in 1934, reviewed the reported cases of both arterial and venous occlusion—some forty cases in number, and concluded that of them only twenty-five were acceptable examples of the condition.

The numerous publications do not sharply distinguish between total occlusion of the main renal artery, multiple occlusions of its smaller branches and venous occlusion. For this reason it is difficult to know the exact character of the vascular occlusion or combination of occlusions that was responsible for the clinical findings in the reported cases.

Consideration of the reports of massive renal infarct makes it apparent that the characteristic onset is one of sudden severe pain, usually localized to the kidney region although at times being epigastric. The pain is without remission or radiation and usually of such severity as not to be relieved by morphine. In the majority of cases gross hematuria occurs. Apparently it may be present with primary arterial as well as primary venous occlusion.

The reports are agreed that there is exquisite tenderness of the affected kidney with or without spasm of the overlying muscles. Albuminuria is the most frequent laboratory finding occurring in roughly 60 per cent of the cases referred to. It tends to decrease or disappear by the sixth day.

The papers to which we have had access disclose only three cases closely analogous to the one here reported—that is embolism or sudden arterial thrombosis with complete occlusion of the whole renal artery. None of these reported cases contains detailed information concerning frequently repeated observations following the event though in two cases subsequent cystoscopy and pyelography are reported with findings similar to ours. The case we have described appears to be the most complete and detailed observation of the condition as clinically encountered.

The meeting adjourned.

Meeting of May 11, 1938

The regular monthly meeting of the Minnesota Academy of Medicine was held at the Town and Country Club on Wednesday evening, May 11, 1938. Dinner was served at 7 o'clock and the meeting was called to order at 8:10 by the president, Dr. R. T. LaVake.

There were forty-nine members and three guests present.

Minutes of the April meeting were read and approved.

The scientific program followed.

NON-TUBERCULOUS SPONTANEOUS PNEUMOTHORAX

E. V. KENEFICK, M.D.
Saint Paul

Abstract

Spontaneous pneumothorax may be caused by tuberculosis, lung abscess, bronchiectasis, emphysema, empyema, carcinoma of the lung, lung cyst, and silicosis. Fracture of the ribs and puncture wounds of the chest were responsible for the first reported cases. Tuberculosis is the most common cause and is present in 70 to 80 per cent of all cases. Another small group without obvious cause are classed together because of a common symptomatology and course. Benign pneumothorax, idiopathic pneumothorax, and non-tuberculous pneumothorax are the various terms applied to this condition. It is this group I wish to discuss.

The various types of spontaneous pneumothorax encountered may be classified according to the degree to which the lung is collapsed. The collapse may be partial or complete, with or without mediastinal displacement. If the pressure continues to increase a tension, pneumothorax may develop. Recurrent attacks are common. Simultaneous bilateral pneumothorax may occur and is much more serious than the unilateral form. Hemopneumothorax is also a serious type, due to the presence of large amounts of blood in the pleural space.

The close relationship of pulmonary tuberculosis to spontaneous pneumothorax has been an accepted dictum for many years. Several reasons may be advanced to prove this is not true in all cases. Spontaneous pneumothorax occurs usually in the late stages of tuberculosis. If it does occur due to the rupture of a solitary focus in the pleura, a pleural effusion invariably results. In spontaneous pneumothorax, pleural effusion is not present and follow-up studies do not reveal the presence of pulmonary tuberculosis. Kjaergard has studied fifty-one cases, some of which were followed for as long as eighteen years, and found only one patient had developed active tuberculosis. Morriss studied twenty-six cases over a period of from three to eleven years, and found no tuberculosis. The more general employment of the tuberculin test and routine x-ray examination of the chest has demonstrated that an antecedent tuberculous infection is not necessary in the development of spontaneous pneumothorax.

The condition occurs most frequently in young males between twenty and thirty years of age. Physical effort or strain does not play any part. Ranking, Pitt, Hayoshii and Fisher have reported finding vesicles at the apices of the lung surrounded by areas of emphysema or retracted areas due to scar tissue. No evidence of tuberculosis was present in any of their autopsied cases, six in number. Fisher and Hayoshii ascribe the pneumothorax to the rupture of a vesicle, usually situated at the apex, which is surrounded by either scar tissue or emphysematous tissue, closed by a valve at the base. The valves develop from inflammatory processes with resulting scar tissue formation, producing a constriction of the lung tissue or bronchiole.

Case histories of seven patients with spontaneous pneumothorax were presented together with the results of tuberculin tests and x-ray studies of the chest. These studies failed to reveal evidences of tuberculosis in any of the patients. The follow-up period was five years in all cases. Mantoux tests were negative except for one patient with a plus reaction three years after the attack of pneumothorax. Fever was not present and there was no evidence of pleural effusion in any case. All patients completely recovered in from two to six weeks with simple bed rest and symptomatic care

CONCLUSIONS

1. Non-tuberculous spontaneous pneumothorax occurs in healthy young adults without demonstrable cause and runs a benign afebrile course with complete recovery in a few weeks.

2. The condition is caused by the rupture of pleural valve vesicle either emphysematous or scar tissue in nature.

3. Tuberculosis is not a factor in this type of spontaneous pneumothorax.

4. Roentgenology and tuberculin tests are extremely valuable aids in the diagnosis and treatment of the condition.

Discussion

DR. E. V. GOLTZ, Saint Paul: I recently had an opportunity of observing just such a case as Dr. Ken fick reports, and his paper has been very interesting to me because of this recent experience, for his cases simulate mine very closely. It seems to me the interesting observation here is the etiologic factor. While it is true that some claim 80 per cent of their spontaneous pneumothorax cases to be tuberculous, I think this probably holds true more in hospitals and sanatoria. In private practice I think one can not claim so high a percentage. The problem is to prove that these young people who have these benign spontaneous pneumothoraces are not tuberculous. Dr. Kenefick has shown very definitely that his group is not tuberculous; and, if this can be proven, it is certainly very much worth while in the prognosis.

Dr. S. Marx White, Minneapolis: One patient of mine at the age of 32 first had a spontaneous pneumothorax in 1928. He had two subsequent recurrences, each after about a year's interval, and two of the three attacks were brought on apparently by riding horseback. At the time of the first attack minor symptoms of a chronic type of arthritis were present, and subsequently a moderately severe extensive Strümpel-Marie type of spinal arthritis has developed. The Mantoux reactions have all been negative, and repeated x-ray films, taken at the time and subsequently, to the present time have been negative to tuberculosis.

A fact of interest is that a paternal uncle had very marked and extensive cystic disease of the lung, found at autopsy. In the x-ray films of this patient, however, we have not been able on careful search to find anything indicative of cystic disease of the lung, even though this was searched for at the time of the attacks.

Dr. Max Hoffman, Saint Paul: In the last two years I have seen three cases of spontaneous pneumothorax. None of them showed much air in the chest and in all cases the symptoms were minimal. There was some pain in the chest underneath the clavicle on the affected side, but there was much less air than in the cases Dr. Kenefick reported tonight. That would make one feel that spontaneous pneumothorax of mild degree is fairly common. The pain may last for a day or two and the condition may heal quite quickly. Last year I read an article in which the author had injected 25 per cent glucose into the thoracic cavity for this condition. He felt it was very effective in preventing a return of spontaneous pneumothorax. I have not had a chance to use this treatment.

Dr. C. M. Carlaw, Minneapolis: I was very glad to hear Dr. Kenefick's paper. It has taken me back many years. About the year 1890 at the Montreal General Hospital, Dr. George Ross, then Professor of Clinical Medicine at McGill, in one of his clinical lectures to the class of which I was a member, explained and demonstrated to us the use of the "Coin Test" in the diagnosis of pneumothorax. The second year after I was graduated I came to Minneapolis. One night shortly after, I was called to see a young man who was suffering with severe chest pain. I could not at first arrive at any diagnosis. Suddenly, however, I remembered Dr. Ross' lecture on the "Coin Test," tried it, and there was a pneumothorax as plain as the nose on his face. I made some inquiry into his family history and found that his mother had died of consumption, also an uncle on his mother's side. The patient looked as though he might have it too. That man got well after about two weeks' rest in bed. He is now an officer in one of our Minneapolis banks, has reared two fine healthy children, and has just been blessed with a fine big grandson; and he (grandpa) still does not show any signs of tuberculosis.

Dr. Kenefick, in closing: I want to thank the members for their kind discussions. There are a few points I wish to mention. Dr. White mentioned the possibility

of lung cysts as a cause of pneumothorax. A number of these cases have been reported. I know of two cases where x-rays taken at the time of the pneumothorax showed a cyst which had ruptured and remained after the lung collapse. I believe in Kjaergard's monograph there is a nice picture of a lung cyst with a pneumothorax.

Dr. Goltz mentioned the differences of opinion as to the incidence of tuberculosis in these cases. I think that is perfectly true. Men who are doing most of their work with tuberculosis in institutions have an idea that these are all tuberculous because they are dealing mostly with tuberculosis. On the other hand, in private practice one probably sees many more cases of the simple type.

Dr. Hoffman mentioned the injection of glucose. This is recommended in cases of hemopneumothorax to cause the blood to clot. The injection of sterile water or glucose, or almost any foreign protein, seemingly causes coagulation and stops the hemorrhage.

These cases are mainly of interest because of the prognosis. If one takes for granted that these patients are tuberculous and keeps them in bed for a long time with the stigma of tuberculosis, naturally they lose much time. With the use of the Montoux test, a large percentage of these cases are proven not to be tuberculosis.

The meeting adjourned.

A. G. Schulze, M.D., *Secretary.*

ACUTE LYMPHATIC LEUKEMIA WITH REMISSION (CASE REPORT)

(Continued from Page 501)

area of consolidation or dulness in the left base had disappeared entirely by April 9, leaving normal breath sounds. The child seemed to gain a little in strength, her color improved, she was brighter, she responded better and on April 6 began to eat rather generous amounts of solid food, the first solid food she had taken for two weeks. Her pulse became somewhat slower, changing from 140 and 150 to 130. The temperature, however, was never less than 100 by axilla and it would rise very easily to 104 by axilla. On April 9, her white count was 64,000, a reduction of almost 100,000 cells per cm. over a period of ten days. The blood smear continued to show the typical picture of acute lymphatic leukemia. From March 30 to April 10 eight injections of liver extract were given. April 9, a pink generalized maculopapular eruption was first observed. This persisted until her demise five days later.

April 10, the patient began definitely to lose ground. Bleeding from nose, mouth, and rectum began. Breathing was rapid and shallow. The pasty pallor returned and the responses were very poor. There were a few scattered leukemic infiltrations in the skin still remaining, but neither did these increase nor did any areas of dulness return to the chest. Indeed, the skin nodules from the time they began to subside until exitus continued to do so although much more slowly the last few days. April 11, the child had a few mild convulsions. General appearance was one of pallor, bloating, extreme toxicity. Exitus occurred April 14.

BOOK·REVIEWS

Books listed here become the property of the Ramsey and Hennepin County Medical libraries when reviewed. Members, however, are urged to write reviews of any or every recent book which may be of interest to physicians.

HANDBOOK OF ORTHOPÆDIC SURGERY. Alfred Rives Shands, Jr., M.D., and Richard Raney, M.D. 593 pages. Illus. $5.00. St. Louis: Mosby, 1937.

I find this an adequate outline covering the subject adapted to the needs particularly of students. The drawings illustrate deformities and bone pathology in many cases better than the average photographs of radiographs. The bibliography is comprehensive and well organized and the index accurate.

S. W. SHIMONEK

MODERN TREATMENT AND FORMULARY. Edw. A. Mullen, M.D. 707 pp., $5.00. Philadelphia: F. A. Davis Co., 1936.

Anyone interested in the essentials of treatment including numerous authenticated prescriptions, and diet lists, tables of differential diagnosis, and other valuable data and tables, will find these compactly embodied in this well-organized and readable volume. It should prove a valuable handbook, particularly for the general practitioner.

THOMAS MYERS, M.D.

MANAGEMENT OF THE SICK INFANT AND CHILD. By Langley Porter and Wm. E. Carter. 5th Ed., 874 pp. $10.00. St. Louis: C. V. Mosby Co., 1938.

This excellent discussion has been justly popular, having gone through six printings in sixteen years. Despite its title, the work is not limited solely to a discussion of treatment, but also devotes ample space to etiology, symptomatology, and description of the various manifestations of diseases. Over two hundred pages are devoted to a well-illustrated discussion of methods of treatment, briefly and simply outlined. Diets in disease and health are competently described, and appropriate recipes and tables are included. A valuable chapter on drugs with appropriate prescriptions and dosage in various conditions completes this volume. The typography and excellent paper used make the book easily readable. Certainly this is an indispensable addition to the library of anyone treating children.

THOMAS MYERS, M.D.

INJECTION TREATMENT OF VARICOSE VEINS HEMORRHOIDS. H. O. McPheeters, M.D., and Kerr Anderson, M.D. 315 pages. Illus. $4.50. Philadel F. A. Davis Co., 1938.

The section on injection of varicose veins by F McPheeters is a very comprehensive treatise on anatomy, embryology, etiology and diagnosis of condition. There is an excellent and clear descri of the physiology involved and of the Trendelen test. The chapters on treatment are extremely and easily followed. The few hours necessary to this is time well spent.

The section on the injection treatment of he rhoids by James Kerr Anderson is the clearest, concise, and most thorough description of this su that one can find. The chapters are written with c ness and brevity that is welcome. Obscure points brought forth in easily understood terms and the no doubt in the reader's mind as to the author's m ing. It is well worth reading by everyone who cor plates injecting or is injecting hemorrhoids. The r ing time is a little over an hour.

WALLACE P. RITCI

IN MEMORIAM
(Continued from Page 513)

(Continued from Page 513)

whom I have ever known. Intolerant of anything the highest type of professional conduct, he was r influenced by anything commercial in his profess life. He maintained in his surgical diagnosis and nic a perfection that few attain.

The life and work of the medical man are brief often too soon forgotten but the great principle ethical conduct to which he was committed are old and permanent. I like to believe that the me of Dr. Wiese will live for all time in these principles.

CLAUDE C. KENNEDY, M

L. G. Wilberton
1853-1938

Dr. L. G. Wilberton, a practicing physician at nona for fifty-eight years, died at his home the May 29. Dr. Wilberton was reared in New State, and was a graduate of Hahnemann Colle Philadelphia, in the class of 1880, coming to W directly after his graduation. Surviving him ar wife and two children, Mrs. Ernest E. Shepa Winona and George L. Wilberton of Seattle, Dr. Wilberton was a member of the American tute of Homeopathy and for a time was vice pre of the Minnesota State Homeopathic associatior was the oldest homeopathic physician in Minr

MINNESOTA MEDICINE

Journal of the Minnesota State Medical Association, Southern Minnesota Medical Association, Northern Minnesota Medical Association, Minnesota Academy of Medicine and Minneapolis Surgical Society

| Volume 21 | AUGUST, 1938 | No. 8 |

CARCINOMA OF THE COLON AND RECTUM*

IRVIN ABELL, M.D.

Louisville, Kentucky

MALIGNANCY of the large bowel is a frequently noted lesion and, as with carcinoma elsewhere, the picture is not a bright one. The age at which its greatest incidence is observed and the relentless character of the disease with its consequent reduction of an already waning vitality combine to make the operative mortality a high one, while the number of patients remaining permanently free from disease following operation is discouragingly small. Unfortunately, with few exceptions, this is the usual history of cancer in other parts of the body; and yet there are certain features about cancer of the colon, notably its slow growth with tardiness of metastasis to readily removable groups of lymph nodes, which should make the outlook more favorable, with the opportunity for radical treatment which an early diagnosis affords. This study is presented as a plea for the early recognition of the disease and its radical removal, the two factors which in the light of our present knowledge offer the only hope of its eradication. The material upon which this paper is based comprises 200 patients with carcinoma of the large bowel, including the rectum, observed since 1915, the growth being in the colon in 125 and in the rectum in seventy-five. Of this number, eighty-nine (sixty-four in the colon and twenty-five in the rectum) were subjected to radical operation. In sixty-nine, some type of palliative operation, colostomy or a short circuiting ileocolostomy or colo-colostomy was done. In three the lesion was removable, but the operation was declined, while in thirty-nine the condition was such as to preclude any advantage from opera-

tive measures. The fact that but 44.5 per cent of patients came under observation at a time when radical measures could be instituted, 34.5 per cent at a time when palliative measures only could be employed and 19.5 per cent when neither method of possible relief was available, indicates a woeful disregard of symptoms on the part of the patient and a failure on the part of the physician to appreciate their significance, meaning that 54 per cent of the series were denied the chance of cure which surgery offers. Of the 125 patients in whom the growth was found in the colon, two were in the second decade, one a boy of seventeen with a colloid carcinoma of the transverse colon, the other a girl of nineteen with the lesion in the cecum; four were in the third, eleven in the fourth, twenty-six in the fifth, thirty-one in the sixth, thirty-five in the seventh and fourteen in the eighth decade, with the age not stated in two. It will be noted that fifty-seven, or approximately 62 per cent, were between the ages of fifty and seventy, a period in which the duration of life alone takes its toll in the wear and tear upon the vital functions. Of the seventy-five in which the lesion was situated in the rectum, two occurred in the third decade, in women of twenty-one and twenty-eight, four in the fourth, sixteen in the fifth, twenty-five in the sixth, sixteen in the seventh and twelve in the eighth decade. It will be noted again that forty-one, or 54.7 per cent, occurred between the ages of fifty and seventy, and fifty-three, or 70 per cent, between the ages of fifty and eighty. This great incidence of the disease in advanced life serves in part to explain both its high operative mortality and the paucity of five and ten year cures.

*Presented at the eighty-fifth annual meeting of the Minnesota State Medical Association, Duluth, Minn., June 29, 1938.

The carcinoma was situated in the cecum in thirty-six, in the cecum and transverse colon in two, in the ascending colon in thirteen, in the hepatic flexure in thirteen, in the transverse colon alone in fourteen, in the transverse colon and right ovary in one, in the splenic flexure alone in ten, in the splenic flexure and right ovary in one, in the descending colon in eight, in the sigmoid colon in twenty-seven, in the rectum alone in seventy-four, and in the rectum and breast in one. Sixty-four were in the right colon, fifteen in the transverse and 121 in the left colon and rectum. It will be noted that five patients are recorded as having multiple foci, two with carcinoma of the cecum and transverse colon, two with carcinoma of the colon and ovary and one with carcinoma of the rectum and breast. Together they present a fertile field for speculation as to whether or not they represent primary multiple foci. The conception that cancer is primarily local in origin, the secondary tumors developing as the result of metastatic transplantation, is so definitely fixed that one accepts the idea of multiple primary foci with a certain amount of reserve. Billroth formulated three conditions to be fulfilled by multiple cancers before their acceptance as individual and independent tumors: (1) there should be histological differences of such degree as to preclude the interpretation of the two growths as representing different stages of development; (2) each growth must spring from its parent epithelium; and (3) each growth must have its own group of metastases. Mercanton adds a fourth condition to the effect that if, after the removal at one operation of two cancers, the patient remains free from disease, it is practically certain that the two growths were independent, since had either been a metastasis it would be entirely reasonable to assume the presence of other metastases, a state of affairs incompatible with life.

Of the two instances in which cancer was noted in the cecum and transverse colon, one probably represents metastasis by transplantation; the other may represent multiple primary foci. The former, a woman of sixty, presented a large carcinoma of the cecum with two polypoid tumors distal to it, one in the hepatic flexure and one in the transverse colon. Both of the distal tumors showed a microscopic structure identical with the parent growth. No other metastases were found. This patient is now living and well six years fol-

lowing operation. The second patient affords a somewhat different picture. A man, aged 40, had a tumor of the cecum 3.2 inches in its greatest diameter, and one of the transverse colon 2.4 inches in its greatest diameter. Microscopical examination revealed the cecal tumor to be a colloid carcinoma, the transverse colon tumor to be an adenocarcinoma. No metastasis to the lymph nodes was found. The size of the tumors, their histological structure and the duration of life following their removal suggest the possibility primary multiplicity. Metastasis commonly occurs by a path leading away from the tumor, but there is always the possibility of metastasis by retrograde or other circuitous routes. Lymphatic metastasis may occur by way of the mesentery to its root, and, finding continued progress in this direction blocked, may extend by retrograde route to another point in the colon. Dissemination or implantation metastasis is recognized in which cancerous cells float off in the peritoneal fluids and produce secondary growths in the pelvic peritoneum. Similarly, cells from a parent growth involving the mucosa of the colon may become implanted and give rise to secondary growths distally situated from it. Such growths are usually smaller, indicating more recent origin, and they present the same histological structure as the parent tumor. This mode of transmission accounts satisfactorily for multiple growths of similar structure which involves the lumen, with the exception of those observed in polyposis. The colloid cancers observed in the colon are fundamentally adenocarcinoma in which the cells, while retaining the power of forming mucin, are nevertheless unable to excrete it properly. Microscopically they differ from adenocarcinoma in that the acini are filled and more or less distended with hyaline or granular basophilic mucin.

It is generally accepted that metastatic tumors from primary ones which produce colloid may continue to produce material like the primary tumor, or may fail to do so; and, in addition, that metastatic tumors very seldom or never produce colloid, if the tumor from which they have arisen does not produce colloid material. The difference in structure and the fairly wide separation of the two tumors argue for primary multiplicity. This patient was operated upon in 1927, the terminal ileum and the right half of the colon being removed to a point beyond the location of the second growth. He remained well for six years, returning in 1933 with an adenocarcinoma involving the descending colon which at that time was removed. At the present time, eleven years after the first operation and five years after the second, he shows no evidence of further growth, affording interesting material for speculation as to whether each tumor represented a primary focus, or as to whether the second and third ones were but instances of mucosal implantation with the third one showing unusually slow development. Both cases could well seem to bear out the hypothesis that carcinoma of the colon originates in polyps and that each growth represented a separate and primary focus.

Of two patients with cancer of the colon, one a scirrhous adenocarcinoma of the transverse colon, the other an adenocarcinoma of the splenic flexure, both presented papillary adenocarcinoma of the right ovary. The difference in histological structure and the widely separated sites of origin in unrelated organs strongly suggest primary multiplicity.

The fifth instance in which multiple foci were noted occurred in a woman of fifty-nine who presented a tumor in the rectum and one in the breast. Microscopical examination showed the rectal tumor to be a colloid carcinoma, columnar cell, arising from the mucosa and not the mucous glands. The breast tumor was an adenocarcinoma, polygonal cell, primary in the mammary gland. The coincident development of the growths in widely distant and non-related organs, the one a polygonal cell, the other a columnar cell colloid carcinoma, together with the similarity between the cells of the neoplasms and those occurring in their respective sites, would argue for their independence, while their basic structure, adenocarcinoma, introduces an element of doubt which cannot be convincingly eliminated.

But one instance in the series showed carcinoma developing in diffuse polyposis. A man, aged 29, gave a history of intermittent bleeding since the age of twelve. Sigmoidoscopic examination showed the presence of multiple polyps in the upper rectum and lower sigmoid, varying in diameter from one-eighth to one-fourth inch. X-ray film of the colon showed a diffuse polyposis with a defect in sigmoid suggestive of carcinoma. The rectal polyps were destroyed by fulguration and the colon excised. It presented extensive polyposis from the ileocecal valve to the rectum with adenocarcinoma in the sigmoid. It has been argued that all cancers of the colon and rectum have their origin in polyps, an hypothesis in which, from our experience, we cannot concur. Doering noted that carcinoma occurred in 43 per cent of cases of polyposis and pointed out that this accounts for some of the cases of carcinoma occurring in early life. It is recognized that polypi are the most frequent precancerous lesions noted in the colon and rectum, but it is not possible to state with assurance that they invariably precede the development of cancer in these situations.

Of the 125 patients with cancer of the colon, eighty-eight were males and sixty-seven were females. The symptoms in this group have shown rather wide variation. Digestive disturbances have been the rule, in some instances constituting the sole complaint causing the patient to seek relief. Weakness and pallor were given by five as the only complaints. Weight loss has been noted in more than 50 per cent, varying from several to ninety pounds. Diarrhea with and without bloody stools has been noted in lesions involving all parts of the colon, the diarrhea being more frequent when the cancer involved the right colon, the bloody stools more frequent when the left colon was the site of the growth.

Constipation and obstipation were noted in but eighteen of the sixty-two cases in which the growth was situated in the right half of the colon, but were frequently present when the lesion involved the left half of the colon. Pain was the chief complaint given by forty-one; in most of these, this symptom was to be attributed to a partial obstruction. Obstruction was noted in fifty-nine, or 62.5 per cent, thirty being of the acute and twenty-nine of the chronic variety; sixty-six, or 57.8 per cent, presented no obstructive symptoms. While obstruction occurs with lesions in all parts of the colon, it was more frequent in the left than in the right half, the explanation being found in part in the fluidity of the feces in the right colon as compared with the solidity of the feces in the left colon. Again the annular, scirrhous or fibrocarcinoma, producing marked constriction of the lumen of the bowel, has been in our series more common in the left than in the right half of the colon. The anatomical arrangement of the angles favors the development of obstruction when these parts are the seat of growths. This is especially true of the splenic flexure, acute obstruction not infrequently being the first subjective symptom of cancer at this point. The cecal and ascending colon cancers as a rule have been either the soft medullary adenocarcinomas or of the colloid type, the former more frequent than the latter. The soft, medullary growths occurring in the cecum and ascending colon produce rather large tumors, the early ulceration and infection of which lead to rather marked anemia, disturbance of digestion and weight loss, although they may still be limited to the bowel and readily operable. The blood picture has been somewhat significant, the greatest percentage of low counts being found in involvment of the cecum and ascending colon. In fifty-one patients with the growth in these situations the lowest hemoglobin was 32, the highest 90, the average being 72 per cent. The red cells varied from three to five million, the average being slightly under four million. The average hemoglobin in growths of the transverse colon was 76.3; splenic flexure, 77.2; and in the sigmoid, 72.8; the red cell average was, respectively, 4,250,000, 4,350,000, and 4,-000,000.

Perforation of the growth with abscess formation was noted in three instances: in two, the growths being of the medullary type situated in the cecum and in one of the scirrhous type in the descending colon. Perforations may occur in any type of cancer and at all points of the bowel, adding greatly to the difficulty and danger of removal, granting its operability. In one of these, nothing more than a palliative colostomy could be undertaken, the patient surviving eight months; in the remaining two, recession of the growth and sinus in the abdominal wall was carried out. One patient died from postoperative peritonitis, the other at the end of four weeks from wound infection. A palpable mass was present in sixty-five, none being detected in sixty. The distention accompanying acute obstruction as a rule effectively hides the mass; in the non-obstructed cases, growths situated at the flexures and the annular, stenosing ones in the descending colon and sigmoid do not readily lend themselves to detection by palpation, particularly in the presence of a thick abdominal wall. The masses in the ascending and descending colons are usually detected in the abdomen at points corresponding

to the usual course of the bowel. Those at the flexures are fairly constant in their situation due to the fixation of the bowel at these points. The mobility of the transverse colon is such, at times, that masses originating therein may be felt at any part of the abdomen; cecal masses usually remain in the right lower quadrant, but in the event of the tumor originating in a mobile cecum quite a range of motion and consequently of location will be permitted. X-ray examination has shown constantly two manifestations, filling defects and obstructions, upon neither of which alone can the diagnosis of cancer invariably be made. Syphilis, tuberculosis, pericecal inflammations and diverticulitis may each and all, at times, give x-ray manifestations indistinguishable from those produced by cancer. The barium enema rather than the barium meal has been employed, since the distention of the bowel wall by the former gives clearer definition both under the fluoroscope and on the film. Sigmoidoscopy will reveal growths too low to be shown by the x-ray and too high to be felt upon digital exploration of the rectum, and should constitute a step of the routine examination. A correlation of the history with the physical, laboratory, x-ray and sigmoidoscopic findings will reduce to a minimum the chance for error in detection and diagnosis. Of the sixty-four patients with cancer of the cecum, ascending colon and hepatic flexure, including two with additional tumors in the transverse colon, thirty-eight were subjected to radical and fourteen to palliative operations, twelve being classified as non-operable. The radical operation has consisted in the removal of six to eight inches of the terminal ileum and the colon from the cecum to the junction of the proximal with the distal two-thirds of the transverse colon. In two patients whose cecum and transverse colon both contained tumors the resection was made to include the proximal two-thirds of the transverse colon.

The reasons for such extensive removal when the growth is situated in the right half of the colon are to be found in the embryological, physiological and anatomical differences between it and the left half. Embryologically, the ileum and right half of the colon as far as the mid portion of the transverse colon are derived from the midgut, whereas that portion of the colon distal to the midportion of the transverse colon arises from the hindgut. The lymphatic drain age of the right colon is relatively scant, whereas that of the left is more abundant. The blood supply of the right half, through the ileocolic artery is very constant; that of the left half is variable. The contents of the two halves of the colon also differ. In the proximal colon the contents are fluid and less septic, whereas in the distal colon the fecal contents are more solid, are formed and contain a larger number of organisms. These factors conduce to the maintenance of a more satisfactory technic and to the safe removal of the ileocolic and right colic glands. In addition, there is greater ease and safety in securing union between the small intestine and colon, as contrasted with resection of the cecum and ascending colon, in continuity. In the earlier cases closure of the ends of both colon and ileum with side-to-side anastomosis, suture method, was done. Later, closure of the end of the colon with end-to-side anastomosis with Murphy button was employed, and latterly, closure of the end of the colon with end-to-side anastomosis with Rankin clamp has been practiced. All three methods are satisfactory, but the latter has the advantage of simplicity, ease of execution and greater freedom from infection.

There were ten operative deaths, three on the fourth day and two on the fifth day from peritonitis. One seventy-six-year-old man died from anuria on the ninth day. A portion of the ureter had been removed on account of its incorporation in the tumor, the proximal end being ligated. One patient died on the twenty-first and one on the thirty-fifth day from myocardial failure. A man whose abdominal wall was resected because of tumor perforation died at the end of the fourth week from infection, and one from bronchopneumonia at the end of the fifth week. Eight of the deaths occurred in twenty-six one-stage resections, a mortality of 30.7 per cent, as contrasted with two deaths in fourteen two-stage resections, a mortality of 14.2 per cent. In thirty-four patients in whom the neoplasm was situated in the splenic flexure, transverse and descending colon, radical operation was done in eighteen, a palliative operation in thirteen, and three were classed as inoperable.

Of the eighteen radical operation, ten were two-stage and eight were one-stage procedures. There were four operative deaths, three following one-stage operations, two on the third day from peritonitis and one on the thirtieth day

from pulmonary abscess following septic infarct, and one following a two-stage operation.

Of the twenty-seven patients with cancer of the sigmoid, thirteen had radical and eleven had palliative operations, three being inoperable. Of the radical operations, seven were one-stage resections, five were two-stage resections, and one consisted of colectomy for diffuse polyposis with carcinoma in the sigmoid. There were four operative deaths, one from myocardial failure eight hours after operation and three from peritonitis, on the first, sixth and eighth day, respectively.

Resection of the left half of the colon in continuity undoubtedly carries a higher primary mortality than the Mikulicz operation and was selected because of the opportunity it affords for removing the mesocolic glands and avoiding the 7 per cent of abdominal wall metastases noted in the latter procedure. It is believed that the added ultimate security given by such removal justifies the primary increased risk. It is generally conceded that in the presence of obstruction a decompression by means of an enterostomy or ileocolostomy proximal to the barrier offered by the growth, followed by rehabilitation before carrying out the resection of the involved segment, will greatly enhance the safety of the secondary procedure. The absorbed toxins lower the resistance of the patient, the thickening and edema of the obstructed intestine interfere with its vitality and render asepsis difficult to maintain, while the abdominal distention hampers both technic and manipulation. Decompression and rehabilitation will save lives that would be lost if the radical operation were attempted under such adverse conditions. The same principle has been widely applied in all resections of the left half of the colon. Our experience leads us to the belief that the application of this principle in the treatment of all cancers of the colon, regardless of their location, is a necessary factor in the further reduction of operative mortality.

Of the seventy-five patients with cancer of the rectum, twenty-nine were males and forty-six were females. The symptoms were pain, tenesmus, constipation, bleeding and discharge with secondary disturbances of digestive function and obstruction appearing late in the course of the disease. The average duration of symptoms was fourteen months; the shortest, one month; and the longest, six years. The blood picture varied with the stage of the disease and the extent of the bleeding. Little need be said about the diagnosis since the rectum is susceptible of both palpation and visual examination In sixty-two of the seventy-five, a mass could be palpated upon digital examination, while but thirteen required the proctoscope for detection. It is only when one fails to employ these two measures that the lesion can be overlooked. The microscope may be required for the positive determination of malignancy, the eye and the finger being sufficient for the determination of the presence of tumor. Some excuse may be offered for delay in recognizing cancer of the colon, none for failure to recognize cancer of the rectum. The one in a closed cavity may elude any but the most careful examination, the other sufficiently near the surface to be seen and felt will be detected if looked for. The so-called conservative operations for cancer of the rectum in which an attempt is made to retain the sphincter muscle have been disappointing in that recurrence frequently follows. Conservatism, when dealing with malignancy, conserves the disease, not the patient. There are two potent objections to the Kraske operation in that it does not afford access to all of the lymph nodes to which the rectal lymphatics pass and in that it leaves the artificial anus in a most inconvenient site. The two-stage operation evolved by Coffey, in which a permanent colostomy is first made and later followed by removal of the distal portion of sigmoid, mesosigmoid, rectum, perirectal fat and lymph nodes, appeals as being based on sound principles in that it removes the rectum and cancer-bearing lymphatics that drain it. The first stage affords opportunity for accurately determining the operability, enabling one to avoid unnecessary resections. The Miles one-stage operation offers the same opportunity of recognizing inoperability, insofar as removal of the growth is concerned, and of selecting a palliative procedure based upon the pathology revealed upon abdominal section. Of the seventy-five patients in this group, twenty-five had radical operations, twelve two-stage and thirteen one-stage; twenty-eight had palliative colostomies, nineteen were inoperable and three, while operable, refused operation. In the twenty-five radical operations there were six deaths, one at the end of twenty-four hours following the first stage, cause

unknown; two from peritonitis at the end of fifty hours following the second stage, one on the ninth day from cardiorenal failure, and two from broncho-pneumonia.

Operations done for cancer of the colon and rectum, as is true of all operations for cancer, must be complete in that the tissue involved and the tissue apt to be involved must be removed in all cases if a satisfactory percentage of cures is to be expected. This necessitates a knowledge of the characteristics of the growth, the methods of spread and the paths it takes as well as a thorough knowledge of the anatomy and physiology of the part involved. The blood supply and lymphatic distribution of the colon and rectum necessitate and permit of radical removals, the loss of such part or parts being readily physiologically compensated. The operability of the growth, except in advanced cases, cannot be accurately forecast until the incision is made; it will then be determined by the local attachments and visible spread of the growth and by distant metastases. Attachment to adjacent organs does not always contraindicate the radical ablation if the attached and involved organ is susceptible of removal. Such extension militates against the probability of permanent cure, but the prolongation of life and comfort thereby obtained makes the removal worth while. We have resected the ureter, the ileum, the uterus, the vagina, and the abdominal wall without influencing the immediate result. The enlargement of adjacent lymph nodes often presents a problem not soluble without microscopic examination. The nodes tributary to the right colon are commonly enlarged when the cecal growth is ulcerated and infected. Microscopical examination has shown both metastatic deposit and toxic lymphnoditis, it having been impossible in some instances to make the distinction on other grounds. In view of such findings the presence of enlarged lymph nodes at this point should not deter one from doing a radical removal. This is true in far lesser degree in cancers of the left colon. In our experience the hard dense nodular enlargement indicative of metastatic deposits has been more frequently noted.

A summary of the results in the 200 cases coming under observation before 1938 shows that eighty-nine were subjected to radical operation and sixty-nine to palliative operation, while

534

in forty-two the lesion was so advanced that surgery offered no relief, or was refused. The eighty-nine radical operations done during this period show a total operative mortality of 27.4 per cent. There is, however, an appreciable difference in the mortality of operations done during the first fifteen years of this period, contrasted with those done during the last decade. In the first period, one-stage operations without utilization of modern methods of rehabilitation was the rule, while in the latter period multiple-stage operations with decompression, transfusions and other methods of increasing resistance have reduced the total mortality to approximately 12 per cent. As an immediate cause of death, bronchopneumonia takes first place, with peritonitis and uremia accounting for an equal number in

the second division; shock was a cause of death in two instances and pulmonary embolism in one. Of the patients surviving the operation, approximately 60 per cent have survived for five years and 24 per cent for ten years or longer. The percentage of five and ten-year cures, 60 and 24 per cent, respectively, is gratifying, but the saving of life has been pitiably small when the total number of cases under observation is taken into consideration. It is to be hoped that the widespread interest manifested in the cancer problem today, together with the reassuring knowledge that the disease within certain limitations is curable, may result in bringing an increasingly greater number of patients under professional scrutiny sufficiently early to give them the chance for cure which surgery offers.

PROBLEMS ASSOCIATED WITH THE CLINICAL RECOGNITION OF PULMONARY HYPERTENSION

THOMAS J. DRY, M.B.

Rochester, Minnesota

A VARIETY of pathologic conditions, some of which are admittedly rare, result in increased pressure within the pulmonary circuit. Since there is no practical method of determining the blood pressure of the lesser circulation, the clinical recognition of pulmonary hypertension depends on the recognition of secondary effects resulting from its presence and on a knowledge of the different etiologic factors capable of producing pulmonary hypertension.

In some instances the primary disease of which pulmonary hypertension is a part or a consequence may somewhat obscure and distort the picture, but, if a deliberate attempt is made, the essential findings can usually be readily elicited. Since the presence of pulmonary hypertension affords information of prognostic importance, its recognition is of more than mere academic interest.

Physiologic Considerations

In discussing conditions affecting the pulmonary arterial tree it is important to visualize clearly the functional continuity and the anatomic relationship that exists between the systemic and

pulmonary circulations (Fig. 1). The physiologic purpose of the right side of the heart is to convey venous blood to the alveolar system of the lungs, where gaseous exchanges occur. The physiologic purpose of the left side of the heart is to distribute the same blood after oxygenation to the systemic circulation. These two units are inseparable and a disturbance of function in one will sooner or later influence the other.

Another important consideration in understanding pulmonary arterial disease is the concept of a "vascular reserve." The pulmonary arterial tree, like the remainder of the vascular system, is endowed with a vascular area and a capillary bed greater than ordinary functional demands can exceed.

Among experimental subjects, Haggart and Walker have shown that 52 to 66 per cent of the pulmonary circulation could be cut off without significant variation in the general circulatory condition. The point at which failure occurs is sharply defined, and beyond this point circulatory collapse is precipitated by even a minute increase in the arterial obstruction. Underhill sums up the position as follows: "The healthy heart, therefore, can accommodate itself with-

*From the Section on Cardiology, The Mayo Clinic, Rochester, Minnesota.

out difficulty to sending the same volume of blood through one lung only, in a given time, as it previously sent through both."

The presence of structural changes in the

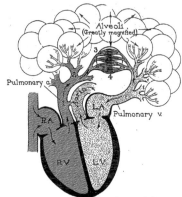

Fig. 1. Showing anatomic and functional continuity of the systemic and the pulmonary circulation. Pressure in the pulmonary circuit is increased when the left ventricle fails, when there is obstruction either at the mitral orifice or within the pulmonary circuit itself and when an extra quota of blood is shunted into the pulmonary circulation. This diagram further suggests the conception of a "vascular reserve."

pulmonary circuit, therefore, does not imply necessarily that there has been any limitation of function. As long as the "reserve" is not encroached on to a serious extent, symptoms may be in abeyance and the cardiorespiratory apparatus may adapt itself to new conditions and remain compensated.

The Results and Effects of Pulmonary Hypertension

Any mechanism which leads to increased pressure in the pulmonary circuit, irrespective of its mode of production, increases the work of the right ventricle and, if sustained, as it usually is, will lead to hypertrophy of that chamber. As secondary effects on the pulmonary vessels themselves, there follow arteriosclerotic changes in the main pulmonary arteries and added obstructive effects in the arterioles. Over a period of time, when the reserves are exhausted, failure of the right side of the heart may ensue with resultant dilatation, venous congestion and edema. When pulmonary hypertension is the result of

obstruction within the pulmonary circuit, the interference with ventilation and the resulting anoxemia eventually exert deleterious effects on the nutritional status of the left side of the heart, and so set up a vicious cycle. As Waring and Black point out, the collateral circulation which may be afforded by the bronchial arteries cannot, in any way, compensate for the respiratory difficulties, inasmuch as those vessels carry oxygenated blood.

Etiologic Factors and the Manner in Which Each Causes Pulmonary Hypertension

The conditions resulting in increased pressure within the pulmonary circuit are varied, but they can be arranged conveniently into two groups, depending on the mechanism involved: (1) obstruction to the pulmonary circuit either beyond or within the pulmonary system and (2) arteriovenous shunts in certain cases of congenital heart disease.

Obstruction of the pulmonary circuit.—Obstruction beyond the pulmonary circuit. Mitral stenosis constitutes the classic example of a mechanical obstruction to the circulation beyond the pulmonary circuit. This results in increased pulmonary pressure. Oxygenation is not interfered with until compensation fails, because the obstruction is beyond the alveolar system. Enlargement of the left auricle eventually results.

A failing left ventricle, for any cause, be it systemic hypertension, aortic disease or myocardial degeneration, results in a similar train of events. With rise in pulmonary pressure, the right ventricle is compelled to contract against an increasing load. Dilatation of the left ventricle in the process of failure may be associated with two events which further embarrass the right side of the heart, namely, mitral insufficiency and bulging of the interventricular septum into the right ventricle, constricting its capacity and thereby interfering with emptying of the right auricle. Thompson and White have shown that the effects on the right side of the heart resulting from left-sided strain alone may proceed to preponderant hypertrophy of th right ventricle and, in some cases, electrocardio graphic examination gave evidence of right axi deviation. Accentuation of the second pulmoni sound in the course of hypertensive heart dis ease represents the clinical counterpart of suc a state of affairs.

536

Obstruction within the pulmonary circuit. The obstruction may be at various levels of the pulmonary arterial tree.

I. The main pulmonary vessels.

A. Acute cor pulmonale. The sudden closure of a large pulmonary branch results in an equally sudden pulmonary hypertension, presumably because of arterial spasm in the associated pulmonary radicles. If the accident is not fatal, the evidence of strain of the right side of the heart usually can be elicited clinically and electrocardiographically.

B. Thrombosis of the pulmonary artery. A number of cases have been reported which presented clinically a picture of pulmonary hypertension and culminated in hypertrophy and failure of the right side of the heart. At necropsy, multiple thrombosis, the origin of which was obscure, was found occluding many of the larger pulmonary branches. The reader is referred particularly to the reports of cases of Means and Mallory, Montgomery, Jump and Baumann, and Barnes and Yater exemplifying this group. In the last named case, the history suggested that the arterial occlusions were of embolic origin.

II. Small and medium-sized pulmonary branches.

A. Sickle-cell anemia. The occurrence of cardiac enlargement, systolic murmurs and a palpable liver simulating rheumatic heart disease, has been noted frequently in association with sickle-cell anemia, when, at necropsy, evidence of valvular heart disease was not discoverable.[6] The assumption that these findings were the result of the anemia of itself has been questioned by Yater and Hausmann, who have reported illustrative cases in which the picture of failure of the right side of the heart was shown to have been caused either by thrombotic occlusion of the small and medium-sized arteries of the lungs or by thickening of the walls of the small and medium-sized arteries and the arterioles of the lungs with reduction in the size of their lumens, but without thrombotic occlusion. Capillary stasis, owing to distortion and agglutination of erythrocytes, was felt to be the essential factor in producing these arterial lesions.

B. Carcinomatous lymphangitis associated with obliterative pulmonary arteritis resulting in failure of the right side of the heart was described by Girode as early as 1889 according to Greenspan, who, in addition to reporting four such cases, gives an excellent and extensive review of the literature. The essential picture consists of widespread occlusion of arteries and arterioles apparently secondary to perivascular lymphatic infiltration with carcinomatous cells and proliferation of connective tissue incidental to this. Carcinomatous emboli occur within the vessels but play a relatively unimportant rôle in the obliterative process. By far the majority of cases result from a spread by way of the lymphatic vessels from a primary lesion in the stomach. The clinical course in such cases is much less protracted than in all other forms of chronic cor pulmonale, and, thus, the term subacute cor pulmonale, as applied by Brill and Robertson, seems entirely justifiable.

C. Schistosomiasis (Mansoni) has been shown to cause granulomatous pulmonary lesions within or related to the blood vessels. On examination, many small arteries gave evidence of extreme concentric thickening of the intima with diminution of the size of the lumen and hypertrophy of the media in the case reported by Clark and Graef. Right ventricular hypertrophy and congestive heart failure were present and there was no other ascertainable factor which might have caused pulmonary hypertension. It will be recalled that infection occurs through the skin and that the parasites are carried by the bloodstream to the lungs, through which they are carried to be distributed by the systemic circulation, but ending mainly in the portal system. However, residual infestation in the lungs apparently can occur with secondary effects in the pulmonary vessels sufficiently widespread to cause pulmonary hypertension.

III. Pulmonary arterioles.

A. Secondary pulmonary arteriolar sclerosis occurs in association with a wide variety of conditions such as those already discussed, in certain cases of mitral stenosis, emphysema and pulmonary fibrosis, but these changes are not always sufficiently widespread to cause pulmonary hypertension in themselves.

B. Primary pulmonary arteriolar sclerosis is a rare and interesting entity in which no cause for these widespread arteriolar changes is ascertainable in either the pulmonary system or the cardiovascular apparatus. (Fig. 2).

IV. Capillary system. When obstruction occurs to radicles of the pulmonary artery at levels proximal to the capillary bed, it is apparent that the corresponding sets of capillaries also are put out of commission automatically. Similarly, when the left side of the heart fails, capillary function is interfered with even if the capillaries are not

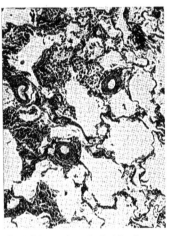

Fig. 2. Pulmonary tissue; sclerosis of the pulmonary arterioles with considerable diminution in the size of their lumens.

altered structurally. Obliteration of portions of the capillary bed results further as a consequence of a group of pulmonary diseases, chief among which are emphysema (through destruction of the interalveolar walls) and widespread pulmonary fibrosis (which destroys portions of pulmonary tissue). Both these conditions, as a rule, are associated with chronic bronchitis, also asthmatic bronchitis and emphysema coexist in many instances. It is apparent that obliteration of the capillary bed must be much more widespread and extensive in order to exhaust the vascular reserves and to cause pulmonary hypertension than when the larger radicles of the pulmonary arterial tree are involved in such a process. This is an important point to grasp because it has a direct bearing on the controversy concerning the rôle of emphysema in the production of pulmonary hypertension.

The association of emphysema and asthma with hypertrophy of the right side of the heart

and congestive heart failure finds expression in the literature of the later Eighteenth Century and out of these observations the term "emphysema heart" was born. The historical background of our present conception of emphysema and its effects on the heart was adequately described by Parkinson and Hoyle in a recent article. This problem cannot be pursued without incorporating two important observations in the discussion. The first is that advanced pulmonary emphysema may not be attended by hypertrophy of the right ventricle, increased venous pressure or other evidence of congestive heart failure and the circulation time through the pulmonary circuit may be within normal limits even in the terminal stages of the disease. There may actually be some venous engorgement associated with emphysema without any increase in venous pressure; however, this venous engorgement is the result mainly of increase in the intrapleural pressure which interferes with drainage of the venous blood into the right auricle. The second observation is that whenever pulmonary arteriolar obliterative changes are found, irrespective of the circumstances, hypertrophy of the right ventricle is present in a high percentage of cases with or without congestive failure.

It would seem that, if emphysema of the so-called obstructive type, which is a relatively frequent disease, were obstructive in the sense that it always impedes the pulmonary circulation, there should be a far closer correlation between the degree and duration of emphysema on the one hand and evidence that the right ventricle has worked against resistance on the other. Most of the literature relative to the subject has failed to take into consideration the part which vascular changes (apart from capillary destruction) may have played in these cases in which hypertrophy of the right ventricle was found and was accompanied by congestive failure. One ventures to predict that when representative surveys of cases of emphysema are completed, results will show that emphysema of itself does not cause pulmonary hypertension, for, although the obliteration of capillaries is extensive in cases of advanced emphysema, it is extremely unlikely that it ever reaches a degree capable of exhausting the vascular reserve. In addition, evidence of failure of the right side of the heart, when it occurs, is usually owing to a second factor. This factor is either pulmonary arteriolar

the venous side is not enough to cause any circulatory embarrassment unless a secondary factor supervenes which increases the arteriovenous shunt. A classic example of this type is so-called Lutembacher's disease consisting of a combination of mitral stenosis and a patulous foramen ovale. In such cases, extreme degrees of pulmonary hypertension with dilatation of the pulmonary artery to aneurysmal proportions may result.

III. Tetralogy of Fallot and other congenital anomalies associated with pulmonary stenosis result in a chronic cor pulmonale. Although an admixture of venous and arterial blood usually occurs in this group through imperfect septa, the pulmonic stenosis is the main etiologic factor concerned.

Acquired arteriovenous shunt. In rare instances a condition analogous to patency of the ductus botalli is created by the gradual rupture of an aortic aneurysm into the pulmonary artery. Such an event may be associated with the roentgenologic and electrocardiographic evidence of pulmonary hypertension and with a bruit simulating that caused by a patent ductus botalli.[5]

A Discussion of the Clinical Picture of Chronic Cor Pulmonale With Special Reference to Differential Diagnosis

In short, the clinical picture of chronic cor pulmonale is that of pulmonary hypertension plus the features contributed by the factor responsible for the pulmonary hypertension. In cases of so-called primary pulmonary arteriolar sclerosis, the distinct syndrome of pulmonary hypertension occurs without the presence of any such discoverable factor to obscure or to distort the clinical picture. There is usually a history of gradually increasing dyspnea as the obliterative process progresses. The resulting interference with ventilation gives rise to cyanosis, which also increases as the disease advances. The striking symptom, then, is dyspnea, which is prominent even in the absence of congestive heart failure. and is out of all proportion to other evidence of congestive heart failure, when the right side of the heart does fail. In short, it is the dyspnea of interference with ventilation and this in itself immediately should suggest its pulmonary origin. It is a characteristic of all pulmonary diseases in which the function of oxygenation is limited.

By the time these patients present themselves

for examination, the secondary manifestations of pulmonary ·hypertension usually can be elicited. The individual often looks older than his chronologic age would·imply,·and this is accentuated by

a, b, c). Finally, the characteristic electrocardiographic pattern indicative of predominant right ventricular strain affords corroborative evidence (Fig. 4 a, b). This consists of right axis devia-

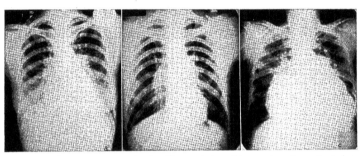

Fig. 3. Chronic cor pulmonale, representing three different mechanisms which can produce pulmonary hypertension: a, Obstruction beyond the pulmonary circuit by mitral stenosis (proved at necropsy); b, obstruction within the pulmonary circuit by pulmonary arteriolar sclerosis (proved at necropsy); c, arteriovenous shunt in widely patent foramen ovale (proved at necropsy). Points in common to all three types of chronic cor pulmonale are an aortic knob which is less prominent than normal, an enlarged conus shadow. There is enlargement through the auricles, especially the left auricle, except when the obstruction is within the pulmonary circuit when the left auricle is normal.

the cyanosis which is present. The striking auscultatory finding is an accentuated second pulmonic sound. The clinical evidence of a hypertrophic right ventricle is afforded by a systolic pulsation to the left of the sternum best elicited by firm palpation in this region. This is accounted for by the fact that, as the right ventricle becomes hypertrophic, it comes to form, more and more, the anterior surface of the heart and approximates the anterior wall of the thorax more closely. On auscultation, the lungs are likely to be clear even in the presence of congestive failure, because the obstruction is proximal to the alveolar system. It is only when the left side of the heart fails secondary to the effects of anoxemia that congestion of the bases of the lungs comes into the clinical picture.

Confirmatory evidence is afforded by laboratory procedures. Roentgenologic examination reveals a prominent pulmonary conus, an enlarged right ventricle and auricle and unusually clear pulmonary fields. Pulsation of the vessels in the pulmonary hilus sometimes can be elicited. An important distinguishing feature is the absence of enlargement of the left auricle which distinguishes it from obstructions beyond the pulmonary circuit, as in cases of mitral stenosis (Fig. 3,

tion which is usually definite and if changes in the T wave occur, they will consist of inversion in the second, third and fourth (standard) leads. There may be secondary polycythemia, the result of anoxemia.

With failure of the right side of the heart, venous congestion, hepatic enlargement, peripheral edema, ascites and increasing cyanosis are added to the picture and it is characteristic of this disease that, when congestive failure supervenes, the subsequent course is invariably rapidly downhill, a type of congestive failure unusually refractory to therapy.

This description holds essentially for pulmonary hypertension owing to any cause, the provoking disease, either in the pulmonary system or cardiovascular apparatus, adding its quota to the symptoms and findings described. Pulmonary hypertension secondary to diseases of the left side of the heart and to the congenital lesions enumerated needs no special comment because the corresponding clinical picture in each case bears hallmarks sufficiently well recognized to establish a diagnosis.[7]

The ability to distinguish between the various processes which cause pulmonary hypertension by obstructing various levels of the pulmonary

540

arterial tree depends on (1) a knowledge of the possible pathologic conditions which are capable of producing such obliterative vascular disease, (2) an understanding of the mechanism involved in each case, that is, the life history of the disease, and (3) a deliberate attempt to elicit evidence of pulmonary hypertension when diseases are encountered which are known to be capable of producing pulmonary hypertension. Because some of these diseases are likely to obscure the characteristic findings of pulmonary hypertension, valuable prognostic data may be overlooked unless a special effort is made to search for such evidence.

In short, these general principles are essentially the same as the methods employed in distinguishing between conditions which obstruct other hollow muscular viscera. The clinical course and the speed with which symptoms and signs develop often give a clue to the pathologic nature of the obstructing mechanism.

With special reference to the pulmonary circuit, we may lay down three principles which afford indirect evidence of the nature of the obstructing lesion: (1) The more proximal the obstruction, that is, the larger the vessels that are occluded, the more profound are the effects. (2) The more rapidly progressive the primary disease, the equally more rapid will the picture of failure of the right side of the heart supervene. Thus, in cases of carcinomatous lymphangitis, the course of failure of the right side of the heart is so much more rapid than in other cases of chronic cor pulmonale, that the term subacute cor pulmonale has aptly been applied to it. (3) Multiple factors which individually may place an inconsequential burden on the right ventricle, when acting together can become a serious threat to the integrity of the right side of the heart. Frequently, mitral stenosis of minimal degree that has been tolerated perfectly well terminates in congestive heart failure because a disturbance of ventilation such as that caused by emphysema, which in itself would not be incapacitating, is superimposed on it. The term Ayerza's disease purposely has been omitted from the discussion because this name has been linked with so many varied pathologic and clinical entities that it contributes neither etiologic nor differential diagnostic information.

Summary and Conclusions

Pulmonary hypertension is a secondary manifestation of a wide variety of conditions which exert their effects either by obstruction of the

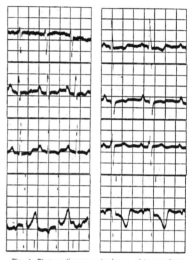

Fig. 4. Electrocardiograms: showing a, right ventricular strain resulting from pulmonary hypertension with right axis deviation, inversion of the T waves in leads II and III, and a positive T wave in lead IV (Wolferth) and, for comparison, b, left ventricular strain with left axis deviation and inversion of the T waves in leads I and II. The fourth lead (Wolferth) is normal.

lesser circulation in or beyond the pulmonary circuit, or by shunts of arterial blood into the pulmonary circulation in certain cases of congenital cardiac anomalies.

The pulmonary circulation is endowed with a rich vascular reserve. Lesions obliterating the larger radicles of the pulmonary arterial tree curtail this reserve and produce pulmonary hypertension more readily than do lesions affecting its more peripheral elements. By the same token, exhaustion of vascular reserve to the extent of causing pulmonary hypertension requires an extremely widespread, obliterative process, if the obstruction is at the capillary level. Thus, emphysema of itself seldom, if ever, causes pulmonary hypertension. Failure of the right side of the heart in the presence of capillary obstruction may be assumed to be associated with a second factor, either an associated obliterative process, proximal to the capillary level, or independent cardiovascular disease throwing an added burden of "back pressure" on the pulmonary circulation and on the right side of the heart. The increased incidence of both emphysema and degenerative cardiovascular disease after middle life must be kept in mind.

Irrespective of the mechanism responsible for its production, pulmonary hypertension is recognized by the secondary effects on the cardiorespiratory system, eventuating in right ventricular hypertrophy, characterized by accentuation of the second pulmonic sound, prominence of the pulmonary artery and conus roentgenologically and the electrocardiographic pattern of right ventricular strain. Absence of enlargement of the left auricle places the obstruction within the pulmonary circuit. Dyspnea is the prominent symptom and is usually progressive. When the obstruction is situated within the pulmonary circuit, dyspnea is caused by interference with ventilation and is usually prominent even in the absence of congestive features and out of all proportion to other evidence of congestive heart failure, when the right heart does fail. Under these circumstances, too, the pulmonary fields are likely to be unusually clear.

The final syndrome depends on the symptoms and signs that are contributed to this picture by the disease provoking the pulmonary hypertension. The differential diagnosis depends on a knowledge of the possible pathologic conditions

capable of producing obliterative pulmonary vascular disease, a knowledge of the clinical behavior of these conditions, and on a deliberate attempt to elicit evidence of pulmonary hypertension when diseases are encountered which are known to be capable of producing pulmonary hypertension.

References

1. Bachmann, M. O.: Die Veränderungen der innern Organen bei hochgradigen Skoliosen und Kyposkoliosen. Stuttgart, E. Nagle, 1899, pp. 172.
2. Barnes, A. R., and Yater, W. M.: Failure of the right ventricle due to an ancient thrombus in the pulmonary arteries. Med. Clin. N. Amer., 12:1610-1613, (May) 1929.
3. Brill, I. C., and Robertson, T. D.: Subacute cor pulmonale. Arch. Int. Med., 60:1043-1057, (Dec.) 1937.
4. Clark, Eugene, and Graef, Irving: Chronic pulmonary arteritis in schistosomiasis mansoni associated with right ventricular hypertrophy: report of a case. Am. Jour. Path., 9:693-705, (July) 1933.
5. Delp, M. H., and Maxwell, Robert: Rupture of an aortic aneurysm into the pulmonary artery: report of a case. Jour. Am. Med. Assn., 110:1647-1649, (May 14) 1938.
6. Diggs, L. W., and Ching, R. E.: Pathology of sickle cell anemia. South. Med. Jour., 27:839-845, (Oct.) 1934.
7. Dry, T. J.: An approach to the diagnosis of congenital heart disease. Am. Heart Jour., 14:135-154, (Aug.) 1929.
8. Greenspan, E. B.: Carcinomatous endarteritis of the pulmonary vessels resulting in failure of the right ventricle. Arch. Int. Med., 54:625-644, (Oct.) 1934.
9. Haggart, G. E., and Walker, A. M.: The physiology of pulmonary embolism as disclosed by quantitative occlusion of the pulmonary artery. Arch. Surg., 6:764-783, (May) 1923.
10. Jump, H. D., and Baumann, Freida: Large thrombus of the pulmonary artery with chronic cyanosis and polycythemia. Pennsylvania Med. Jour., 32:754-756, (Aug.) 1929.
11. Means, J. H., and Mallory, T. B.: Total occlusion of the right branch of the pulmonary artery by an organized thrombus. Ann. Int. Med., 5:417-427, (Oct.) 1931.
12. Montgomery, G. L.: A case of pulmonary artery thrombosis with Ayerza's syndrome. Jour. Path. and Bacteriol., 41:221-230, (Sept.) 1935.
13. Parkinson, John, and Hoyle, Clifford: The heart in emphysema. Quart. Jour. Med., 6:59-86, (Jan.) 1937.
14. Thompson, W. P., and White, P. D.: The commonest cause of hypertrophy of the right ventricle—left ventricular strain and failure. Am. Heart Jour., 12:641-649, (Dec.) 1936.
15. Underhill, S. W. F.: An investigation into the circulation through the lungs. Brit. Med. Jour., 2:779-782, (Nov. 12) 1921.
16. Waring, J. J., and Black, W. C.: The syndrome of obstruction in the lesser circulation. Am. Jour. Med. Sc., 187:652-662, (May) 1934.

UTERINE CANCER*

ROLAND S. CRON, M.D., F.A.C.S.

Milwaukee, Wisconsin

E VIDENCE is gradually accumulating to prove that cancer in the United States is increasing. The cancer death rate, the number of deaths per 100,000, has increased from 63 per 100,000 in 1900 to 108 per 100,000 in 1935. A part of this increase may be related to the lengthened span of life and also to more accurate diagnosis, but most of it is due to its more frequent appearance. Its increase is viewed

with alarm and by many it is considered our greatest menace. Further analysis of the situation shows that not over one out of every four treated cases of genital cancer in women remains cured for five years or more. This is not a very encouraging showing. It has not changed even with the lowered mortality resulting from the introduction of x-ray and radium therapy. Is it any wonder that, with the general instruction of the public, so many women have become cancer conscious and not a few developed a definite

*Presented at the eighty-fifth annual meeting of the Minnesota State Medical Association, Duluth, Minn., June 29, 1938.

542

phobia? Even so, there is no object in throwing up one's hands in horror, but, instead, let us do as Te Linde suggests, continue to hew away at the problem and thereby reduce the mortality little by little. Cancer of the cervix is the most common variety of uterine cancer, occurring about eight times to each fundal cancer. It is a disease of middle life, but has no respect for age periods. It has been seen in the first and last decades of life but its greatest incidence is in the years immediately preceding and including the menopause, the menopausal period being assumed to occur between the ages of forty and forty-five. The writer, however, has been impressed with the frequency of the disease during the second and third decades. He is of the opinion it is making its appearance at earlier ages. Cancer of the corpus in contrast is distinctly a disease of the menopause and postmenopausal period.

Etiology

Formerly, we considered cervical cancer a rarity in the woman who had never experienced pregnancy. This is not true. Cervical and especially fundal carcinoma are frequently found in the nonparous uterus. Cervical lacerations and erosions have never been proven to be precursors of cancer, but a lacerated, eroded and discharging cervix is not only a definite focus of infection but also a menace. Cautery, repair or excision of such a lesion will act as a prophylaxis against cancer and make detection of any malignant lesion in the future much easier. Vaginal pessaries when worn for correction of retroversion or prolapse of the uterus do not cause cancer. For hygienic reasons, they should be removed and cleansed at frequent intervals. It is also wise, at that time, to inspect the vagina and cervix and to treat any lesion present. That so-called chronic irritation of the cervix is not the cause of cancer is well borne out by the infrequency of its incidence in prolapse of the uterus. In a study of 200 cases of uterine prolapse not a single cancer of the cervix was found.

Cancer appearing in the cervix following subtotal hysterectomy is frequently the result of a faulty diagnosis before or at the time of operation. It is often present in the cervix at that time and is either not recognized by the operator because of his inability to do so, or not diagnosed because of his negligence to visualize and study the cervix. The argument that such errors could be rectified by performing total instead of subtotal hysterectomies is an unsound one. True, such a procedure will cure early cervical cancer and prevent the subsequent development of one, but it will also increase the operative mortality. There is no question but that, in the hands of operators doing the large majority of hysterectomies in this country, the supravaginal operation is the safer and simpler of the two. Also the reduction in morbidity, injured intestines, bladder, and ureters will compensate many times over for any increase in cervical stump cancer. And finally an eroded, infected, degenerated or lacerated cervix can be treated very satisfactorily through the vagina.

Uterine fibromyomata and strictures of the uterine canal are occasionally associated with corporal cancer. Oesterlin and the author found that 20 per cent of fundal cancers were associated with myomata. In the majority of cases, it was coincidental, but in at least one uterus a calcified nodule impinged upon a malignant area directly opposite to it. Strictures by damming back infected secretions may also be factors in the etiology of cancer.

Evidence is accumulating to show that heredity is a factor in the appearance of cancer. There is a greater incidence in brother and sister relationship than in husband and wife. Cancer families are a definite entity. Experimentally, Maud Slye has proved that cancer susceptibility in rodents is hereditary. The least one should do is to speculate on the possibility that this is a recessive Mendelian characteristic.

Hormones have been suggested as the cause of cancer. There is an amazing similarity in the chemical formula of estrogenic and carcinogenic substance. One has only to switch a few radicals of the chemical formula of estrin and one has the stimulus necessary for carcinoma. It has also been observed that hyperplasia of the endometrium during the menopause is associated with the excretion of estrin in the urine. Novak states that a postmenopausal endometrium subjected to persistent estrogenic stimulation is predisposed to adenocarcinoma. Such observations have opened an entire new lead in cancer investigation. It may not be a mistake to bring up the problem of the indiscriminate use of the endocrines in the treatment of the many ailments of women. The long continued substitutional administration of any glandular product may result in atrophy of the organ treated.

Pathology

Cervical cancer is most commonly epidermoid. Early in its metamorphosis it appears as a circumscribed, easily bleeding, slightly elevated lesion. Only very occasionally it is seen or recognized at this stage. Later, it is an excavated ulcer or a cauliflower-like mass. These three types of lesions make up 90 to 95 per cent of all cervical cancerous lesions. The other 5 to 10 per cent are adenocarcinomata. They arise in the canal and cannot be distinguished macroscopically from epidermoid cancer. They are almost always far advanced when diagnosed, due to the fact that the vaginal portion of the cervix remains intact, while the growth extends into the neighboring structures.

A few pertinent facts in regard to the grading of malignant tumors are worthy of presentation. Broders, in 1920, was the first to correlate the different microscopic pictures of similar cancers with their clinical course. Thus, he was able to divide histologically, all cancers into four groups or grades. This also covered the clinical outcome from those which could be cured to those which were hopeless. The principle of grading is based upon an estimation of the ratio of mature to immature cells within the tumor. In Broders' classification, a grade one carcinoma contains 0 to 25 per cent immature or undifferentiated cells. This is the least malignant lesion. A grade two cancer has 25 to 50 per cent immature cells; a grade three 50 to 75 per cent immature cells and a grade four 75 to 100 per cent immature cells. This last is the most malignant lesion.

A study of the incidence of cervical cancer has shown that very few if any can be classified as grade one where most of the cells are mature or differentiated; that only 15 per cent are of grade two; and that 85 per cent are grade three and four, where the cells are for the most part immature or undifferentiated. The chief characteristic of these immature cells is that the chromatin of the nucleus is deep staining and granular and stands out most prominently. Mitosis is very active. The nucleolus is also proportionately greatly increased in size. Fundal cancer can be graded in a similar way, but there are many more that can be classified as grades one and two than is the case in cervical cancer.

Correspondingly, more than 60 per cent of fundal cancers remain cured five years or longer. Ewing has divided corporal cancer into adenoma malignum and adenocarcinoma. The incidence of the two are about equal but the percentage of three-year cures is about ninety-three for adenoma malignum against thirty-nine for adenocarcinoma. Fundal cancer, in either case, has a much better prognosis than cervical cancer. It remains confined to its site of origin much longer than does cervical cancer.

A correlation of the grade of cervical cancer and end-results of treatment shows that, independent of the stage or advancement of the disease, grade two cancers when treated by x-ray, radium, surgery or a combination of any of the three have resulted in .53 per cent of five-year cures. On the surface this result appears encouraging, but on further analysis one finds that only 15 per cent of cervical cancers are grade two cancers. Grade three cancers, when treated, result in 21 per cent cures and grade four in 9 per cent five-year cures and since 85 per cent of all cervical cancers are in these two groups the average of five-year cures has never advanced much beyond 25 per cent.

Diagnosis

The early diagnosis of uterine cancer depends upon two factors. First, the consulting of the physician by the patient. Even in spite of the immense amount of publicity and propaganda that has been carried on during the past years many women, suspecting or having cancer, still prefer to remain in ignorance of their condition. Then, they report to their physician only long after their doom has been sealed. Stovall, in an editorial, summarized the situation as follows: "This is due to the public's fear of cancer. They are aware of the fatality of the disease commonly recognized as cancer and cancer is commonly recognized as a late process. The public thinks of the doctor in connection with critical illness only. The way to change this attitude is to give them the basic facts on which to diagnose early cancer. The thoughtful consideration of this will lead them to the acceptance of the advice that early cancer is curable."

The part the physician plays. He must be able to recognize the disease in its incipiency or, at least, before it has involved adjacent structures or metastasized. To accomplish this he must obtain a thorough and complete history. The earliest symptom of uterine and cervical cancer is bleeding. It may be only a show or it may be profuse. It may occur before, during, or after the menopause. Its outstanding characteristic is that it frequently follows trauma such as coitus, douching, or instrumentation. Bleeding after the menopause in over 50 per cent of cases is due to cancer. It may be associated with a watery and foul discharge, but this is usually a complaint of a more advanced stage. Pain is a late symptom.

Every woman consulting a physician for a health examination or because of any illness should have a gynecological examination. This examination should consist in not only bimanual palpation (single finger) but also visualization of the cervix. The examination is then completed only after tissue from any questionable area has been removed for microscopic study. Thus, one may be able to diagnose incipient and very early cervical cancer. No gynecological examination is complete without rectal palpation. The number of anal and rectal cancers casually diagnosed by this procedure is surprising. More important is the assistance it affords the examiner in determining the extent of involvement of the broad and sacro-uterine ligaments and rectum by an inflammatory reaction or carcinoma. Occasionally, it is the only means of ascertaining the size and mobility of the uterus and adnexa. It is always a great help in evaluating one of these problems.

Hinselman and others by magnification of the cervix have described the characteristics of early cancerous lesions. These are: (1) leukoplakic patches; (2) slightly elevated prominent pale areas with uneven surfaces and richly supplied with blood vessels; (3) a slightly irregular area with a tendency to bleed readily and having appearance of an erosion; (4) very small ulcerations, shallow with slightly elevated margins and friability detected on palpation.

Schiller uses the iodine test to aid in the detection of early cancer. The cervix is painted with Gram's iodine solution. Cancerous and all other tissue deficient in glycogen will not take the stain, while the rest of the epithelium takes on a chestnut brown. Unfortunately, inflammatory areas, erosions, nabothian cysts, hornified areas and cervical canal epithelium fail to take the stain.

Whether one uses the colposcope, Schiller's test or the naked eye the final diagnosis must be accomplished by removing tissue and examining it under the microscope. When obtaining tissue it is wise to remove a generous piece including suspected cancerous as well as healthy tissue. One may obtain this with the knife followed by cauterization of the cut surface or by the use of surgical diathermy. There is very little if any danger of disseminating cancer by curettage or biopsy. Squeezing or manipulating a growth is much more likely to produce metastases. Endocervical and fundal carcinoma is diagnosed by examination of tissue obtained by curettage.

Treatment

The greatest opportunity in treatment of cervical cancer still lies in the field of prophylaxis. Thorough eradication of benign cervical pathology by whatever means indicated, be it cauterization, conization, plastic repair, amputation or total hysterectomy, will prevent the development of cervical cancer. The author does not know of a single case of malignancy developing in a healthy cervix. Infection and inflammation are more important predisposing causes of cancer than are lacerations and scars. It is even conceivable that prophylactic treatment may cure very early unrecognized cancer.

Epidermoid cervical cancer is most successfully treated by x-ray and radium. Experience has proven that preliminary high voltage deep therapy x-ray followed by topical and intracavitary radiation produces the best end-results. Initial x-ray exposures through six ports with cross firing brings about amazing shrinkage of the tumor, reduction in the amount of infection and sealing of the lymphatics. It is also more effective if administered before the cancer becomes radioresistant from the influence of the radium.

Radium can be administered either in one or two doses or frequent small ones. In either case, it should be well distributed and applied where it will accomplish the most good. It should be carefully screened and the adjacent structures well protected. This is especially true when using massive doses.

Fundal and early cervical adenocarcinoma is most successfully treated by complete extirpation of the uterus, followed by roentgen-ray therapy.

When surgery is not feasible, treatment with x-ray and radium has afforded good results.

Injuries to bladder, bowel, ureters and small intestines have resulted from x-ray and especially radium therapy. Many times, these injuries do not appear until later in the disease or after an apparent cure. Swelling of the broad ligaments, the result of local inflammatory reactions, produce difficulty with elimination. Temporary or permanent bowel obstructions and interference with ureteral function are common. Occasionally, rectal and ureteral dilatations are indicated. Bladder injuries are distressing. Various fistulas are usually the result of malignant tissue destruction but many times the radium therapy is unjustly blamed. Cancer fistulas are generally irreparable.

Prognosis

The grade of the malignancy of uterine cancer is by far the most important factor to consider in prognosis. Tumors of low grade mean slow growth, late metastases, less radiosensitivity and a greater percentage of cures. On the other hand, tumors of high grade have a faster growth, earlier metastases, more radiosensitivity but a shorter length of life. Other factors being equal, the more immature the cell in the tumor (higher grade), the more radiosensitive is that tumor. It is this type of lesion that one should treat most intensively, first with x-ray, and then radium.

Of course, there are other factors which influence the outcome of treatment. The younger the patient the more virulent the disease. Epidermoid cancer of similar grade in a woman of sixty is not as serious a lesion as if it were present in a woman of thirty. The local extent of the lesion is likewise of great importance. Cancers involving only the portio vaginalis of the cervix or the endometrium of the fundus in adenocarcinoma are lesions most amenable to treatment. Metastases and extension, of course, are most important determining factors. Finally, it is up to the clinician to combine his knowledge of all of these factors and after that to give a fairly accurate prognosis.

SULFANILAMIDE IN UROLOGY*

EDWARD N. COOK, M.D., and HENRY A. BUCHTEL, M.D.

Rochester, Minnesota

SULFANILAMIDE (p-amino-benzene-sulfanilamide) is a new drug which is proving its value in the treatment of many and varied diseases. A certain skepticism has accompanied its introduction, and rightly so; but when it is used under the careful and diligent supervision of the physician, a minimum of serious complications has developed.

The antecedent of sulfanilamide was discovered in 1908, but it remained for Domagk, in 1935, to revive interest in it. He was able to demonstrate its therapeutic activity and in a very short while many other investigators had corroborated his work with the various forms of this drug.

Sulfanilamide has been tried in all fields of medicine, and urology is no exception. During the past five years, the treatment of infections of the urinary tract has been taken from its place in the hit or miss file and assigned to a respectable position in the scientific therapy of disease. We have learned the value of frequent and careful bacteriologic investigation in every case of infection of the urinary tract. Depending on the results of Gram's stain and culture of the urine, we have planned our treatment, and sulfanilamide is a welcome addition to our armamentarium. The importance of this drug to the urologist is becoming well known.

Mode of Administration and Dosage

When sulfanilamide is given to man, it is practically entirely eliminated in the urine in a free state and in a conjugated form, as paraacetyl amino benzene sulfanilamide. When given orally, the rate of absorption of the drug varies somewhat in different cases; two or three days usually are required to establish equilibrium between the amount ingested and the amount excreted. Following the taking of this drug, concentrations which are but slightly lower than

*From the Section on Urology, The Mayo Clinic, Rochester, Minnesota.

those in the blood occur in the prostatic secretion, pleural and peritoneal effusions, and spinal fluid.

The dosage of this drug in urologic conditions varies and is greatly different from the dosage in its general use. When treating infections of the urinary tract, we feel it advisable to begin with the maximal dosage in order to build up an adequate concentration of the drug in the body as quickly as possible. What this initial dosage will be depends on the age of the patient, the general condition of the patient, and the nature of the disease. Clinically, in a series of more than 600 cases, we have observed that the elderly patient rarely will tolerate a dosage greater than 40 grains (2.59 gm.) daily. Fortunately this dosage is frequently sufficient to sterilize the urine, and an increase is not necessary. In cases in which the patients are debilitated, the drug must always be given with care. In certain cases in which it is not advisable to give this dose, even smaller doses have produced some benefit, and it is wise to limit the dose. In cases in which the patients are young and strong, daily doses of 60 to 75 grains (4 to 5 gm.) of sulfanilamide are well tolerated and are advised. Our usual procedure is to give 60 grains (4 gm.) each day for two or three days and then reduce the dose to 40 grains (2.59 gm.) daily; the latter dose is maintained for the entire period of treatment, which usually lasts eight to fourteen days. Administration of the drug should be stopped at the end of this time, regardless of the condition of the urine. If sterilization of the urine has not taken place, a similar course of therapy is repeated in ten to fourteen days. When treating gonorrhea, we usually use a dose of 75 grains (5 gm.) daily for two or three days, then 60 grains (4 gm.) daily for a similar period, and then 40 grains (2.59 gm.) daily until a period of fourteen days has elapsed since the beginning of treatment. A second course of treatment may be necessary after a rest of ten to fourteen days without medication.

Clinically, the effectiveness of this drug is attended with many of the limitations which attended the use of the ketogenic diet or the administration of mandelic acid in the treatment of infections of the urinary tract. Nevertheless, the drug is of great value in a few cases in which these latter forms of medication failed entirely.

We will consider the use of sulfanilamide in a variety of urologic conditions.

Uncomplicated Infections

When the causative organism is any one of the bacilli usually found in the urinary tract, the use of this drug is attended with great success. Even in cases in which organisms of the genus Proteus are found, the results have been good, as we have not had to contend with the factor of pH, as we did with mandelic acid.

In cases of infection of the urinary tract in which there is no complicating factor, such as obstruction to the flow of urine, stone, tumor, or cicatricial deformity of the renal pelvis and calices, sulfanilamide is of great value. Eighty-two patients who had uncomplicated infection of the urinary tract and who were treated at The Mayo Clinic were followed in great detail. In seventy of these cases a bacillus was the causative organism, and in twelve cases a coccus was found. In sixty-four cases in which the infection was caused by a bacillus, the urine became sterile while the patients were on sulfanilamide therapy. In two cases there was definite improvement, and in four cases no benefit was noted. Of the twelve patients who had infection caused by a coccus, nine were definitely cured and three did not obtain benefit at all.

Complicated Infections

When a bacillary infection of the urinary tract is associated with chronic prostatitis, our experience in the past has been that the efficacy of mandelic acid or the ketogenic diet was definitely reduced. Fortunately, this is not equally true when sulfanilamide is used. In our earlier work, we were able to show that the concentration of sulfanilamide in the prostatic secretion is only slightly less than that reported in the blood of patients taking the drug. We feel that this is the explanation for the increased efficiency of this drug in cases in which bacilluria is associated with marked chronic prostatitis. In almost all instances the same bacillus can be isolated in pure culture from the prostatic secretion. We feel that prostatic massage is clearly indicated in conjunction with the administration of sulfanilamide and have carried out the procedure in all our cases. There were ninety-eight cases of this type in our series: in sixty-two of these cases the infection was caused by bacilli and in thirty-six cases it was caused by cocci. In the cases of bacillary infections, fifty-two patients had sterile urine at the end of the period of treatment and obtained a very marked improvement in the degree of prostatitis. Eight patients were improved, but the urine was not sterile, and in two cases there was no improvement. In the thirty-six cases of coccal infection, eighteen patients experienced very marked relief and the urine became sterile, eight were improved, but ten were not benefited by the administration of sulfanilamide. In more than half of the cases in which the patients were not benefited, the organism was the Streptococcus fæcalis, which, we knew, experimentally and clinically, would not usually respond to sulfanilamide therapy. More striking than the improvement in the urine or in the symptoms was the improvement of the prostatitis in this group of cases. Under the usual prostatic treatment, which consists of massage, heat, and urethral irrigations, it is very unusual to see an appreciable change in the number of pus cells in the prostatic secretion in less than six to eight weeks. When this local regimen was combined with the administration of sulfanilamide by mouth, a very definite change in the cell count was frequently noticed in seven to ten days. However, in the group of cases of nonspecific prostatitis in which there was no bacteriuria, sulfanilamide has had little or no effect on the degree of prostatitis.

Renal infections without any complicating factor, such as stone, obstruction, or cicatricial deformity, respond very well to this drug. There were eighteen cases of this type, and in sixteen cases the urine was rendered sterile. When the pyelonephritis is associated with any of the complications mentioned, the results are not nearly so good. In fifty-eight of the eighty-two cases of complicated renal infection, bacilli were found in the urine. In twenty-two of these cases the urine became sterile, and a similar number of patients noted improvement; in fourteen cases there was no change. Of twenty-four patients who had a coccal infection, only four had sterile urine after treatment, and ten did not improve. The same number, however, did experience relief of symptoms with some improvement in the urine, although the cultures remained positive.

In cases of prostatism, sulfanilamide must be given with care because of the age of the patients. When the drug is administered as a pre-

liminary measure, before any surgical procedure is directed to the relief of obstruction at the neck of the bladder, it rarely will produce a sterile urine. In a considerable percentage of cases, some improvement may be noted, but there usually is not much benefit. However, the drug is worthy of trial when the urine is very cloudy. Gaudin, Zide and Thompson have carefully studied the value of giving this drug postoperatively to patients who have undergone a transurethral prostatic resection. As a general rule the drug was usually poorly tolerated by the patients. However, there seemed to be less infection in the urines of these patients at the time of their dismissal from the hospital than there was in the urines of a group of patients who were not taking the drug. Again, the raw healing surface of the prostatic bed will preclude sterilization of the urine, and it seems advisable to postpone administration of sulfanilamide or any other strenuous attempts to eradicate the infection until healing has taken place. This seems to correspond with our experience with mandelic acid or the ketogenic diet, as previously reported.

Gonorrhea

In cases of gonorrhea our results have been just as good. From time immemorial the medical profession has sought some drug which, when given by mouth, would be destructive to the Neisseria gonorrhoeæ. Following the work of Dees and Colston, many workers have used this drug in treating gonorrhea with variable success. In our rather small series of cases, we discontinued all local treatment when giving the drug, in order to ascertain its true worth. However, we insisted on abstinence from alcohol and any form of sexual excitement. In twenty-one cases the patients were males and in twelve they were females. All but two of the males responded nicely to the drug. In some of these cases a second course of sulfanilamide was necessary before the cultures became negative, and each one had a follow-up course of the drug two weeks after the cultures became negative. Eight of the females obtained negative cultures within one month after the treatment was started, but in the other four cases repeated courses of sulfanilamide were ineffectual and fever therapy was resorted to. In one case this failed, and it was finally decided to give the patient large doses of sulfanilamide. When the concentration of the drug in the blood was high, the patient was given a ten-hour treatment in the Kettering hypertherm and diathermy was applied to the pelvis for five hours during the period of elevated temperature. Following this procedure, the cultures became negative and have remained so since treatment was stopped seven months ago. Unquestionably, in this case we were dealing with a very resistant strain of the Neisseria gonorrhoeæ.

In a second group of thirty-eight cases of gonorrhea observed in the city dispensary, there were thirty males and eight females. Seven males had clear urine, no urethral discharge, and negative smears in twelve days. Fifteen of the patients showed very definite improvement during the first course of sulfanilamide, but the urine was still hazy and the smears were positive. In these cases a second course of sulfanilamide, however, produced negative smears and negative cultures in an additional twelve days. In eight cases there was little or no change in the symptoms or in the objective findings after the first course of treatment. We then used local treatment which consisted of instillations of mild silver protein (5 per cent solution of mild protein silver and 5 per cent solution of neo-silvol) or 1:3000 solution of merthiolate. Later, the patients again were given sulfanilamide and in all instances the symptoms were relieved and the smears became negative. In this group of cases the shortest period of treatment was two months and the longest was three months. All of these patients were seen at intervals of one week for a month after the smears and cultures became negative.

Of the eight females, two did not complete the treatment. In four cases the cultures became negative within three weeks after administration of the drug was started, and the cultures remained negative for two months, at which time the patients were dismissed. In two cases local treatment was instituted and the administration of sulfanilamide was repeated. In these cases all cultures were negative at the end of an additional eight weeks.

In regard to complications, one man had a swollen, tender right epididymis at the time of admission; within twenty-four hours after administration of the drug was started, the swelling had decreased a fourth, the tenderness was practically gone, and the urethral discharge had stopped completely. Another patient had a swollen, reddened left epididymis; this resulted in fluctuation, which necessitated incision and drainage in spite of sulfanilamide and fever treatment. We have seen a few cases of gonorrheal arthritis, and the results have been variable. If there is not a very marked decrease in the pain and swelling of the gonorrheal joint within three to six days after starting sulfanilamide treatment, we believe the patient should be subjected to fever treatment, as this method of therapy has been of the greatest value in such cases.

Complications

In reviewing our cases we have noted few untoward results with sulfanilamide therapy. Approximately 8 to 10 per cent of our patients have been unable to take the drug for any appreciable period. Some of these will have to stop taking it after the first few doses and others will have to discontinue taking it later because of marked cyanosis or skin reactions. We do not believe that tinnitus, headache, nausea, or a mild cyanosis necessitates discontinuing administration of the drug, but we do feel that these symptoms should demand close observation of the patient. If the physician will insist on frequent, regular visits of the patient, we feel certain that any probably serious reaction can be averted. Prolonged or intensive administration of sulfanilamide may produce methemoglobinemia or sulphemoglobinemia. The latter condition is of serious consequence and must be watched for. Granulocytopenia and acute hemolytic anemia have also been reported as occurring after sulfanilamide administration. If the drug is used extensively, it is well to examine the blood microscopically for evidence of destruction of the corpuscles.

Comment

Within a relatively short period, sulfanilamide has proved itself of inestimable value in the treatment of infections of the urinary tract. The drug is more efficacious in the treatment of bacillary infections than it is in the treatment of coccal infections. It has little or no effect on the Streptococcus fæcalis. The Neisseria gonorrhoeæ is definitely killed by the drug in the majority of instances.

The limitations of its use in treating infections of the urinary tract are well recognized, and when complications of infection occur, such as stone, tumor, or obstruction, the effectiveness of the drug is greatly reduced. The use of the drug is not without danger. At least 10 per cent of patients will not tolerate the drug, and this is particularly true of elderly patients. Definite

toxic signs do appear and must be watched for. The drug should always be administered under the diligent supervision of the physician, who should note any untoward reaction. This will practically always avert any serious reaction to the administration of sulfanilamide.

THE PRESENT STATUS OF GASTROSCOPY*

NORMAN GIERE, M.D.

Minneapolis, Minnesota

MUCH has been written concerning the procedure of gastroscopy since the introduction of the flexible instrument in 1932 by Schindler. Most of the literature has concerned itself with the phase of gastroscopy in which the worker was especially interested. Since so much was promised at its inception by the enthusiasts of the procedure whereas by the skeptics it was thought to be little more than an ultra refinement in gastro-intestinal diagnostic procedures, it might be well at this time to take stock as to what the experience of the various workers in this field has been, and thus to gain some conception of its present status in medicine.

Schindler[21] has said that in the field of gastritis gastroscopy will find its greatest usefulness. This statement is undoubtedly true for the reason that gastroscopic examination alone can accurately diagnose this condition in the usual case. Much work has been done by roentgenologists in attempting to diagnose gastritis by relief method,[8,16] and in the hands of experienced and critical examiners certain cases may be correctly diagnosed. It is safe to say, however, that the present consensus amongst radiologists is in agreement with Berg, who stated at the fifth international congress of radiology in Chicago that even careful study of the mucosal relief would often fail to indicate the presence of chronic gastritis. This disease entity has previously been a very indefinite thing. Acute gastritis was clearly shown by the famous observations which Beaumont made on his Canadian, St. Martin, through an open gastric fistula. Chronic gastritis, however, could not be shown to exist in such an objective and dramatic way

and thus after a period of great enthusiasm the disease disappeared from routine diagnosis. Many pathologists[5] at various times thought they had found sections of gastric mucosa which demonstrated gastritic changes. In most instances, however, it was found to have been due to post mortem changes. Knud Faber was the first to inject a ten per cent solution of formalin directly into the abdominal cavity immediately following death, thus fixing the tissues and establishing the histological entity of gastritis. We are indebted to pathological specimen study and the gastroscope for not only definitely establishing the disease as an entity, but also for allowing us to conclude that it is very probably the most frequent cause of gastric disturbance.[6,7,17] Gutzeit[6] has stated that in his clinic gastritis was observed twelve times as frequently as was gastric ulcer and three times as frequently as was duodenal ulcer. Henning[15] stated that because of the frequency of gastritis he believes no diagnostic investigation of the stomach to be complete without gastroscopic examination. It is not the purpose of this paper to discuss the pathology of gastritis, but merely to suggest that experience has borne out the predictions as to the value of gastroscopy in diagnosing this condition. Observation of gastritis is important not only in order to manage the existing condition but because of the possible complications. If we are to agree with the gastritic theory as advocated by Hurst,[8] Konjetzny[10] and Knud Faber[5] as to the etiology of ulcer it is to be expected that by treatment of the gastritis many potential cases of ulcer might be prevented, and in cases where the ulcer process has already begun that treatment will be instituted earlier. If we believe with Schindler[20] that ulcer originates from a mucosal hemorrhage

*From the Department of Surgery, University of Minnesota College of Medicine.

either as a result of stasis due to protracted irritation of the vasomotor nerves or of traumatic origin, it can still be said that observation of these early mucosal changes will allow earlier and thus more satisfactory control of gastric ulcer. Hurst[9] and Konjetzny,[11] among others, also believe that atrophic gastritis generally precedes the development of gastric carcinoma. Hurst[9] has shown that anacidity is present not only in 75 per cent of gastric cancer as a result of chronic gastritis, but that it was present for years before the carcinoma developed. Thus, it seems reasonable to suppose that periodic observations of cases of atrophic gastritis may result in earlier diagnosis of gastric carcinoma. Recently, two cases were reported from the Mayo Clinic in which carcinoma developed within fifteen and four months respectively from a hypertrophic gastritis, which had been examined microscopically from biopsy taken at the first operation and which was seen to have been free from carcinoma at that time. In the report of these cases,[4] the statement is made: "The conception that chronic gastritis is the soil in which cancer develops in a large percentage of cases, if finally accepted, will influence greatly the methods used in the prophylaxis and early diagnosis of cancer."

In any branch of medicine it is usually conceded that the most satisfactory and exact means of studying the progress of treatment of a gross lesion is by direct inspection; this applies as definitely to gastric lesions as to those of other parts of the body. It may be added that since there is the possibility of a malignant change developing from a benign mucosal lesion the importance of direct inspection may be even greater than in some other cases. As a diagnostic procedure, gastroscopy is probably not as valuable in ulcer cases as is x-ray.[4] Both have their advantages and each can demonstrate the ulcer in certain cases where the other fails. In those cases where the lesions are visualized by gastroscopy we find the procedure to be of value in following their therapeutic management. Both Gutzeit[6] and Schindler[14] are of the opinion that clinically and roentgenologically the ulcer is apparently healed at a time that gastroscopic examination can clearly demonstrate its existence. Gutzeit believes this to be of great importance in the correct management of gastric ulcer and in the prevention of recurrence. Schindler[19] has

stated that complete epithelialization of ulcer can be determined only by gastroscopy and that this completion may require as long as two months after refined x-ray compression has failed to visualize any abnormality.

At the international congress of gastro-enterology held in Paris this past September the question for consideration was early diagnosis of gastric carcinoma. Many speakers were enthusiastic about the value of gastroscopic examination in this respect. It must be stated, however, that practically all these statements were based on clinical impressions rather than on controlled study. Schindler states:[18] "There is much reason for thinking that a differential diagnosis between a benign and a malignant ulcer can be made much more easily by gastroscopy than by any other procedure." Other gastroscopists are not so sure that a correct differential diagnosis can be made in such a high percentage of cases (Moutier, Rodgers, Henning, Friedrich).[18] It is true that the circulating blood seems to facilitate the differentiation between benign and malignant ulcers. The floor of the carcinomatous ulcer is not the usual dull yellowish gray of the benign ulcer, but is rather dark brown or violet in color.[7] The edge is generally ragged and irregular instead of giving the sharp punched out appearance of the benign ulcer.[18] In addition, the transition from the ulcer to normal tissue is more gradual in cases of malignancy than is usual in benign ulcers. A controlled series of cases for differential diagnosis was studied by Schindler and the author in 1936 with the conclusion that in this particular series gastroscopic examination gave more correct and detailed information concerning differential diagnosis than did roentgen examination.[22] More controlled work must be done to determine the exact value of gastroscopy in differential diagnosis of benign and malignant lesions, but that it is of value can at this time be safely stated.

Up to the present time exploratory surgery has been very frequently carried out in cases of advanced gastric carcinoma. The end-results have, of course, been very poor. This fact not only makes surgical mortality figures for cancer cases as a whole unreasonably high, but helps to instill in the mind of the layman the attitude that surgery in all cases of gastric cancer is hopeless. It is reasonable to believe that all surgeons would welcome a method which would give the needed information without the operative risk. It is possible that gastroscopy will to a large extent fill this need. Nine case of gastric carcinoma were studied in which the question of operability arose. The accuracy of gastroscopic examination in these cases as to demonstrating the operability of the lesion was not only found to be greater than by x-ray, but was, in fact, correct in every instance.[22] Inoperability of a gastric tumor may become evident by gastroscopy;[1,12,22] it may be shown that the tumor is not sharply defined and that the infiltration extends too high to allow even a radical operation.[10] Certainly, if these cases of obvious inoperability as shown by gastroscopy could be saved from exploratory operation, it is reasonable to suppose that the surgical mortality from gastric carcinoma would be lowered, which in turn might convince medical men and laymen that the prognosis of an early carcinoma of the stomach is a very different thing from that of an advanced case. They would understand that early cancer may be cured by surgery whereas it is not even attempted in cases of advanced cancer. It is possible that this would result not only in more operations in cases of gastric carcinoma, but particularly in a higher percentage of early cases in which definite cure is most likely to be brought about. By way of bringing about this end the following simple suggestions have been made:[22]

a. Patients over thirty-five years of age who have anorexia and loss of weight should be examined roentgenographically and gastroscopically.

b. All patients suffering from a gastric carcinoma, which is not diffusely infiltrating but is sharply limited, should be advised to undergo operation regardless of the location of the neoplasm, unless it is at the extreme cardiac end. On the other hand, a diffusely infiltrating tumor should be operated on only if it is small and if it is strictly confined to the pyloric region.

c. Exploratory laparotomy should be done only in those cases in which gastroscopy cannot definitely decide the operability of the lesion.

In addition to the above instances in which gastroscopy has proved its value, we have the further consideration of its potential value in investigative work of stomach diseases in general. Since it allows direct visual study we may hope

to arrive at an understanding of disease processes which will ultimately prove to be of great practical value. In this connection we may speak of gastritis, which lamentably has no specific treatment. It is conceivable that the objective study which gastroscopy permits may disclose an understanding of the condition which may eventuate in control of the disease. Another great field for gastroscopic investigation is found in the study of cases which have undergone gastric surgery. The importance of this work lies in the attempt to determine the cause of the poor clinical results which frequently follow. In a study of the condition, it was found that the four principal morphological changes which may cause postoperative trouble following gastroenterostomy or gastric resection were the following:[22]

1. Recurrent or gastrojejunal ulcer. This condition was long thought to be the only complication in the postoperative stomach.

2. Chronic gastritis. This is now thought to be by far the most frequent cause.

3. Erosions and irritation caused by silk sutures remaining from operation and which have cut through the mucous membrane.

4. Carcinoma which develops at the stoma —very rare. Since gastroscopists[2,6,12,13] agree that chronic gastritis is a frequent and important cause of postoperative trouble, gastroscopy becomes important not only in the differential diagnosis but again in allowing an objective study of the condition.[2] The gastritis causes at least as much discomfort as recurrent ulcers and may even cause massive hemorrhages.[7,10,22] Some interesting findings have already come to light in this connection. In a series of thirty cases, four were found which did not present gastric changes, and in each case it was noted that the artificial stoma had developed a pylorus-like activity in contrast to the patent nonactive stomas of those cases showing gastritis.[22] It may be supposed that this pylorus-like functioning of the postoperative stoma may be a factor in inhibiting the development of this condition; it may be thought that the intestinal juices flowing into the stomach through this patent opening is in some way responsible. It is not known what the surgeon can do in resections to favor the development of this pylorus-like activity of the new stoma, but Schindler believes that in

cases of gastroenterostomy those carried out on the posterior wall near the greater curvature close to the pylorus are most likely to show this adaptability. More work is being done on this important question at the present time.

It seems then that on the basis of the experience of gastroscopists since the introduction of the flexible instrument the following points may be fairly stated by way of determining the present status of the procedure:

1. Gastroscopy offers a practical and safe objective method of gastric examination.

2. Gastroscopy offers the best method available in determining the presence of gastritis or other mucosal changes of the stomach.

3. Gastroscopy allows direct visual control of therapeutic progress during treatment of gastric lesions.

4. Gastroscopy gives valuable information in differential diagnosis of benign and malignant lesions.

5. Gastroscopy is of value in determining operability of gastric carcinoma, thereby making less frequent the necessity for exploratory surgery.

6. Gastroscopy has great potential value in investigative work of stomach diseases in general.

Bibliography

1. Benedict, E. B.: Gastroscopic observations in neoplasm. New Eng. Jour. Med., 214:563, 1936.
2. Benedict, E. B.: Gastroscopy in surgical diagnosis. Amer. Jour. Surg., 40, 5-11, 1938.
3. Berg, H. H.: Röntgenunters., am Innenrelief d. Verdaungs-kanals 2 Aufl. Leipzig, Thieme, 1931.
4. Comfort, W. W., and Butsch, W. L.: Proceedings Mayo Clinic, 13:151-154, 1938.
5. Faber, Knud: Gastritis and Its Consequences. New York, Oxford Univ. Press, 1935.
6. Gutzeit, Kurt: Die Bedeutung der Gastroskopie. (Unter besonderer Berucksichtigung der Gastritis.) Die Ergebnisse der Gastroskopie. Verhandl. d. deutsch. Gesellsch. f. innere Med., 47:368-378, 1935.
7. Henning, Norbert: Lehrbuch der Gastroskopie. Leipzig, J. A. Barth, 1935.
8. Hurst, A. F.: Gastric and duodenal ulcer. New York, Oxford University Press, 1929.
9. Hurst, A. F.: Lancet, 1023, 1929.
10. Konjetzny, G. E.: Die entzundliche Grundlage der typischen Geschwursbildung im Magen und Duodenum. Berlin, 1930.
11. Konjetzny, G. E.: Über die Beziehungen der chronischen Gastritis mit ihrem Folgeerscheinungen und des chronischen Magenkrebses. Beitr. z. Klin. Chir., 85:455, 1913.
12. Moersch, H. J., and Snell, A. M.: Gastroscopy in diagnosis of gastric disease. Amer. Jour. Surg., 39:521-526, 1938.
13. Moutier, Francois: Traite de gastroscopie et de pathologie endoscopique de l'estomac. Paris, Masson et Cie, 1935.
14. Palmer, W. L., Templeton, F., and Schindler, R.: Roentgen and gastric study of gastric ulcer. Tr. Assn. Am. Phys., 52:264-271, 1937.
15. Personal communication.
16. Reinberg, S. A.: Fiftieth anniversary Pub. Med. Post-Grad. Inst. Leningrad. 1936, pp. 493-507.
17. Rossi, C.: Practical value of gastroscopy. Policlinico, 40: 1207-1209, 1937.
18. Schindler, R.: Diagnostic gastroscopy. Jour. Am. Med. Assn., 105:352-355, (Aug. 3) 1935.
19. Schindler, R.: Gastroscopy and gastroduodenal ulcer. Surg., 2:692-709, 1937.
20. Schindler, R.: Gastroscopy, University Chicago Press, 1937.
21. Schindler, R.: Gastroscopy with a flexible gastroscope. Amer. Jour. Dig. Dis, and Nut. 2:11, 656-663.
22. Schindler, R., and Giere, N.: Gastric surgery and gastroscopy. Arch. Surg., 35:712, 1937.

TUMORS OF THE LARYNX*

FREDERICK A. FIGI, M.D.
Rochester, Minnesota

TUMORS of the larynx constitute some of the most interesting and at the same time most serious of the pathologic conditions that affect this structure. A number of different types of benign and malignant neoplasms occur. Some of these are met with frequently, and accordingly are of great clinical importance. Others are so rare that a laryngologist of even wide experience is not likely to see more than one or two during many years of practice. Early recognition and proper treatment of these growths is extremely important, since the likelihood of cure, particularly in cases of malignant tumor, is directly dependent on these two factors.

The possibility that a tumor of the larynx

present must be ruled out in every case in which chronic hoarseness, labored breathing, persistent cough, difficulty in swallowing or any symptoms referable to the lower part of the throat are encountered. These tumors may occur at any period of life but are most common in middle age. At times they are present at, or shortly following, birth. With few exceptions, those which occur among patients less than twenty years of age are benign. Malignant neoplasms at times are met with in the first and second decades, however. Since malignant disease is much more prevalent during the degenerative period of life than earlier, an increasing proportion of malignant tumors of the larynx is encountered with advancing age. Males of all ages are much more frequently affected by both benign and malignant tumors of the larynx than are females. The most

*From the Division on Laryngology, Oral and Plastic Surgery, The Mayo Clinic, Rochester, Minnesota. Read before the meeting of the North Dakota Academy of Ophthalmology and Otolaryngology, Bismarck, North Dakota, May 17, 1938.

common benign laryngeal growths are, in the order of their frequency, papillomas, myxomas, cysts, inflammatory masses, epithelial hyperplasia and leukoplakia, angiomas and amyloid tumors. Fibromas, chondromas and xanthomas occur rarely. Among the malignant neoplasms, carcinomas (epitheliomas) are by far the most common. Sarcomas, hemangio-endotheliomas and adenocarcinomas comprise a small proportion of such growths.

Benign Tumors

The symptoms of benign tumors of the larynx depend on the situation, attachment and size of the growth. These neoplasms may be present for years and become large without producing symptoms sufficiently severe to cause the individual to seek medical aid. Many of them are, in fact, discovered in the course of routine examination of the throat while patients are undergoing a general physical examination. This is particularly true of the cysts which develop on the anterior aspect of the epiglottis. If these originate on the free border of the vocal cords, however, symptoms are noted promptly. Discomfort in the larynx, effort in speaking, hoarseness, dyspnea, cough and complete aphonia are commonly present. A small, sessile growth may impair the voice more than a large, pedunculated one, especially if it is situated on the anterior portion of a vocal cord. Repeated efforts at clearing the throat at times are made. Attacks of glottic spasm and a sensation as of a foreign body being present in the throat may be experienced. Severe paroxysmal dyspnea may be produced by a pedunculated neoplasm, but more frequently the respiratory difficulty associated with benign tumors in this situation is constant.

The diagnosis of benign tumor of the larynx usually can be made from inspection of the tumor, together with consideration of the history and the age of the patient. When there is any doubt concerning the nature of the mass, biopsy should be done.

Treatment and prognosis in these cases depend largely on the nature of the tumor and its extent, and will be considered individually for the different groups.

Papillomas of the larynx are usually multiple. They are the most common of the benign neoplasms which occur in this situation, and may be met with at any period of life from infancy to old age. They may even be congenital. If individuals are of middle or advanced age the growths may be malignant. They may occur in any portion of the larynx but are most commonly situated on the true or false vocal cords and in the subglottic region. Frequently they extend well down to, or beyond, the bifurcation of the trachea. This extension may occur while they are still present in the larynx, or after the larynx has been entirely freed of the growths. At times they fill the upper portion of the larynx and a large part of the hypopharynx, extending well up on the base of the tongue and pharyngeal wall, so that they are visible on looking directly back into the mouth.

Papillomas may appear as single, but usually as multiple, warty growths, often presenting as grape-like clusters. At times they form an almost flat, verrucous surface, again a large, irregular cluster of a whitish, pinkish or reddish color. They may be fibrous or very friable, and they range from 1 or 2 mm. to 2 or 3 cm. in diameter. Usually they grow slowly, but following incomplete removal or if an inflammatory process is present, growth may be very rapid. There is no associated pain and no invasion of the surface to which they are attached. They frequently produce respiratory obstruction and necessitate tracheotomy. Recurrence is likely following removal, especially if individuals are young. At times papillomas will become engrafted on traumatized portions of the larynx or pharynx and they may become malignant, even when the patients are small children. I have seen epithelioma develop on the basis of recurring papillomas in the larynx of a girl five years of age and, in several other cases, they developed in the first and second decades of life.

Removal of papillomas and electrocoagulation of their attachment by means of direct, indirect or suspension laryngoscopy offers the best chance of cure. This latter procedure is usually most satisfactory as it permits of a very good view and the surgeon is enabled to use both hands. Treatment by means of radium tubes held directly in contact with the growth in the larynx, or by means of externally placed radium packs, formerly was used a great deal, but has been discarded by most laryngologists because of the danger of perichondritis. Roentgen therapy is in more general favor at present, although it does not offer the possibility of cure that is offered by

554

electrocoagulation. While multiple papillomas at times disappear following infectious diseases, subsequent to a single external application of radium or after tracheotomy, more frequently they are extremely persistent and require repeated removal and electrocoagulation, especially if patients are young. With persistence and patience the prognosis is usually good, however.

Myxomas of the larynx are encountered frequently in our experience at The Mayo Clinic, next in frequency to papillomas. The patients usually are adults and the tumors most commonly are attached by a broad base to the free border or upper surface of the anterior portion of the vocal cords, where they exert the greatest interference with voice production. In most cases a tumor of this sort presents as a single, small, discrete nodule, measuring only 3 or 4 mm. in diameter, but the tumor may be diffuse and widespread, involving the entire length of both vocal cords and rarely the ventricular bands as well. The color is usually grayish, pink or deep red. At times the nodule is hemorrhagic and its appearance very strikingly resembles that of an angioma. Microscopic examination of the majority of these tumors discloses some inflammatory reaction in the myxomatous tissue.

Treatment of myxomas consists in removal and electrocoagulation of the base by means of either direct or indirect laryngoscopy. There is very little tendency for the growths to recur, providing they are cleanly removed. If involvement is diffuse, it is difficult entirely to eradicate the growth.

Cysts of the larynx are usually smooth, translucent tumors situated on the anterior aspect of the epiglottis, but they may occur on the ventricular bands, the aryepiglottic folds, the pharyngeal surface of the larynx, or, rarely, on the vocal cords. They most often have broad, sessile attachments and the color may be yellow, grayish, pink or red. At times they strikingly resemble lipomas. Their size varies from 1 to 4 cm. in diameter. While usually single, they may be multiple.

Unless cysts are of sufficient size to produce symptoms, treatment is often not necessary. Situated as they commonly are, in the vallecula, and attached to the anterior aspect of the epiglottis, they rarely cause trouble. When removal is necessary, the wall of the cyst should be excised and the base electrocoagulated.

Fibromas are said by Thomson to be next to papillomas in order of frequency of benign laryngeal tumors. This has not been true in our experience at The Mayo Clinic. Fibromas are encountered chiefly among adults and are usually attached to the middle or anterior portion of the vocal cords; however, they may spring from any part of the larynx. In color they vary from whitish or grayish to pink or even deep red. While they usually are firm, smooth, round, sessile growths, they may be soft, pedunculated and, at times, nodular. Tortuous blood vessels often stand out prominently on the surface of the growth. The diameter ranges from a few millimeters to 3 or 4 cm. We have encountered fibromas which had broad sessile attachments covering almost the entire laryngeal aspect of the epiglottis. In one such case the tumor completely concealed the glottis and produced moderate respiratory obstruction so that preliminary tracheotomy was necessary prior to electrocoagulation, using laryngeal suspension.

Singers' nodes should be mentioned in this connection for they are frequently assumed to be neoplasms. Actually they are merely the chief feature of a form of chronic laryngitis. The nodules are usually bilateral, localized portions of hypertrophic epithelium, but they may be fibrous. They are situated at the junction of the anterior and middle thirds of the vocal cords and are caused by faulty voice production. Often they develop promptly following strain of the voice, and they may disappear spontaneously in the course of some months with rest of the voice. They frequently require removal, however.

True angiomas of the larynx are rare; a total of only fifty-five cases had been reported up to 1919. These included forty-seven hemangiomas and eight lymphangiomas. They may occur primarily in the larynx but more often they are associated with similar conditions about the face, mouth or upper air passages. Cavernous hemangioma is the most frequent type. It usually involves the true or false cords and appears as a smooth, soft, compressible, dark bluish or purplish mass.

Unless angiomas are producing severe symptoms, no treatment other than irradiation should be carried out because of the danger of hemorrhage and secondary infection.

Amyloid tumors of the larynx are rarely encountered. They may occur either as part of general amyloidosis in which other organs of the body are involved, or as a local condition. They are not true neoplasms. In the larynx the condition may exist as a diffuse subepithelial amyloid infiltration, localized amyloidosis with tumor formation or amyloid degeneration of a preexisting tumor. The clinical picture of the condition is rarely sufficiently characteristic to permit of positive recognition without microscopic confirmation. The vocal cords, ventricular bands and subglottic region are most often involved.

Treatment of amyloid tumors consists in removal and irradiation if the involved portion is sufficiently localized, otherwise radium or roentgen therapy alone is employed.

Chondromas are among the more unusual of the benign tumors of the larynx. During the period of fourteen years preceding 1932, only six such tumors were seen at The Mayo Clinic, while approximately 600 malignant neoplasms were encountered. These six cases increased to seventy-seven, the total number reported up to that time. Most of these cartilaginous tumors arise from the cricoid and thyroid cartilages and more frequently from their inner aspects than elsewhere. A few originate from the epiglottis and arytenoid cartilages. Laryngoscopic examination of tumors of this type which arise within the larynx usually reveals a smooth, sessile mass covered with normal mucous membrane in which the blood vessels stand out prominently. This feature is especially striking, and of itself is strongly suggestive of chondroma. The tumor is hard on palpation and may be pedunculated, although it is more often sessile. Mechanical interference with the mobility of one or both vocal cords is commonly present.

The diagnosis of chondromas of the larynx at times can be made from the history, together with the physical findings and roentgenographic demonstration of the tumor; microscopic examination of the tissue, however, as a rule is necessary for confirmation.

Treatment of chondromas depends on the situation and size of the growth, the character of its attachment to the laryngeal cartilages and its activity. Surgical removal is, of course, necessary, but the usual benign character of these tumors justifies decided conservatism. Laryngectomy is indicated only in case the growth is so extensive that its complete removal would leave a nonfunctioning, collapsed larynx. Prompt re-

currence is likely to follow incomplete removal.

Tumors of the thyroid gland are at times present in the larynx and are attributable to abnormal distribution of thyroid tissue. They grow slowly, are covered with normal mucous membrane and usually appear very vascular. Attempt at removal is, as a rule, inadvisable unless they are producing severe symptoms, for they may contain the only thyroid tissue that the patient possesses.

So-called prolapse of the laryngeal ventricle probably is not an eversion of the ventricle of Morgagni, as the name implies. The smooth, pinkish, fleshy tumor indicated by this term apparently results from hypertrophy of a portion of the mucous membrane of the ventricle. Electrocoagulation of the mass, using either direct or indirect laryngoscopy, is the most satisfactory form of treatment.

Certain infectious processes at times produce tumor-like masses in the larynx which must be distinguished from true neoplasms. Most important among these are tuberculosis, syphilis, blastomycosis, leprosy and rhinoscleroma. Solitary tuberculoma and gumma of the larynx at times strikingly simulate neoplasms. As these conditions are not neoplasms, however, they need not be considered here.

Malignant Tumors

Malignant tumors of the larynx alone present a big subject for discussion and only a brief consideration of them can be given here. These neoplasms are, with few exceptions, squamous-cell carcinomas and a discussion of these latter growths accordingly will suffice for the entire group.

Carcinoma of the larynx, while not a common disease, is encountered more frequently than are benign tumors in this situation. This, together with its seriousness, makes carcinoma of great clinical importance. An average of approximately sixty patients who had this condition have been examined at The Mayo Clinic in each of the past twelve years. The disease is about ten times as common among males as among females. The majority of these tumors affect patients between the ages of forty and seventy years and most of them occur when the patients are between fifty and sixty years of age. The disease, however, not infrequently is encountered in examination of patients who have not

556

reached forty or who have passed seventy years of age. I have carried out laryngectomy for squamous-cell epithelioma of the larynx which affected two boys, aged sixteen and nineteen years, respectively, and have met with the condition in several other instances in which the patients were in the second, or even in the first, decade of life.

Carcinoma of the larynx most commonly originates on, or in close proximity to, the vocal cords, usually on the upper surface of the anterior two-thirds of these structures. Extension, then, as a rule takes place along the length of the cord, and as this is at times a slow, gradual process, the lesion may remain operable for a considerable time, possibly for several years.

These tumors generally have been classified as intrinsic and extrinsic. The intrinsic tumors consist of those lesions which spring from the vocal cords, ventricular bands, ventricles, interarytenoid region and subglottic region. The extrinsic growths are those which develop about the epiglottis, aryepiglottic folds, arytenoid cartilages, pyriform sinuses and postcricoid region. In our experience it has seemed more logical to designate tumors of the epiglottis, aryepiglottic folds and arytenoid cartilages as "supraglottic" lesions, and those of the pyriform fossæ and postcricoid region as "laryngopharyngeal" or "hypopharyngeal" lesions. The supraglottic growths, with the exception of those which spring from the arytenoid cartilages, are less active, metastasize later, and offer a much better prognosis than do tumors of the laryngopharynx. In addition, surgical considerations in the two groups are vastly different. The majority of supraglottic growths spring from the epiglottis, especially its posterior aspect, and secondarily involve the aryepiglottic folds. They are usually fungating rather than infiltrating and commonly appear as cauliflower-like masses. Tumors of the laryngopharynx are prone to metastasize very early; this is in marked contrast to most of those tumors which originate within the larynx.

The earliest and most common symptom of carcinoma of the larynx, in the majority of cases, is hoarseness. Change in the voice of an adult, which persists for more than a few weeks, particularly if the patient is a man, always should arouse suspicion. Progression is gradual and usually painless until the lesion is well advanced.

The symptoms of advanced laryngeal carcinoma, that is, dyspnea, dysphagia, pain and hemorrhage, vary in their time of onset, depending largely on the situation and activity of the growth.

To an experienced laryngologist the picture of laryngeal carcinoma is recognizable on clinical examination in the majority of cases. Recent treatment or an acute inflammatory process will alter the picture to such an extent as to cause considerable difficulty and delay in diagnosis. In any event, even though the diagnosis appears obvious on clinical examination, it should always be confirmed by biopsy before treatment is initiated. Failure to obtain such confirmation has resulted in needless removal of more than one larynx.

The prognosis in carcinoma of the larynx depends on the situation, extent and activity of the growth, as well as on the thoroughness of treatment and the general condition of the patient. A fatal termination is inevitable without treatment and, as a rule, takes place in from one to three years. Death is usually the result of suffocation, dysphagia, hemorrhage, cachexia, sepsis or some intercurrent complication. Early intrinsic carcinoma of the larynx offers a very favorable prognosis. Lesions on the posterior aspect of the epiglottis and on the aryepiglottic folds also offer a satisfactory outlook.

Generally speaking, carcinoma of the larynx should be dealt with by means of radical operation, as only through an open operation can the majority of laryngeal carcinomas be clearly visualized. Lesions situated in the supraglottic portion of the larynx, especially those which spring from the epiglottis or the aryepiglottic folds, and which are commonly of an inactive type, often can be treated satisfactorily by suspension laryngoscopy; the lesion is electrocoagulated directly through the mouth. Pharyngotomy is at times necessary in this group of cases because of the extent, situation and activity of the growth. Preliminary tracheotomy may be required also. Thyrotomy, or laryngofissure, is the most satisfactory procedure for dealing with early, intrinsic carcinoma of the larynx. Laryngologists, however, hold widely divergent views concerning the usefulness of this procedure. One group, of which Sir St. Clair Thomson is the leading proponent, recommends laryngofissure "so long as the disease appears limited to the soft parts lining one-half of the larynx." The other group, headed by the late Dr. Mackenty, has taken a much more radical stand, holding that the operation is indicated only for "middle third cord growths involving only the surface of the vocal or ventricular bands circumscribed and small in extent and of slow growth"; in all other cases, laryngectomy is advised. My own inclination is to reserve thyrotomy for cases of laryngeal carcinoma in which the tumor is inactive and not fixed, or, if active, the tumor must be in a very early stage and well localized.

Thyrotomy is decidedly preferable to laryngectomy if its use is consistent with safety, for it leaves the patient with a very useful and often an almost normal voice and does not alter the upper air passages. Thyrotomy consists in dividing the thyroid cartilage, usually in the median line, although when the lesion extends into the anterior commissure it is safer to open the larynx a little to the opposite side. The growth is then excised and the open wound thoroughly electrocoagulated. A cannula usually is introduced into the trachea at the same time because of the possibility of respiratory obstruction resulting from the local reaction following the operation. In properly selected cases laryngofissure offers an excellent chance of curing the disease. Of thirty-four patients whom we were able to trace following this operation at the clinic, twenty-eight (82.3 per cent) were living and well five years later.

When the malignant process involves both sides of the larynx or extends onto the arytenoid cartilage on one or both sides, especially if it is active or if there is fixation, complete removal of the larynx alone offers a reasonable chance of controlling the disease. Even though many of these tumors are highly malignant, laryngectomy will result in cure in a high percentage of cases, providing the disease has not spread beyond the larynx. In cases in which perforation or metastasis of a highly malignant tumor has occurred, especially if the patient is young, the prognosis is so poor that operation rarely is indicated.

Laryngectomy gradually has been perfected during the years until at present the mortality following the operation is remarkably low. Tapia, of Spain, a few years ago reported a series of 106 consecutive cases in which laryngectomy was performed without an operative death. At The Mayo Clinic the longest series without a fatality was sixty cases.

As is true of most of the other major operations on the upper part of the respiratory tract, laryngectomy is best carried out under cervical block anesthesia because of the lessened danger of pulmonary complications as compared with general anesthesia. We routinely perform preliminary tracheotomy, as we feel that this renders the operation much safer than it is when the preliminary procedure is omitted. While laryngectomy permanently deprives the patient of his normal voice, satisfactory speech is possible in all cases with the use of one of the several mechanical contrivances now on the market. With one of these, most of the patients suffer comparatively little handicap and are able to resume their original calling even though it entails considerable speaking. Moreover, with speech training many patients develop satisfactory speech by swallowing air and utilizing the pharyngeal muscles for production of the voice as the air is regurgitated. The exposed tracheal opening causes comparatively little inconvenience, and patients who have such an opening are no more subject to infections of the respiratory tract than are normal individuals. The marked mental depression following laryngectomy, described in some of the older textbooks, rarely has been seen at the clinic.

The end-results with regard to control of the carcinoma are very gratifying. Seventy-three patients who were subjected to laryngectomy were traced, and forty-one (56.1 per cent) of them were found to be alive and well after five years.

Radium and roentgen rays often are of considerable value as supplementary measures in the treatment of malignant tumors of the larynx. They rarely should be used to the exclusion of other measures, however, in the treatment of malignant laryngeal lesions that can be removed surgically. In recent years the Coutard fractional dosage method of roentgen therapy has been used a good deal in the treatment of advanced laryngeal carcinomas. Encouraging primary results have been obtained in some of the cases, but the results do not warrant substitution of this form of therapy for surgical measures in cases of operable carcinoma of the larynx.

FUTURE AIMS OF THE HOSPITAL LIBRARY*

GORDON R. KAMMAN, M.D., F.A.C.P.

Instructor in Neurology and Psychiatry, University of Minnesota
Saint Paul, Minnesota

IF there is any phase of the care of the sick in which our European contemporaries surpass us, it is in providing our hospitalized sick with suitable reading material and properly supervised reading programs. In this respect some of the Europeans are years in advance of us. One of the reasons probably is that here the medical profession is not fully aware of the therapeutic possibilities of reading when directed and supervised by one who is especially trained in that field of endeavor. Possibly the hospital administrators or even the librarians themselves are equally responsible for lack of interest in this field; but, regardless of on whom the responsibility lies, effort along this front several years ago would have resulted in significant advances. Proof of this assertion lies in the fact that in the comparatively brief time that the subject has been receiving attention in this country, great progress has been made in the field of hospital librarianship.

The first formal get-together of persons in the American Hospital Association and affiliated groups interested in hospital libraries was held in Philadelphia in September, 1934. At this meeting it was pointed out that the hospital library is a very important accessory service in the complete and rounded out care of the patient. It was further pointed out that in the minds of hospital people there was not the proper appreciation of the importance of this fact. I was honored by a request to address this meeting. In preparing my address I found that practicing physicians as a whole had even less appreciation of hospital library service than did anybody else. At the meeting there were papers on various aspects of hospital librarianship and in every one of them the need of hospital librarians and of trained librarians to supervise them was stressed. It also was pointed out that there exists a fundamental difference between public and hospital libraries. In the former, scientific accuracy and literary merit are the criteria of a book. In the latter, thera-

peutic effectiveness is the only criterion of a book. Thus a book may be a literary masterpiece and yet have little therapeutic value. It may even be harmful to the patient. By the same token, a book may be very inferior as a literary work, yet it may be very effective from a therapeutic standpoint.

The next meeting was held at the time of the American Hospital Association meeting at St. Louis, in September, 1935. There the meeting was much better attended than at Philadelphia, and in the transactions of the American Hospital Association for that year the discussion on hospital libraries covers ten more printed pages than the one at Philadelphia. There it was pointed out that in twenty-five States of the Union, there were 386 hospitals with library service, but that there were only forty-two trained librarians. At this meeting also, the necessity was mentioned for a scientific study on the reading habits of patients. Dr. Magnus Peterson, who is now superintendent of the State Hospital at Willmar, Minnesota, gave a very fine paper indicating how it is possible to establish reading curves for patients and in this way obtain insight into some of their psychodynamics, and also to evaluate the results of planned reading programs on controlled groups of patients.

By September, 1936, when the American Hospital Association met in Cleveland, the hospital library movement had grown, and this meeting was attended the best of all. By this time, under the stimulation and guidance of Miss Perrie Jones and her very able committee, the Quarterly Book List had been issued and been put on a subscription basis. Then there were 134 paid subscriptions, and I am informed by Miss Jones that there are now more than 250 paid subscriptions, a gain of nearly 100 per cent in less than two years. This is a very healthy sign. In this list are published each quarter fifty annotated titles each of fiction and nonfiction, plus scores of titles of inexpensive reprints, specially illustrated material, and a few entries for professional reading. At this Cleve-

*Delivered before Association of Hospital and Medical Librarians, Minnesota Hospital Association, Minneapolis, Minnesota, May 20, 1938.

land meeting, which was the last one I attended, it was also pointed out that somebody was necessary to establish contact between books and patients. This meant a trained librarian.

In this same year the American College of Surgeons recognized the hospital library movement, and at its meeting that year in Philadelphia there was a formal round table discussion of hospital libraries. This was led by Miss Perrie Jones.

The present situation here in Minnesota is, I believe, a healthy one. Here the Minnesota Association of Hospital, Medical and Institution Librarians is doing pioneer work. It is engaged in what is the first step of any new investigation. It is gathering together all of the available factual data having to do with hospital libraries in this state. This kind of survey is the first requisite of any intelligent approach to the consideration of a new project. One of the many things discovered is the fact that we have in this state 3,148 hospital patients who are without library service of any kind. My guess is that the incidence of patients who are not so supplied in other states is much higher. In order to supply the demand for trained hospital librarians, the Division of Library Instruction at the University of Minnesota now offers a course for training hospital librarians. To show the demand for people so trained, one need only to be reminded of the fact that every student taking this course last year (the first one given) was offered a position as hospital librarian within a very short time after she had finished the course. I feel that the ground work is being well laid here in Minnesota, and now a few remarks might be pertinent concerning the future aims of the hospital library.

The first question to be considered is: "Should each hospital have its own library?" I believe that the answer is: "Yes," unless in Saint Paul, Minneapolis and other large towns in the state, the public or municipal library is able to furnish adequate hospital library service. Even then it would be preferable for the larger hospitals to have their own libraries independent of the municipal library. This is especially true in the case of the hospital for tuberculous patients. We all know how reluctant people are to send books to tuberculous people, and we also know how difficult it is to induce anybody to use a book which is known to have been in the hands of somebody suffering from tuberculosis. Furthermore, a hospital owning its own library has many advantages.

1. The Reading Room.—If a hospital owns its own books and keeps them in its own library, it is more likely that there will be a reading room set aside for the use of the patients. This promotes a community spirit among the patients and is conducive to an atmosphere of goodwill and of cheerfulness. I might add in, passing that it is my firm conviction that the reading room should be kept absolutely separate from the room for occupational therapy, the room for social service, and the room for physiotherapy. Each of these activities is an important adjunct to the treatment of the hospitalized sick, and each one is an integral part of the hospital. However, while they are part of an integral whole, they should be separate departments within the hospital itself.

2. Equipment.—If each hospital had its own library, it could also have its own distinctive book carts and other equipment. This equipment could be designed to serve the particular class of patients cared for in each particular hospital. Every physician knows the importance of having meals served in an attractive manner on trays tastily arranged. By the same token it is necessary in order to interest patients in reading, to serve the books in an attractive manner. The book carts should be designed to excite the curiosity and to please the taste of the type of patient cared for in the hospital under consideration.

3. Planning.—If the hospital owns its own library, it is easier for the librarian to work out a reading program for each patient. She knows exactly what books are available and where they are. She can correlate that patient's reading with various other projects in the treatment program and can always calculate what books will be available to any particular patient at an approximate time. Furthermore, she can organize programs of group reading and of project reading. Group discussions, research reading, and reference reading are much more easily planned if the library is part of the hospital itself instead of being a separate institution.

4. A Resident Librarian.—If the hospital owned the library, the librarian could be a resident member of the hospital staff. She could live in the hospital, be available at all times for

560

consultation with the attending or the resident staff, and also supervise evening group reading activities.

This brings us to the second question: "What should be the relationship between the hospital librarian and the rest of the hospital staff?" In my opinion, the hospital librarian should be considered the same as any other therapist. The librarian should be a consultant in the same sense as the occupational therapist, the physiotherapist, or the medical social service worker. We frequently consult with the dietitian about the patient's diet, so why not consult with the librarian about the patient's reading? I like the idea of considering the hospital librarian as an expert in psychologic dietetics. The librarian should be known as the bibliotherapist. She should consult with the attending staff whenever possible, and in certain hospitals and under certain conditions sit in on staff conferences. This, of course, will vary with the kind of hospital and the particular set-up under consideration.

Everything that I have discussed thus far will necessitate launching a very active educational program among physicians. Dr. MacEachern says that doctors are very quick to take up anything once they are convinced that it is for the good of the patient. Doctors must be taught the importance of professional supervision of the reading programs of their patients. They must be taught the difference between recreational, educational and therapeutic reading, and the value and place for each one of them. They must be taught that it requires experience, training and skill to fit the right book to the right patient. They must be taught that a skilled bibliotherapist can help materially in reducing the patient's morbidity and in shortening his convalescense in a great number and variety of illnesses. This means that at medical meetings more papers should be read dealing with this phase of the care of the sick. Any well rounded plan for the care of the sick must contain bibliotherapy as well as occupational therapy, physiotherapy, dietotherapy and medical social service.

I may be visionary and very speculative on this subject, but I can conceive of a plan by which the patient could be furnished with a program of supervised reading even after he leaves the hospital. The day may come when the bibliotherapist will make regular visits to the patient's home after he has left the hospital, and, like the social service worker, aid in his rehabilitation. I am firmly convinced that today bibliotherapy is in the same stage of development as medical social service was a generation ago. As medical social service has grown into a major adjunct to the care of the sick, so will bibliotherapy grow in a like manner.

MELANOSIS COLI*

LOUIS A. BUIE, M.D.

Rochester, Minnesota

MELANOSIS coli of Virchow cannot be considered a pathologic disorder but one in which a form of pigment is deposited, chiefly in the tunica propria of the mucous membrane of the colon, as a result of some disturbance of its function, accompanied by slowing of its activity, development of a condition commonly classified as constipation or colonic stasis and the laxative habit. The condition may occur also in the colons of individuals who harbor obstructive lesions.

Although melanosis coli has been recognized since it was first described by Cruveilhier a full century ago, all studies which have been devoted to the subject had been based on postmortem investigations until Bockus, Willard and Bauk published their report in 1933. It remained, therefore, for these investigators to provide the first and, as far as I know, the only comprehensive record of the condition as it appears in vivo and of its clinical interpretation.

Virchow's description in 1847 followed that of Cruveilhier, and the report of C. T. Williams, twenty years later, was next in order. According to Stewart and Hickman, a description of a case of melanosis coli, in which the patient was a lead worker who died of chronic Bright's disease, was provided by G. N. Pitt in 1891, and Rolleston reported a similar case the following year. Noth-

*From the Section on Proctology, The Mayo Clinic, Rochester, Minnesota.

ing further of interest appeared until 1930, when Pick and Brahn furnished the first account of the morbid anatomy of melanosis coli. Stewart and Hickman, when referring to the study made by Henschen and Bergstrand in 1913, stated that they showed that "while gross examples of the disease are comparatively rare, microscopic pigmentation of the colon is of frequent occurrence."

Various ideas as to the source of the pigment and its method of entry into the mucous membrane of the colon have been advanced, but thus far there has been little agreement on these subjects, and it is doubtful if plausible explanations have been advanced. Some believe that the pigment is hematogenous; some maintain that metals such as mercury and lead are the causes, while others adhere to the conception that the deposit is melanin and occurs as a result of the action of a tyrosinase-like ferment on aromatic products of degradation of protein.

Incidence

Most estimates of the incidence of this condition are based on postmortem examinations and are, therefore, unsatisfactory as far as clinical value is concerned. Bockus, Willard and Bauk provided the only exception to this and I employ their figures for comparison with those which I have obtained from a study of similar cases at The Mayo Clinic. They found an incidence of 2.7 per cent in examination of 960 routine "office" patients. Among those patients who gave definite evidence of "colon stasis," they found that the incidence was 5.1 per cent. They also found that the incidence by age was practically the same as that observed among individuals who complained of constipation. Of their patients, 88 per cent were females. Of the patients who were subjected to proctoscopic examination at the clinic, from 1925 to 1934, inclusive, about half complained of constipation. About 25 per cent of those who were constipated were able to control their sluggish colonic function by dietetic measures or by taking only an occasional laxative, so that for comparison with the series of Bockus, Willard and Bauk, there are left 75 per cent of the constipated patients, and these represent, to a certain degree, the type of patient which Bockus, Willard and Bauk studied. In this group we found 571 patients with melanotic deposits in the lining of the colon, or an incidence of about 3.5

per cent, which compares favorably with 5.1 per cent found by Bockus, Willard and Bauk in examination of those patients who evidently had the more severe form of constipation termed "colon stasis." The incidence of melanosis coli in our entire series of patients was 1.3 per cent, which strikingly corroborates the estimate of 1.0 per cent furnished by Lockhart-Mummery (quoted by Bockus, Willard and Bauk). The age incidence in our study was also found to parallel the age at which constipation appears, and 74.1 per cent of our patients were between the ages of thirty and sixty years. The distribution by sex also agreed with that of individuals who suffer with constipation; 381 (66.7 per cent) of the patients who had melanosis coli were females, and 190 (33.3 per cent) were males.

Gross and Microscopic Appearance

One who sees this melanotic deposit in the rectal mucosa for the first time may be confused as to its nature, but once it has been observed and identified, there does not seem to be any reason why such difficulty should be experienced again. There is rather wide variation in the intensity of the color but its appearance otherwise, and its arrangement, are unmistakable and if the mucosal surface is rubbed with a cotton applicator, inflammatory or ulcerous change, with which the condition may be confused, will not be found. If inflammatory reaction is present, the pinkish stain of serosanguineous exudate will appear on the cotton applicator when the diseased mucous membrane is traumatized. If there is no such stain, the condition may be melanotic. The pigment may be light brown, dark brown or black. It may be scattered in the mucous membrane, or it may leave no part of the lining of the bowel uninvolved; it is rare for the condition to extend beyond the confines of the colon. On closer scrutiny it will be observed that the coloring is not solid but is divided by linear, yellowish markings, into small segments, usually several millimeters in diameter (scarcely ever as large as a centimeter). According to Pick and Brahn, the yellow striations are owing to the vascular pattern of the superficial blood vessels of the colonic wall, an idea which accords with Pope's description of the vascular arrangement of the colonic mucosa, and the lymph follicles account for the spots of yellow at the angles of the yellow lines. The segments may be square or irregularly polyhedral.

562

Grossly, it appears that the deposit is in the surface of the mucous membrane but on microscopic examination it will be found that there is no pigment in the epithelial cells. Instead, the entire deposit of pigment accumulates in the tunica propria of the mucous membrane, where it lies chiefly within the large mononuclear cells. Rarely it extends to the muscularis, and lymphatic involvement has been reported.

Etiology

In attempting to determine the source of these deposits, my reasoning is in accord with that of Bockus, Willard and Bauk, who expressed the belief that the pigment is derived from ingested food which is "phagocytized" by the cells of the intestine. I never have seen melanosis coli in examination of an individual who was not constipated and the frequency with which such a person habitually takes cascara is too striking to be disregarded. Bartle first called attention to the possible relationship between the constant ingestion of cascara and melanosis coli. And in Bockus' review, a complete record is given of the views of various authors on the significance of anthracene and other derivatives of anthraquinone, all of which "contain emodins or trioxymethylanthraquinone" and which, according to Sollman, Tappeiner and Brandl, act largely on the colon. My opinion in regard to the hypothesis that the condition arises as a result of phagocytic action of the mucosal cells agrees with that of Bockus only in so far as it applies to substances which may be picked up by this phagocytic action and does not relate particularly to foodstuffs as such. I believe that this pigment is obtained either directly from elements within laxative agents or from the products which develop as a result of the action of these chemicals on the intestinal content. When it is considered that practically all patients who have melanosis coli are constipated, the likelihood that colonic stasis and its effect on metabolism of foods may play significant rôles in the production of this condition becomes impressive. However, when it is recalled that more than 95 per cent of persons who are constipated, many of whom are not in the habit of taking cascara, show no sign of melanosis of the colon, one leans more toward the belief that this drug, or one of its constituents, or one of its effects, is of significance as a causative factor. With such a large number of constipated patients who do not have melanosis,

it seems that the factor of stasis alone is not of great importance but that the limited group with melanosis represents those who ingest some particular chemical which causes deposits in the walls of the colon. Investigations are now being made in an attempt to discover the chemical nature of the material deposited in the colonic wall and its relationship to various laxatives, but unfortunately they will not be completed in time for inclusion here.

Clinical Significance

There is no evidence that the physician should be concerned over the presence of melanotic pigment in the walls of the colon. I never have observed features which suggested pathologic tendencies. The condition has been seen in examination of patients with carcinoma of various parts of the colon, but on each occasion it appeared to have developed as a result of the obstructive effect of the lesion, the consequent stasis above it and the necessity of taking laxatives; it has not seemed that melanosis coli was a cause of the carcinoma. Until the exact nature of the pigment is known, however, justifiable conservatism forbids that one should adopt the arbitrary position that it cannot produce harmful effects, either of a toxic nature or otherwise. But if clinical experience can be relied on, it can at least be stated that those symptoms experienced by patients in examination of whom the condition is found are owing to those disorders such as constipation, colonic stasis, laxative habit, and so forth, which probably are responsible for the presence of the pigment in the colonic mucous membrane.

References

1. Bartle, H. J.: The sigmoid. Med. Jour. and Rec., 127: 521-524, (May 16) 1928.
2. Bockus, H. L., Willard, J. H., and Bauk, Joseph: Melanosis coli: the etiologic significance of the anthracene laxatives: a report of forty-one cases. Jour. Am. Med. Assn., 101:1-6, (July 1) 1933.
3. Cruveilhier, Jean. Anatomie pathologique du corps humain ou descriptions avec figures lithographiées et colpriées, des diverses altérations morbides dont le corps humain est susceptible. Paris: J. B. Ballière, 1829-1835, vol. 2e, p. 6.
4. Henschen, Folke, and Bergstrand, Hilding: Studien über die Melanose der Darmschleimhaut. Beitr. z. path. Anat., 56:103-174, 1913.
5. Pick, L., and Brahn, B.: Das Pigment der Melanosis coli und seine chemische Darstellung aus dem Organ. Virchow's Arch. f. path. Anat. u. Physiol., 275:37-49, 1930.
6. Pitt, G. N.: Colon pigmented black throughout with lead. Tr. Path. Soc. London, 42:109, 1891.
7. Rolleston, H. D.: Colon pigmented from mercury. Tr. Path. Soc. London, 43:69-70, 1892.
8. Sollman, Tappeiner and Brandl: Quoted by Bockus, H. L., Willard, J. H., and Bauk, Joseph.
9. Stewart, M. J., and Hickman, Ella M.: Observations on melanosis coli. Jour. Path. and Bacteriol., 34:61-72, (Jan.) 1931.
10. Virchow, Rud.: Die pathologischen Pigmente. Virchow's Arch. f. path. Anat. u. Physiol., 1:379-402, 1847.
11. Williams, C. T.: Black deposit in the large intestine from the presence of mercury. Tr. Path. Soc. London, 28:111-114, 1867.

HINTS ON THE USE OF THE MEDICAL INDEXES*

THOMAS E. KEYS, A.B., M.A.

Reference Librarian, The Mayo Clinic

Rochester, Minnesota

SOME outstanding physicians and surgeons have recommended from time to time that instruction be given to medical students on the use of the library and the indexes that synthesize the medical literature. Dr. John Shaw Billings felt that a course in medical bibliography was important from a practical point of view to teach the younger men the use of the implements of their profession. Dr. Harvey Cushing suggested that short talks on the use of the library for the benefit of the younger men might be made obligatory. And Dr. Bayard Holmes maintained that if medical students were trained in the use of the library they would read with a better sense of discrimination in the active years of a busy practice.

Librarians and editors have similarly felt that both the undergraduate and graduate student need instruction about library tools and library methods. To this end a few medical schools and special libraries have set up brief educational programs. When administrators realize the full value of bibliographic research more time will be spent by more schools on this fundamental instruction.

The medical indexes are the first library tools that the reader should be acquainted with for from them he can find what has been written, by whom, and where the material has been published. In the first place the reader should know how to use the library catalog. In medical libraries, generally the textbooks and monographs the library has are listed in the card catalog. These cards are filed alphabetically, similarly to the arrangement of words in the dictionary. If the reader's primary interest were pathology, for example, and he wished to know what editions the library had of Bell's *Textbook of Pathology*, he would look in the catalog under the B's and under Bell, Elexious Thompson, would be found the required information, one card for each edition of the book in question. If the reader wished to know what textbooks the library had on pathology he would look under the subject heading, pathology, in the catalog and there in alphabetic order would be listed the textbooks contained in the library.

Readers are interested in the articles found in periodicals chiefly for three reasons: 1. The new developments in medicine and surgery are first published in periodicals. 2. The investigator contemplating a new research problem needs to know what has been published in order to avoid duplication, as well as to provide a suitable background for his study. 3. The general practitioner and medical student desire to know at first hand the literature on particular phases of medicine. The chief sources of illumination for such readers are: The Quarterly Cumulative Index Medicus, The Index Medicus, The Quarterly Cumulative Index to Current Medical Literature, and The Index-Catalogue of the Library of the Surgeon General's Office, United States Army (Army Medical Library). Most medical libraries have these indexes and they should be studied carefully.

The best source for the recent literature is the Quarterly Cumulative Index Medicus. This is published by the American Medical Association. Since 1931 the entire cost of publishing this invaluable index has been borne by the association. It is published at a deficit of about $45,000 a year. In making this index available, the American Medical Association is rendering an inestimable contribution to international medicine and its scholarship. The subscription price is only $12.00 a year. More practitioners might well subscribe to this index, for their perusal of it will pay many times over the small initial cost.

The Quarterly Cumulative Index Medicus (here often referred to as the Q. C. I. M.) is issued four times a year. The January to March issue is paper bound and indexes the medical literature for the three-month period. The January to June issue is bound in cloth and is a permanent record. It incorporates the material included in the January to March index. The second half of the year is treated similarly to the first half, with the unbound numbers cover-

*Submitted for publication June 8, 1938.

ing material issued from July to September, and the bound volume covering material from July to December. Because of the large number of periodicals indexed and the mechanical problems of indexing, it is impossible for the bibliographers and publishers to keep the Index up to date. It will be noticed, therefore, that the Q. C. I. M. lags from two to four months. However, compared to other indexing tools, this is of little consequence.

The Q. C. I. M. includes the following items: 1. New books listed (a) according to author and (b) according to subject. 2. List of medical publishers. 3. List of journals indexed. 4. Index to the periodical literature. In the list of journals indexed the accepted abbreviations are given, and these abbreviations should be followed when it is necessary to make reference to the literature. Biographical notes and sketches are indexed under Biographies and also under Obituaries.

The reader consults the Q. C. I. M. as he would the dictionary or the library card catalog, for the index is arranged in one alphabet. This is much more convenient than having the index of authors and subjects at the end of the volume. Articles are listed under subject and also under author. Cross-references and "see also" references help guide the reader to the subject heading under which the articles are listed. It is true that some skill is required to extract all of the required references from the Q. C. I. M. Practical experience should develop an ability to use the index properly. Occasionally it is necessary to use the "trial and error" method before the material can be found. If the material is not listed under the accustomed heading, another heading should be tried. Of one thing the reader can be certain, nine times out of ten, there are good data available. Articles may be listed under general headings with more specific subheadings, for example, spondylolisthesis is listed under Spine—Dislocations. The literature is usually indexed under the simpler form of the name. For example, cancer is used instead of carcinoma. Cancer of an organ of the body is listed under the organ. Example: Breast—Cancer. Diseases that can be classed under the organs are so listed. Example: Eyes—Diseases. The heading, Ophthalmology, is used for the theory of diseases of the eye, apparatus, history and so forth. Some subjects are from necessity

grouped under broad subject headings. Example: Acids, Bacteria, Hospitals, Instruments. If the approximate title is known, a good plan is to look under the key word that most adequately describes the paper. In case an article is to be used as a reference, for which correct bibliographic form is necessary, it must be remembered that the complete bibliographic reference is listed only after the author's name. Under the subject heading will be found an incomplete title. Often, for the purpose of ready reference, the title is reversed in form. Titles to foreign articles are translated for the convenience of the reader under the subject. If the title of an article is in a language other than English, French, German, Spanish, Italian, or Portuguese, it appears in translation under the author entry.

The Index Medicus, another important library tool, preceded the Quarterly Cumulative Index Medicus. It was started in 1879 by Dr. Robert Fletcher with the coöperation of Dr. John Shaw Billings, both of the Library of the Surgeon General's Office. The publication was issued monthly and was arranged according to medical subjects. The volumes were bound annually and an index both of authors and subjects was included in each bound volume. This index is hard to use because the numbers were not made cumulative, and consequently, the yearly indexes must refer to articles in twelve separate issues. However, the Index Medicus is very useful in locating an author's work for a particular year between 1879 and 1916; at the end of that period a new index made its appearance.

This new bibliographic tool, The Quarterly Cumulative Index to Current Medical Literature (1916-1926), was published by the American Medical Association. The bound numbers were cumulative and the references by both author and subject were brought together. Accordingly the Index Medicus was combined in 1927 with the Quarterly Cumulative Index to Current Medical Literature to form the Quarterly Cumulative Index Medicus, which has been discussed in detail.

The last bibliographic tool to be discussed is the Index-Catalogue of the Library of the Surgeon General's Office, United States Army (Army Medical Library).

The making and publishing of this index has been called, by some of the most distinguished physicians of the world, America's greatest contribution to medicine. The "Index-Catalogue" is an analysis of the largest, and in many ways the finest, collection of the medical literature in the world.

The "Index-Catalogue" was begun by Dr. John Shaw Billings, father of the Army Medical Liabrary.[4] The first series of the catalogue (sixteen volumes) was completed by 1895. Two more series were completed by 1932. The fourth series of the index (1936-) is now being published at the rate of one volume a year. The advantage of the "Index-Catalogue" over the other indexes is that each series contains the medical literature for a great number of years instead of the literature for a short period. Books, chapters of books, pamphlets and theses are listed under subject and also under author. Under the author entry may also be found references to biographical information if this is available. The disadvantage in using this catalog is that references to articles are not indexed directly under the author's name but are found under the subject only. Because of the tremendous scope of the "Index-Catalogue" it would be hardly possible to list the articles as does the Quarterly Cumulative Index Medicus. The Index Catalogue is more complete than the Quarterly Cumulative Index Medicus, listing more books and journals, and is cumulative for a period of many years. It is ideal for a review of the literature. With the four series in front of him, the reader looks under the appropriate subject in four places (Series I, Series II, Series III, and Series IV), notes the date of the last article and completes the references from that time on by use of the Q. C. I. M.

In compiling a list of references to the periodical literature, the following suggestions are offered. For brevity they are stated imperatively. First of all, limit your subject as specifically as possible. If, for example, you are interested in therapy for pleurisy, consult only the heading: Pleurisy—Therapy. Do not bother with the other headings. However, if you are reviewing such a subject as sulfanilamide in all its different aspects and you desire a total bibliography, consult all the headings under Sulfanilamide and Sulfanilamide Derivatives. Besides this, consult all the "see" and "see also" references. In volume 22 (July to December, 1937) of the Quarterly Cumulative Index Medicus the "see" and

"see also" references on this subject alone refer the reader to the following places:

Sulfanilamide and Sulfanilamide Derivatives

Effects: See also Meningococci, infections; Puerperal Infection, prevention.

In blood: See Blood, sulfanilamide and sulfanilamide derivatives.

In urine: See Urine, sulfanilamide and sulfanilamide derivatives.

Therapy: See also Abortion, criminal; Abscess, peritonsillar; Appendicitis, therapy; Arthritis, gonorrheal; Bladder, inflammation; Erysipelas, therapy; Gangrene, gas; Gonococci, infections; Gonorrhea, therapy; Infection, therapy; Jaundice, therapy; Lungs, abscess; Malaria, quartan; Malaria, tertian; Malaria, therapy; Meningitis, influenzal; Meningitis, meningococcic; Meningitis, pneumococcic; Meningitis, streptococcic; Meningitis, therapy; Meningococci, infections; Otorhinolaryngology, therapy in; Penis, gangrene; Pneumococci, infections; Pneumonia, therapy; Poliomyelitis, therapy; Puerperal Infection, therapy; Pyelitis, therapy; Pyelocystitis, therapy; Scarlet Fever, complications and sequels; Septicemia, therapy; Skin, diseases; Staphylococci, aureus; Staphylococci, infections; Streptococci, hemolytic; Streptococci, infections; Streptococci, viridans; Syphilis, therapy; Tonsils, infection, Undulant Fever, therapy; Urinary Tract, infections.

All the references must be consulted if a complete bibliography is desired. From the above examples it can readily be seen that the bibliographic problems for different subjects may vary widely. Experience with the indexes and personal judgment help a good deal in this bibliographic work. Generally the literature is so exhaustive that not everything can be read. The literature for the past five years should be enough to read for an ordinary article. The reader also should decide whether he wants the literature in all languages and should make his selections accordingly. Being acquainted with the outstanding men in a given field also should be of help in making a bibliography selective. Experience teaches that the caliber of certain journals is better than that of others. The journals that are official publications of societies and those of national reputation should be read first; only then, if at all, journals that accept questionable advertising. Attention to the above points probably will save the reader and the library a great deal of unnecessary work.

I have found that the best way to use indexes is to start with the newest index and work backward. In so doing the reader occasionally picks up a good review article which may save him considerable time. References to the literature are generally more accessible when made on standard bibliographic cards, and they are convenient for filing for future needs. When bibliographic cards are filled out the entries should be complete. They should include: 1. The name of the author and his initials (if he has two or more Christian names; otherwise, his full name. The full name always is written out if the author is a woman.) 2. The complete title entry. It should be remembered, here, that the complete title is filed only under the name of the author in the Quarterly Cumulative Index Medicus. 3. The name of the journal. This may be in the abbreviated form suggested by the Q. C. I. M. 4. The volume number, the inclusive pagination, the month and the year. This information is necessary if the bibliography is to be helpful to anyone else.

It is well to remember that the scientific quality of an original work can be judged somewhat by the excellence of its bibliography; that is, if the references are incomplete and inaccurately cited, the results of the author's original work may be thought to be unreliable. Of course, a great scientist may be a careless bibliographer, but the bad impression made by carelessness in any field is one good reason for taking pains in the first place and for verifying the references when a bibliography is compiled.

References

1. Billings, J. S.: Methods of research in medical literature. Tr. Assn. Am. Phys., 2:57-67, 1887.
2. Cushing, Harvey: The doctor and his books. Am. Jour. Surg., 4:100-110, (Jan.) 1928.
3. Holmes, Bayard: The medical library and its influence on medical culture and remuneration. Am. Med., 16:480-483 (Sept.) 1910.
4. Hume, E. E.: The centennial of the Army medical library coincident with the beginning of the fourth series of the index catalogue. Med. Ann. District of Columbia., 5:159-164, (June) 1936.

THE USE AND MISUSE OF MEDICAL TERMS: SOME SUGGESTIONS FOR IMPROVEMENT

H. E. Robertson, M.D., Section on Pathologic Anatomy: There is an old saying to the effect that those who live in glass houses should hurl stones with considerable discretion. . . .

With this in mind . . . I am proposing that we modify our employment of certain terms.

First I am advocating a change in the words "lymph gland" to "lymph node." "Gland" was perhaps permissible when no one knew the nature of these collections of lymphocytes. Now, whatever they really are, we feel certain they are not glands. Your first answer may well be, that the term "lymphadenitis" means "inflammation of a gland" but we use it exclusively to mean "inflammation of a lymph node." Right at the start I am in a bad position for I do not like "lymph noditis." But I still persist in suggesting the change to lymph "nodes."

My next proposal is concerned with the term "epithelioma," by which we usually mean a "squamous cell carcinoma." The word is illogically used, as all kinds of carcinomas are epitheliomas and hence the word loses its specific signification. Whatever term is employed to characterize carcinomas of squamous epithelial surfaces (and I suggest the name I have just used), "epithelioma" has no place in the nomenclature of tumors and should be dropped.

The adjective "colloid" which qualifies some of the carcinomas in our writings is inappropriate and inaccurate. It refers to the gelatinous appearance which some tumors possess, almost wholly owing to the presence of large quantities of mucus secreted by the epithelial cells of some cancers. A much better term would be "mucous" (not mucoid) carcinoma.

The word "mucus" brings to mind a much more debatable word, "myxoma," which we employ to designate certain connective tissue tumors which contain appreciable quantities of interstitial mucin. This form of mucin is found in all sorts of tissues other than tumors. It is a normal constituent of the walls of the arteries, it is the basis for the various myxedemas, elephantiasis and other chronic edemas and is often found in leiomyomas, so-called fibroma sand other fibrous tissue masses. There is probably no such entity as a "myxoma" in the sense of a specialized tumor. Instead we should describe such tissues, whether neoplasms or not, as "myxedematous."

In considering the "adenomas," I at once am in deeper water. Without entering too far into a discussion of this complicated group, I would suggest that we restrict this term as much as possible to neoplastic conditions. This would exclude its use for "nodular repair" of the liver in cirrhoses, for "nodular goiter" and "nodular prostate" in focal hyperplasias of these organs and limit the term largely to new growths of the pituitary, and adrenal glands and pancreatic "islands."

A favorite of even our more cultured confreres is the word "fibroid" meaning a leiomyoma of the uterus. When the true nature of these smooth muscle collections was not known, perhaps fibroid was permissible, but now it is, at its best, medical slang. Even the combination "fibromyoma" is probably not correct. Leiomyomas may partially be replaced by fibrous connective tissue, which in turn may be myxedematous, calcareous, osseous, or necrotic. Hence the correct designations might be fibrous, calcareous, and so forth, leiomyoma of the uterus, stomach, esophagus or other organs.

Medical slang is perhaps, as in all languages, a forerunner of future correct usage, but to these old ears much of it is, and probably always will be, an anathema. "The surgical abdomen," "he had a gallbladder" or "I did his gallbladder," "he had no temperature," "round cell infiltration" for collections of lymphocytes, "the liver showed malignancy" and so on with a list that has no ending, and against which medical editors thunder loud and often.

May I pause over one particular pet aversion—namely, the wrong use of the word "pathology." For example, often I hear the expression, "There was no pathology in the abdomen," or "the specimen showed (sic!) no pathology" or "the surgeon found pathology in the liver." Here the word is employed to mean "lesion," "disease condition" or "pathologic condition." When it is used in this perverted sense, it indicates to my mind, a distinct pathologic complex in the user's mental makeup, education, or mode of thought.

—Proceedings of the Staff Meetings of the Mayo Clinic, March 3, 1938.

HISTORY OF MEDICINE IN MINNESOTA

MEDICINE IN WASHINGTON AND CHISAGO COUNTIES

(Continued from July issue.)

Beginning with the seventies, the history of the counties is easier to trace. Records of the Board of Health and of local medical societies, available periodicals of various sorts, some early directories, and the Transactions of the State Medical Society all supply bits of information.

The newcomers of the seventies were numerous. In 1870 Taylors Falls gained Dr. A. J. Murdock, and Stillwater Dr. B. G. Merry. Although Dr. Merry was a dentist, he did much research in mouth infections and wrote an excellent article on that subject which was published in the *Northwestern Medical and Surgical Journal.* He also served on the first Board of Dental Examiners for four years, the last year as president. In 1871 Drs. W. H. Pratt, Th. Roehrig, and David Sime, settled in Stillwater. Sime had graduated with honors from Glasgow University, and had attended both Glasgow and Edinburgh hospitals, being for some time resident physician and surgeon at the former. He stayed in Stillwater only a few months, however, before leaving for his former home. In 1872 Dr. Perry H. Millard arrived at Stillwater. Millard had studied chemistry at the University of Michigan, and after graduating had gone to Rush Medical College. He then settled in Chicago to practise, but left after the Chicago fire, which destroyed his office and everything in it. He came to Stillwater then, and stayed for many years, finally moving to Saint Paul. The same year three others arrived: Drs. George A. Lambert, R. F. Goodwin, and E. Cooley; the two latter were homeopaths. In 1873 Dr. Wm. A. Bentley and Dr. Q. C. Thompson settled at Rush City, Chisago County; as far as records show, they were the first physicians there. In the same year Dr. F. Hefti, a "practical physician," announced his presence in Stillwater. In 1874 Dr. A. H. Steen settled in Cottage Grove; Drs. Edson R. Wait and R. A. Livingston in Stillwater. All three of these were Rush graduates. Dr. F. L. Puffer, a graduate of the University of Michigan, came to study under Dr. Murdock of Taylors Falls. The year 1875 was rather uneventful. Two physicians, Drs. G. H. Hawes and C. Adams Sheeley, came to the valley but stayed only a few months each. Sheeley later moved to Pine City, then to Grantsburg, Wisconsin. At Harris, there was a Dr. Wilkes, but nothing is known of him save his name, and that he left in February at the request of his wife, who financed his departure on the condition that he never return. In 1876 Dr. E. A. Umland, a German, settled at Franconia, but a year later moved to Rush City where he became one of the most prominent physicians. Also a Dr. Zuercher settled at Stillwater and Wm. Olding, a Swedish cancer specialist who guaranteed a cure in every case, moved into Chisago County. In 1877 Dr. T. R. Austin came to North Branch; a Dr. Ogden to Center City, Dr. W. H. Caine to Stillwater, and Mrs. Sorenson, who specialized in female diseases, to Taylors Falls. The latter two were both homeopaths. In 1878 Dr. J. Reginald DeCousens moved to Rush City. He had been practising for some time before this in Isanti County, and was well known along the valley. He stayed at Rush City only a short time. A Dr. Lamb also came to Rush City in 1878, but stayed only a year. A Dr. J. N. Allen practised a short while in Stillwater. In 1879

MINNESOTA MEDICI

Drs. Woodling and Chapman came to North Branch, Dr. Oscar Hallberg to Marine, a Dr. Hunter to Center City and Dr. C. F. McComb to Rush City. Dr. McComb later moved to Duluth and at one time was mayor of that city. These, then, were the newcomers of the seventies; they included in their number some of the most prominent physicians who ever practised in the valley.

The health of the people of the two counties during the seventies was in constant danger from a great variety of epidemics which were always present and showed remarkable persistence in spite of the many physicians. In addition to the smallpox alarm in March, 1870, there was a severe typhoid epidemic in all the towns in the valley. One elder at Stillwater was called on to attend six funerals in one week. Dr. Rhodes himself had a slight attack of it. In Volume II of the *Northwestern Medical and Surgical Journal*, in the report of the Committee on Climatology and Epidemics for 1871, Dr. Reiner reported in Washington County during the year sixty-five cases of fevers, twenty-three enteric and the balance entero-malarial; twenty-two cases of scarlatina, nearly all mild and no deaths; twenty-six cases of diphtheria with four deaths; fourteen cases of erysipelas; six cases of cerebro-spinal meningitis, with three deaths; thirteen cases of acute rheumatism. No account was kept of rubeola or dysentery, but all cases were mild and there were no deaths. The year 1872 was somewhat more healthful. Although there is no available report for the year, the newspapers mentioned only smallpox, which was reported prevalent at Taylors Falls in October. However, in April, 1872, an ordinance was passed by the city council of Stillwater as follows:

"Every practising physician or other person attending or having under his care or become directly or personally cognizant of the existence of smallpox, varioloid, cholera or any other infectious, malignant or contagious disease within the city of Stillwater must within 24 hours report to the city recorder or the chairman of the Board of Health the disease, the name of the afflicted person, and the house or place of infection."

The ordinance also provided for a fine of from $75 to $100 for anyone willfully neglecting to do so. It went into effect April 22, 1872. This ordinance and a severe quarantine system, helped but little in keeping down epidemics. The next year there were deaths from diphtheria, measles, spinal meningitis and typhoid. At Chisago Lake and Franconia there were four deaths and several other severe cases of scarlet fever in one month. Apparently, however, this was a comparatively healthful year, for at the State Medical Society's meeting in February, 1874, Dr. Reiner said that they had "a season of immunity from epidemic diseases during the year." The fall of 1874 was marked by measles and whooping cough epidemics at Taylors Falls, and the diseases persisted through the following spring. They were followed by a much more serious visitation of scarlet fever, which was precedent throughout Chisago County and lasted through 1875 and the early part of 1876. It died out for a year, and then in September of 1877 returned and for five or six months was extremely severe. Several schools were closed as a precaution. At one time there were as many as eighteen cases in the small town of North Branch, though most of them were mild. This epidemic was punctuated by smaller, contemporary epidemics of whooping cough and typhoid. By the time these were out of mind an epidemic of diphtheria visited Stillwater during the summer of 1878, and in January and February of 1879 touched North Branch and Rush City at the same time as typhoid, membraneous croup and pneumonia prevailed. When these were over, and the threat of the return of scarlet fever was past, Rush City came down with a severe epidemic of measles which kept Drs. Umland and McComb busy day and night. At the end of the decade typhoid came again to Rush City.

In spite of all these diseases, the physicians seemed to have had plenty of time to take part in other activities besides practicing their professions. Dr. Carli found time to be city physician and chairman of the Board of Health, and in 1876 president of the St. Croix Old Settlers Association. In February, 1878, he bought and reopened the City Drug Store, which he had established twenty-five years before. Dr. Gaskill was one of the first supervisors of Marine, and for many years one of the inspectors of the state prison. Dr. Griswold was treasurer of the library association and chairman of the Republican county convention. Dr. A. J. Murdock was a charter member of the Temperance Society in October, 1877, and examining surgeon for the United States pension department, a member of the school board in 1877, and 1871 county physician. Dr. Reiner was a member of the board of education and prison physician at the time of his death in January, 1874. He was succeeded in this office by Dr. Lambert, who was in turn succeeded by Dr. W. H. Pratt. Dr. Rhodes was a member of the Board of Education and city physician in 1873 and 1874. Dr. Runge started a drug store in 1871. Several other physicians also conducted drug stores, among whom were R. F. Goodwin in 1875, Chapman at North Branch in 1879, and C. F. Forssman at Taylors Falls in 1870. Dr. Whiting was a delegate to the Republican district convention, was president of the St. Croix Bridge Company in 1874, to which position he was re-elected in 1875, and was several times elected president of the library association. Dr. Steen found time to collect a large and well selected medical library. Dr. Lamb was for three years government physician at the Pawnee and Winnebago agencies. The position of county physician was held by Dr. Pratt in 1874, and beginning March, 1875, by Dr. Livingstone, who held it until his death. In 1877 the position was held by Dr. Millard, and in January, 1879, the position was again given to Dr. Millard at a salary of $300 per annum. Millard also frequently served as a delegate to the State Medical Association, and in June, 1876, was delegate to the American Medical Association. Many of the doctors were enthusiastic hunters and fishermen, and Dr. C. F. McComb owned a particularly fine horse which won several races. Dr. DeCousens was a United States pension examiner and Dr. Umland sold insurance.

At Rush City, Dr. Wm. A. Bentley took an active part in civic affairs; he was one of the leading men in the temperance movement, was a United States pension examiner, was chairman of the Republican district convention, and in November, 1876, was elected representative from the district. While representative he introduced a temperance bill, which, though defeated, had the honor of receiving the largest vote any such bill had ever received up to that time. He was a member of the Literary Circle. In 1875 he gave two lectures to the Teachers Institute on "Hygiene in Our School" and "Physical Culture as the Legitimate Base of All Mental and Moral Development." He spoke at the State Medical Association meeting in February, 1876. Like most politicians, Dr. Bentley had enemies, among whom unfortunately was the editor of the *Rush City Post*. The editor was in the most advantageous position; he could say anything he pleased and spread it among the many readers of his paper, and he did so. Finally Bentley called at the editor's office in a fighting mood to settle the affair. He found the editor, Mr. Robie, prepared; the floor was carefully greased and a keg of diluted ink had been placed where it would do the most good. At the first blow the doctor's heels flew up, and the editor "lit on him like a grasshopper onto a cornstalk," at the same time upsetting the keg of ink. Robie got his hands in Dr. Bentley's hair and proceeded to mop up the floor very effec-tively before friends separated the two. Suitable apologies and explanations were made, but Bentley left town not long afterward and never returned.

Mrs. Sorenson, in November, 1877, opened the first hospital in Chisago County. Just what sort of hospital it was is unknown, but she offered homeopathic and electrical treatment and free treatment in the eye and ear department on Thurs-days. This hospital was kept up until Mrs. Sorenson was appointed county phy-sician of Polk County, Wisconsin, and moved to St. Croix Falls. In April, 1879, she established a hospital there. During the seventies another medical society was formed in Washington County. Although it was apparently fully organ-ized and existed for several years, its history is only known by a series of six newspaper items in the *Stillwater Gazette* and the *Stillwater Messenger*. The first item, published June 6, 1871, was as follows:

"We are requested to announce that a meeting of all the regular physicians of Wash-ington county will be held at the office of Doctor Carli on Thursday evening of this week at eight o'clock. The object of the meeting is to take steps for the organization of a 'County Medical Society.' Every physician in the county is earnestly requested to be present."

The second item was published June 20, 1871:

"St. Croix Medical Society"

"The physicians of the St. Croix Valley are requested to meet at the office of Dr. J. K. Reiner on Saturday evening next June 24 at eight o'clock. A full attendance is desired, as it is the wish and intention to perfect the organization at that time."

The third item was a brief letter from Dr. Roehrig, published in the *Gazette* for August 15, 1871, announcing his withdrawal from the St. Croix Medical Society. Evidently there had been a misunderstanding of some sort, for Roehrig left town shortly after. Then on September 16, 1873, there was a report of a meeting at the office of Dr. Millard. A committee to prepare a fee bill was chosen, consisting of Drs. Millard and Pratt, and a resolution was adopted which provided that each member furnish a black list of patients whose bills were not paid, and that no other physician should render any medical service until such debts be settled. At this meeting it was decided to admit Dr. Lambert to the society upon presentation of his diploma. The next report was merely a state-ment that the St. Croix Medical Society of Minnesota meeting was held at Dr. Livingstone's office with full attendance. This was in March, 1875. The last item was the news of a special meeting on September 10, 1875, to adopt suitable resolutions on the death of Dr. Livingstone. These are the only records of this society. There is no way of telling who the officers or members were, but in the obituary of Dr. Reiner in the *Gazette* for January 20, 1874, it was mentioned that he was secretary of the organization.

During the seventies a board of health was organized in Stillwater. It was first appointed on May 5, 1874, and consisted of Dr. Carli, William Casey and Dan Fry. Dr. Carli held the position of chairman for several years. Taylors Falls and Rush City apparently had no boards of health at this time.

Several of the pioneer physicians died during this decade. Dr. B. F. Babcock passed away at Afton on September 19, 1870, and Dr. Henry I. Jordan of Still-water on October 16 of the same year. It is not known what caused either death. On August 2, 1872, Dr. J. N. Ahl died of a paralysis after six days of illness. He was one of the earliest practitioners in the valley. Less than a year later another pioneer, Dr. H. F. Noyes, died at Milwaukee, where he had retired two years earlier, because of his age, to live with his son. Noyes was a skillful surgeon in his day and did most of the surgical work at Stillwater when he was there. Exactly a year later, on January 20, 1874, he was followed by Dr. J. K. Reiner. Reiner had been assisting Millard, Pratt and Carli with an amputation and contracted blood poisoning. In 1875 came the tragic and untimely death of a young physician, Dr. Livingstone. On September 8, after suffering for some time from severe indisposition, he took a hypodermic of morphine. Feeling no relief, he also took five grains by mouth, remarking that he should have "a good night's sleep." About 11 o'clock his wife became alarmed and sent for her half-brother, Dr. Millard. Several other physicians were also called in, but could do nothing, and Livingstone died before morning. Another young physician who died was Edson R. Wait, who died of a severe cold combined with tuberculosis in February, 1877.

Several physicians left the valley during this decade, besides those previously mentioned. Kinkle left in August, 1876, moving to St. Cloud. Lambert left Stillwater—and a number of indignant creditors—behind him in December, 1875, and died the following August "after a protracted debauch." Puffer, after completing his study of medicine with Dr. Murdock of Taylors Falls, and having practiced there for a while, left in February, 1878, to settle at Beaver Falls. The other physicians presumably stayed in Washington or Chisago Counties.

During the early eighties an even greater number of physicians arrived in the valley. In 1880 Dr. Oscar Hallberg, who was a graduate of the Carolinan Institute of Stockholm and who spoke Swedish, German and English fluently, settled at Taylors Falls. Dr. Weiseman, or Wynsma—it may have been two different men, or merely a variation in spelling—came to Center City and stayed a year. A Dr. Jackson, who was also, conveniently, a reverend, came to North Branch. Dr. Chapman also spent the year there. Dr. M. P. Goodwin, physician and dentist, came to Taylors Falls from Hudson, but moved to Stillwater in October, and later to Clear Lake. Several others came to Stillwater: Drs. O. A. Watier, Alfred Fliesburg, Alexander Donald (a homeopath) and A. Chisholm. They were joined the next year by Dr. Mark Edgerton, who came and formed a partnership with Drs. Caine and Hood (both homeopaths) and Dr. Jurden, a "noted chronic physician" who cured cancer, heart disease, syphilis or anything else presented. A Dr. M. Whittier ran a stationery and musical store that year, and Mrs. M. C. Hancock, a nurse, stayed for a while. The most important arrival of that year, however, was that of Dr. T. C. Clark, who settled at Stillwater, where he remained for many years, later becoming surgeon in the State Soldiers Home in Minneapolis. Dr. H. C. Murdock, a brother of A. J. Murdock, came to Taylors Falls at that time to take care of his brother's practice when the latter was absent. Later he took over the practice entirely when his brother moved away. In 1882 Dr. Wm. Jenner stayed for a while at Stillwater. Dr. H. S. Hersey also practiced there until March of that year. Dr. Merrill came from Hudson to form a partnership with Dr. Millard, and in 1883 James Sinclair began to study medicine with Dr. Caine. About that time a Dr. Beardsley settled at Rush City, and a Dr. Robb at North Branch, who stayed about a year. In 1884 Dr. J. G. Hodgkinson, from Saint Paul, located at Taylors Falls, Dr. Geo. B. McGuin at North Branch, Drs. W. D. Bolles and Leonard Pitkin, and again the much-moving Dr. Kinkle, at Stillwater. Dr. T. J. Hutton was at Taylors Falls at this time. The next year Stillwater gained Dr. E. R. Jellison, Dr. Charest (who came from Montreal and stayed only a short time) and Dr. Sinclair, who had once studied medicine with Dr. Caine, and later at the Hahnemann Medical College. A Dr. Carpenter practiced at Marine.

HISTORY OF MEDICINE IN MINNESOTA

If prevalence of disease attracts physicians, there was small wonder that so many new ones came at this time; besides mild annual epidemics of measles, frequent threats of an outbreak of mumps, whooping cough, scarlet fever, small pox, chicken pox and cerebrospinal meningitis, typhoid fever was constantly present and occasionally assumed alarming proportions. In September, 1882, there were some fifty cases of typhoid in Stillwater alone. The most serious disease was diphtheria. This disease, which killed fifty-nine persons out of a population of 7,997 in Chisago County in 1879, appeared as a severe epidemic and lasted until the winter of 1884, after which it very gradually died down until only an occasional case was reported. It was by far the most serious and longest epidemic the valley had ever had. Not only individuals, but often nearly all the children in a family died. In April, 1881, four children in one Taylors Falls family died. A year later the village council of Rush City was moved to order several barrels of chloride of lime and "proposed to disinfect the whole town." In July, 1883, one Stillwater physician alone reported ten cases under his care, and in August at the same place an undertaker reported that he had sold fifty-five coffins within two months. *The Stillwater Messenger* admitted that the disease was increasing. Dr. Carli's house was a regular hospital, two visiting relatives and a servant having contracted the disease. In Taylors Falls in November, 1883, not only were schools closed, but churches and Sunday schools did not meet. In Osceola, across and down the river, even the saloons were closed! In the family of John Ekegren of Stillwater, six children were prostrated at one time; a month later (January, 1884) four children of Jonas Grandstrand, who lived six or seven miles north of Marine, were buried at one time—three of them having died within twenty-four hours, and the fourth a few hours later. In Stillwater, in June, 1885, a girl, fourteen, and her brother six, died; several other members of the family had died during the two previous years, leaving only two children of a large family. Other cases were too numerous to mention. Quarantines were apparently enforced quite strictly at this time, but often the disease spread far before it was recognized. Often a well-meant visit to a friend with "a sore throat" resulted in a spread of diphtheria. In one case several neighbors dropped in to see if they could help care for a sick baby; the next day the baby died of diphtheria, and shortly afterwards the neighbors, and in turn their families, came down with the disease. In February, 1880, there were five cases of diphtheria in one family near Taylors Falls. The entire family lived in a one-room house, which was tightly sealed in the winter, and which had no sanitary arrangements at all. Naturally, if one member of the family contracted a contagious disease, the rest of the family could hardly hope to escape. Another case, which shows how the epidemics were carried, occurred at Fish Lake, Chisago County. A traveling Adventist minister, Mr. Carlson, came from Isanti County, where he had been in an infected house, praying over the body of a boy who had died of the smallpox. Taking no precautions, and without warning his host, he came to Fish Lake and stayed overnight at the home of a Mr. Almquist. That was on the fourth of December; on the fifteenth two daughters of Mr. Almquist were taken ill. The minister, who professed to have some knowledge of medicine, came again and assured them that it was only measles. However, he took the precaution of vaccinating the rest of the family. The vaccinations did not work, and Mr. and Mrs. Almquist and two other children caught the infection, which was, of course, smallpox. One of the girls died, though the rest of the family recovered. Another disease which was especially prevalent in 1885 and 1886 was scarlatina.

Unsanitary conditions, in at least some of the towns, greatly encouraged epidemics. During the earlier winters, before sewers were constructed, refuse of all sorts was merely thrown out on the snow, where it soon sank from sight. Most of the river towns were built on hillsides, so that when spring came and the snow melted, quantities of refuse was washed down the streets and scattered liberally throughout the town, often draining into cellars and remained there in stagnant pools. By the eighties this was partly remedied, but the *Stillwater Messenger* of July 14, 1883, reported that conditions were still "frightful." According to that paper, "Scarcely anything has been done in the way of cleaning up or disinfecting rear yards, alleys, open sewers, water closets, while in many places ponds of stagnant water can be found on which a thick green scum has formed. Unless immediate steps are taken . . . we will soon witness such a harvest of deaths as was never before witnessed in Minnesota."

While mentioning the subject of disease it might be of interest to remark on the sudden increase of cancer noted after the death of Ex-President U. S. Grant in 1885. The quacks, at least, made quite a fad of this disease and used it as the excuse for many operations.

The Stillwater Board of Health was active at this time, and in March, 1883, Taylors Falls established a board of health, which consisted of Dr. H. G. Murdock, E. C. Reynolds, and L. F. Snow. The first official act of this board was announced the next day; it was an order that all persons who had not been, or had not recently been, vaccinated should do so within one week. Rush City also formed a board of health. There is no record of when this was done, but it is known to have existed in March, 1884, at which time Dr. Umland served on it.

In March, 1880, a group of women at Stillwater organized the first hospital at that place. The women managed it themselves, collecting beds, clothing, medicine and money by means of benefit parties and donations. In the *Messenger* for October, 1882, appeared the following request: "The animal which furnished milk for the city hospital strayed away some ten days ago, and our philanthropic citizens are requested to furnish a substitute." In 1890 the city contributed $300 per year, and the county agreed to pay at the rate of a dollar a day for each county charge.

Two other hospitals—one a homeopathic institution—were established about 1881. W. H. Caine was house physician and surgeon, Alexander Donald was oculist and aurist, Drs. Edgerton and Dorion of Saint Paul and Dr. Steek of Minneapolis were the consulting surgeons, and Drs. Hutchinson and Humphrey of Saint Paul and Minneapolis, respectively, were the consulting physicians. This hospital was also supported partly, at least, by benefit parties, records of which appeared in the newspapers of that time. This hospital apparently did not last very long, evidently being closed in the spring of 1883, for at that time Dr. Caine was patronizing the city hospital, which he continued to do until he was excluded from the grounds "for conduct unbecoming a physician and a gentleman." He was permitted to return after he threatened to sue the managers. The managers later quarreled with Drs. Merrill, Marshall, and Millard. The third hospital was established in March, 1885, and was especially devoted to the care of lumbermen and private patients.

(To be continued in September issue.)

EDITORIAL

MINNESOTA MEDICINE

OFFICIAL JOURNAL OF THE MINNESOTA STATE MEDICAL
ASSOCIATION

Published by the Association under the direction of its Editing
and Publishing Committee

EDITING AND PUBLISHING COMMITTEE
J. T. CHRISTISON, Saint Paul   C. B. WRIGHT, Minneapolis
E. M. HAMMES, Saint Paul   T. A. PEPPARD, Minneapolis
WALTMAN WALTERS, Rochester

EDITORIAL STAFF
CARL B. DRAKE, Saint Paul, Editor
W. F. BRAASCH, Rochester, Associate Editor
GILBERT COTTAM, Minneapolis, Associate Editor

Annual Subscription—$3.00   Single Copies—$0.40
Foreign Subscriptions—$3.50

The right is reserved to reject material submitted for editorial
or advertising columns. The Editing and Publishing Committee
does not hold itself responsible for views expressed either in
editorials or other articles when signed by the author.

Classified advertising—five cents a word; minimum charge,
$1.00. Remittance should accompany order.

Display advertising rates on request.

Address all communications to Minnesota Medicine, 2642 University Avenue, Saint Paul, or Suite 604, National Bldg., Minneapolis. Telephone: Nestor 2641.

BUSINESS MANAGER
J. R. BRUCE

Volume 21   AUGUST, 1938   Number 8

Roentgen Therapy

RADIATION therapy during the present century has developed into one of the dominant
therapeutic means available to the medical profession. It is best known as a weapon in combating cancer but its field of usefulness has
gradually extended to almost all medical specialties. Like all new tools it has often been
misused and has occasionally been enthusiastically
hailed as the remedy for a disease which later
was found to be uninfluenced by radiation. This
should, however, not be used as an argument
against the sane use of radiation therapy. Unfortunately conclusions concerning the effectiveness of a therapeutic agent are often drawn too
hastily. An extensive use should not be attempt-

ed until the beneficial effect has been definitely
established by careful tests. It is also important
to have a clear concept of what is supposed to
be accomplished by the treatment. Radiation
therapy is often used to relieve pain or to cause
a temporary improvement of patients suffering
from advanced stages of cancer. Consider for
instance the numerous patients suffering from
painful bone metastasis who by means of roentgen therapy have been relieved of the pain and
from a completely helpless condition have been
able to return to active life for one or more
years. Though these patients eventually succumbed to the cancer, they received all the benefit from the treatments which could reasonably
be expected. It is evident that the patients
should be carefully studied and selected before
any therapy is inaugurated and the treatments
should be planned individually. If it seems possible to obtain a cure the procedure is usually
much more radical than when palliation is the
only hope. Many "five-year cures" have been
obtained with radiation but the percentage cure
is as yet small when the whole group of cancer
patients is considered. The present method of
building up the dose to a very high value in a
period of about one month has led to better
results. The relatively higher cure rate can,
however, not be obtained unless the total roentgen dose is so great that it produces rather severe tissue damage and vesiculation of the skin
is often a necessary stage of the reaction that
the patient has to contend with.

It was mentioned that many diseases besides
cancer can be favorably influenced by means of
roentgen therapy. The treatments of many types
of infections has become an important field in
radiation therapy but it requires careful selection of cases. The dose is as a rule small and
severe reaction should be avoided. Just as radical treatments are essential from the start for
malignant conditions so it is important to use
special caution and to avoid unnecessary damage
for benign conditions.

Due to the fact that the macroscopic changes
following roentgen therapy develop slowly and
may manifest themselves months or even years
afterwards it should be evident that considerable

study and experience must be a requirement for the specialist in this type of therapy. The dose used in each case must be carefully chosen and accurately measured and the distribution of the radiation through the cross section of the body considered. Adequate protection for all who work with or in the immediate vicinity of a roentgen machine is another important consideration.

Radiation therapy compares in several respects to surgery and requires just as intense continued practice and study. It has little in common with radiography except that it utilizes similar machines and that it has become a common practice for one man to specialize in both of these divergent fields. A physician may, however, be an outstanding specialist in roentgen diagnosis without being a roentgen therapist and vice versa.

The sane use and development of roentgen therapy is determined largely by the medical profession as a whole. Specialists in this field have to rely upon the support and coöperation of other physicians. A great step in this direction was taken when the American Medical Association started to coöperate with the American Board of Radiology. The important function of this Board is "to issue a certificate to each candidate who meets the requirements of the Board, to the effect that the holder of the certificate has adequate training in Radiology and has successfully fulfilled the requirements of the Board." Different forms of certificates are issued. Either it is to the effect that the applicant has been qualified to practice Radiology in all its branches or else that he has been qualified to practice Radiology in one or more of the special fields. Among these special fields are included Therapeutic Radiology and Therapeutic Roentgenology.

K. W. Stenstrom, Ph.D.

Anesthesiology: A New Specialty

"ANESTHESIOLOGY," said Stedman, in 1933, is "the science that treats of the various means of inducing local or general anesthesia and of the accidents and complications of this condition." This definition affords an interesting and well-founded contrast to the title of Paluel J. Flagg's book "The Art of Anesthesia," published in 1910.

Ever since its introduction, ninety years ago, efforts have been made to improve the quality of anesthesia, both by trying to lessen its dangers and increase its comforts to the patient. For a long time these efforts were concentrated on making the administration of the three original anesthetic agents safer and less disagreeable. Of the three, ether made much the best showing, for the inherent dangers of chloroform could never be eliminated and nitrous oxide, in those days, was thought of only for the short cases and chiefly in dentistry. Ether became the first choice and when the open drop method came in anesthesia became an art and so remained until the turn of the century and even later. Then began important development in the whole field of local and general anesthesia. The refinement of preanesthetic medication, the introduction of the newer gases and ingenious methods of their administration with intensive study of their peculiarities and the means to prevent any untoward effects, the use of helium as a carrier in certain contingencies and the adoption of procedures to diminish the post-anesthetic sequels are a few of the improvements which have been worked out in this later period. In local and spinal anesthesia similar advances have been made, ensuring safer and surer results, with correspondingly wider applicability to all types of surgery.

Naturally all this has contributed largely to the strides which surgery itself has been able to make in this period. New fields have been successfully invaded and difficult, time-consuming procedures made feasible by the application of these newly found principles in anesthesia. They have done much for all kinds of surgery, but the most apparent is probably in that of the chest, so long hallowed ground for anything but emergency operations but now invaded with relative safety for extensive, premeditated and prolonged efforts.

The anesthetist who is to be in a position to meet all the demands of modern anesthesiology must have had considerable training, in addition to fulfilling all the requirements of the complete course in medicine in all its branches. A great deal of ground is covered by the accumulated knowledge of this new science and one must be prepared to undertake a long period of study and demonstration in proper environment. The number of persons who may be considered to be fully qualified in this field is at present very

576

small and scattered, for naturally enough they are to be found only where there is sufficient demand for service of this highly specialized type. But they are training others and in due time there will be enough to furnish every community where there is the necessary volume of surgical activity with an anesthetist of the requisite ability to comply with the exacting requirements which have been described.

Very wisely, we think, the new American Board of Surgery has established an affiliate which will be known as the American Board of Anesthesiology, an arrangement which has been approved by the Advisory Board for Medical Specialties. Coöperating societies include the Section on Surgery of the American Medical Association, the American Society of Anesthetists, Inc., and the American Society of Regional Anesthetists, Inc. This board, composed of nine members well known for their standing in the field of anesthesia, will hold examinations and issue certificates in much the same way as is done by the other special boards.

G. C.

Dr. E. A. Meyerding

AT the time of the annual meeting of the Minnesota State Medical Association held in St. Cloud in 1924, the idea of having a full time secretary for the Association came to a head. Until that time the secretary was paid a nominal sum for attending to duties which were for the most part in connection with the annual meetings. It was at this time that Dr. E. A. Meyerding, who had proven himself an efficient executive secretary of the Minnesota Public Health Association, was induced to also become secretary of our State Association. With his assumption of the office, the State Association changed its passive attitude to one of widespread activity. Dr. Meyerding furnished much of the drive to the Association's activities since 1924.

Advantageous as it has been in many respects to both organizations to have them closely bound with the link of a common secretary, the job was a man killer, and Secretary Meyerding had expressed the desire to retire before his leave of absence for a year was granted at the 1937 meeting. At the annual meeting this year, his resignation was accepted, not, however, without an expression of the Association's appreciation of his services.

The following resolution was passed by the Council and House of Delegates on June 28 in Duluth:

"RESOLVED, that the Minnesota State Medical Association provide an appropriate token to be awarded on occasion to a member of the Association who has rendered especially valuable and distinguished service to the Minnesota State Medical Association. The Council of the State Medical Association are to select candidates for this award."

On June 29, the Council passed the following resolution:

"BE IT RESOLVED, that the first recipient of the distinguished service medal awarded by the State Medical Association be given to Dr. E. A. Meyerding in recognition of years of faithful and excellent service rendered to the Minnesota State Medical Association."

This is a most fitting way for the Association to express its appreciation of Dr. Meyerding's long and efficient service as secretary.

Human Rabies Doubted by Dr. Brady

THE presence of rabies in the canine population of Hennepin County during the past few months and the finding of an infected dog recently in Ramsey County has brought the disease again into the limelight. The presence of an epidemic makes it incumbent on the health authorities to institute control measures and requires the wholehearted coöperation of the public. As a rule, this is not obtained. Dog lovers oppose the muzzling ordinance and the physiognomy of certain breeds is not conducive to the use of muzzles. Certainly the use of muzzles, leashes and fences will not control an epidemic if stray dogs are not picked up, for it is the stray dog that is the worst offender.

With the announcement in the *Saint Paul Pioneer Press* that regulations would be extended to Ramsey County and of the health officer's request for coöperation in carrying out the ordinance on the part of the public, the same article quotes from the columns of its medical advisor, Dr. Brady, which appeared July 17 as follows:

"I do not doubt that rabies occurs in animals. I merely doubt that it occurs in man. . . . If I were bitten, whether the animal was suspected of having rabies or not, I should want first aid treatment by a competent physician (*good judgment*), and in view of the chance for tetanus infection, an immediate injection of tetanus antitoxin five to seven days later (*whatever that means*). . . . That would be all. I wouldn't care how mad the animal was before or after he bit me." (Italics ours).

All the medical literature on rabies in human beings from the time of Pasteur to the present has not convinced Dr. Brady. Pasteur's outstanding contribution in providing a method of immunizing human beings bitten by mad dogs and preventing a sure and horrible death is of questionable value in Dr. Brady's mind. Let him be a "doubting Thomas" as far as he personally is concerned. Few physicians have seen cases of human rabies and none wants to, for there is no specific treatment and death is sure. But, Dr. Brady assumes a grave responsibility when he gives advice publicly which no conscientious practitioner would dare to follow if confronted with a patient bitten by a rabic animal. We doubt whether a jury would acquit a physician who failed to use the Pasteur treatment even though he might refer to Dr. Brady as an authority.

The attitude of a newspaper in spreading doubt as to the existence of danger to human beings in a rabies epidemic in dogs is not cooperating with the health department. Wholehearted coöperation of dog owners, as well as health department ordinances, is necessary to stamp out this real menace.

Government Activity Against Poisonous Contaminants

Recently the Food and Drug Administration has been issuing monthly news releases concerning its actions. Under the subheading "Other Food Seizures" (March 22) reference is made to "54 gallons and 310 small bottles of flavors and solvents containing poisonous glycols; and 515 bushels of apples carrying excessive spray residue." Similar seizures are reported also for April. The recent Elixir of Sulfanilamide-Massengill incident focused attention on diethylene glycol. Toxic glycols have been used in the food and drug industry, such as "Carbitol," which is the mono-ethyl ether of diethylene glycol; this apparently is more acutely toxic than diethylene glycol. The dosages containing "Carbitol" were so small that deaths apparently occurred rarely if at all. From time to time THE JOURNAL has warned against the potential harm of sprays for fruits containing lead or arsenic. The government deserves considerable encouragement in having reduced this hazard by requiring careful removal of spray residue from fruits sold in interstate commerce. The hazard of lead cannot be attributed to any one industry or source. Whether the source of lead is contamination of drinking water, the increasing amount of lead of exhausts from automobiles, fruit sprays from lead solder or other sources, it is a hazard. (J.A.M.A., June 4, 1938, p. 1929.)

Communication

SIMPLE TREATMENT FOR MAGGOTS

TO THE EDITOR:

July 20, 1938.

Ever since reading about the case of "Wohlfartia Vigil Cutaneous Myiasis in Minnesota" in your June, 1938, number by Drs. Vandersluis and Whittemore of Bemidji, I have wanted to write you about my experience with maggots. Little did I realize that my experience might in any way be unique or of interest to any one. My principal reason for writing is to inform those who may have cases, of a very simple and effective treatment.

About 25 years ago I was called twelve miles out in the country to see a baby about six months old. When I arrived I found a much agitated mother and a squirming baby. The mother informed me that she had noticed maggots crawling out of a tiny opening in the skin of the baby's neck. I was a bit skeptical but not for long. A little massage of the neck produced a real live maggot and there was no room for doubt as to where it came from. The skin about the opening was practically normal and the opening so small that it was hard to locate after the maggot emerged. But the maggot found it readily enough. Knowing the family not to be very clean in their habits I thought nothing much of the cause, but I was stumped what to do for treatment. A 95 per cent alcohol bath seemed to agree with the wiggler to perfection. I tried all the antiseptic lotions I had with me, all to no avail. Then I recalled, as a boy, I had seen my father pour some turpentine into a maggot infested wound in the leg of one of our cows. With a cotton swab I painted a bit of turpentine on the skin about the hole and to my great amazement, maggots immediately emerged as fast as they could until eight husky maggots, about 1 cm. long, hustled away from their home with no attempt to return. The maggots were white with black heads and segmented. The remedy proved effective in one application.

My second experience with maggots came three years ago when I was called by the sheriff to see a prisoner in jail. The man had been picked up by the police while sleeping in the railway yards. Too much alcohol had made him dead to the world for several hours. It was summer and a hot sun had brought many flies to him. He had complained persistently that he had "crawlers" in his ear and they were killing him. On arrival, inspection was sufficient to convince me that maggots in numbers had invaded his ear, as frequently one would come to view at the external opening. The jailor had turpentine on hand. Two drops produced complete evacuation of the maggot home in the ear. Swabbing completed the cure.

After reading the article in MINNESOTA MEDICINE I recalled an experience that came to me when, as a cowboy, one afternoon I chanced to sit down close to a clump of recent discharge from one of the animal's bowels. A gray fly, a bit larger than a housefly, lit on the heap and after a few restless wiggles of her rump a small maggot emerged from her "distal end," much to my amusement and amazement. Then came another and another and still another, until eight or ten had thus emerged to disappear on the soft mass of droppings.

Thus endeth my tale of the maggots. Will any one duplicate it?

G. H. LUEDTKE, Fairmont, Minn.

MEDICAL ECONOMICS

Edited by the Committee on Medical Economics
of the
Minnesota State Medical Association
W. F. Braasch, M.D., Chairman

SURVEY INVITATION—
PENNSYLVANIA

Re personal complaint of lack of medical care:

The Pennsylvania State Medical Society is one of the most active in the country in pushing its own state Survey of Medical Facilities, under the guidance of the State Secretary, Dr. Walter Donaldson.

An interesting move designed to bring to light any public complaint against doctors, hospitals and medical care has been taken by Chairman Frederick M. Jacobs of the Committee on Public Relations of the society with the approval of the society's Committee on Medical Economics in charge of the Survey.

Pennsylvania newspapers are to be asked by the doctors to publish a public invitation from the local county medical society to register with the secretary or other representative of the society any complaint anyone may have concerning medical care.

Says Doctor Jacobs in a recent issue of the *Pittsburgh Medical Bulletin:*

". . . . We urge you to contact the editors of all newspapers in your county—daily and weekly—asking them to publish your county medical society's invitation to anyone in your county to register with the secretary or other representatives of your county society the fact that he or she is NOT receiving medical care.

"The American Medical Association and your state medical society have, for many years, endeavored to reply to individual communications from such individuals, but for the first time this invitation is to be brought through the newspapers urgently to the attention of the people in each county.

"Your earnest support of this, our own endeavor, to uncover facts and to institute corrective measures is solicited."

Secretaries of Minnesota societies might consider this matter carefully with a view to the advisability of adopting it in Minnesota.

MEDICINE ON THE MARCH

When the Minnesota State Medical Association brought to a close its eighty-fifth annual meeting in Duluth, July 1, some 1,500 doctors in Minnesota held a clearer conception than ever before of the peculiar problems and responsibilities that belong to the physician alone in the social readjustments of our time.

Probably there was never a meeting of the association at which the responsibility for leadership in public health and social problems was so frequently and so definitely pointed out, even in the scientific sessions.

The clear cut conclusion is that Minnesota physicians are on the march toward a practical, well considered public policy and that they are prepared to act in accordance with this policy as leaders in community effort to improve the distribution of medical care to all the people in each community wherever, as public spirited men, they see the need for such improvements.

Need for Medical Leadership

There was a time, perhaps, when the text of typical exhorters at the economics sessions and the House of Delegates' sessions of most medical meetings was jingoistic. An enemy with a deep animosity to the medical profession was abroad in the land; we must fight the enemy. When we had vanquished the foe, sometimes called the social worker, sometimes the Foundations—why then we should have preserved intact the house of medicine and nothing further need be done. There was truth in much of what the exhorters had to say; but soberer statesmen of medicine know that it is not enough for medicine to defend itself against unjust criticism. There is a definite need for leadership in the social adjustments of the times. If medical men do not supply that leadership insofar, at least, as these adjustments involve the prevention and control of disease and the care of the sick, then America will inevitably flounder through a costly and futile period of ill-judged social experiment in the course of which our cherished leadership in medicine may be lost for many years.

Problem Complex

To go out and fight a known and ticketed enemy is a simple matter. The problem of the doctor is much broader and more complex than that. The profession of medicine now looks behind and beyond its critics knowing that their vituperations are of no moment so long as medical men are awake to their public job and honestly at work at it.

In their careful study of the relief problem in Minnesota; in their active coöperation with relief and welfare officials to provide adequate medical care without sacrifice of standards to the needy; in their current extensive study of medical needs and supply in every community of the state, leaders of the Minnesota State Medical Association showed, at this meeting, that they are assuming this broader responsibility. They are not fighting critics; they are doing their utmost to see that the people of Minnesota have the benefit of the best that medicine has to offer. They are clearly conscious that as physicians they must keep clear before legislators and welfare officials the relation that poverty and a low standard of living bears to disease.

New Officers

Administrative responsibility for the conduct of medical association affairs will shortly rest in new hands, though only one new name is added to the roster of councilors.

Dr. George Earl of St. Paul is president-elect of the association and in line to succeed Dr. J. M. Hayes of Minneapolis as president in January, 1939. In his place as councilor of the fifth district, the House of Delegates elected Dr. E. Mendelssohn Jones of St. Paul.

Dr. B. B. Souster of St. Paul will succeed Dr. E. A. Meyerding of St. Paul, whose resignation as secretary of the organization was accepted by the delegates.

First Service Award

A report of fourteen notable years in medical organization history in Minnesota was submitted with the resignation of Doctor Meyerding and the Council voted unanimously to present him with the first distinguished service award

ever bestowed upon any member for his services to the organization. This award will be bestowed, in the future, upon other members judged worthy of the honor by the Council of the organization.

It is fitting that the first award should go to Doctor Meyerding, whose service as secretary and executive secretary contributed so largely to the establishment of the Minnesota State Medical Association in its present high standing among the medical societies of the country.

The active administration of the state office of the association will remain in the capable hands of Mr. R. R. Rosell, executive secretary since leave of absence was granted to Doctor Meyerding last September. As formerly, he will carry on his work under the direction of the Council and officers of the association and in conformity with established policies of the association.

The new vice presidents of the organization are Drs. J. C. Jacobs of Willmar and Adolph M. Hanson of Faribault. Speaker W. W. Will of Bertha was reëlected; Doctor Meyerding will serve as vice speaker.

Dr. W. H. Condit of Minneapolis was reelected treasurer and Drs. H. Z. Giffin, L. L. Sogge and B. S. Adams were reëlected councilors of the first, second and ninth districts, respectively.

The delegates to the American Medical Association remain as before except that Dr. Joel C. Hultkrans of Minneapolis will act as alternate for Doctor Coventry in place of Doctor Earl.

Two major addresses made at this meeting will greatly affect the thinking of many physicians in Minnesota.

Notable Addresses

One was the presidential address of Dr. J. M. Hayes of Minneapolis which sketched in terms of exact figures the immensity of the welfare and relief problem that faces Minnesota today. Also the status in general of medical participation in the handling of medical care for thousands of people—running very close to a half million—for whom some degree of care is provided.

The other was the banquet address of Dr. Howard W. Haggard, associate professor of applied physiology at the Sheffield Scientific School to every member through the secretaries of county and district societies.

Form No. 2 on hospital facilities and activities is in charge of Mr. A. M. Calvin, secretary of the Minnesota Hospital Association. Forms have been sent to all of the members of the association and we understand that a satisfactory return is coming in.

Form No. 3 is concerned with nursing in general. To secure the information required concerning public health nursing, forms were sent to all public health nurses under the jurisdiction of Miss Olivia Peterson, director of public health nursing for the Minnesota State Department of Health. Returns were reported from 35 counties this week by Miss Peterson's office. (It will be remembered that only a limited number of counties support public health nurses.) To secure information concerning private duty nurses, forms were sent out by the Minnesota Registered Nurses Association to the nine districts of the organization. To date, the information has been received from four districts.

Form No. 4 on official public health activities is in the charge of Dr. A. J. Chesley, executive officer and secretary of the State Board of Health and member of the American Medical Association's advisory committee on the Survey, who sent it to all community and county health officers in the state. To date returns have been received from 68 counties and 7 communities.

Form No. 5 on public welfare activities is in the charge of officials of the State Relief Agency, who have sent the form to relief workers in every county. To date 65 counties have returned properly filled in forms.

Form No. 6 on health activities in the schools is in charge of the State Department of Education for the public schools. To date 80 per cent of city and town schools and all county superintendents of the state have returned their forms. Forms were sent direct from the state office to the 300 parochial schools in the state and of these 150 have already been returned.

Form No. 7 on health services in the colleges went from the state office to the 25 colleges and universities of the state. Of these 22 have been properly filled and returned.

Form No. 8 concerning medical services arranged for or provided by industrial, fraternal, mutual benefit, group hospitalization, community health and other similar organizations or by the county medical society is being handled direct by the state office.

Form No. 9 on activities and experience of wholesale and retail druggists was received at a much later date than the other forms. The forms are now in the hands of the state pharmaceutical association, however, and are being distributed by districts all over the state. Group meetings are being held by the association in the various districts for the purpose of stimulating interest among members and securing accurate information.

Returns from Physicians

Said Doctor Braasch:

"No comprehensive information is available as yet as to the progress made by county and district medical society secretaries in securing the information on Form No. 1 from the individual doctors.

"The return is close to one hundred per cent in some counties. In others, forms are coming in slowly. Your committee would ask that every delegate here take it upon himself to see that the survey is carried out in his county as completely and as rapidly as possible.

"Without doubt, the information asked for in Form No. 1 is the crux of the Survey, and other data, no matter how comprehensive, cannot be evaluated properly without the testimony of the doctors themselves. It is of greatest importance that questions No. 7 and 9 be answered. It is of fundamental importance to know what the practitioner thinks about methods for improving the distribution of medical care.

"The forms were sent to the secretaries of the local societies and are to be returned to them and a special appeal to all members who have not yet made their returns should be made at this meeting.

Accurate Estimates Will Serve

"The committee in charge appreciates the fact that exact information may not be available in all cases and for all questions. In general, however, an appropriate estimate is possible and will serve to answer the questions. It has been suggested that an accurate record of the number of charity patients and other specific data be made for a definite period as a check on the estimates furnished. The American Medical Association will soon forward blanks for this purpose. These blanks are to be filled out during a period of one week during two or three specific months of the ensuing year. They will soon be distributed by the state secretary.

"The physicians' forms are to be sent unsigned to the local secretary and he, in turn, with the assistance, if necessary, of the state office will tabulate them on a

form provided by the American Medical Association. The original forms returned by the physicians will remain in the possession of the local societies concerned.

Not a Statistical Exercise

"It goes without saying that the Survey will be of small value either as a picture of conditions in Minnesota or as a basis on which to build improvements and readjustments where they are needed unless the information secured is representative of all districts and classes.

"This effort is not a statistical exercise but an honest attempt to evaluate our medical service in every county in Minnesota. As such, it is of personal importance to every physician. Upon the accuracy and honesty with which it is carried on may well depend the future of medical practice in Minnesota."

Public Health Committee

Public health education is the greatest problem that faces the doctor today, Dr. L. R. Critchfield, chairman of the Committee on Public Health Education, told the House of Delegates in the annual report of his committee.

It is the crux of much of our economic and social difficulty and the foundation for good medical care.

According to this report, people in the low income groups who fail to get good care, go uncared for, often, because they did not know how or where to go for help; or because they did not know the importance of getting help before their trouble progressed to a stage where medical care was unavailing.

This interpretation of the problem facing physicians prefaced an appeal to the individual practitioner of medicine all over Minnesota, not only to be alert to every accepted means of disease prevention and control but to be a teacher of good hygiene to the general public and also to be thoroughly informed as individuals on every community resource for helping the unfortunate.

"When the neglected illness is thoroughly investigated," Doctor Critchfield said, "it usually develops that ignorance and carelessness and not actual absence of medical facilities was the cause of the neglect.

"The conclusion seems to be inescapable that public health education is the fundamental health need in this country rather than federal subsidies to physicians or new laws and new taxes.

"It becames increasingly clear to members of this committee that it is the doctors and not the nurses, social workers or lay health agencies who must assume the responsibility for direction of this work. A concentration upon a more extensive and far-reaching

ing program of public health education should be a cardinal objective in our program for better medical care for all the people in Minnesota; but this program must not be delegated to a single committee or group. It must be the individual responsibility of every practicing physician in the state."

Low Income and Indigent Problems

Dr. W. A. Coventry of Duluth, chairman of the Committee on Low Income and Indigent Problems, concurred in the above recommendation as one of the fundamentals of meeting the problem of care for the sick poor in the report for his committee.

"The United States leads the world in emphasis on prevention of disease," he said. "But even the United States has taken only the first steps in preventive medicine.

"The ultimate objective of all our efforts should be to lessen sickness rather than to lower costs of medical care.

"At the same time, physicians, knowing well the burden placed upon people of small income in time of illness, are morally and socially bound to coöperate with the proper authorities to the fullest extent so that competent care can be made available to all who need it."

The Doctor's Side

Delegates were urged by Doctor Coventry to do their part toward making the nation-wide study of medical facilities (reported above by Doctor Braasch) accurate and representative.

"Many surveys of medical care have been conducted by government and private lay agencies," he said. "It is well for us to have their side of the story; but, as in all stories, there is another side. And this side, which is the doctor's side, is absolutely essential to an accurate evaluation of needs.

"The medical profession will never oppose any adjustment of our system that careful studies may show to be necessary for the good of all. The doctors will insist, however, that government agencies shall not be in complete control of services that cannot be administered properly except by trained medical men. They will also insist that the sick man be allowed to apply to his own physician when he seeks medical aid."

Praise for State Officials

Resolutions of appreciation to officials of the State Board of Control and the State Relief Administration for their sound handling of medical phases of welfare and relief work in Minnesota were passed by the delegates at their Tuesday night session.

A résumé of the participation of the state medical association in framing plans for care

of the needy in the state was given to the delegates in the report of R. R. Rosell, executive secretary of the association. Mr. Rosell's report included warm praise for the readiness of state officials in all departments to coöperate closely with the doctors in order that the best possible service may be given to relief clients and recipients of assistance aids.

Marked Gains This Year

"Definite and marked gains have been made during the past year," Mr. Rosell said, "in the firm establishment among all official welfare agencies of accepted medical procedures in the care of the sick.

"Fundamental to all of them was the inclusion in the Extra Session Laws of 1937 of the 'choice of vendor clause' which guarantees to the relief patient the right to select his own physician.

"Equally important was the ruling of the Attorney General on the clause which establishes this right."

The obligation upon the individual physician, particularly in the rural districts, to know all of the official sources of aid for needy patients was reiterated by Mr. Rosell in his report.

"The doctor's individual relationship to the community appears to have changed considerably during the last ten years," he pointed out. "It is generally agreed, now, that it is as much a part of medical practice to know how to direct needy patients as it is to know how to treat them medically. It is obvious, also, that the physician who is thus informed will be able to lay his finger upon weak spots when they present themselves and take the lead in his community in correcting the difficulty" . . .

"The result of the confidence and mutual understanding which characterizes all of our relations with official agencies, is that no hasty proposals for state supported sickness insurance or politically inspired reforms have emanated from any of the leaders in politics or welfare in Minnesota. Such alternatives have been relinquished altogether in favor of an honest attempt to deal with medical problems fairly and realistically and with no motive except the public good."

* * *

Recommendations made by the scientific committees of the organization and accepted by the delegates were noticeably framed upon public interest and public welfare.

For Better Handling of Fractures

The Committee on Fractures of which Dr. O. W. Yoerg of Minneapolis is chairman urged the appointement of a special committee in each county to study methods of first aid and transportation of accident cases in their own counties.

The adoption of standard splints for handling of fracture cases all over the state was asked also, and a public education campaign to eliminate the damage done by untrained bystanders who are first at the scene of an accident.

Reducing Asphyxial Deaths

The Committee on Asphyxia and Asphyxial Death, of which Dr. A. E. Cardle of Minneapolis is chairman, asked the especial interest of the association in reduction of the mounting death and disability rate from gas poisoning. The increasing use of automobiles and of gas in the home has brought asphyxia into the domain of everyday medical practice according to this committee. Special studies, on the one hand, and a special public campaign of caution, on the other, are necessary to handle the situation.

Insulin Substitutes

A special effort to acquaint the public of the danger of nostrums as substitutes for insulin in the treatment of diabetes was specially urged by the Committee on Diabetes, of which Dr. H. B. Sweetser, Jr., of Minneapolis is chairman. Two other projects received the sanction of the delegates: one is an effort to secure employment from relief funds of a dietitian or nurse dietitian to help in the instruction of relief patients who are receiving insulin; the other is a study to determine the attitude of industry in general toward employable diabetics, looking to better employment arrangements for otherwise normal people who suffer from diabetes.

The Child Who Does Not Hear Well

The need of concerted effort on the part of the physicians, the State Board of Health and the State Department of Education to find and help the child who does not hear well at school was brought to the attention of the delegates once more by the Committee on Deafness Prevention and Amelioration, of which Dr. Horace Newhart of Minneapolis is chairman. Every city having a population of 2,000 or more should own its own equipment for testing hearing, in the opinion of the committee.

Praise for Minnesota

Praise for the program of venereal disease control carried on in Minnesota by the State Board of Health was voiced by the Committee on

Syphilis and Social Diseases before the delegates.

Minnesota's program is one of the best established and most thoroughgoing in the United States and there is no immediate need for expansion according to Dr. S. E. Sweitzer, Minneapolis, chairman.

There is danger, however, that the widespread campaign of publicity about syphilis and gonorrhea may be exploited by fakers and commercial opportunists. A recent questionable promotion in Minneapolis is a case in point (see "Social Hygiene Institute" elsewhere in these columns).

Cancer Campaign

Every member of the association should be informed on the objective and organization of the Women's Field Army which is working closely with the Committee on Cancer, of which Dr. Martin Nordland of Minneapolis is chairman. Every member should be ready, according to the report of the committee, to assist in the educational program of the Field Army. Each society should have a regularly constituted and trained speakers bureau on the subject of cancer.

Cancer control lies largely in the hands of the individual patient and his physician and the effort of the Field Army to bring people early to their physicians should have the closest assistance, in the opinion of the committee, from the physicians themselves.

Military Affairs

Among other recommendations made by the Committee on Military Affairs, of which Dr. F. L. Smith of Rochester is chairman, was the appeal to all medical reserve officers to participate as frequently as possible in army maneuvers.

The military committee also urged extension of opportunities to flight surgeons for observation of pilots under flying conditions. A recent war department ruling grounded all but five of the 285 flight surgeons in the regular army and the ruling is likely to prove a decided handicap to adequate examination, according to the committee.

SOCIAL HYGIENE INSTITUTE

A new lay educational organization was formed in Minneapolis last spring to promote a program of venereal disease education in Minnesota.

This organization was incorporated under the name of the Minnesota Social Hygiene Institute as the first step. Then an elaborate program, including a "five year plan" for public health education on syphilis and gonorrhea and vague future legislative activity, was drawn up and the backers were ready to go to prominent citizens for subscriptions and backing.

With the widespread educational campaign on venereal diseases sponsored by Surgeon General Thomas Parran in mind, and with the impressive program of the Minnesota State Board of Health under the able direction of Dr. A. J. Chesley before them, many prominent persons were easily persuaded to lend their names to the undertaking.

To date one public meeting of the organization has been held. This was in Mayor Leach's office on June 6 and prior to the meeting several prominent persons had already withdrawn their names from this organization.

Inadequate Medical Advice

The reason was that nowhere in this birth of a promotion had the medical advice been obtained of those persons who for many years have specialized in this field.

At no time had any of the constituted health authorities been consulted as to the need for the organization in the first place or as to its conduct and printed material.

The objects of the organization as outlined in letters seeking prominent sponsorship were stated as follows: to secure and supply reliable information regarding social diseases; to disseminate such information both to its members and the public; to aid in bringing knowledge regarding health and disease to the citizens of Minnesota.

When at length the health authorities and the physicians were informed about the matter, they pointed out to the backers and to potential subscribers who inquired, first, that there was an inadequacy of responsible medical leadership in the new organization; second, that a sound, well established and vigorous campaign for venereal disease control has already been in operation under the State Department of Health for many years; third, that the American Social Hygiene Association, an old, authorized and medically approved organization for public education is thoroughly qualified to provide any additional public education on venereal disease that may be necessary. There is, therefore, no need for any new organization. As a result, the Institute has been refused approval by the Minneapolis Civic and Commerce Association. Needless to say, the Minnesota Social Hygiene Institute does not have the endorsement of the Minnesota State Medical Association.

LAWS OF EXISTENCE

(Monthly editorial prepared by the Medical Advisory Committee.)

That man in intelligence is a higher order of animal than the so-called lower mammal easily accounts for the fact that he is not only controlled by the laws of nature but is subject to the laws of economics, and one of his chief concerns, as well as most perplexing problems, is to adapt himself to the changes in economic laws after he has recognized them.

The higher the degree of brain development, the more the individual is subject to economic laws and the more influence he should exert in their control. We as doctors have a deep-seated obligation to those among whom we work, as well as a profound responsibility to our confreres, and we should acknowledge our duty one to the other.

Any one who has attended recent medical meetings and noted the deep, sincere and thoughtful attitude of the discussions and the general concern evidenced in our economic problems, as they affect the medical profession as a whole, must return to his home with a desire to know more of these changing times as they affect not only himself, as an individual, but each person whether a practitioner of medicine or not.

The laws of nature center around the survival of the fittest. Petty bickerings, misunderstandings, misrepresentations of facts and quarrels ending in malpractice suits are but the urge of our lower animal instincts and should be beneath the dignity of the members of our Association.

To the thinking man in this world of change, the greatest sport is the Game of Life. Play it in such a way that you will increase, not destroy, your faith in humanity, or humanity's interest in the good works and progress of medicine.

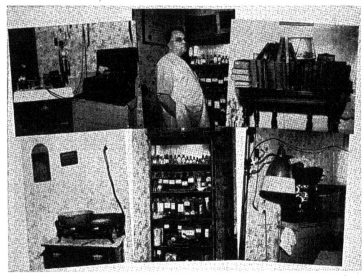

"DR." FRANK DAHLMAN AND VIEWS OF HIS EQUIPMENT

MINNESOTA STATE BOARD OF MEDICAL EXAMINERS

Minneapolis Naturopath Pays $200.00 Fine

Re: State of Minnesota vs. Frank Dahlman

"Dr." Frank Dahlman, sixty-three years of age, entered a plea of guilty on July 7, 1938, before the Honorable Levi M. Hall, Judge of the District Court, of Hennepin County, to an information charging him with practicing healing without a basic science certificate. Judge Hall ordered the defendant to pay a fine of $200.00 or serve six months in the Minneapolis Work House. Dahlman elected to pay the fine and Judge Hall ordered it deducted from his cash bail.

Dahlman was arrested on June 18, 1938, following an investigation that disclosed he was maintaining an office in his home at 2507 Emerson Ave. N., Minneapolis. Although Dahlman holds no license to practice any form of healing in the State of Minnesota, he represented himself to the public as a naturopath. On the walls in his office he had a diploma from the so-called American University, Chicago, Illinois, dated January 21, 1920, conferring upon Dahlman the degree of Doctor of Chiropractic. Dahlman stated, at the time of his arrest, that he did not attend this school and that he received the diploma by mail on the payment of $50.00. He also had a diploma from the Kellberg Institute in Chicago, in massage and hydro-therapeutics. This diploma is dated April 27, 1920. He had a certificate from the National College of Obstetrics and Midwifery in Chicago, dated June 2, 1924. In addition to a membership certificate in the Minnesota Naturopathic Association, he also had a postgraduate certificate from

the Minneapolis College of Naturopathy, dated December 27, 1928. Prior to entering the field of healing, Dahlman had worked at one of the flour mills in Minneapolis; he also had been employed as a tailor. At the time of his arrest Dahlman had, in his office, medicine bottles that would contain, when full, approximately 40,000 tablets of medicine; he had on his person the sum of $1,042.00 in cash. He stated that he had no confidence in banks, which caused him to keep such a large sum of money in his home. The investigation disclosed that many of Dahlman's patients came from Shakopee, Chaska, Carver and Norwood, Minnesota, in addition to a few from Frederic, Wisconsin.

On various occasions Dahlman had represented himself to the public as a chiropractor, chiropodist, electropath, masseur and naturopath. In 1927 he obtained a massage license from the old Minnesota Massage Board but did not renew this license in 1929 when the masseurs were placed under the Minnesota State Board of Medical Examiners. Dahlman, at one time, was chairman of the Membership Committee of the Minnesota Naturopathic Association.

Very fine coöperation was received in this case from Ed I. Goff, County Attorney, his assistant, Mr. Peter S. Neilson, and the Minneapolis Police Department.

License of Minneapolis Physician Suspended for Three Months

In the Matter of the Revocation of the License of Lewis Van Deboget, M.D.

The license of Lewis Van Deboget, M.D., Minneapolis, was suspended by the Minnesota State Board of Medical Examiners on July 16, 1938, for a period of three months. Dr. Van Deboget was charged with "immoral, dishonorable and unprofessional conduct," and particularly with the fraudulent issuance of over 4,000 prescriptions during January, February, March and April, 1938, all of the prescriptions calling for alcohol, whiskey, brandy, gin or wine.

This is the first license suspended by the Medical Board for violation of the liquor laws of this state. In the past, the Medical Board has reprimanded the physicians and has given publicity to that fact. However, there are still a number of physicians who apparently have little or no realization of why their medical licenses were issued to them. The Board hopes that it will not be necessary to discipline other physicians, and the Board also wishes to state that unless this unlawful practice stops, a permanent revocation of the medical license will be ordered.

Saint Paul Physician's License Suspended for Two Years

In the Matter of the Revocation of the License of Nels G. Mortensen, M.D.

The Minnesota State Board of Medical Examiners, at its regular meeting held on July 16, 1938, suspended, for two years, the license to practice medicine held by Nels G. Mortensen, M.D., Saint Paul. Dr. Mortensen was found guilty by the Board of "immoral, dishonorable and unprofessional conduct," and specifically with "procuring, aiding and abetting a criminal abortion."

In Memoriam

Dr. Henry A. Schneider

1875-1938

DR. H. A. SCHNEIDER, who formerly practiced at Jordan, Minnesota, but who had been making his home since the fall of 1934 with his sister, Mrs. F. A. Rosenthal, in Owatonna, died May 7, 1938, from a heart affliction.

Dr. Schneider was born July 25, 1875, in Baden, Germany, and came to this country as a boy in 1881 with his mother and sister, settling on a farm near Deerfield, Minnesota.

Graduating from Pillsbury Academy in 1896, he attended the University of Minnesota, receiving his M.D. in 1901. After a year's practice in Stillwater, he entered a partnership with Dr. James at Jordan, which continued for twenty years. Dr. Schneider continued to practice alone in Jordan for another thirteen years, when he retired and moved to Owatonna.

It had been the practice of Dr. Schneider to spend part of each winter in Florida, but this winter he spent at Laredo, Texas. He had returned to Owatonna about a month before his death.

Dr. Schneider was always very active in the Masonic Order. He leaves, besides many friends, a sister, Mrs. Fred Rosenthal of Owatonna, several nephews and nieces.

OF GENERAL INTEREST

Dr. A. J. Button, formerly of Pine River, has opened an office at Walker.

* * *

Dr. Willard Akins of Eveleth was recently married to Miss Lila Koivisto.

* * *

Dr. A. R. Ellingson of Detroit Lakes has been appointed county coroner.

* * *

Dr. Earl Ellis of Elgin was recently married to Miss Marvel Magner of Shafer.

* * *

Dr. George J. Halladay has opened an office at Brainerd for the practice of medicine.

* * *

Dr. M. P. Virnig, of Wells, was married on June 20 to Miss Genevieve Kelly of Minneapolis.

* * *

Dr. L. N. Casmey, formerly at Moorhead, has located in Crookston for the practice of medicine.

* * *

Dr. Clifford Wadd of Waseca has become associated with Dr. O. J. Swenson in the practice of medicine.

* * *

Dr. S. J. Raltz, formerly of Racine, Wisconsin, has become associated with Dr. F. T. Brigham of Watkins.

* * *

Dr. Arthur Ecker of Rochester was awarded an M.S. degree in neurology from the University of Minnesota in July.

* * *

Dr. A. A. Giroux, formerly of Duluth, has been appointed Assistant Physician at the new Moose Lake State Hospital.

* * *

Dr. John E. Boysen, son of Dr. Peter Boysen, has opened an office in Pelican Rapids, his home town, for the practice of medicine.

* * *

Dr. Marie K. Bepko has opened offices in Cloquet for the practice of medicine. She is associated with her husband, Dr. R. H. Puumala.

* * *

Dr. Carl Coombs, a graduate of the University of Minnesota, has recently become the assistant of Dr. R. C. Radabaugh at Hastings.

* * *

Dr. D. Howard Rolig, formerly at the Ancker Hospital, Saint Paul, has taken over the practice of Dr. L. J. Hoyer at Howard Lake.

* * *

Dr. Carl H. Mattson, formerly of the Olson Clinic, Duluth, has returned to Saint Paul, with offices at 411 Lowry Medical Arts Building.

Dr. Baldwin Borreson, Superintendent of Oakland Park Sanatorium at Thief River Falls, was recently elected president of the Rotary Club.

* * *

Dr. G. H. Adkins, formerly of Grygla, has purchased the St. Matthew Hospital at Pine River, which was formerly operated by Dr. A. J. Button.

* * *

Dr. Byron Cochran of Saint Paul has joined the staff at the Rood Hospital at Coleraine. Dr. Cochran was formerly at the Miller Hospital in Saint Paul.

* * *

Dr. A. A. Schmitz, who has just completed an internship at the Minneapolis General Hospital, is now associated with Dr. E. G. Nethercott of Pine City.

* * *

Dr. V. D. Thysell of Hawley and Miss Nanette Abt of Minneapolis, were married in June. After an eastern trip, Dr. and Mrs. Thysell are now at home in Hawley.

* * *

Dr. Frank A. Grawn of Northome, formerly of Duluth, has retired after 42 years of practice and left for Traverse City, Michigan, where he will establish the family home.

* * *

Dr. H. J. Kurtin, formerly of Cudahy, Wisconsin, has become associated with Dr. S. T. Kucera of Lonsdale. Dr. Kurtin will also assist Dr. Kucera in the office which Dr. Kucera has opened at New Market.

* * *

Dr. and Mrs. S. Z. Kerlan have gone to California, where they expect to make their home. Dr. Kerlan, who has practiced at Aitkin, is retiring from active practice. Dr. R. A. Murray of Duluth has taken over the practice.

* * *

The Minnesota Academy of Medicine held a stag party at the country home, Rippleside, of Dr. Archa Wilcox, on July 12. Some forty members enjoyed the hospitality of their host and hostess, some indulging in cards, and all enjoying to the utmost the informal get-together.

* * *

Dr. Philip Rains Beckjord of Duluth, who was recently married to Miss Margaret McGilvray, also of Duluth, has located in Willmar for the practice of medicine. He is associated with the Willmar Clinic. Dr. Beckjord is a grandson of the late Dr. John M. Rains, a pioneer Willmar physician.

* * *

Dr. F. M. Feldman of Mankato, who has been director of the rural health district in that vicinity, will be transferred, September 1, to Rochester to organize a new district health unit there. The Rochester unit will be the third district established in Minnesota under the State Department of Health.

* * *

In our July number the statement was made that Dr. L. J. Leonard of Minneapolis is the only individual in

the Northwest licensed to practice both law and medicine. Our attention has been called to the fact that another Minneapolis physician, Dr. W. K. Foster, has also been admitted to the bar. Are there any others?

* * *

Dr. and Mrs. C. G. Oeljen of Waseca sailed July 27 on the Europa for Vienna, where Dr. Oeljen expects to take a course in eye, ear, nose and throat work. Dr. Clifford Wadd, who recently became associated with Dr. O. J. Swenson of Waseca, will have charge of Dr. Oeljen's practice during the six months he will be away.

* * *

The Board of Regents of the University of Minnesota has accepted gifts from the Trustees of the Stevens Avenue Home of Minneapolis and the Commonwealth Fund of New York for the establishment and maintenance over a five-year period of a Children's Psychiatric Clinic. This Clinic will be affiliated jointly with the Department of Pediatrics and the Department of Psychiatry. Its primary purpose is to integrate the teaching of preventive psychiatry with pediatrics for senior medical students and for graduate students registered in Psychiatry and Pediatrics.

* * *

The Post Graduate Medical Institute's courses which have been offered to practicing physicians during the past two years in connection with the Center for Continuation Study, at the University of Minnesota, have evoked such enthusiastic responses on the part of physicians and have seemed to meet such a definite need that the Commonwealth Fund of New York is providing a subsidy for the further development of this program over the next five years. This will make possible a study of the need for and the effectiveness of the courses offered, and experimentation with various types of instruction. Dr. William A. O'Brien has been transferred from his other duties to the Directorship of Post Graduate Medical Education on a full-time basis.

* * *

Dr. and Mrs. A. E. Henslin, Le Roy, Minnesota, were given a testimonial dinner on June 23 at the Odd Fellows Hall in recognition of the doctor and his forty-seven years of professional service rendered the community. Mr. J. A. Schneider, acting as toastmaster, eulogized the guest of honor as a doctor and friend, and Mr. Frank Young spoke in behalf of the older generation who had known Dr. Henslin since he first came to Le Roy. Other speakers recalled the activities of the doctor as one of the organizers of the First National Bank of Le Roy, as a founder of the local telephone company, as a former mayor of Le Roy, and as a member of the school board. Others who took part in the program were Dr. M. P. Morse of Le Roy, and Dr. J. J. Morrow of Austin, who spoke of the medical progress achieved during the years Dr. Henslin had practiced in Le Roy. Most satisfying must have been the tributes paid Dr. Henslin as a fine type of general practitioner.

◆ REPORTS and ANNOUNCEMENTS ◆

MEDICAL BROADCAST FOR AUGUST

The Minnesota State Medical Association Morning Health Service

The Minnesota State Medical Association broadcasts weekly at 9:45 o'clock every Saturday morning over Station WCCO, Minneapolis and Saint Paul (810 kilocycles or 370.2 meters).

Speaker: William A. O'Brien, M.D., Associate Professor of Pathology and Preventive Medicine, Medical School, University of Minnesota. The program for the month will be as follows:

August 6—Trichinosis
13—Growth and Illness
20—Dyspepsia
27—Dental Disease.

AMERICAN ASSOCIATION FOR THE STUDY OF GOITER

The annual meeting of the Association will be held in Washington, D. C., September 12-14, in conjunction with the Third International Goiter Conference. Members of the profession are cordially invited to attend. Dr. W. Blair Mosser, Kane, Pa., is the secretary of the organization.

AMERICAN CONGRESS OF PHYSICAL THERAPY

The 17th annual scientific and clinical session of the American Congress of Physical Therapy will be held coöperatively with the 2nd annual convention of the American Occupational Therapy Association, September 12, 13, 14, and 15, 1938, at the Palmer House, Chicago. Preceding these sessions, the Congress will conduct an intensive instruction seminar in physical therapy for physicians and technicians—September 7, 8, 9, and 10.

The convention proper will have numerous special program features, a variety of papers and addresses, clinical conferences, round table talks, and extensive scientific and technical exhibits.

The instruction seminar should prove of unusual interest to everyone interested in the fundamentals and in the newer advances in physical therapy. The faculty will be comprised of experienced teachers and clinicians; every subject in the physical therapy field will be covered. Information concerning the convention and the instruction seminar may be obtained by addressing: The American Congress of Physical Therapy, 30 North Michigan Avenue, Chicago.

INTER-STATE POSTGRADUATE MEDICAL ASSOCIATION

The Twenty-third International Assembly of the Association will be held in the public auditorium of

Philadelphia, October 31, November 1-4, 1938. The program will include some eighty prominent teachers and clinicians and the facilities of this large center of population will provide an abundance of clinical material. Pre- and post-assembly clinics will be held at the local hospitals on the Saturday before and that following the meeting.

Hotel reservations should be made in advance through Mr. Thomas E. Willis, Chamber of Commerce Building, 12th and Walnut Streets, Philadelphia. All members of state and provincial societies are cordially invited to attend the meeting.

Officers this year are: Dr. Elliott P. Joslin, Boston, president; Dr. George W. Crile, Cleveland, chairman of program committee; Dr. William B. Peck, Freeport, Illinois, managing director.

NORTHERN MINNESOTA MEDICAL ASSOCIATION

The annual meeting of the Northern Minnesota Medical Association will be held in Crookston on August 29 and 30.

Dr. Richard Bardon of Duluth is chairman of the program committee. A feature of this year's program will be a surgical clinic conducted by Dr. Arthur A. Zierold of Minneapolis, and a medical clinic conducted by Dr. Moses Barron of Minneapolis. Dr. E. M. Hammes of Saint Paul will speak on the newer aspects of neurology and psychiatry. Dr. E. L. Tuohy of Duluth will speak on the present status of vitamin and hormone therapy. The Mayo Clinic will be represented. Fractures, obstetrics and traumatic surgery and medical economics will be presented by men prominent in their respective fields. A complete program is being mailed to members of the profession.

The local committees have made plans for an enjoyable visit. The ladies will be entertained, golf will be played and the annual banquet will include an address by the president-elect of the State Medical Association, Dr. George A. Earl of Saint Paul.

Present officers of the Association are Dr. J. F. Norman, Crookston, president; Dr. O. W. Parker, Ely, vice president; and Dr. Clarence Jacobson, Chisholm, secretary-treasurer.

WABASHA COUNTY SOCIETY

Dr. A. J. Chesley, secretary and executive officer of the Minnesota Department of Health; Dr. R. N. Barr, epidemiologist and director of Rural Health Units; Dr. Gaylord Anderson, professor of Medicine and Public Health at the University of Minnesota; Dr. Floyd M. Feldman, district health officer for District No. 2, and Dr. Vern Irwin, superintendent of Dental Health Education, Division of Child Hygiene, State Department of Health, addressed a special meeting of the

(Continued on Page 600)

HEMANGIOMA AND ITS TREATMENT

WILLIAM PEYTON, M.D.

Hemangioma is rather a common lesion when considered in all of its forms, and occurs in practically every part of the body. It is unexpectedly encountered at times at operations for supposedly benign tumors. It may be easily diagnosed, or it may be very difficult to diagnose. The treatment of hemangioma will always have to be varied to suit the form and location of the lesion, but at the present time, certainly, there is no uniformity of opinion concerning the treatment of hemangioma.

Hemangiomas are classified as cavernous or capillary. The capillary type appears chiefly in the form of the port-wine stain and the hypertrophic form or the strawberry type. The cavernous type with which we are primarily concerned, in its typical form, resembles the corpora cavernosa of the penis, that is, there are large venous spaces lined with endothelium separated by connective tissue septa. These connective tissue septa are of variable thickness and the venous spaces are of variable size. It also occurs in mixed form; especially does it occur with lymphangioma and it may also occur in association with lipoma or with neurofibroma.

It is obvious that the tumor with large blood spaces and little connective tissue stroma will be most compressible and that the one with small spaces and much connective tissue or the mixed tumors will be relatively noncompressible. This is of practical importance in selecting a form of therapy to fit the individual tumor.

Cavernous hemangioma is most common in the skin and subcutaneous tissues and it is usually present at birth. Some 83 per cent are recorded as being present at birth, and another 13 per cent occur in the first three weeks of life. Usually, the diagnosis is easily made from the compressibility and from the discoloration of the skin. Cavernous hemangioma of the mucous membranes occurs most frequently about the oral cavity, where, as a rule, it is rather easily diagnosed. It occurs more rarely in the gastro-intestinal tract and in this location it is very difficult to diagnose. There have now been some forty-four cases reported and most of them have not been diagnosed before operation. The story is usually that the child from birth has had repeated gastro-intestinal hemorrhages and as a rule no other signs. Sometimes the diagnosis can be made from the history and findings. A polypoid type occurs that may give symptoms of obstruction and this type of lesion may be demonstrated on x-ray examination. X-ray may also show phleboliths within the lesion that is not polypoid in type. If the hemangioma is in the lower part of the bowel it can be visualized with the proctoscope and so diagnosed.

We have had only one experience with cavernous hemangioma of the intestinal tract and this was in a boy about fifteen years of age who had had no symptoms from birth except that he had always been weak and tired more easily than other children of his age, until some eighteen months before he entered the hospital, when he developed measles. At that time he became very pale, his hemoglobin dropped to 15 per cent and red blood cells to 900,000. Just before he entered the hospital he had a sudden collapse. All examinations, including gastro-intestinal examinations, were negative, and he was explored with the diagnosis of a Meckel's diverticulum with an ulcer at the base. At the exploration an hemangioma was found involving all of the jejunum and possibly some of the ileum.

A rather uncommon form of hemangioma is so-called sinus-pericranii, which is a hemangioma of the pericranium communicating through one or more abnormal openings with the dural sinuses. This lesion was described by Percival Pott in 1760. It was again described by Pellatan in 1810. Strohmeyer, in 1850, first called it sinus pericranii and since that time it has been known as sinus pericranii of Strohmeyer. It is a soft, fluctuant tumor mass overlying one or other of the cranial sinuses. It is compressible and the characteristic thing about it is that when some maneuver is carried out which increases the intracranial venous pressure this tumor mass becomes distended. Not infrequently, therefore, the diagnosis of meningocele is made. The diagnosis should be readily made. X-ray examination will frequently show phleboliths and it shows the abnormal openings in the skull, when aspirated blood is obtained.

Up to the present time, some eighty-five cases of sinus pericranii have been described in the literature. They may be either congenital or traumatic.

Hemangioma of muscle is a more common form of cavernous hemangioma. It may be either circumscribed or diffuse, involving other tissues, especially subcutaneous tissues, tendons and joints. In an experience with five cases that we have had, two involved the subcutaneous tissues, and probably also tendon, and two involved the knee joint. These hemangiomas of muscle have all, in our experience, occurred below thirty years of age. In the literature, 95 per cent have occurred below thirty years of age, and 42 per cent of the total group of 270, that have been reported, have occurred in the thigh. The symptoms resulting from these tumors are weakness, especially a tendency to tire easily, pain, and later functional impairment and even contracture deformities may develop. All of these symptoms have occurred in one or other of the patients that we have observed. Curiously enough, this diagnosis is rarely made before operation, only 12 per cent of the cases reported having been so diagnosed.

The treatment of hemangioma has been varied. Many of the methods tried have been discarded, some because they were unsuitable for the type of lesion and others because they were unsound in principle. However, some successes have been reported with almost all methods. Even in most ancient times vascular tumors including hemangiomas were cauterized or excised. Other types of therapy that have been introduced in more ancient times (about 1835) were the introduction of hot needles; and of setons with threads. These methods were effective, in all probability, because they produced scar tissue. About 1845, the injecting of sclerosing solutions in the treatment of hemangioma was introduced or at least popularized by Pravez. The treatment was not limited to hemangiomas since no distinction at that time was made between hemangioma, aneurysm and arterio-venous aneurysm. All of these lesions were treated by the injection of ferric chloride solution, a caustic. Very serious complications and deaths occurred as a result of this treatment and it apparently fell into disregard after several years of popularity. Vaccination was introduced in the treatment of hemangiomas about this time and it was revived by Friedjung in 1933. It does destroy some small superficial hemangiomatas by scar tissue formation. The injection of hot water was introduced by Wyatt in 1902 and has been used quite extensively since that time. Alcohol injections were introduced in more recent times. Gallant, in 1903, reported sixty-seven cases so treated, and in general he considered the results satisfactory. At the present time, this method is used at the General Hospital under the supervision of Dr. S. E. Sweitzer with very satisfactory results in properly selected cases. Galvanocautery, introduced by Middledorff in 1854, was soon used for the treatment of hemangioma and more recently high frequency current has been used. Figi, in 1936, considered high frequency current the preferable method of treatment for cavernous hemangioma about the face. Irradiation, of course, has been introduced in rather recent times and is satisfactory in hemangioma of the skin of children.

Excision, of course, has been utilized throughout this period and is still the favorite method of many. It is a satisfactory type of treatment in properly selected lesions, that is, well circumscribed lesions, where the resulting scar will not be disfiguring.

The injection of sclerosing solutions was revived in the treatment of hemangioma by Babcock in 1917 when he injected quinine hydrochloride and urethane. Dowling, in 1929, reported five cases treated by the injection of sclerosing solution and it is now frequently referred to as the treatment of Dowling. That the injection of sclerosing solutions is still not an accepted form of treatment by many, is evident in the literature. It is much more frequently mentioned than recommended in the treatment of hemangioma.

At the University Hospital, we began the injection of sclerosing solutions in properly selected cases in April, 1929. Since that time, I have found the records of 132 patients that have been treated by x-ray therapy, 109 of which were treated by superficial therapy, and in the traced cases (fourteen not traced), 51 per cent had excellent or good results. Twenty-three were treated by high voltage therapy and in the traced cases

(three not traced) 48 per cent had excellent or good results. The records of thirty-three cases treated by the injection of sclerosing solution have been reviewed and of the traced cases 82 per cent obtained an excellent or good result. Five cases were either not traced or are still under treatment so that the end-result cannot be determined.

In mucous membranes we have treated two cases involving the tongue, both with very satisfactory results. We have had one case of sinus pericranii which was treated with the injection of sclerosing solution with a very excellent result. It might be objected that there is danger of embolism when you inject and coagulate blood spaces which directly communicate with the dural sinuses. This may be a legitimate criticism if the lesion overlies one of the more important sinuses, but in our case the sinus pericranii was over the forehead and if thrombosis had extended into the anterior part of the sagittal sinus it probably would not have produced any serious trouble. It would seem that this fear of extensive thrombosis following injection of hemangioma is much over-rated. The same objection has been raised to cauterization of hemangioma about the face but apparently no embolism has ever occurred as a result of this, at least none have been reported. In all of the injections which we have now made, perhaps 300 or 400 individual injections, I have never seen a case of extending thrombosis as a result. It is not like injecting varicose veins where you may have an extension of the thrombosis. It seems to me the reason for this is that the spaces are large and have small communications with each other. At the present time, we are having some wax reconstructions made to determine this question. Our experience with the injection treatment of hemangioma of the muscle is not great and the results have not been excellent but they have been so promising that we feel it is well worth continuing.

The technic is very simple. If the hemangioma is large, one plunges the needle into or through the blood-filled tumor and then on withdrawing the needle with suction applied one gets blood when the point of the needle is within a blood space. The spaces are then emptied if possible by elevation or pressure and the solution injected. Sodium morrhuate in amounts up to 3 c.c. is the solution used. A pressure dressing is applied. We have used this treatment both with and without pressure and do get thrombosis without pressure but the patient complains of more pain when a pressure dressing is not applied. There is a tendency to over-distention of the hemangioma immediately after the injection is made. This reaction, following some of the early injections, was rather alarming. This is now avoided by injecting smaller amounts of solution and the application of a pressure dressing. (Slides were shown.)

Discussion

DR. ORWOOD J. CAMPBELL: While my own experience with hemangiomata has not been large, I have followed with considerable interest, the work which Dr. Peyton has been doing with such cases at the University Dispensary. When he first told me what he was at-

591

tempting I thought the method was quite irrational, but I was thinking of hemangiomata as being neoplastic in nature.

The evidence, however, is strongly in favor of the view that these tumors are not neoplastic in nature but represent a persistence of an embryonic form of circulation into later life. Viewed in this light, the injection with sclerosing agents is an entirely reasonable procedure.

It is probable that the same principles hold here as in the injection of varicose veins. An adequate concentration of the sclerosing agent must be maintained in contact with the vessel intima for a sufficient period to produce damage.

Most hemangiomata lend themselves well to these conditions. Riebert has shown that the connections between hemangiomata and the normal circulation are not very plentiful and the blood velocity is not great. Dr. Peyton has pointed out how pressure applied to a hemangioma assists in accomplishing obliteration of venous spaces.

I would expect that the more generous the connections between hemangiomata and the normal circulation and the greater the blood flow through the tumor, the greater will be the difficulty in obtaining obliteration.

I want to congratulate Dr. Peyton for interesting himself in a group of cases which heretofore have been treated in rather desultory fashion and for encouraging us in the use of a method so simple and so safe.

DR. CARL WALDRON (by invitation): I haven't had very much experience with hemangiomata from the standpoint of their initial treatment, except that I have followed with great interest many of the patients that Dr. Peyton showed on the slides, in whom the face was involved. I think it is pretty well agreed that in the infants and very young children x-ray or radium therapy is probably the procedure of choice. In older individuals with involvement of the skin of the face and the lips, or of the mucous membrane of the mouth, Dr. Peyton's results are certainly much superior to many that I have seen in other parts of the country, and I see them at times at clinical meetings. I know that this method is very much simpler and more satisfactory than the repeated use of diathermy in the coagulation form even with special protected electrodes, and the patients seem to be much more comfortable and more happy about their treatment.

Quite a number of these cases, of course, have a resultant scarring or remains of connective tissue that calls for plastic surgery at a later date. In those that I have followed I feel that many times the plastic surgery is a very minor procedure. It can readily be undertaken to bring the result up from 90 per cent to the 100 per cent from a cosmetic standpoint. Many of them require the removal of but a little bit of mucous membrane to make, for instance, the vermillion border of the lip symmetrical with that of the other side.

As for the other group, the capillary forms, it is unfortunate that many of them are treated by all sorts of methods that are not satisfactory. I think it is pretty well conceded that excision with plastic restoration is the method of choice in these cases where the cosmetic appearance is such that it would interfere with the patient's happiness and ability to get along with associates and perhaps, later on, the ability to gain a satisfactory livelihood and desirable occupation. These patients are treated by different methods, depending largely upon the part of the face involved. Certain of them near the eye can be treated best by the removal of the entire lesion and the substitution of perhaps a full thickness graft, or occasionally a flap may be used. The question of matching the skin is a problem to the plastic surgeon but, after all, any kind of satisfactory skin is usually much better than the lesion. If the

lesion, however, is away from the eye where there will not be so much danger of distortion, the men who are doing a great deal of plastic surgery now feel that fractional removal and stretching of the neighboring skin adjoining the lesion over a period of perhaps three, four or five years, may make a better looking ultimate result than a patch of skin from a distant part, be it brought there as a full thickness graft or as a pedicle flap.

I had occasion to see several very fine cases of this type of treatment at a recent meeting our plastic surgery group had in Texas. The width of the lesions may amount to two and one-half to three inches and more, yet, by fractional removal and resuturing at intervals of four, five or six months, in a period of two or three years it is possible to advance the skin from the neck the entire distance and have a good matching skin with a single scar line that is not at all disfiguring. This method is very painstaking; it demands a lot of coöperation on the part of the patient, a lot of massage, a lot of stretching of the skin, the use of odds and ends of elastic apparatus in connection with adhesive in order to stretch out skin, but finally the eventual result is usually more satisfactory than skin flaps brought to the area from the chest or further down from the lateral abdominal wall or a full thickness graft from the leg or the arm.

The plastic problem in some of these cases, of course, is very much complicated by the previous treatment, the type of caustic solutions that may have been used, carbon dioxide snow or the use of x-ray and radium, et cetera, but with care, usually, it can be taken care of nicely.

The case that Dr. Peyton showed of the rather massive hypertrophic type of capillary hemangioma of the face, of course, was quite a plastic problem. In a case of that extent, one has to resort to quite a massive flap from the chest or from the lateral wall of the chest and abdomen such as the thoracic-epigastric type. The forehead flap, of course, when available, is very fine. It matches well, but, on the other hand, in America the men and women do not want their forehead skin used. In Europe it is different, the surgeons use them almost everywhere they can because they feel they can tell the ladies to wear the hair down to the eyebrow level and in the men the forehead scar and the skin graft may not be at all prominent. On this side of the water, the women wear their hair way up high and they want to show their foreheads and we can't talk them into using a forehead flap even though it will match the skin texture or the color of the nose or face better than almost any other skin.

The skin from other parts of the body, of course, sometimes makes a very satisfactory match, after a period of two or three years have elapsed, but ordinarily it takes that length of time. At other times, it doesn't match; at least, a part of the area doesn't match. It may sunburn quite differently from the rest of the skin, but now we have plenty of aids in a cosmetic way in the type of powders and creams that can be used, so that variations in color really can be disguised pretty satisfactorily.

I want to again thank you for asking me to discuss this paper and I want to compliment Dr. Peyton on the simplification of the problem of many of these cases that he has been able to offer us by his careful and cautious handling of the cases he has had under his care. Thank you.

DR. WILLARD WHITE: Dr. Peyton has mentioned that these lesions may occur in any of the tissues. I wish to call attention to the fact that similar and also allied lesions may occur in bone. Hemangiomata are not so very rare in bone. A condition sometimes confused with hemangioma is hemangio-endothelioma. I recently saw an autopsy on a patient at the General Hospital in Minneapolis where this lesion occurred in the body of one of the vertebræ and had extended by pressure so that the cord was completely destroyed. It had also extended outward into the thoracic cavity and made a very large lesion. In the discussion of this case at the General Hospital it was, brought out that hemangio-endotheliomata in bone is very rare.

DR. KENNETH BULKLEY: Nothing has been said about hemorrhage in the treatment of these hemangio-mata, particularly, of course, during the operative treatment. I would like to say a word in regard to those that occur in the extremities. I would also like to ask Dr. Peyton the strength of his sodium morrhuate, and also the relation, if any, of these to trauma. I had a man, just under thirty years old, who had done hard labor all of his life and who, in hitting the end of a screw driver, developed pain in his thenar eminence. Within twenty-four hours he developed a mass. When I saw him the thenar eminence was fully twice the size of the thenar eminence on the other hand. I operated on him with the diagnosis of lipoma. It turned out to be a hemangioma involving the muscles of the thenar eminence. I did the operation, of course, using a tourniquet. It was imposible, at first, to control hemorrhage. I dissected out practically the entire thenar eminence, tying off everything I could see and we controlled his hemorrhage, finally, only by packing. I left the packing in four days, gave him an anesthetic and attempted to take the packing out with just as much hemorrhage as I had originally. I finally left the packing in three weeks before I could take it out without hemorrhage. I am wondering if there is any definite established relationship between trauma and these hemangiomata.

DR. HARVEY NELSON: I would like to ask Dr. Peyton what his recommendations are in some of these smaller capillary types of hemangiomas. I have had occasion to refer some of them to the x-ray men and they advised using carbon dioxide snow rather than x-ray, saying that the x-ray doesn't affect them very much.

DR. CYRUS HANSON (by invitation): The small hemangiomata in children do respond in a very large percentage of cases, very nicely. As the patient gets older we do not get the results with the x-ray and radium that we do in the younger people because of the tissue becoming more adult and not being as sensitive as it is at first and the blood spaces have become larger. We know, of course, that in the lymphatic type of hemangioma where the vessels are largely lymphatic in character rather than blood vessels, the response is very poor to x-ray therapy.

DR. WILLIAM T. PEYTON (closing): As to the origin of hemangiomata, I think what Dr. Campbell said about their being a congenital anomaly is entirely true, although there is still considerable discussion in the literature, at least some write as though they still considered them a new growth. They are probably an anomalous development of the capillary beds that occurs early in the embryo. The extension which occurs later is either enlargement of individual spaces or opening up a new bed.

Perhaps this would be the best place to take up the question that Dr. Bulkley asked about trauma. I think that most vascular lesions which occur following trauma are not hemangiomata but are arterio-venous aneurysms, and yet it seems that occasionally a hemangioma does occur following trauma. Sinus pericranii is said to sometimes appear following trauma. It is hard to explain these unless one admits that there are abnormal vascular spaces present that are broken into and then fill, or some such explanation. I think in general that vascular lesions which follow trauma are arterio-venous. However, Dr. Bulkley's case may have been a traumatic hemangioma and I presume it was from what he has said.

This leads to the question as to how one distinguishes between arterio-venous aneurysms and hemangioma. Arterio-venous aneurysm has increased head and often growth changes due to increased circulation to the part. These hemangiomata are of normal temperature, may even be colder than normal because their circulation is not increased. Growth changes due to hemangioma, if they do occur, should result in a decrease in growth or development in the part affected. The bones of the forearm in one of our cases were demonstrated by x-ray to be smaller than normal. The most important symptoms, of course, are bruit, thrill, and pulsating veins. If any of these signs are present, it is surely an arterio-venous aneurysm. If in doubt, one can draw blood from the vein that is returning blood from the involved part and one gets an increased oxygen content in this venous blood if an arterio-venous aneurysm exists. In hemangioma the venous blood oxygen content will be normal.

Dr. Campbell mentioned the extension of the thrombosis. Our greatest difficulty in injection treatment is that we cannot get extensive thrombosis. The thrombosis is always localized and that is the reason one has to make so many injections to destroy a large lesion. Recently, I have been trying to inject two different places at one sitting, by putting the needle way through, getting one place where I can draw blood back through the needle, inject, and then draw back farther and get into another blood space.

This brings up the question asked about how you get these blood spaces. It is very easy to get into them if one is dealing with a cavernous hemangioma. All you have to do is plunge the needle in, withdrawing it until one gets blood. In a vein, on the other hand, you have to have some technic, but in this all you do is to plunge the needle through. If the spaces are very small, of the capillary forms, then it is difficult or impossible. We have not had any success with an injection that was not made within venous spaces. We have tried injecting some of the capillary type that were mentioned by Dr. Nelson, and made some interstitial injections but all we got were sloughs, not cures, and I have very little to offer in the treatment of the capillary type except x-ray therapy.

Hemangioma of the vertebræ have been described by Makrycostas[3] and by Bailey and Bucy.[1] They find that it is a more frequent lesion than is generally appreciated (on routine postmortem examination, 12 per cent). They are usually, however, small and do not give symptoms unless they grow back into the cord.

Hemangio-endothelioma which was mentioned is an entirely different lesion. It is a neoplastic lesion and most of them are radio-sensitive.

Hemorrhage is the principal cause of death in cavernous hemangioma. Bowers[2] recently reported one in the lung that caused death by hemorrhage. Fatal hemorrhages occur in the intestinal tract and even the superficial ones may rupure, and if the patient does not know how to stop it, it may cause death.

Dr. Bulkley asked about the percentage of sodium morrhuate. We use 7 per cent.

Carbon dioxide snow was introduced by Pusey in 1907 and it is satisfactory in the destruction of the superficial lesions like the capillary ones that Dr. Nelson mentioned, except that it leaves a white scar. I think, under certain circumstances, the use of carbon dioxide snow is justifiable but I do not use it. All I know about it is what I read and see following its use by others.

References

1. Bailey, P., and Bucy, P.: Cavernous hemangioma of the vertebrae. Jour. Am. Med. Assn., 92:1748, 1929.
2. Bowers, W.: Rupture of visceral hemangioma as cause of death. Nebraska State Med. Jour., 21:35, 1936.
3. Makrycostas, K.: Ueber die praktish klinische Bedeutung des Wirbelangioms. Arch. f. Klin. Chir., 155:663, 1929.

LOW BACK PAIN*

R. E. Hultkrans, M.D.

For the purpose of discussion, this paper has been divided into two parts: acute back pain and chronic back pain. In view of the recent and numerous explanations of chronic ·and intractable back pain, noted in the literature of the past year or two, this particular paper will be limited largely to the consideration of acute back pain. Numerous attempts have been made to classify symptoms concerning the lower back. "Low Back Pain and Associated Conditions" is ·the name given to no less than several thousand articles between 1929 and 1938.[18] Many of these articles attempt some sort of a classification of back symptoms and advise some sort of treatment or other. This writer was surprised to find that very few of these articles went into certain fundamental considerations such as anatomy, physiology, and definitions of terms. One also notes a definite lack on the part of most authors to classify low back pain into an acute or chronic condition, a differentiation which I feel is very important.

Just what is low back pain? Magnuson[19] presents an interesting discussion of backache as follows: "From time immemorial we have been talking about backache as something to treat instead of regarding it only a symptom, sometimes only a very small portion of a complete picture which can be ascertained only by the history and in the physical examination. It is true that backache is a very frequent symptom and undoubtedly a very irritating one. We know that in acute infectious diseases, backache is one of the symptoms of which the patient complains most. Whereas, from the standpoint of the doctor, where the disease is fully developed, it is not of major importance because he knows that the backache will clear up when the condition causing it has been removed. But where there is no well developed disease to account for the complaint, the fact that this is only part of the picture may escape attention entirely."

His discussion then continues with the indication that fully 80 per cent of people with chronic pain in the back are over forty. He discusses factors of posture and weight, occupation, and the fact that perhaps physical makeup seems to give little clue as to the cause. No definite conclusions are drawn in this particular paper by Magnuson, as in most other papers, and we find that both the acute and chronic symptoms are discussed together.

These introductory remarks have been made particularly with the idea of establishing the fact that low back pain, after all, is a symptom and of itself not a pathological entity. So numerous are the classifications of low back pain as noted by this author in the review of the literature that any attempt to present them here would be quite futile and would add to the confusion which already exists concerning this subject.

Regardless of the questions concerned in acute or chronic low back pain, certain fundamental considerations are necessary before any definite conclusions can be drawn. First, let us consider some of the general anatomical structures involved, along with a discussion of certain terms commonly used. In the hope of simplifying a conception of the muscle structure in the back,[3] we may say that there is a large group made up principally of the sacrospinalis, or more commonly called the erector spinæ group, lying on each side of the spinous processes and attaching at various levels all the way up the spine. Next, we have the flat group of muscles consisting of quadratus lumborum, serratus posterior, along with the termination of the abdominal muscles which come way around into the back. In the external layer we have the trapezius in the dorsal and upper lumbar regions, and the latissimus dorsi with its lumbo-dorsal fascia making its principal attachment at its lower margin. The lumbo-dorsal fascia is somewhat quadrangular in shape and has its principal tendon insertion down over the sacrum. Both gluteal muscles exert their influence on the back through the lumbo-dorsal fascia. There are numerous smaller· intrinsic muscles which may be factors in the development of back pain, but their detailed review does not appear necessary at this time. The structure and physiology of the intervertebral disc was very carefully worked out by Schmorl.[5] Space does not permit a more detailed discussion of the other structures involved. The spinal canal, of course, encloses the spinal cord and the intervertebral foramen permits exit of the spinal nerve on either side. The ligamentum flavum covers the cord posteriorly along with the laminæ and the interspinal ligament. Again, space does not permit a detailed description of the anatomy concerning the ligaments in the lower back, particularly the sacro-iliac, ilio-lumbar, and lumbo-sacral ligaments, but reference to any standard text in anatomy will give a full review of these structures.

In discussing low back pain, it seems that certain fundamental terms must be considered. A description of common terms follows:

Muscle Spasm: Muscle spasm really means an increase in muscle tone. We must consider first then muscle tone. Muscle tone normally consists of a certain state of contraction of skeletal muscles. From embryology, we learn that there is a segmental development of the musculature with a corresponding segmental division of the nervous system. The nervous system has both the somatic and splanchnic divisions all located to each corresponding segment.[14] Normal muscle tone exists as the result of proprioceptive stimuli acting upon a spinal reflex. If the path of the reflex is interrupted, a loss of tone follows. Stimulation of this reflex produces an increase in tone or ·muscle spasm Zierold[17] points out in his article on ·"Morphine as Diagnostic Agent," that if the stimuli affecting the spinal reflex overwhelm the reflex, then the excessive stimuli are carried upward along the spinal thalam tracts to the cortical centers, spreading to the sensorium. From here, conscious, purposeful, voluntary contractions of a protective nature occur and many time are falsely interpreted as true muscle spasm. Kunt

*Inaugural Thesis

written following the White House Conference on child health, and protection, in which the question of body mechanics and posture is gone into very thoroughly. This book is a result of the work of a large group of consultants and very worthy of review. It does not definitely establish itself as the final authority on posture, but at least makes an attempt to begin with a definite working standard.

In considering posture, we find that the center of gravity of the body is located as low as the first and second lumbar vertebra at the beginning of the lumbar curve.[7] It becomes quite evident that with the center of gravity located at this point the muscles below this area attaching to the sacrum have a tremendous leverage to overcome.

The following classification seems logical as far as acute low back pain is concerned.

Acute Back Pain, resulting from (1) trauma; (2) infection (including toxemias); (3) posture; (4) congenital defects.

Under trauma, we do not wish to include any of the injuries which affect the bony structures of the back. We wish to include only sprains, strains, contusions, overstretching of the muscle groups or individual fibers, minute tearing of tendons, ligaments, and muscle fibers, small hemorrhages and so forth.

Under infectious conditions, one has but to refer to the article on "Myofascitis" of Albee[1] in which this particular question is most ably handled except that no mention of the pathology is made. I doubt if one could find a better definition of lumbago than that given by Osler[12] in his first text book published in 1892. He says that lumbago is a form of muscular rheumatism limited to the lumbar region of the back.

Sciatic neuritis is not to be confused with sciatica, the former representing a typical neuritis, localized to the sciatic nerve, whereas a sciatica simply means pain along the course of the sciatic nerve and may be due to other causes than inflammation.

Arthritis is always a factor which must be contended with in cases of the infectious type. Numerous forms of arthritis are described, but probably the most commonly used names are osteoarthritis, atrophic arthritis, acute articular arthritis. Here, again, time does not permit an extensive discussion of a term about which volumes have been written.

Posture as a cause of back pain is open to a wide difference of opinion. The term is so commonly used, however, in practically all articles that it can scarcely be eliminated here. It is interesting to note that the survey on posture indicated that most students fall into a class of C or D, and yet after taking postural exercises over a period of two or three or four years, still show no improvement.

The last under this classification concerns congenital anomalies. Undoubtedly, congenital anomalies lead to structural weaknesses which make an individual's back with such anomalies more susceptible to strains or stresses than that of a normal person without such anomalies. Brailsford,[2] in his book on "Radiology of Bones and Joints" gives an excellent résumé of the various types of congenital anomalies occurring in the lower back. Probably more skeletal congenital anomalies occur in this region than elsewhere in the body combined.

All of the foregoing discussion may seem rather elementary, but unless we have a common foundation from which to start, one becomes hopelessly bogged down with a mass of confusing opinion. As a result, the examination is oftentimes made without keeping in mind these certain fundamental ideas. It is difficult to improve upon the outline offered by Webb[18] for the examination of back cases. This outline may be found in "Minor Surgery" by Christopher.[8] One notices here that particular attention is paid to a careful history. One essential part which I feel has been omitted in this outline, is again, the non-division of symptoms into the acute or chronic stage. I believe that the duration and variation of symptoms is of prime importance in the taking of a history. A diagram of bony structures of the back is furnished with these blanks with instructions to the physician, to indicate with an "X," the location of the spot indicated by the patient where the pain occurred. I feel that this is important because persistent pain in one location is more indicative of some definite pathological condition than pain which moves from one spot to another at various times during the examination or at subsequent examinations.

Another factor is often overlooked in the examination of a back case. Too often the examiner feels that a diagnosis must be made when the individual is seen first. This particular circumstance undoubtedly accounts for numerous mistaken diagnoses. At one examination, symptoms of backache may appear to be due to trauma, whereas subsequent examinations may show, definitely, that they are of an infectious or toxic origin. If you are not sure of your diagnosis do not hesitate to have the individual return for subsequent examination and further history, and a checking of the findings noted at the time of the original examination. Surprising variations may occur between two examinations, as was the experience of this particular examiner.

A man was sent in with a history of acute back pain sharply localized to the right sacro-iliac joint. He was seen by his local physician whose examination and report was thorough, and what treatment was appropriate for a sacro-iliac sprain, on the right side. When seen by this examiner, eight weeks later, the diagnosis of the examining physician was confirmed and continued supportive treatment advised. Three months after this examination, the individual returned because his compensation had been terminated. In going over the history, he began explaining how his symptoms had improved for a while but then became worse. On this subsequent examination, his symptoms were entirely on the left side. His description of the symptoms and his response to the various tests readily indicated that he had some knowledge of the tests used for diagnosing a sacro-iliac sprain. When he was confronted with the fact at a hearing before the In-

dustrial Commission, that his original symptoms had occurred on the right side and that his subsequent symptoms had occurred on the left side, even though he had had no other accident, he became terribly confused and was disclosed as a malingerer, quite obviously.

Another case in point was that of an individual who had a definite accident resulting in a contusion to the back, immediate disability followed, and he was treated by his local physician. As his disability stretched out, he was referred to us for treatment and after a period of eight weeks, we were unable to show any improvement in his condition. Then, an orthopedist was given an opportunity to treat him and some temporary improvement followed. His compensation was stopped and he went to the University Hospital where further examination was made. The case finally came up for a hearing and the general consensus of opinion was that the man should have a back fusion, because of findings in the lumbo-sacral joint both clinically and upon x-ray. The x-ray findings had shown no change from the time of the original examination up to a period of six months later, but did disclose evidence of an atrophic type of arthritis involving the lumbo-sacral joint. This particular individual did not wish to have any surgery done. The case was settled out of court for a sizable sum of money, and three days later one of the representatives of the insurance company saw this particular individual weaving down Washington Avenue certainly enjoying his settlement to the fullest and exhibiting no evidence of pain or disability.

It is not the purpose of this paper to present any specific type of treatment. We feel that we can make certain suggestions, however, which we have found of particular value in practical experience. Consider the patient first. What is his attitude? What is his ability to stand pain? Does he have confidence in you? If these factors are within normal limits and the examination has disclosed no evidence of any severe pathology or injury, even though some objective findings may be present, the treatment, with recovery, should be simple. Attempt to explain to the individual what has happened in his back. Allay his fear of pain and his fear of a chronic back condition. Avoid strapping or splinting of the back in acute back strains since it limits the exercise so necessary to maintain circulation, and decreases the ischemia which follows even with prolonged muscular contractions of a voluntary nature. Advise him to exercise to overcome the spasm in his back. Show him how to exercise to avoid undue straining or increased pain.

Recent preliminary work done by Caron[14] on the use of novocaine in the back appears to offer a tremendous opportunity in the handling of cases of acute back pain. Fear of pain, undoubtedly, is one of the biggest factors in the development of muscle guarding or subconscious voluntary muscle spasm. If this can be overcome in the acute case, a recovery is very prompt within a few days or not more than a few weeks.

X-ray therapy is being used with almost sensational

results in some cases, yet the x-ray therapists are unable to say why.

The second part of this paper dealing with chronic back pain will be very brief. At present, we are hearing much about a protruding or herniated intervertebral disc. Not long ago, we heard about articular facetitis. Prior to that we heard of taut ilio-tibial band and prior to that any number of other causes. Perhaps the best discussion of the situation is given by Ryerson[11] of Chicago in which he states: "Again, there is offered a solution for low back pain and sciatica. In the years in which I have been coming to these meetings, I have seen many new procedures advised and adopted. What is the reason that it is so difficult to find out the pathological conditions underlying low back pain and sciatica? Obviously, these people don't die of low back pain and sciatica. No specimens are obtained, not any scientific evidence as to what is causing these troubles except in those few who are subjected to laminectomies, and in whom the foramina of the fourth or fifth lumbar nerve is exposed, or who can be seen postmortem in rare instances after accidents or the results of intercurrent disease. We do not have a good pathologic scientific foundation for most of our work on the low back and sciatic region."

In conclusion, it seems that a tremendous number of things can happen to cause pain in the back. Perhaps our evolution from quadrupeds to bipeds may have something to do with the situation. It may be that the race is deteriorating physically because of the changing social order. The author feels that a more careful observation of fundamental principles both as to examination and treatment may be of some value, but when all is said and done the actual pathology of low back pain remains largely unknown.

References

1. Albee, F. G.: Myofascitis. Am. Jour. Surg., 23:70, (Jan.) 1934.
2. Brailsford, J. F.: Radiology of bones and joints. London, Churchill, 1934.
3. Callander, C. L.: Surgical anatomy. W. B. Saunders, 1933.
4. Caron, R. P.: Personal communication.
5. Christopher, Frederick: Minor Surgery. Philadelphia, Saunders, 1929.
6. Crohn, B. B.: Pain sensibility: A variable human factor. Am. Jour. Surg., 7:474, (Oct.) 1929.
7. Davis, G. G.: Applied anatomy. Philadelphia, Lippincott, 1929.
8. Geist, E. S.: Intervertebral disc. Jour. Am. Med. Assn., 96:1676, (May 16) 1931.
9. Kuntz, A.: Autonomic nervous system. Philadelphia, Lea and Febiger, 1929.
10. Magnuson, P. B.: Backaches: a symptom. Jour. Kansas Med. Soc., 36:89, (March) 1935.
11. Ober, Fred R.: Relation of fascia lata to conditions in the lower part of the back. Jour. Am. Med. Assn., 109:554, (August 21) 1937. Discussion by E. W. Ryerson—p. 557.
12. Osler, Sir William: The principles and practice of medicine. New York, Appleton, 1892.
13. Quarterly Cumulative Index, 1929 to 1938.
14. Sherrington, C. S.: Integral action of the central nervous system. London, 1906.
15. Webb, R. C.: Personal communication.
16. White House Conference on Child Health and Protection (Committee on Medical Care for Children), Body mechanics: edition and practice, New York, Century (1932).
17. Zierold, A. A.: Morphine as a diagnostic agent. Mayo Clinic, Staff Meeting Proceedings. Vol. 10:297, (May 8) 1935.

Discussion

Dr. R. P. CARON: The subject of low back pain, including acute and chronic back strains and industrial accidents, has been exceptionally well presented by Dr.

Hultkrans. It brings to our attention all of the problems we must consider in this type of case. To my mind, so far as treatment of acute back strains is concerned, treatment comes under two important factors. First, the anatomical findings and, second, the psychological aspect of the patient. I believe that the beginning of the treatment is most important. In other words, in addition to careful history and physical examination, one must institute prompt relief, both physiologically and psychologically. For the last few years, I have used the novocaine injection treatment by injecting a one per cent novocaine solution, without adrenalin, into the most painful area, the one which usually shows most muscle spasm. In most instances within five or ten minutes relief of pain and spasm is observed. The patient, thus, gains confidence in his doctor and in himself. He is then told to bend forward and backward as far as he can. In some cases the spine is then manipulated in order to break up any muscle spasm which may persist. The patient is then advised to return home and to use external heat. The following day, the back may be reinjected if muscle spasm persists. I should like to add, however, that usually the injection and manipulation treatment is done only after x-rays have been taken, expecially in the industrial accident type of case. This type of treatment, in most instances, shortens the convalescence.

Another peculiar thing is in reference to industry. The type of industry in which the patient is employed and the compensation which he receives are definite factors in determining the period of recovery. Those who receive the least compensation return to employment sooner. This would lead one to conclude that the compensation factor has something to do with the prolonging of an acute back strain into a chronic one, that is, if there are no positive bony or neurological findings. It would appear that the employer can help a great deal by allowing the employe with an acute back strain to go to work on light duty and gradually return to regular duty rather than have him wait until he is completely well.

Dr. WM. PEYTON: I don't know just how much credit Dr. Hultkrans gives to prolapse of intervertebral disc as a cause of pain. I think that perhaps some people, at the present time, are too enthusiastic about this but I think it would be unfortunate if this group were left with the idea that there is no such thing as pain due to intervertebral disc. I have operated upon people for pain supposedly due to an intervertebral disc and I don't believe they had it, at least results were not entirely satisfactory, but I have operated upon some with very satisfactory results. I have seen intervertebral discs that were so prolapsed that a portion could just be picked out and certainly that is evidence that there is something wrong with the disc. The only reason for my making this discussion is that I wouldn't want to leave the impression left that there is no such thing as pain due to intervertebral disc. Perhaps, Dr. Hultkrans didn't mean to put it so strongly, but I got the impression that he considered it a very minor cause of back pain.

One of the most difficult things for me to decide, at the present time, is when to inject lipiodol to make this diagnosis. If you do inject lipiodol, I think you can pretty definitely say that the patient has or has not prolapse of an intervertebral disc, but one does not like to fill a lot of spinal canals with lipiodol which is retained a long time. I don't know just what the indications are, at the present time. I think they are something like this, that you have a good thorough examination for every other cause of back pain, including all of the things that Dr. Hultkrans has mentioned tonight and then, if nothing is found, spinal puncture is done. If it shows increase in the protein content, that is an indication for injection of lipiodol. On the other hand, if you do not get a change in protein content, then you still are faced with the question of whether you should or should not inject lipiodol. Some discs will be prolapsed and still you will have normal spinal fluid content. I think, if the pain is severe enough and persistent enough and you cannot find some other cause after sufficiently thorough search, then lipiodol injection is justified.

DR. KENNETH BULKLEY: What is the life history of lipiodol if it is left alone and the patient is not operated upon? Is it absorbed, and have any of these cases been traced?

DR. WILLIAM PEYTON: Lipiodol in the spinal canal apparently is not absorbed. As far as one can tell from repeated examinations that have so far been made, it remains there indefinitely. Some patients do have irritation from it; many of them do not.

DR. R. E. HULTKRANS (closing): A discussion of chronic back pain was avoided purposely. I do not believe that anyone has shown that acute back pain results from a protruding disc. The Mayo Clinic reports a series of 100 cases in which spectacular results have been obtained for the relief of chronic back pain by the surgical removal of the protruding portion of the offending intervertebral disc. My feeling is that it is still too early to draw any definite conclusions concerning the work on the protruding disc. One such operation was performed in Minneapolis just recently for severe intractable pain in the dorsal region of the back, causing the patient to threaten to commit suicide. Lipiodol injections followed by x-ray revealed a definite protruding disc which was removed surgically and resulted in a complete relief of symptoms. Whether all of these cases will remain cured over a period of three or four or five years remains to be seen.

One wonders, in reviewing the literature, why there have been so many numerous types of operations advised for the relief of relatively similar symptoms. Fusions of the lumbo-sacral and sacro-iliac joint have been commonly done, cutting the ilio-tibial band, cutting the pyriformis muscle, stripping the fascia, and numerous other surgical procedures have been done and each author reports results which show over 75 per cent cures.

The pathological condition in these cases most likely remains unknown. About six years ago, I went to Dr. Bell and asked if there would be an opportunity to obtain autopsy specimens of backs. He said that there would not be, and I might just as well forget about it for two reasons. The first was, that it meant doing an autopsy other than the routine autopsy and immediately one would be open to liability for doing anything but the routine autopsy; the second was, that the undertakers would not permit it. If you take out the spine, you injure the large vessels and embalming becomes quite a problem. Schmorl's work of several years ago was a very carefully done piece of research. Fresh autopsy specimens of the entire spine were obtained and examined in various ways. He took out the nucleus pulposis and even measured the pressure within the nucleus. He described a ruptured nucleus pulposis with the rupture occurring into the bodies of the vertebra either above or below the particular disc involved. If we could obtain such autopsy material and review the findings in the light of our present surgical experience, perhaps much would be added to the picture.

As stated before, I had hoped to avoid a discussion of chronic back pain in this paper. I wish to call attention particularly to the voluntary element in the contraction of muscles occurring in acute back sprain. I wish, also, to call attention to the necessity of overcoming this element before relief of the acute symptoms can be obtained. If these acute back strains or

sprains can be treated and relieved of symptoms in a short period of time, I believe that many of the chronic cases of low back pain will be prevented.

The meeting adjourned.
HARVEY NELSON, M.D., Secretary.

BOOK REVIEWS

Books listed here become the property of the Ramsey and Hennepin County Medical libraries when reviewed. Members, however, are urged to write reviews of any or every recent book which may be of interest to physicians.

ESSENTIALS OF OBSTETRICAL AND GYNECOLOGICAL PATHOLOGY. Marion Douglass, M.D., F.A.C.S., Assistant Professor of Gynecology, Western Reserve University, and Robert L. Faulkner, M.D., Senior Clinical Instructor in Gynecology, Western Reserve University. 187 pages. Illus. Price, cloth, $4.75. St. Louis: C. V. Mosby Co., 1938.

MEDICAL WRITING. The Technic and the Art. Morris Fishbein, M.D., Editor of the Journal of the American Medical Association. 212 pages. Illus. Price, $1.50, flexible binding. Chicago: American Medical Association Press, 1938.

DIE THERAPIE DER THROMBOSE. Dr. Ernst Friedlander. 117 pages. Illus. Price, paper cover, 5.40 K. Leipzig and Vienna: Franz Deuticke, 1938.

STANDARDS FOR THE DIAGNOSIS AND TREATMENT OF CANCER. By the Executive Cancer Committee, Iowa State Medical Association. 168 pages. Price, $1.00, paper cover. Iowa City: Athens Press, 1938.

SYMPTOMS OF VISCERAL DISEASE. Fifth Edition. Francis Marion Pottenger, A.M., M.D., LL.D., Medical Director Pottenger Sanatorium & Clinic for Diseases of the Chest, Monrovia, California, Professor of Clinical Medicine University of Southern California, etc. 442 pages. Illus. Price, $5.00, cloth St. Louis: C. V. Mosby Co., 1938.

HERNIA. Anatomy, Etiology, Symptoms, Diagnosis Differential Diagnosis, Prognosis and the Operative and Injection Treatment. Second Edition. Leigh F. Watson, M.D. Member of Attending Staff o California Lutheran Hospital and Methodist Hospita of Southern California. 591 pages. Illus. Pric $7.50, cloth. St. Louis: C. V. Mosby Co., 1938.

A CHALLENGE TO SEX CENSORS. Theodore Schroeder 159 pages. Privately printed in New York to pro mote the aims of the Free Speech League. 193

HEMORRHOIDS. Marion C. Pruitt, M.D. 170 page Illus. Price, $4.00. St. Louis: C. V. Mosby, 1938. This monograph on hemorrhoids by Dr. Pruitt exceptionally well formulated and written. It has n been my pleasure to read a more excellent treati on this subject.

BOOK REVIEWS

This monograph should be readily available for any and all physicians who attempt to treat hemorrhoids. The operative detail is so well illustrated and explained that any physician can easily learn how to make hemorrhoidectomy a clean, physiologically correct operation.

I cannot praise the author too highly for his excellent treatment of this subject.

E. E. SCOTT.

METHODS OF TREATMENT. 6th edition. Logan Clendening, M.D., 879 pp., Illus., $10.00. C. V. Mosby Co., St. Louis, 1937.

This justly popular text, now in its sixth revision, is attractively printed, on good paper, and with large uncrowded type. Its well-known author has succeeded in introducing his characteristically informal style into the discussions, and thus makes such chapters as those on psychotherapy, and the psychoneuroses, readable and enjoyable. One is inclined to accept his attitude toward psycho-analysis with sympathetic approval.

The chapters on drugs are excellent, practical and complete. The subject of digitalis medication receives comprehensive and valuable treatment. Frequent historical references, and brief quotations from original writings add to the value of this work. Excellent descriptions of methods of hydrotherapy, physiotherapy, and dietetic advice are given simply and succinctly. Aside from its lack of information about sulphanilamide, and anti-pneumococcus serum, obviously due to their more recent development, the book makes an excellent addition to any physician's library.

THOMAS MYERS, M.D.

EMOTIONAL ADJUSTMENT IN MARRIAGE. Le Mon Clark. 261 pages. $3.00. St. Louis: Mosby, 1937.

Some thirty years ago a Minnesota physician went to prison because he sent through the mails a book which undertook to teach the art of sexual intercourse so as to elicit from it the highest enjoyment. The then President, Theodore Roosevelt, was appealed to for a pardon, but refused after reading a few extracts from the book. Such has been the change in attitude towards sex literature that Dr. Clark need fear no indictment, although his work is much more erotic than was that by the Minnesota doctor.

This is as it should be, provided the circulation of this kind of literature is kept strictly in the hands of the medical profession, by them to be entrusted to engaged or newly married couples. No one can practice medicine for any length of time without encountering numerous marital misfits because of faulty sexual relations, a condition that can be met only by the fullest and frankest discussion. A spade must be called a spade, and in order to be understood it may be necessary sometimes to lay aside purely scientific terms and resort to some of those current on the street; there must be no uncertainty in the minds of those to be instructed as to what is meant.

Dr. Clark bases his thesis on the claim that there can

be no perfect union without bringing together both the physical and the psychical elements of love, consummated by sexual intercourse that satisfies both the participants. He describes the gradual approach by which this objective may be attained. Repeatedly he asserts that anything which is pleasurable to both is desirable. How to get this pleasure is minutely described, as also how to avoid the pitfalls into which many stumble. This calls for highly sensuous descriptions and he gives them, but his object is laudable and for the end in view he does not go beyond the limits of decency, although as intimated before, it would be most objectionable to put the work into the hands of those who would read it only from prurient motives.

Do doctors need the kind of information and instruction given in these pages in order to give the best and most intelligent advice to those who consult them on sexual matters? Yes, many of them do, and there are few who will not get some valuable points. The subject is seldom dealt with so intelligently and understandingly.

A chapter on birth control adds nothing new.

Some very erotic though classical poetry does not really belong in a serious medical book.

W. DAVIS

THE COMPLEAT PEDIATRICIAN. PRACTICAL, DIAGNOSTIC, THERAPEUTIC AND PREVENTIVE PEDIATRICS. Second, completely rewritten, edition. By W. C. Davison, Professor of Pediatrics, Duke University School of Medicine, formerly acting pediatrician in charge, The Johns Hopkins Hospital. Duke University Press, 1938, pp. 250.

For more than eight years on trains, steamers and planes from Helsinfors to Houston, the author of The Compleat Pediatrician read, rummaged and ransacked 147,359 cases of 329 different diseases among 80,000 children admitted to the Johns Hopkins Hospital from 1912 to 1932. The result is a book, not a textbook but an almanac, whose compressed 250 pages contain a vast collection of facts.

In this one volume encyclopedia, you will find: (1) one hundred and sixty-four signs and symptoms peculiar to childhood; (2) a concise summary of the differential diagnosis of 329 diseases of children; (3) the grain separated from the chaff in pediatric treatment (drugs and prescriptions especially valuable); (4) 213 practical laboratory tests that have stood the test of time; (5) the best facts in the growth, development, and guidance of children, which every non-medical health worker as well as physician should know; and (6) excellent instruction for taking histories and making physical examinations.

If you want leisurely reading, do not buy this book, but if you want accurate, precise, practical, up-to-date pediatrics be sure to get a copy and make a constant companion of it.

One final word, the author urges that the reader follow the instructions on page 5 explicitly in order to understand the arrangement and the cross index.

M. SEHAM.

BOOK REVIEWS

NEW PATHWAYS FOR CHILDREN WITH CEREBRAL PALSY. Gladys Gage Rogers and Leah C. Thomas. New York: Macmillan, 1935, 167 pp., illus., $2.50.

This is a practical, concise, readable discussion of the authors' experiences and observations in the education and development of the handicapped children at their summer camp, Robin Hood's Barn.

It is a book that the parents of a child with cerebral palsy should read, as it affords them a sane approach to their problems of education and the adjustment necessary in their lives to assure the maximum development of these children.

To the physicians it may serve as a manual in outlining toys, suggesting games and developmental exercises, both direct and indirect. It offers suggestions for construction of simple supportive apparatus. The physician can well afford to read further and develop the general approach to the education of these children that the authors have learned to be a fundamental part of their success.

HAROLD F. FLANAGAN, M.D.

WABASHA COUNTY SOCIETY

(Continued from Page 589)

Wabasha County Medical Society and the Wabasha County Dental Society at Lake City, Tuesday evening, July 8. About twenty-five were in attendance.

These officials explained the newly inaugurated system of having divisional health districts in the state. There are three such districts now, and the intention is to establish a fourth in Southeastern Minnesota, including Winona, Olmsted, Goodhue, Fillmore, Mower, Houston, Dodge, Dakota and Wabasha Counties, provided these counties qualify by employing a County Public Health Nurse and otherwise fulfilling the requirements of the State and Federal laws and regulations in this respect. It was unanimously voted by the organizations present to favor, advocate, and promote this measure.

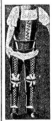

MINNESOTA MEDICINE

Journal of the Minnesota State Medical Association, Southern Minnesota Medical Association, Northern Minnesota Medical Association, Minnesota Academy of Medicine and Minneapolis Surgical Society

| Volume 21 | SEPTEMBER, 1938 | No. 9 |

PHASES OF BRONCHOSCOPY AND ESOPHAGOSCOPY OF IMPORTANCE IN GENERAL PRACTICE

VIRGIL J. SCHWARTZ, M.D.

Minneapolis, Minnesota

THE DAY has long since passed when the practice of bronchial and esophageal endoscopy consisted only of the removal of foreign bodies from the air and food passages. It has become one of the most important procedures now in use for the examination and treatment of certain chest conditions. True, a major portion of the field is still devoted to the foreign-body problem; but more and more it has been enlarged to include the study and treatment of such conditions as primary carcinoma of the bronchi, malignancy (sarcoma or carcinoma) of the esophagus, lung abscess, tuberculosis, diphtheria, bronchiectasis, and tracheal stenosis or displacement due to thyroid enlargement, mediastinal gland involvement, or aortic aneurysm. Also to be considered are cicatricial stenosis, scleroma, asthma, unexplained vomiting of blood or regurgitation of food, and atelectasis due to thick lung secretions. Any unexplained interference with the function of swallowing, or of the stomach, and unexplained cough, dyspnea, hemoptysis, and expectoration call for appropriate investigation. Furthermore, marked advances in gastroscopy are also being made.

The mechanical problems associated with foreign-body extraction are naturally interesting. A few foreign-body cases which present particular points of interest will be discussed briefly. The esophageal foreign bodies encountered in this series include coins of various kinds (pennies, quarters, nickels, coin slugs), food in large masses, meat bones, pheasant bones, chicken bones, fishbones, open safety pins, straight pins, advertising buttons, wire rings, a thermometer, tin whistles, a peach stone, buttons, a dental bridge, and so on. Bronchial foreign bodies include nuts of various kinds, diphtheritic casts, a thumb-tack, an acorn, a steel screw, fine pieces of carrot, a metal clasp from a dress, a broken portion of an intubation-tube obturator, beads, and others.

Until recently, one of the most tragic situations in the entire field of medicine was our comparative helplessness in the treatment of primary carcinoma of the lung. From a diagnostic standpoint, great advances had been made: a piece of tissue obtained through the bronchoscope settled the diagnosis immediately. Sometimes the patient may have been in splendid condition so far as general operative risk was concerned, and the process may still have been at an early stage of development; yet the danger of operation was so marked that it was generally not advised. In fact, even now a patient who is still in what he considers comparatively good health will not readily entertain the idea of submitting to an operation which has had such a high mortality rate. We have had, therefore, to resort to radium and deep roentgen-ray therapy. The latter had, in fact, given much encouragement. Yet, in general, this treatment is only a palliative measure, as most patients thus treated live considerably less than a year after the diagnosis is made.

Within the past few years, however, marked advances have been made in the surgery of carcinoma of the lungs. Reports of successful lobectomy and pneumonectomy are beginning to appear in the literature, and, if substantial progress continues, it is to be hoped that before long a reasonably safe procedure will be developed for use in all cases which are not too far advanced.

Mrs. A. P., aged sixty-four, was a typical case. She had complained of shortness of breath for four or five years. A year previously she began to have a dry cough, with a little clear sputum. She noted some blood in the sputum, and expectorated small quantities resembling "cherry-pits" —small, round and sticky. There was no pain, but there was mild dyspnea. The appetite was good; there was no fever nor loss of weight. Anteriorly, on the left side the breath sounds were heard faintly, but the percussion note was almost normal. This is usually the case. Roentgenograms revealed some fluid which was removed. Bronchoscopy and biopsy showed a carcinoma. The patient left the hospital and it was reported that six months later she died.

Mr. W. J., aged sixty-four, was bronchoscoped and a similar condition was found except that instead of presenting a small tumor which only partly filled the bronchial lumen, as in the preceding case, the mass here was so large as to occlude completely the left bronchus.

Carcinoma of the esophagus is an even more discouraging and challenging disease. A common offense in this case is erroneous diagnosis through inferring that the patient's trouble is one of several benign or "nervous" conditions, such as esophageal spasm, cardiospasm, neurasthenia, hysteria, globus hystericus, refusal to swallow, et cetera, instead of doing an early esophagoscopy and giving the patient the benefit of such relief as radium and deep-ray therapy may offer. A still worse offense is the practice of blind bouginage. It is often the immediate cause of death in the presence of an ulcerated, weakened esophageal wall, and is greatly to be condemned, except possibly after esophagoscopy, when the operator is thoroughly familiar with the shape and condition of the particular esophagus in question. Even so, it is a dangerous procedure.

A striking case was Mrs. G. M., who had had increasing difficulty in swallowing for about seven weeks until at the time she was examined she was unable to swallow even liquids. This patient was only twenty-three years old; yet by means of the esophagoscope a carcinoma was found involving the entire circumference of the wall of the upper esophagus and causing almost complete obstruction.

Cancer is found most frequently in the middle

third of the esophagus, somewhat less often at its lower end and least of all in the upper third. Jackson states that strangely enough the most frequent site in women is at the upper end as was the case in the patient just mentioned.

M. K., aged sixty-five, had been unable to swallow solids for weeks and fluids for many days. She was so weak and emaciated that she could not even sit up, yet esophagoscopy was not suggested to her until she came to the clinic. She, too, had a complete ring carcinoma of the upper end of the esophagus.

Another patient, Mrs. C. S., aged thirty-three, had complained of moderate dysphagia for a few weeks. By means of the esophagoscope there was found, in the right pyriform sinus, and extending downward from this for a short distance into the mouth of the esophagus, a sarcoma which was extensively and carefully treated by operation, radium and deep-ray therapy. The patient lived for about eighteen months. All except three of the men and two other women in this series of esophageal cancer showed lesions in the middle or lower third.

In conditions in which tracheal compression, due to goiter, mediastinal glands, tumors, aneurism or other lesions is suspected or evident, tracheoscopy is urgently and sometimes immediately indicated. Unfortunately, this is often delayed until it is too late. The writer received an emergency call to do a tracheotomy upon a patient who was in the operating room, and who was about to have a goiter removed, but became cyanotic on the table. She was found to have a scabbard trachea, which was so markedly compressed on each side by two enormously enlarged thyroid lobes, that it was difficult to understand why she had not suffocated long before. Tracheotomy was done and the patient recovered, but there were some trying moments. Tracheoscopy is easily and quickly done and frequently gives so much information that it should be resorted to much more often. It is frequently possible to tell by the pushed-in appearance of the tracheal wall just which of the two thyroid lobes is enlarged, and to exactly what degree it is encroaching upon the tracheal lumen. It is a well known fact that a patient may go for a long time with slowly increasing tracheal compression and not show any symptoms until sudden dyspnea and cyanosis set in.

Unexplained vomiting of blood in the pres-

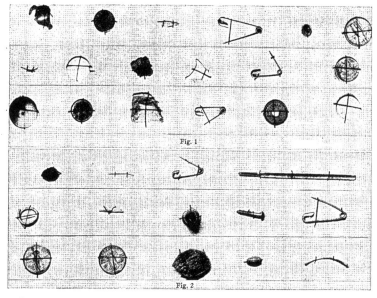

Fig. 1. First row: Dental bridge, penny, bone, open safety pin, bead in bronchus, quarter.
Second row: Fish bone in root of tongue, advertising button, meat bone, chicken bone, open safety pin, nickel.
Third row: Tip whistle, penny, meat bone, open safety pin, coin machine slug, nickel.
In all illustrations, unless otherwise indicated, foreign bodies were removed from the esophagus.

Fig. 2. First row: Acorn in trachea, steel wire, safety pin, thermometer.
Second row: Wire ring, chicken bone, thumb tack in bronchus, steel screw in bronchus, safety pin.
Third row: Quarter, quarter, peach stone, bead in bronchus, pheasant bone.

ence of a normal stomach, normal chest findings and a normal nose and throat may be due to a simple esophageal erosion or benign ulceration. Mrs. M. S., aged fifty, had vomited about 1,200 c.c. of bright blood two weeks previous to her admission. It was impossible to find the source of this bleeding, so esophagoscopy was done and an ulcer was found on the posterior wall of the esophagus, thirty-one centimeters from the teeth, possibly due to food or bone trauma. This was cauterized and she has had no bleeding since that time. This type of bleeding is occasionally due to a small dilated vessel, usually a small varicosity, but while these are common in the hypopharynx and on the posterior surface of the root of the tongue, they are comparatively infrequent in the esophagus itself.

Grim as is the aspect in the matter of malignancy, it is exceedingly bright in the foreign body field. In this connection there are some points which warrant mention. First of all, it cannot be too strongly emphasized that the blind insertion of a finger, whether by a doctor or a layman, into the throat for the purpose of pushing down a foreign body is often a disastrous procedure. It is very rare that the finger can actually hook itself around a foreign body, and if the attendant states that he can "feel" it with the finger tip, it is possible that he himself may have pushed it down into an incarcerated position. The old saw that nothing smaller than an elbow should be put into an ear by one not qualified, applies almost equally well to the throat. The only thing that should be used for the removal of a foreign body in the throat is a pair of forceps, of one kind or another, and under inspection.

The writer was called to see Mrs. C. S., who complained of sudden dyspnea and severe pain in the throat, evidently due to a bone which had just become lodged. The patient was carefully examined with the mirror and no bone was seen, so an x-ray plate was taken and that seemed to show nothing wrong within the photographed field. The only finding of any importance was a small, flat swelling, seen with the laryngeal mirror in the posterior wall of the hypopharynx which could easily have been due to trauma. However, the patient was observed closely and told to report immediately if she felt anything sharp in her throat. On the fourth day she phoned and reported such a sensation, and upon looking into the lower part of the pharynx there was found a bone protruding from the swelling which had previously been noticed on the posterior wall. She then stated that when she first had a choking sensation, her excited son-in-law put his finger in her throat and feeling something there pushed it down hard. In this case he evidently pushed it through the mucous membrane of the posterior wall, but he could just as easily have pushed it into the anterior or lateral wall, in which case the result might have been fatal.

A. R., a year and a half old infant, had a coin slug in his throat which was forced down by a parent so that it was firmly embedded in the upper end of the esophagus. It was removed by esophagoscopy, but this procedure should not have been necessary because it could undoubtedly have been removed with a pair of simple forceps from the pharynx. In another instance a doctor pushed a piece of bone, loose in his own hypopharynx, down into his esophagus, inflicting severe trauma.

Grasping a child by the feet and holding him upside down while trying to have him cough out a foreign body may also be a fatal mistake. This happened in the case of M. N., a child of three. He was brought into the hospital after having stopped breathing about seven or eight minutes before. Tracheotomy was done immediately and an acorn was found firmly wedged in the subglottic space and between the vocal cords. It was impossible to restore breathing. The child had told his parents that he had inhaled an acorn. This had doubtless lodged in the upper part of

one of the main bronchi, and had left him only one lung for breathing, but the parents immediately turned him upside down and forced him to cough, whereupon the acorn fell into the trachea and lodged in the subglottic space, causing spasm of the glottis, a completely blocked trachea, and suffocation.

In view of the common practice of leaving thermometers in the mouths of patients, it is surprising that these do not more frequently enter the esophagus or bronchi. The writer had the unique experience of removing intact a thermometer from the esophagus of M. A., a man with bulbar paralysis. This case was recently reported elsewhere as being the first, or among the first, of its kind on record.

An unusual case was that of H. T., aged seventy-one, who swallowed some food which became stuck in his esophagus. Upon entering the esophagus we found in about its middle third the major part of an entire peach, including the stone. This was removed by the exercise of considerably more pull than is usually applied, yet the patient apparently suffered no ill effect from his experience.

Some foreign bodies are not actually so large, but when the esophagus contains, for instance, a lye-burn stricture, certain foreign bodies are caught which might otherwise pass through. This was the case with G. G., aged 9. He swallowed some lye when a year and a half old and the resulting stricture had been repeatedly dilated since. On January 1, 1932, he swallowed a prune stone which stuck in the esophagus, but was removed without difficulty. In the absence of the stricture the stone would have gone through easily.

A distressing condition with which bronchoscopists have to deal is laryngeal and tracheal diphtheria. It is astonishing to see how frequently children, and occasionally adults, are allowed to go without antitoxin, either through neglect or through failure to make a diagnosis. The patient may be brought into the hospital moribund or so dyspneic and cyanotic that life is a matter of only a few minutes. In such cases immediate laryngoscopy and tracheoscopy, with removal of the obstructing membrane by suction or forceps, will very frequently accomplish what any other method will not. In some cases intubation is indicated, while in others even tracheotomy may fail because often the membrane or diphtheritic

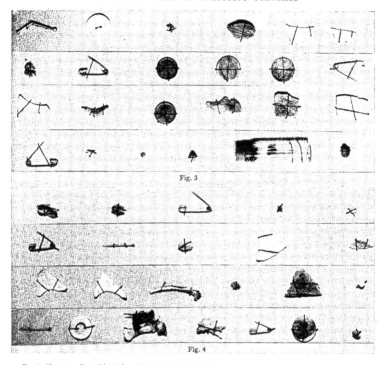

Fig. 3

Fig. 4

Fig. 3. First row: Part of intubation obturator in left bronchus, button, peanut in bronchus, prune pit, chicken bone, chicken bone.
Second row: Peanut in bronchus, safety pin, penny, zinc plate from battery, tin disc, open safety pin (in infant aged two months).
Third row: Chicken bone, meat bone, penny, meat bone, meat bone, meat bone.
Fourth row: Safety pin, concretion from mouth, bead from ear, cork from nose, piece of carrot in left bronchus (mounted in vial), stone in right bronchus.

Fig. 4. First row: Pistachio nut shell in bronchus, peanut in bronchus, safety pin, peanut in bronchus, egg-shell in trachea.
Second row: Safety pin, straight pin, watermelon seed in bronchus, chicken bone, meat bone.
Third row: Chicken bone, chicken bone, chicken bone, sand-burr in left ventricle of larynx, meat bone, glass bead in left ear.
Fourth row: Pin in larynx, aluminum washer, chicken bone, chicken bone, safety pin in esophagus (open end foremost), nickel, peanut in bronchus.

cast extends downward into the main bronchi. G. K., aged 17, was brought into the hospital fighting so hard for breath that a fatal issue seemed unavoidable. This patient had been sick for about twelve days with gradually increasing dyspnea, yet no medical attention was sought. Through a tracheoscope a long diphtheritic cast was removed by suction. The patient's breathing immediately became easier and she eventually recovered. There was, of course, a great amount

of edema of the laryngeal and tracheal mucosa, but this gradually subsided. This procedure is a well established practice in contagious hospitals, and deservedly so.

It must be borne in mind that many things may happen between the time that the x-ray plate is taken in any case of suspected foreign body, and the time of bronchoscopy. A. N., aged four, was brought into the hospital and the x-ray showed a thumb tack in the right main bronchus.

Within a half hour the thumb tack was found on bronchoscopy in the left main bronchus instead of the right. In other words, while lying on his left side, he had coughed the tack up into the trachea and promptly aspirated it into the left main bronchus.

Similarly J. L., aged eleven months, had definite x-ray evidence of a small dress clasp, such as is used in women's dresses, in his right main bronchus. At bronchoscopy within fifteen minutes nothing was found in the bronchial tree and a second x-ray showed it lodged in his stomach, it having been coughed up and swallowed.

A more interesting case is that of R. G., aged four. X-ray showed definitely a long bead in the right main bronchus. Within a few minutes she was on the operating table and while the instruments were being prepared she suddenly became cyanotic. We suspected the probable cause of her trouble and changed her position a little, with the result that her color improved at once. Within two or three minutes, however, her color again became bad, but by this time the bronchoscope was ready for introduction and the bead was removed from the trachea. It had been coughed from the right main bronchus up into the trachea, and so long as the lumen of the bead was in the long axis of the trachea she was able to breathe through the hole, but when the bead tilted to one side or the other, the air was shut off and the patient became cyanotic.

An unusual accident occurred during the insertion of an intubation tube in a case of laryngeal diphtheria. F. M., aged four, was deeply cyanotic, and upon attempting intubation the attendant was unpleasantly surprised to find that he was not able to insert the tube and that the distal portion of the metal obturator was missing. An x-ray plate was immediately taken and showed this piece to have been broken off and lodged in the bronchus to the left upper lobe. The foreign body was removed and the intubation then proceeded without trouble.

M. B., an infant of twenty months, was admitted with a clinical diagnosis of peanut in the right lung. The child experienced a severe bronchitis, as was to have been expected, but made a good recovery. The bronchial walls normally dilate during inspiration and collapse during expiration; therefore a piece of nut which lies in the lumen often will admit air during inspiration into the area distal to it, but in expira-

tion the walls collapse and the air is imprisoned, causing emphysema. If the foreign body fills the bronchus completely during both inspiration and expiration, atelectasis results. In passing, it is well to repeat again that children under the age of three or four should not be given nuts to eat, but this injunction is rarely heeded.

A man, aged sixty-two, evidently of low mentality, was found to have an entire esophagus full of food. A great piece of meat and cartilage, measuring approximately 4 to 5 inches in length, 1.5 inches in width and 0.5 inch in thickness was removed. A great degree of traction, perhaps the equivalent of 3 or 4 pounds, was required. Upon removal the mass was found to have been literally strangled at the lower esophageal constriction; a deep groove encircled the mass at its middle, as though a heavy rope had been tied about it. This experience may throw considerable light upon the degree of spasm which the cardiac end of the esophagus may develop, for these constrictions must occur at times in people who do not have a foreign body at this point. From a general diagnostic and therapeutic angle, therefore, this case is important. Some careful work has been done by various investigators on the actual, measured degree of contraction or constriction possible at the lower end of the esophagus. This is often due to diaphragmatic compression.

Another case of peanut in the bronchus is mentioned only to emphasize the great necessity of correlating a very careful history with seemingly insignificant symptoms and physical signs. This six year old child had had a very slight coughing spell four days previously, while eating an ordinary candy bar. When first seen by a doctor she had a slight occasional cough with a few râles. There were no other complaints. Roentgenogram showed an almost normal chest on inspiration, but a slight emphysema of the right middle and lower lobes on expiration. A peanut was found not quite filling the lumen of the right bronchus, below the opening of the bronchus to the upper lobe.

A man, aged fifty-nine, had complained of difficult swallowing for some time, but there were no clinical or roentgenologic findings of any kind. Despite this, we found, on esophagoscopy, a ring of pathologic tissue at the cardiac end which, on biopsy, showed adenocarcinoma. This case again emphasizes the need for endoscopic examination when an adequate explanation of persistent symptoms is not possible.

Cases of straight pins and safety pins in the esophagi of infants have been seen rather frequently. An uncommon foreign body, however, was a piece of egg-shell in the trachea which was producing symptoms through irritation and spasm out of all proportion to the size of the foreign body. These symptoms disappeared following removal of the egg-shell. Several cases of watermelon seed in the bronchi have been seen, all in young children three to five years of age.

A boy, aged eight, developed atelectasis and emphysema (in different lobes) following an abdominal operation. Bronchiectasis developed after a time and became very troublesome, but it was interesting to note that an injection of lipiodol yielded so much improvement that the boy was able to go about his customary duties, including attendance at school and work following school hours without any appreciable discomfort. Frequently bronchiectasis can be prevented by repeated aspiration of residual pus in the lungs or bronchial tree, the result of an acute suppurative inflammation in this area.

We do not usually expect to find more than one major foreign body in the same patient. Recently a child was brought in with a foreign body in the esophagus which was of the exact size of a five-cent piece. However, we noted that there was hardly enough shadow cast by this foreign body on the roentgenogram to enable us to call it a coin. At esophagoscopy we found a round, very sharp piece of tin which had been swallowed one month before, and had, in the meantime, produced a great deal of trauma in the esophageal wall. The interesting fact in this case is that the child had at the same time also swallowed an open safety pin which the local

doctor was able to remove from the pharynx without much trouble. He did not suspect the presence of more than one foreign body. The case, therefore, indicates the advisability of an x-ray in all cases of foreign body in the air or food passages.

The foregoing reports are only a few which illustrate some general principles. Space does not permit a consideration of the entire series. However, on the basis of some of the experiences cited, a few important rules may be listed, as follows:

1. Never diagnose "nervous" (so-called) conditions in the esophagus without endoscopic examination, if symptoms persist.

2. Never practice "blind bouginage."

3. Never allow the age of your patient to influence your diagnosis unduly.

4. Never "push down" blindly a foreign body in the throat.

5. Never turn a child upside down to cough out a foreign body.

6. Never leave thermometers in the mouths of unattended children or mental incompetents.

On the other side:

1. Always examine early the bronchi or esophagus if malignancy or foreign body is suspected. The earlier this is done the better.

2. Always repeat roentgenologic examination if a known foreign body cannot be found.

3. Always be prepared for tracheotomy.

4. Always be on guard for non-opaque foreign bodies in the chest.

Bronchoscopy and esophagoscopy are in themselves safe, quickly-performed procedures. Do not fear them. If doctors and the laity can be impressed with the necessity of caution and precaution, as above outlined, it will mean the saving of lives which are even yet unnecessarily sacrificed.

Did you know that twenty-five million cows are milked daily in the United States and that the output of dairy products is estimated at three and one-third billion dollars annually? That Wisconsin headed the list in 1937 for cash farm income from the sale of milk with $168,255,000 and Minnesota fourth with $95,330,000? That Minnesota headed the list for butter production in 1936 with 289,830,000 pounds? That Wisconsin produced in 1936 over half of the 642,551,000 pounds of cheese manufactured in the country, while Minnesota rated far down the list with only 12,643,000 pounds production? That in 1908, Chicago enacted the first compulsory pasteurization law? That New York followed in 1912 and that since that date no milk-borne epidemics have been recorded in that city and it is estimated that yearly several thousand babies are saved there annually from cholera infantum?—From *Milk Facts*, Milk Industry Foundation, July, 1938.

THE USE OF PEDICLE MUSCLE GRAFTS IN FACILITATING OBLITERATION
OF LARGE, CHRONIC, NONTUBERCULOUS, PLEURAL
EMPYEMA CAVITIES*

HOWARD K. GRAY, M.D.

Rochester, Minnesota

THE obvious problem in the treatment of chronic nontuberculous pleural empyema is to obliterate the cavity or cavities as rapidly as possible with the minimum risk and deformity, and to restore to as nearly normal as possible the physiologic activities of the chest. With adequate treatment during the acute or subacute stage, most chronic empyemas can be avoided. Unfortunately, however, many cases are encountered in which inadequate drainage has been instituted and in which a chronic process therefore persists.

As is true of many pathologic conditions of the chest, time is an important factor, for the lesion may have produced widespread general effects and it is a constant source of potential danger. Not the least of such a patient's worries may be financial, and for this as well as for physical reasons, it is important that the period of rehabilitation be terminated as rapidly as possible.

Before resorting to any of the more extensive operative procedures, adequate drainage with appropriate local treatment of the chronic empyema cavity should be instituted. By so doing, the general condition of the patient will be improved, and the cavity may diminish appreciably in size or become completely obliterated. If the cavity is not too large, the "roof" may be removed subsequently in multiple stage operations. That further surgical treatment will be necessary and that extensive "unroofing" is inadvisable in an appreciable number of cases is readily admitted, and it is with special reference to the use of pedicle muscle grafts in facilitating obliteration of such cavities that this paper is primarily concerned.

With the exception of Lilienthal's "major noncollapsing thoracoplasty," most of the procedures advocated for the obliteration of large empyema cavities from within have been characterized by extensive deformity. The chief advantage of a modified decortication operation, such as

was originally described by Fowler and Delorme, is the reinflation of the lung which occurs to a limited extent and in so doing may partially obliterate the cavity and restore a greater degree of vital capacity. Unfortunately, however, the procedure is applicable only in a very limited number of cases because of the frequent association of marked fibrosis in the underlying pulmonary tissue and it cannot be carried out without appreciable risk.

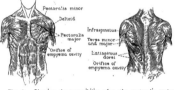

Fig. 1. Showing the accessibility of a, the pectoralis major muscle, and b, the latissimus dorsi muscle for pedicle muscle grafts in facilitating obliteration of large, chronic nontuberculous pleural empyema cavities.

Similar criticism of the marked deformity and unwarranted risk imposed may be directed at most procedures designed to obliterate the empyema cavity by collapsing the thoracic wall. This can be accomplished only after the bony framework has been removed, whether it be by the radical thoracoplasty of Schede or the many modifications of this procedure in which the soft tissue is preserved.

If obliteration of a large empyema cavity by permitting the lung to expand is impracticable, and if by collapsing the wall of the chest too great a risk and deformity are imposed, the only method by which obliteration may be accomplished is to assist the natural healing processes by filling the cavity with some foreign substance. In order to conform to accepted surgical principles, it is essential that this substance be viable. Because of their accessibility, the pectoralis major and the latissimus dorsi muscles are ideally suited for the purpose (Fig 1).

*From the Division of Surgery, The Mayo Clinic, Rochester, Minnesota. Read before the meeting of the Minnesota Surgical Society, Minneapolis, Minnesota, May 20, 1938.

According to Gray, the latissimus dorsi muscle "arises by tendinous fibers from the spinous processes of the lower six thoracic vertebræ and from the posterior layer of the lumbodorsal fascia (by which it is attached to the spines of the lumbar and sacral vertebræ, to the supraspinal ligament, and to the posterior part of the crest of the ilium)." It is inserted into the bottom of the intertubercular groove of the humerus and receives its blood supply through the subscapular artery, a branch of the axillary artery. Impulses pass to the latissimus dorsi muscle along the sixth, seventh, and eighth cervical nerves through the thoracodorsal (long subscapular) nerve. The pectoralis major muscle arises "from the anterior surface of the sternal half of the clavicle, from half the breadth of the anterior surface of the sternum as low as the attachment of the cartilage of the sixth or seventh rib, from the cartilages of all the true ribs, with the exception, frequently, of the first or seventh or both, and from the aponeurosis of the obliquus externus abdominis." The muscle ends in a flat tendon, which is inserted into the crest of the greater tubercle of the humerus and receives its blood supply chiefly through the thoraco-acromial and lateral thoracic arteries, both of which are branches of the axillary, and through the perforating branches of the intercostal and internal mammary arteries. Impulses pass to the pectoralis major muscle along the medial and lateral thoracic nerves. Through these nerves the muscle is to receive filaments from all the spinal nerves entering into the formation of the brachial plexus.

The origin and insertion of these two muscles make them particularly suitable for pedicle muscle grafts. The base of the pedicle in both instances is preferably the insertion of the muscle, for in preserving the tissues in this region there will be no interference with the nerve and blood supply. Although the origin may be changed by transplanting the bulk of these muscles into some intrathoracic cavity, the major portion of their function will be retained if there is no interference with the points of insertion.

Report of Cases

Case 1.—The first patient, a youth aged seventeen years, registered at the clinic on March 11, 1936. Five weeks previously a diffuse bronchopneumonia had developed on the right; this was complicated by a hemolytic streptococcic empyema. Multiple thoracen-

teses were performed between March 11 and April 7, and open drainage was instituted by removing a portion of three ribs in the region of the most dependent portion of the empyema cavity. The capacity of the cavity at this time was approximately 750 c.c. and it

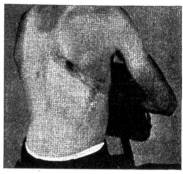

Fig. 2 (Case 1). Showing the line of incision which was made at right angles to the thoracotomy incision in order to mobilize as much as possible the intact portion of the latissimus dorsi muscle.

extended nearly to the apex of the right hemithorax, compressing the lung medially. The patient was dismissed from the hospital on the fourteenth postoperative day and for the next two weeks returned for daily irrigations and dressings. On May 6 (one month after the open operation) the skin flap on the outer portion of the thoracotomy wound was dissected back and a perpendicular incision was made from the outer third of the lower flap in the direction of the fibers of the latissimus dorsi muscle. A pedicle graft of the latissimus dorsi muscle, approximately 20 cm. in length, was dissected free, leaving the pedicle attached above. This was inserted into the empyema cavity and held in place with one suture. Plastic closure of the skin, where it was dissected free, was then made, along the line of the new incision. The capacity of the cavity at this time was approximately 500 c.c. The wound was packed lightly with vaseline gauze. The patient's convalescence was uneventful and he was dismissed from the hospital on the fourth postoperative day (Fig. 2). Final surgical dismissal was granted two weeks later, and the patient was permitted to return home. His local physician continued to irrigate the residual cavity and complete healing occurred within three months after his dismissal.

Case 2.—The second patient was another youth, also seventeen, who registered at the clinic on September 2, 1937. In April, 1934, a right pleural empyema had developed following pneumonia. Drainage of the empyema cavity had been instituted (elsewhere) a week later but the wound had continued to drain at intervals in spite of several operations for osteomyelitis of the ribs. There had been considerable loss of weight and, since the operation, the patient had noticed definite curvature of the spine. On physical examination the patient appeared to be poorly developed and poorly nourished; he had a moderately sallow

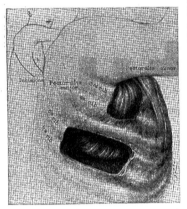

Fig. 3 (Case 2). A window has been made in the thoracic wall near the uppermost portion of the empyema cavity. The pectoralis major muscle has been separated from its origin and the bulk of the muscle has been placed within the cavity through the opening, thus obliterating the apex of the cavity without waste of muscle substance.

complexion. Dulness and diminished breath sounds were noted over this entire right side. A roentgenogram of the thorax revealed a large amount of fluid on the right and evidence that partial resection of the eighth, ninth, and tenth ribs had previously been carried out. Moderate scoliosis was seen in the roentgenograms of the thoracic and lumbar spine.

A needle was inserted in the seventh interspace in the posterior axillary line on the right and a large quantity of thick, yellowish-green pus was found. Staphylococcus aureus was cultured from this material.

On September 10 open operation was carried out. After removing a portion of the ninth rib posterolaterally, the empyema cavity was entered. It was found to extend practically from the diaphragm to the apex of the right hemithorax. The lung was compressed medially. The cavity held approximately 1,000 c.c. of thick, yellowish-green pus containing very large clots of fibrin. A portion of what appeared to be regenerated eighth and ninth ribs was removed and also a portion of the tenth rib, leaving an opening into the thoracic cavity approximately 20 cm. in its longest diameter and 12 cm. in width. The cavity was packed lightly with vaseline gauze. The patient was dismissed from the hospital on the thirteenth postopera-

tive day and returned for daily irrigations and dressings.

On October 8 (one month after the open drainage), the patient reëntered the hospital for further surgical treatment. A large empyema cavity still persisted which extended medially and upward approximately 15 cm. from the anterior and superior border of the edge of the opening to the cavity. A long, slightly curved, linear incision was made along the fifth rib, and a skin flap over the pectoralis major muscle was reflected as far as the midsternal line. The pectoralis major muscle was then dissected from its points of origin and reflected upward and laterally. Portions of what appeared to be the fourth and fifth ribs anterolaterally were removed with the intervening muscle bundle, and by so doing a window was made in the uppermost part of the empyema cavity. Through this window and also through the lower opening, the visceral pleura was cross-hatched according to the method of Ransohoff. The pectoralis major muscle was then brought through this opening into the empyema cavity and held in place by several sutures to the thickened visceral pleura (Fig. 3). The incision over the pectoralis muscle was then closed tightly. Following this procedure the patient was dismissed from the hospital on the thirteenth postoperative day, final surgical dismissal being granted on November 12, slightly more than a month after the second operation. Following the patient's dismissal the wound was irrigated and dressed by his mother, as the patient lived in a sparsely settled part of one of the western states. In her last letter (dated May, 1938) she said that the cavity would hold only a 5-inch strip of gauze. Her son had attended school all winter and felt well.

Comment

These two cases illustrate circumstances in which the use of muscle pedicle grafts are of value in facilitating obliteration of large, chronic, nontuberculous empyema cavities. The procedure is not new, as it was advocated more than twenty years ago by Robinson. As is true of so many worth-while procedures, however, it has gradually fallen into disuse and in recent years has been mentioned only briefly by those interested in this field of surgery. It should not be looked on as a procedure intended to supplant others but rather as one to supplement the surgical armamentarium of those whose responsibility it is to rehabilitate these unfortunate persons as rapidly as possible, and with the minimum deformity and interference with normal function.

References

1. Gray, Henry: Anatomy of the human body. Ed. 21, New York, Lea and Febiger, 1930, pp. 434-435; 430-432.
2. Robinson, Samuel: The treatment of chronic non-tuberculous empyema. Surg., Gynec. and Obst., 22:557-571, (May) 1916.

ACUTE UPPER RESPIRATORY INFECTIONS WITH
GASTRO-INTESTINAL SYMPTOMS*

EDWARD DYER ANDERSON, M.D.

Minneapolis, Minnesota

THE purpose of this paper is to discuss from a strictly clinical standpoint, the gastro-intestinal symptoms which so frequently occur in children with respiratory infections, and in particular the condition which is commonly called "intestinal flu."

It has been known for many years that in children, gastro-intestinal symptoms may be the predominant complaint in various respiratory diseases. In general, the younger the child, the more marked the intestinal symptoms. A child or infant may have anorexia, abdominal pain, vomiting, diarrhea or a combination of these symptoms. They may be mild or severe. A child suffering from an upper respiratory infection ranging in severity from a simple head cold to a lobar pneumonia may show any or all of these gastro-intestinal symptoms.

Whereas in the past, it was assumed that a child showing marked intestinal symptoms had an infection directly involving the gastro-intestinal tract, today we realize that in the majority of instances there is no actual intestinal infection, but rather that the symptoms are brought about by the absorption of toxins from a parenteral infection.

In the most common type of respiratory infection, namely, the simple head cold, the intestinal symptoms vary greatly with the age of the child. In children over two years of age, anorexia is usually the chief and in most instances the only one found. The lack of appetite may be extreme and last for the duration of the cold. If the mother does not force or urge the child to eat more than it wants, the appetite returns when the cold is over and no harm is done. However, if feeding is forced, it may cause a more serious gastro-intestinal disturbance or as so frequently happens, the child may develop a chronic anorexia. I am convinced that many children with persistent poor appetites and poor feeding habits can trace the beginning of their trouble to a simple upper respiratory in-

fection, at which time they were forced and urged to eat when they had no desire for food, by an over-solicitous mother. Their appetite was never allowed to return to normal because of continued forcing of food.

In babies and small children, anorexia is usually a marked symptom accompanying a simple head cold. This is probably due to both absorption of toxins and to the mechanical obstruction of breathing with resultant difficulty in taking food.

Besides anorexia, babies frequently have vomiting, diarrhea and abdominal pain. Allowing the child's appetite to determine the amount of food taken and removing laxative foods from the diet in cases of diarrhea, are usually the only measures needed other than those used for the treatment of the cold. As soon as the cold clears up, the gastro-intestinal symptoms disappear quickly.

In the more severe respiratory infections, such as tonsillitis, grippe, influenza, scarlet fever, measles and pneumonia, the intestinal symptoms are more frequent and severe in all ages of childhood. Abdominal pain is the most frequent symptom. This may vary in intensity from mild abdominal distress to extreme pain which may simulate the pain of appendicitis or even that of intestinal obstruction. The importance of never operating upon a child for appendicitis until one is convinced that the pain is not the result of an upper respiratory infection has been so well and frequently called to our attention by Brennemann and others that I do not feel it necessary to discuss it further in this paper.

I do, however, wish to speak of the opposite phase of this subject. Although much has been written about the danger of operating unnecessarily when the abdominal symptoms are the result of respiratory infections, comparatively little has been said about the great danger of overlooking a surgical abdomen due to a false sense of security when a respiratory infection is present in the patient. When there is evidence of respiratory infection it is very easy for us

*Read before the annual meeting of the Minnesota State Medical Association, Duluth, Minnesota, July 1, 1938.

to become careless and miss an acute appendix or obstruction, because we assume the abdominal symptoms are due to the respiratory infection and we either do not examine the abdomen at all, or, if we do so, do it inadequately. In other words, we must constantly remember that just because a cold, sore throat or other respiratory infection is present, it does not rule out the possibility of a surgical condition also being present in the abdomen. This is particularly true when we realize that there is considerable evidence that acute appendicitis may occur as a direct complication of an upper respiratory infection. Also, the fact that intussusception occurs frequently when diarrhea is present should put us constantly on guard against careless diagnosis.

Although many children have been operated upon unnecessarily for abdominal conditions which did not exist, and in whom an upper respiratory infection was the cause of the symptoms which led to a mistaken diagnosis, nevertheless, I am convinced that many more have been allowed to die because either the parents or physician, or both, have been lulled into a feeling of false security because an upper respiratory infection was present, and have neglected to recognize that an acute abdominal condition also existed. Certainly, every child who has persistent abdominal pain should be examined thoroughly and carefully with the possibility of the presence of both an upper respiratory infection and a surgical condition of the abdomen always in mind.

During the last few years a gastro-intestinal condition has been prevalent at various times which is called by the laity and often by ourselves, "intestinal flu." I am sure we all have a peculiar feeling about this term. When a mother tells me that she thinks her child has intestinal flu I unconsciously squirm, and when I use the term myself I consciously squirm. Undoubtedly, this feeling of apology which most of us have when this term is used is due to the fact that we realize that the name is a misnomer, and also that we of the medical profession know so little about the true etiology, bacteriology and pathology of this condition. Perhaps one should hesitate to discuss a disease about which so little can be offered from a purely scientific standpoint. The fact that one meets it so frequently makes me feel that a clinical discussion is warranted. Although intestinal flu is the most commonly used term, many others have been given to this clinical picture, such as, "intestinal cold," "intestinal grippe," "gastro-enteritis," and finally the one which is perhaps the most accurate but certainly too cumbersome for practical purposes, namely, "an upper respiratory infection with gastro-intestinal symptoms."

In this paper I shall use the term "intestinal flu," simply because it is the one most commonly used, and not because I think it is a scientific or good one. Although we do not definitely know what organism is the cause of this symptom syndrome, what evidence we do have would indicate that it definitely is not caused by the influenza bacillus. The term would also imply that the infection is one of the gastro-intestinal tract itself. There is considerable doubt as to whether there is any actual infection of the intestinal tract but rather that the intestinal symptoms are brought about by absorption of toxins from the upper respiratory tract. Many clinicians and pathologists do not think that the condition is a separate entity in itself but rather that it is an ordinary upper respiratory infection. At the present time I do not think we can say positively that it is a separate entity caused by a specific organism, but nevertheless, the symptoms are so definite and often so severe, and the physical findings so uniform, that from a clinical standpoint it does seem an entity. Whatever the name and whatever the etiology, the fact remains that we are dealing with a disease that is common, troublesome to the patient and one which offers problems both in diagnosis and treatment to the physician. Personally, I feel that it probably is due to a virus closely related to that of the ordinary cold. Until the etiology is definitely determined, this symptom-complex will probably continue to be called "intestinal flu" by the laity and by the majority of physicians.

The symptoms of intestinal flu are varied and give us several types of the disease. The most common type is that in which vomiting is the outstanding feature. Although the onset of the vomiting may be preceded by symptoms of a head cold or a mild sore throat, nausea and vomiting are the first and predominant symptoms in the majority of cases. The onset is sudden and the vomiting severe and frequent Retching continues long after the stomach is empty. This retching will often continue for hours and in some instances for two or three days. The taking of any food or fluid usually aggravates the vomiting. Even small sips of water cause immediate emesis. The child becomes markedly exhausted and if the condition persists long enough may develop dehydration and, in severe cases, acidosis. In the majority of instances the children do not complain of sore throat, but they do have severe headache and often have abdominal cramps, which are particularly severe just before vomiting. Extreme restlessness is frequently present and sleep is fitful and broken. Anorexia is invariably present and is usually extreme. Temperature is generally present and may be high but in the majority of cases is low, varying from 100 to 101 (rectal). The white blood count is usually within normal limits or slightly elevated. Physical examination shows a child with a distressed facial expression and with marked pallor. However, if the vomiting has persisted long enough to cause dehydration the skin may appear flushed. The physical finding almost invariably present is the injection of the veins along and about the pillars of the throat. These dilated veins are also on the back of the pharynx but are particularly noticeable about the pillars. When vomiting persists for several hours one usually finds generalized soreness of the abdominal muscles.

In some cases the course of the disease is short and within a few hours the child feels well, wants to play and his appetite returns. In most instances, however, the nausea and vomiting last from twelve to forty-eight hours. After the nausea stops, anorexia and weakness persists for several days and occasionally the child remains languid, tired and has no appetite for several weeks.

Complications

Acidosis must be watched for and guarded against by the giving of adequate fluids which necessitates at times rectal or subcutaneous administration.

I believe that appendicitis may and does occur in some instances as a direct complication of intestinal flu. In three cases I have seen, I am convinced that acute appendicitis developed on the third or fourth day from the onset. Both because intestinal flu may simulate acute appendicitis and because appendicitis may develop

as a complication, it is imperative that every child with abdominal pain and vomiting should be carefully watched.

Various forms of treatment are advocated in the vomiting type of intestinal flu. Personally, I have found the following the most satisfactory procedure. All food is withheld until the child acts hungry and demands food. Until there has been no vomiting for twenty-four hours the only food given is gelatin, jello, dry toast or soda crackers, dry puffed rice or wheat or unbuttered popcorn. The youngster is also allowed to suck pure stick candy.

When there has been no vomiting for twenty-four hours, broth, soft boiled or poached egg, and cooked cereal are added. If no vomiting occurs for another twenty-four hours, the child is allowed to have his regular diet if he desires. At no time is he urged to eat.

In small infants breast milk or milk mixtures diluted to half of the regular strength are given at the regular feeding intervals if the baby wants food.

When the child cannot retain plain water, the only liquids given by mouth are French Vichy water or ginger ale until there has been no vomiting for twenty-four hours. These are given cool and in small amounts. When there has been no vomiting for twelve hours, plain water is given if the child prefers. Milk is not given until vomiting has ceased for at least forty-eight hours. If there is considerable dehydration or any evidence of threatened acidosis, fluid is given rectally or subcutaneously.

The drug which has been found most useful in combating excessive vomiting is chloral hydrate given by rectum. If given long enough and in dosage sufficient to keep the child quiet and resting for twenty-four hours, in the majority of cases the chloral can be discontinued and the vomiting will not recur if the proper diet is given and no effort is made to force the child to eat. Chloral hydrate per rectum is also very effective in relieving the abdominal pain which is so often present.

There are a considerable number of children suffering from the vomiting type of intestinal flu who get over the acute nausea after two or three days, but who do not seem to completely recover. Their appetite does not come back, and they appear languid and tired. Many of them will have abdominal cramps from time to time.

This chronic condition may go on for weeks. In these children the giving of acidophilus bacilli in the form of acidophilus milk or as a straight culture will usually quickly restore them to their normal condition. The child is kept in bed until all acute symptoms have subsided. This chronic type so frequently develops as a sequel of the acute form, that I routinely give my patients some form of acidophilus bacilli for a week, starting as soon as the nausea has stopped.

A second type of intestinal flu is that in which diarrhea is the outstanding feature. The diarrhea may vary greatly in severity. The majority of children have frequent stools for from twelve to thirty-six hours, at the end of which time the stools return to normal in a comparatively short time. In some instances the diarrhea may be severe, last for several days and may lead to marked dehydration and even severe acidosis. The stools may vary in number from four to twenty in twenty-four hours. They are watery and have considerable mucus. Blood is rarely seen and, if present, is in the form of small flecks. The stools are usually light in color. They have a foul odor and tend to cause marked excoriation of the buttocks. Cramps are almost invariably present and are severe. Tenesmus is a frequent symptom. Anorexia in most instances is severe. Headache is more common than in the vomiting type. Weakness and restlessness develop in the severe cases. The outstanding physical finding is the same as in the vomiting type, namely, injection of the veins about the pillars of the throat and pharynx. Generalized abdominal soreness is usually present. Temperature may be absent or may be high, but in most instances is from 100 to 102 (rectal).

The treatment I have found most satisfactory is as follows: The child is kept in bed until all acute symptoms have subsided. If nausea is not present, fluids, with the exception of fruit juices, are given by mouth in large amounts. If unable to retain fluids by mouth or if an adequate amount cannot be given to guard against excessive dehydration and acidosis, subcutaneous fluid is given. Food is given if the patient is not

nauseated and wishes to eat. Any simple food is given with the exception of those which are laxative. If chloral hydrate can be retained by rectum it is given to relieve the abdominal cramps. If it cannot be retained and no nausea is present, paregoric by mouth is usually effective. If neither of these can be retained, and the cramps are severe, codeine is given hypodermically. Because of a marked tendency for these children to develop a chronic condition of poor appetite and fatigue following the diarrheal type of intestinal flu, I routinely give them some form of acidophilus bacilli for at least one week. This seems to prevent the occurrence of a prolonged convalescence.

In a considerable percentage of cases of intestinal flu, the patient has both nausea and diarrhea. In these cases the prostration tends to be greater and the danger of acidosis is increased. Subcutaneous fluid often has to be given. The dietary regime is the same as outlined above and codeine by hypodermic may be used to control the restlessness, pain and excessive vomiting. Acidophilus bacilli given by mouth as soon as the nausea stops seems to hasten complete recovery.

Another type of intestinal flu is occasionally seen in which neither vomiting nor diarrhea are present, but in which abdominal cramps, which may be frequent and severe, are the only symptoms. The cramps may persist for many days. The throat findings are the same as previously described. There is usually temperature, and chloral hydrate per rectum is the most effective way of controlling the pain. Acidophilus bacilli given by mouth for several days is of value.

Summary

Attention is called to the frequency with which gastro-intestinal symptoms occur in children who have respiratory infections. The importance of examining all children having abdominal pain or vomiting, for both respiratory infections and surgical conditions of the abdomen, is emphasized. The symptomatology, physical findings and treatment of the condition called "intestinal flu" are discussed.

SOLITARY DIVERTICULITIS OF THE CECUM*

W. N. GRAVES, A.B., M.D., F.A.C.S.

Duluth, Minnesota

IT is not my intention to discuss diverticulitis of the colon in general but rather to confine my remarks to inflammatory conditions of solitary diverticuli of the cecum, an entity confused with and encountered in the operation for that most common surgical emergency, appendicitis. I have been able to find only twenty-three such cases in the accessible literature, to which I wish to add the accounts of two cases occurring at identical sites on the cecum in two members of one family, a father and daughter.

Case 1.—Mrs. R. L. C. was seen on December 29, 1936, complaining of pain in the right lower abdomen. This began two nights before as generalized abdominal pain and became localized the following morning. The pain was dull and intermittent and was aggravated by change of position, walking, etc. There was no nausea or vomiting. For two or more years there had been soreness in the right loin but there had never been any severe attacks. She did notice, however, that the pain was worse on fatigue. Constipation was never a prominent symptom but she had been troubled for some years with "gaseous indigestion." Otherwise her past and family history were irrelevant except that eight years prior to this I operated upon her father for suppurative diverticulitis of the cecum, which case will be included in this report.

Physical examination revealed an adult female aged forty-nine. Findings were limited to a marked tenderness at McBurney's point extending upwards along the crest of the ilium. Muscle spasm was present over this area. No mass could be definitely outlined though there was a suggestion of it above the iliac crest. Vaginal examination was negative except for tenderness high in the right fornix. The temperature was 100 degrees F. Blood examination revealed 20,000 leukocytes. The urine examination was negative.

The pre-operative diagnosis was acute gangrenous appendicitis. Under cyclopropane and ether anesthesia, a right rectus incision was made. Upon opening the peritoneum free fluid was encountered. The appendix was markedly injected and edematous. It was removed in the usual manner and the stump invaginated. On the lateral surface of the cecum, opposite the ileocecal valve, was a severely injected, hard mass about one-half the size of a golf ball, covered with adherent omentum. No dimple could be palpated in this mass and it was thought to be either a phlegmon, diverticulum, or tumor. The attached omentum was ligated and transected and the mass delivered into the wound. There was

marked edema of the greater portion of the cecal wall and because primary excision would have necessitated removing almost all of the anterior and lateral walls, it was entirely extraperitonealized by suture of the visceral and parietal peritoneum. Vaseline gauze was applied and the wound left open. Six days later the mass was removed by means of the endotherm knife. In cutting through edematous serosa and muscularis, the mucosa appeared normal and uninvolved. Therefore, the dissection was carried just outside the mucosa until the center of the mass was reached, when it was found that the mucosa invaginated into the mass. At this time a definite diagnosis of diverticulitis was made. The mucosa was ligated and invaginated with a purse-string suture. The muscularis and serosa were sutured over the stump and the wound closed with drainage. Convalescence was normal except for mild infection of the wound and no fistula resulted.

The pathological report as given by Dr. G. L. Berdez was as follows: "This is a specimen measuring 5.4 by 5 by 3 cm. The external surface is quite congested and shows in places fibrino-purulent deposits. The surface shows also a somewhat irregular opening measuring up to .4 cm. in diameter leading into a diverticulum; the cavity of the diverticulum is almost spherical, measuring up to 1.2 cm. in diameter, and is filled with fecal material and fetid purulent exudate. The internal surface of the diverticulum is lined by mucosa; in the distal extremity the diverticulum shows a small perforation which leads into the surrounding adipose and scar tissue. A large mass of quite edematous and congested adipose tissue, which shows several scar-like areas, is connected with the external wall of the diverticulum and forms the main part of the specimen.

"Microscopically the internal surface of the diverticulum is lined by mucosa having the structure of the mucosa of the large intestine. The lumina of some of the glandular tubules are dilated and filled with polymorphonuclear leukocytes. At one place the mucosa is ulcerated; the defect is lined with a mass of fibrino-leukocytic exudate. The deeper layers of the wall of the diverticulum are formed mainly by a mass of moderately cellular, partly new formed, connective tissue. The muscularis mucosæ can still be recognized in those parts of the diverticulum which are still represented in places. At other places of the wall of the diverticulum, the muscular layers cannot be demonstrated.

"Diagnosis: Diverticulum of the cecum with chronic inflammatory changes and acute exacerbation."

Gross and microscopic examination was also made of the appendix, which showed marked, diffuse congestion. The proximal half of the lumen contained purulent mucous material and the mucosa was congested and edematous. The distal half was thickened and

*Read before the Duluth Surgical Society, November 18, 1937.

fibrous and obliterated by a mass of scar-like fibrous tissue. Dr. Berdez' diagnosis was "chronic appendicitis with acute exacerbation."

Since her recovery, Dr. J. R. McNutt, radiologist, examined the colon fluoroscopically and by radiograms and no other diverticuli or abnormality was found in the entire large bowel.

Case 2.—Mr. W. R. S. was seen August 30, 1929, because of pain in the right lower quadrant which had persisted for thirty-six hours. There was no nausea or vomiting. He had many complaints which were not referable to his abdomen but were due to degenerative changes accompanying old age.

Physical examination revealed a white male, aged 69, very obese, and apparently suffering considerable pain. Essential findings were in the right lower quadrant, where there was a marked tenderness and rigidity of all the muscles. There was a suggestion of a mass but it could not be definitely outlined due to the large amount of adipose tissue present. His temperature was 100.8 degrees F.; pulse 100; leukocytes numbered 19,200.

Under spinal anesthesia, with a pre-operative diagnosis of acute appendicitis, the abdomen was opened through a right rectus incision. A mass the size of a baseball was delivered which involved the cecum, appendix and omentum. In the center of this mass was an abscess surrounding an inflamed, perforated diverticulum on the lateral surface of the cecum. The appendix was removed but was intact. Drains were inserted to the site of the diverticulum and also extraperitoneally. Convalescence was marred by development of fecal fistula and other complications incident to his heart and other organs, but he eventually recovered.

The postoperative diagnosis was intra-abdominal abscess due to suppurative diverticulitis. The pathologist reported only fibrous appendicitis.

Unfortunately, there was never a colon study made to prove that this was a solitary diverticulum but none were seen at the time of operation.

In summarizing the twenty-five reported cases, thirteen were in females averaging in age 44.1 years, the most common age incidence in this group being between 45 and 60. Twelve were males averaging 38.1 years in age. The condition occurred most commonly between the ages of twenty and thirty-five. The youngest was a female, aged 3, and the oldest a male, aged 69. The pre-operative diagnosis was acute appendicitis in all cases except one, which from previous barium study was diagnosed carcinoma of the cecum. In analyzing the symptoms of the reported cases, the chief complaint in all the patients was pain in the right lower abdomen of a few hours to a few days duration, accompanied by nausea and vomiting in 50 per cent of the cases. Two of these patients gave histories of almost continuous aching in this region and four

had complained of flatulent dyspepsia for years. The findings common to appendicitis which were noted in this series were: fever varying from 99 to 102 degrees F. in 74 per cent of the cases; rigidity and tenderness, either together or singly, in all but three cases. The average leukocyte count taken in six cases was 18,381, a somewhat higher average than is usually seen in acute appendictis.

The operations done were as follows:

Primary diverticulectomy........ 9
Delayed diverticulectomy......... 1
Invagination 2
Ileocolectomy or cecectomy....... 12
Drainage of abscess............. 1

In the cases in which primary diverticulectomy was done, the condition was recognized as a diverticulum by palpation of a dimple within the bowel, or by noting a concretion, or the mass was assumed to be a small tumor or inflammatory area surrounding an ulcer. The delayed operation was explained in my case above.

In the two cases in which invagination was done, the diverticulum in one was pea sized; the other was three-fourths of an inch in diameter and after extruding a concretion there was little induration present, making invagination the most logical procedure.

The more radical operations of ileocolectomy or cecectomy were done because the condition was mistaken for carcinoma, tuberculosis, tumor or ulcer. The case in which drainage was done has already been explained.

Mortality: All patients recovered except that of Portier, in which it was thought pre-operatively that there was a carcinoma of the cecum present and a resection of the right colon was done, the patient dying from gangrene of the gut.

Comment: There is much conjecture about the cause of solitary diverticuli of the cecum. Greensfelder and Hiller theorize on the origin as follows: "We should like to suggest another possibility, though a congenital one, as a factor; namely, the retention in some residual form of the appendix, which appears early in embryological life but normally disappears before the true appendix develops." In a study covering 5,385 major operations and 400 adult autopsies, they were able to find four cases of small traumatic diverticuli occurring after purse-string suture during appendectomy.

One must allow the possibility that solitary diverticuli of the cecum may be congenital in origin rather than acquired, which is the generally accepted opinion. In twenty-three of these twenty-five cases found in the literature no diverticuli were evident in other parts of the colon. According to Bargen, diverticulosis of the colon occurs most commonly between the ages of fifty-five and fifty-nine and rarely under thirty. The average age of this series was 41.2 years with 36 per cent under thirty. He also states that the incidence ratio of diverticulitis of the colon of males to females is 2.75:1. This series shows slightly greater occurrence in the female. All muscle layers were found microscopically in nine of the fourteen above cases in which studies were done, and the appendix was present in all cases. To the reported cases may be added the two here reported with diverticuli occurring opposite the ileocecal valve in two members of the same family, a father and daughter.

Summary

1. Many solitary diverticuli of the cecum are probably congenital but acquired diverticuli may follow ulcerative processes or surgical trauma.

2. They occur in a much younger age group than does diverticulosis of the colon in general.

3. Solitary diverticulitis of the cecum presents practically the same symptoms and findings as acute appendicitis.

4. The condition should be sought for and when found, invagination or primary diverticulectomy performed if possible.

5. In the presence of marked induration of the cecum delayed extraperitoneal diverticulectomy is a safe and desirable procedure.

6. Suppurative diverticulitis of the cecum may be mistaken for appendiceal abscess.

7. The fact that Bennett-Jones found three cases in one hospital within three months, that Weible was able to report two cases, that I have encountered two cases, leads me to believe that solitary diverticulitis of the cecum is not as rare as a review of the literature would suggest.

Bibliography

1. Bargen, J. A.: Diverticulosis and Diverticulitis of Colon. Cyclopedia of Medicine. Revision Service F. A. Davis Company, pp. 109-112, 1937.
2. Bennett-Jones, M. J.: Primary solitary diverticulitis of cecum: Report on 3 cases with review of 17 recorded cases. Brit. Jour. Surg., 25:66, 1937.
3. Epstein, S. E.: Diverticulitis of the cecum. Am. Jour. Surg., 22:276, 1933.
4. Greensfelder, L. A., and Hiller, R. L.: Cecal diverticulosis with special reference to traumatic diverticula. Surg., Gyn. and Obst., 46:786, 1929.
5. Klages, F.: Akute Entzündung eines isolierten Blinddarmdivertikils unter dem Bilde der Wurmfortsatzentzundung. Zentralbl. f. Chir., 64:1090-1093, (May) 1937.
6. Portier, M. F.: Enteroliths and diverticula. Surg., Gyn. and Obst., 45:185, 1925.
7. Weible, R. E.: Diverticulitis of the colon. Minnesota Medicine, 20:21, 1937.

FUNDAMENTALS IN THE SURGICAL TREATMENT OF COLON DISORDERS*

LAWRENCE M. LARSON, M.D., F.A.C.S.
Clinical Instructor in Surgery, University of Minnesota
Minneapolis, Minnesota

SURGICAL procedures on the large bowel remain some of the most difficult of all operations in which not only to obtain satisfactory end-results but also to establish a definite standardization of technic to fit all cases. Many factors tend to produce such a condition. In colonic malignancies the concomitance of obstruction, debilitation, cachexia, anemia, and the imminence of infection, peritonitis, and hemorrhage makes any surgical attack on the large bowel an extremely hazardous maneuver. In recent years, following studies of the physiology and pathology of the large intestine, the actual technic of colon surgery has been proved to be of no more importance than the pre-operative and postopera-

tive management these individuals receive. It is with this factor in mind as well as with accurate conception of the anatomy, pathology, and physiology of the lesions that affect the colon that this paper is concerned.

Several points in the anatomy and physiology of the colon are worth of emphasis. When one considers the function of the large bowel it becomes apparent that the organ is distinctly a double one. The proximal half is an absorptive organ and it acts in a manner similar to the small gut. Embryologically this is in keeping with the fact that the proximal half of the colon of the adult, along with that portion of the small bowel distal to the papilla of Vater, is derived from the mid-gut of the fetus. Furthermore, the superior mesenteric artery supplies the proximal

*Presented before the Upper Mississippi Medical Society at Cass Lake, July 31, 1937.

half of the colon while the inferior mesenteric artery supplies the distal half of the colon. These factors operate to produce a definite bilaterality to the colon which is furthermore reflected on the physiology of the organ. The left or distal half of the large gut has little to do with absorption, a function which is possessed by the right half, but here the bowel is concerned entirely with storage, propulsion, and expulsion of the feces. Evolution of the form and contour of the walls of the colon give further substantiation of this fact, since the proximal colon has thin walls, its lumen is large and movements here are rapid, small, churning ones. In the left side the walls are thick and muscular, the lumen is small and movements are strong, prolonged contractions which propel the contents onward to empty the colon. When disease, such as a malignant growth, attacks this organ there is consequently a difference in the effects which the lesion produces, depending on its location in the bowel. Therefore when we find an individual harboring a carcinoma of the right colon, the symptoms are most likely to be those of disturbance of physiologic equilibrium, resulting in anemia, weakness, loss of weight and so forth, yet accompanied by no visible loss of blood. The exact explanation of this anemia and weakness is not known but it probably is due to a perverted function of the mucous membrane so that abnormal absorption of toxic products in the bowel takes place.

In the left half of the colon, obstruction is the predominant symptom and this symptom results from a combination of three factors. Here the bowel content is hard and relatively incompressible, the majority of carcinomata in this location are the scirrhous encircling type and consequently obstruction takes place early. Lastly, here movements are strong and prolonged. The symptoms, therefore, are pain, tumefaction, and alternating periods of diarrhea and constipation along with flatulence and borborygmi. Finally one of the phases of complete obstruction takes place. Thus it is seen that the anatomical and physiological differences in the two arms of the large bowel play a part in determining the type and extent of the surgery which one may safely do in various parts of the colon. Probably of no less importance are these differences in making decisions as to details of pre-operative and postoperative management.

First of all it should be emphasized that malignant lesions of the bowel are, in general, slow growing, they metastasize late and, if obstruction, exhaustion or concomitant disease does not supervene, good results may be expected from removal of the lesion. This fact has been proved by studies in which individuals dying of malignant tumors of the bowel at autopsy show metastases in surprisingly few cases. In fact, of 210 cases so studied, extension or metastases was found in only half of them, and liver metastases in only a third.

Another point of importance to remember is that diagnosis of these lesions is not, in the majority of cases, difficult. The use of the barium enema, especially with the aid of the double contrast method, has resulted in great accuracy as to the type and location of the lesion as well as its size and operability. Roentgen-ray methods along with the use of the proctoscope and sigmoidoscope should render diagnosis possible in most cases. More than half of the carcinomata involving the entire colon can be visualized by direct inspection through the sigmoidoscope or proctoscope, a fact which has been substantiated by necropsy studies of 210 individuals who died of this disease. Thus by simple means, which can be carried out in the office, it is possible to actually visualize a large percentage of these tumors.

In the pre-operative and postoperative management of individuals harboring diseases of the colon, all measures are directed toward producing and maintaining physiologic rest of the bowel so that healing without complications may be facilitated. Pre-operatively, a diet low in residue, emptying of the bowel of gas and fecal content by properly controlled cathartics, cleansing enemas, and final intestinal sedation along with supportive measures intended to improve the patient's general condition, are all intended to have the bowel at the time of the operation empty, collapsed, quiet and clean. Postoperatively, we have routinely employed, to very great advantage, continuous nasal catheter suction siphonage to prevent the entrance of air into the intestinal tract, a procedure which eliminates, to a large extent, any gaseous distention and consequent aggravation of peristalsis. After distention, nausea and vomiting have occurred, they can be relieved by this suction method but ileus is much more easily prevented than relieved. It should be kept in mind that the extent of surgical trauma within the peritoneal cavity, the length of anesthesia and the general condition of the patient are other factors which determine the degree of ileus to be expected postoperatively. Morphine in frequent moderate doses has a beneficial effect because of its property of relieving pain, restlessness, thirst and apprehension, as well as its ability to increase intestinal tone. Its tonic effect results in maintainance of the proper absorptive function of the bowel so that toxemia is definitely lessened, since it has been proved that distention of the gut is notably accompanied by absorption of toxic products. Constipation often accompanies the use of morphine and is most likely the result of inhibition of the defecating reflex, accompanied by increase of tone of the sphincters. A compensatory diarrhea frequently develops after withdrawal of morphine and its mechanism is obvious. The most important factor in prevention of intestinal activity is the withholding of food and fluids by mouth. In our opinion, with the act of swallowing, even though it may be only a small amount of water, and especially with the ingestion of any solid food, a peristaltic wave is initiated which usually travels the entire course of the intestinal tract down to the anus. This increased activity is prone to spread any inflammatory process which may be present in the peritoneal cavity. When the propulsive power of the bowel has been regained—as evidenced by motility of gases in the abdomen, gurgling, movements, and so forth—fluids and, later, food may be administered orally. These measures, along with heat to the abdomen, are an excellent stimulus to complete recovery of normal bowel activity.

It is best, in any patient who goes without ingestion of fluids and foods for any length of time, to stimulate flow of saliva, especially from the parotic gland, by use of chewing gum, or the sucking of a lemon. This definitely lessens the incidence of postoperative parotitis. In brief, the less the swallowing, the less the peristaltic activity initiated.

Fluids, combined with saline or glucose, or both, in these cases are best administered through the intravenous route, less satisfactorily by means of hypodermoclysis. Proctoclysis, of course, in any type of colon operation is contraindicated since fluid given by this method can only be absorbed by being carried into the right colon. This could only be accomplished by reverse peristalsis, which, of course, would delay healing.

The factors mentioned have for their purpose primarily the promotion of local healing in the bowel by quieting peristalsis and increasing the tone of the bowel, but, of course, measures which increase the general resistance and condition of the patient must not be neglected, such as transfusions, large amounts of parenteral fluids, and so forth. In the immediate convalescence of the patient, after four or five days, it is wise to start, very judiciously, the use of clear fluids, then soft foods and finally, as determined by the tolerance of the patient, a diet high in calories and vitamins, but low in residue. As time goes on, the patient will find out for himself the type of food best suited to his needs.

It is thus evident that, because of the bifunctional nature of the large intestine, most diseases, especially those of a surgical nature, should be regarded differently, depending upon the location in the colon of the lesion. This especially is true when one comes to a consideration of problems involved in resections of the colon. In the distal portion of the large gut, it is usually much more dangerous to resect a segment and make a primary anastomosis in one stage than it is to first employ a drainage operation, such as a colostomy or cecostomy, and sidetrack the fecal current. On the other hand, it is relatively safer, in right colon lesions, to do a short-circuiting operation and in addition to resect the diseased area at one sitting, depending, of course, to a large extent, on the general condition of the patient and characteristics of the lesion. The factor of obstruction is rarely encountered when considering the treatment of lesions in the proximal colon. Aside from the question of relieving obstruction in left colon lesions, and of doing graded operations where the general condition of the patient comes into consideration, there still is another factor of which cognizance is not often taken. This is as described as follows.

Peristaltic movements of the distal colon, as well as anatomical conformations of this portion of the gut, are of a distinctly different nature than those of the right colon and small bowel. In the distal large bowel, the thick muscular walls have for their purpose forceful, strong movements which are distinctly prolonged and are made under considerable tension. In fact, tonus waves here may last as long as ten to fifteen minutes. In addition there are superimposed on these long contractions smaller contractions often lasting one to two minutes. Thus it is evident that, with such prolonged tension on an anastomosis, healing would be very difficult, largely because of the local ischemia which is produced. This is further evidence as to the value of preliminary colostomy (Larson and Bargen). Furthermore, the contents of the left colon are rather hard and incompressible, and this condition, combined with relative fixation of the mesentery, tends to favor pulling apart the suture lines of an anastomosis. The blood supply in this region is not as abundant as it is in the small bowel, another factor tending to retard healing, since any tension on suture lines results in further ischemia of anastomosed margins and gives increased chance for infections to gain headway. Consequently there is a greater possibility of failure of the tissue to heal. If a preliminary drainage has been done, resection of a segment of bowel followed by anastomosis is more liable to heal satisfactorily for several reasons. The first, of course, is the side-tracking of the fecal current and the decompression of the bowel. Secondly, since a certain amount of peristaltic motion of the bowel is due to impulses traveling along the muscular layers, interruptions of these muscular fibers by cutting across the bowel in making a colostomy results in many of these waves being stopped and they cannot jump from the proximal to the distal bowel. This has the effect of keeping the side-tracked loop of gut much more quiet with consequent avoidance of tension on suture lines. It is, of course, true that the latter segment contains no fecal material and that it can be cleansed readily

so that inflammatory reactions may subside and exudates may be absorbed, but the factor of inactivity is, likewise, an important one in successful promotion of healing.

It is true that the mesenteric nerves (sympathetic fibers), which run along the blood vessel, do reach the bowel wall regardless of interruption of continuity of the gut, as demonstrated in a previously published communication (Larson and Bargen). However, the main motor nerve to the colon, the pelvic nerve (or nervi erigentes), supplies only the distal portion of the left colon and this nerve plexus lies on the surface of the bowel wall between the muscular layers. Consequently, it is readily understandable why motor impulses through the gut are interrupted by section of the bowel. When reëstablishment of the continuity of the bowel is again made, coördination of the intestinal movements is usually resumed in a relatively short time with no particular difficulty, although it is rather common to find some difficulty in bowel habits is experienced for some time. A parallel situation exists in many cases of local pain occurring postoperatively after appendectomy. It is usually true, when recurrent pains are present for a time after removal of the appendix, that adhesions are considered to be the source of this embarrassing discomfort, and this is no doubt possible in many instances. On the other hand, I am convinced that, in many instances, this pain is due to interference with conductivity of nerve impulses through muscle tissue, resulting from the removal of the appendix. This has the effect of temporarily producing stasis in the proximal cecum, or at least an incoördinated motility in this region, so that pain, flatulence and other symptoms result. These symptoms frequently continue for varying lengths of time, until reëstablishment of normal motility has been made.

Dangers of Protamine Insulins

Reports of reactions following the use of protamine zinc insulin have appeared in considerable number. In one of the earlier discussions of protamine zinc insulin it was reported that hypoglycemia from this type is more subtle in onset and on the whole subjective symptoms are less severe than with soluble insulin. Preliminary symptoms of shakiness, sweating and palpitation may be absent; thus severe hypoglycemic symptoms may appear without warning. Ample evidence is now available that protamine zinc insulin is not a foolproof substitute for the older preparation. Although reactions to it seem to appear with less frequency, they also are often characterized by the suddenness of onset, delayed and therefore unexpected appearance, and symptoms precipitated by exercise at such a distant time as also to be wholly unexpected. Although the development of protamine zinc insulin is an advance of unquestioned value to many diabetic patients, the possibilities of delayed severe reactions cannot be ignored. (J.A.M.A., July 16, 1938, p. 254.)

PRACTICAL PHYSIOLOGY OF THE NOSE*

HAROLD I. LILLIE, M.D.

Rochester, Minnesota

W HEN it is realized that the nose is the
only portion of the body that cannot be
appropriately protected from the environment
to which it is subjected, it will be appreciated
that in order to withstand the exposure to which
it is subjected, it must have a wonderfully adaptable functional mechanism. For that reason it
is important that fundamentals of the physiology
of the nose be known, because in daily practice
many patients are encountered who complain of
symptoms referable to the upper part of the
respiratory tract, which, on final analysis, are
not symptoms of pathologic change, but may be
explained as evidences of normal physiologic
response of the structures to changes in environment.

The details of the function of these structures
are not thoroughly understood by many practitioners, and apparently are not known by the
laity. This is largely attributable to the fact
that, in medical curriculums of the past and
present, very little mention is made, and little
attention paid, to the part that the upper portion
of the respiratory tract plays in respiration and
to the effect of this function on the general
well-being of the individual. Careful study has
been made by research workers on the physiologic processes referable to the special senses,
olfaction, taste, and so forth, and, in turn, this
knowledge has been passed on to patients. Patients do not understand how the nose and throat
would be expected to function under certain environmental conditions, and they, therefore, complain of symptoms which, in reality, are of no
more consequence than other physiologic bodily
reactions which seem commonplace to them, such
as sweating, chilling, sunburning or tanning.
Usually, when the symptoms are explained on
this basis, the patients are relieved and satisfied.

It is generally considered that the first serious
attempt accurately to describe the anatomy and
physiology of the nose can be credited to Galen,
who lived in the second century A.D. Hippocrates and Aristotle had thought that the reason
the nasal interior was moist was that the secre-

tions came from the brain through the cribriform
plate of the ethmoid bone. Galen subscribed to
this idea. He thought that the nasal membranes
were bloodless but he recognized that they were
continuous with those of the pharynx and mouth.
That the nasal membranes contained secreting
glands was not recognized until the time of
Schneider. To his credit, Galen said that the
function of the nasal interior was to prevent the
air from entering the trachea, directly, "First,
because the air surrounding us is at times quite
cold and the lungs then would be chilled; and,
secondly, because small particles of dust or of
ashes or anything of this kind may not fall into
the trachea."

It was in the sixteenth century that open revolt against the previously accepted ideas of Galen
occurred. Among the revolters was Vesalius, a
Belgian, who had that attribute of genius described by Carlyle as the ability to see with one's
eyes and the inability not to believe what one
sees. However, Vesalius, in his observations of
the anatomy of the nose and throat, committed
more errors than he corrected.

Contemporaneously with Schneider, Willis felt
that the fluids in the nose came through the
nerves, which he considered to be tubes coming
from the brain. Van Ruysch believed that nasal secretions came directly through arterioles
and he did not accept the ideas on intermediary
effect of glands. Schneider, in the middle of
the seventeenth century, wrote voluminously. He
showed that secretions in the nose could not
come from the brain, through the cribriform
plate of the ethmoid bone or lacerated foramina,
or through the nerves because they are imper-
vious. He found that mucus could be squeezed
out of living or dead membranes but did not
mention glands. It was Steno who first described mucous glands. Following introduction
of the microscope and discovery of methods of
preparing tissue for microscopic study, great
strides were made.

Rhinology has made great progress in the past
quarter century and, fortunately for patients,
is now practiced on a more conservative and
scientific basis than before. Formerly it

*From the Section on Otolaryngology and Rhinology, The
Mayo Clinic, Rochester, Minnesota.

was largely practiced on a purely anatomic basis, and, in consequence, many patients underwent very destructive intranasal operations without their symptoms being relieved. This practice led, as Stein[16] said, to adding many new symptoms to the old. In the future, we may look for the application of more physiologic facts and, as experience grows, we may learn to see the patient as a whole rather than through the "hole" of the nasal speculum.

The function of the nose has been said to be fourfold: to warm, to moisten and to filter the inspired air, and to smell. The efficiency of each of these processes depends, largely, on the function of the vasomotor control. The special sense, olfaction, will not be considered.

General Fundamental Aspects

Certain individuals can be identified easily by the particular conformation of their noses. In fact, in police work, the nose has been used for this purpose. A well-functioning nose may not necessarily be a thing of beauty but it is a joy forever. It would be difficult to describe the external appearance of the nose in words, and rather difficult to describe its position on the face. All noses of men have one common characteristic: the openings are more nearly on the horizontal than on the vertical plane, when one lives an upright life. There seems to be a natural reason for this, the directing of the air currents into the intranasal structures, or real functioning region. To be sure, a person may live his allotted life breathing through the mouth, but he will not live so comfortably under all environments. Patients are also known to have lived twenty years breathing through a tracheotomy tube.

The indications of the nasal fossa in the embryo appear as pits, situated on either side of the anterior portion of the head, and are first seen at about the twenty-first day, the same time that the eyeball and ear vesicles appear. As development takes place, these nasal pits fuse.[10] Intranasally, the nose is divided by the septum, which is scarcely ever perfectly straight, into nearly equal cavities, opening anteriorly through the vestibule and posteriorly into the pharynx through the choana. From the lateral wall project the three turbinate bones, thereby enlarging the available surface exposure, and helping to direct the air currents within the nose. Beneath each turbinate is situated the so-called

meatus, of which the middle meatus is the most important because in it, protected by the middle turbinate, is situated the hiatus semilunaris, with the openings to the paranasal sinuses. The inferior turbinate is normally the largest and tapers toward each end. Under it is the opening for the lacrimal duct. The intranasal cavity narrows as it approaches its upper extent. That portion of the nose which is below the level of the superior border of the middle turbinate may be said to be respiratory in function, and that above, olfactory. From the choana, the air enters the pharynx.

Histologically, the upper part of the respiratory tract may be said to be lined by the same type of membrane and substructures, except that in certain situations certain characteristics predominate. For instance, the mucosa is relatively thicker over the turbinates than it is in any of the other portions of the tract, and in the ethmoid cells it is relatively very thin. The lining mucous membrane is very vascular and is inseparably united with the periosteum and perichondrium over which it lies.

The blood supply comes largely from the sphenopalatine artery, which anastomoses with the ethmoidal, external nasal, septal and palatine arteries and with those which supply the lower part of the nasolacrimal duct. This network of vessels occupies the deepest regions of the mucosa and the periosteum. The veins empty into the facial veins largely but from the ethmoidal region they communicate with the venous plexus through the cribriform plate. The veins which arise around the lacrimal sac and duct empty into the orbital veins, and into those of the face around the orbit. The lymphatics are subepithelial and large.

The respiratory membrane is supplied with cavernous blood spaces of erectile tissue. The arterioles are supplied with a muscular layer and, from their deep situation, take a corkscrew course toward the surface and the venous sinuses, the latter of which may be of considerable size and so much enlarged in the mucosa when it is the site of inflammatory change, that it is often difficult to judge what is abnormal Development of the erectile tissue has a close relationship with the beginning of sexual life since it is seen in its full extent only after adolescence has been established, and it begins to atrophy after middle life. This fact is of definite clinical importance in everyday practice.

The capillaries are distributed everywhere through the connective tissue of the mucosa. Tiny capillary twigs are in contact with the basal layer of the glandular epithelium, and Wright[17] has said that it is possible to see direct diapedesis of the leukocytes through the capillary walls and between the gland cells, into the lumina of the acini. There is every reason to believe that in this way the blood vessels may empty the serous and leukocytic elements of the blood directly into the glands. Vasomotor dilatation, therefore, means not only exudation of the serum of the blood vessels into the stroma, and consequent swelling of it, but simultaneously a direct discharge into the glands and onto the surface of the mucosa. Around the ducts of the glands, the mouths of which usually lie in some sulcus of the surface epithelium, there is a more or less thick network of capillaries. It is seen, then, that vasomotor dilatation of these capillaries would mean considerable constriction of the outlets of the glands. As the vasomotor excitement subsides, this constriction is released and free discharge of the content of the seromucous glands is afforded.

The contractile elements of the stroma are composed of elastic tissue and smooth muscle fibers. It will be recalled that attention was drawn to the erectile tissue and to sexual development, and it becomes clinically important that this be recognized, for it accounts for many of the so-called "stuffy noses" so often seen in adolescence and newly married couples. Innervation of these substructures comes from the parasympathetic nerves through the sphenopalatine ganglion and, as knowledge of the sympathetic nervous system and its substructures increases, it will be possible to deal more intelligently with the various syndromes that are attributable to derangement of the vasomotor control. The elastic elements are important because of the effect that repeated inflammatory reactions may have on them. Thick interlacing bundles, running parallel with the planes of the one, are demonstrable. In the same manner, the smooth muscle cells of the blood vessels are important because of the effect that repeated inflammatory reactions, resulting in enlargements, may have on the caliber and function of the blood vessels.

The sensory nerve supply comes largely from the fifth cranial nerve. The activating nervous

impulses that control what might be called the automatic responses of the nasal membranes, come through two sets of antagonistic autonomic nerves, the vasoconstrictors and the vasodilators. The vasoconstrictor fibers arise from the preganglionic fibers from the central nervous system and the postganglionic fibers from the cells of the sympathetic ganglions. These nerves exert a constant tonic effect. The efferent fibers which cause vasoconstriction are called "pressor" fibers and those that cause vasodilatation are called "depressor" fibers. The vasoconstrictors arise chiefly from the cervical sympathetic nerves. Hempstead[7] has observed marked congestion of the nasal membranes of patients who have been subjected to removal of the cervical ganglions for certain vasospastic conditions of the upper extremities.

It is known that the caliber of the blood vessels is influenced by agents other than the vasoconstrictor and vasodilator fibers. Chemical substances, carbon dioxide, histamine and lactic acid, Bayliss[2] has shown, may produce vasodilatation. Internal secretions, such as epinephrine, may cause vasoconstriction.

Whether the cells of the surface layers of epithelium are of the columnar or of the pavement variety, those of the basal layers, except for the olfactory region, are cuboidal in shape, resembling closely the fixed connective-tissue cells with which they mingle, for there is no limiting membrane between them. It is often difficult to determine where the epithelium leaves off and the stroma begins. In the olfactory region, the epithelium is nonciliated and columnar, and does not possess the glandular elements seen elsewhere. In the respiratory portion, the membrane is covered with columnar, ciliated cells and a mucous film.

In recent years, action of the cilia and movement of the mucous film have received much attention in rhinologic circles. Elucidation of these phenomena has called the attention of observers to the importance of normals and thus has had good effect. However, it can be said, without detracting from the interest of these phenomena, that the action of the cilia is only one phase of the general physiology of the nasal membranes. It has been shown that cilia, fortunately, are present in newly formed membrane following operations. It has been clearly shown by Hilding,[8] Proetz,[12] Yates[19] and others how the mucous film and the movement of the cilia perform their function. In the sinuses the cilia have the important function of directing flow toward the ostia. The greatest good has come from exposition of the facts that the normal presence of mucus and the activity of the cilia are great barriers to infection. It is only when this mechanism is deranged that infection gains a foothold.

The Bowman type of gland prevails in the olfactory region. These glands secrete a much less viscid fluid than the racemose glands in the respiratory membrane. Although it may be true that these cells secrete a peculiar fluid which aids in the function of olfaction, its watery character is especially adapted to extend over the olfactory surface and to cause the fluid to drip down as sterile irrigation for the respiratory region below. It is not bactericidal in action.

The racemose glands of the respiratory region differ in no way from the structure of racemose glands elsewhere in the body. Not infrequently the acini are imbedded in the tissue, but, as a rule, they lie more superficially than the cavernous sinuses, varying greatly in their distribution. In the paranasal sinuses there are very few. It is said that the secretion from the respiratory part of the membrane is in itself considerably bactericidal, at least bacteriostatic.

Under normal conditions the secretions of the nose maintain a certain physiochemical composition which fluctuates within a limited range, depending on the demands of physiologic activity. This is an involved subject and the details have no place in a discussion such as this. The secretion is composed of mucin, solids, minerals and an aqueous portion. The mucin originates in the racemose glands and probably acts as a deterrent to the rapid absorption of the serous portion of the secretion; in additon to having a protective influence on the sensitive ciliated cells it has been shown that the mucus has a bacteriostatic effect.

The activity of the secretory mechanism may be observed clinically. If a patient whose nasal interior is apparently normal can be observed over a period of time, at short intervals, it will be noticed that the appearance and relative position of the membrane within the nose changes. At first one nostril may be filled because the membranes are swollen; the surface is smooth and relatively dry. In a moment or two, the sur-

face is seen to be studded with little discrete drops of moisture. Soon the droplets increase in size and the surface begins to be covered with a film. Now it is noticed that the swelling of the membrane is less and gradually becomes much less, so that the membrane does not fill the nostril as it did. The membrane in the opposite nostril, if examined, may be found to be increasing in size. What has happened is that the blood spaces in the membrane have filled; the involuntary muscle, through stimulation of nerves is causing contraction of the blood spaces, forcing the blood into the glands and stroma, and in turn the content of the glands is expelled through the ducts onto the surface, producing the droplet that can be seen. As the activity is increased, the secretion increases until the cycle is completed. The watery, or predominant, portion of the secretion comes from the tubular, Bowman type of gland. This automatic flushing of the surface cannot be imitated by sprays and douches. Denuding of the surface subjects the sensitive epithelium to changes that are not consistent with normal conditions.

It can be observed clinically that nasal respiration is an adaptive reflex mechanism, lessening resistance when respiratory need is increased, and vice versa. Dilatation of the vessels, when it is not carried to the point of rendering insufficient the amount of air supplied to the lungs, renders the air, when it reaches the pharynx, not only warmer, more moist, and more free of dust and bacteria, but by filling the unnecessary space in the respiratory region of the nose, it directs a more copious supply of air toward the olfactory region. Wright and Smith[18] said:

"The internal configuration of every nose, even of those we would pronounce normal, varies so greatly that every nasal chamber is a law to itself. Anterior and posterior rhinoscopy are often incapable of furnishing us with trustworthy information as to the efficiency of the nasal chambers in the performance of these functions. The statements of patients are still more untrustworthy. Some fail to appreciate even extreme grades of nasal obstruction. Others complain of it when manifestly it does not exist. The clinical experience, the common sense of the physician, and his ability to judge the patient's temperament are more important guides to the appreciation of how these functions are in reality being performed, than the help his technical skill or the instruments of precision at his disposal furnish him."

Paget[11] has said that he believed the function of the nose to be to filter the air and that the other ascribed functions are entirely subsidiary. He expressed the belief that nearly every healthy man has lost the power to breathe through the nose because of the tendency to alar collapse, that if more respiration was nasal there would be less pulmonary disease.

Chepmell,[4] in discussing Paget's annotation, quoted Catlin's book entitled, "Shut Your Mouth," written in the early forties of the nineteenth century. Catlin was impressed by the healthiness of the American Indian children, whose mothers insisted on their breathing through their noses. Hagemann[5] expressed the belief that the function of the nose may be emunctory to a large extent. Wright has said, "Vasomotor phenomena answer to every demand of physiologic need only so far as the mechanism is undamaged in all its parts. Repeated temporary exaggerations of physiologic response lead gradually to the graver forms of polypoid rhinitis and atrophic states." Thus it is seen that the function of the nose is carried on by virtue of its internal configuration and the mechanism of its mucous membrane. As the air enters the vestibule, it takes an upward course, passes over the superior surface of the inferior turbinate, over both surfaces of the middle turbinate, and enters the pharynx. The membrane of the pharynx is essentially like that of the nose, except that it is not so specialized. In the pharynx, however, there is lymphoid tissue; such tissue is not encountered in the nose. In passing over these structures, the air currents take up the moisture from the surface, and are thus warmed, moistened, and filtered. In expiration, the air currents are directed largely through the inferior meatus by the posterior tip of the inferior turbinate. What function is served by the accessory sinuses of man is a question, but it is apparent that they are ventilated by the negative pressure effect exerted by the passing streams of air. The function of the tonsillar tissue in the pharynx is also uncertain; that it has a function in early childhood, even though it is not understood or known, I am willing to admit.

Symptoms referable to the upper part of the respiratory tract are less common and are less often complained of when persons live where the climate is warm and equable. This is because there is less necessity for the nose to overfunction in order to prepare the air for the lower part of the respiratory tract. Such a

climate, however, has its definite drawbacks, as it has been shown that mental and physical productivity are at lower levels than in less equable environments. Huntington,[6] in his "Civilization and Climate," proved that the output of factory workers increases with change in temperature, and that no other elements of weather seem to have a real influence on such productivity. He explained the physical superiority of persons who live in hard, rugged climates by the subjection of their bodies to frequent and extreme alternations of temperature. The reasonable physiologic explanation of this phenomenon seems to be stimulation of the tonus of the vasomotor system.

Sewall[15] said:

"Climate is the summation of atmospheric conditions as recorded for a long period of time, or, in other words, it is the totality of the weather, while weather is the physical condition of the atmosphere at a given time, or during a limited period.

"It was formerly thought that the atmosphere affected the body only, or chiefly, through the absorption of its elements by the lungs, but it has been found that this is not the case, and that these symptoms are caused by the effects of the atmosphere on the surface of the body. . . . . In this connection, the various respiratory membranes are to be thought of as internal body surfaces, which are also brought in direct physical contact with the atmosphere. Heat, humidity, and stillness are the essentials in a bad atmosphere; coolness, dryness, and motion of the air constitute good ventilation."[1]

From what has been described as the normal physiologic reaction of the nose, it can be seen how, with a perfectly acting mechanism, particularly the vasomotor mechanism, the nose would be called on to function in different atmospheres. In the variable, rugged climate of the Northwest, with frequent changes in weather, one might expect that the membrane of the upper part of the respiratory tract would become hypertrophic, whereas, in the warm, equable climate, where the nose is not required to function excessively, there might be very little change. It is easy to understand, then, that in the north, in adolescent and early adult life, many symptoms might arise from the physiologic activity of the respiratory membrane, particularly as it is at this period of life that the function of erectile tissue is at its height. This is why many adolescents and young adults complain of nasal obstruction and excessive secretion. It has been variably estimated that the respiratory membrane might secrete anywhere from a pint to a quart

(500 to 1,000 c.c.) a day. Patients often complain of obstruction on alternate sides, but as a matter of fact this is normal. Scarcely ever would both sides of the nose be open to the same extent, for the reason that there appears to be a cycle of reaction; that is, while the mucous membrane of one nostril is filling to a point approaching obstruction, the other nostril is opening and throwing off its secretion, and by the time the nostril that is filled has completed its cycle, the other nostril has completed the opposite cycle. The reverse is also true. The cycle may not always take place to the extent described, but nearly to that extent.

At my suggestion, Heetderks[6] made observations on reactions of the nasal membranes of apparently normal persons in each of the first six decades of life, when the persons were subjected to various atmospheric conditions. It was observed that the nasal membranes of adolescents were much more responsive to environmental changes than were the nasal membranes of older persons. In about 80 per cent of cases a definite cycle of activity such as has been alluded to previously, occurred. Also, even though the environmental condition remained the same, a cycle of activity occurred; that is, while the membranes on the turbinates were filling on one side, the membranes on the opposite side were throwing off secretion. Heetderks found that when the subjects were subjected to cold air the secretion was abundant, while in warm air it was less copious and the membrane appeared duller in color.

Patients often complain of obstruction at night on the side on which they are lying. This is the result of passive congestion from gravity and is a normal condition. Complaint is also made of the accumulation of a considerable amount of secretion in the pharynx during the night. Really, the accumulation occurs because it has not been involuntarily disposed of, as it would have been during the day by involuntary swallowing and by eating and drinking. Many persons feel that this condition is detrimental to their health, but I have seen no evidence of this; it is usually the most robust type of patient who makes this kind of complaint. The laity call this condition "catarrh." With the condition of hypertrophic rhinitis superimposed on nasal obstruction caused by anatomic defect, such as a crooked septum, symptoms are naturally aggravated. In other

words, there is an anatomic obstruction and physiologic hyperactivity. Often, in this type of case, correction of the anatomic obstruction by some operative measure which conserves the membrane, will largely relieve the symptoms. If the symptoms are not relieved in this manner, a change to a high, dry climate often will effect the change by natural processes. The dryness and equability of such a climate will take up the excess secretion that the hypertrophic condition is producing, and there will be little or no variation to cause the excessive physiologic responses. It is in this type of nose that destructive intranasal operations were often performed formerly; these, I believe, are contraindicated.

Occupation has a great deal to do with the physiologic responses of the membrane of the upper part of the respiratory tract. It has been shown that examination of workers in steam laundries, who have been engaged in this type of work a long time, invariably discloses rather definite grades of atrophy of the membrane of the nose. This can be explained on the basis of climatic conditions, already discussed.

Stark[15] made observations on the nasal membranes of patients who were forced to use a tracheotomy tube because of laryngeal obstruction. During the first several days the nasal membrane was congested and the patient had a sense of fullness. After physiologic rest had been established, the congestion disappeared and the membranes were merely moist and duller in color. One patient, who had been troubled by crusting in the nose previous to the use of the tracheotomy tube, was relieved of the crusting after about a week's time. The explanation of this phenomenon must be that because there were no passing air currents to absorb the moisture, the air did not have a drying effect on the mucous constituent of the secretion.

The lumberjack, the farmer, the delivery man, and others who are constantly out-of-doors in all kinds of weather, are not so much troubled with infection of the upper part of the respiratory tract, or with symptoms encountered so often among persons who live a sedentary, indoor life. Attention to personal hygiene will, in some measure, relieve the symptoms. The city dweller has found that he must protect his face from becoming wet or cold, or have a "cold in the head." "The man clad all day in the same kind of clothing finds that he cannot remov any part of this clothing without the risk of taking cold. His wife wears high shoes or spats during the day, when it is warm, and has her neck and chest protected, but in the evening, attending a social function, she apparently disregards all sane principles of dress; yet it is observed that she is less disposed to catch cold than the man." This is another example of the hardening process. The vasomotor tone is better developed if one exposes the surfaces of his body and changes his clothing to suit the occasion than if one constantly dresses in the same manner. Susceptibility to the physiologic changes can be largely controlled by training; that is, the city dweller can become a farmer or a rural delivery man, and gradually acquire the same physiologic reactions, and the reverse is true.

Much has been written and said recently about the effect of relative humidity and ventilation in the home. At first, attention was given to these matters because of the economic factor; it was noticed that the furniture began to creak and come apart in the winter and that by evaporating water in the rooms this was overcome. In addition, a feeling of greater general physical comfort was obtained at a lower temperature. It has been observed that acute infections of the upper part of the respiratory tract resolved more readily when the temperature was warm and the air moist than when the environment was cold and dry, and that when inhalations of steam were used to saturate the inhaled air with moisture, pharyngeal and laryngeal coughs could be largely controlled. During the cold weather the relative humidity of the air is very low. Sleeping out-of-doors on sleeping porches has been advocated as a health-producing habit, probably because of the wonderful health of those who live out-of-doors and sleep out-of-doors; but it is not taken into account that people in the city live, during at least two-thirds of the day, in a temperature sometimes 100° F. above that to which they might be subjected at night. The change causes too great a physiologic response to be endured by a respiratory membrane not accustomed to such changes.

There is another type of physiologic reaction within the nose which is attributable to some derangement of the sympathetic nervous system, and which results in what is called "vasomotor rhinitis." It may be caused by allergy, endocrine disturbances, avitaminosis or the effect

of severe inflammation, and can sometimes be controlled by removing the causal factor if that factor can be ascertained. If the causal factor cannot be ascertained readily, topical applications to the region of the sphenopalatine ganglion, as shown by Sluder,[14] are beneficial; now ionization is advocated by some observers. Brubaker[3] called attention to the physiology of sneezing. Sneezing may be the manifestation of vasomotor rhinitis. Sneezing is the normal manner of clearing the nose externally. It is customary for the human being, in order to clear the nose, to blow it in some manner, and he usually closes the open nostril and blows against the opposite nostril. It is granted that this method is effective. This creates a strong, positive pressure in the nasopharynx, and may produce untoward results, because it may cause the forcible spreading of infections to the ear or paranasal sinuses. Patients often indicate that pain in the ear followed blowing of the nose. Animals are seldom affected because their only method of clearing the nose is by sneezing.

Finally, it can be inferred, from what has been said, that in the daily management of patients it is important that an understanding of the mechanism of the function of the nasal membrane and its reaction to various environmental conditions be common knowledge and that such knowledge be considered of fundamental importance in the practice of rhinology. Only in this way can the variations caused by pathologic conditions be evaluated.

The prime purpose of any form of treatment should be, as nearly as possible, to establish the parts in a condition of "restitutio ad integrum." The patient, in this way, would be relieved of symptoms and would not have to contend with the discomfiture of having had new symptoms added to the old. Conservation of the functional mechanism of the nasal membrane can be effected in many instances if therapeutic measures are applied with this end in view.

References

1. Barker, L. F.: Environment and its relation to health and disease. Oxford Medicine. New York, Oxford University Press, vol. 1, chap. 19, 1920, pp. 729-738.
2. Bayliss, W. M.: Die Innervation der Gefässe. II, Die Regulation die Blutversorgung. Ergebn. d. Physiol, 5:319-346, 1906.
3. Brubaker, A. P.: The physiology of sneezing. Jour. Am. Med. Assn., 73:585-587, (Aug. 23) 1919.
4. Chepmell, I. D.: The functions of the nose. (Editorial.) Lancet, 1:278, (Jan. 24) 1914.
5. Hagemann, J. A.: The upper respiratory mucous membranes as emunctories. Med. Rec., 85:296-297, (Feb. 14) 1914.
6. Heetderks, D. R.: Observations on the reaction of normal nasal mucous membrane. Am. Jour. Med. Sc., 174:231-244 (Aug.) 1927.

7. Hempstead, B. E.: Unpublished data.
8. Hilding, Anderson: The physiology of drainage of nasal mucus. I. The flow of the mucus currents through the drainage activity. Arch. Otol., 15:92-100, (Jan.) 1932.
9. Huntington, Ellsworth: Civilization and climate. New Haven, Yale University Press, 1915, 333 pp.
10. McMurrich, J. P.: The development of the human body; a manual of human embryology. Ed. 6. Philadelphia: P. Blakiston's Son and Co., 1920, 501 pp.
11. Paget, O. F.: The functions of the nose. Lancet, 1:192-193, (Jan. 17) 1914.
12. Proetz, A. W.: Nasal ciliated epithelium, with special reference to infection and treatment. Jour. Laryngol. and Otol., 49:557-570, (Sept.) 1934.
13. Sewall, Henry: Climate in relation to health and disease. Oxford Medicine. New York, Oxford University Press, vol. 1, chap. 11, 1920, pp. 453-500.

14. Sluder, Greenfield: Concerning some headaches and eye disorders of nasal origin. St. Louis, C. V. Mosby Company, 1918, 272 pp.
15. Stark, W. B.: Unpublished data.
16. Stein, O. J.: The treatment of intranasal and accessory sinus diseases. Illinois Med. Jour., 34:202-204, (Oct.) 1918.
17. Wright, Jonathan: The relation of the biophysical laws of osmosis to nasal vasomotor processes. New York Med. Jour., 94:861-865, (Oct. 28) 1911.
18. Wright, Jonathan, and Smith, Harmon: A textbook of the diseases of the nose and throat. Philadelphia, Lea and Febiger, 1914, 683 pp.
19. Yates, A. L.: Methods of estimating the activity of the ciliary epithelium with the sinuses. Jour. Laryngol. and Otol., 39:554-560, 1924.

SYNCOPE

BAYARD T. HORTON, M.D.,* L. McKENDREE EATON, M.D.

and

LODWICK S. MERIWETHER, M.D.

Rochester, Minnesota

SYNCOPE, or fainting, is usually described as a sudden loss of consciousness, which probably is the result of an acute anemia of the brain. However, as to just what happens in these cases, we do not know. In this article, we shall make no attempt to consider all of the possible causes of syncope but rather shall report representative cases of the more common types of syncope in order to make the article of practical value. One could list innumerable causes of syncopal attacks but such a list would serve no useful purpose in this article. We are concerned not only with the patient who has had a transient loss of consciousness and promptly recovers, but also with patients who have had recurring attacks. Usually, the history of the case, if carefully taken, will furnish a definite lead as to the nature of the attack, especially if some relative or friend has observed the patient during an attack and can describe it accurately. The mode of onset and character of the seizure, the presence or absence of an aura, the history of injury during a seizure as well as the concern which the patient himself has with reference to the attack represent important points to be observed in recording the history. Patients almost invariably demand, from the physician, knowledge regarding the nature of their attacks and, particularly, the outlook for the future. It is with these thoughts in mind that the following cases are presented.

*Dr. Bayard T. Horton, Division of Medicine, Dr. L. McKendree Eaton, the Section on Neurology, The Mayo Clinic, Rochester, Minnesota, and Dr. Lodwick S. Meriwether, Fellow in Medicine, The Mayo Foundation, Rochester, Minnesota.

Simple Syncope

Case 1.—A man, fifty-eight years of age, was being used as a blood donor for his wife, who had recently undergone an operation. Following the taking of his blood, he became emotionally upset and fell unconscious. He was put to bed and advised to stay in the hospital over night. The next morning he was dismissed; at this time he felt perfectly well.

Comment on Case 1.—Fainting is a functional circulatory disturbance which can easily occur if a person has an unstable vasomotor system. As a rule, it is induced by pain or the sight of blood. It is characterized by a feeling of weakness which is followed by some dimness of vision and finally by unconsciousness. The most characteristic feature of such an attack is its slow onset. The patient recovers consciousness in a few minutes and in an hour or so he feels normal.

Simple Fainting Versus Hypoglycemia

Case 2.—A minister, aged forty-eight years, came to the clinic on February 3, 1938, because of the fact that in April, 1937, while he had been brushing his teeth early one morning, he suddenly had lost consciousness and had fallen to the floor; he had struck his chin against the tiles, which had caused a rather severe laceration. He apparently had regained consciousness in ten to fifteen minutes and had felt well enough to walk back to his bed. During the attack of unconsciousness, he had had incontinence of the bowels. He had remained in bed for a week as a matter of precaution, but he had felt perfectly well. He never had had an attack of this sort before or since that time. During the following summer he had worked hard and had not taken his usual vacation. In August, he had begun to note transient periods of complete exhaustion; these usually had occurred after breakfast and had consisted of a "let-down" or exhausted feeling. This sensation had lasted for ten to fifteen minutes, after which he had felt all right. He never had noted this disturbance before breakfast. These attacks of exhaustion had seemed to increase in frequency when he had been subjected to nervous tension. They had not been associated with physical exertion. In October, 1937, he had had a dizzy spell which had lasted for one and a half hours; during the attack he had felt weak and unsteady but had not had any definite vertigo. It was at this time that he had collapsed completely while he had been attending an important meeting where he was to have given the main address. His address had to be read by one of his assistants. After a day's rest, he had felt entirely normal.

Physical examination at the clinic revealed a powerfully built man who was 6 feet and 3 inches (190.5 cm.) in height and who weighed 225 pounds (112 kg.). He had no excess flesh. At the time he came to the clinic the values for the systolic and diastolic blood pressures were 130 mm. and 80 mm. of mercury respectively while the patient was in the recumbent position. Immediately after he had assumed the standing position the respective values were found to be 110 mm. and 80 mm. On the following day, when he was in the supine position, the respective values were 120 mm. and 84 mm. As soon as he stood up, the respective values were found to be 100 mm. and 80 mm.; after he had stood for one minute, the values were found to be 108 mm. and 80 mm. Routine physical examination and neurologic examination did not reveal any abnormality. The value for the uric acid was 5 mg. per 100 c.c. of blood and that for the sugar was 73 mg. per 100 c.c. of blood. At a previous visit to the clinic, in October, 1935, a diagnosis of gout had been made and since that time he had been following a rather strict regimen because of this condition. In the interval between his first and second visits to the clinic, the values for the uric acid in the blood had been determined at various times; these values always had varied between 6 and 6.4 mg. per 100 c.c. of blood.

Comment on Case 2. In this case the patient was primarily concerned with an explanation for the previous loss of consciousness. This was uppermost in his mind and was the reason why he made a hurried visit to the clinic. He had been seen by numerous physicians; practically every one of them had suggested that his attacks were the result of hypoglycemia. However, the value for the blood sugar during his previous attacks of exhaustion always had been 70 mg. or more per 100 c.c. He had noted that the taking of sugar or food had not prevented these attacks of exhaustion and he had not felt better after he had taken food. At the clinic the value for the blood sugar was found to be 73 mg. per

100 c.c. This determination was made at 10:00 a. m., and the patient had not taken any food since 2:00 p. m. the previous day; yet he felt normal at the time the value for the blood sugar was determined. It seems obvious that one can rule out hypoglycemia as the cause of his attack of unconsciousness. In our experience, in cases in which syncopal attacks are the result of hypoglycemia, the value for the blood sugar usually is about 35 to 40 mg. per 100 c.c. during the attacks. The patients almost invariably respond promptly to the ingestion of sugar or food and frequent feedings between meals usually will prevent the attacks. Such had not been this man's experience. The presence of an intracranial lesion has not been ruled out entirely but we are inclined to regard the condition as a simple attack of fainting, which probably was the result of an associated postural hypotension. For this reason we advised the use of ephedrine and benzedrine to see if this would not maintain the blood pressure at a more constant level. However, this patient should again be examined in the course of three to six months to see if there is any additional evidence to suggest an intracranial lesion.

Carotid Sinus Syndrome

Case 3.—A man, aged sixty-two years, registered at the clinic in June, 1937, complaining of rather unusual attacks of "dizziness" which had developed two months previously. Careful questioning disclosed that he had had a similar attack in 1931. For a short time before the patient came to the clinic these attacks had occurred three to four times a week. He described an attack somewhat as follows: Suddenly, without any particular warning, he had noted a dizzy feeling and a sensation as though he were going to fall; he had to steady himself by grasping some supporting object in order to keep from falling. He was not sure whether he had completely lost consciousness or not but he thought that if he had become unconscious it had been for only a moment or two. Most of the attacks had occurred after the patient had assumed an erect posture after he had been in a sitting or recumbent posture for some time. In one of the attacks he had vomited and diarrhea had developed. He had not been aware of the fact that moving the head in one direction or another had precipitated these attacks. He had not had any disturbance of vision or headaches.

Physical examination revealed a man who appeared normal for his age. He weighed 158 pounds (71.7 kg.). The results of general physical examination were essentially negative, while he was in the supine position, were 150 mm. and 85 mm. of mercury, respectively. When he was standing, the value for the systolic pressure dropped to 130 mm. and that for the diastolic pressure dropped to 80 mm. No abnormal sensations were experienced as a result of this drop in blood pressure. Digital pressure over the right carotid sinus caused the patient to become unconscious immediately. After he regained consciousness he said: "That's the type of attack I've been having." The rate of the radial pulse was markedly decreased and the pulse was almost imperceptible. This man had been a patient at the clinic on two previous occasions. In 1931, a diagnosis of chronic cholecystitis and chronic cholelithiasis had been made. A cholecystectomy had disclosed multiple stones in the gallbladder. He had made an uneventful recovery from that operation. His second admission had been in November, 1936. At this time there had been clinical evidence of periarticular changes in both shoulders; infected tonsils and chronic prostatitis also were discovered. The periarticular arthritis apparently had followed a septic sore throat. At his third, or last, visit there were no arthritic symptoms.

Comment on Case 3.—The diagnosis was a hypersensitive carotid sinus reflex on the right side. We are of the opinion that his previous attacks of vertigo and syncope had been due to the hypersensitive carotid sinus. It is interesting to note that digital pressure over the right carotid sinus produced a typical attack, and that the patient said that it corresponded to the spontaneous attacks which he had been having. In view of the fact that the attacks had been present only for two months and that he had not been incapacitated, surgical denervation of the carotid sinus was not advised. The patient was advised to refrain from wearing tight collars and to avoid sudden turning of the head, so as to avoid pressure or strain on the sensitive carotid sinus. Smith and Moersch have pointed out that the effects of medication are not very satisfactory as far as prophylaxis is concerned. Anyone interested in this syndrome should read their reports.

Syncope Caused by Hypersensitiveness to Cold

Collapse caused by exposure to cold or which occurs while swimming has been observed in a number of instances. Horton has reported a number of cases of this condition. It usually affects subjects who are otherwise healthy. This phenomenon is illustrated by the following case:

Case 4.—A man, aged forty-two years, was under observation at the clinic in November, 1935. During the previous year, he had noted urticarial swelling of his hands when they had come in contact with

630

cold water or cold objects. When he had been out on a cold day, an urticarial rash had developed over the exposed surfaces of the skin. On one occasion, he had collapsed while he had been swimming and had had to be rescued from the water. Physical examination revealed nothing of significance and the routine laboratory tests did not reveal any abnormality. When his left hand was immersed in cold water at 10° C. for five minutes, no swelling of the hand occurred while it was in the water, but approximately three to four minutes after the hand was removed from the water it began to swell, and in ten minutes after it had been taken from the water it was swollen so much that the patient was unable to make a fist. With the swelling of the hand, the patient felt dizzy, but syncope did not actually develop. The blood pressure had decreased from its original level of 118 mm. of mercury for the systolic and 80 mm. for the diastolic to 114 mm. for the systolic and 70 mm. for the diastolic, respectively. This drop in blood pressure was not sufficient to produce symptoms. Shortly after the patient returned home he had a most unusual experience. One morning, when the outside temperature was about 30° F. below zero, he left his home and walked or partially ran a distance of four blocks to catch a bus. After he had got off the bus, a few minutes later, he walked a distance of about one block, when he collapsed and did not regain consciousness until forty minutes later, when he found himself in a hospital with a nurse holding a bottle of medicine for him to inhale. He vomited three or four times. He remained in the hospital one day but did not regain his full strength for about one week. As soon as he regained consciousness, he explained to the attending nurse and later to the physician that his collapse had been due to hypersensitiveness to cold. We previously had warned him against undue exposure to cold and, so far as we know, he has never had a similar attack. At one time he had collapsed while he had been swimming, but he had recovered completely in twenty-four hours.

Comment on Case 4.—One of us (Horton) previously introduced a test for hypersensitiveness to cold, which was employed in this case. The test is as follows: The hand is immersed in ice water at 8° to 10° C., for five minutes. Prior to immersion of the hand in ice water, observations on the blood pressure and pulse rate are made and observations are continued at intervals of one minute while the hand is immersed in the water and for a period of twenty minutes after the hand is removed from the water. If swelling of the hand occurs after it has been removed from the water, the indication is that the patient is hypersensitive to cold. A systemic reaction is indicated by a drop in blood pressure, an increase in the pulse rate, and flushing of the face. We are of the opinion that in all cases in which this systemic reaction occurs symptoms of collapse would develop if the patient swam in cold water.

In 1936, one of us (Horton) reported twenty-two cases of hypersensitiveness to cold, which represented the total number of such cases previously observed at the clinic. With few exceptions, the patients appeared to be in good health. Hypersensitiveness to cold constitutes a grave menace to the unwary swimmer who is the victim of this malady, but the danger can be eliminated by adequate desensitization. In Minnesota alone, since 1920, 3,000 persons have drowned while swimming. One cannot help but wonder if some of these persons were not victims of this condition. Of the twenty-two patients who were hypersensitive to cold, fourteen had systemic reactions and eleven of the fourteen had had attacks of syncope; in nine cases the syncope had occurred while the patients had been swimming and four of the nine patients had to be rescued from the water. More than twenty-four cases in which syncope occurred following swimming have been reported in the literature, and at least nine of these persons had to be rescued from the water. Fortunately, patients who are hypersensitive to cold are amenable to treatment. Systemic desensitization to cold can be accomplished in at least three ways: first, by having the patient immerse the hand in water at 10° C. for from one to two minutes twice a day for three or four weeks; second, by the subcutaneous injection of 0.1 mg. of histamine, or less, twice daily for two to three weeks; and third, by the oral administration of histaminase.

Syncope Associated with Postural Hypotension

Case 5.—A married woman, aged thirty-three years, came to the clinic in October, 1934, for a general examination. She had symptoms of vague indigestion and said that on various occasions she had fainted, particularly if she had been lying down and had got up suddenly. This had occurred frequently when she had had to get up suddenly to answer the telephone. By the time she had reached the telephone and had said "Hello," she had collapsed on the floor. Consciousness had returned promptly and she had never hurt herself when she had fallen. Physical examination did not reveal any abnormality. Her blood pressure was taken on numerous occasions for a period of ten days, but the values for the blood pressure did not fluctuate to any very marked extent. The systolic and diastolic blood pressures were 103 mm. and 78 mm. of mercury

respectively while the patient was in the horizontal position. As soon as she assumed the erect posture, the values were 100 mm. for the systolic pressure and 70 mm. for the diastolic pressure. Readings of this character were made over a period of ten days, but the greatest drop in the systolic pressure was only 5 mm. and that in the diastolic pressure also was 5 mm. The routine laboratory tests did not reveal any abnormality.

Comment on Case 5.—It seems reasonable to assume that the attacks of syncope probably were due to circulatory asthenia and postural hypotension, but we could not demonstrate marked postural changes during the short period of observation. She did not have any attacks of syncope during this period of time. She was advised to return home and to take ⅜ grain (0.024 gm.) of ephedrine sulfate two to three times a day if she had additional attacks of syncope. She is unlike the patient in Case 6 as she had had frequent attacks of syncope but there were no demonstrable changes in blood pressure when she changed posture.

Case 6.—A woman, aged forty-three years, came to the clinic in March, 1937, because of frequent attacks of dizzy spells which had been recurring at frequent intervals for the past year. These attacks had been precipitated when she suddenly had arisen from a sitting to a standing posture. Attacks of syncope apparently had not been noted, although on many occasions she had felt as though she were going to faint. When she came to the clinic the value for her systolic blood pressure was 130 mm. of mercury and that for the diastolic pressure 85 mm. No record was made as to whether the readings were observed while the patient was in the recumbent or sitting posture. Two days later, the systolic blood pressure was 98 mm. and the diastolic pressure was 60 mm. while she was in the recumbent position. As soon as she assumed the standing position, the systolic blood pressure was 95 mm. and the diastolic pressure was 58 mm. for a few seconds, but the respective pressures gradually dropped within a period of two minutes to 82 mm. and 58 mm. Slight vertigo developed at this point. As a result of the administration of 10 mg. of benzedrine sulfate three to five times a day, all of the symptoms of vertigo disappeared and she was able to walk around without any discomfort. Previous to her admission to the clinic, she had not gone out without an escort for she frequently had become so dizzy that she had been unable to walk. There are a number of features about this case which we cannot adequately explain but we are of the opinion that the attacks of vertigo were due to the low blood pressure and the associated postural hypotension. Routine laboratory studies did not reveal any abnormality. She continued the use of benzedrine and we have heard from her on a number of occasions; she has continued to be free from symptoms.

Postural Hypotension Associated with Syncope, following Operation

Case 7.—A woman, aged forty-four years, came to the clinic in August, 1935, complaining of urinary symptoms which had been present for six to seven years. During this time she had not had any attacks of dizziness or syncope. A cystoscopic examination did not reveal anything of definite significance. The capacity of the bladder was 200 c.c. A moderate cystocele was present. Under anesthesia, the bladder was overdistended to a capacity of 600 c.c.; three days later, she underwent an operation for the repair of the cystocele. After she had recovered from this operation and had been dismissed from the hospital, on more than one occasion when she had arisen suddenly from a sitting to a standing posture, she had collapsed and had fallen to the floor. Each time, she had regained consciousness promptly. It seems reasonable to assume that a postural hypotension developed following the surgical operation and that she promptly recovered from this after she had regained her strength. At no time were we able to demonstrate postural changes in the blood pressure but she did have a relatively low blood pressure following the operation; the average values were 95 mm. of mercury for the systolic pressure and 68 mm. for the diastolic pressure. The transient drop in blood pressure, which accounted for the attacks of syncope no doubt lasted for only a few seconds so that we were never able to obtain readings quickly enough to demonstrate the postural changes. The attacks ceased before she left the clinic and she has not had attacks since that time.

Comment on Case 7.—Postural hypotension is not a disease, but an expression of an inadequate vasomotor control of the arterial system, which may be associated with numerous diseases. In the average case, there is always a sharp drop in systolic and diastolic blood pressure, when a patient arises from a recumbent to a standing posture. In addition, in well advanced cases, hypohidrosis or anhidrosis, is usually present. Also, there is a loss of reflex acceleration of the cardiac rate when the patient assumes an erect posture.

Postural changes in the blood pressure are almost invariably noted after extensive sympathectomy, such as that performed by Adson, Craig and Love, at the clinic, for the relief of essential hypertension. These changes always are most marked when patients first get out of bed. They have been described by Adson in numerous articles on the surgical treatment of hypertension.

In the cases which we are reporting the postural changes in the blood pressure were relatively mild and changes in sweating, as well as

the excretion of large volumes of urine at night, were not observed. When one suspects the presence of a postural hypotension, the blood pressure should be taken while the patient is in the recumbent as well as in the standing posture. We recommend that this method of taking the blood pressure should be a routine part of all physical examinations.

Arteriosclerosis of the Central Nervous System and Hypertension Associated with Dizziness and Syncope

Case 8.—A woman, sixty-five years of age, came to the clinic August 26, 1937, because of attacks of dizziness and fainting. She previously had undergone a thyroidectomy at the clinic in 1930 and had remained well until one week before her last admission. At that time she had had several attacks of dizziness which had lasted from a few minutes to two hours and she had lost consciousness on three occasions. She had never fainted before in her life. Physical examination revealed generalized arteriosclerosis and a systolic pressure of 200 mm. of mercury and a diastolic pressure of 110 mm. The results of routine laboratory tests were negative. A diagnosis of general arteriosclerosis, arteriosclerosis of the central nervous system, hypertension, vertigo and syncopal attacks was made.

Comment on Case 8.—In cases in which hypertension is associated with arteriosclerosis of the central nervous system or in cases in which arteriosclerosis of the central nervous system occurs alone, the patients not infrequently have attacks of transient unconsciousness which may be of the nature of a syncopal, petit mal, or grand mal attack. In cases in which arteriosclerosis of the central nervous system is associated with the hypertension the attacks may be the result of a vasospastic phenomenon but in cases in which arteriosclerosis occurs alone the attacks are most probably the result of destruction of the brain, which is caused by closure of smaller vessels and infarction.

Paroxysmal Tachycardia Associated with Syncope

Case 9.—A woman, aged fifty-six years, came to the clinic on May 30, 1936, complaining of pain which had occurred intermittently over the cardiac region for thirteen years. The attacks had begun with a feeling of faintness and sinking sensation; the patient had felt as though she could not get her breath. There had been some associated pain in the thorax and left arm; at first, the attacks had occurred only two to four times a year and had lasted ten to fifteen minutes, but they gradually had increased in frequency and duration until at the time of her registration at the clinic she was having one or more attacks a day. The longest attack had lasted for three hours. Dr. A. R. Barnes said that the patient was unconscious at times during the attacks. He observed her during one of the attacks and found that the heart rate was 180 to 200 per minute; the pulse was feeble and barely perceptible. His diagnosis was paroxysmal tachycardia associated with anginal pain and syncope. Dr. Barnes said that attacks of unconsciousness associated with paroxysmal tachycardia are not a common occurrence, but that they occur often enough to be of importance from the standpoint of differential diagnosis.

Heart Block

Case 10.—A man, aged fifty-eight years, first came to the clinic on February 28, 1935, complaining of spells of unconsciousness, arthritis, and an injury of the head. The attacks of unconsciousness had first occurred in November, 1935; since then they had occurred irregularly; the frequency had varied from one attack every three to four months to one attack weekly. The attacks of unconsciousness had been of brief duration and had seemed to occur immediately after the patient had turned his head toward the left or after he had arisen from a stooping position. He had had a feeling as though a stocking cap were slipping over his head, and then he had become unconscious for a few moments. On one occasion slight muscle twitching had been noted and at another time urinary incontinence had occurred. A diagnosis of petit mal had been made and phenobarbital sodium (luminal) had been prescribed. This had not affected the attacks although he had taken as much as 6 grains (0.4 gm.) of the drug daily and had become very sluggish mentally. Routine general examination revealed that the patient had received a fracture of the skull as a result of an injury which had occurred one month before he came to the clinic, but the neurologic examination did not disclose any other abnormality. In view of the history and type of the attacks, an electrocardiogram was made and a complete auriculoventricular dissociation was noted.

Comment on Case 10.—Such transient attacks of unconsciousness may be easily confused with petit mal. The fact that the attacks had been initiated by turning the head would lead one to suspect a carotid sinus syndrome, but the diagnosis was made by the electrocardiogram. The carotid sinus syndrome is also accompanied by a slowing of the heart; therefore, one cannot be definitely sure of the diagnosis by merely counting the pulse rate.

Epileptic Seizures

Petit mal.—The petit mal seizure typically consists of a sudden loss of consciousness that lasts for a few seconds. It may or may not be preceded by an aura. Automatic activity, such as walking, may continue throughout the attack.

The patient may or may not fall. When petit mal alternates with grand mal, the diagnosis of the minor seizure is obvious.

Grand mal.—Little difficulty is experienced in differentiating the typical grand mal type of epileptic seizure and other types of unconscious attacks. About 57 per cent of grand mal attacks are introduced by an aura. The aura manifests itself in many ways, but it most often is of the visceral type. The patient frequently describes it as an "all-gone feeling in the stomach" or a "hot (or cold) wave starting in the stomach." Unconsciousness quickly follows; it is prompt and complete; therefore, the patient falls and often injures himself. Unconsciousness usually is followed by a tonic phase in which the muscles are contracted, the patient is rigid, and cyanosis occurs and the veins become engorged. Generalized convulsive movements then occur. Biting the tongue, foaming at the mouth, micturition and defecation not uncommonly occur. As the convulsive movements abate, the muscles become flaccid. Examination at this stage almost always reveals that the pupils are dilated and unresponsive to light; the tendon reflexes are absent, and the Babinski's reflex is positive. In about three to ten, or even thirty, minutes after the onset of the attack, the patient gradually regains consciousness. He may then complain of headaches and somnolence. A deep sleep of several hours may follow the attack.

If the typical grand mal attack is witnessed or well described by a competent observer, little or no doubt remains as to the classification of the seizure. Often the witness is too terrified to observe accurately the sequence of events. It is always helpful and at times necessary for accurate diagnosis to observe a seizure. Attacks can usually be induced by hydration within a short time. The patient is placed in a hospital under the constant scrutiny of a trained observer. The fluid intake is increased considerably above normal, and the elimination of fluid is decreased by the subcutaneous injection of solution of posterior pituitary. This method of inducing seizures is of value when they are normally far apart and the patient is desirous of an immediate diagnosis.

Failure to realize that epileptiform seizures vary greatly from the common types leads to diagnostic errors. In our experience, atypical seizures are believed to be hysterical more often than hysterical seizures are mistaken for epilepsy. In the following case the condition was wrongly believed to be hysterical because of the uncommon precipitating factor.

Case 11.—A young man described vaguely seizures which had followed startling situations. For example, the unexpected explosion of a firecracker at his feet had been followed promptly by loss of consciousness and convulsive movements which he could describe only from hearsay.

From previous experience, the patient expected physicians to frighten him in an attempt to produce an attack for observation. Consequently, the attempts were not genuinely startling. However, when an attempt was finally successful, dilated pupils which were unresponsive to light, and the presence of a positive Babinski's reflex, left no doubt as to the correct diagnosis.

Atypical epileptic seizures without prompt loss of consciousness, with so-called dream states in which loss of consciousness may be incomplete, with bizarre motor contortions instead of the usual tonic and clonic phases frequently lead the physician, who is unaware of these variants, to the wrong conclusion.

Classification of the type of seizure is difficult but discovery of the cause of the epileptic seizure is usually more difficult. The physician must not accept too readily the diagnosis of idiopathic epilepsy. Often, such a diagnosis is reversed by careful clinical and laboratory study.

We choose to look upon the epileptic seizure as a symptom of organic disease. True, there may be an underlying hereditary predisposition to the attack. Even so, if the precipitating cause can be detected and eliminated the patient may be relieved of seizures. The organic disease may be intracranial or extracranial. Intracranial causes include cerebral tumor, abscess, or an acute inflammatory focus. A small scar that is the result of some previous injury to the brain, may act as the epileptogenic focus. Cerebral arteriosclerosis and senile atrophy of the brain may produce convulsions. The organic disease may not be primarily intracranial. Generalized metabolic disturbances, such as tetany, pernicious anemia, and spontaneous hyperinsulinism, may produce seizures that readily are mistaken for idiopathic epilepsy. Consequently, an awareness of, and a careful clinical search for, possible etiologic factors must be undertaken. The following cases are examples of the practical importance of such a search.

634

Grand Mal Seizures Produced by a Meningioma

Case 12.—A professional man, fifty years of age, had had recurrent convulsive seizures for six years. They had been characterized by a sudden, complete loss of consciousness and a generalized clonic convulsion. He previously had been treated with phenobarbital sodium, which apparently had reduced the frequency of attacks. Physical examination of the head, which was almost completely bald, disclosed that the veins of the scalp were abnormally enlarged and radiating from a point which was situated to the right of the midline of the vertex. At this point the bone could be seen and could be felt to be abnormally thickened over an area which was about 5 cm. in diameter. Roentgenograms of the skull revealed thickening of the internal and external tables and increased vascularity of the skull in the region to the right of the midline of the vertex. Surgical exploration and successful removal of a parasaggital meningioma resulted in relief from the convulsive attacks.

Grand Mal Seizures Associated with Tetany

Case 13.—A boy, aged fourteen years, had had convulsive seizures for six years. They had been introduced by a tingling sensation in the left foot, which had been followed by prompt loss of consciousness and generalized convulsive movements. At times, the tingling sensation had occurred without the usual subsequent events. Roentgenograms of the head revealed symmetrical cerebral calcification of the basal ganglions. The results of pneumo-encephalography were essentially negative. Although Chvostek's and Trousseau's signs could not be elicited, the concentration of serum calcium was 6.8 mg. per 100 c.c. and that for the phosphorus was 7.2 mg. per 100 c.c. of serum. Oral administration of powdered calcium lactate and cod liver oil increased the values for the serum calcium and serum phosphorus to, and maintained these values at, normal levels. The patient has had no convulsive seizures for eighteen months and no sedative drugs have been given. Previous to the treatment of the tetany, the seizures had occurred about every four weeks in spite of the adequate dosage of phenobarbital sodium.

Pernicious Anemia Associated with Attacks of Petit Mal

Case 14.—A woman who was in the sixth decade of life was brought to the clinic for examination because of failing memory and falling attacks of several months' duration. The attacks had occurred at irregular intervals without warning and had caused the patient to fall without protection. No serious injury had resulted but the relatives had anticipated it if the attacks were not relieved. The periods of unconsciousness always had been less than one minute and no convulsive seizures had been observed. Although the concentration of hemoglobin and the erythrocyte count were only slightly decreased, a study of blood smears disclosed a macrocytosis and a tendency to increased lobulation of the polymorphonuclear leukocytes. The gastric contents contained no free acid after the administration of histamine. These findings led to a tentative diagnosis of pernicious anemia. The mental symptoms and petit mal-like attacks were tentatively attributed to the pernicious anemia. An expanding intracranial lesion could not be excluded definitely. It was decided to treat the pernicious anemia and determine the effects of such treatment on the symptoms. After one month of intensive administration of liver extract intramuscularly, the unconscious seizures stopped and the mental symptoms improved greatly.

Hysteria

Hysterical attacks of coma are recognized by both the positive findings characteristic of the hysterical personality and the negative findings of other diseases which they may simulate. Frequently, the patient is known to have parents who are emotionally unstable. The patient frequently lives under an environmental situation that is not conducive to good mental health or he previously has been frankly psychoneurotic. This information may be helpful, but it must be remembered that such patients also are subject to organic diseases and that the symptoms of these diseases may be masked or complicated by psychoneurotic manifestations. The hysterical attacks are unlikely to occur when the patient is alone or in any situation in which serious injury is probable. The seizure is usually bizarre and histrionic; it often is accompanied by apparently purposeful movements. Friends or relatives may notice that the attacks occur only when some situation unpleasant to the patient is to be avoided. The seizures often vary from time to time, and unless the patient has witnessed epileptic seizures, the characteristic organic progression of epilepsy is not evident. A confident physician may alter the character of an attack that is in progress or he may induce an attack at will by proper suggestion. The ability to induce zones of anesthesia or paralysis by suggestion attests to the hysterical personality of the patient and allows for deductions as to the hysterical nature of the spontaneous seizures. During the attacks the patient incurs no serious injury, does not soil himself, the pupils are not fixed to light, and Babinski's reflex is negative.

We believe that emphasis on the necessity of careful clinical study to exclude organic disease

is justified. Judgment made with incomplete study is often fallacious. We have seen the neurologic manifestations of diabetic acidosis, hyperinsulinism, tetanus, lobar pneumonia, and other conditions, mistaken for hysteria. Pitfalls exist in the opinion arrived at by apparently effecting a restitution of consciousness by the time-honored procedures of painful pressure upon the supraorbital nerves, a dash of cold water in the face, and vigorous slapping of the patient. Such effects may be coincident with the normal recovery from an organic seizure.

The safest criterion for diagnosis is the ability to end the attacks of hysteria by psychotherapy. Suggestion alone may be effective in relieving symptoms. If the unconscious conflicts are discovered and if the patient is led to an awareness of them, cure is likely to be much more durable than it otherwise will be.

Case 15.—An unhappily married woman, twenty-eight years of age, had had unconscious attacks and convulsions for four years. Her mother had never been strong and had been considered by herself and daughter to be gifted in divining the future. The patient believed that her seizures had been precipitated by close proximity to electric apparatus. The first seizure had followed a thunder storm, during which lightning had struck a tree near the patient. The patient had not been injured by the lightning. Since the onset of the convulsive seizures the patient had lived with her mother, to whom she was greatly attached. The mother obviously had been alarmed by her daughter's spells. The mother had done all of the cooking, as proximity to the light meter in the kitchen was believed to have induced attacks. Incidentally, the patient was a poor cook, disliked that type of work, and much of the marital difficulty had been based on the husband's dissatisfaction with the food she had prepared. The seizures could be induced at will by bringing into the room the electric apparatus used in testing for reactions of degeneration and setting it so that the oscillator made a humming sound. Although the patient writhed vigorously on a narrow examining table she did not fall off. She forcibly closed her eyes more tightly when attempts were made to open them. The pupils were of normal size and reacted normally to light. The deep reflexes were present and the plantar responses were normal. After we had explained confidently to other physicians, who were present, that the abdominal muscles were contracting and that the patient would soon sit up, such a posture was immediately assumed. The attacks ended a few seconds after the audible oscillations were eliminated, although the current still was traversing the coils.

EXFOLIATIVE DERMATITIS AS A MANIFESTATION OF MONOCYTIC
LEUKEMIA (SCHILLING)

HAMILTON MONTGOMERY, M.D.* and CHARLES H. WATKINS, M.D.

The Mayo Clinic, Rochester, Minnesota

WE HAVE emphasized recently the distinction between the so-called Naegeli type of monocytic leukemia (which may be regarded as a variant of myelogenous leukemia with predominance of monocytes) and the true Schilling type (monocytic leukemic reticulo-endotheliosis) in which the cells are derived from the reticulo-endothelial cells (reticular cells[8]). Either type of monocytic leukemia may have a primary, autochthonous, cutaneous origin and either type may start out with the clinical and histopathologic features of mycosis fungoides.[4,8,11] In our previous paper we emphasized the close relationship of monocytic types of leukemia to other forms of leukemia and, in fact, to any of the so-called lymphoblastomas.[12] Two cases of exfoliative dermatitis attributable to the monocytic leukemia of Schilling were included, the first of such cases to be reported in the literature.

In the last six months of 1937, we encountered four additional cases of monocytic leukemia of Schilling associated with exfoliative dermatitis.[9] In these latter cases, changes in the blood may have preceded changes in the skin. It is becoming increasingly apparent that cutaneous manifestations, and especially exfoliative dermatitis, are a frequent occurrence in cases of monocytic leukemia of Schilling, as high as 50 per cent of the cases reported (Doan and Wiseman quoted by Lynch) having been associated with cutaneous lesions either specific or nonspecific in type. This is in contrast to the relative rarity of specific cutaneous lesions associated with myelogenous leukemia, of which Goldhamer and Barney found only seventeen instances in the literature up to 1936, including only two of a generalized eruption. We wish, therefore, to give the history of two of the six cases of monocytic leukemia associated with an exfoliative dermatitis that we have encountered

at The Mayo Clinic and to discuss the cutaneous, histologic and hemocytologic findings in cases of monocytic leukemia of Schilling.

Report of Cases

Case 1.—A man, aged seventy-six years, was seen at the clinic July 1, 1937, because of an exfoliative dermatitis. In September, 1936, a vesicular lesion had developed on the palm following a game of golf. A scaling dermatitis developed over the entire hand and spread gradually to other parts of the body. Within the last month before coming to the clinic an exfoliative dermatitis had developed involving the entire trunk, extremities and face. In December, 1936, a diagnosis of lymphatic leukemia had been made elsewhere, based on the finding of 21,850 leukocytes per cubic millimeter of blood. Seventy-five per cent of these were lymphocytes. He had received superficial roentgen therapy and various types of applications locally.

Examination at the clinic revealed the presence of a generalized exfoliative dermatitis. In addition, there were diffuse infiltrations in the skin, including small nodules on the legs and areas of lichenification. Hemorrhagic bullæ were present on the hands and feet. There were impetiginous lesions about the mouth and nose and a very noticeable, diffuse, bronze-like pigmentation of the skin. Hemorrhagic lesions were not present in the mucous membranes nor was there any bleeding of the gums. General examination, including roentgenologic examination of the thorax, gave essentially negative results. Enlargement of the spleen or liver was not present. Hemocytologic studies revealed that the concentration of hemoglobin was 14.2 gm. for each 100 c.c. of blood; erythrocytes numbered 3,410,000 and leukocytes 67,400 in each cubic millimeter of blood. Eighty per cent of the leukocytes were of reticulo-endothelial cell origin. The hemocytologic picture was definitely that of monocytic leukemia of Schilling. A specimen for biopsy from the right heel showed a definite picture of lymphoblastoma and contained many monocytes, including typical grooving of many nuclei, which latter picture is characteristic of the Schilling type of monocytic leukemia. Similar findings were noted in a specimen removed from the region of the shoulder for biopsy. Repeated determinations of the number of leukocytes while the patient was under treatment varied from 67,000 to 16,000 in each cubic millimeter of blood, the proportion of reticulo-endothelial cells reaching as high as 90 per cent.

*Dr. Hamilton Montgomery, Section on Dermatology and Syphilology, and Dr. Charles H. Watkins, Division of Medicine, The Mayo Clinic, Rochester, Minnesota.

The patient showed a definite response to two courses of local and systemic roentgen therapy. The last of December, 1937, Dr. Henry Michelson of Minneapolis reported that the patient was gradually failing. The hemocytologic diagnosis remained that of monocytic leukemia of Schilling (monocytic leukemic reticulo-endotheliosis). The number of leukocytes had increased to more than 500,000 in each cubic millimeter of blood. Enlargement of the prostate gland with symptoms of obstruction developed. Ulcers appeared on the cutaneous surfaces. The patient died January 22, 1938. Postmortem examination was not performed.

Case 2.—A young man, aged twenty years, was seen at the clinic November 29, 1937, because of an exfoliative dermatitis. This had started as an area of scaling dermatitis on the thigh five years previously and had gradually spread to involve the entire skin of the body. During the past twenty months he had experienced a generalized exfoliative dermatitis. Examination revealed a universal exfoliation of the skin and, in addition, there was a generalized lymphadenopathy. He gave a history of having had a lymph node removed for biopsy some two years previously and a course of two treatments with roentgen rays had subsequently been given. Because of his age, however, it was felt that he had an atopic eczema. Various intracutaneous tests were performed with negative results. General examination revealed a slightly enlarged and tender liver. Albuminuria, grade 2, was present and a few erythrocytes were noted in the urine which could be explained most readily on a toxic basis. The hemocytologic findings on admission to the hospital were as follows: the concentration of hemoglobin was 8.4 gm. per 100 c.c. of blood; erythrocytes numbered 3,150,000 and leukocytes 16,800 in each cubic millimeter of blood; the percentages of the various types of leukocytes were as follows: lymphocytes, 8; monocytes, 5.5; neutrophils, 32; and eosinophils, 54.5. The high eosinophilia together with monocytes possessing nuclei suggesting a reticulo-endothelial cell origin suggested the possibility of Hodgkin's disease.

A specimen for biopsy from the region of the right shoulder revealed a definite picture of lymphoblastoma. There was a very definite eosinophilia. There were many large cells, some with notched or indented nuclei and others with longitudinal grooving. Although it was recognized that the presence of grooved cells suggested that the leukemia was of the Schilling type rather than of the Naegeli type, the tremendous increase in eosinophils seemed to fit in better with the Naegeli type, which most hemocytologists regard as a variant of myelogenous leukemia. True Dorothy Reed cells of Hodgkin's disease were not demonstrable nor was the infiltrate like that encountered in cases of mycosis fungoides. Further hemocytologic studies showed that the number of leukocytes varied from 16,000 to 25,000 per cubic millimeter of blood; monocytes varied from 2 to 5.5 per cent; the percentage of eosinophils present on two occasions was 54.5. There were definite immature cells of the reticular cell series developing to monocytes and further hemo-

cytologic studies by one of us (Watkins) established the diagnosis of monocytic leukemia of Schilling. The disease ran a febrile course with a septic type of temperature reaching as high as 100.8° F. (38.2° C.). He was given a course of treatment with filtered roentgen rays, directed toward the axilla and inguinal lymph nodes and he was sent home to take further treatment. Dr. A. C. Barry, of Norfolk, Nebraska, reported that the patient died on Ferbuary 11, 1938, the result of cardiac decompensation. Shortly after his return home from the clinic, swelling of the feet and abdomen occurred. The cutaneous condition improved but the inguinal glands became larger and more tender than they had been previously. It was believed that the mediastinal lymph nodes had become involved but circumstances prevented the carrying out of further roentgenologic studies.

Cutaneous Manifestations

Mercer emphasized that two elementary types of cutaneous lesions are seen in cases of monocytic leukemia: "(1) macules and papules which, when seen early, simulate a secondary syphilid but later become slate blue and (2) pale, shotty papules which may lie deeper in the corium and are felt more easily than they are seen." In our experience, as well as in that of others,[4,5] these two types of cutaneous lesions are not specific for monocytic leukemia of Schilling, but may be encountered in other forms of lymphoblastoma. Purpuric, hemorrhagic and bullous lesions are frequently encountered early in the course of the disease, in contrast to their usual appearance as a terminal manifestation in cases of other forms of lymphoblastoma. They may result from specific infiltrations of the skin. Ulcerative gingivitis and bleeding of the gums, which appear to be frequent manifestations of monocytic leukemia, were not associated with exfoliative dermatitis in our six cases. The development of ulcers and furuncle-like lesions is usually a late or terminal manifestation of the disorder. Loveman was the first to emphasize that the disease may begin with indurated, eczematoid plaques similar to those seen in the early stage of mycosis fungoides.

Epstein and MacEachern have recently stated that the characteristic cutaneous lesion of Hodgkin's disease is the so-called exfoliative erythroderma (dermatitis). In our experience, however, exfoliative dermatitis may be a cutaneous expression of any one of the lymphoblastomas, including mycosis fungoides, Hodgkin's disease, lymphosarcoma and various types of leukemia.

637

It may be either a primary or a secondary manifestation. A third to a half of all instances of exfoliative dermatitis encountered among patients more than forty years of age are the result of lymphoblastoma, but a lymphoblastomatous etiology in cases of exfoliative dermatitis must be suspected at any age, as is exemplified by Case 2. Fortunately, the histopathologic picture of exfoliative dermatitis remains that of the original benign dermatosis or lymphoblastoma causing the exfoliative dermatitis,[7] although it may not be specific as to the type of lymphoblastomatous involvement. It may be necessary, therefore, to correlate clinical, histopathologic, roentgenologic and hemocytologic data. At times, removal of a lymph node for biopsy is necessary in order to determine the type of lymphoblastoma present.

Histopathology

The cutaneous, histopathologic changes were specific for monocytic leukemia of Schilling in four of the six cases associated with an exfoliative dermatitis, and were suggestive in the other two cases. Touch smears made from the specimen for biopsy at the time of excision presented a picture identical with that of the blood smears in two cases. In the earliest lesions of monocytic leukemia of Schilling the histopathologic picture may duplicate that of mycosis fungoides, which is not surprising in that in both conditions there is involvement of the reticulo-endothelial system of the skin together with increase in Gitterfäsern (lattice fibers).

If a specimen for biopsy is taken from a well-developed nodule, plaque, or zone of exfoliation, characteristic histopathologic changes are seen. There is an infiltration ranging from a diffuse to a dense nodular character limited at times to the upper part of the cutis, but often extending to the subcutaneous tissue. The epidermis may be involved in the process as in mycosis fungoides or there may be a grenze or border zone separating the epidermis from the infiltrate. The infiltrate occurs especially about the smaller blood vessels, which show proliferation of the endothelium and adventitia. The infiltrate is composed chiefly of monocytic cells of varying degrees of maturity. Indented, kidney-shaped nuclei and notching of nuclei are seen, but diagnosis rests on the demonstration of many monocytes which show a longitudinal

grooving of the nucleus.[2] This longitudinal grooving is actually the result of the arrangement of the chromatin but in slides for histopathologic study appears as a hyperchromatic longitudinal groove of the nucleus.

Monocytes with longitudinal grooving of the nuclei may occasionally be seen in cases of mycosis fungoides and Hodgkin's disease of the skin. In cases of mycosis fungoides, however, there is a multiplicity of cellular types with pyknosis and karyorrhexis of individual cells and clumping of cells to form pseudo-giant cells, whereas in true cases of Hodgkin's disease of the skin, Dorothy Reed cells characteristic of this disorder are usually present. In cases of lymphatic leukemia of the skin the lymphocytic cells composing the infiltrate are smaller in size than the monocytes and lack the morphologic features of the latter. Histopathologic or even hemocytologic distinction between the Naegeli and Schilling types of monocytic leukemia may at times be difficult, especially when there is a pronounced degree of eosinophilia in both tissue and blood, as exemplified by Case 2. Histopathologic diagnosis of the Schilling type is dependent on the demonstration of numerous monocytes with longitudinal grooving of the nuclei and must be corroborated by hemocytologic studies. Because of distortion in shape and character of the cells, the result of fixation and imbedding in paraffin, a final diagnosis of monocytic leukemia of Schilling is dependent on the result of touch smears from a specimen for biopsy or on hemocytologic studies.

Hemocytology

Monocytic leukemia of the Schilling type is distinguished from monocytic leukemia of the Naegeli type by the fact that the monocytes in the former develop directly from endothelial cells, whereas in the latter they develop from the myeloblast or stem cell. The Schilling type of monocytic leukemia, like the Naegeli type, may occur in acute, subacute, chronic, and even rarely, in aleukemic phases, depending on the degree of immaturity present. In the acute Schilling type, it is often difficult to distinguish this condition from an acute leukemic reticuloendotheliosis. The distinction depends on finding a great majority of the circulating leukocytes showing a tendency to develop into cells with the characteristics of the monocyte, whereas in leukemic reticulo-endotheliosis the predominating cell is more lymphocytic in character. Unless the predominating cell is of the monocytic type, the disease should be regarded as a leukemic reticulo-endotheliosis.

In the more chronic cases of leukemia, this distinction is readily made. In practically all cases of the Schilling type of monocytic leukemia, true reticular cells may be found in the circulating blood (Fig. 1). These cells are large, are usually much larger than the average leukocyte and have an eccentric nucleus that is almost spherical. The chromatin strands usually originate from the nuclear membrane and usually run transversely across the nucleus. These strands are very thin and are sharply distinguished from the parachromatin. Under a high power of magnification these strands are found to be made up of small granules, which when stained with Wright's stain, take a blue color. The nuclear membrane is very smooth in outline and is sharply defined. Usually one or more nucleoli are found. The nuclear pattern is so clear cut that the nucleus stands out prominently from the remainder of the cell. The cytoplasm is usually abundant, is blotchy in appearance and usually takes on a grayish-blue color when Wright's stain is applied.

During differentiation of this cell toward the monocyte, the chromatin strands become thicker and seem to bend on themselves slightly, producing what appears as a groove, running across the nucleus, which has usually become slightly elongated at this time.[8] Because grooving is so distinct and because it persists almost to the stage of complete maturity of the monocyte, it becomes a great aid in distinguishing the Schilling type of monocytic leukemia from the Naegeli type. In very acute forms of the Schilling type of monocytic leukemia most of the cells will be reticular cells with only a few of the cells approaching mature monocytes in character, whereas in the more chronic forms, only an occasional very immature cell will be found. The grooving tendency persists throughout the intermediate and mature stages. This is not usually associated with the more frequent forms of leukemic reticulo-endotheliosis.

The Naegeli type of monocytic leukemia is often regarded as one form of myelogenous leukemia because of its tendency to terminate usually as a typical myelogenous leukemia with

large numbers of intermediate forms and some mature forms of all types of the granular leukocytes. The parent cell in this type of leukemia is the myeloblast and the diagnosis may be made by the recognition of this cell and the inter-

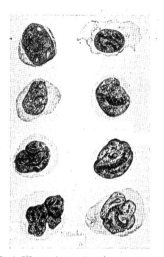

Fig. 1. Differences between the various types of cells in monocytic leukemia; the left column, Naegeli type, from top to bottom illustrates the changes from the myeloblast to the relatively mature monocyte. The right column, Schilling type, represents stages in development from the reticular cell to the mature monocyte. (Reduction of colored illustration from first article on monocytic leukemia. Arch. Int. Med., 60:51-63, (July) 1937.)

mediate stages through which it must pass in its development into the mature monocyte. The myeloblast is a relatively large cell, containing a large nucleus which makes up a great portion of the entire cell, the cytoplasm being a relatively thin band of substance around the nucleus, if compared to the much more abundant cytoplasm of the reticulo-endothelial cell. The nucleus of the myeloblast has a very thin nuclear membrane, the chromatin is usually granular, but it may occur in very fine strands. With Wright's stain, the chromatin is blue and is in very sharp contrast to the pink-staining parachromatin. The chromatin is usually in a sieve-like arrangement and is somewhat in the background, the parachromatin predominating.[2] This sieve-like chromatin structure is very characteristic of the myeloblast and differs greatly from the pattern seen in the nucleus of the reticulo-endothelial cell. Several nucleoli are present. During the stage of differentiation, the nucleoli disappear, the chromatin becomes more prominent and there is a gradual development of the string-like clumps of chromatin that are so typical of the mature monocyte. Concomitantly, the cytoplasm gradually loses its bluish tint and becomes slate gray in color, so characteristic of the mature monocyte.

One is not justified in making a diagnosis of the Naegeli type of monocytic leukemia unless the myeloblast has become differentiated into monocytes to the practical exclusion of the other myeloid leukocytes. In an occasional case, there may be only a slight predominance of monocytes, and in such a case it would be better to make the diagnosis of myelogenous leukemia. It is probable that the Naegeli type of monocytic leukemia is a variant of myelogenous leukemia but it seems, in the light of our present knowledge, that the diagnosis of the Naegeli type of monocytic leukemia is justified when differentiation of the myeloblasts through intermediate forms into monocytes occurs, to the practical exclusion of other myeloid leukocytes.

Prognosis and Treatment

Any type of leukemia eventually proves fatal, but it is the impression of one of us (Watkins) that the Schilling type is a more benign form than the Naegeli (myelogenous) type of monocytic leukemia. The two patients referred to in this paper have died, but the other four patients who had exfoliative dermatitis associated with a monocytic leukemia of Schilling were still living in February, 1938. In all six cases there was a history of cutaneous lesions of various types appearing on the extremities, including the face, months to years before the disease was recognized. Thus, in Case 3 of our first paper, cutaneous lesions developed on the arms and thighs in March, 1931. When the patient was seen at the clinic in April, 1935, the clinical and histologic picture was that of mycosis fungoides, although in retrospect many monocytes typical of the Schilling type of leukemia were demonstrable. The characteristic picture of exfoliative dermatitis and of monocytic leukemia of Schilling was present when the patient was seen in June, 1936. There has

been some improvement in the cutaneous condition since then.

In Case 4 of our first paper, the patient, a young woman, has had a generalized exfoliative dermatitis since April, 1933, which was diagnosed elsewhere as lymphatic leukemia, and then on examination at the clinic in April, 1935, as a monocytic leukemia. The patient has recently shown features of both conditions. The long duration of the dermatitis in these two cases might possibly be explained on the basis that the condition started out as mycosis fungoides and lymphatic leukemia, respectively and, later, evidence of monocytic leukemia of Schilling developed. It does seem, however, that these six patients who have exfoliative dermatitis tend to run a relatively benign course. Case 2 (Case 3 in a previous report[9]) is the only one in which there was any evidence of enlargement of the liver or spleen or a febrile course, all of which signs are frequently encountered in cases of monocytic leukemia of Schilling and may occur independent of any cutaneous lesions.[10]

The treatment of monocytic leukemia of Schilling, like that of other forms of leukemia, is only palliative and consists essentially of radiotherapy. High voltage roentgen therapy or radium therapy is indicated if the process is not too acute, but the dosage should be given with careful observation of the hemocytologic changes in order to determine the resistance of the cells to treatment. Moderate rather than intensive dosage usually gives the best results. The cutaneous lesions frequently involute temporarily, after superficial local roentgen therapy, or indirectly as the result of systemic high voltage roentgen therapy. In the cases of very acute leukemia, treatment is of no avail.

Summary and Conclusions

Exfoliative dermatitis in our experience is a rather frequent cutaneous manifestation of monocytic leukemia of Schilling. It has not been emphasized as such in recent articles in the literature. There are various other types of cutaneous manifestations of monocytic leukemia. The clinical, histopathologic and hemocytologic findings in six cases of exfoliative dermatitis associated with monocytic leukemia of Schilling are briefly referred to. A specific cutaneous pathologic picture is frequently encountered. The hemocytologic distinctions between the Schilling and Naegeli types of monocytic leukemia, however, are diagnostic. It is important to distinguish between these two types of monocytic leukemia because of their different prognosis and response to treatment.

References

1. Epstein, Ervin, and MacEachern, Katherine: Dermatologic manifestations of the lymphoblastoma-leukemia group. Arch. Int. Med., 60:867-875, (Nov.) 1937.
2. Giffin, H. Z., and Watkins, C. H.: The distinction between splenic anemia and subleukemic splenic reticuloendotheliosis. Am. Jour. Med. Sc., 188:761-767, (Dec.) 1934.
3. Goldhamer, S. M., and Barney, B. F.: Myelogenous leukemia with cutaneous involvement. Jour. A.M.A., 107:1041-1043, (Sept. 26) 1936.
4. Loveman, A. B.: Monocytic leukemia cutis; report of a case with biopsy studies. South. Med. Jour., 29:357-364, (April) 1936.
5. Lynch, F. W.: Cutaneous lesions associated with monocytic leukemia and reticulo-endotheliosis. Arch. Dermat. and Syph., 34:775-796, (Nov.) 1936.
6. Mercer, S. T.: The dermatosis of monocytic leukemia. Arch. Dermat. and Syph., 31:615-635, (May) 1935.
7. Montgomery, Hamilton: Exfoliative dermatosis and malignant erythroderma; the value and limitations of histopathologic studies. Arch. Dermat. and Syph., 27:253-271, (Feb.) 1933.
8. Montgomery, Hamilton, and Watkins, C. H.: Monocytic leukemia; cutaneous manifestations of the Naegeli and Schilling types; hemocytologic differentiation. Arch. Int. Med., 60:51-63, (July) 1937.
9. Montgomery, Hamilton, and Watkins, C. H.: Exfoliative dermatitis as a manifestation of monocytic leukemia (Schilling). Proc. Staff Meet. Mayo Clinic, 13:294-297, (May 11) 1938.
10. Osgood, E. E.: Monocytic leukemia; report of six cases and review of one hundred and twenty-seven cases. Arch. Int. Med., 59:931-951, (June) 1937.
11. Wayson, J. T., and Weidman, F. D.: Aleukemic reticulosis; an additional member of the group of so-called cutaneous lymphoblastomas. Arch. Dermat. and Syph., 34:755-770, (Nov.) 1936.
12. Wile, U. J., and Stiles, Frank, Jr.: Clinical mutations in lymphoblastomas. Jour. A.M.A., 104:532-536, (Feb. 16) 1935.

ARTIFICIAL IMPREGNATION

R. T. SEASHORE, M.D.

Duluth, Minnesota

ARTIFICIAL impregnation is fertilization resulting from the artificial transfer of active semen from the male to the female.

The literature on this subject is chiefly foreign. Since 1902 there have appeared only twenty-four articles in the American literature, and among these the case reports are not numerous. With this in view it was considered worthwhile to present a brief review of the available literature, and also to present a case in which artificial impregnation was successfully carried out.

The first reference to mammalian artificial impregnation is that of a 15th century Arab chieftain who desired to sire his mare by an enemy chieftain's prize stallion. Unable to do so, his men managed to steal some semen from the stallion, which was then inserted into the mare's vagina. Successful impregnation is said to have occurred.[6]

However, the first authentic and recorded report came from Spallanzani, in 1780. He recorded an artificial impregnation of a Spaniel bitch, as a result of which she bore a litter of four pups.[1]

John Hunter, early in the 19th century, made the first recording of artificial impregnation in the human. In his case the husband suffered from hypospadias, and coitus was impossible. The semen was collected artificially and transferred to the wife's vagina, conception resulting.[2]

From 7 to 10 per cent of marriages are reputed to be sterile. With that in mind, the procedure as here described is occasionally justified to bring family happiness to an otherwise childless couple who have the requisites of good parents.

Who should be submitted to this procedure? First, we should use this opportunity to practice good eugenics, and encourage the procedure only in those who are apt to improve society. Second, it should be done only in those cases where both the husband and wife are desirous of the procedure after due consideration.

Biologic indications include male infertility due to hypospadias or other abnormality, or to aspermatogenesis from any cause. Indications from the female standpoint, assuming that the tubes, ovaries, and uterus are normal, include stenosis of the cervix, dyspareunia, abnormal vagina, and chemical incompatibilities with the sperm.

An effort must first be made to procure, if possible, a normal impregnation by correcting any abnormalities, improving the general health, changing the vaginal flora and chemical reaction, stimulating spermatogenesis with hormonal therapy, and by whatever other means are indicated. Of course, the procedure should never be carried out in the presence of tubal or cervical infection.

And, we may add, the unfit from a social or eugenic standpoint should not be submitted to this procedure.

Legal Aspects

The attorney, who served in the case to be presented, found no mention of any ruling or any discussion of this subject in the legal literature. Consequently moral dictates must be our guide in handling these cases. Also, it is advisable to use the utmost legal precaution for all concerned.

When the husband himself is the source of the sperm, the legal aspects are not great, but even so it is wise to have a signed statement acknowledging understanding of the procedure and willingness to comply. However, in the case of the sterile husband, where the sperm is obtained from a donor, obviously legal entanglements of a greater variety can arise. Anyone contemplating this procedure should certainly read the excellent article of Seymour and Koerner in *The Journal of The American Medical Association* for November 7, 1936, in which they discuss the legal, moral, and psychologic aspects of the procedure very thoroughly.[9]

Among the entanglements that may arise are accusations of adultery. The husband, having proof of his sterility at the time of conception, may use his wife's pregnancy as grounds for divorce. He may refuse to accept the responsibility of supporting the child. The donor might claim the custody of the child. The child's status in the settlement of an estate might be questioned. The child could even claim a share in the donor's estate.

The procedure, of course, should not be done unless there is an intense desire for a child on the part of the wife, and the husband is entirely agreeable. It is wise to delay several months in order to be certain that it is not merely a hasty and transient desire on their part. During this time the husband and wife could be treated in an attempt to establish normal conception.

For the protection of everyone concerned, legal papers should be drawn in which the wife and the husband accept full responsibility for the procedure, and also accept the child as their legal offspring. Seymour and Koerner, in the above mentioned article, present this excellently worded consent statement to be signed by the husband and the wife:

"I, ..., residing at .... of my own free will and volition have requested Dr. .... to inseminate my wife artificially with the sperm of a male selected by Dr. .... This request has been made with the full knowledge and consent of my wife, whose authorization is hereto annexed. I am making this request, because it is not possible for me to procreate and because both my wife and myself are extremely anxious to have a child and because our mutual happiness and the well being of my wife will be best served by this artificial insemination.

..................................(LS)

On this ...... day of .... 19...., before me came ...., to me known and known to me to be the person described herein and who acknowledged to me that he executed the foregoing consent.

..................................(LS)

I, ..., join in my husband's request above stated and hereby authorize Dr. .... to inseminate me artificially with the sperm of a male selected by Dr. ....

..................................(LS)

On this ...... day of .... 19...., before me came ...., to me known and known to me to be the person described herein and who acknowledged to me that she executed the foregoing consent.

..................................(LS)

If the people involved are strangers to the physician they also recommend that the thumb prints be placed alongside their signatures to further identify them, thus further reducing the possibility of trickery through false identification. These consent records, made in duplicate, are then sealed and filed away in separate safe places, to be available and unsealed only in case of legal complications.

It is well to have a separate consent statement signed by the donor accepting release of the child from his custody, and waiving all claims to it. It also is then filed away separately. If the donor is married, his wife should also sign the document to prevent her from later accusing him of adultery, and to minimize any possible family discord which might result.

Will the child be a legal heir, or must he be adopted by the father through court procedure? Inasmuch as no legal ruling states that he is not a legitimate heir, it is fair to assume that the consent signatures of the husband and wife are sufficient to legalize him.[9]

Psychologic Aspects

The process should be kept as secret as possible, the minimum number of people knowing of the affair, and after conception nothing should be said about it in order that the couple may more readily forget the artificial character of the conception. Likewise the donor should be one who is unknown to them, and one who is not apt to encounter them in any way. They should be told that the donor is in excellent health, and that he resembles the husband in appearance and temperament, all this to encourage the association of the child with the husband rather than the donor and thus to diminish the possibility of estrangement of affections.

Psychologic influences of a lesser degree may rest on the donor also. If he knows who the child is he may develop affection for the child, and even to some extent for the mother. Even if he does not know the child, his thoughts may wander in that direction and influence his mental makeup.

For the good of the child, he should be kept in ignorance of the affair, at least until he is able to meet the knowledge with intelligent understanding.

Selection of the donor should be done carefully. He should be someone of the same nationality, physique, appearance, and temperament as the husband, so that if the donor's characteristics are dominant in the child they will resemble the husband's as nearly as possible. Naturally, he should be in good health, both physically and mentally, and of good family heritage. The donor should be advised to keep the affair secret so that it will not arise on later occasions to plague him.

Objections to the procedure may be esthetic, psychologic, and moral attitudes. However, any couple really desirous of a child will willingly overlook these things after they are fully explained. Objections on the part of prospective donors may be even harder to handle. Finding a good donor may be the hardest part of the task. Other objections are complications such as infection and tubal and abdominal pregnancy which might conceivably occur. However, careful technic should make this risk no greater than normal impregnation. Mental shock after the pregnancy occurs must be thought of as a possibility, which suggests that the procedure should

not be carried out in any individual who might be subject to mental unrest.

Technic

The semen is collected from the husband or donor either by frictional ejaculation or by vesicle massage into a sterile vessel. It could be collected also by coitus interruptus or by condom specimen but these methods are less aseptic. The semen should be examined to be certain that the spermatozoa are present in large numbers (about 1,000,000 per c.c.), active, and not over 20 per cent are dead or abnormal.[2] Attempts at placing the donor's semen into the vas or vesicles of the husband have not proven successful.[10]

The woman prepares herself with a cleansing douche and is placed in the lithotomy or the knee chest position. The spermatic fluid is then instilled by means of a Eustachian catheter and a syringe into the vagina, cervical canal, or uterine cavity, the latter probably being the most effective. Various authors recommend the use of from 0.1 to 1.00 c.c. of the spermatic fluid. It should be done slowly and gently, observing aseptic precautions carefully. The patient is kept lying down for a short while afterward.

Just before or at the time of ovulation is the time of choice for carrying out the procedure. The methods for determining this will not be mentioned here except to state that in the twenty-eight day cycle, anywhere from the tenth to the fourteenth day after the onset of menses will probably be right in most cases.

If failure occurs it is justifiable to repeat the process several times inasmuch as ovulation may have failed to occur within the few days following insemination, due either to delay or failure of the descent of the ovum.

Case Report

The case to be presented is that of a couple who were childless after six years of married life. No pregnancies had occurred. The wife had been in good health except for scarlet fever when thirteen years old, complicated by acute nephritis which cleared up, and for three attacks of rather severe cystitis. The husband had always been in good health except that he was sterile as a result of orchitis complicating mumps. Attempts to stimulate spermatogenesis in him by general care and Antuitrin "S" over a six months period had failed only an occasional dead spermatozoön being found in the specimen.

At their suggestion it was decided to impregnate her artificially with the sperm of a donor. I delayed them for several months, giving them plenty of time to think it over. Legal papers were drawn and filed away in safe places that they know of and will have access to only if necessary. A donor of good health and family was selected, with the precaution that he was unacquainted with the patient or her husband.

A specimen of spermatic fluid was collected by the frictional ejaculation method into a sterile container, and was then examined and found to have an adequate number of active spermatozoa and a minimal number inactive and abnormal.

The recipient, having prepared herself with a cleansing douche before coming to the office, was placed in the lithotomy position, the cervix exposed in the usual manner and painted with a mild antiseptic. One-half c.c. of the spermatic fluid was then instilled into the uterine cavity with the aid of a syringe and a Eustachian catheter. She was kept lying down for a half hour and then sent home. She promptly became pregnant and has since that time been delivered of a normal child.

Since the time of the insemination not a word has been said about it to this couple. To all appearances they are a happy father and mother and betray no evidence of regret on their part.

Bibliography

1. Brewer, H.: Artificial insemination. Marriage Hygiene, 2: 420-427, (May) 1936.
2. Cohen, J.: Artificial insemination. New Orleans Med. and Surg. Jour., 85:817-822, (May) 1933.
3. Cohen, J.: Artificial insemination. New Orleans Med. and Surg. Jour., 86:730-731, (May) 1934.
4. Dickerson, R. L.: Artificial impregnation; essays in tubal insemination. Am. Jour. Obst. and Gynec., 1:255-261, 1920.
5. Lifvendahl, R. A.: Tubal pregnancy following insemination. Am. Jour. Obst. and Gynec., 25:733-735, (May) 1933.
6. Loessl, H.: Practical use of artificial impregnation in animals. Vet. Med., 29:441-443, (Oct.) 1934.
7. Seymour, F. I.: Viability of spermatozoa in cervical canal. Jour. A.M.A., 106:1728, (May 16) 1936.
8. Seymour, F. I.: Eugenics in practice. Marriage Hygiene, 3:44-48, (Aug.) 1936.
9. Seymour, F. I., and Koerner, A.: Medicolegal aspects of artificial insemination. Jour. A.M.A., 107:1531-1534, (Nov. 7) 1936.
10. Stepita, C. T.: Physiologic artificial insemination. Am. Jour. Surg., 21:450-451, (Sept.) 1933.

MODERN TREATMENT OF BURNS

An Evaluation of Various Methods Used in 968 Cases in the Cook County Hospital

KARL A. MEYER, M.D., F.A.C.S., and J. LESTER WILKEY, B.S., M.D.

Chicago, Illinois

SINCE Davidson[7] suggested that tannic acid applied to burns forms a protective crust, the treatment of burns has been greatly simplified. When treating burns, whether they be severe or moderate, a definite program must be maintained if success is to be achieved. Regardless of the program decided on, we must plan to:

1. Treat the initial shock
2. Prevent absorption of toxins from the burned surfaces
3. Combat fluid loss
5. Shorten the period of disability by promoting healing
6. Avoid permanent deformity.

During the past decade various types of treatment have become popular, and many different dyes, antiseptics, and escharotics have been used.

In the Cook County Hospital we treated 968 burns from 1933 to 1937 inclusive. Some were superficial burns, others second degree burns, but a greater number were severe third degree burns, widespread over the body. We have had

occasion to use almost every type of treatment. In this paper we shall attempt to evaluate the various treatments as used by the surgical services of this hospital.

Treatment of the Initial Shock and Toxemia

The patients that we see, or at least a great percentage of them, are in shock and are very toxic. One of our great problems is to bring the patient out of the shock and to lessen the toxemia. This brings up the great present day controversy as to whether the morbidity and the mortality that occurs in patients with burns is due to the absorption of a toxic substance formed at the site of the burn, to the loss of body fluids through the open skin surfaces causing gradual dehydration, or to the toxemia from absorbed products of infection which occurs in the burned areas.

Underhill,[15] in 1923, showed that patients with extensive superficial burns might have a blood concentration of 209 per cent of the normal. He felt that all of the symptoms following severe

*Read before the annual meeting of the Minnesota State Medical Association, Duluth, Minnesota, June 30, 1938.

burns could be accounted for by this marked blood concentration.

Davidson[7] claimed that a toxin was formed at the site of the burn, the absorption of which caused a constitutional reaction.

Rosenthal[12, 13] in a series of experiments showed that a substance was present in the blood of burned humans, a burn toxin, which was capable of lowering blood pressure, and he demonstrated that this burn toxin could be neutralized by the serum of healed burned shoats, pigs, and humans.

Kapsinow's[9] experiments, on the other hand, showed that toxins are probably not absorbed from the burned site. He was not able to find evidence of absorption after applying strychnine and phenolphthalein to burned areas.

Wells[16] states that there is increasing proof that bacterial infection rather than proteolytic toxins is the cause of death in the severely burned.

Aldrich[1] popularized the rôle of infection in burns and showed that the toxemia of a burned patient was not due to the absorption of a burn protein, or a shifting of the water balance, but to an invasion of the body by virulent forms of streptococci which entered through the burned areas.

Regardless of whether it is a toxin, an infection, or loss of vital tissue fluids, the possibility of the presence of one or all of these factors must be considered and combated.

A rule that we adhere to strictly is that any patient who has had one-eighth or more of the body surface burned is treated for shock whether it is present or not. Regardless of the local care of the burn, the shock must be combated first.

We find that shock following burns is best treated by:

1. Administration of morphine for control of pain.
2. Intravenous administration of saline and glucose.
3. A heat cradle to the body, with enough light to maintain constantly a heat of 90 degrees.
4. Blood transfusion.
5. Stimulants, when necessary.

The morphine is given in sufficient quantity to control pain and restlessness. The saline and glucose mixture is given to replace the lost blood chlorides and to bolster the liver. We give, as a

rule, 1,000 c.c. of saline and glucose per 25 pounds of body weight in twenty-four hours. Some of the members of our staff add gum acacia to the saline and glucose mixture.

Blood transfusion is a routine procedure for patients in shock. The blood bank system in the Cook County Hospital makes it possible for the patient to receive blood as soon as thirty minutes after admission to the hospital. We feel that the immediate accessibility of the blood to these patients who are severely burned, has materially aided in lowering our morbidity as well as the mortality rate.

The Control of Fluid Loss

The loss of blood plasma and the concentration of blood is probably the cause of death in the first twenty-four hours. The dressing of choice must be the one that will prevent the loss of fluid from the blood stream by adequately sealing the open surfaces.

The Tannic Acid Treatment

In 1925, Davidson suggested the use of tannic acid in the treatment of burns. He showed that tannic acid would precipitate the broken down tissue proteins and close off the capillary beds, thereby preventing the loss of body fluids.

In the past ten years, tannic acid has been used very successfully in the Cook County Hospital in the treatment of burns.

When the patient comes out of the initial shock the wounds are cleansed of grease, dirt, and grime. Most of the burns that we see are covered with oils and grease. If the patient is not in shock, he is placed in a bath tub of warm water containing sodium bicarbonate. The bath tub is scrubbed daily and kept covered to prevent further contamination of the burns. The surgeon and his assistants wear caps, masks, sterile gowns and gloves. Fat solvents, such as benzine and ether, are used to remove the grease and oil without undue scrubbing. The unburned skin surrounding the wound is scrubbed with soap and water. The burns are washed with white soap and a solution of boric acid. We use white soap instead of green soap, because green soap was found to be more irritating (Koch).[10] The burned area is thoroughly débrided after the initial cleansing. In a majority of the cases the blisters and blebs are widely opened under aseptic technic using sterile instruments, and the loose areas of skin are removed. We believe that opening of these blisters removes the fluid which contains the organisms that may later cause infection. The patient is placed on sterile sheets.

The burned areas are then sprayed with a 5 per cent aqueous solution of tannic acid every fifteen minutes until a dark mahogany colored coagulation is obtained. The heat cradle with enough light to produce a heat of 90 degrees is then placed over the body. Sheets are placed over the cradle. The coagulum is allowed to remain in place until it becomes loose or its edges curl up as healing occurs. When this happens it is cut away. If serum collects underneath the crust, as may occur when there has been complete destruction of the tissues, or should infection cause its loosening, the coagulum is removed sufficiently to allow for drainage or subsequent treatment.

From the latter part of 1933 to 1937 inclusive, 272 patients were treated by this method. Of this number thirty-four died, giving a mortality rate of 12.1 per cent. One hundred and eight showed infection.

The Compound Aniline Dye Treatment

In 1929, Aldrich[2] took cultures from the burned areas and from the serum of the blisters following burns. In all patients who were severely burned, he found growths of streptococcus hemolyticus as well as other organisms. He found that the persistent presence of these organisms was in direct proportion to the severity of the toxemia, as well as the signs of sepsis.

Aldrich felt that the success of tannic acid depended on whether or not the burn to which it was applied was sterile. He stated that if a burn is to be sealed and if this sealing is to carry out its function of preventing fluid loss, infection beneath this sealing must be avoided. A great number of infections beneath the tannic crust were being reported. So Aldrich looked for a new escharotic that would be antiseptic and nontoxic. He finally decided on gentian violet. Gentian violet is a specific antiseptic for gram positive organisms but its weakness is that it has no effect on the gram negative organisms. He developed a compound of aniline dyes using gentian violet, three parts by weight, brilliant green, 2 parts by weight, and neutral acriflavine, one part by weight. This mixture is known as "Aldrich Dye Mixture." Two grams of this mixture are dissolved in 100 c.c. of water and used in the form of a spray.

We have used the Aldrich treatment in 104 cases. Our routine is as follows:

No preliminary clean-up is done unless the patient has been treated previously with grease, oils, or ointments. If so, then these are removed by soft sponging with ether. Under strict asepsis the blebs are opened and the loose skin cut away, but no extensive débridement is done. The patient is placed under a heat cradle and sprayed every hour by means of an atomizer. An eschar develops in about eight hours.

Continual watching of the crusts are necessary. This crust does not hide infection as does tannic acid but becomes moist if there is any underlying pus.

If infection develops, the softened areas are excised, the underlying area is dried with a sterile sponge and the dyes reapplied. This technic is continued until good granulations form. One annoyance is that the dyes stain the bed linen which necessitates frequent changes.

We used this treatment in 104 patients with second and third degree burns of the abdomen, trunk and extremities. Of the 104, nine died (a mortality of 8.7 per cent) and only ten became infected.

The Gentian Violet Treatment

Following the suggestion of Aldrich,[1] we treated 125 burns with a 1 per cent aqueous solution of gentian violet. Most of the burns treated by this method were second degree burns of the extremities. It was used on both clean and contaminated burns after sufficient débridement and removal of greases and oils was done. Strict asepsis was adhered to. The gentian violet was applied by means of sterile cotton pledgets. The patient was then put under a heat cradle. Of the 125 cases treated by this method, there were only two deaths or a mortality of 1.6 per cent. There were twenty-two infections.

The Tannic Acid-Silver Nitrate Treatment

In 1935, Bettman[3, 4] introduced the tannic acid-silver nitrate treatment of burns. He believed that while the tannic acid treatment of Davidson was the height of advancement in the treatment of burns, it was not entirely satisfactory because

1. It takes the solid coagulum of tannic acid hours to form, while with silver nitrate added, it take minutes.

2. As the coagulum slowly forms, the loss of circulating body fluids continues, and this loss

must be made up by repeated administration of parenteral fluids, thereby disturbing the patient frequently. With tannic acid followed by silver nitrate, one thorough application of the medication is all that is necessary for a good solid coagulum to form, and the loss of body fluids is stopped immediately.

3. By preventing dehydration, shock is minimized, and this tends to carry the patient safely through the most critical period, the first twenty-four hours following a serious burn.

This treatment is used to a great extent in the children's surgical division and Hedin[12] used this treatment in eighty-two consecutive cases with six deaths (a mortality rate of 7.3 per cent).

To effect a good result with this treatment, all grease and oil must be removed. This is accomplished by benzine. The burns are then dried by an electric dryer. Then, under strict asepsis, and with the patient on sterile sheets, a 5 per cent tannic acid solution is sprayed on by means of an atomizer. Immediately following the single spray, silver nitrate in 10 per cent solution is applied to the surface by means of cotton pledgets. The formation of a crust is accomplished in a few minutes and the crust is a flexible one. The patient is placed under a heat cradle. Fluids are forced orally and parenterally. Blood transfusion is given routinely.

If the crust becomes loose it is removed. Unhealed areas are treated by the application of oxyquinoline sulfate (scarlet red) as suggested by Bettman.[4]

The cases in which this treatment was used were severe second and third degree burns. Since January, 1938, we have treated 220 burns by this method. There were nineteen deaths (a mortality of 8.6 per cent). Of the 220, only eighteen became infected. Our records show that the period of hospitalization with this treatment is definitely shorter than that of patients treated by other methods. We also noted that the amount of scarring and deformity is reduced to a minimum by this treatment.

The Methyl Rosaniline-Silver Nitrate Treatment

In 1937, Branch[6] introduced the methyl rosaniline-silver nitrate treatment of burns. He used a 10 per cent solution of silver nitrate, which acts on the proteins of the burned area, to immediately lay down a milky white coagulum. This took

the place of tannic acid in coagulating the proteins and preventing fluid loss. The methyl rosaniline stained this coagulum violet and aided in destroying and preventing infection.

After the application of the methyl rosaniline which is sprayed on in 1 per cent solution, the patient is placed under a heat cradle. The patient is resprayed five times at fifteen-minute intervals. If necessary, the spray is used once or twice daily following the initial treatment. If any coagulum remains at the end of two weeks, it is soaked off by the warm sodium bicarbonate bath. When the crusts are soaked off, epithelial islands are present in many of the cases. Scarlet red ointment is then applied.

Skin grafts were not needed in any of the cases on which this treatment was used. We used this treatment in twenty-six cases of second degree burns of the extremities. There were no deaths and only two became infected.

The Cod Liver Oil Treatment

Steel[14] of England found that crude cod liver oil, when used from the beginning of the treatment on burns, caused speedy recovery and it transformed indolent areas into healthy granulations.

We used this treatment on thirty-eight cases of first and second degree burns. These burns were not very extensive. The crude cod liver oil was applied after the burns were debrided and cleansed with warm boric acid solution. In the first degree burns, healing was fast, and the results were gratifying, but on the second degree burns, of which there were twenty-six, eight became infected, and in a large number, healing was delayed. A disadvantage of this treatment is the persistent presence of the fish odor about the patient. There were no deaths with this treatment.

Treatment of Severely Contaminated Burns and Those Over Ten to Twelve Hours Old

It is a rule in the Children's Surgical Division to treat burns which are ten to twelve hours old, or those severely contaminated with greases, oils, and dirty clothing, so that infection is assured, with moist saline dressings, or moist boric acid dressings. This establishes drainage and cleans the burned area. These dressings are changed three to four times daily and the burn is washed at each changing with white soap.

In many cases Xeroform* strips are used. These are strips of gauze treated with sterile vaseline containing 3 per cent Xeroform. These strips are changed daily. The burns are cleansed at each changing with boric acid and white soap. The strips are covered by sterile dressings and a sea sponge is placed over these dressings so that the burn only will receive the benefit of the dressing. This is done to prevent maceration of the surrounding healthy skin. The sponge is held in place by a binder. The sponge pressure is also useful in preventing the formation of excess granulation tissue.

We used this treatment in 186 cases with two deaths (a mortality rate of about 0.6 of 1 per cent). With this treatment the period of hospitalization is definitely much longer than that with other treatments, but the morbidity and mortality rates are much lower. The scarring and deformity are not of a high degree.

We have also used Amertan† on many first degree burns and some second degree burns. The results were satisfactory in that infection was not commonly seen with this drug and healing seemed to be quite rapid.

General Care of Burn Patients

At this point we must stress the importance of adequate nursing care. The outlook for a burn patient, like that of a patient following a major surgical procedure is dependent, in a great part, on the nursing care. She must see that the fluid intake is maintained, that the patient is comfortable and has adequate rest. The dressings are kept clean so that infection can be minimized.

Daily urine examinations are made on all burn patients. Blood chemistry examinations are made twice weekly to determine the blood chloride content and kidney function.

If, in spite of all precautions, infection develops, and it does in some, the patient is placed in a clean tub of warm water with sodium bicarbonate added. This is a daily procedure. Moist boric acid or saline dressings are then applied following the suggestion of Blair and Brown[5] who stated that these dressings arouse the resisting and fighting forces of the neighboring tissues, alleviate pain, and promote drainage. These dressings are moistened frequently, but not ex-

cessively so that they do not dry in place. Excessive moisture causes maceration of the surrounding tissues.

Excessive granulation is combated by the use of adhesive strips placed across the burn.

Nourishing food and tonics are given to all patients, and if the response of the patient is not as quick as expected, a blood transfusion is given to speed up the powers of healing and hasten recovery.

Skin grafts are done frequently when indicated. The burns are grafted early if the surfaces are clean and suitable for a graft.

Summary and Conclusions

1. The morbidity and mortality of burns are definitely determined by: (1) the absorption of a toxin or toxic substance from the site of the burn; (2) the loss of body fluids; (3) infection; or (4) by a combination of these factors.

2. The initial shock must be treated by proper methods as soon as a burn patient is seen. This is as important as the local treatment of the burn.

3. Blood transfusion is of great value in severe burns.

4. We believe that the Bettman tannic acid-silver nitrate treatment is the treatment of choice in severe burns not contaminated or infected, especially if the patient is seen in less than twelve hours after the burn occurred.

5. The aniline dye treatment has been quite successful in our hands where infection is imminent.

6. In severely contaminated burns, moist saline dressings and cleansing with white soap is the treatment of choice.

7. Rigid asepsis must be maintained in the treatment of all burns.

8. If infection occurs, in spite of precautions, the patient is given daily sodium bicarbonate baths and moist saline dressings are applied.

9. Good nursing care is of the utmost importance.

Bibliography

1. Aldrich, R. H.: Role of infection in burns, theory and treatment with special reference to gentian violet. New Eng. Jour. Med., 208:299-309, (Feb. 9), 1933.
2. Aldrich, R. H.: Treatment of burns with a compound of aniline dyes. New Eng. Jour. Med., 217:911-914, (Dec.) 1937.
3. Bettman, A. G.: The tannic acid-silver nitrate treatment of burns. Northwest Med., 34:46-51, (Feb.), 1935.
4. Bettman, A. G.: The rationale of the tannic acid-silver nitrate treatment of burns. Jour. Am. Med. Assn., 108:1490-1494 (May) 1937.
5. Blair, V. P., and Brown, J. B.: Use and uses of large split skin grafts of immediate thickness. Surg., Gynec. and Obst., 49:82-97, (July) 1929.

*Tri-bromphenol plus bismuth.
†A 5 per cent tannic acid plus 1:5000 merthiolate in a jelly base.

6. Branch, H. E.: Extensive burns, treatment with silver nitrate and methyl rosaniline. Arch. Surg., 35:478, (Sept.) 1937.
7. Davidson, E. C.: Tannic acid treatment of burns. Surg., Gynec., and Obst., 41:202-211, (Aug.) 1935.
8. Hedin, R. F.: The immediate and subsequent treatment of burns. Minnesota Med., 21:229, (April) 1938.
9. Kapsinow, R.: Rate of absorption from extensive superficial burns. New Orleans Med. and Surg. Jour., 85:597-599, (Feb.) 1933.
10. Koch, Sumner L.: From the Children's Surgical Division.
11. Lueck, A. M.: Personal communication. Children's Surgical Division.
12. Rosenthal, S. R.: The toxin of burns. Ann. Surg., 106:111-117, (July) 1937.
13. Rosenthal, S. R.: Neutralization of histamine and burn toxin. Ann. Surg., 106:257-265, (Aug.) 1937.
14. Steel, J. P.: Cod liver oil treatment of wounds. Lancet, 2:291, (Aug. 10) 1935.
15. Underhill, F. P., Carrington, G. L., Kapsinow, R., and Pack, G. T.: Blood concentration changes in extensive superficial burns and their significance for systemic treatment. Arch. Int. Med., 32:31;49, (July) 1923.
16. Wells, D. B.: The aseptic tannic acid treatment of diffuse superficial burns. Jour. Am. Med. Assn., 101:1136-1138, (Oct. 7) 1933.

◆ CASE REPORT ◆

SUPPURATIVE PAROTITIS AS A COMPLICATION OF MUMPS

EVERETT C. PERLMAN, M.D.

Minneapolis, Minnesota

IN MOST of the current textbooks of medicine, pediatrics or contagious diseases, little mention is made of suppuration in the parotid gland as a complication of acute epidemic parotitis. Differential diagnosis between the epidemic and the suppurative types is very definite and suggests to the reader that one never occurs with the other. Suppurative parotitis occurs, more than rarely, as a sequel to operative procedures, notably those for suppurative abdominal conditions, and also as a sequel to certain infectious diseases such as typhoid fever, scarlet fever, diphtheria, and pneumonia. Those following surgical procedures are attributed by Berndt[1] to general dehydration from vomiting, reflex diminution of the salivary secretion from the anesthetic and from surgical manipulation, as well as from actual trauma to the gland by unskilled anesthetists. Those occurring as complications of infectious diseases are due to a locus minoris resistantia rather than to a metastatic invasion of the gland, except in the case of typhoid fever, wherein the typhoid organism has been recovered from the infected glands. Various other factors in the incidence of this complication have been well reviewed by Lewis.[2]

That suppurative parotitis does occur as a complication of epidemic mumps, although rarely, seems evident in a few case reports scattered through the literature. It is therefore necessary to report this case, to the end that other similar cases may be recognized. In 1920 and 1921, Bernstein[4] saw three such cases in the School-Polyclinic, Odessa, all of which terminated by spontaneous rupture of the abscess into the external auditory canal. He thought that the tendency to abscess formation was enhanced by the marked exhaustion and the deficient oral hygiene of the children during the blockade and the typhus epidemic of those years. Alexander[3] also reported such a case in 1927 with a similar spontaneous rupture into the external auditory canal. Bader,[2] in 1931, reported a case of acute suppurative parotitis as a complication of mumps, with rupture into the canal, but this swelling was secondary to an otitis media of three weeks' duration.

Case Report

D. F., female, aged eleven, had a past history which was essentially negative with the exception of pertussis at six months and rubeola at four years. On February 26, 1938, the patient came into her home after play, with a swelling in the left parotid region, and announced to her mother that she had mumps. Several children, playmates, had had the same infection during the past few weeks. She complained of nothing else, and was not ill enough to be confined to bed. The swelling disappeared gradually during the next four days.

On the evening of the fourth day she complained of dizziness. She went to bed, slept all night and arose the next morning feeling well. In the afternoon she complained of pain in the right cheek. Her mother noticed that there was a swelling on this side of the face and that the child had a fever. That night she complained a great deal of pain in the ear and cheek and slept poorly. The next morning she was seen by a physician who told her that she had mumps. She was seen by the writer that evening and at that time she had a marked swelling over the right parotid gland with exquisite tenderness over the gland, under the jaw, and extending around to the right ear. There was no tenderness over the mastoid, but marked trismus was present. On slight pressure over the gland a thick yellow, purulent material escaped from Steno's duct. Her temperature at this time was 103.8 by mouth, and her pulse rate was 128. The right ear drum was not visible because of the swelling in the canal from pressure of the swollen gland. The orifice of Steno's duct on the left side also was swollen and surrounded by a red areola, but no pus was expressed. She was given supportive treatment at home and when seen, two days later, there was definite evidence of extensive suppuration in the gland, with an area of beginning fluctuation inferior to the helix of the right ear. Purulent material continued to exude from Steno's duct during all of this time. The next morning there was a spontaneous rupture of the abscess into the anterior wall of the external auditory canal, with profuse discharge of purulent material from the ear canal. There was also, by this time, definite fluctuation of the abscess below the ear. The temperature, by mouth, varied each day from 101 to 102.5.

At this time the patient was transferred to a hospital where the fluctuant area was treated with very small hot packs for twenty-four hours in order to localize the suppuration, and then it was incised. The incision,

(Continued on page 670)

HISTORY OF MEDICINE IN MINNESOTA

MEDICINE IN WASHINGTON AND CHISAGO COUNTIES

(Continued from August issue.)

Besides their practice, the physicians found plenty of other things to do. In 1880 Dr. A. J. Murdock was elected treasurer of the Union of the Towns of the St. Croix Valley, secretary of the Chisago County Bible Society, and (in December) president of the town council. Dr. Millard was Washington county physician; Drs. Weiseman, Hallberg and Olding sold liquor (unfortunately, without licenses), which caused them to be arrested. Dr. Comfort was for many years editor of a *Thompsonian Medical Journal.* Where and when this journal was published is unknown. In 1881 the office of Washington county physician passed to Dr. Caine. Dr. T. C. Clark was Stillwater city physician, and Dr. Millard took a long and very interesting trip abroad. Dr. Hallberg was physician for the Scandinavian Relief Association, a position he held for several years. Dr. A. J. Murdock served on the Board of Education, and was second vice president of the State Medical Association. In 1882 Dr. Olding ran a mercantile business. Drs. Murdock, Fliesburg and McComb shared the position of Chisago county physician, while Dr. Pratt was made county physician of Washington county, despite much opposition from the local homeopaths. Upon his return from abroad in June, Millard was elected president of the State Medical Association. Clark served as deputy coroner. Edgerton ran an eye and ear infirmary; Gaskill owned and managed a drug store. Zuercher proved his versatility by winning a $100 prize with a poem he had written. In 1883 Caine was elected one of the censors at a homeopathic convention. Watier was one of the incorporators of "Le Canadian" publishing company of St. Paul. Murdock was again president of the council of Taylors Falls; Millard was a member of the first State Board of Medical Examiners, and Umland was appointed county commissioner in the place of McComb, who had left for Duluth.

In 1884 Umland was nominated for the state legislature and Caine was reappointed surgeon for the Milwaukee road. Pratt was second vice president of the State Medical Association, as well as prison physician and member of the state legislature. Jenner left in February for a year's study in the hospitals of Berlin and Paris, and Watier turned from his publishing business to the job of running a drug store. At least two of the physicians had very interesting hobbies: Hodgkinson collected old medical books and owned a large library, and Umland was a very talented musician. In 1885 Caine was a delegate to the national homeopathic convention, and secretary of the association of sergeants of the first regiment. Merrill became county physician; Gaskill moved to South Stillwater and opened a drug store there, while McGuire opened one at North Branch. Among the pastimes which the doctors enjoyed was hunting, especially Umland, who got the first and finest buck of the season. Cooley, who at this time lived in South Stillwater, amused himself by constructing a large astronomical telescope, seven feet long, with a five and a half inch lens. He also made magic lantern outfits which he sold for $150 each. Apparently some one of the physicians who was in Stillwater at this time was a pretty good story teller, for in the *Stillwater Messenger* of September 30, 1882, appeared the following hoax:

"A physician of this city, whose name we are not at liberty to divulge, was one of a party of four students in the medical college from which he graduated who had shoes made from the skin of human beings which they purchased of dealers for dissection. His pair were made from the skin of a young lady eighteen years of age, and lasted him a year. The leather took a handsome polish, was very soft, but did not keep out the weather. . . ."

An unusual event, which deserves to be mentioned here, was the reception at Stillwater tendered the delegates of the American Medical Association on June 9, 1882. The convention that year was at Saint Paul, but all the delegates were invited to spend the day at Stillwater, at the home of Hon. and Mrs. Sabin. The guests were variously estimated at from seven hundred to over a thousand; they filled sixteen coaches. Three steamers—the Jennie Hays, the G. M. Knapp and the Sam Atlee—had been chartered, and the guests were given an excursion on the river. They then returned to the Sabin residence, where a grand dinner awaited them. The grounds were beautifully illuminated with Japanese lanterns; incidentally, upon this occasion electric lights were first used in the valley. A ladies' committee of arrangements waited on the guests. After the feast Dr. Millard called the meeting to order and Judge Murdock made the address of welcome. The delegates stayed until a late hour before returning to Saint Paul, and all declared they had never had a finer time.

Probably under the impetus of this meeting, another local medical society was formed. It was better organized than the preceding ones, and its constitution and the minutes of its meetings have been preserved. The first meeting was held May 31, 1882; officers were elected, consisting of W. H. Pratt, president; Carli, vice president; T. C. Clark, secretary; W. Jenner, treasurer, and Carli delegate to the State Association. The constitution was signed by P. H. Millard, C. B. Marshall, W. C. Voigt, O. A. Watier, T. C. Clark, B. J. Merrill, E. R. Jellison, W. H. Pratt and D. W. Jenner. Drs. J. R. M. Gaskill, A. H. Steen and J. C. Rhodes were elected members. The name chosen was the Washington County Medical Society. The next meeting was held some time later, on January 19, 1884, and officers were again elected. This time Pratt was president, Merrill vice president, Clark secretary, and Voigt treasurer. Censors were appointed by the president, and motion was made and carried that Pratt act as a committee of one to see that the "State Medical Act be complied with in the county, and to enter any necessary complaints before the State Examining Board." From this time on, meetings were held irregularly until the summer of 1885. Several papers were read by the members, and discussions were held on various subjects. After this society became defunct, another was formed, the Stillwater Medical Society. There are no records of its membership or meetings, and apparently it was chiefly a social organization. After this, there were no other local societies until 1902, at which time the present Washington County Medical Society was formed. This society has functioned, with only a few brief periods of inactivity, until the present time.

By the middle of the eighties many of the early pioneers had left the valley or had died. Dr. A. J. Murdock had moved to Saint Paul following the death of his father, Dr. Thaddeus Murdock. Dr. Comfort died in 1881; little is recorded of his history, but he had lived and practiced in Wyoming, Chisago county, for over thirty years. In March, 1884, Dr. Olding, who had also lived in Chisago county for many years, was found dead one morning in his bed. Dr. E. D. Whiting, another of the pioneers, died in 1882, after suffering for six months from a softening of the brain, and in 1885 Dr. Otis Hoyt died at his home in Hudson. Hoyt and Carli had often joked about which would attend the other's funeral, and the margin was not a very wide one, for a little over two years later Carli also died. At the time of his death he was the oldest inhabitant of the city. There remained of the early pioneers only Rhodes and Gaskill.

The places left by these men were filled by a large number of new arrivals. A great many physicians came during the last fifteen years of the century, most of whom stayed only a short time, though some are still practicing in the valley. In 1887, when another medical practice act was passed by the state legislature, affidavits were signed by Drs. Maisch, Cooney, and Coats, stating that they were practicing in Woodbury, Afton, and St. Paul Park, respectively. The same year a Dr. F. H. Mitchell practiced for a while in Stillwater and St. Paul Park. A Dr. Freligh settled at Stillwater and Dr. Thomas Zein at Rush City, both of whom remained several years. In 1888 there were no new arrivals, but in 1889 Dr. S. O. Francis moved to White Bear, Dr. Oscar F. Thomas to Lakeland, Dr. George A. Carpenter to Marine, and Drs. C. M. Lee and A. J. Howe (or Stowe) to somewhere in Chisago county. A Dr. E. Carleys practiced at South Stillwater, Dr. Philip Muller returned to practice for a while in Stillwater, and Dr. E. Y. Arnold settled at St. Croix Falls. Although he resided in Wisconsin, Dr. Arnold had many patients in Taylors Falls and its vicinity. Many of the physicians practiced on both sides of the river, in both states.

In 1890 the Official Register of Physicians listed the following other physicians in Washington county: George G. Barnett of Lakeland, H. L. Brynildson of Vasa, Arthur De Voe, Albert Fenner, C. E. Hoveland, Julia M. Jacobson, James G. McCoy, Mary Reis Melindy, Leonard F. Pitkin, James Sinclair, and Eindred Viks, all of Stillwater, and Andrew Soderlind of Marine Mills. Directories of that year added E. M. Lundholm, N. Amherst Nelson and Lemuel P. Wetherby of Stillwater, and C. R. Keyes, who was hospital steward at the state prison at this time. Besides these, four midwives offered their services to the Stillwater public: Ursula Bauman, Mrs. Henry Hagen, Annie Tobisch, and Mrs. Cornelia Tozendine.

In 1891 F. Van Waters practiced in Stillwater, W. O. Tessier at Franconia, J. G. Erickson at Marine, and W. S. Fullerton at Rush City in Chisago county. In 1892 a Dr. Wilbur was mentioned as having a patient in the Stillwater hospital. In 1893 Dr. F. H. Hall served as steward at the prison hospital until he was obliged to resign to care for his wife, who had contracted typhoid fever, and in June, 1894, has place was filled by Dr. E. Sidney Boleyn, from Minneapolis. After holding this office for a year, Dr. Boleyn resigned also, but remained in Stillwater, where he is still practicing today. Several other newcomers also made their appearance in 1894: Drs. S. O. Watkins, E. P. Ryan and Joseph Legault of Stillwater, J. F. Gemmel of Rush City, and E. E. Krogstad (or Krogblod) of somewhere in Chisago county. In 1895 A. J. Teiten practiced at Harris, Daniel G. Beebe was steward at the prison hospital, and J. G. Erickson settled at Lindstrom—probably the same Dr. Erickson who had been at Marine a few years earlier. In 1896 four new physicians were reported to be practicing in the two counties: F. J. Bedard and E. A. Edholm of Stillwater, C. L. Clark of White Bear and R. W. Getty of North Branch. In 1897 G. N. Watier, F. G. Landeen, J. H. Haines and a Dr. Lenox moved to Stillwater. Dr. M. E. Withrow arrived to fill the again vacant post of prison hospital steward. In 1898 came Drs. J. W. Rulien, C. M. Anderson and E. S. Fowler, all of whom practiced in Chisago County for several years, and F. L. Puffer, who lived on Bird Island. There were no new arrivals in 1899, but in 1900 Drs. P. C. Bjorneby and A. Lyon settled somewhere in Chisago county, and Dr. E. A. Riley at Willow River.

These, then, were the physicians who practiced in the two counties up to 1900.

Probably there were others whose names are not recorded, and certainly many of those listed are forgotten, since most of them stayed only a year or so. However, each one must have added something to the welfare and the history of the county in which he lived.

In the last fifteen years of the century there were few epidemics or diseases of much historical interest. This was probably due to the activities of the boards of health, which worked under the guidance of Dr. Merrill and several other physicians. In Stillwater the first of a series of thorough sanitary inspections was begun in 1885, which must have been quite an undertaking. Dr. Merrill's description, in the board's report, is interesting. "A house to house inspection," he wrote, "was begun as early as the weather permitted, and continued two months. The citizens in general were helpful, though others were arrested and brought before the municipal court. Thousands of loads of garbage and contents of privy vaults were taken from every part of the city to the dumping grounds. The city never underwent such a general cleaning before. The death rate has gone down in a remarkable manner (only one death from acute disease among 16,000 people in the month of June) and the health of our community is second to no other city or section in the entire country."

However, the best of cleaning could not have remedied for long the condition of the town, for the report continues: "The city is practically without sewerage, except that which its hilly conformation provides. Instead of the constant and efficient drain of a sewer, the householder is obliged to resort to the sluggish and terribly inefficient soil about his dwelling for the deposit of his slops and their drainage. This absence of systematic drainage has greatly impeded the work of the Health Board. We need some method for the daily removal of garbage, kitchen refuse and night soil, especially in the hot months, to complete our system of keeping clean. We also need a permanent sanitary inspector."

It seems amazing that a city over forty years old and as large as Stillwater was at that time had gone without these things for so many years, but it must be remembered that it grew so quickly and spontaneously that it was a large city before anyone had time to plan such a thing as a sewerage system, and, of course, people became accustomed to the lack of one. At that time cleanliness and health were not as closely associated in the average mind as they are today. These conditions were all later remedied, and until then the annual clean-ups were well conducted.

In 1888 Rush City followed Stillwater's example by having a sanitary inspection and general clean-up. Dr. Zein, the health officer, reported in the "Public Health": "During the past year the board of health has found it necessary to urge a lot of cleaning up; citizens generally were very helpful but we need a lot of cleaning. There was slight cause to resort to legal means. . . . The past year has been an unusual one for sickness and death. Diphtheria is a constant dread and a persistent visitor, and in a very malignant form; it seems to defy all attempts of the board to stop it. It has, in the past year, visited twenty-one families in the valley, all of whom have been quarantined. There have been fifty-three cases and twenty deaths, ten male, ten female, the youngest three years seven months old, the eldest twenty-one years three months."

"The Board has spent four hundred dollars cleaning up the village of nuisances, sources of filth and causes of disease, in maintaining quarantine and furnishing nurses and disinfectants for the poor." He added that slaughter houses required much attention, and concluded that the village was, finally, in good sanitary condition.

Despite the improving conditions, disease was still prevalent. In 1885 epidemics of scarlatina were reported at South Stillwater and diphtheria at Franconia and Schafer. In 1887 more complete reports show that in Washington County there were six deaths from measles, five from scarlatina, fourteen from croup, nineteen from diphtheria, thirteen from typhoid, eighteen from diarrheal diseases of infancy, twenty-four from phthisis, five from bronchitis and twenty from pneumonia. Chisago county, that same year, had one death from measles, eighteen from diphtheria, five from typhoid, twelve from diarrheal diseases of infancy, twelve from phthisis, three from bronchitis and eight from pneumonia. In 1889 the only epidemic of interest in Chisago county was a mild outbreak of scarlet fever at Taylors Falls. In Washington county the health officer reported that the city had an unusually healthy year; the drinking water was good, the city was kept cleaner than ever before, and the citizens were "becoming habituated to the notion of cleaning up at least once a year." Possibly the citizens were a little too satisfied with their work, for in July a sanitary conference which had been planned nearly fell through because of public apathy and lack of interest; only the exertions of the clergy and the vigorous comments of the mayor finally made it a success. The report continues that a sewerage system had been started but should be extended, and some means of dealing with kitchen refuse was still needed. However, the quarantine system was well developed.

Another item of interest in 1890 was the discovery of a leper in Rush City. One had been found nine years before in Washington county by Dr. Caine, but this was the first to be reported in Chisago county. It was discovered by Consul Christenson and identified by Dr. Gronvald. Both of these patients were Scandinavians. In the last decade of the century there were no serious epidemics reported, nor any particularly interesting diseases in either county.

Even in the state prison conditions were much improved, though still rather far from a modern conception of perfection. Arrangements were made for clean water, meals were eaten outside of the cells, new cells were built to relieve crowding, zinc night-buckets replaced the old wooden ones, and a sewer was constructed. The prison hospital was enlarged, and the use of antiseptics was introduced, and a graduate physician employed as hospital steward. A laboratory with a microscope and other instruments necessary for physical and chemical analysis was instilled, and a medical library was begun. All prisoners were given a thorough physical examination upon entering, and contagious diseases were isolated. These reforms were not introduced until 1893. Tuberculous prisoners were put in a separate wing. All of these changes were brought in slowly over a period of many years after much urging by the prison physicians, wardens, and various boards. That the city and village lockups could use some similar reforms was shown by a report made in 1890 by the secretary of the State Board of Corrections and Charities. The secretary had sent out a questionnaire which asked, among other things, what sort of beds and bedding were provided, and how often this bedding was washed and the lockup scrubbed. Marine Mills and North Branch performed both duties twice a year, White Bear and Franconia when needed, and Rush City, Stillwater and Taylors Falls made no report. Two other towns in the state replied once in ten years and never.

Besides attending to their practice most of the physicians served the community in some official capacity. Drs. H. G. Murdock, Stowe, Krogstad, Gemmel, Teitin, Rulien, Anderson, Fowler, Werner, Erickson, Zein, Bjorneby, Lyon and Robb all served as Chisago county physician at one time or another, while Dr. T. C. Clark held the same office in Washington county. Drs. Robb, Erickson and H. G.

Murdock served as coroners. Dr. Voight was city health inspector of Stillwater, and Drs. Cooley, Merrill, Fliesburg and Zein were health officers of South Stillwater, Stillwater, Fish Lake and Rush City, respectively. Dr. Merrill was also prison physician for a time, as was Dr. Pratt. Physicians who served as stewards in the prison hospital included Drs. Keyes, Hall, Boleyn, Beebe and Withrow. Dr. Keyes also made a study of cestodes, which was printed in the Transactions of the State Medical Association for 1890. Dr. George E. Clark was professor of homeopathy at the state university. Dr. T. C. Clark and Dr. Hallberg were both commissioners in the counties in which they lived. Dr. Marshall ran a drug store, and Dr. Watier manufactured a cough syrup. Several physicians travelled, Dr. Jellison going to China and Dr. Erickson to Sweden.

Dr. Beardsley was president of the village council of Rush City; Dr. Umland was appointed receiver of public monies at Taylors Falls, and later was postmaster at Fosston. Dr. H. G. Murdock was on the board of pension examiners, and at a meeting of the literary society he "entertained as soloist" though the nature of his solo was not described in the report of the meeting. The doctor was a "woodsman," and must have been quite a fisherman, too, for a news item in 1895 credits him with a morning's catch of two hundred trout. Dr. Caine, in 1894, had the honor of being mentioned as candidate for the office of Grand Exalted Ruler of the Elks, and the same year Dr. Mitchell, then of St. Paul Park, had the "honor" of a coat of red paint and feathers from the citizens of that town. Many of the physicians took an active part in the State Medical Association. Dr. McComb, then a resident of Duluth, was president in 1887, Drs. Rhodes and Stone served many years as censors, and Drs. Millard and Stone were delegates to the national convention. Dr. Merrill was essayist, his subject being "Medical Iconoclasm," and chairman of committees on finance, medical jurisprudence, legislation, and medical education. Dr. Pratt was also very active on many committees, and Dr. Millard's services are too well known to be repeated.

The last fifteen years of the century saw the passing of the last links with the early pioneer days: the deaths of Drs. Hoyt and Carli in 1885 and 1887, and Dr. Gustaf Colins, of Franconia, in 1889. Dr. Colins was over eighty years of age and according to his obituary had practiced for over forty years in the county, and was one of its oldest settlers. The obituary explains that he "had a natural gift for surgery, and was called the 'handy man' in that connection, being noted in his way for operations. He had no instruction, but always attended to dislocations and broken limbs without charge, even during his old age when he sometimes made mistakes." In 1891 the valley suffered the rather more serious loss of Dr. O. A. Watier of Stillwater. In April, 1894, Dr. J. R. M. Gaskill died at Danville, Ill., from the effects of poison administered in his coffee, evidently by accident. Several other persons in the same hotel were made very sick, but the doctor was the only one to die, probably due to the fact that, being fond of coffee, he drank more than the others, and also because he was in poor health at the time because of a recent operation. Three years later Dr. C. B. Marshall, who had practiced for many years in Stillwater, died following an operation for appendicitis, and in 1900 Dr. Umland also passed away, at Fosston, Minn. Umland had spent much of his time in the valley, though he had moved away some time before his death. One other event which should be mentioned was the passing of Dr. J. C. Rhodes. He was one of the earliest and the most prominent physicians in the valley, and the time of his death, in May, 1903, is an appropriate place to end this history of medicine in the St. Croix valley. The last of the pioneer physicians was gone, and the new century was on its way.

(To be continued in the October issue)

EDITORIAL

MINNESOTA MEDICINE

OFFICIAL JOURNAL OF THE MINNESOTA STATE MEDICAL
ASSOCIATION

Published by the Association under the direction of its Editing
and Publishing Committee

EDITING AND PUBLISHING COMMITTEE

J. T. CHRISTISON, Saint Paul   C. B. WRIGHT, Minneapolis
E. M. HAMMES, Saint Paul   T. A. PEPPARD, Minneapolis
WALTMAN WALTERS, Rochester

EDITORIAL STAFF

CARL B. DRAKE, Saint Paul, Editor
W. F. BRAASCH, Rochester, Associate Editor
GILBERT COTTAM, Minneapolis, Associate Editor

Annual Subscription—$3.00   Single Copies—$0.40

Foreign Subscriptions—$3.50

The right is reserved to reject material submitted for editorial
or advertising columns. The Editing and Publishing Committee
does not hold itself responsible for views expressed either in
editorials or other articles when signed by the author.

Classified advertising—five cents a word; minimum charge,
$1.00. Remittance should accompany order.

Display advertising rates on request.

Address all communications to Minnesota Medicine, 2642 University Avenue, Saint Paul, or Suite 604, National Bldg., Minneapolis. Telephone: Nestor 2641.

BUSINESS MANAGER
J. R. BRUCE

Volume 21   SEPTEMBER, 1938   Number 9

Group Hospital Association, Inc.

IF THE contemplated grand jury investigation of the District of Columbia Medical
Society instigated by Assistant Attorney General
Arnold materializes, the trial will hinge on
whether the local medical society had grounds
for expelling a member for accepting employment from the Group Health Association, Inc.
There should be no question of the right of
a medical society to determine its own membership. From a practical standpoint, it is a simple
matter for a society to decline election to membership. On the other hand, a physician already
a member suffers injury by being expelled and
generally cannot be expelled without cause. Was
employment by the Group Health Association

sufficient cause for expulsion from the District
of Columbia Medical Society?

The Group Health Association filed articles
of incorporation at Washington, February 24,
1937. It provided for medical and hospital care
for any employe of the Federal government
(the army and navy excepted) for $26.40 per
year for a single person or $39.60 for a married
person or one with dependents. Although really
an insurance company, it was filed under the
heading of benevolent, charitable, educational,
literary, musical, scientific, religious and missionary organizations. The source of the capital
necessary to launch the Association was, for a
time, obscure. Eventually it became known that
the Home Owners Loan Corporation had appropriated $40,000, which appropriation was ap-
proved by the Legislative Council of the Senate
in February, 1938, and by the House Appropriations Committee, which, however, stated that it
was the Committee's unanimous opinion that
the expenditure was not authorized by law. The
United States District Attorney for the District
of Columbia has held that the Association is
engaged unlawfully in the practice of medicine,
and the insurance commissioner that it is unlawfully carrying on the business of insurance.

It would seem that the case for the District
of Columbia Medical Society is rather strong.
The Group Hospital Association, Inc., threat-
ens to entirely disrupt private practice in the
District of Columbia. Incorporated to give medical and hospital care to Federal employees,
who number about 840,000, and with their dependents some 2,500,000, irrespective of income,
the effect on medical practice in Washington,
D. C., particularly, is evident. So far its membership, we understand, has been limited to
employes of the Home Owners Loan Corporation, a government agency.

Newspaper comment has been made to the
effect that organized medicine has made a mistake in opposing a new method of meeting medical bills. Was the District of Columbia Medical Society to sit idly by and ignore an organization which threatened to annihilate private practice and which the society had good reason to
believe would furnish inferior medical care to

its members? The Association had little experience whereby it could estimate membership fees and the medical staff required. The undertaking abolished any choice on the part of members as to medical adviser. Knowing the preference for doctors of their own choice manifest by most Americans, we wonder how the membership has reacted to the set-up.

Desirable as the equal distribution of the cost of sickness it, the Group Hospital Association, Inc., is a good example of just the form of group medicine which most doctors oppose. The Association has been backed by the Government, and presumably any deficits will be paid by taxpayers; free choice of medical advisers does not exist; membership is not restricted to the low income group, and in all probability the medical care offered will be of an inferior quality.

Has it come to the point where the Government can dictate the membership of a medical society when the activities of a member are disapproved by the society but approved by the Government? We think the Department of Justice has made a poor selection as a test case and that the Department has work cut out for it in the case of the Group Hospital Association, Inc.

Recommendations of the National Health Conference

THE National Health Conference, held in Washington in July, supposedly to discuss ways and means to meet the medical needs of the country, resulted in the recommendation by the technical committee of the Federal Government, that 850 million dollars be appropriated yearly for the next ten years, half by the Federal Government and half by the states, for what, in the opinion of the Committee, are much needed medical activities. These include an expansion of public health activities to the amount of 200 million yearly to combat tuberculosis, venereal disease, malaria, pneumonia, cancer and mental disease; 165 million for more maternal and child health service, to include the provision of medical and nursing care of mothers and newborn infants, medical care of children, services for crippled children, consultation services of specialists, and postgraduate training (for all income groups); 146 million for

building more hospitals to provide 360,000 more hospital beds and 500 health and diagnostic centers; 400 million to provide medical care for the medically needy.

There is evidence in the proposed huge appropriation of nearly a billion dollars a year, half in the form of a Federal subsidy to the states, of entrance to a much greater degree by the Federal Government into activities heretofore conducted largely by the states themselves, and in addition provision for payment of medical bills for those considered medically needy and apparently in certain instances for those in the higher income brackets.

In considering the need for any such appropriation, it is interesting to note that, except for the years of the influenza epidemic, each year for the past twenty-five years has shown a reduction in the mortality rate of the country which has continued into 1938. Recent statistics published by the Metropolitan Life Insurance Company show that the death rate for the first six months of 1938 is much below that of any previous like period. Further, the recent survey of the Council on Medical Education and Hospitals of the American Medical Association shows that 98.5 per cent of our citizens live within thirty miles of a hospital. While there is doubtless need in certain areas for medical aid, no evidence has come to our attention of any general medical need not at present supplied.

Whether Congress will make this enormous appropriation is perhaps not problematic. Whether the states will appropriate dollar for dollar is, in the light of past experience, quite likely.

It should be remembered that this proposal comes at a time when some eleven million are unemployed, a situation which it is to be hoped and expected will not persist the next ten years.

Minnesota's need for the expenditure of several millions along the proposed lines is not apparent. There is no doubt but that the state would have to go further into debt to raise its share of the sum. It is to be hoped the state legislature will be able to resist the temptation to accept Federal subsidy for this great increase in government medical activity.

Aside from the question of whether Federal and State governments can afford such a great increase in appropriations of this sort, desirable as they may be for certain scattered localities, the question resolves itself into what type of government we are developing in our country. What are the functions of the Federal government and what are distinctly those of the individual states? Is it the function of government to enter into competition with its citizens? Should private industry be called upon to make up deficits in government business activities? Do our citizens want government medical activities aside from those concerned with Public Health and medical care in general subject to politics? In short, do we want socialism?

The private practice of medicine is apparently about to receive another blow just as industry has received blow after blow from government intrusion. The wild appropriation of government funds, of which the proposal of the National Health Conference is another example, cannot go on indefinitely. It is to be hoped that our representatives will exert their prerogatives and call a halt before all government becomes bankrupt.

C. B. D.

Tact Toward the Sick

WHEN one is laid up at home or in the hospital and is bored with existence, nothing is more welcome or of greater aid in convalescence than the visits of friends. To feel that one has friends who are interested in one's recovery is an urge to get well. And yet there are friends who are totally lacking in what is called "tact," who cannot limit their calls but stay on and on; others who through the association of ideas relate similar or dissimilar cases of illness in which the outcome was not so favorable, leaving the patient exhausted and depressed.

The acutely ill need special consideration. While a friend can be a friend indeed in helping organize the medical care in an emergency, a seriously ill person has no energy to spend on visitors. The attending physician should lay down the rule "no visitors" and in certain instances even the nearest relatives should be limited as to duration and frequency of visits. The persistence with which some so-called friends insist on seeing an acutely ill friend, ferreting out the hospital room and showing a lack of consideration for hospital rules, is astounding. Even a telephone call was recently

put through by an unwary hospital operator after bed-time, disturbing the patient's rest.

Sympathy is often due the wife of a man acutely ill in the hospital. Telephone calls keep her busier than a down-town central, and frequent and prolonged calls from solicitous friends only too often lead to exhaustion.

Even the attending physician deserves compassion at times when a patient with a large circle of friends happens to be acutely ill. During his moments of relaxation he is likely to be barraged with questions only serving to keep a subject already the source of much worry the more before his mind.

The obstetric patient should be mentioned. The long expected event has taken place and family and friends seem to think that mother and infant are eager to celebrate the occasion at once by holding a reception. Too often the inexperienced mother has this same attitude and the attending physician sometimes finds the recently delivered mother surrounded by relatives and friends who have long overstayed the proper time limit for such a visit, apparently awaiting the next nursing hour and a view of the newly arrived citizen-to-be. Nothing in hospital management has been harder to enforce than the exclusion of friends and relatives from the nursery of the hospital.

Then there is the hospital hound. A friend goes to the hospital and she (as is usually the case) trots down to the hospital and sits by the hour, often making several trips each day to keep posted on the progress of events. The more gruesome details she can learn the more a certain almost morbid pleasure is derived and the telephone wires are kept hot during spare moments with the latest bulletins.

There is one friend who should never be visited in the hospital. This is the type of neurotic woman who often with the connivance of a certain type of physician goes periodically to the hospital quite unnecessarily. With the room full of flowers and arrayed in her best and telephone at hand, she is prepared to greet the friends she has notified of her predicament.

After all, the matter of sick room visitors is of great importance to any patient and should receive the most thoughtful consideration on the part of the attending physician.

MEDICAL ECONOMICS

Edited by the Committee on Medical Economics
of the
Minnesota State Medical Association
W. F. Braasch, M.D., Chairman

SURVEY LAGS

Form No. 1 for physicians, most important source of information for the Survey of Needs and Supply of Medical Care, is coming in very slowly.

From the response to a recent inquiry, it appears that no county in the state has yet been able to report a 100 per cent return. Only a few are able to report 50 per cent or over.

Furthermore, the meager returns thus far submitted by the secretaries show that questions seven and nine, most important of all for the purposes of this study, have been too frequently omitted altogether.

Secretaries should canvas their members immediately to spur laggards and secure as complete a return as possible.

Organized medicine has cast doubt upon the reliability of statistical studies used to back up the government program for increased health protection, building of hospitals and possible grants in aid for establishment of state systems of health insurance.

This Survey is acutely needed NOW to provide facts and figures upon which physicians may rely and upon which sound programs of improvement can be built. They are equally needed to prevent the foisting of elaborate and expensive services unnecessarily upon the American people.

Medicine is being challenged daily in the magazines, on the radio, in the newspapers.

A complete and reliable presentation of the facts through the Survey is the answer to that challenge.

IMPRESSIONS GAINED FROM THE RECENT NATIONAL HEALTH CONFERENCE IN WASHINGTON

IN THE first place the gathering in Washington was no conference at all—at least in the generally accepted meaning of that term. As I understand it, the term conference implies an attempt to arrive at a solution of some problem by a group of individuals who might have different opinions but who possess authoritative information concerning the subject in hand. The problem should have free and frank discussion from all sides in order to obtain as much information as possible, and the only objective in mind should be to arrive at conclusions which would be mutually agreeable.

Cleverly Pre-arranged

Instead of a conference, a cleverly pre-arranged program was set up, with the sole objective of publicizing and supporting a program of health reform inspired by federal officials. Invited to the "conference" was a carefully selected group of some 150 individuals, most of whom were known because of their so-called liberal views toward medical care, and who had either written or spoken in behalf of these views. In the group were men and women with a wide assortment of occupations, including many social and welfare workers, magazine editors, newspaper men, and labor union representatives.

To give it an atmosphere of fairness, a small group of physicians representing the American Medical Association was invited. They were quite overwhelmed by the mass of hostile propaganda—and for all practical purposes, they might better have stayed at home. *Conspicuous by their absence were representatives of banking, investment activities, and of industry and manufacturing, who might have been interested in the financing of the vast expenditures involved.* Neither were there any economists or educators who had ever been guilty of entertaining any theories which might be called conservative or reactionary.

Discussions Released in Advance

Much of the time scheduled for the program of the conference was spent in reading the report and recommendations of the governmental health forces. These had been typed previously and had been read and studied by some of the delegates present. They also had been released by previous arrangement for national newspaper publicity from day to day. The discussion which followed was largely pre-arranged and the remarks made by many of those who took part in the discussion were also previously written and dated for publication.

For the most part those who were called upon to discuss the problem were sympathetic with the government program and in most cases urged that even more radical steps be taken.

Emotional Well-wishing

It is difficult to understand the psychology of many of those who were assembled in the conference. One fact stands out above everything else, however, and that is that when it comes to opinions regarding the care of health, many intelligent people base their ideas more on emotion than logic. One wonders how intelligent men and women could make statements which were largely without factual basis and governed purely by emotional well-wishing.

It was surprising as well as discouraging to hear well-meaning representatives of such supposedly well informed organizations as the Farm Bureau Federation, Parent-Teachers Association; General Federation of Women's Clubs, and League of Women Voters get up and urge various phases of health socialization without acquainting themselves with all phases of the problems involved. It is to be hoped that these splendid organizations, usually well informed and unbiased, will in the future get their information on matters of health from all sources, including that storehouse of information available at the headquarters of the American Medical Association.

Lay Confusion

One feature of much of the laymen's barrage was a curious confusion of the indigent with the low income groups. Apparently many of the lay speakers failed to realize the fundamental differences in the problems involved in their health supervision. They did not seem to know that the health of the indigent was supposed to be under municipal, state, or federal control. It was rather ironical to hear their outspoken criticism of the failure of government agencies to look after this group properly when governmental control was supposed to be the objective of their arguments.

Doctor Ridiculed

The physicians present were placed in a curious position. One almost felt like a social outcast in the group, and a guilty conspirator to block justice and progress. We were placed in

the role of selfish, narrow-minded individuals, having no vision or ability to sense reform and incapable of managing affairs of health as they should be managed. A jibe or sally at the unfortunate doctor was greeted with a round of laughter or applause. On the other hand, a calm statement showing what the physician or medical societies had already done and were trying to do to improve medical care received scant attention or was greeted with silence.

Sensational Publicity

Another feature of the conference was the sensational publicity of the proceedings by the daily press. Liberal space was given to the Federal Health program as released by the Interdepartmental Committee. Only the sensational features of the discussion were publicized, which were largely radical and in support of the proposed reforms. The remarks made by Dr. West and Dr. Abell, which stated that the medical profession was in sympathy with some features of the federal program, while others were regarded as objectionable, and their statements showing how much already had been accomplished by physicians along these lines, received only abbreviated notice in the press. The contribution of Dr. Cabot, in which he ridiculed the present methods of medical care, and the well merited rebuke by Dr. West, received more headlines than any other feature of the entire conference.

Unfortunately, the introductory remarks made by Dr. Cabot received but little notice but, in all fairness, should be repeated. Before reading his paper he spoke as follows: "I wish to have it distinctly understood that the views I hold in this controversy are my own and in no way represent the attitude of the Mayo Clinic." Instead of publicizing this statement, the newspapers gave the impression that Dr. Cabot spoke as a representative of the Clinic, which was quite contrary to the truth.

A Few Tricks of Their Own

It must be said that the skill with which the proponents of medical socialization have inoculated an increasing circle of the laity with their ideas is most impressive. They have learned all of the tricks practiced by other governmental activities marvelously well and added a few of their own. The way otherwise intelligent lay-

660

men mouthed the oft-repeated but incorrectly founded statements concerning lack of medical care is a startling illustration of what skillful propaganda can accomplish.

Purpose

The purpose of the conference was discussed in the introductory remarks of Miss Josephine Roche, the able General Chairman of the Interdepartmental Committee. The federal program for medical reform was discussed in general terms by its progenitor, Dr. Parran, Surgeon General of the United States Public Health Service. His sententious remark to the effect that medical care promises to be the main issue, both political and social, before the American people in the immediate future would seem to give clear warning of the purpose of the government to invade the promising field of medical care, both therapeutic and preventive, and use it for any political advantage that it may possess. The report of the Technical Committee and the agenda of the conference have been published in detail in recent issues of the *Journal of the American Medical Association*. A synopsis of the recommendations made, with a few random comments, may be of interest.

Program

The Technical Committee's study of health and medical services in the United States indicates that deficiencies in the present health services fall into four broad categories:

1. Preventive health services for the nation as a whole are grossly insufficient.

2. Hospital and other institutional facilities are inadequate in many communities, especially in rural areas, and financial support for hospital care and for professional services in hospitals is both insufficient and precarious, especially for services to people who cannot pay the costs of the care they need.

3. One-third of the population, including persons with or without income, is receiving inadequate or no medical service.

4. An even larger fraction of the population suffers from economic burdens created by illness.

The Committee submitted a program of five recommendations to meet these problems which are as follows:

I. **Expansion of public health and maternal and child health services.**

A. Expansion of general public health services. It is recommended that Federal participation in the program of preventive health service should be increased and, furthermore, that Federal participation be increased to promote a frontal attack, to (1) eradicate tuberculosis, venereal disease and malaria; (2) control mortality from pneumonia and cancer; and (3) promote mental and industrial hygiene.

B. Expansion of maternal and child health services. This includes provisions for medical and nursing care of mothers and newborn infants; medical care of children; services for crippled children; consultation services of specialists; and more adequate provision for postgraduate training of professional personnel. It includes, also, recommendations for the establishment of numerous health and diagnostic centers for these purposes. The total cost of taking care of the recommendations under A. is estimated at $200,000,000, and under B. $165,000,000, or a total of $365,000,000.

II. **Expansion of Hospital Facilities.** The Committee found hospital facilities inadequate and recommends a ten year program providing for expansion of the nation's hospital facilities by provision of 360,000 beds, and by construction of 500 health and diagnostic centers. Averaged over a ten year period the total cost of such a program was estimated at $146,000,000.

III. **Medical Care for the Medically Needy.** The Committee finds that, based on a National Health Survey, one-third of the population which is in the lower income levels is receiving inadequate general medical service. This applies to (1) persons without income supported by general relief; (2) those supported through old age assistance or work relief, and (3) families with small incomes. Current provisions to assist these people by any local and voluntary organizations and by physicians are not equal to meet the need. The Committee recommends that the Federal government, through grants-in-aid to the states, implement the provision of public medical care to these groups. It is estimated that on the average ten dollars per person annually would be required to meet the minimum needs for essential medical care, hospitalization, and emergency dentistry. This part of the program would probably reach an estimated level of $400,000,000 annually.

No statement was made as to how this money was to be spent, nor to whom it would go.

IV and V include a general program for medical care and insurance against loss of wages during sickness. The Committee states that without great increase in the total national expenditure the burden of sickness cost can be greatly reduced, through appropriate devices to distribute these costs among groups of people and over periods of time. The cost of the insurance and allied program has been estimated at approximately $2,600,000,000 annually.

To finance the program, two sources of funds could be drawn on: (a) general taxation or special tax assessment; (b) specific insurance contributions. The Committee recommends consideration of both methods.

Cost: 30 Billions

The role of the Federal Government would be principally that of giving financial and technical aid to the states in the development of procedures largely of their own choice. The maximum annual cost to Federal, State and local governments of all recommendations, other than the insurance features, is estimated at about $850,000,000. Over a period of ten years this would mean $8,500,000,000. If compulsory health insurance is added to this at an estimated annual expenditure of $2,600,000,000, the ten year expenditure for this and the other program would amount to more than thirty billion dollars.

The manner in which the inspired health reformers referred, without batting an eye, to the expenditure of billions was most impressive. If the government is actually called on to meet these demands, it will make the cost of old age and unemployment insurance look like a mere side issue. No doubt the alleged lack of business ability and financial sense in the medico accounts for his inability to disregard, in like manner, the stupendous sums involved.

Some Are of Value

Although it would be impossible to make a detailed review of these proposals in these columns, their comparative value may be summed up as follows: some of the recommendations are well founded and should prove to be of benefit to public health; others are either unnecessary or are not practical; and the rest would do more harm than good. Many features of those recommendations which are largely of a preventive nature will meet with approval by the medical profession, provided that the program can be carried out in close coöperation with and under the control of medical organizations.

Would Alter Medical Practice

Many of the recommendations which would alter if not transform the practice of medicine require careful study and investigation before they can be endorsed by the medical profession. Outstanding among these proposals may be mentioned the establishment of at least 500 health centers throughout the land for the control of tuberculosis, cancer and other lesions, and several thousand centers for the control of child health. These centers will, in order to be complete, necessarily require the services of a host of physicians in various capacities as specialists, technicians, and administrative officers, which, together with allied dental, nursing and technical services, will lead to complete modification of the present methods of medical practice.

It would be quite impossible for any nationwide plan of this kind to escape eventual lay and political control, with leveling and deterioration of service, not to mention professional regimentation and suppression of individual professional initiative.

Based on WPA Figures

Most of the information and recommendations made in the Report of the Technical Committee and most of the statements made by the three introductory speakers on the program regarding the incidence of illness and lack of medical care were based on statistics obtained from the National Health Survey. This survey was made largely by WPA workers over a period of six months under the supervision of the Public Health Service. The resulting statistics are based on a house to house canvass of 740,-000 urban and 36,000 rural families. Much of the reported illness and type of disease had no medical confirmation. The fact that the diagnosis and evaluation of reported disease was made without medical training would in itself make the survey of doubtful value.

A review of the survey reveals many other data which might be questionable. For example, statements made by persons on relief or with low incomes as to disease being the cause of their economic status may be biased. The frequency and severity of illness reported by this survey so greatly exceeds that reported by the Committee on Cost of Medical Care and that of the Metropolitan Life Insurance Company, and differs widely in so many other respects with these surveys, that the accuracy of the entire report is open to question.

Open to Question

Many broad conclusions were made from the survey statistics which are open to question, such as the statement that 40 per cent of the persons canvassed were receiving too low an income to maintain them in a healthy condition. This certainly is not true in most sections of the country—and even if it were true the problems involved are more economic than medical. The situation would be changed very little by giving this group more medical care without correcting the economic factors.

The statistics purporting to show the percentage of individuals who receive no medical care are not even probable, furthermore. Most similar studies have shown that about 50 per cent of the population suffer no illness requiring medical care during any given year. The statistics in regard to relative need and distribution of hospitals in relation to the population have been proved to be quite erroneous by the careful survey carried out under the supervision of the Council on Medical Education and Hospitals. These are random examples but they show how statistics can be made to fit preconceived ideas and used to prove them.

Said Dr. Goldwater

Space will not permit a detailed review of the discussion which followed the reading of the various sections of the Committee Report. I have already indicated the general tenor of the remarks of those who took part. Among those few who discussed the problems from a more conservative angle was Dr. Goldwater of New York City and his remarks deserve special consideration. Unfortunately, space permits only a few quotations from his address, which are as follows:

"The objectives stated by spokesmen for the Interdepartmental Committee are commendable, but the program submitted arrives at its results by methods of calculation that are too simple to be reliable. Neglected illness is not always convertible by means of money grants or administrative measures into illness effectively prevented or cared for. A substantial fraction of increased government expenditure is almost certain to be used for more custodial care. ·

"Sincere enthusiasts who, thirty years ago, were sure that tuberculosis would be abolished by 1935, are still writing optimistic tuberculosis programs in glamorous terms of hundreds of fresh millions of dollars.

Self-help Preferable

"In health-protection, self-help is preferable to outside aid; government intervention in medicine is desirable as a last, not a first, resort.

"For similar reasons the efforts of county medical societies and of medical coöperatives sponsored by ethical physicians should be encouraged. These efforts are of primary importance in relation to home care, which is of concern to a greater number of individuals than actual or theoretically required institutional care.

"Medical care should be locally, rather than nationally, administered. The effective and economical administration of medical aid for the masses by huge Federal agencies is well nigh impossible."

The vigorous defense by Dr. Fishbein of the methods employed by the American Medical Association and organized medicine, ex-cathedra and also in the abbreviated time allotted him for discussion, should be mentioned. Also among those who contributed from the conservative side Dr. McCormack should be mentioned and Dr. Paullin, Father Schwitalla, Dr. Veeder, and Dr. Meyer.

In the summing up of the evidence for the plaintiffs by E. E. Witte, Professor of Economics, University of Wisconsin, the liberal cohorts were urged to press their cause even more than in the past. He pointed out that in order to obtain real progress action by the separate states would be necessary. He predicted that the honor of being the first state to support a health insurance law would probably go to New York, but that the immediate opportunities in Wisconsin appeared most promising. It would seem that our brethren in Wisconsin will be in for a hard winter and it is up to medical organizations in the surrounding states to give them all the support, both moral and actual, that we can muster.

W. F. BRAASCH, M.D.

FRONT PAGE ATTENTION

Reverberations from the National Health Conference had scarcely died down in the press when an investigation of the American Medical Association and its affiliate in Washington, D. C., the District of Columbia Medical Society, to determine whether or not their activities constituted a monopoly in restraint of fair competition under the anti-trust laws, claimed front page attention.

The investigation is the next step in the contest that has been going on for some time (résumé in these columns, May, 1938) between the District of Columbia Society and the Group Health Association of employees of the Federal Home Loan Corporation.

The Group Health Association was set up by a federal appropriation of $40,000 and is operated by monthly contributions of members with a hired medical staff. Both the original grant and the method of operation have been declared illegal and unconstitutional by various authorities and, on those grounds, physicians who associated themselves with it were threatened with expulsion from the society and were denied the privilege of taking their Group Health Association patients into the hospitals.

Question at Issue

The District of Columbia Medical Society is not open to the charge of lagging in the provision of medical care to low income groups in Washington. Its bureau to assist in providing care for these people and in suiting fees to their ability to pay has been in successful operation for some time. The question at issue is whether or not the federal government may step in to finance a type of medical service which encroaches on the rights of physicians and holds grave possibilities for establishing a low standard of medical care in the District of Columbia.

To Be Tested in the Courts

According to a recent dispatch from Washington, three prominent Washington physicians have taken legal steps to bring the issue to a head and possibly force a Supreme Court decision on the legality of the whole matter. They have asked the district court to restrain the Group Health Association from practising medicine.

The likelihood that the federal charge of monopoly in violation of the anti-trust laws can be made to stick against the American Medical Association and its affiliate is extremely doubtful.

Physicians have nothing to fear from the law. Their problem is to prevent a swing of public opinion to a general unthinking endorsement without trial of compulsory health insurance.

PUBLIC ASSISTANCE

Figures for May, 1938, on case loads and payments to recipients of Public Assistance indicate a steady increase in the number of recipients and in the amount of money expended for it in Minnesota.

On December 31, 1937, the case load for Old Age Assistance in Minnesota was 62,357. On May 31, 1938, the case load had risen to 64,717. On December 31, 1937, the case load for children receiving Aid to Dependent Children was 11,512 in the state. In May, 1938, it was 14,688.

The same increase is apparent throughout the

record. At the end of May there was an increase of almost 600 on WPA certification lists waiting for assignments, over the number on the waiting list at the end of April.

The *Monthly Review of Public Assistance* in the State of Minnesota issued by the State Board of Control provides complete graphs and tables showing case loads and amounts expended by counties for Old Age Assistance, Aid to Dependent Children, Aid to the Blind and certain limited data on WPA.

They should be of profound interest to physicians especially as a gauge of the welfare situation in Minnesota.

IF I HAD KNOWN

(Monthly Editorial Prepared by the Medical Advisory Committee)

If I had only known—. One of our members so expressed himself after a Summons and Complaint had been served on him recently in an alleged Malpractice suit.

If he had only known what? That many times your friends are the source of your most disagreeable lawsuit. You have confidentially told them of a case of yours. The news spreads. An unscrupulous lawyer hears of it. The patient is interviewed, and the story must be told in Court.

If he had only known what? That good records, not too meticulous, but covering the essential points from day to day, written, if possible, and, if dictated, read and signed by the attending physician on the case are a most necessary means of defense in Court. That these records are confidential, should never be altered, and are for the use of the doctor himself. They should be filed in such a way that only the Court can make them public property.

If he had only known what? That his fellow medical confrere down the street should be his most valued friend and that a good lawyer is a source of much peace of mind when a cloud of prejudice appears on the horizon.

If he had only known these things, your Medical Advisory Committee is sure he would have had less cause for worry.

and Mr. A. B. Anderson and Mr. Charles Stones, county attorney and assistant county attorney, respectively, of Steele county. White waived extradition and was returned to Owatonna, where he was released on the bond furnished by Mr. Brown and Mr. Briese.

White came to Steele county in the latter part of March, this year, driving a Packard car with Georgia license plates. Because of a bad snowstorm White asked for shelter at the home of farmers a few miles west of Owatonna. He represented himself as "Professor" White and also as "Dr." White; he claimed to be a psycho-analyst and in a few days was diagnosing ailments and suggesting pills, tablets, capsules, etc. He charged from $6.00 to $40.00 per patient. The medicine was purchased by White at drugstores in Owatonna for a mere fraction of the amount he charged.

Sheriff Helgeson sent White's fingerprints to the Federal Bureau of Investigation at Washington and was promptly advised that White was wanted at Jesup, Georgia, for swindling and practicing medicine without a license. White, in the meantime, had secured his release at Owatonna on bond and started for parts unknown. White also had been arrested in Detroit, Michigan, in 1918 on a charge of "larceny by trick." White claims to have been born in 1858 but appears to be sixty to sixty-five years of age; he is accompanied by Mrs. White. Judge Alexander issued a bench warrant for White's arrest and it is hoped that he will be apprehended somewhere.

The Medical Board wishes specifically to mention the splendid work done by Sheriff Helgeson and Mr. Anderson and his assistant, Mr. Stone; quackery cannot exist in a county where public officials give the whole-hearted coöperation and timely effort that was given in this case.

PHYSICIANS LICENSED BY THE MINNESOTA STATE BOARD OF MEDICAL EXAMINERS MAY 13, 1938

April Examination

Ahl, Carl Willard, U. of Minn., M.B. 1937, Minneapolis, Minn.

Ansprenger, Aloys Georg, U. of Munich, M.D. 1933, Rochester, Minn.

Berman, Abe E., U. of Minn., M.B. 1937, Minneapolis, Minn.

Brown, Hugh Osborne, Northwestern U., M.D. 1937, Rochester, Minn.

Burkhart, Roger John, U. of Minn., M.B. 1938, Chaska, Minn.

Campbell, Donald Clarence, U. of Neb., M.D. 1935, Rochester, Minn.

Chalek, Jack I., U. of Minn., M.B. 1937, St. Paul, Minn.

Cochrane, Ray Fleming, U. of Minn., M.B. 1937; M.D. 1937, Minneapolis, Minn.

Colyer, George Edward, U. of Ill., M.D. 1936, Rochester, Minn.

Cronin, Thomas Dillon, U. of Texas, M.D. 1932, Rochester, Minn.

Darling, John Pendleton, Rush Med. Col., M.D. 1937, Rochester, Minn.

Doehring, Paul Christoph, Jr., Rush Med. Col., M.D. 1937, Rochester, Minn.

East, John, U. of Okla., M.D. 1937, St. Paul, Minn.

Feinstein, Julius Yale, U. of Minn., M.B. and M.D. 1937, Minot, N. Dak.

Fischer, Verrill John, Rush Med. Col., M.D. 1937, St. Paul, Minn.

Flink, Edmund Berney, U. of Minn., M.B. 1937, Minneapolis, Minn.

Gordon, Martin Norton, U. of Minn., M.B. 1937, Minneapolis, Minn.

Gorman, William Ambrose, Western Reserve, M.D. 1932, Duluth, Minn.

Greene, Laurence Francis, Harvard U., M.D. 1936, Rochester, Minn.

Hauge, Erling Trygve, U. of Minn., M.B. 1937, Clarkfield, Minn.

Hoffbauer, Frederick William, U. of Minn., M.B. and M.D. 1937, Minneapolis, Minn.

Hollinshead, William Henry, Jr., U. of Minn., M.B. 1937, Minneapolis, Minn.

Holmstrom, Emil Gustave, U. of Minn., M.B. 1937, Minneapolis, Minn.

Holzapfel, Fred C., U. of Minn., M.B. 1937, Minneapolis, Minn.

Hudec, Elwyn R., U. of Minn., M.B. 1937, Silver Lake, Minn.

Hughes, Bernard J., U. of Minn., M.B. 1937, Duluth, Minn.

Jones, Herbert William, Jr., Harvard U., M.D. 1937, Minneapolis, Minn.

Katzovitz, Hyman, U. of Minn., M.B. 1937, St. Paul, Minn.

Kendrick, Marvin Hayne, Harvard U., M.D. 1935, Rochester, Minn.

Kershner, Calvin Myles, U., of Pa., M.D. 1936, Rochester, Minn.

Knutson, Lewis Arthur, U. of Minn., M.B. 1937, Minneapolis, Minn.

Kremen, Arnold James, U. of Minn., M.B. 1937, Minneapolis, Minn.

Lamin, Bernard G., U. of Minn., M.B. 1937, Mabel, Minn.

Leary, William Vincent, U. of Minn., M.B. 1937, St. Paul, Minn.

Leitschuh, Linus Frederick, U. of Minn., M.B. 1937, M.D. 1938, Minneapolis, Minn.

Mavrelis, William Peter, U. of Minn., M.B. 1936; M.D. 1937, Chicago, Ill.

McCullough, John Andrew Lawson, U. of Toronto, M.D. 1934, Rochester, Minn.

McKean, Frank Flanders, U., of Minn., M.B. 1938, Minneapolis, Minn.

Merrill, Robert William, U. of Minn., M.B. 1937, Starbuck, Minn.

Mickelson, John Charles, U. of Minn., M.B. 1938, Mankato, Minn.

Moren, Leslie Arthur, U. of Minn., M.B. 1937, St. Paul, Minn.

Moss, Arthur James, U. of Minn., M.B. 1937, Minneapolis, Minn.

Munn, Elizabeth L., U. of Ore., M.D. 1936, Rochester, Minn.

Murphy, James Edward, U. of Minn., M.B. 1937, Minneapolis, Minn.

Nesheim, Martin Otto, U. of Iowa, M.D. 1937, Duluth, Minn.

O'Brien, John Patrick, Jefferson Med. Col., M.D. 1935, Rochester, Minn.

Overpeck, Darrell O., Indiana U., M.D. 1934, Rochester, Minn.

Parson, Edwin Irvine, U. of Minn., M.B. 1937, Duluth, Minn.

Pastore, Pietro Nicolino, Med. Col. of Va., M.D. 1934, Rochester, Minn.

Plotke, Harry Louis, U. of Minn., M.B. 1937, St. Paul, Minn.

Pollock, George Angus, U. of Glasgow, M.B. and Ch.B. 1923, Rochester, Minn.

Rein, Gerald Norman, U. of Mich., M.D. 1933, Rochester, Minn.

Roberts, Lewis Joshua, U. of Minn., M.B. 1937, St. Paul, Minn.

Robertson, Frank O., U. of Ore., M.D. 1937, St. Paul, Minn.

Ross, Alexander Joseph, U. of Minn., M.B. 1937, Minneapolis, Minn.

Rousseau, Maurice Cyprian, U. of Minn., M.B. 1937, St. Paul, Minn.

Rudin, Harry N., U. of Minn., M.B. 1938, Minneapolis, Minn.

Schroder, John Richard, U. of Minn., M.B. 1938, Duluth, Minn.

Schweiger, Lamont R., Rush Med. Col., M.D. 1937, Rochester, Minn.

Sherman, Alfred Gustav, U. of Minn., M.B. 1938, Minneapolis, Minn.

Simonson, Donald Bennett, Rush Med. Col., M.D. 1937, Minneapolis, Minn.

Squire, Everett Wayne, Rush Med. Col., M.D. 1937, Rochester, Minn.

Strassmann, Erwin Otto, Friedrich-Wilhelms U., M.D. 1922, Rochester, Minn.

Tingdale, Carlyle, U. of Minn., M.B. 1937; M.D. 1938, Minneapolis, Minn.

Tudor, Robert Bruce, U. of Minn., M.B. 1937, Minneapolis, Minn.

Uihlein, Alfred, Jr., Johns Hopkins U., M.D. 1935, Rochester, Minn.

Welte, Edwin Joseph, U. of Minn., M.B. 1937, Minneapolis, Minn.

Wil, Charles Bishop, U. of Minn., M.B. 1938, Duluth, Minn.

By Reciprocity

Elliott, William, Rush Med. Col., M.D. 1927, Virginia, Minn.

Laney, Howard John, U. of Wis., M.D. 1935, Prescott, Wis.

Lipp, Frank Edward, Creighton U., M.D. 1934, Appleton, Minn.

Thompson, Harlow B., U. of Ore., M.D. 1935, Park Rapids, Minn.

National Board Credentials

Morrison, Charlotte Jean, U. of Minn., M.B. 1933; M.D. 1934, Minneapolis, Minn.

Neff, Walter Scott, Jefferson Med. Col., M.D. 1932, Virginia, Minn.

Schmitt, George Fredrick, Jr., U. of Maryland, M.D. 1935, Rochester, Minn.

PHYSICIANS LICENSED JULY 16, 1938
June Examination

Anderson, Robert Edward, U. of Minn., M.B. 1935, Minneapolis, Minn.

Arey, James Blanding, U. of Minn., M.B. 1937, Excelsior, Minn.

Arko, Joseph Lawrence, U. of Minn., M.B. 1938, Chisholm, Minn.

Biorn, Carl Ludvig, U. of Minn., M.B. 1938, Jackson, Minn.

Borowicz, Leonard Ambrose, U. of Minn., M.B. 1938 Strandquist, Minn.

Breslow, Lester, U. of Minn., M.B. 1938, Staten Island N. Y.

Buehler, Martin Stowell, U. of Minn., M.B. 1938, Minneapolis, Minn.

Cameron, John Hugh, McGill U., M.D. 1937, Bagley Minn.

Ceplecha, Stanley Francis, Marquette U., M.D. 1938 New Prague, Minn.

Childs, Theron Baker, Northwestern U., M.D. 1938 Duluth, Minn.

Clarke, William O., U. of Minn., M.B. 1937; M.D. 1938 Hibbing, Minn.

Cohen, Ephraim Bernard, U. of Minn., M.B. 1938 Minneapolis, Minn.

Condon, William B., McGill U., M.D. 1933, Rochester Minn.

Danstrom, John Richard, Northwestern U., M.D. 1938 Duluth, Minn.

Demo, Robert Anthony, U. of Minn., M.B. 1938, Blu Earth, Minn.

Farkas, John Victor, U. of Minn., M.B. 1938, St. Pau Minn.

Frank, Harold Joseph, U. of Minn., M.B. 1938, Ne Prague, Minn.

Freedland, Morris, U. of Minn., M.B. 1938, Minnea olis, Minn.

OF GENERAL INTEREST

Dr. E. I. Parson, who has just completed his internship at St. Luke's Hospital in Duluth, has located in Askov for the practice of medicine.

* * *

Dr. Dwight Martin, son of Dr. and Mrs. T. P. Martin of Arlington, was married recently to Miss Evelyn Kienitz of Saint Paul. Dr. and Mrs. Martin will make their home in Saint Paul.

* * *

Dr. George T. Ayres of Ely was elected president of the Vermilion Range Old Settlers' Association at the twenty-fourth annual reunion of the group, held at Eveleth in July.

* * *

Dr. Duane Olson of Gaylord was recently married to Miss Lyndis Iverslie of Delano. Dr. Olson is associated with his father, Dr. Duane O. C. Olson, in the practice of medicine at Gaylord.

* * *

Dr. W. G. Benjamin, of Pipestone, has recently been selected as a new member of the board of education at Pipestone. Dr. Benjamin is also president of the Pipestone Civic and Commerce Association.

* * *

Dr. C. E. Anderson, who has practiced medicine in Brainerd for the past thirteen years, has gone to Great Falls, Montana, where he will continue his medical practice. Dr. Anderson has disposed of his practice in Brainerd to Dr. W. E. Fitzsimmons of Saint Paul.

* * *

Dr. R. A. Glabe has become associated with Dr. J. A. Slocumb of Plainview for the practice of medicine. Dr. Glabe, who obtained his medical degree at the University of Minnesota, recently completed his internship at St. Luke's Hospital in Duluth.

* * *

Dr. Robert D. Mussey of Rochester is Vice Chairman of the Executive Committee and Chairman of the Educational and Scientific Exhibit Committee of the American Congress on Obstetrics and Gynecology, which is to be held in Cleveland, Ohio, in 1939.

* * *

Dr. T. J. Bloedel has become affiliated with the Bratrud Clinic at Thief River Falls, where his work will be limited to internal medicine, diagnosis and treatment. Dr. Bloedel graduated from the University of Minnesota, and served his internship at the Minneapolis General Hospital.

* * *

Dr. S. D. Wolstan has become associated with Dr. Oscar Daignault, of Benson, in the practice of medicine. Dr. Wolstan is a graduate of the Faculty of Medicine of the University of Paris. He served his internship at St. Louis Hospital in Paris and at the Swedish Hospital in Minneapolis.

667

◆ REPORTS and ANNOUNCEMENTS ◆

MEDICAL BROADCAST FOR SEPTEMBER

The Minnesota State Medical Association Morning Health Service.

The Minnesota State Medical Association broadcasts weekly at 9:45 o'clock every Saturday morning over Station WCCO, Minneapolis and Saint Paul (810 kilocycles or 370.2 meters).

Speaker: William A. O'Brien, M.D., Associate Professor of Pathology and Preventive Medicine, Medical School, University of Minnesota. The program for the month will be as follows:

September 3—Premature Care
September 10—Birth Marks
September 17—Tularemia
September 24—School Dentistry.

INTERSTATE POSTGRADUATE MEDICAL ASSOCIATION

The International Assembly of the Interstate Postgraduate Medical Association of North America will be held in the Public Auditorium of Philadelphia, October 31, November 1, 2, 3 and 4, 1938. The Assembly will be preceded and followed by clinics in the various Philadelphia hospitals.

This well known medical meeting aims to present the newer developments in medicine and surgery with particular emphasis on their practical use from a clinical standpoint. The five-day program, which will occupy morning, afternoon and evening, except for Wednesday evening, which will be devoted to the annual banquet, will be presented, for the most part, by professors from medical schools of the United States and Canada. One European guest speaker appears on the program, Professor Dr. V. Eicken of the Medical Faculty of the University of Berlin, whose subject will be "Osteomyelitis of the Frontal Bone."

Philadelphia, with its wealth of clinical material, fine hospitals and excellent hotel accommodations, offers an ideal city for the Assembly meeting. The Philadelphia County Medical Society, the Pennsylvania State Medical Association, the College of Physicians of Philadelphia, and the Philadelphia Chamber of Commerce, will all coöperate to make the Assembly a success.

A cordial invitation is extended to all physicians in good standing in their state and provincial associations. Physicians are urged to bring their ladies, for whom an excellent program has been arranged. Philadelphia holds many places of historic interest which will make a visit to Philadelphia particularly attractive.

Attention is called to the list of distinguished Assembly speakers, which appears on page xxi of the advertising section of this issue.

Registration fee is $5.00.

This year's officers of the Association are: Dr. El-

liott P. Joslin, President, Boston; Dr. George W. Crile, Chairman of Program Committee, Cleveland, and Dr. William B. Peck, Managing Director, Freeport, Illinois.

MEDICAL CORPS OF THE U. S. NAVY

Graduates of Class A medical schools between twenty-one and thirty-two years of age are eligible to take the examinations which will begin November 7, 1938. Applications should be filed at least one month prior to that date. Successful candidates will be commissioned as Assistant Surgeons with the rank of Lieutenant (junior grade) and assigned to the Naval Medical School, Washington, D. C., for a postgraduate course of instruction. Upon completion of the internship competitive examinations will be held for permanent appointment, the right to return to civilian practice being retained. The rank of Lieutenant affords compensation of $2,699 per year for those without dependents and $3,158 for those with dependents. Applicants must be American citizens.

For further information address the Bureau of Medicine and Surgery, Navy Department, Washington, D. C.

MILITARY TRAINING FOR MEDICAL RESERVISTS

The tenth annual training course for Medical Department Reservists (Inactive Status) of the Army and Navy will be held at the Mayo Foundation Rochester, Minnesota, October 3-15, 1938.

Special clinical and hospital work will be given mornings and subjects in military medicine morning, afternoon and evening.

The program for the last three days will be merged with that of the Association of Military Surgeons of the United States. Surgeons General of the Army, the Navy and the Public Health Service will attend and participate.

All Medical Department Reservists are eligible for enrollment. Applications should be made to the Headquarters of the Seventh Corps Area, Omaha, Nebraska.

GRADUATE FORTNIGHT OF THE NEW YORK ACAMEDY OF MEDICINE

The eleventh annual Graduate Fortnight will be held this year from October 24 to November 1938. The program consists of daily afternoon clinics at the various New York hospitals, evening lectures at the Academy headquarters, and scientific exhibits. The profession is invited and a registration fee of $3.00 admits bearer to all three groups

MINNESOTA MEDICINE

meetings. For further details those interested should communicate with Dr. Mahlon Ashford, The New York Academy of Medicine, 2 East 103rd Street, New York City.

MISSISSIPPI VALLEY MEDICAL SOCIETY

The fourth annual meeting of the Society, which includes in its membership physicians of Illinois, Missouri and Iowa, will be held at Hannibal, Missouri, September 28 to 30, 1938.

The program will consist of over fifty lectures, clinics, short courses and round table discussions. An All-Chicago program will occupy the first day of the meeting with a Stag Buffet Supper in the evening. A banquet and entertainment will be held the second evening. Dr. I. C. Brill, Assistant Professor of Medicine at the University of Oregon Medical School, winner of the Prize Essay Contest, will read his winning essay on Failure of the Circulation; Types and Treatment.

Physicians are cordially invited to attend. Harold Swanberg, M.D., 209 W.C.U. Building, Quincy, Illinois, is secretary.

CENTER FOR CONTINUATION STUDY

The Center for Continuation Study announces a fall program of six postgraduate medical courses. The subjects are Proctology, September 19 to 24, Diseases of Genito-urinary Tract, September 19 to 24, Diseases of Infancy and Childhood, September 26 to October 1, General Medicine, October 10 to 15, Diseases of the Skin, October 31 to November 5, and Tuberculosis, November 14 to 19.

The tuition for each course will be $25.00. Registration may be made by sending in a registration fee of $3.00, which will apply on the tuition. The enrolment in the course in Proctology is closed.

Physicians will find it to their advantage to live at the Center for Continuation Study, where delightful accommodations will be found. Members of physicians' families may accompany them and stay at the Center for the same living rates.

Physicians planning on attending the home football games with the Universities of Washington, Nebraska, Michigan, and Iowa which will take place during the medical programs should make their ticket applications directly to the Football Ticket Office, 108 Cooke Hall, University of Minnesota, Minneapolis.

As in the past, the faculties will be recruited from the staff of the Medical School, Mayo Foundation, and members of the Minnesota State Medical Association. In addition, distinguished clinicians from other centers will lead discussions. Among others Dr. Curtice Rosser, Professor of Proctology, Baylor University, Dallas, Texas; Dr. Hobart A. Reimann, Magee Professor of Practice of Medicine and Clinical Medicine, Jefferson Medical College, Philadelphia, Pennsylvania; Dr. Lloyd G. Lewis, member of the Urology Staff of Johns Hopkins Hospital, will appear on the programs.

Physicians planning to attend should make their reservations early as enrolment in each course is limited.

CENTRAL ASSOCIATION OF OBSTETRICIANS AND GYNECOLOGISTS

The annual meeting of the Central Association of Obstetricians and Gynecologists will take place in Minneapolis, October 6-7-8, Radisson Hotel. Dr. J. C. Litzenberg will be the honored speaker. All physicians are invited to attend as guests.

HOMECOMING CLINIC OF MEDICAL ALUMNI

The Minnesota Medical Alumni Association will hold its annual business meeting at a luncheon at the University Hospital on Friday, October 14. This is the day preceding the Homecoming game with Michigan. The president of the Association, Dr. Robert L. Wilder of Minneapolis, has appointed Dr. Harold G. Benjamin as chairman of the program committee for the clinical presentations at the hospital on Friday morning. The details of this program will be announced at a later date.

In Memoriam

W. P. Ross
1893-1938

DR. W. P. ROSS died suddenly of a heart condition in his home at Ottertail County Sanatorium, Battle Lake, Minnesota, on June 25, 1938.

Dr. Ross was a Canadian by birth, having been born in Woodstock, Ontario, 1893. He became a citizen of the United States in the summer of 1937. He moved with his parents to Saskatchewan when a boy and obtained his preliminary education in that province. His medical education was obtained in the Manitoba Medical College, Winnipeg, where he graduated in 1923. His internship was obtained in one of the hospitals of Winnipeg. He was in general practice at Brandon, Manitoba, several years, following which he served as one of the assistant physicians at Ninnette Sanatorium, Ninnette, Canada.

Dr. Ross came to Minnesota in December, 1929, as assistant physician at the Southwestern Minnesota Sanatorium, Worthington. He held the position until November, 1937, when he resigned to take over the duties of Superintendent and Medical Director of the Ottertail County Sanatorium, Battle Lake, Minnesota. This position he was holding at the time of his death.

He was faithful to his duties and held high the ideals of his profession. The past ten years of his life were devoted to tuberculosis work, a phase of medicine in which he was intensively interested and to which he contributed much of value. He was a member of the Minnesota Sanatorium Association and the Minnesota State Medical Association.

He was married to Rita Brooks of Winnipeg on August 11, 1926. She, together with two sons, William and James, survives him.

BOOK REVIEWS

Books listed here become the property of the Ramsey and Hennepin County Medical libraries when reviewed. Members, however, are urged to write reviews of any or every recent book which may be of interest to physicians.

THE VITAMINS AND THEIR CLINICAL APPLICATIONS. Prof. Dr. W. Stepp, Doz. Dr. Kühnau and Dr. H. S. Schroeder, University of Munich. Translated by Herman A. H. Bouman, M.D., Minneapolis. 173 pages. Price, cloth, $4.50. Milwaukee: Vitamin Products Co., 1938.

OUTLINE OF ROENTGEN DIAGNOSIS. Leo C. Rigler, B.S., M.B., M.D. Professor of Radiology, University of Minnesota, Minneapolis. 212 pages of text. 254 illustrations. Price, student's edition without illustrations, paper cover, $3.00; complete edition, cloth, $6.50. Philadelphia: J. B. Lippincott Co., 1938.

THE HORSE AND BUGGY DOCTOR. Arthur E. Hertzler, M.D., of Halstead, Kansas. 322 pages. Illus. Price, cloth, $2.75. New York: Harper & Bros., 1938.

THE TECHNIQUE OF CONTRACEPTION. Fourth Edition. Eric M. Matsner, M.D., 50 pages. Illus. New York: National Medical Council on Birth Control, 1938.

THE STORY OF LUCKY STRIKE. Roy C. Flannagan, Staff Commentator of the Richmond News Leader, Richmond, Va., 71 pages. Illus. 1938.

THE ROCKEFELLER FOUNDATION, ANNUAL REPORT 1937. 506 pages. Illus. Paper cover. New York: The Rockefeller Foundation, 1938.

CANCER—WITH SPECIAL REFERENCE TO CANCER OF THE BREAST. R. J. Behan, M.D., Dr. Med. (Berlin), F.A.C.S. Cofounder and formerly Director Cancer Department of the Pittsburgh Skin and Cancer Foundation, Pittsburgh. 844 pages. Illus. Price, cloth, $10.00. St. Louis: C. V. Mosby Co., 1938.

ZUR ENTDECKUNG DER INSULINSCHOCKTHERAPIE BEI AKUTEN GEISTESKRANKHEITEN, INSBESONDERE BEI DER SCHIZOPHRENIE. Dr. Julius Schuster, Gewesener I. Assistant der Pazmany Peter-Universitat Psychiatrisch Neurologischen Universitatsklinik in Budapest. 90 pages. Paper cover. Budapest: Druckerei der Pester Lloyd-Gesellschaft, 1938.

THE MANAGEMENT OF FRACTURES, DISLOCATIONS, AND SPRAINS. John Albert Key, B.S., M.D., and H. Earle Conwell, M.D., F.A.C.S. Second edition, 1246 pages, illustrated. St. Louis: C. B. Mosby Co., 1937.

This book is one of the best and most complete, as well as concise descriptions of the principles, general aspects, diagnosis and treatment of specific injuries of the skeletal system that one could desire.

The chapter dealing with general considerations of fracture equipment desirable for any general hospital treating fractures is excellent. The authors are to be commended upon their inclusion of a chapter relating to first aid in fracture and automobile injuries, and also for their clear discussion concerning workmen's compensation laws affecting fracture cases and medical-legal aspects of fracture cases.

Discussion concerning diagnosis and treatment of injuries to specific portions of the skeletal system are clear, concise and complete. Illustrations are profuse and adequate. The index is complete and well organized. The book is practical in its entirety, relatively devoid of extraneous material, and should be a very useful tool to the medical profession.

C. H. MEAD, M.D.

DISABILITY EVALUATION; PRINCIPLES OF TREATMENT OF COMPENSABLE INJURIES. Earl D. Mcbride, M.D. Octave of 623 pages, illustrated. Cloth $8.00. Philadelphia: J. B. Lippincott Company, 1936.

This book is valuable in pointing out the factors that should be considered before an estimate of disability in industrial cases is to be made. The author suggests what he terms a functional measuring rod, composed of one hundred units. On this rod he assigns values to the factor of function in the following way: delayed action—10%; awkwardness—20%; weakness—20%; insecurity—10%; diminished endurance—20%; lowered safety factor—10%, and averse influence of conspicuous impairment. He states that many examiners may not agree with him on the relative values of the factors concerned. His functional measuring rod suggests the consideration of factors of function often overlooked in making estimates.

The author presents a good synopsis of the Workmen's Compensation Laws in operation in the United States. The chapter on "Industrial Back" is very interesting and instructive.

R. M. BURNS, M.D.

SUPPURATIVE PAROTITIS AS A COMPLICATION OF MUMPS

(Continued from page 649)

two centimeters long, was made just through the skin, along the lines of the natural skin folds at the angle of the jaw. The underlying tissues were then separated by blunt dissection. About forty cubic centimeters of greenish-yellow pus was evacuated, which showed pure staphylococcus aureus on culture. Two days later there appeared below the incision, in the region of the submaxillary gland, another fluctuant area which was emptied by blunt dissection through the previous incision. After a convalescence, uneventful except for the profuse drainage, the patient was discharged in about ten days. When seen one month later there was complete closure of the operative wound, with a normally functioning parotid gland and all the symptoms had disappeared, including the trismus.

Conclusion

An unusual case is presented of suppurative parotitis complicating epidemic mumps, with spontaneous discharge into the external auditory canal.

Bibliography

1. Alexander, G.: Mumps mit Abszessbildung und Spontandurchbruch inden Ausseren Gehörgang. Monatschr. Ohrenh., 61:785, (July) 1927.
2. Bader, George: Acute suppurative parotitis with rupture into the external auditory canal, occurring as a complication of mumps. Jour. Am. Med. Assn., 97:929-1931.
3. Berndt, A. L., Buck, R., and Buxton, R.: The pathogenesis of acute suppurative parotitis. Am. Jour. Med. Sci., 182:639, (Nov.) 1931.
4. Bernstein, S. K.: Mumps mit Abszessbildung und Spontandurchbruch inden Ausseren Gehörgang. Montaschr. Ohrenh., 62:212, (Feb.) 1928.
5. Lewis, Geo. V.: Acute suppurative parotitis. Jo. Ark. Med. Soc., 25:58, (Aug.) 1928.

MINNESOTA MEDICINE

Journal of the Minnesota State Medical Association, Southern Minnesota Medical Association, Northern Minnesota Medical Association, Minnesota Academy of Medicine and Minneapolis Surgical Society

| Volume 21 | OCTOBER, 1938 | No. 10 |

THE SOCIAL SIDE OF MEDICAL PROGRESS*

HOWARD W. HAGGARD

Director, Laboratory of Applied Physiology
Sheffield Scientific School, Yale University

New Haven, Connecticut

IN DISCUSSING the social side of medical progress, I shall deal not so much with factual matters as with interpretations. Interpretations are inevitably opinions. And you may not agree with my interpretations. My excuse for presenting them on this occasion is simply this: it is as well at times to draw back a little from the details of immediate and practical projects and in contemplation to view medical and social situations in broad perspective, to see trends, directions and dimensions. Such a procedure serves to bring these matters to the front so that for a few minutes we may think about them in a way that is essentially detailed and philosophical.

Viewed in this way the feature that shows as peculiar to the present period is the rapid shift and change of long established social institutions. As we watch these changes, the realization is forced upon us that the body of society is a delicately integrated entity just as is the body of man—so closely knit and interdependent in its parts that a change in any one must necessarily result in a change in all other parts, in a total readjustment.

Thus if medical discovery is made and applied to the saving of lives, there must follow a reorganization of society as a whole. The saving of life results in a change in the age structure of the population. The change in the age structure of the population upsets the balance of established institutions and necessitates social and economic readjustments.

*Banquet address at the annual meeting of the Minnesota State Medical Association, Duluth, Minnesota, June 30, 1938.

The consequences of somewhat less than a hundred years of not too intensively applied preventive medicine—mostly an impersonal sort of medicine—have been the enormous diminution in the diseases and deaths of early life—the acute infectious diseases and infant mortality. As a result, the average length of human life has nearly doubled in this period. The age structure of the population has shifted and is still shifting. The facts and figures are familiar to you: In 1900 there was one person of sixty years of age or over in every twenty members of the population; in 1930 there was one in every twelve; and by 1960 there may be one in every six—one-sixth of the population sixty years of age or over. Here is the greatest change of its sort that has ever affected civilization. In the past there have been changes from war and pestilence but they have been from loss, not saving, of life. Here, growing from medical advancement, is a social and economic problem of vast magnitude in which the first efforts toward solution have taken the forms of social security legislation and old-age pensions; but these efforts do not touch upon the real problems of old age and retirement in an industrial civilization. They do not touch upon the consequences to medicine.

It is axiomatic in our field that as one disease diminishes, others rise to take its place. As the incidence of tuberculosis, typhoid, dysentery and smallpox go down, cancer and diseases of the circulatory system rise correspondingly. The change in the leading causes of death in the last thirty-eight years is commonplace knowledge.

So far the physician sees clearly; but sometimes I think he fails to see that medicine itself is one of the institutions affected by. the changes that are brought about. Completing its circuitous course through the social structure, the change eventually comes back to medicine. A readjustment must be made there. Medicine does not stand alone; it is an integral part of society. It must either make the necessary adjustments to change or be swept aside. Readjustment—continual readjustment—of medicine is the inevitable consequence of medical progress.

Readjustment is disturbing. We tend to resist it; and resisting it we sometimes get out of step with progress and are left behind. Such resistance is futile; its consequences are destructive.

In the face of such change there appears one of the peculiarities of medicine: the failure to realize that it must change as society changes. It has been one of the most characteristic features of the physician of all ages—and the present is no exception—to hold in a certain arrogance the belief that the form of medicine, the principles of medicine and its practice, are vastly superior to those of all preceding ages; that they are the ultimate, beyond which there can be no constructive change.

In short, the progress of medicine has always showed this: Medical thought has crystallized on a line of endeavor. This line has been followed long after its usefulness has passed. Medicine has then, to the great cost of the doctor, been stopped and redirected to move in another line until that in turn has lost its usefulness—until the form of medicine was no longer suited to the time and was therefore discarded by the public. This same process occurs in government as well as medicine; a regimen goes along getting more and more out of step with social needs. Then there is a war, a revolution, and a new start is made. This process repeats itself over and over.

Now what I say tonight is essentially an indictment of the inertia of modern medicine. And in so doing I ask you to remember that inertia does not apply alone to things that are stationary; there can be inertia also of movement. Medicine and the physician, following a course that has been set, stay fast to the direction with fixed attention and dogged disregard of the fact

that goals may shift, that situations may that the direction of the movement m. longer lead to the desired goals. In the pa phenomenon has occurred time and time and medicine has dwindled out to futility. same situation is, I think, developing toda} medicine, for all the apparent progress of ical science, can dwindle out again to f The medicine of today may be vastly di from the medicine of the past but the fa mains that the social and sociological force guide it, operate upon it today just as th in the past.

The great danger that I see to the pract medicine today lies in the very thing th: given medicine its modern preëminence that is science. The physician has com: himself to science. He stands or falls w My indictment tonight is against this sci a science that has led the doctor to negle equally fundamental and non-scientific soc pects of medical practice—those things th sometimes sum up as the art of medic thing about which the younger generati physicians knows so little. The doctor, in ing a fetish of science, may find himself shipping alone. He will unless his m practices are changed continually to sui cisely the society in which he lives.

The doctor of America in the eighteen early nineteenth centuries was not a sc He was a public-spirited man whose me suited the times. He was a social leade bodying the rare combination of medical p and sociology. He was arrogant wh thought of the lack of knowledge of his cessors—sometimes of his own contempo But this temporal arrogance is always a acteristic of the doctor. We today loo pity, mingled with contempt, on the pract Benjamin Rush. It was Rush, you will ber, who made that pathetic statement: cine is my wife and science my mistre was Oliver Wendell Holmes, with the ar of the succeeding generation, who comm "Medicine may be his wife and science h tress, but it cannot be shown that this of the Seventh Commandment was of a vantage to the legitimate recipient of hi tions." Yet, in spite of his lack of scienc as practitioner and medical leader has n today.

a far more accurate diagnosis is made by a technician in the laboratory. When—and if—medicine becomes an exact science we shall no longer need the practicing physician. Until it does become an exact science, then we not only need him, but we should grant him his due and proper importance.

The practicing physician is not a scientist. He is, if he really practices medicine, more, far more, than a scientist. He is an artist. He does not deal with the controlled and limited matters of the laboratory; he deals with human beings. So long as the human mind in its full ramifications remains beyond an evaluation with scientific precision, then the practice of medicine must remain an art. So long as medical practice involves the personal contact of physician and patient then it is the art of the physician which must establish the necessary bond. This is very different from medical research. It is, in many ways, more difficult. It involves not only intelligence and skill, but also qualities of personality unnecessary to the research worker. This personality element in medical practice has been—if not openly at least by indirection—scoffed at by the scientist or ignored.

There are two sides of medicine and we tend to confuse them. On one side is the medical research worker searching for knowledge; on the other is the practicing physician applying that knowledge. Far oftener than not the research worker is a poor physician. There is more to medical practice than the mere knowledge of medical fact. There is the old and true adage that "you can't carry an experiment bleeding from the laboratory to the bedside." The medical research worker and the practicing physician each has his proper and equally important place.

And yet with the emphasis placed upon science, with the public believing in the marvels of science, with the kudos of science, the physician has very naturally wished to believe that he was a scientist.

In the first flush of the triumphs of the application of science to medicine, it appeared that all the problems of medicine were to be answered and that medicine at last was destined to become as exact and impersonal as engineering. In consequence, to the eventual great detriment of the practice of medicine, our medical education was changed. It adopted the precise

673

methods of science. It built its structure on the laboratory as a foundation.

Trace with me the broad steps in the change in American medical education. A century and a quarter ago French medicine went through one of the periodic changes of direction—a drastic change in a revolution. The old staid and formal dogmatic teaching broke down to give way to an active clinical investigative type of medicine. In Germany the change came a little later but it was mainly German medicine that ours followed. A little over a century ago Germany, following the Napoleonic wars, was in the throes of a wave of idealism and romanticism that denied in the medical schools factual investigation and permitted only speculation. It was one of the extremes of the pendulum movement of education. Then it swung the other way; by the middle of the century German preclinical medicine had been founded by Johannes Müller. It was around him that the great school of Berlin was developed. His pupils, including Virchow, give the roster of the famous teachers and investigators of Germany. Almost without exception, and this includes Müller, they were men with enormous social interests. Virchow, you will remember, was as fearless and fiery in his political activities and his denouncements as he was in the classroom. The best of German medicine was gradually brought to America. The part that caught and held attention was the research aspect. At first the leading schools in this country were famous for their clinical teachers. The preëminence of Johns Hopkins in the closing years of the last century, and the early years of this century, was based on its great clinicians. Today, with the continual swing of the pendulum toward research, the preëminence of a school is judged, not by how well it trains doctors for the practice of medicine, but upon the eminence of its researches. The chairs once occupied by great clinicians with wide social interests and wide social influences are too often filled by scientists out of touch with the real problems of the practitioner. Few great scientists have been outstanding physicians. Harvey, who described the circulation of the blood, was a bad therapeutist; Koch, to whom we owe the conception of the bacterial cause of disease, gave up practice; and Pasteur was not even a physician. Formerly, students in our schools were trained to be social-

ly beneficial. Now they are trained too often with the apparent intention of making laboratory investigators out of them and that in spite of the fact that medical practice is a social application. Today we train too often, not physicians with all the significance of the term, but instead, we train bedside pathologists.

Medical training is being divorced from medical practice; preclinical training is being sold out to educators who are not even physicians. There are those who wisely think that the student from the first to the last of his four years of training should be in contact with physicians and be taught clinically. Instead, there has grown up the whole division of subjects called preclinical. If they are preclinical they should be premedical. If they are taught in medical schools they should be taught, not as if in training for the Ph.D. degree, but instead constantly from the medical point of view and by physicians. Our grandfathers had only two years of medical training; it was almost entirely clinical; we are contemptuous of their deficient education. Today we have four years in our schools, but mostly we still have only two years of actual training in medical practice. The expansion has come from the addition of preclinical subjects taught in a detail and with a detachment wholly unnecessary to medical practice.

The emphasis upon science, upon the laboratory, has extended down even into the premedical field in the college. The selection there is made upon the basis, not of socially-minded individuals who would make good practitioners, but upon the basis of aptness in the laboratory subjects. The class of men who enter our medical schools, at least from our large Eastern colleges, are today, as potential material for social leadership, distinctly inferior to the young men from the same colleges entering law and business. We are turning away good men because no matter how great their ability might be as practitioners—they show no aptitude for the technic of medical research.

There is today a greater need for socially-minded, public-guiding physicians than at any previous period in medicine. The application of sanitation are wiping out the infectious diseases of early life. In consequence, as I have mentioned, the average length of life has changed and with it the leading causes of mortality. The diseases that come to the front in the modern medical readjustment cannot be cured or prevented by impersonal science. They can be controlled only ·by the close and intelligent coöperation of the individual members of the public with the physician. Obtaining this coöperation is a vastly different matter from acquiring the knowledge of how to prevent or treat the diseases. It is not medical research or science; it is the practice of medicine in its broadest service of a social leadership.

All achieved medical advancement consists of two distinct parts—and they are distinct. One is medical research in the acquisition of the knowledge of means by which suffering can be assuaged and diseases cured or prevented. That is the part today that receives the interest and the emphasis both in most of our schools and certainly in the minds of the public. But this part alone, this knowledge gained from research, accomplishes none. of these things. They are accomplished and true advancement achieved only when the second necessary part is fulfilled. And the second part is putting the knowledge into application. Application is then for all practical purposes as important as discovery. Application belongs to the practice of medicine. Today unquestionably, with our enormous accumulated knowledge, there exists a wider gap between what can be done to control and prevent disease and what is being done than at any previous time in history. This fact is a grave indictment against the practice of medicine. It is the result of following a set direction of medical progress with no consideration of changing social conditions.

The great resultant danger to medical practice lies here. The public is beginning to realize the gap—the failure of application. The recognition will grow as long as these matters of application—crying in their need today—remain, if not in the contempt of the physician, at least not in his highest regard.

The social worker of today knows that the greatest, indeed probably the only possible field of social betterment, is offered by medical application. Some aggressive lay groups stand ready to raid the medical field for its unapplied potentialities. With the natural reaction of newcomers to the field—unacquainted with its ramifications, but sensing its deficiencies—they assume that there is something basically wrong with the form of medical practice. Their first

inclination is to remake the form of medicine. Today the doctor must take his choice—lead or be led.

There is tremendous danger from this direction. Public opinion determines the condition and future of medicine. Today the public has an influence on social affairs and upon medical affairs greater than at any other time in history. But the actions of the public, unless guided, are always destructive, never constructive. People tend to pull down everything to the average level. Advancement, construction, is not made by great numbers, but by great individuals.

The only chance for medical leadership from the physician is to cultivate throughout our public a realization of what medicine can do; and to cultivate a coöperation between the public and the physician to do the things that medicine can do. In the last analysis it comes down to this: the shaping of public opinion to a high regard of medicine and of the practicing physician as its prophet. Unfortunately too much of the shaping has been to divert attention to the marvels of medical science and the deficiencies of medical practice.

It isn't what medicine does, it isn't what science discovers, that gives the necessary high public regard to the physician. It is what the public thinks and believes. And the public attitude reflects the doctor's own opinion of himself. If he thinks of himself as a scientist, he will be treated as one; he will be held in the same regard in which the physicist, the chemist, and the engineer are held. If he believes, as he should believe, and shows that he is a leader toward social betterment, worthy of public regard, he will receive that regard. These are matters of emotion and not of reason.

The physician, in casting his lot with scientific research, stands and falls with it. And he has chosen an uncertain support. We have grown to believe in the ruggedness, the permanence, the necessity of medical research. In so doing we delude ourselves. As a matter of fact, medical science is one of the most highly cultivated aspects of civilization. It can flourish, even exist, only under the most favorable conditions of civilization. A social disturbance destroys first of all medical science. It has happened in other countries and it can happen in our own just as easily. A little over a hundred years ago, as I said, there was no medical science in Germany.

The country was in the throes of a wave of romanticism and mysticism. Then in half a century Germany raised herself to world preëminence in medical science, set the course which we follow today. And then in the present century, under changing social conditions, medical science declined in Germany—it is disappearing; it has already gone in Russia, Italy and Spain. We still have it in our country. But it remains at the mercy of social change.

The permanent basis of medicine is not its research, but its social application—its practice. That has persisted in every age; it will endure in spite of our neglect of it. It can and will rise up to great importance if our public is taught to respect it.

In looking toward shaping public opinion we see today a situation such as has never existed before. We have a tremendous literate but uneducated public bound together by the marvels of modern communication—the radio and the printed page. The means for shaping public opinion exist as they have never existed before. The consequences are, at one and the same time, enormous dangers and enormous possibilities for doing good. The good or bad will depend upon the leadership and the ideas and ideals of the propagandists in medicine.

This field of propaganda is one in which I have been particularly interested for the last ten or twelve years. And here again as in the matters about which I have been talking I have definite ideas which are contrary to many of the present tendencies. These ideas are based on the belief that I have reiterated here, that the regard in which the physician is held is engendered in emotion—not in reason. The general tendency in medical propaganda by the physician and his organized groups is to tell of the glories of medical research—the new discoveries in medicine—to tell of medical knowledge. Years ago the physician carefully hid his knowledge from the public—made a mystery of his arcanas—wrote his prescriptions in Latin. He surrounded his calling with a glamor. Then there came a change, a reaction. The physician put aside the mystery. The measures of public sanitation could be put into effect only by the intelligent aid of the public, particularly in passing laws. He had no secrets left from the public—and he shouldn't have. But he went even further—he not only let the bars down, he let his hair down as well, and began in his new and rigorous scientific attitude to debunk the art of his own calling, to divest it of all its appealing emotional qualities. Instead of shaping public opinion he attempted to give the public medical information. Medical discoveries have become news, news about which lay writers express opinions, news which the public discusses from the factual point of view critically. It is a case of the dangers of a little knowledge. Far too often the propaganda lacks the one thing that propaganda should have and that is the cultivation of a public regard of the physician and of his calling—a regard that makes him something more than a scientist in search of novelty—that gives a veneration that the physician deserves and must have if he is to guide the American people.

My talk tonight is rambling in spots; it lacks the vigor and directness of the legal brief. It does so because these are things over which I am emotionally aroused. To my mind what I have been discussing is the decline of American medicine. On one side is research commanding public veneration; on the other is medical practice, a fair target, unprotected by public regard from the economic experimenter, the sociological reformer and the political opportunist. What I ask is not any decrease in medical research, indeed every increase, but that medical research and medical practice be recognized as distinct but equally important, equally skilled, equally valuable parts of medicine as a whole. I ask that we may recognize that a physician may be a great doctor without doing original and basic laboratory investigations; that such research belongs to the research investigator and practice to the practitioner. And most of all I hope that we will go back to training our medical students clinically by great clinicians to be great clinicians.

MEDICINE AND THE LAW*

THE HONORABLE JOHN M. GALLAGHER

Chief Justice of the Supreme Court of Minnesota

Waseca, Minnesota

THE privilege of addressing this distinguished gathering is one that any citizen would welcome. It is one that any member of the bench or bar should appreciate. It affords the opportunity of exchanging views with the members of a great profession upon questions concerning which you, as members of the medical profession, and I, as a member of the legal profession, are similarly interested.

We speak of law and medicine as learned professions. We have learned lawyers and learned physicians of whom we are justly proud. Law and medicine are professions, which mean the common obligation of work to be done under the domination of the idea of excellence. The financial reward, if any, acceptable as it may be, is not the dominating idea. Law and medicine alike lure us on with those ideals of excellence, that we may well give them the best that any man can give.

Fate seems to have thrown the professions of law and medicine into fruitful contact, almost since their very beginning. The contact arises from the fact that both deal with the ills of human beings. And while the art of science of medicine is the older and has existed ever since organized society came into being, law, as a form of social control, has affected medicine.

In the modern legal world, the contact between law and medicine is greater, because of the limitations imposed by society, through law, upon the exercise of the profession, the manner of its exercise, and the use which law makes of medicine in the solution of some of its problems.

A trite definition of the physician or surgeon states "that he is one who is experienced in the art of healing or curing the disorders of the human body."

We need not discuss the historical development of the medical profession, or the constant broadening of social control over it. The profession itself has been chiefly instrumental in securing, in its own interest, and in that of hu-

manity, the strictest regulations. It aims to weed out charlatanism and quackery. From the earliest times, courts have upheld the right of society, through its legislative bodies, to regulate the practice of medicine and surgery. These regulations have had as their chief aim the protection of public health—which is always a matter of social concern. The methods of achieving this, which courts have upheld, have dealt with educational requirements and standards, aiming to establish a minimum standard of skill and learning, as a prerequisite to the exercise of the science or art of healing.

The Court of this state, as early as 1889 (State vs. Fleischer, 41 Minn. 69), held constitutional an act passed by the 1887 Legislature regulating the practice of medicine, the licensing of physicians and surgeons and providing punishment for violations of the act. Holding the law constitutional, Justice Collins speaking for the court said:

"From the spirit and object of the act, plainly seen in its several sections, it is obvious that the lawmakers intended to establish a high standard of qualification and fitness for the medical profession, whereby the people might be protected from ignorance and quackery."

Later in State vs. Broden (181 Minn. 341, decided Oct. 10, 1930), the Supreme Court of this state held that the basic science act is not violative of any constitutional provision, either state or federal. Only recently in State v. Mielke, (277 N. W. 420, decided Feb. 4, 1938), the court sustained an information against a person who was endeavoring to circumvent the provisions of the basic science act by means of advertising and other quackery holding that the practice resorted to was a violation of the law.

Generally, the law has protected the public by holding the practitioner to a high degree of professional and ethical responsibility. This applies to the practice of medicine, or any of the other schools of healing, whose graduates are entitled to the license of physician and surgeon.

The law provides that the medical board may

*Read at the annual meeting of the Minnesota State Medical Association, Duluth, Minnesota, July 1, 1938.

refuse to grant a license to or may revoke the license of any person guilty of "immoral, dishonorable, or unprofessional conduct" but subject to the right of the applicant to appeal to the court on questions of law and fact. The words "immoral, dishonorable, or unprofessional conduct" are defined in the act to mean:

    (a) Procuring, aiding or abetting a criminal abortion,

    (b) Advertising in any manner either in his own name or under the name of another person or concern, actual or pretended, professional superiority to or greater skill than that possessed by fellow physicians or surgeons . . . ,

    (c) The obtaining of any fee or offering to accept a fee on the assurance or promise that a manifestly incurable disease can be or will be cured,

    (d) Wilfully betraying a professional secret,

    (e) Habitual indulgence in the use of drugs,

    (f) Conviction for wilfully violating any narcotic law,

    (g) Conviction of offense involving moral turpitude,

    (h) Conviction of a felony.

It is evident, therefore, that while the standard of ethical conduct is high, it is not rigorous or unfair. Certainly no layman would want to trust a healer who did any of the acts denounced by the statute. It is also fair in allowing the courts to review the acts of the Board of Examiners, who, after a hearing, have deprived a physician of his right to practice. In reviewing the evidence presented before the board, the courts adopt the principle which applies to all bodies exercising quasi-judicial functions. Their findings will be upheld if there is any substantial evidence to support them. When there is conflict of evidence, the courts will not endeavor to resolve the conflict in a manner different from that of the Board.

When the law steps in to hold the physician accountable, in damages, for negligent acts in the exercise of his profession, it is also fair. It requires no impossibilities. It does not even require an abstract standard of skill. It requires a skill limited in time, and in character. Briefly stated, the fundamental principles governing liability for negligent acts on the part of the physician or surgeon are as follows: The physician is not a guarantor or insurer of cure. By accepting employment, he merely undertakes to use the average skill of other physicians in the same or similar localities. A mistaken diagnosis

does not constitute malpractice, in the absence of negligence.

The following quotation from a case recently decided by the Supreme Court (Yates v. Gamble, 198 Minn. 7) is a good summary of the law on the subject:

"A physician and a surgeon is not an insurer of a cure or a good result of his treatment or operation. He is only required to possess the skill and learning possessed by the average member of his school of the profession in good standing in his locality, and to apply that skill and learning with due care."

This summary indicates that in modern times, the law takes a reasonable attitude towards the practitioner of the healing act. It does not punish him for failure to cure, in the absence of negligence. The law has not always been so charitable. The oldest code of the world, the Code of Hammurabi of Babylon (dating from 2250 B. C.) while doing nicely by the physician by regulating his fees, punished him severely for his failures. Here are some of the provisions of that famous code, taken from a new translation (J. M. Powis Smith: The Origin and History of Hebrew Law, pp. 211-212):

"215 If a physician makes a deep incision upon a man (i.e., perform a major operation) with his bronze lancet and save the man's life: or if he operate on the eye socket of a man with his bronze lancet and save that man's eye, he shall receive ten sheckles of silver.

"216 If it were a common man, he shall receive five sheckels.

"217 If it were a man's slave, the owner of the slave shall give two sheckels of silver to the physician.

"218 If a physician make a deep incision upon a man with his bronze lancet and cause the man's death, or operate on the eye socket of a man with his bronze lancet and destroy the man's eye, they shall cut off his hand.

"219 If a physician make a deep incision upon the slave of a common man with his bronze lancet and cause his death, he shall substitute a slave of equal value."

The physician is a valuable man to the court. This fact was recognized early in our jurisprudence. Physicians like to quote the following statement made by Mr. Justice Saunders in an English case in 1553, justifying the employment of a medical expert:

"If matters arise in our law which concern other sciences, we commonly apply for the aid of that science which is concerned therein, which is an honor rable and commendable thing in our law, for thereby t appears that we do not despise all other sciences han our own but we approve them and encourage hem as things worthy of commendation."

Thus the help of the physician has always been 'elcome in courts. That prejudice has arisen gainst the testimony of the physician, when he ppears as an expert, is common knowledge. I ʰink the prejudice may be traced to the great ivergence between the opinions of experts in ental diseases. They occur in important will ises, and in criminal cases—under the plea of sanity. The difficulty in criminal cases is often aceable to the difference between legal and edical concepts of insanity. In law, insanity ʰplies inability to recognize the wrongfulness ' an act. Our concept is based upon outmoded ental science or psychology. And when the hysician and the lawyer speak of insanity they o not speak of the same thing. With the phy-ician and psychologist, mental derangement may e entirely unconnected with any doctrine of re-ponsibility. Moreover, according to the tenets f modern psychology, an ability to distinguish etween the rightfulness and wrongfulness of an ct, does not necessarily imply either wilfulness r responsibility. The psychopathic personality, which expresses itself in criminality, is the very embodiment of irresponsibility to the physician. And yet, in law, we hold him responsible.

I believe that in a great majority of cases dif-ference of opinion between medical men arise for the same reason that differences arise be-tween other experts. Lawyers are proverbially in disagreement, not only as to the meaning of decisions, and such differences are easily explain-able when we consider how laws are enacted, en-forced and interpreted. A legislature composed ɔf two branches and consisting of men gathered

from every nook and corner of the state as-semble every two years for the purpose of en-acting new laws, repealing old ones and amend-ing others. It is not strange that errors and in-consistencies occur. The drafters have different political, economic and social views. Occasion-ally, a joker goes in. Is it a wonder that con-fusion and uncertainty exists? Is it a wonder that errors are made? To me the only wonder is that more errors are not made, that greater inconsistencies do not result.

Some of these laws eventually reach the courts for interpretation. The courts are as a rule made up of men of different political, economic and social views. They are even composed of a varied degree of ability and intelligence. It is only natural therefore, if they are honest, that they should sometimes disagree as to interpre-tation. And, fortunately, under our system of government each has a right to express his views as to such interpretation.

I hope that the time may come in this state when medical experts may become "arms of the court" rather than "aids to partisans." That is partially possible now under our compensation law. And still in such cases the expert must testify with full knowledge that his compensation must eventually come from the coffers of the employer.

Law both through legislation and court inter-pretation will continue to coöperate with the physician, as it has done in the past, to help him to carry on his noble calling. It will call upon him for aid when necessary and will aid him when occasion calls. Each profession needs the other. The public needs both. Each should, and, I am sure, will, in the future as in the past, aid the other.

PROFESSIONAL CO-OPERATION IN THE PUBLIC INTEREST*

STANLEY B. HOUCK†

Minneapolis, Minnesota

I HAVE been wondering why my talk to you has been placed between that of the Chief Justice of Minnesota and that of my very good friend, the president of your Association. I am not entirely clear whether I am intended to be the valley between the hills or the heights between the valleys.

I am especially pleased to be here this morning and to have an opportunity to speak to you. Before I say anything else I want to express the pleasure I have had during the past year, as a member of a committee of the Minnesota State Bar Association, in working with your Committee on Coöperation with the Bar, of which Dr. Branton of Willmar is chairman. These two committees of the Bar and of your Association have not only had a most delightful series of personal contacts and conferences but have laid the foundation and done much of the spade work for a more healthy relationship between the two associations and for a better regard by each profession for its obligation to the public and for the basic public interest. The work of these two committees is just begun. I do not know what you have done to continue your committee for another year. I hope you have made the necessary arrangements to do so.

I like to think of the medical and legal professions as representative of the highest possible type of professional existence. Each is, I am confident, freer from the taint of commercialism than any of the other so-called professions. In saying this I am not disparaging other professions, since they are usually by the very nature of things more intimately and inherently associated with commercial undertakings. The relationship of the medical and of the legal profession to the public is usually a more directly personal relationship than can be true of the other professions. This is true of the medical profession even more than it is of the legal profession. You deal only with persons and their ailments. The legal profession deals also with the problems and difficulties of natural persons but in

addition deals with those of artificial persons such as partnerships, associations and corporations.

What the courts have said regarding the basic characteristics of the legal profession is likewise true in most respects of the medical profession.

The Supreme Court of Washington has said:

"The practice of the law is a personal right, and, that the public may not be imposed upon by the unworthy, the law requires that those engaged in practice shall be men of good moral character and with certain qualifications and a degree of learning to be ascertained by the agents, not of the courts, but of the whole people speaking through the legislative body. The right to practice law attaches to the individual and dies with him. It cannot be made the subject of business to be sheltered under the cloak of a corporation having marketable shares descendible under the laws of inheritance. One engaged in the practice of the law is subject to personal discipline for misconduct and to penalties for violating the ethics of the profession that could not possibly attach to a corporate body."

Justice Cardozo of the U. S. Supreme Court, when he was a member of the highest court of New York, said:

"Membership in the bar is a privilege burdened with conditions. The appellant was received into that ancient fellowship for something more than private gain. He became an officer of the court, and, like the court itself, an instrument or agency to advance the ends of justice. His coöperation with the court was due, whenever justice would be imperiled if coöperation was withheld."

From this, the conclusion is inescapable that our professional existence depends upon the public need. The license given us to practice our professions is not given to confer an advantage upon us as individual members thereof but to afford to the public whom we serve a necessary protection from exploitation and other abuses. The requirements of education and character are similarly imposed. They become more exacting as the public need for greater knowledge, greater training and greater skill develops.

I may summarize the fundamentals of our professions by saying that the prerequisites to a license to practice law or medicine are those

*Address given at the annual meeting of the Minnesota State Medical Association, Duluth, Minnesota, July 1, 1938.
†Chairman of the Committee on Unauthorized Practices of the Law of the American Bar Association.

680

MINNESOTA MEDICINE

things which the public conceives to be necessary from time to time for its protection. The problem which confronts the members of each of our professions is how to so conduct ourselves in our professional relations that we shall supply what the public needs and demands without allowing such evils to arise as will cause the public to relax and liberalize its requirements preliminary and prerequisite to license to practice.

There is, of course, a distinction between the place of the legal profession and that of the medical profession in relation to the processes of government.

The principal, the effective distinction, between a lawyer and all others, whatever their walk in life, lies in the lawyer's relationship to the judicial department of our government and is largely a matter of his morals and character and his special education and training in the field of the law and his resulting knowledge of the rules of law, the principles of justice and the means and manner of their suitable administration. To round out the difference, the lawyer is an officer of the court and a direct agency and instrumentality—an integral part—of the judicial department. There is imposed upon the lawyer certain inescapable duties and obligations not placed upon anyone else, in respect of his every act and conduct, whether it affects himself, his client, the general public, or the court.

I pause, to digress momentarily. I hope you will not think, because of what I have just said, that each of you, as members of the medical profession, has no public duty to perform in respect of the administration of justice. The original basic obligation to do justice rests upon each of us without regard to the existence of courts or what it may be their province to do. It rests in the first instance upon each of you in the conduct of your profession and upon every other business and professional man. If all of us in our contacts and transactions with those with whom we deal did mere justice, as we are so obligated and in duty bound to do, there never would arise the occasion to apply to the courts for their aid to see that there is done the justice we have failed to do.

You are not a public agency, nor a part of any of the divisions or the departments of our local or national governments. You are not an instrumentality concerned with the administration

of justice; nor licensed to practice law as an officer of any courts.

However, to an increasing degree, especially of late, members of the medical profession are coming more directly into contact with the processes of justice. The more intelligent administration of the criminal laws is making more frequent and continuing demands upon the medical profession for a saner determination and appraisal of the causes and degrees of criminal culpability and the suitability of the punishments and restraints about to be imposed or released. The astounding increase in personal injury litigation has made similar rapidly expanding demands in the field of civil litigation.

As the lawyer functions as a part of the judicial machine and as an aid to the court and to the public in the administration of justice, so does the doctor contribute to the doing of justice by the character of testimony and other forms of evidence he presents both before courts and before our administrative tribunals such as Workmen's Compensation Commissions.

As I have said, there is a basic duty on the part of each citizen to do justice. That duty, obviously, is not less in the case of members of either of our professions than in the case of the ordinary citizen. It can only be a greater obligation imposed because of our professional status. This imposes an added responsibility for seeing that the processes of justice, so far as we have anything to do with them, are not distorted, exploited or turned to the public injury or disadvantage.

Because members of the legal and medical professions are having more frequent dealings with each other in matters legal in character, the two professions inevitably must concern themselves more seriously with the problems arising therefrom.

The lawyer for the plaintiff and the lawyer for the defendant each turns to a doctor for testimony. With the plaintiff attempting to establish one state of facts and the defendant to prevent the establishment thereof, or to establish a different state of facts, a situation exists which provides fertile ground for serious abuses and presents problems calling for action not only by the individual members of the two professions but for the coöperative attention of both professional groups.

Probably the most common problem which

arises is the all too prevalent alliance between attorney and doctor. A continuing relationship —sometimes almost in the nature of a partnership or joint adventure—between lawyers who usually serve the plaintiff and a doctor who usually testifies on behalf of the plaintiff represented by the particular lawyer, cannot be viewed with equanimity by either profession. Nor, of course, is the relationship between the lawyer for the defendant and the doctor ordinarily and customarily appearing as a witness on behalf of the defendant in any better case. There are many abuses in this relationship. Certain attorneys almost invariably send all of their clients to certain doctors for treatment, for observation, all in anticipation of litigation and testimony. Attorneys for defendants do substantially the same thing.

It seems unnecessary to state that doctors employed under such circumstances are confronted with conditions not favorable to proper and ethical conduct either as doctors or as witnesses. If we add another factor and let the doctor's compensation be contingent or its amount depend upon the outcome of the case we have cause for the gravest concern.

Not only do lawyers send their clients to particular doctors but frequently the process is reversed and doctors urge their patients to go to particular lawyers for the purpose of collecting damages for physical injury. Sometimes doctors indicate that only thereby will they collect their bills.

In addition are the various forms of misconduct and abuse of the public of which individual members of each profession are guilty. Just as there are many lawyers who are known as "plaintiffs' lawyers" and "defendants' lawyers" so there are doctors who are generally known in the community as those from whom can be obtained testimony most appropriate to the plaintiff's case or most appropriate to the defendant's case. The eradication of such individuals from both professions is an obligation of each profession which calls for prompt action.

Nothing can be more serious in its effect upon the public than to have witnesses, and especially expert medical witnesses, participating in the "build-up" of a case, and interested in the amount recovered either because of participation in its planning or because their compensation depends upon a successful outcome.

The responsibility for such things can not be assigned alone to the individual. They can not be passed off by a shrug of the profession's shoulders and an attitude of indifference.

Both professions have imposed upon them the obligation to treat in confidence all communications from the patient or the client which are necessary to enable the member of the profession to deal with or treat the particular case. These are called, in the law, privileged communications. The reason for the obligation is known to all members of both professions. It is, of course, imposed solely in the public interest and to enable the better treatment of medical cases and the more certain assurance that justice will ultimately be done.

The development of medical science and the great changes which have occurred within recent years in the making of medical records and the use of hospitals as a part of medical treatment have resulted in substantial disregard of the patient's right to have his necessary communications kept scrupulously privileged.

There is the problem of the extent to which the privilege extends to hospital records. The position of the interne and the nurse in respect of these communications may be doubtful unless it can be said that they are at all times the representatives, the *alter ego*, of the doctor himself. Even then this does not cover all situations.

In the public interest the medical profession must concern itself at once with the protection of the privileged communications of patients. Doctors must themselves be more discreet and circumspect. They must either refrain entirely from communicating such disclosures to their representatives or must find some means of controlling these representatives so as to prevent disclosure thereof by them. Since hospital records are at least in an uncertain zone and are sometimes brought into court, practically as a public record, the profession must give consideration to the extent to which privileged matters may appropriately be entered upon those records. I have had clients tell me that because confidential and privileged matters communicated to doctors apparently become public property very speedily and very readily, they have felt compelled to go to a remote city for medical and surgical attention. Whether or not this be an exaggeration, it is not in the public interest that such a condition be allowed either to grow up to any extent or to continue.

Perhaps the most delicate of all of these subjects is the malpractice case. I have heard doctors say that at least 95 per cent of these cases are "frame-ups." I know very well the attitude of the members of the medical profession toward this type of action. I can sympathize wholeheartedly with that attitude. You need not tell me the reprehensible part that all too many lawyers have had in these cases. Here again is a problem concerning both professions. The legal profession must do what it can to prevent lawyers from seeking out, "building up," or exaggerating cases of this nature against doctors. But when a meritorious malpractice case exists, the plaintiff is entitled to the testimony necessary to the presentation of his case conformable to the processes of justice. The abuse which exists today may be more imaginary than real. I hope it is; but I am constrained to say that, rightly or wrongly, there prevails, both in the legal profession and in the minds of the public generally, the belief that one doctor will not testify in a malpractice case against another, regardless of the facts. If this be true, and I know it is true to some extent, there has been created a condition which the legal profession and the public must take prompt means to correct. However unjustly individual doctors may be treated when made defendants in malpractice cases, the answer is not a concerted effort on the part of the medical profession to suppress evidence and to interfere with and obstruct the administration of justice. Nor, in the public interest, can it be the province of a committee of the medical profession to review and pass upon such cases and determine whether they "should be settled" or tried. Together with the feeling to which I have already adverted, is the further belief that even in meritorious malpractice cases the medical profession has combined and conspired and united to force settlements on its own terms with the express or implied threat that unless such settlement is made no doctor will testify in favor of the injured person.

From what I have said it is apparent that there is much for each profession to do within its own ranks and much for both professions to do working together, coördinating their efforts and coöperating for the incidental benefit of each and both professions but with the primary objective of serving the public.

Abuses, such as I have referred to, do exist. They do not exist to anything like the extent believed by the public. The danger is not lessened in any way by the fact that the public believes it has been injured to a degree which has been greatly exaggerated. As I said at the outset, the excuse for our existence as professions is the public belief that it is necessary for us to exist in the manner in which we now exist in order that the public interest be thereby better served. Just as soon as we fail to accomplish the purpose and objective set for us by the public, or, what is more important, just as soon as the public thinks and believes either warrantably or not that either profession is not attaining the goal prescribed for it, there will be further attacks such as those to which each profession is now being subjected and these attacks, unless steps are taken to correct the public impression causing them, will result in measures which will seriously restrict and limit each profession.

I can not be too emphatic in saying that each profession must see to it that its individual members place the public welfare and the public interest above personal individual advantage and gain. I am not speaking idealistically. I am stating blunt facts. The public will not be idealistic about the matter. It will demand that the individuals making up each profession so conduct themselves as to serve the public interest and, if they do not, they will probably ruthlessly, recklessly, and perhaps unwisely, sweep the boards clear of everything characteristic of our present day professions and substitute something in their place which will not at all be to our liking.

HERMAN M. JOHNSON*

Past and Present Medical Problems

THE HONORABLE ELMER A. BENSON

Governor of the State of Minnesota

Saint Paul, Minnesota

Introduction

J. M. HAYES, M.D., President, Minnesota State Medical Association: Members of the State Medical Association, honored guests, ladies and gentlemen.

We are assembled here in this large dining room of the Hotel Duluth at the largest luncheon meeting in the history of the organization to do honor to the name of our departed friend and servant, Dr. Herman M. Johnson.

To me one of the most important duties of any organization is the commemoration of the names of those who were the most important factors in the success of that organization.

No man ever made greater personal sacrifices for any organization[1] than did Doctor Johnson for this one.

Not only did he make great personal sacrifices, but no man ever had a keener, clearer and more plausible insight into future medical policy than did this same Doctor Johnson.

One of the most remarkable traits of this man in all his work was that no one could ever, justly, accuse him of promoting any selfish interests. Everything he did was in the interest of the people and the profession.

By doing honor to such a man we are doing honor to the association, and to the profession. Honoring such men should inspire younger men, at least to some degree, to attempt to follow in his footsteps.

Those who did not have the good fortune to be brought into close contact with Herman or closely associated with him in his work, will never realize or appreciate the value of his work to this association.

Fortunately, his Honor, the Governor, was a friend of Dr. Herman Johnson and quite closely associated with him in his work for many years. This association, I believe, has been a benefit to the medical profession. This association, I believe, at least to some degree, has taught the governor that the practice of medicine cannot, in justice to all, be made a political football. This profession knows no political bounds.

I am pleased to say that my experience has taught me that the Governor knows and recognizes the fact that the practice of medicine must be controlled and administered by the practicing physician.

It is my pleasure to present, now, his Honor, the Governor, who will give the first memorial lecture in honor of our departed friend and servant, Dr. Herman M. Johnson.

His Honor, the Governor of Minnesota.

*First address given under the Herman M. Johnson Lectureship at the annual meeting of the Minnesota State Medical Association, Duluth, Minnesota, July 1, 1938.

Address

THIS gathering today is a memorial to the late Dr. Herman M. Johnson, of Dawson, Minnesota. Two years ago, his sudden and unexpected death brought forth, from people throughout our state and nation, expressions of regret at his passing and praise for his work and memory.

One of his life-long friends, former Governor and Congressman Theodore Christianson, paid him a personal tribute from which I quote the following:

"He was the very soul of honor. . . . He was direct, outspoken, sincere. If he ever lacked in tact, it was because he was so honest that he preferred to tell the truth even when it hurt, rather than to keep silent and have his own conscience accuse him of insincerity.

"He had keen perception, and an analytical mind. The ability to note symptoms and diagnose causes, to trace effects to their source, which made his professional career notable . . . he carried into fields outside that of medicine. Ofttimes I have been with him when as with a surgeon's skill, he dissected the social body and probed for the causes of its ailments. When so engaged, he showed that mingling of courage and caution that characterizes the true scientist. . . ."

In this tribute by Theodore Christianson, I concur with all my heart; for, like many of you who are here today, I had the good fortune to know Doctor Johnson personally.

Soon after Doctor Johnson's death, the House of Delegates of the Minnesota State Medical Association, adopted a resolution declaring their grateful remembrance of his aid to their organization and their profession. "We can, but hope," they said, "that the memory of him which is ours, and his spirit which abides, will carry us all on to higher and greater achievements."

In that spirit, his friends created a trust fund to perpetuate his work and memory. One means of doing so will be these annual Herman M. Johnson Memorial Lectures, of which my address today is the first.

I think it is extremely important to bear in mind that when we commemorate significant work and noble men of the past, we do not have our eyes only upon the past; we have them also upon the present and the future.

A famous British scholar and scientist once pointed out that the present'is, after all, merely the shifting point at which the past and future meet. We can have no quarrel with either the past or the future, he said. "There can be no world without traditions; neither can there be any life without movement. . . . There is never a moment when the new dawn is not breaking over the earth, and never a moment when the sunset ceases to die. It is well to greet serenely even the first glimmer of the dawn when we see it, not hastening towards it with undue speed, nor leaving the sunset without gratitude for the dying light that once was dawn."

In that spirit, we seek to perpetuate the memory and work of the late Dr. Herman M. Johnson. We do not want to forget his achievements; we want to look back upon them, and remember them with gratitude. At the same time, we do not wish to rest merely in the memory of such achievements; rather, we seek to take from them fresh inspiration to press forward to meet the challenging new problems of the future into which we are now entering. We seek to make the present not merely the twilight of a fortunate past, but also the dawn of a hopeful future.

Notable Achievements

In that spirit, we turn our eyes backward today for a few moments, to examine the notable and exceptional achievements of Dr. Herman Johnson.

Part of Doctor Johnson's distinction is the realism with which he adjusted himself to the special conditions of the period in which he lived.

He was born in the eighteen seventies. Up until then, changes in our economic and social conditions had taken place so slowly, that one could reasonably assume a man's children would live under conditions about like those under which he himself had lived. Since the eighteen seventies, however, owing largely to discovery and invention, change has taken place so rapidly that the very face of society has altered from one generation to the next.

Doctor Johnson began life in a pioneer community in Ottertail county, into which his parents had traveled in ox wagons from Wisconsin,

about the time of the Civil War. As a child, he heard from the lips of his father many interesting stories of the first settlers in that region. When he himself began to practice medicine in western Minnesota, in the opening years of the twentieth century, rural calls were made with a horse and buggy. Between then, and the year when he died, nineteen thirty-five, there occurred sweeping changes in human knowledge, in the organization of human society, and in the problems confronting members of the medical profession.

Dr. Hugh Cabot, of the Mayo Clinic in Rochester, is authority for the statement that during the past forty years the development of scientific knowledge has given us more new knowledge, some of which is applicable to the treatment of disease, than the whole previous period of recorded history put together. The accumulation of scientific fact in that period, he declares, is so extensive as to stagger the imagination. As a result, during the past thirty-five or forty years, adjustments between professional activities, such as the practice of medicine, and current social and economic conditions have had to be made with a frequency and constancy which have challenged the caliber of men in the professions.

Doctor Johnson met that challenge. The record shows that he kept constantly abreast of the rapidly developing needs and opportunities of the medical profession during his lifetime.

Thus, one of the needs of Minnesota was a well organized and effective state-wide association of physicians and surgeons. Only by means of such an organization could the medical men of this state direct their influence fully toward developing programs of public health and promoting high professional standards in a highly complex society which was daily changing and becoming more complex.

Formerly, the Minnesota State Medical Association was only a loosely linked collection of county scientific societies. It exercised little influence in legislative councils. It assumed little responsibility for leadership in the protection of public health. Today, however, this association is generally spoken of by men in the medical profession as one of the best organized and most efficient medical societies in the United States. A great deal of the credit for this achievement belongs to the wisdom and ability which Dr. Herman Johnson exercised in aiding that organization by his services, his contributions, and his counsel.

Outstanding Service

When the state medical association elected him president in nineteen twenty-six, they were indeed paying recognition to his medical scholarship and his skill as a physician and surgeon; but they were also honoring him for his faithful and important work, over a period of years, in behalf of the state medical association and the profession as a whole.

Doctor Johnson's outstanding service in that capacity was rendered as chairman of the Minnesota State Medical Association's committee on public policy and legislation.

In that position, he gave every effort to securing adequate appropriations for the equipment and maintenance of a first-class medical school at the University of Minnesota, which would meet the new needs for longer and more specialized training, and for wider and more extensive scientific research.

He gave every effort to securing adequate appropriations for our State Board of Health, whose record of achievement in public health programs is envied in many states of the union.

For the Public Welfare

He took part in achieving Minnesota's outstanding piece of medical legislation, namely, the Basic Science Law, enacted in nineteen twenty-seven, and generally regarded as a model of basic science legislation.

To Doctor Johnson, perhaps more than to any other person, should go credit for making the Minnesota State Board of Medical Examiners a self-supporting body.

Furthermore, he worked to have the Medical Act amended, so that when vacancies occurred on this Board, recommendations for filling them should be made to the governor by the Council of the Minnesota State Medical Association. He believed that recommendations made by organized medicine would be helpful to the governor in making these appointments. Here today, I have the privilege and honor of publicly acknowledging that we have kept faith with Doctor Johnson in this matter. The two most recent appointments to the State Board of Medical Examiners have been made in accordance with the recommendations of the Council of the

State Medical Association, as he hoped they would be.

One of Doctor Johnson's most important and humane contributions to the people of this state was the coöperation he rendered, in nineteen thirty-four, when the state emergency relief administration was being set up. He spent many days conferring with relief administrators, and helping to organize the work, in an effort to insure that those who were unfortunate enough to be out of work and in need of relief would be able to secure the services of their own family physician when needed.

These achievements which I have been enumerating, are only a fragment of the long role of Doctor Johnson's public services.

They were prompted by his recognition of the fact that the medical profession, like all other human occupations, must constantly readjust its practices and organization to meet the intricate needs of today's complex conditions of life.

They were prompted by the social idealism which causes men like Doctor Johnson to labor wholeheartedly and with unfailing optimism for the achievement of the highest excellence in human skill, in human character, and in the organization of human activities.

They were prompted by the true spirit of liberalism, which, possessed of abundant and realistic knowledge of the facts and a sense of social perspective, seeks to find creative, rather than repressive, measures for liberating men from the diseases and scourges which afflict them.

How the work and memory of this man may best be perpetuated lies, after all, in the hands of the medical profession of this state. Speaking as a layman, I venture to suggest that the best way to do so is to apply his combination of social vision and a practical spirit to the facts and issues of the present.

From that point of view, let me try to outline for you what seems to me the next great field for organized medicine to tackle in the spirit of the late Dr. Herman Johnson.

Progress in Public Health

The province of caring for human health covers two fields. One field, the field of general medicine, is concerned with restoring sick persons to health. The other field, the field of preventive medicine, is concerned with maintaining healthy conditions of living in our highly complex and artificial mode of living and working.

In this second field, the field of public health programs, the medical profession has been more than abreast of public demand. True, our programs of public health have not been entirely satisfactory; they have been marked by confusion, overlapping, and inadequacy—especially in the rural sections. This condition, however, is chiefly the result of inadequate legislation and lack of public understanding. Scientists and physicians have done their part in seeking to rouse people to the importance of adequate legislation and appropriations to carry on programs to protect the public's health by promoting sanitary living conditions, by checking the interstate transmission of disease, by preventing the pollution of public streams which flow from one community to another, by officially inspecting foods and drugs, by warding off occupational diseases and the effects of overwork in today's factories and mines, and by the collection of uniform vital statistics. In all these matters, medical knowledge has usually preceded that of the laity.

As a result, the field of preventive medicine and public health is beginning to be conquered. There already exist in the federal government, for example, at least two dozen agencies concerning themselves with the problems of public health, such as the United States Public Health Service, the Children's Bureau, the Women's Bureau, and the Bureau of Chemistry.

The Next Great Field

In the other and older field of medicine, however—in the field of general medicine, concerned with restoring sick persons to health, the medical profession is falling behind the public demands of the moment. As everybody knows, this is not because of any lack of scientific knowledge, skill, or devotion to the highest professional standards. It is owing to the fact that the present organization of our medical services does not provide for the widest possible application of those services to all our people.

In the year that Doctor Johnson died, in 1935, the President's Committee on Economic Security reported that "nearly one-half of the individuals in the lowest income group receive no professional medical or dental attention of any kind." The Committee also reported that millions of American families live in dread of sickness be-

cause when illness strikes one of their members they are compelled to sacrifice other essentials of decent living, or go without needed medical care, or depend upon the charity services of doctors and hospitals. Such a condition leaves large sections of our population without adequate medical service, and at the same time fails to provide adequate employment for large numbers of potential physicians and nurses.

Now, you and I both agree that it would be wrong to lay the blame for this state of affairs upon the medical profession. If blame belongs anywhere, it is upon the economic arrangements of our society. The important thing, however, is not to blame anybody, but rather to recognize that the problem exists, and then to seek methods of coping with it.

How will the problem be solved? I, as a layman, can scarcely venture an answer to such a question. The answer must come from the medical profession itself. *I may say, however, that I do not believe our people favor a government-dominated medicine.* On the one hand, they hold the medical profession in great esteem, owing to its traditions of learning, skill, and personal integrity; on the other hand, they lack faith in the arbitrary centralization of power which they fear would come from government-dominated medicine. Furthermore, the medical profession itself would not tolerate such an approach to the question.

Medicine's Problem

Nevertheless, we must recognize that the problem of providing all our people with some semblance of equality of opportunity for adequate medical service is one of the insistent problems of our time. This first memorial lecture, in commemoration of Dr. Herman Johnson, is the most fitting occasion possible on which to draw clear-cut attention to this problem, whose solution is the next step in the advance of organized medicine.

We laymen have confidence that the profession which produces and pays tribute to men of the caliber of Doctor Johnson, has also in its ranks the social vision combined with the practical capacity to grapple with this problem, and work out a solution which will neither mar the integrity of the profession itself, nor leave the medical needs of our population unmet.

Surely the time is not far distant when our people may expect government to aid them in guaranteeing minimum standards of economic well-being, including medical attention of the kind they receive from the physician and surgeon whom they know and confide in. The people of this state would, I believe, be willing to consider favorably legislation designed toward this end, provided it came from the state medical association and represented their best judgment and matured experience. Such legislation would be one of the ways of keeping alive the memory and work of the late Dr. Herman Johnson. It would be evidence that his spirit abides, and is carrying us all on to higher and greater achievements. It would proclaim to all the world that we in Minnesota do not only rest in the twilight of a fortunate past, but also move forward serenely and without undue haste to greet the dawn of a more hopeful future.

FRACTURES—GENERAL PRINCIPLES*

CLARENCE JACOBSON, M.D.

Chisholm, Minnesota

THE treatment of fractures has its origin in the Neolithic age. Specimens have been discovered in sufficient quantities to justify statistical statements. Karl Jaeger found 53.8 per cent of good unions as against 46.2 per cent bad unions in prehistoric fractures, indeed a credit to Neolithic intelligence. Immobilization was practiced in the 4th Dynasty, about 2500 B. C. by means of well padded palm branch splints. Hippocrates, 460-377 B.C., describes mechanical extension for fractures of the thigh and leg. He advised treating fractures of the jaw by binding the teeth together with gold or linen thread. Fundamental principles adhered to by the ancients are still in use and to a great extent form the basis of modern treatment.

The first consideration in the treatment of fractures is to save the patient's life. Treatment begins the moment he is touched at the scene of accident and not after the arrival at the hospital. Preparatory to transportation, the patient is kept warm, morphine administered if necessary to control pain. The application of the Thomas Splint in fracture of the long bones is often a life saving measure and should be done before the patient is lifted from the ground. If possible, traction thus maintained should be fixed throughout the remainder of the treatment. This procedure combats shock, prevents further serious injury at the site of fracture, and adds materially to the comfort of the patient during transportation. Many hospitals make it compulsory to transport acute fractures of the long bones with some form of traction. The use of the Thomas Splint during the World War reduced the mortality from 80 per cent in 1916 to 15.6 per cent in 1917 in compound fractures of the femur alone.

Patients with fractures of the spine should be gently rolled on to a blanket face down and lifted by means of the blanket onto the stretcher, and kept lying on the abdomen during transportation. Cervical spine fractures are best transported with some form of extension. In case of a suspected skull fracture the patient should receive no morphine and should be transported to the nearest hospital. If found in a home where favorable surroundings exist, transportation may well be postponed, a capable nurse secured to record the pulse, respiration, temperature and blood pressure. Emergency operative treatment in acute skull fractures should be limited to compound fractures, those showing marked depression of the skull, cases of extradural hemorrhage, and those exhibiting constant recurring convulsions.

Life is threatened in elderly patients who are suddenly compelled to lie in bed. Pneumonia and bed sores are often immediate complications. In the absence of shock it is imperative to free these people from pain and compel them to sit up. Recent fixation treatment with the Smith Peterson nail and other similar metal devices for fracture of the femoral neck have proven a boon to elderly people in whom these fractures so frequently occur.

Having assured ourselves that life is not in danger, our attention is centered on saving the injured part and to return in the shortest time the fullest capacity of function. Careful exam-

*Read before the Annual Meeting of the Minnesota State Medical Association, Duluth, Minnesota, June 30, 1938.

ination of the injured limb is important, taking note of contusions and skin abrasions, injuries to tendons, muscles, nerves and vessels. Musculospiral paralysis is often missed in fractures of the humerus on first examination because of the attention being centered on the fracture. Amputation other than for the purpose of saving life should be based upon the extent of gross injury to the tissues and the question of adequate blood supply to the distal part. A more conscientious appraisal of these aspects has led to fewer amputations in late years.

Physiological principles are concerned with the healing of bone as well as the restoration of the injured limb to normal function. Immediately following a break, an orderly process of repair is begun. An interlacing mesh of fibrin derived from the blood clot, lymph and inflammatory exudate begins to bind the bone and adjacent lacerated tissues together. Within a few hours fibroblasts appear in the fibrin clot and granulation tissue formation begins. Cells from the endosteum, marrow, reticulum and periosteum enter into this formation as well. Organization takes place within forty-two to ninety-six hours. The manner in which calcium is deposited is not understood other than it makes its appearance as early as seventy-two hours after fracture, being deposited in the granulating tissue. This constitutes what is known as early callus formation. Denser deposits gradually appear, the concentration becoming sufficient to cause hard bone formation. Subsequent use of the limb causes the return of the normal architecture of the bone. A year or more is required to complete the process.

Interference with this normal process results in non-union. Among the common causes are poor apposition of fragments, early massage and passive motion, interposition of tissue even though it be periosteum, infection, extensive damage to soft parts at the site of the break, and, for purpose of emphasis, manipulation of the slow healing fracture. Failure to note callus formation on the x-ray plate lead many to unnecessary manipulation. It should be remembered that firm union often takes place without visible evidence of callus on the x-ray plate. Non-union can often be prognosticated on a history of violent injury such as having a limb caught in revolving machinery carrying the body with it, or in an auto accident where the car

has turned several times with the occupant within. In these types the force producing the fracture has continued to act over a period of time. Cubbins states, "It is the continuation of force that has caused the interposition of tissue, that injures and destroys the periosteum, that causes its twisting and being torn to bits, as well as injury to the blood supply of the bones and adjacent tissues."

Principles governing the treatment of fractures are concerned with the best means of obtaining union in good functional position. Proper reduction is first to be desired. Perfect anatomical reduction should be attempted, but not at the expense of destroying possibilities of good function. Boehler, known for his exacting procedures, often allows up to one centimeter overlapping of fragments providing the alignment is correct. Actual lengthening of the lower limb has been noted by Magnusson and others after two years in femur fractures in children where no shortening was demonstrated at the time of discharge. The methods of reduction are many. Traction, manipulation and open operation are fundamentally the only three. Boehler states that every fracture should be reduced by traction and counter-traction. Manipulation, when used, should be reduced to the fewest number of movements and not over longer periods than absolutely necessary. Delayed healing and non-union may be attributed to this procedure. There is much wasteful controversy over the merits of the open and the closed method of treating acute fractures. Whichever method gives the best results in function in the individual surgeon's experience should be used. All are agreed that there are certain fractures where open operation is necessary for maximum restoration of function. These compose the fractures involving joints where fragments are in poor apposition, some of the fractures of the mid forearm involving both bones, fractures of the patella and olecranon process, in fractures where there is known to be interposition of tissue between the fragments and in instances where fragments are widely separated. The optimum results are obtained in open reduction when the cases are selected and operated upon immediately. Henderson advises not to limit its use to cases in which the closed method has failed. Often in cases seen late where the closed method would have been satisfactory, he chooses to use the open method. Skeletal traction by the use of Kirschner wire serves as an excellent method in obtaining proper reduction and in maintaining adequate retention. The Steinmann pin is likewise used. Some claim bone infection is more apt to take place when the latter is used. Boehler, however, blames infection upon the rotation of the pin within the bone, and has devised bearings on the tractors attached to the pin preventing it from rotating, and has had no further trouble. Maintaining reduction by means of a Steinmann pin incorporated within a cast as advocated by Roger Anderson has produced excellent results. Experience in this method and maintenance of aseptic surgical technic is imperative, not only in this method but in all methods involving entrance into bone with foreign material.

The means of retaining a properly reduced fracture is often the most difficult problem in fracture management. Fractures are maintained in their abnormal positions by muscle pull, gravity playing a part as well. When properly reduced anatomically and placed in a neutral position, the muscles of the limb resume a balanced pull and render a comparatively easy retention with the ends of the bones locked. Boehler has gone to great length in explaining the various neutral positions which must be maintained in proper retention. Thus, in fractures of the upper end of the humerus, the arm must be abducted 90 degrees, externally rotated 90 degrees and brought anteriorly 30 to 40 degrees. Correct alignment and anatomical apposition is thus attained. In fractures of the neck of the femur, we find that abduction with internal rotation produces the neutral position. In supracondylar fractures of the humerus, assuming the flexion and varus (adduction) position often interferes with the circulation and innervation to the forearm. Early recognition of vessel injury must be noted to prevent the dreaded Volkmann's ischemic paralysis. This was formerly thought to be due to tight dressings alone. We now know that blood from a severed or torn vessel has infiltrated the fascial planes which, not being elastic, causes enough tension to produce ischemia. The blood must be evacuated immediately. The radial pulse must return before the danger is passed. Boehler is not in accord with the usual practice of reducing and maintaining this fracture with the forearm in supi-

nation, for the simple reason that in so doing the pronator muscles, which are also flexors, being on the stretch, are in a state of spasm and tend to maintain adduction of the distal fragment causing impingement on the radial nerve. This is corrected by pronating the forearm, thereby bringing it into a relaxed position correcting the varus or adduction deformity. Being also flexors of the elbow joint, relaxation of the pronators brings about reduction of the flexion deformity. Retention is maintained by means of traction on an abduction splint in adults, either by plaster cast, aluminum or wire airoplane splints. The Jones sling and adhesive may suffice in children following satisfactory reduction. The same principle of neutral position with balance muscle pull holds for all fractures of long bones.

Operative retention by means of metal bone plates and screws may be necessary. The Lane technic must be strictly adhered to. Venable has shown that the metals commonly used are not suitable. When two different metals were used in plating a fracture, the difference in potential of these metals thus placed in the tissue acted like plates in a storage battery causing electrolysis to take place. Thus the screws were seen to loosen with consequent loss of retention. Certain alloys acted similarly. The best metal was found to be an alloy composed of cobalt, tungsten and chromium, called vitalium, which resists both electrolytic and chemical action of the body fluids.

Immobilization of the fracture is necessary until firm union takes place. This varies in individuals, and to a great extent in the type and location of the fracture. Firm union is best determined by the x-ray, although, as previously stated, union can take place without visible callus formation. The rule is, nevertheless, not to permit weight bearing or lifting without mature callus formation. Tenderness over the site of fracture means immature callus formation, and is, therefore, a warning to withhold use of the limb. Early removal of the cast for passive motion and massage is to be condemned. Non-union as well as myositis ossificans has resulted in these cases. Active motion is safer and is to be encouraged.

Restoration by functional treatment as advocated by Boehler is a distinct contribution to the industrial surgeon. He defines functional treatment as "the complete uninterrupted fixation of the fragments in good position with the simultaneous active movements of all the joints, or as many as possible, and with the avoidance of pain." In short, this means immobilization with a cast placed upon the unshaven skin of an extremity and immediate use of the limb. A metal heel is incorporated in the cast in fractures òf the lower extremities, and the patient made to walk as soon as the plaster-of-Paris is hardened. Circulation is thus made more active, atrophy of bone is avoided and the joints return to full function in a much shorter time. Fixation can thus be prolonged with safety. Compression fractures of dorsal and lumbar vertebræ are immediately reduced, guided by x-ray films and retained in a body cast, pressure being applied to three points, the upper portion of the sternum, pubic bone and at the site of fracture on the spine, thus maintaining the spine in lordosis. Patients without paralysis are encouraged to be up in twenty-four to thirty-six hours and are given weights to carry on their heads and such exercises as are necessary to keep up good muscle tone. Caution should be undoubtedly exercised in immediately adopting all these methods. We have had occasion to use this form of treatment in a sufficient number of cases to justify our continuing doing so. Experience gradually acquired will undoubtedly reveal the fact that the principle is physiologically sound, and that the future will see wider adoption of this method of treatment.

Needless to say, the keeping of accurate records and progress notes is as important in proper fracture management as in any other field in medicine. Many an unjust lawsuit has been won because of the poor record submitted at court. Litigation must be kept in mind in every fracture case. Failure to produce x-ray films before and after reduction has led to the same sad end. Plates taken in anterior, posterior and lateral planes suffice for the majority of cases. Plates at various angles may be necessary before ruling out fracture in instances where it is strongly suspected. Follow-up plates are necessary and should be taken every eight days until firm union takes place.

The general principles applicable to the proper management of fractures have been briefly alluded to. The best results will be obtained if whatever method is being employed proves to be physiologically sound. Perfect anatomical result should not be at the expense of optimum

functional result. Most of the estimated 1,500,-000 fractures occurring yearly in the United States are first seen by the practitioner and general surgeon. Smaller communities are being better equipped to care for these emergencies. We find that adequate consultation in complicated cases is of great value, not only for self protection, but for the welfare of the patient and his continued coöperation through a trying period of convalescence.

Summary

1. Some of the fundamental principles of present-day fracture treatment were used in ancient times.

2. The first consideration in dealing with fractures is the saving of life. Treatment begins when the patient is first seen at the place of accident. Proper first aid is of paramount importance as a life saving measure.

3. The use of the Thomas splint affords the necessary traction for fractures of the long bones and should be used in the transportation of patients with fractures of the long bones.

4. Interference with the normal process of healing by unnecessary manipulation and by early massage and passive motion is the cause of non-union. Cases of myositis ossificans have been reported by Boehler as a result of these measures.

5. Reduction is best produced by traction against counter-traction.

6. Retention in the neutral position of balanced muscle pull is necessary.

7. Longer periods of immobilization are to be desired for better bony union. Keeping the fracture immobilized and at the same time keeping the muscles and uninvolved joints active will prevent bone atrophy, and shorten the period of disability.

8. Adequate fracture and follow-up records, as well as proper x-ray plates during the healing period, are important aids to both patient and surgeon.

Bibliography

1. Adams, Bertram S.: Notes taken at the Boehler Clinic, Vienna, Austria. February, 1938.
2. American College of Surgeons: General Principles. An Outline of Treatment of Fractures, 1938.
3. Clark, Arthur William: History of fracture treatment up to sixteenth century. Jour. Bone and Joint Surg., 19:47-63, (Jan.) 1937.
4. Cubbins, W. R., Callahan, J. J., Scuderi, C, S.: The causes of non-union bone growth and regeneration. Surg., Gyn. and Obst., 62:427-433, 1936.
5. Henderson, Melvin S.: Acute fractures. Surg., Gyn. and Obst., 60:535-539, 1935.
6. Kennedy, Robert Hayward: Our responsibility to the fracture patient. Bull. Am. Coll. Surg., 21:169-172, (Sept.) 1936.

7. Key, J. A., and Conwell, H. E.: The Management of Fractures, Dislocations, and Sprains. St. Louis: Mosby, 1934, Chap. 3.
8. Sinclair, Meurice: The Thomas splint and its modifications in the treatment of fractures. London, Oxford Univ. Pr., 1927.
9. Venable, C. S., Stuck, W. G., and Beach, Asa: The effects on bone of the presence of metals; based upon electrolysis. Ann. Surg., 105:917-938, (June) 1937.

Discussion

DR. E. E. CHRISTENSEN, Winona: Dr. Jacobson has presented a very comprehensive review of the general principles of fractures.

His statements relative to the values of the open and closed method, I believe, are very fair. The open method should not be reserved for only those cases in which reduction has been impossible after repeated manipulations, but rather a method of choice when the surgeon recognizes the fact that he has to deal with a particularly difficult reduction and when the proper facilities are at hand. The failure to recognize these cases often leads to repeated manipulations and consequent permanent damage to the tissues.

Skeletal traction when properly applied has been of untold value in the treatment of fractures. However, these cases must of necessity be watched very closely and checked repeatedly by x-ray studies to avoid an over-correction or the pulling apart of the bony fragments with a resulting delayed or non-union. I believe this is more apt to be true when the Roger Anderson method of fixed skeletal traction is used in fractures of the neck of the femur, or in fractures of the long bones where there has been fixation by pins according to the method of Boehler. Of course in the hands of these men the results obtained encourage the contention that their methods are the ones of choice. However, the average practitioner, with a limitation of experience and perhaps limited facilities, should proceed, I believe, along more conservative lines.

I would like to bring to mind the so-called compensatory fracture, the majority of which occur in the leg due to the powerful action of the leg muscles. Here we encounter a fracture of the lower end of the tibia and our attention is centered on this one area. Unless we keep in mind the possibility of a fracture of the upper third of the fibula we may often overlook this point. The same holds true of the bones of the forearm but to a lesser degree, due to the free rotation of the latter. This type of fracture was brought to my mind very forcibly about four months ago when I completely missed the fractured upper fibula. It was only because of repeated complaints on the part of the patient that I had further x-ray studies made on the third day, and you can imagine my embarrassment when the second fracture was found. It is true that in most fractures of this type the end-result would not be appreciably, if at all, effected, if the second fracture were missed, but it is because of the medicolegal angle that we must keep this in mind.

My experience in immobilizing fractures with a cast directly upon the unshaven skin has not been satisfactory. I have noted a much greater tendency toward development of areas of pressure necrosis with this method than when using sufficient padding, particularly over the bony protuberances.

In the past four years we, in our group, have treated with very good results a series of thirty-nine compression fractures of the spine. Following reduction and the application of a cast, those in which there was no evidence of paralysis were allowed to be up as soon as they were free of pain and abdominal distention. This usually took between one and three weeks, depending upon the severity of the fracture. Most authorities are agreed that this type of fracture should be in a cast or brace and in the recumbent position for a period of from six to eight weeks. Dr. Jacobson has adopted the Boehler method, that of making this type of patient ambulatory in from twenty-four to thirty-six hours. This is even a greater departure from the time honored methods than what we have been using. If this treatment is correct, it will revolutionize the treatment of fractures of the spine in this country.

I thoroughly agree with Dr. Jacobson that follow-up records and frequent x-ray studies are necessary during convalescence, for it is the one means that the surgeon has of knowing just what is going on. Failure to do this may result in a disability that affects the patient's earning capacity, which, in turn, assumes an economic and a medicolegal importance.

RECOGNITION AND TREATMENT OF REFRACTIVE ERRORS IN CHILDREN*

EDWARD JACKSON, M.D., Sc.D.

Denver, Colorado

ALL animals that move on the land, or in the sea, or air, have eyes to guide their movements. But these eyes differ greatly, to meet the special requirements of the animal. The eyes of a puppy are closed after birth; perhaps to keep him from running away from his source of food until he has learned to stay with it. The eyes of the colt are open from the start. With sight, his long legs can save him from wolves, or other enemies. The eyes of the infant open at once, to begin the long training in their use that they must have before they will be ready for the tasks of school and labor.

Human eyes differ from the eyes of the lower animals. Most lower animals need to see clearly at a distance, to keep away from their enemies, and to know where to seek their food. Men, too, need to see clearly at a distance; but they also need to see things held close to their eyes. They can see far away, but they also have a focussing muscle, that enables them to see small objects held very close to the eyes. Nearly all babies' eyes are hyperopic (far-sighted), and the average amount of hyperopia would unfit the eyes for use in school work.

Young children, with short arms, use their eyes for looking at small things held close to

*Read before the Annual Meeting of the Minnesota State Medical Association, Duluth, Minnesota, June 29, 1938.

their eyes. By this they get less and less far-sighted. At school age, six years, the average amount of hyperopia is not much over 2D.; and a few eyes have grown near-sighted. If the child strains its eyes, by holding things too close to them, they will become more and more near-sighted. They thus become subject to the dangers that may bring blindness from atrophy of the choroid, separation of the retina, or cataract. The wearing of glasses that enable the scholar to read print farther from the eyes, is the one important thing to prevent increase of myopia, and its consequences.

Astigmatism is a defect in the refraction of the eye, that prevents the light, which should be focussed to one point in the eye, from being so focussed. It causes the blurring of images formed on the retina, and causes straining of the eye to get the best image it can. It affects the seeing at all distances, and at all times. It usually continues throughout life but is liable to change from time to time. These anomalies or errors of refraction are so common and so serious in their effects during school life, that their early recognition and correction is very important.

Human vision is different from that of the lower animals. The human eye has the same powers of refracting light and forming images on the retina, the wide field of vision, and power of adaptation to light or darkness. But it also has greater power in detecting separate points of light, coming to it from different points of viewed objects that are close together. The cerebral coördinations of vision in man are far wider and more important than those of the lower mammals. The dog knows his master and recognizes other animals by his sense of smell. Man recognizes and discriminates by sight. His memories of persons and objects, animate and inanimate, are visual memories. In all our memories and coördinated thought, visual impressions predominate. Only what we learn by hearing may be compared with what we learn through vision.

The vision of the human eye is different because of the macula developed in the retina. The general retina is one of the first parts to become recognizable in the fetus, and it is well developed at birth. The macula cannot be recognized until the middle of fetal life, and continues to develop for months after birth. It may not reach its full functional capacity until the child is six or eight years old. Macular vision enables us to distinguish letters or small figures and to follow the mechanical trades that depend on "good vision." The education secured at school through use of books, exact drawing, fine needle-work, and all the more accurate handicrafts, depend on macular vision. This is the kind of vision that makes possible human usefulness, successful living, and rational pleasure. Good macular vision is what is generally meant by "good vision." Our common tests of vision are tests of vision at the macula. Visual acuity is the visual acuity of the macula. In all normal eyes the visual acuteness rapidly decreases in the retinal field away from the macula. The vision, as usually tested and recorded, depends on the sensitiveness and accurate focussing of the light falling on the macula. This determines the ef-fectiveness of the eyes in all kinds of school work. No scholar who has an uncorrected defect in vision should be expected to compete with others whose vision is perfect. Justice in the school room demands equal vision for the performance of visual tasks. So far as is possible, this should be brought about. Progress in learning is the purpose of schools, and it depends on seeing and hearing.

The school curriculum should provide first for the building of a strong, efficient body. The value and efficiency of our schools would be greatly increased, if the first two years of school life were devoted strictly to the building of bodily health. This could be effected by supervised playground exercises, directed to developing the power and control of the body. During this health education, the defects of sight could be detected, and refractive and motor defects of sight could be corrected before the most important employment of vision had to be entered upon.

How Are Refractive Errors Known?

Many children have been puzzled by defective vision, but have not understood what was the matter. Often, parents have thought that the child was simply inattentive, or stupid, or was not trying to see. But there is no excuse, except ignorance, or indifference, for not knowing how well, or how poorly, a child can see. Many charts have been devised for testing the vision of children and illiterates. The easiest and most efficient is the incomplete square, proposed by Snellen, when he found that his test letters were not a good test for people who did not know their letters. Such a test may be turned in either of four directions, and the child asked or told to point in which direction the opening is turned. With this, a dozen children may be tested together, and in less time than for the same number of adults to be tested with letters. If a child does not have standard, or par, vision, some error of refraction should be thought of, as the most common cause of poor sight.

In the presence of refraction errors, perfect sight may be possible but more difficult. Children in this class are slower to see than those with good sight; or they do not like to study, seem in poor health, tire easily; or they have some nervous symptoms, as headache, restlessness, or nausea, or vomiting, when they use their eyes much for reading. These symptoms may come from other causes, but in school children who are having difficulty in keeping up with their classes, refractive errors should be first considered. The same troubles may be brought on by other things, such as poor light for reading, impaired health by loss of sleep, poor diet, lack of outdoor exercises, excessive home duties; or chronic disease, as malaria or tuberculosis. But the excessive demand of school studies with eye strain is obviously the first thing to be thought of by school authorities, parents, school physicians, or nurses, when they recognize any such departure from health in school children.

Defects of vision are so important to school children that their presence should not be left to accidental discovery. They should be kept in mind and looked for in every child coming under the care of school authorities. Parents do not expect such defects in their own children and have very little knowledge of how children with ordinary sight may be entirely unable to meet the requirements of school tasks. The playground supervisor and the grade teacher have ideal opportunities for observing such defects.

The indications of defective vision, such as holding the book too close to the eyes, or quickly getting tired of reading and letting the attention wander to more distant objects, may need to be explained to teachers and parents. This, the properly trained school nurse, or school physician, or the principal should be prepared to do. The assumption that the understanding of such things will come by nature is on a level with the explanation that reading and writing come by

nature. Provision should be made to teach children what is good health and how to have it. This is the most important subject that can be taught in schools.

The campaign for health may well begin with the better lighting of homes and school rooms. Light, by contracting the pupil, is a universal corrective for all refractive errors. Try the small pupils for yourself. Take a +4. D. lens from the trial set, or grandmother's spectacles, too, strong to see clearly with across the room. See how much blurring results. Then take the pinhole disk from the trial case, or a pin hole in any thin card, and hold it in contact with the glass, and look through the pin hole across the room. A few seconds will convince you of the effect of a contracted pupil in correcting the blurring due to refractive errors of the eye. The real need of corrective glasses can only be known by measuring the ocular refraction, knowing what the eyes are expected to do, and carefully considering the symptoms and the general strength and nutrition of the child. The absurdity of turning over health problems and health maintenance to the advertising claimants of skill in measuring eyes who in general call themselves "optometrists," may be easily appreciated.

There is a general feeling that this subject of optics is complex and beyond the average physician. In the cities, where certain young men are looking forward to making ophthalmology their life work, the proper examination of the eyes of all school children can be easily provided. In the country there are physicians in general practice who have time to read and study the methods of examining eyes for congenital defects including those of refraction. Any young physician might use his spare time in this way while waiting for a full practice, and thus improve his own fortune and render a very important service to his community. The practical points of visual optics are not so abstruse as might be supposed from looking over the classical books on the subject. And a training in medical diagnosis is the best preparation for the recognition and measurement of the refractive errors and motor anomalies of the eye. Experts in salesmanship, radio and newspaper advertisers, and the manufacturers of instruments and lenses, have profited by confusing the general public as to visual defects and their correction. Any well trained physician may quickly train himself to give optical corrections to school children or patients.

For detection of optical defects in school children, a few schools have every child's eyes examined by a school physician. Others have the vision tested by a school nurse. This discloses myopia and high astigmatism. But other defects, such as high degrees of' hyperopia, causing eyestrain, headaches, lack of attention and dislike of reading, can be only suspected by a teacher from daily observation. The essential point is that some one who knows of the existence of such defects, should be on the lookout for evidence of their presence. The presence of refractive errors, or their absence, may be determined in each child only on examination by an oculist.

Good lighting and correction of refractive errors supplement each other, but one is not a substitute for the other. In every school room will be found pupils who need correction of their refractive errors; and in most school rooms are children with desks poorly lighted. An exact light-meter, or sight-meter, should be used in every school room, to test the light available for use on the desk of each child.

The treatment of the refractive errors of the eyes of children is a most important, forward-looking step in preventive medicine—the medicine of the future. It is a great duty of parents to children, of one generation to the next. It is a duty of the State which demands the education of the young, to make them better citizens. It is the duty of the medical profession, to maintain and live up to its claim of leadership, in providing for the health of all the people. The service rendered to the child will last longer, and do more for the general welfare than anything that can be done for older people. All the knowledge and skill of the oculist of today should be applied in this developing branch of preventive medicine.

MEDICAL CARE

A wave of publicity regarding medical care is going over the entire country at the present time. Magazine articles, editorials and special syndicate articles are to be found in almost every periodical one picks up. We offer the following, reproduced with thanks by special permission of the *Minneapolis Journal* and United Features Syndicate, holders of the copyright, from the pen of the well known writer, Mr. Westbrook Pegler:

"The problem of medical and surgical treatment for the masses is cluttered with undeserved pity for people who have convinced themselves they can't pay the doctor for easing their pains or saving their lives, but could do so if they tried.

"The doctors of this country give away more free goods off their shelves than the members of any other profession, including actors and musicians, who come next.

"They have their gyps and rotters, their publicity-crazy hams and ignoramuses, but they do more good for suffering humanity and in critical moments than the members of any other calling.

"Of course, it will be argued that they should do this because they are in a position to. That is their job. But the fact is, nevertheless, that they do give this service, and it is a further fact that society doesn't appreciate the good they do.

"People overemphasize their mistakes of judgment or negligence, forgetting that a doctor's mistake is more likely to have fatal, or, anyway, dreadful consequences than a mistake by a plumber, a grocer, or a journalist.

"If the work of the plumber springs a leak, if the grocer sends Snookies instead of Snackies, or if the reporter names W. C. Smith as corespondent in the divorce story when it should have been W. G. Smith, that means very little paint off anyone's fenders.

"But, let a doctor make a comparable mistake and there is all hell to pay, on top of the fact that maybe he stood to be swindled out of his pay—or most of it, anyway—even if he had done a bang-up job.

"There are many phases of the question, but I mean to stick to this one for today's lesson. I am thinking of those who think that a couple of hundred dollars is an outrageous price to pay for the removal of an appendix which has developed the menacing nature of a bomb in the patient's inwards.

"The surgeon gets the victim into a hospital as quickly as possible, gives him a jab of something to relax him and in a very short time is delving around in his giblets without 50 cents on the line to pay for laundering his smock.

"So the patient gets well, and when the bad news comes he forgets that feeling as of a litter of porcupines frisking about in his abdomen, forgets how scared he was and his alarm for the security of his dependent family, and calls the doctor a burglar.

"Why, he makes only $25 a week, and so, instead of paying the doctor a dollar a week, as he would pay for a radio or sewing machine, his policy is to skip it entirely.

"He forgets also that if the surgeon hadn't done his stuff promptly and well, specialized stuff that nobody but a surgeon could have done, his family would be on the town right now.
* * *
"If a patient can pay small amounts to a coöperative over a spell of years for treatment which he may need in the future, he can just as well pay a doctor a stated amount each week over a long term for treatment which he has already received.

"But, in too many cases he just won't, and the doctor is accused of bearing down on a man who can't afford to pay for the saving of his life but can manage somehow to come up with the price of many non-essentials.

"Many doctors nowadays serve patients in the public clinics who are able to pay reasonable professional rates for their treatment.

"There is more or less larceny in all the human race and this problem of medicine for the masses would be less difficult if those who can pay were prevented from appealing to public sympathy at the doctor's expense by mingling with the truly destitute."—Copyright, 1938. Reprinted from *Bulletin of the Hennepin County Medical Society*, August 25, 1938.

◆ CASE REPORT ◆

TRIPLET PREGNANCIES—TWO CASE REPORTS*

MILTON ABRAMSON, M.D., Ph.D.

Minneapolis, Minnesota

TRIPLET pregnancies because of their rarity and because of the greater possibility of the development of complications for the mother should be regarded as definitely pathological.

Dr. J. C. Hirst in a recently published paper reports on a series of 48,357 viable pregnancies with delivery at the Philadelphia Lying-In Hospital, the University of Pennsylvania Hospital, and the Preston Retreat with an incidence of only four sets of triplets. Of these triplets, two sets survived. Complications present in one or more of these triplet pregnancies were unusual weight gain, hypertension, slow labor, "vague labor," puerperal endometritis, and abruptio placentæ between the second and third infants. The two cases I shall report are interesting in that both sets of triplets survived, both mothers exhibited hypertension and albuminuria (true toxemias of pregnancy), and in both cases the placenta separated between the births of the second and third babies, necessitating extraction of the third baby to save it from asphyxiation. Diagnosis of triplets was made in each case by x-ray study.

Case 1.—Mrs. M. R., a multipara, aged thirty-seven, gravida V, para IV, was seen at regular intervals during her pregnancy until December 7, 1929. At this time the patient was sent into the hospital for observation and study because of loss of 8.5 pounds in weight in one week, albuminuria 2 plus to 4 plus, excessive swelling of ankles, hypertension, and orthopnea of two weeks' duration. Patient's last menstrual period was on April 28, 1929, and her estimated date of confinement was February 5, 1930. The last menstrual period was slight in amount. Patient's past history was essentially negative. She had had four previous full term normal pregnancies and deliveries, labors averaging two hours or less.

General physical examination on admission to the hospital was essentially negative except for the fact that the patient appeared extremely emaciated, and that her blood pressure during her stay in the hospital varied between 192/106 during labor to 126/70 at the time of discharge. Eyeground examination was negative. Urine examination showed albumen varying from 0.4 to 3.5 grams per litre. Blood examination showed a hemoglobin of 77 per cent, 4,270,000 red cells, and 6,950 leukocytes. The Van Slyke estimation was 59 per cent. The blood urea was 7.7 milligrams, blood sugar .07, and creatinin 1.3 milligrams. X-ray taken on December 9, 1929 (Fig. 1) showed the presence of triplets with the head of one fetus in the fundus, the head of the second overlying the pelvic inlet, and the head of the third in the left upper quadrant. The size of the babies was approximately that of an eight months' gestation.

Labor began about 5 p. m. on December 25, 1929.

*From the Department of Obstetrics and Gynecology, University of Minnesota.

Pains at first were quite weak but rapidly became stronger. Rectal examination at 5 p. m. showed a dilatation of 3 cm. and 50 per cent effacement with the head of the first fetus well below the spines. The membranes were intact and the fetal heart tones were good. The cervix dilated and effaced very rapidly with complete dilatation at about 6 p. m. The first baby was delivered in the OLA position at 6:40 p. m. Rectal examination after the birth of the first baby showed the second head presenting. The second baby was delivered in the OLA position at 7:07 p. m. There was an excessive amount of bleeding at this time and rectal examination revealed that the placenta had separated and was lying in the vaginal canal. A large bag of waters was present and the presenting part of third baby was not felt. A hand was inserted vaginally, the bag of water was ruptured, a foot of the third baby found, and the baby extracted in the SLA position at 7:12 p. m. Two placentæ were expressed immediately after the birth of the third baby. Birthweight of the babies were 2,100 grams, 1,650 grams, and 1,620 grams. They were all females. The mother made a normal uneventful afebrile convalescence. Blood pressure rapidly came down to normal, and the urine cleared of albumen. The patient weighed 112 pounds and was in good physical condition when discharged from the hospital.

Case 2.—Mrs. M. L., a primipara, aged twenty-six, was first seen on December 10, 1937. Her past history was essentially negative. She had had an appendectomy at nine years of age. There was no family history of any multiple pregnancies. Menstruation began at 13.5 years, was always regular every twenty-eight to thirty days, lasting for four to five days. She passed no clots and had no pain. The last menstrual period was on August 27, 1937, and the estimated date of confinement was June 4, 1938. She weighed 108 pounds at the time of her first examination. She stated that she was having moderate nausea and vomiting and that her breasts were enlarged and sore. She had no urinary symptoms. Her general physical examination was negative. Blood pressure was 120/80, urine entirely negative. Measurements were adequate. Notation on chart at the time of first examination was: "Fundus to level of umbilicus, unusually large for 3.5 months' pregnancy—cannot hear fetal heart, patient has felt no fetal motion." Patient was seen at regular intervals and because of the size of the uterus an x-ray was taken on February 25, 1938 (Fig. 2) and a diagnosis of triplet pregnancy made.

On March 26 the patient had a blood pressure of 136/90 and the urine was normal. She was given instructions as to her diet, rest, etc. On April 9 the blood pressure was again 138/90 and the urine normal. On April 16 the blood pressure was 138/92 and the urine showed 1 plus albumen. The patient was sent into the hospital on April 18 for observation and treatment. Blood pressure fluctuated between the above readings and 170/110, the urine, however, showed an increasing amount of albumen varying from .5 to 1.3 grams per litre. There were occasional casts and an occasional blood cell. Eyeground findings were normal. The patient gained a total of twenty-six pounds during her pregnancy. On April 29 at 2 a. m. labor started spontaneously, pains being moderate in severity and intensity.

At about 11 a. m. when the cervix was 5 to 6 cms.

the birth of the third baby. There was no abnormal bleeding, the patient being under careful observation for some time following the delivery. The patient had an uneventful afebrile convalescence and was discharged from the hospital at the end of ten days.

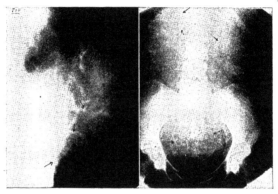

Fig. 1. Case 1.   Fig. 2. Case 2.

dilated, it was felt that the bag of waters was hindering the descent of the presenting part and it was ruptured artificially at 11:10 a. m. Patient continued in labor and delivered a normal female infant weighing 4 pounds, 5 ounces at 12:23 p. m. An episiotomy was done to prevent any undue pressure on the premature heads and to facilitate the subsequent breech delivery. The second bag of waters was ruptured artificially at 12:35 and the second baby delivered at 12:54 p. m. Following rupture of the membranes the presenting part came down with the cord prolapsed in front of it. The cord was pulsating and the second fetal heart was good so no concern was felt. The second baby was delivered as a persistent occiput posterior with a hand prolapsed beside the face. Following the birth of the second baby, the patient started to bleed abnormally and a diagnosis of premature separation of the placenta being assured, a hand was inserted and the third baby delivered by breech extraction. All the babies cried spontaneously. The two placentæ present were expressed immediately following

Blood pressure at the time of discharge was practically normal, 130/80, and the urine showed only a trace of albumen.

The clinical course of multiple pregnancies when more than two infants are present seems to be particularly hazardous for both mother and babies. There have been a large variety of complications reported in the literature. The commonest complications reported in the mother are toxemias of pregnancy, premature delivery, hydramnios, premature separation of a normally implanted placenta, placenta previa and postpartum hemorrhage. In a number of recently reported cases of triplets, the presence of one or two papyraceous feti with only one of the three a normal baby has been observed several times. Malpresentations are common, interlocking in the course of delivery has been reported and placental anomalies are not unusual.

Prostigmine.—Pharmacologic experiments indicate that the prostigmine component of prostigmine compounds possesses some of the properties of the closely allied drug physostigmine. Its actions and uses are similar, but it has the advantage of being more stable. Apparently, it is as active as physostigmine in stimulating intestinal peristalsis and has a similar but somewhat diminished myotic activity. There is no satisfactory evidence that the symptoms produced by toxic doses of prostigmine salts are any less severe than those produced by comparable doses of physostigmine or its salts. Atropine is the antidote to prostigmine. Prostigmine preparations have been used experimentally for the prevention of atony of the intestinal and bladder musculature, and for the symptomatic control of myasthenia gravis. Prostigmine is available only in the form of its salts.—*New and Non-Official Remedies.*

HISTORY OF MEDICINE IN RAMSEY COUNTY

BY J. M. ARMSTRONG; M.D.

I N the year 1835, the Rev. Thomas S. Williamson, M.D., with other missionaries, arrived at Fort Sneling. Dr. Williamson was a graduate of Jefferson
College, Canonsburg, Pennsylvania, in 1820, and of the Yale Medical School, in
1824. He was born in the Union District of South Carolina in March, 1800.
Previous to his ordination as a Presbyterian minister he had practiced medicine
at Ripley, Ohio. He, with others, was appointed by the Presbyterian and Congregational Churches through their joint Missionary Society to visit the Dahcotas
with a view of ascertaining what could be done to introduce Christian instruction.
Williamson was stationed at various points in Minnesota, or Michigan Territory
as it was till 1838, when Wisconsin Territory was established. In 1846, he was
at Kaposia, an Indian village located somewhat up river from the present site
of South Saint Paul, and was still stationed there in 1851. As he was sent there
to administer to both the spiritual and the physical needs of the Indians, it is probable that his medical services were required and used by residents of this vicinity;
in fact, his account book shows memoranda of charges for services and medicines
to residents of this vicinity during those years. Until 1838, however, the present
site of Saint Paul was part of the government reservation and there were no settlers here except squatters until after that time. In his ministerial capacity Williamson performed on the 27th of May, 1835, at Fort Snelling the first marriage
service in which a clergyman officiated within the present State of Minnesota,
and, one may perhaps add, the first performed by a physician. It is not necessary
to go further into Dr. Williamson's career here except to state that he played
an important part in the early years of our history, as is evidenced by the frequency with which his name and letters appear in our histories, and the numerous
papers he read before the Minnesota Historical Society. He also translated the
Bible into the Sioux language. An interesting paper by him on "Diseases of
the Dakota Indians" may be found in Volume IV of the *Northwestern Medical
and Surgical Journal,* Saint Paul, 1874.* He died at St. Peter, Minnesota, June 24,
1879. To refer to his account book, one sees that his charges for medical services
were modest and that he seldom received money for them, being paid mostly in
beef, potatoes, and grain. An item for the year 1843 is of interest as it shows
that Dr. Turner, of Fort Snelling, apparently was away on leave. This item is as
follows:

"For attending on the Garrison and Indians for Dr. Turner, three months and eight days,
$229.00. For private practice while living near Fort Snelling, $110.06."

The six cents must have come in some way through the price charged for drugs.

Fort Snelling, at first called Fort St. Anthony, was established as a military
post in the year 1819, though the present site was not occupied until 1821. There
have always been one or more army surgeons there, and their services were often
sought by our early residents. Surgeon Edward Purcell was with the troops

*See also Sibley Letters in the Historical Society library.

that established the post. He was a Virginian, though Irish by birth, and entered the army in 1813, dying at Fort Snelling, January 28, 1825. He was the first United States officer to die in Minnesota, and again, perhaps one may say, the first physician. Purcell's activities will be taken up in a separate chapter. Purcell was succeeded at Fort Snelling by Surgeon B. F. Harney (entered the army in 1814, died 1858) with Robert C. Wood (1800-1869) as assistant surgeon. The latter became surgeon in 1829 and was married that year at Fort Crawford, now Prairie du Chien, to the oldest daughter of Col. Zachary Taylor (later President). Jefferson Davis (later President of the Confederate States) was his brother-in-law. Both Taylor and Davis, then a lieutenant in the army, were stationed at Fort Crawford. During the Civil War, Dr. Wood was Assistant Surgeon-General.[†] Other surgeons stationed at Fort Snelling were Nathan S. Jarvis (entered the army in 1813 from New York, died 1862), Fitch, in 1837, and George F. Turner, in 1843 (entered the army from Virginia in 1825, died 1854), Joel Martin, who was succeeded in 1849 by Adam N. McLaren (entered the army 1833, died 1874). Whether any of the last named attained to fame as physicians or surgeons is not known. Turner, however, is of particular interest, as his report on an epidemic of scarlet fever at Fort Snelling appears to be the first contribution to a medical periodical from Minnesota. One army surgeon, not yet mentioned, stationed at Fort Snelling was John Emerson (entered the army in 1833, discharged 1842), the owner of Dred Scott, the negro slave whose suit for freedom, because of his residence here, was carried to the Supreme Court of the United States and settled by the decision of Chief Justice Taney. Dr. Turner cared for the pioneer settler, A. L. Larpenteur, in 1847 or 1848, for typhoid fever, which is stated to have been very prevalent here then, as it was up to some thirty-five years ago. Perhaps another man is worthy of note here, though he played no part in the medical history of this state. In October, 1823, one John Marsh, a Harvard graduate of the preceding spring, arrived at Fort St. Anthony as tutor for the colonel's children and conducted the first school in Minnesota. While at the Fort, he studied medicine under Doctor Purcell; in fact at college he had taken courses in anatomy and some medical instruction with Dr. John Dixwell of Boston. It was Marsh's intention to return to Harvard at the end of two years and obtain an M.D. degree; but fate willed otherwise, for instead of returning to the East, he followed the frontier as it moved westward and finally, in February, 1836, found himself in Los Angeles. Being without funds, the most convenient occupation to adopt seemed to be that of a physician. So we find Marsh the first American to practice medicine in California. He had a colorful career and occupied a somewhat prominent place in early California history.[‡]

In 1838, the land east of what is now Seven Corners, Saint Paul, was opened for settlement and a few white people and half-breeds settled there, most of them engaged in supplying the soldiers and Indians with whiskey. In 1840, the commanding officer at Fort Snelling, in an effort to stop this nefarious trade, expelled from the military reservation, then extending to our present Seven Corners, those squatters still on the government land. Among those driven from the reservation was an Abraham Perret (Perry), a Swiss, who came here as early as 1827. He came from Lord Selkirk's unfortunate settlement on the Red River of the North. Perret lived about where the Ancker Hospital now stands. His wife, Mary Anne, who had seven children, enjoyed quite a reputation as a midwife, and it is stated that she was employed in that capacity several times by the army women at Fort Snelling, who for this reason urged the Commandant

†For biography see *Medical and Surgical Reporter*, Phila., 20;275, 1869.
‡John Marsh, Pioneer, by Dr. George D. Lyman, Charles Scribner's Sons, 1930.

not to expel the Perrets with the other squatters. One of Mrs. Perret's daughters, Adele, who became Mrs. Vetel Guerin (died December 21, 1914, aged eighty-seven years), also was called upon in the early days to serve her sex in the same capacity. The Guerin cabin was on the bluff side of Kellogg Boulevard just below Wabasha.

The first white child born within the present limits of Saint Paul was Bazille Gervais, born September 4, 1837 (died in Saint Paul, 1926). Who was the accoucheur there is now no means of knowing. The first white female child born within the present limits of our city was Cleopatra A. Irvine (Mrs. Richard L. Gorman), daughter of John R. Irvine. She was born March 1, 1844, in a log cabin which stood a few feet from the present northwest corner of Kellogg Boulevard and Franklin Streets. Here an Indian squaw and Mrs. Scott Campbell, a half-breed woman, acted as obstetricians. Mr. A. L. Larpenteur's first child, Mrs. Harris, was born there September 22, 1847, and Mrs. Scott Campbell was again the attendant. The Irvines were the second American family to settle there and the Larpenteurs the fourth, so that births could not have been frequent in the early forties. Mrs. Harris was the first female child born in Saint Paul after the town was plotted and received the name Saint Paul (July 25, 1847). Before that time the general locality was successively known as Kaposia, Pig's Eye, the nickname of Pierre Parrant, and later more specifically as Saint Paul's Landing, Saint Paul's, and finally Saint Paul.

From this time on perhaps the best plan of procedure for continuity will be to take up the medical history of the county by years, as it is easier to follow in that way.

1847

In this year, two physicians arrived in Saint Paul's; one came on July 15 to look over the ground and returned on October 15 to remain there the rest of his life. He was Dr. John Jay Dewey.

Dr. Dewey was born September 9, 1822, in Butternuts, now Morris, Otsego County, N. Y. His parents were Ebenezer and Lucy Webster Dewey, and the family, a Connecticut one, had lived in Lebanon till 1814 when they moved to New York state. Dewey's parents were neighbors of the parents of Dr. William Beaumont, at Lebanon. The father, in his day, was a lawyer of some note and it is said at one time tutored in Greek in Yale College. Doctor Dewey received his education at Hamilton Academy, which later became Madison University, and after completing his course there entered Albany Medical College at Albany, New York, where he graduated early in the year 1847, having attended the school for a period of three years, and having had Drs. Joel Lull and A. P. Strong of Laurens, N. Y., as preceptors for thirty-two months. Several years prior to this time his elder brother, Nelson Dewey, had removed to Wisconsin Territory, and he became the first governor of the state. Through his brother's influence, young Dewey came west after his graduation and went to Lancaster, Wisconsin, then the capital of that state, where he remained till he came to Saint Paul's. When Wisconsin was admitted to statehood it was obvious that a new territory would be organized to the west, and that the seat of government would be a desirable place to locate; still better would it be if one could arrive early and become established. It was surmised correctly that Saint Paul's would become the capital, and no doubt this circumstance induced Dewey to go there. In 1848, Dr. Dewey, with Charles Cavileer, opened the first drug store in Saint Paul's and the first in the area which became Minnesota Territory the next year. In 1849 he was elected to the first territorial legislature. He retired from the drug business about 1854 and continued to practice medicine, though, having accumulated a sufficient amount of property to satisfy his needs, he never attempted to extend his clientele. On December 20, 1862, he was commissioned Assistant Surgeon, Ninth Minnesota Volunteer Infantry; he resigned September 11 of the following year and returned to Saint Paul. In 1852, he married Elizabeth Ann Barbour (nee Cannon). The late General Wm. G. LeDuc, of Hastings, who knew Doctor Dewey in 1850, said:

"Dewey was an excellent, quiet, undemonstrative man of sense, medium sized, stocky is the word, dark eyes and hair, and clean shaven in the early days."

About 1870, he retired from all business activities and led a quiet life till his death from pneumonia, April 1, 1891. His residence in the Directory of 1856-7 is given as "Saint Paul Street (now Olive) below Somerset," where he also had his office, and in this neighborhood he lived till the time of his death. He was a cousin of the late Admiral Dewey, U.S.N., and his son, Dr. James J. Dewey, who was born in Saint Paul in 1855. Dr. James Dewey graduated in medicine from Rush Medical College but retired from practice some forty or more years ago (died January 2, 1934). Dr. Dewey, Sr., retired from practice before the present Ramsey County Medical Society was formed. By the kindness of Dr. James J. Dewey and his sister, Mrs. George Bell, of Saint Paul, the Ramsey County Society possesses a photograph and autograph of Dr. John J. Dewey, his medical diploma, some of his instruments, matriculation cards from the Albany Medical College, and his military commissions.

Sometime in the year 1847 there arrived a young Virginian by the name of Wm. C. Renfro, a cousin of Henry Jackson (our first American settler, who came to Saint Paul in 1841). Renfro is said to have been a man of ability and education with pleasant and affable manners. He had studied some medicine but probably never graduated from a medical school and had never practiced medicine. Unfortunately, he was too convivial in his habits. On January 3, 1848, his body was found clothed only in his undergarments under a tree near the present northwest corner of Ninth and Locust Streets. It seems he rose in the night and started to town for another drink and was frozen to death. Nothing further seems to be known about Renfro. Possibly, one might say that he was the first physician who died in Saint Paul.

Since we have just recorded the first death of a physician in Saint Paul, we might also record the name of the first physician born there. Newspaper records state that Dr. John George Kittson died in Saint Paul, May 10, 1884. One paper gives his age as forty years and another as thirty-eight. The records at McGill University, however, show that he gave the date of his birth as August 16, 1844, and the place Saint Paul's, which was the name of Saint Paul at that time. He entered the medical school at McGill in 1864, but for some reason did not attend the session of 1867-68 and graduated with the class of 1869. He practiced medicine at Berthier, Canada East (Quebec). In 1875, he became the first chief surgeon for the Royal Northwest Mounted Police. He returned to Saint Paul broken in health, in 1882, and died at the home of his father, Norman W. Kittson. It is known that Norman W. Kittson did not take up his permanent residence in Saint Paul until 1854. Dr. Williamson's account book contains no record of Dr. Kittson's birth, so one might presume that Mrs. Abraham Perret or Mrs. Scott Campbell, who were here at that time, were present when he was born.

To divert again from the narrative, it may be stated that the first resident of Saint Paul to graduate in medicine was Freeborn F. Hoyt. The Hoyts came to

Saint Paul in 1848. Hoyt attended Rush Medical College in 1850, and after graduation established himself in Red Wing, where he practiced till he retired, some years before his death.

As previously stated, the army surgeons at Fort Snelling were frequently called upon professionally by the residents of Saint Paul's. There were other physicians available, notably Dr. Christopher Carli, of Stillwater, who settled there as early as 1841. Dr. Carli was frequently called over to Saint Paul. Mr. A. L. Larpenteur has related the following incident:

"In the fall of the year when my infant daughter was about a year old, she was taken with fits. We were much alarmed. Doctor Dewey was away so I sent to Stillwater for Doctor Carli. He came. It was cold weather and it took him two days, sometimes, to make the round trip, as it did this time. He came in, looked in the child's mouth, took a lancet from his pocket and lanced the child's gums. In twenty minutes the child was asleep. I could have done it myself had I known enough. Sometime in the sixties we had a reunion at the Sawyer House, in Stillwater, of the old settlers and I sat next to Doctor Carli. I said to him, 'You damned old rascal (we old fellows do not care what we say to each other) you robbed me.' On his wishing an explanation, I said, 'You charged me twenty-five dollars for lancing the gums of my baby.' He replied, 'It was twenty-five cold miles over there and I forgot I had to go home again, it should have been fifty dollars.' In those days there was no direct road to Stillwater and the so-called road was mostly covered with hazel bushes at that."

1848

Only one physician, Charles William Wolf Borup, settled in Saint Paul in 1848. He never practiced medicine in Saint Paul, but when in the employ of the American Fur Company as a clerk he practiced medicine. A paragraph written by one of the missionaries follows:

"Dr. Borup, to whom our family is indebted for much kindness, requests—that you would procure and send in a box with the things for the mission, the following books—Bourgery, A Treatise on Lesser Surgery translated by W. C. Roberts and James B. Kissam, Essays on some of the most important articles of the Materia Medica by George Carpenter, W. E. Tuson, Dissector's Guide—Wood and Bache's Dispensatory of the U. S., latest edition. Also inquire the price of Lizar's Anatomical plates. It is difficult for him to obtain these books."

(S. Hall to David Green under date of February 12, 1835. From Archives of the American Board of Congregational and Presbyterian Missions.)

Dr. Borup was born at Copenhagen, Denmark, in 1806 and graduated in medicine in Copenhagen. He left Denmark, March 24, 1827, and went to the Danish West Indies, but did not like the climate there, having contracted yellow fever. He came to the United States in 1828. In 1831 he came west in the employ of the American Fur Company and resided at different times at Mackinaw, Fort Snelling, Leech Lake, Yellow Lake, and La Pointe. He was an accomplished musician, the Borup home being the social and musical center of the town in the early days. In 1852, he, with Charles H. Oakes, who came west in 1825, established the first bank in Saint Paul and the first in the territory. Dr. Borup died in Saint Paul, July 6, 1859. Several of his descendants are well known residents there.

1849

In 1849, Minnesota Territory and Ramsey County were organized and the town of Saint Paul incorporated. Many settlers flocked to the capital of the new territory and by the end of the year the population of the city was about 250 to 300. There were thirty dwellings by actual count on April 23. E. S. Seymore, under date of June 18, says:

HISTORY OF MEDICINE IN MINNESOTA

"I could count 142 buildings including shanties and those under construction; all except a dozen were perhaps less than six months old—at that time there were five physicians."

These five men were John J. Dewey, already mentioned, David Day, Christopher Caldwell, Thomas R. Potts, and Nehemiah Barbour. However, in addition to these five there were two others who came to Saint Paul sometime during the year and may be regarded as more than transient visitors. Biographies of Dr. Day and Dr. Potts will appear later. For the present, we shall narrate only the occurrences relative to medical men and affairs as found in the *Pioneer* for this year. In the second issue of that paper, dated May 5, 1849, in addition to Dr. Dewey's card and an advertisement of Dewey and Cavileer, druggists (who sold tasteless castor oil, among other things), there appears the simple announcement —"Dr. Christopher Caldwell, Physician and Surgeon." This seems to be all that is known about Caldwell. Research and inquiry have revealed nothing more except that a man named Caldwell married a Miss Pierson in Saint Paul, that year. His name does not appear on the census rolls in 1850, so it is presumed that he must have left before that time. Perhaps he had the announcement placed in the paper intending to locate in Saint Paul but did not do so. In the issue of May 12 (third issue) the following notice may be found:

Dr. N. Barbour

The undersigned would respectfully notify the citizens of St. Paul and vicinity that he has opened a

Drug Store

and will keep on hand a good assortment of Drug Medicines, Paints and Dye Stuffs and will also Prescribe Medicines for all those who wish it according to the Eclectic practice, as taught in the Cincinnati Reformed College of Medicine.

This advertisement ran somewhat over a year, and in 1851 a similar announcement appeared stating that he had returned to Saint Paul and would resume practice. There is very little further to be found out about Barbour. He was known to the old settlers as a "root and herb" doctor. He was apparently still living in Saint Paul in 1854, but no more information concerning him is available.

The other two men referred to as being in Saint Paul that year appear to have been unpopular, at least with the editor of the *Pioneer*, as appears from the following items:

Run Away

From Saint Paul, without paying his honest debts, a person in the shape of a man calling himself Doctor Snow, formerly of Prairie du Chien. This is to warn all persons against this man's rascality.
Prairie du Chien *Patriot* please copy.

George Wells.

Sometime later a rumor became current that Dr. Snow had started for Germany, where he had received a handsome legacy, but the Prairie du Chien *Patriot*, noting this, remarked that it was generally understood there that Snow had gone to California. The *Pioneer's* next jibe was sharp:

"We all expected Snow to liquidate before running off, it seems quite evident from all we can learn that the Doctor has not been properly understood here."

This closed the record of Dr. Snow so far as it is recorded or remembered.

(To be continued in next issue.)

EDITORIAL

MINNESOTA MEDICINE

Official Journal of the Minnesota State Medical Association

Published by the Association under the direction of its Editing and Publishing Committee

EDITING AND PUBLISHING COMMITTEE

J. T. Christison, Saint Paul   C. B. Wright, Minneapolis
E. M. Hammes, Saint Paul   T. A. Peppard, Minneapolis
Waltman Walters, Rochester

EDITORIAL STAFF
Carl B. Drake, Saint Paul, Editor
W. F. Braasch, Rochester, Associate Editor
Gilbert Cottam, Minneapolis, Associate Editor

Annual Subscription—$3.00   Single Copies—$0.40

Foreign Subscriptions—$3.50

The right is reserved to reject material submitted for editorial or advertising columns. The Editing and Publishing Committee does not hold itself responsible for views expressed either in editorials or other articles when signed by the author.

Classified advertising—five cents a word; minimum charge, $1.00. Remittance should accompany order.

Display advertising rates on request.

Address all communications to Minnesota Medicine, 2642 University Avenue, Saint Paul, or Suite 604, National Bldg., Minneapolis. Telephone: Nestor 2641.

BUSINESS MANAGER
J. R. Bruce

Volume 21   OCTOBER, 1938   Number 10

The A.M.A. House of Delegates Meeting

TO ONE who has never before witnessed the deliberations of the House of Delegates of the American Medical Association, the special session held September 16 and 17 at Chicago was a revelation. The appointment of committees to consider the resolutions submitted to the House, and the hearings of the committees which could be attended and taken part in by the delegates, assured opportunities for all delegates to be heard. The reports of the various committees later presented to the House were then accepted, modified or rejected. The final action of the House thus represented the majority opinion of the delegates from the states as well as is humanly possible. The idea, often

expressed, that policies of the A.M.A. are dictated by a small group of officers, is untenable.

The final action of the House of Delegates has already appeared in *The Journal* of the American Medical Association and should be carefully studied by all physicians. The delegates handled a complicated subject very well. The newspaper reports gave the impression that the profession had stepped into line with the recommendations of President Roosevelt's Technical Committee on Medical Care. As so often happens, the lay press gave the wrong impression. Although the House of Delegates showed throughout its deliberations a desire to coöperate with government agencies in the wise expenditure of funds for the medical care of the needy, it does not recognize the need for a yearly appropriation of any 850 million dollars recommended by the President's Committee, and they reiterated their strenuous disapproval of compulsory state-controlled health insurance.

The House of Delegates again recommended the establishment of a federal department of health to consolidate the twenty-seven different public health activities of the government, with a secretary who shall be a doctor of medicine and a cabinet member. They also approved the expansion of Public Health and Maternal and Child Health activities along prevention lines only, and with due regard to economy.

Hospital expansion was recommended where need exists. The wise suggestion is made that the so-called private hospitals be subsidized for the care of the needy rather than that new hospitals be built. It has been shown that private hospitals throughout the country are only 60 to 70 per cent occupied and many are having financial difficulties.

The principle was announced that medical care of the indigent is a local problem and should be handled by local government from tax funds and with the coöperation of the local medical profession. Doubtless some communities and states may require federal assistance in the form of financial and technical aid, but no general federal subsidy is advocated. It is not difficult to appreciate that higher taxes only depress business and increase the burden of the medical care of the indigent. It is wiser for the states to use every endeavor to improve economic conditions which affect the health of our citizens.

Heretofore the various hospital service insurance organizations have received little official support from our national organization. At this meeting, however, the movement which has shown a mushroom-like and healthy growth throughout the country was approved and, providing it does not include doctors' fees, its expansion is urged. Cash indemnity insurance plans to cover in whole or in part the costs of emergency or prolonged illnesses were deemed practical. It is not the occasional need for a doctor that proves a burden for the low income group, but the serious accident or prolonged illness which as a rule requires hospital care. One wonders whether insurance to cover this contingency would not be as popular as that covering hospital bills.

It can be seen that the recommendations of the House of Delegates agreed with the statements submitted by Dr. Braasch on the standpoint of the House of Delegates of the Minnesota profession as expressed at its special meeting September 11.

Pneumococcic Meningitis

THE invasion of the meninges by the pneumococcus is attended by a high mortality rate. This type of meningitis occurs most commonly as a complication of pneumonia, middle ear infections, and skull fractures. Rarely, the meninges may be attacked without any demonstrable primary focus. Until recently, all therapeutic procedures have yielded disappointing results.

Recent reports indicate that, with the introduction of sulfanilamide into the treatment of bacterial infections, a promising therapeutic approach for patients with pneumococcic meningitis has been made possible. Allan and his associates at the Johns Hopkins Hospital have had three patients with pneumococcic meningitis who recovered following the administration of sulfanilamide. Finland and his colleagues at the Boston City Hospital have also presented an important report concerning the use of sulfanilamide alone or in combination with specific antipneumococcic serum in the treatment of ten patients with pneumococcic meningitis, six of whom

recovered. In contrast to these results, before the introduction of sulfanilamide, ninety-nine patients were treated at the same institution between November, 1929, and June, 1936, and none recovered. Many of these patients had been treated with specific antipneumococcic serum. These workers believe that a combination of sulfanilamide and specific antipneumococcic serum is more effective than either one alone. The principles of treatment which they have adopted at present include the administration of large doses of sulfanilamide by mouth or subcutaneously; the intravenous injection of specific antipneumococcic horse or rabbit serum; the intrathecal injection of the patient's own serum obtained after he has received the specific serum intravenously; and frequent drainage by lumbar puncture. Sulfanilamide need not be given intraspinally since it appears quickly in the spinal fluid in adequate amounts when given orally or subcutaneously. On the other hand, the specific serum must be introduced into the spinal canal, since it cannot be demonstrated in the fluid when given intravenously. Fresh human serum also must be introduced intraspinally in order to provide complement, which is necessary for the destruction of the pneumococcus. If the patient's serum is not available, small amounts of normal fresh human serum and specific antipneumococcic serum may be given. In one patient treated successfully in this manner, there were 20,000,000 colonies of pneumococci per cubic centimeter in the spinal fluid prior to treatment.

Although the number of patients treated by these workers is small, the results warrant the trial of their methods by others. It will be important to determine in the future whether a combination of sulfanilamide and specific antipneumococcic serum is not more effective in the treatment of cases of pneumoccic pneumonia than sulfanilamide or serum alone.

The paper of Finland and his associates[*] merits the attention of anyone interested in careful clinical investigation. The protocol of each patient is included with a discussion of the clinical, bacteriological, and immunological studies employed.

WESLEY W. SPINK, M.D.

*Finland, Maxwell, Brown, John W., and Raugh, Albert E.: Treatment of Pneumococcic Meningitis: A Study of Ten Cases Treated with Sulfanilamide Alone or in Various Combinations with Specific Antipneumococcic Serum and Complement, Including Six Recoveries. New England Journal of Medicine, 218:1033, (June 23) 1938.

President Coffman

THE sudden passing of Lotus Delta Coffman, president of the University of Minnesota, ended the career of one who had reached the top in his chosen profession—that of an educator.

President Coffman was born on a farm near Salem, Indiana, January 7, 1875; graduated from the Indiana Normal School at Terre Haute, Indiana, in 1896; received his A.B. degree in 1906, and his A.M. degree in 1910, both from the University of Indiana. In his younger years he taught in country schools, acted as superintendent of schools, director of teacher training, and university teacher, until he took his Ph.D. degree at Columbia in 1911. From then on he taught,—first at the University of Illinois, from 1912 to 1915, when he came to the University of Minnesota. Here he was Dean of the College of Education for six years, until he was named fifth president of the University in 1921, to succeed Dr. Marion Leroy Burton.

During President Coffman's seventeen years as president, the University has shown tremendous development. The enrolment has doubled and the annual budget nearly so. Many new buildings, as well as several new departments, have been added to the University.

The qualifications of a university president have changed in recent years. Whereas formerly scholastic attainment in the dead languages used to be considered a prime consideration in selecting a university president, now he must be not only an educator but an administrator. President Coffman's training, first as teacher and later in administrative capacities, prepared him for the larger task of presiding over a university when the opportunity presented itself. Interested primarily in education, he still possessed an appreciation of the value of extra-curricular activities. His ability as an educator was recognized during his lifetime by honorary degrees from a number of universities. Minnesota has sustained a great loss in his sudden departure at an age when many more years of usefulness might well have been his lot.

We live worthily when we do work that
helps to improve conditions of
life for everyone.

STATUS OF THE GLEN LAKE SANATORIUM*

Donald C. Balfour, M.D., Director, Mayo Foundation
Rochester, Minnesota

I appreciate the privilege of being here on this occasion. It is most appropriate that those who have contributed to the growth of a great institution such as this should receive the recognition which is being given here this evening. I feel honored that I have the opportunity of joining in this tribute to Mr. Gale and Mr. Kingman and to those who have given such unselfish support to Glen Lake.

The control of such a devasting disease as tuberculosis is one of the great triumphs of medical science, and if one traces the history of this achievement he will be struck with the fact that it has paralleled the development of sanatoria. It is true that sanatoria for the care of tuberculous patients have been in existence for over a hundred years, because it was in 1791 that an infirmary for such patients was first founded in England, and up to the time of Koch's discovery of the tubercle bacillus thirteen sanatoria for the treatment of the disease had been established in England. In Germany the first hospital for the treatment of the disease was founded in 1853, and the earliest institutions in this country were "inspired by religious and humane motives as early as 1857." The beginning of modern sanatoria for the treatment of the disease in this country, however, is usually dated from the founding of the sanatorium at Saranac, New York, by Trudeau in 1885.

The change in the physical character of sanatoria during the past thirty years is evidence of the general improvement which has taken place in hospitals, but particularly emphasizes that the treatment of tuberculosis is on as scientific a basis as any other disease. Not so long ago the type of sanatoria was represented by a series of small, shack-like structures, and the treatment of the disease was largely a question of isolation, fresh air, and good food. That rest is the first principle in the treatment of tuberculosis was far from being generally recognized. It was found in later years that the principle of isolation was not necessary, and the tendency subsequently has been to construct sanatoria on the same general plan as any general hospital. As a matter of fact the modern sanatorium, as exemplified here at Glen Lake, with its laboratories and operating rooms and facilities for research and for the training of nurses, is so well constructed and equipped that little change would be needed to convert such an institution into a general hospital.

It has been interesting, too, to find that climate is not as important a factor in the treatment of the disease as was once thought, and it has become possible to construct sanatoria throughout all parts of the country so that those afflicted with the disease can obtain the best possible care without the serious disadvantage of going far from home.

The particular functions of a sanatorium, in contrast

*Presented at the dinner to honor the 25th Anniversary of the Hennepin County Sanatorium Commission held at Glen Lake Sanatorium, September 9, 1938.

to home treatment of the tuberculous patient, are the prevention of the spread of infection, the education of the patient and family and friends, the cure and arrest of the disease, particularly in advanced cases, the training of physicians and nurses for specialization in this field, the economic rehabilitation of the patient, and usefulness as a diagnostic center, furnishing facilities for preventorium care as well as for research and development of surgical methods of treatment of the disease. In all these functions the modern sanatorium has no superior and should continue to lead the way in further advances in our knowledge of this disease.

The control of tuberculosis has been accomplished to a great extent through methods of education and in this the sanatorium has had such a large part that public support and approval have been freely given. The fact that the majority of tuberculosis hospitals are community projects and have been developed with very little assistance from the federal government, which has limited its aid in tuberculosis largely to those patients who are direct wards of the government, will always be an example of what can be done by the community itself. As an example of the extent to which support by public funds is given, it has been shown that in 1908, 34 per cent of the sanatoria were supported by public funds, whereas in 1931 the figure had risen to 78 per cent. In other words, it is obvious that if the public can be convinced of the desirability of a program for the control of a disease and can see that the program is being satisfactorily carried out public support will not be lacking.

No better example of what a sanatorium should be and how it should be run in the estimation of both the public and profession can be found than here at Glen Lake, for it is generally agreed, among those who know, that in Glen Lake, Minnesota has a sanatorium which is unexcelled. The growth of Glen Lake has been steadily toward more scientific management of the disease, and the publications of the staff are recognized as being the observations of men of authority because of high scientific training and experience. An example of the standard of medical practice here is the accomplishment of the staff in carrying out successfully, for the first time in Minnesota, the complete removal of a diseased lung. The influence of such an institution on medical thought and practice is of the greatest importance, and I am glad at this time to express on behalf of the Mayo Foundation our appreciation of the opportunities which Glen Lake has afforded the members of our staff and the Fellows of the Foundation to study here. From the standpoint of graduate medical education we believe that no better opportunity can be found for scientific study of tuberculosis and its treatment than at Glen Lake.

Minnesota can well be proud of those who have made Glen Lake so outstanding. The tribute this evening to Mr. Gale and Mr. Kingman is significant since it is evidence of what can be accomplished when an institution is directed by men who have no other motive than to see that the highest possible medical service is rendered. I consider it an honor to join in the tribute to Mr. Gale and Mr. Kingman, who have had such a large part in the development of this institution.

In Memoriam

Axel W. Swedenburg
1873-1938

DR. AXEL W. SWEDENBURG, of Thief River Falls, died at his home August 20, 1938, from a stroke, at the age of sixty-five. He was born April 6, 1873, at Maiden Rock, Wisconsin. After finishing high school he acquired a Bachelor of Science degree from Valparaiso University. In 1903, he began the study of medicine at the Chicago College of Medicine and Surgery, and received his M.D. in 1907. The same year he married Elfrida Ericson, who passed away in 1913.

After finishing his internship, Dr. Swedenburg practiced at Ellendale, Minnesota, until 1910, when he moved to Thief River Falls. In 1914, he moved to Ashland, Oregon, where he practiced two years with his brother, Dr. Francis Swedenburg, returning to Thief River Falls in 1916.

On October 1, 1917, Dr. Swedenburg was commissioned first lieutenant in the Army Medical Corps and served at Jefferson Barracks and Fort Riley, being honorably discharged December 29, 1919. Since then he continuously practiced at Thief River Falls until two years ago, when he was forced to retire because of ill health.

Dr. Swedenburg was active in local affairs in his home town. He was one of the organizers and the first president of the local Rotary Club. He was affiliated with the local Masonic lodge and was a member of the Elks and Odd Fellows. He was a member of the Lutheran Church and was also a member of the Elmer J. Eklund Post No. 117 of the American Legion, which conducted a military service at the cemetery at the time of his funeral.

Dr. Swedenburg had practiced for over twenty-five years at Thief River Falls and was a member of the Red River Valley Medical Society, the Minnesota State and American Medical Associations. He also belonged to the American Railway Surgeons Association.

In 1919, Dr. Swedenburg was married to Mina Rock at Iowa City, Iowa. He is survived by his wife; one daughter, Mrs. Dorothy O'Connor of Saint Paul, two sons, Carl W. of Saint Cloud and Donald of Thief River Falls.

Fannie Kimball Fiester
1866-1938

Dr. Fannie Kimball Fiester died at her home in Austin, Minnesota, May 6, 1938, after a day's illness.

Dr. Fiester was born in West Randolph, Vermont, May 6, 1866. She received her early education in the city of her birth, and graduated from Northwestern University Women's Medical School in 1891. She received her M.D. from Hahnemann Medical College in 1893 and served her internship in the Iowa State Hospital at Independence, Iowa.

Locating in Austin in 1893, Dr. Fiester practiced continuously until the day before her death.

MEDICAL ECONOMICS

Edited by the Committee on Medical Economics
of the
Minnesota State Medical Association
W. F. Braasch, M.D., Chairman

LAST STEP IN THE SURVEY

Form 1-F, last step in the survey, went to all members of the Minnesota State Medical Association, September 24.

This form was designed to provide a check on the facts reported previously on Form No. 1. A careful record was to be made on it each day for the week beginning September 26 of the number of patients given care without charge, or those referred to agencies and from agencies for service.

This check is an essential part of the survey. Every member is urged to keep the record carefully and send it promptly to the secretary of his county or district society.

The American Medical Association has recommended that new appropriations for extensions of public health and medical programs be governed by the need in each community. It is the business of physicians to show where that need is.

THE SPECIAL SESSION OF THE HOUSE OF DELEGATES

THE recent special session of the House of Delegates of the American Medical Association was an epoch-making event in the annals of that representative body. There was much speculation on the eve of the gathering as to what action would be taken. Vague rumors were circulated that radical plans would be proposed by some of the members.

A plan for the spending of the 850 millions of federal money included in the National Health Program had already been adopted by one state medical society. Several of the state societies had encouraged the establishment of local health insurance plans.

New Plans Blossomed

In fact, during the last six months new plans for medical care have blossomed out almost daily in county medical societies throughout the land. The threat of governmental action, claims that many physicians were leaning toward socialized medicine, and criticisms of the attitude of organized medicine appearing in countless newspapers and periodicals all conspired to make some of us conservatives rather jittery as to what might happen on the morrow. That these influences affected the reactionary attitude previously held by many of the delegates is undoubtedly true.

Wisely Guided

However, as so often has happened in previous meetings of the House of Delegates, apparent crises were smoothly compromised and the action taken was generally satisfactory. The modus operandi for consideration of the problems confronting the delegates was well conceived and functioned exceedingly well. A general committee of twenty-five was appointed which was subdivided into groups of five. Each one of the subcommittees was assigned to the consideration of one of the five sections in the National Health Report. The choice of the general chairman, Dr. Walter Donaldson, was a wise and happy one, and he guided the deliberations of the various committees in a wise and masterly fashion.

The personnel of the subcommittees included many men who had given much previous time and thought to the subjects under discussion. The various subcommittees met separately to consider the subjects involved in the sections assigned to them. Opportunity was given to any delegate who so desired to appear before them and express his views.

The results of the deliberations and the final resolutions adopted undoubtedly represented the opinion of an overwhelming majority of the members present.

Sympathetic Attitude Adopted

Although the government health program was based on inadequate information and was not well considered and in spite of the fact that many of the members objected to many of its proposals, nevertheless they adopted a sympathetic attitude towards the "magnificent" objectives. Although the House of Delegates endorsed the spirit of the proposals embodied in Sections I and II of the Health Program, important reservations were made which did not appear in the press. *These reservations included, `first, that medical services should be expanded only in areas where they were needed, and, second, that those measures should be taken in coöperation and with approval of local medical societies.* These two very important reservations should make the proposals acceptable to the medical profession without hampering their application.

Insurance Principle Accepted

Another outstanding feature of the program adopted by the delegates is the acceptance of the principle of health insurance. While certain features of insurance never have been opposed by organized medicine, nevertheless its present attitude toward the subject permits more liberal interpretation than formerly. Reservations were made, however, which limit insurance to voluntary insurance and under the guidance of the local medical societies. *The resolutions definitely stated opposition to compulsory insurance with government aid.*

The approval of the wide expansion of the hospital facilities and the establishment of numerous diagnostic centers as suggested by the National Health Program was qualified. While the need of greater hospitalization was recognized in certain areas and in the care of certain diseases, nevertheless the hit-and-miss expansion as proposed was disapproved. A plea was made for more intelligent employment of facilities already existing and that any expansion be limited to rural areas and other fields as specified.

It is of interest that the Committee approved the principle of hospital insurance, which is being widely adopted throughout the country, and recommended it as a community project.

The Committee recognized the soundness of the principles of workmen compensation laws and recommended the expansion of such legislation to provide for meeting the cost of illness resulting from industry.

It is of interest that the Committee endorsed the principle of compensation for loss of wages during sickness.

3,000 Medical Society Plans

In the course of discussion, Dr. Leland called attention to the fact that over 3,000 plans are now filed in the Bureau of Medical Economics which have been proposed by medical societies and other medical agencies to provide for more adequate distribution of medical care. It is to be hoped that these plans and the action of the House of Delegates will refute insinuations which have appeared in many publications that the medical profession is not doing all it can to give the public the best possible medical care.

The sympathetic attitude of the delegates toward the National Health Program should refute accusations which have been made that the medical profession is opposed to health reform because of selfish motives. It should emphasize the fact that they had only one object in mind and that is the protection of the best traditions of medical practice.

In order to show their desire to coöperate with the federal authorities in carrying out the National Health Program, a standing committee was appointed by the speaker of the House for the purpose of conferring with them. It remains to be seen whether they will be met by the federal representatives with a similar spirit of coöperation.

W. F Braasch, M.D.

ACTION BY THE DELEGATES

The Board of Trustees was definitely instructed by the House of Delegates in Chicago to oppose the attempt initiated by Attorney General Thurman Arnold to convict the American Medical Association of monopoly. Monopoly was charged by Attorney General Arnold on the strength of opposition to illegal aspects of the Group Health Association of Washington, D. C., employees of the Home Owners Loan Corporation and an investigation threatened.

Any action that may fix upon the association this charge will be fought, if necessary in the courts of last resort.

The Delegates also unanimously rejected a resolution which would have encouraged medical societies to set up group plans and advertise them to the public.

A committee of seven physicians including Dr. Irvin Abell, Louisville, Ky., president; Dr. Henry A. Luce, Detroit; Dr. Frederic E. Sondern,

New York; Dr. Walter E. Vest, Huntington, W Va.; Dr. Walter F. Donaldson, Pittsburgh; Dr. Fred W. Rankin, Lexington, Ky.; and Dr. Edwin H. Cary, Dallas, Texas, was appointed to confer with federal authorities on methods of coördinating health and welfare activities of private practitioners and government health and medical workers.

AS MINNESOTA SEES IT

County officers, delegates and committees met in special session at the St. Paul Hotel, Sunday, September 11, to discuss the government health program and instruct Minnesota delegates to the Chicago session.

It is interesting to note that Minnesota's action anticipated in a general way the more detailed action taken at Chicago.

The Minnesota officers and committees—130 in all from all parts of the state—went on record to the effect that:

Minnesota's Platform

We in Minnesota are in sympathy with all intelligent efforts to help indigents and the people with low incomes.

We insist, however, that any plan adopted or any program proposed leave to the medical and health authorities of each state the exact form and extent of the program from that state.

We insist, also, that the right of freedom in choice of physician be preserved.

We are opposed to any form of tax-supported compulsory health insurance.

This action was taken after a day of discussion by state officers, by representatives of the State Board of Health and the State Board of Control now in charge of Social Security aids to public health and medical care, and others.

Excerpts from important talks made at the Sunday meeting follow.

Important Epoch

DR. J. M. HAYES, Minneapolis, president of the Minnesota State Medical Association and presiding officer at the conference:

We have reached an important epoch in our history. Are we or are we not going to let the politicians tell us what to do?

We have an arrangement in Minnesota whereby the medical profession is consulted on the expenditure of nearly all relief and welfare funds devoted to medical care and the

public health. Our close coöperation with the official agencies has made it possible for any indigent person in Minnesota to receive excellent medical care when he needs it.

Our great problem is to fight false impressions created in the public mind by backers of the so-called National Health Program.

Doorbell Survey

This program is built largely upon statistics gathered in the W.P.A. "doorbell survey." And, in this connection, I would like to say a word about that survey. I had occasion, myself, to follow up the work in several families and I found that even where the people interviewed had been under the care of a naturopath they were listed as having received medical care. In many instances the people interviewed had answered carelessly and without any attempt whatever at truth or exactness. It is on the basis of such a study that the President's Inter-departmental Committee is now claiming the low income class lacks adequate medical care.

The public is easily deceived, however. Mr. Paul Kellogg declares in a recent issue of *Survey Graphic* that the W.P.A. survey was "the greatest medical survey in the history of American Medicine."

It is clear that we must find some way to counteract such statements in the public mind.

DR. W. F. BRAASCH, Rochester, chairman of the Committee on Medical Economics: The program of the National Health Conference (where the President's committee proposed its program) was definitely a "set-up." The atmosphere was radical and antagonistic. When the representatives of organized medicine, Dr. Abell, Dr. West and Dr. Fishbein, told the conference what medicine has already done and what it proposes to do, they were greeted with silence. The doctors were outcasts and no representatives of banking or industry were present.

A number of different plans will be under discussion in Chicago next week. One, at least, will be very liberal. I hope you will instruct your delegates to carry down to Chicago a conservative, well considered program.

Successful Relationship

DR. GEORGE EARL, Saint Paul, president-elect of the State Medical Association: Most successful relationships in life are dual relationships. Notable among these dual relationships is that between doctor and patient which the politicians are trying, just now, to make into a triangular relationship of doctor, politician and patient.

We are of one mind, I believe, on the importance of maintaining the dual character of the doctor's relationship to his patient and also of maintaining the freedom of the patient to choose his physician.

We must remember that the public is not very intelligent on any program involving medical care. Also that the politician and social worker are its favorite teachers.

State Medicine Implied

Among other things, the new government program proposes establishment of 500 government-supported health and diagnostic centers in the United States. All of the elements of tax-supported state medicine are implicit in this proposal.

It is probable that we need very few such units in Minnesota because our level of practice is very high. It seems to me, therefore, that the government might rationally assist and enlarge our present facilities instead of building new hospitals and centers here.

Our problem is to present a rational plan that will provide adequate care and still not fasten upon us, unnecessarily a costly system of state-supported medical units.

Inference Untrue

I want to go on record here on the importance of counteracting the inference, attendant upon National Health Conference publicity, that physicians are opposed to the extension to everybody of good medical care. Nothing could be further from the truth.

We believe in the extension of public health services and we believe in insurance. We do not believe in tax-supported, government-controlled compulsory insurance because it will lead to medicine by politically controlled bureas with an overhead cost that may run to 50 and 60 per cent as it has in other countries.

In my opinion we must assure the public that we do stand for the best possible medical care for all the people. Let us show the public a positive program and a true leadership.

Let us show them, further, that the doctors and not the politicians are their friends.

Minnesota's Record

Dr. E. C. Hartley, Saint Paul, director of Maternal and Child Welfare, State Department of Health: Since 1915 the maternal mortality in Minnesota has been cut in half. In 1937 the infant mortality was three for every 100 live births and more than 98 per cent were delivered by doctors—a record for the entire United States. Certainly the situation in Minnesota with regard to maternal and child health is an example for the rest of the nation.

If the laws suggested go through, considerable sums of money will undoubtedly be available for this work. I can assure you that any methods that may be adopted will be adopted in consultation with the state medical association. We have always assumed that our function in this respect was purely educational. I am sure that Dr. Chesley as executive officer would offer no other kind of service.

Dr. C. A. Stewart, Minneapolis: We have already a well-rounded public health program in maternal and child health, in nutrition, in prevention of crippling conditions, under Dr. Hilleboe of the State Board of Control, in our school health services, including vaccination and immunization with vaccines and toxoids supplied by the State Board of Health when they are requested. In the main, our child health program is adequate and additional funds would scarcely be needed in Minnesota except to supplement already existing services.

Sufficient Sanatoria

Dr. H. E. Hilleboe, Saint Paul, director of the Division of Tuberculosis and of services for Crippled Children, State Board of Control: There are now sufficient sanatoria to take care of all tuberculous patients in Minnesota. Additional funds for construction of sanatoria will not be needed in this state. Funds are needed, however, to supplement the follow-up care already instituted by the State Board of Control. There is need for further medical supervision of discharged patients, also for funds to provide the necessities of life for the families of patients. There is also a need for facilities to segregate tuberculosis patients among the insane.

There is no need to bring in federal funds to build additional hospitals for crippled children. At the present time social security funds are being used, temporarily, to hospitalize some crippled children in private hospitals. Within two years, however, there will be sufficient beds available at Gillette, the Shriners' hospital and the University hospital to care for the load.

Convalescent Home Needed

The Board of Control is especially interested, now, in providing domiciliary care and convalescent homes for indigent children. There are now 1,300 children in the state who were crippled from birth who need such care. Also there are a number of children with heart disease who should have convalescent care. There is a problem which we as physicians must face in time.

The chairman of the Board of Control has instructed me to inform the members of our association that he and the board will continue to follow the policies that have guided us for the past two years with regard to both the tuberculosis and the crippled child programs.

DR. PAUL O'LEARY, Rochester, member of the Committee on Syphilis and Social Diseases: Our Minnesota program for control of venereal disease has been functioning for 18 years and it has functioned so well that it has been set up as a model all over the United States. Some $43,000 has been devoted by the state to the program outlined by Dr. Chesley. Only about 177 doctors have taken advantage of the offer of free drugs which is a part of that program, an indication of the healthy condition that prevails in most communities.

A meeting like this should be of a constructive type. It is our business, now, to present a program for the health situation as a whole that will serve as a model just as our venereal disease program has served as a model in Minnesota.

Cancer Facilities Adequate

DR. MARTIN NORDLAND, Minneapolis, chairman of the Committee on Cancer: Control of cancer depends mainly upon early diagnosis and, certainly, there are ample facilities for early diagnosis of cancer in Minnesota. The importance of the cancer problem should be brought to the physicians, of course, and this

has been a large part of the work of our committee.

DR. H. E. ROBERTSON, Rochester, member of the Committee on Cancer: I am strongly opposed to the carrying out of the recommendations concerning control of cancer which were included in the report of the technical committee and submitted as part of the program of the Inter-Departmental Committee.

Three Phases

The cancer problem resolves itself into three phases: one, research concerning the pathogenesis and cause of malignant growths; two, early and appropriate treatment of these growths (this point involves extensive education of both the layman and the doctor); three, the care of advanced cancer cases, particularly among the indigent.

The stimulus for the study of the pathogenesis and cause of cancer is sufficiently strong so that no urge by government agencies will ever be necessary. The reward of solid contributions in this field is sufficient in itself to keep every worker on his toes. The slightest hint that steps toward the solution of this problem are in sight has produced and would produce adequate funds from private resources to finance fully any such undertaking.

The early diagnosis and treatment of cancer involves a problem that must be solved wholly by the medical profession. In the education of doctors and laymen for the early handling of cancer cases, a program has been established for years by the American Society for the Control of Cancer. It is satisfactorily organized and evidences definitely good results. The establishment of centers throughout the United States for the exclusive study and treatment of cancer might need support from government agencies. But to turn over to these agencies the organization of such an intricate problem in education of doctors and patients and in the medical and surgical handling of cancer cases is distinctly a backward step. One has only to point to the thoroughly inadequate care given in the Veterans' Hospitals of this country to demonstrate the waste and uselessness of such a move.

"Cancer Asylums"

The care of advanced and largely indigent cases of cancer is likely to prove the final development of most government plans in this field.

The demands of relatives of cancer-afflicted people and of the patients themselves, for free hospital care, especially when their condition is incurable, would make overwhelming inroads into funds established for cancer control. The result would be the establishment of cancer asylums throughout the country without material benefit to anyone except insofar as they provided free living for these unfortunate people. The resources now available in city hospitals and special cancer clinics are fairly adequate for handling this phase of the cancer problem. These are organized and controlled by medical men and no other lay substitute could be developed which would do a better job.

Supplement Hospitals

DR. PETER WARD, Saint Paul, superintendent of Miller Hospital and president of the Minnesota Hospital Association: The effect upon the private hospitals of further building of federal hospitals could probably be compared to the effect upon business in general of government interference. Hospital facilities in Minnesota today are sufficient, I believe, to take care of the needs of patients and doctors. There may be isolated communities where facilities are not ideal and government funds can be used as Dr. Earl suggests to supplement and amplify existing facilities.

Incidentally the Minnesota Hospital Association enjoys a membership of 98 per cent of all the hospitals in the state. In the Hospital world this is a unique record and evidence of the general excellence of our hospital facilities.

DR. ORIANNA MCDANIEL, Saint Paul, director of the Division of Preventable Diseases, State Board of Health: About one-third of the 2,000 or more pneumonia deaths that occur on the average each year in Minnesota could be prevented by use of serum. This would mean a saving of at least 340 lives each year.

Since federal money became available our board has set up a state-wide program of pneumonia control. The objectives were to assist physicians in diagnosing pneumonia and to furnish serum to needy persons. Typing centers have been set up in various parts of the

state, 67 of them in the hospitals and others at the health unit districts. It is left to the physician to determine whether or not the patient is needy and should have the serum furnished by our board. Before serum is sent, sputum must be typed and a report telephoned to the Board. This work is in its infancy and much still remains to be done in the way of publicity both to the public and the doctors.

DR. A. J. CHESLEY, Saint Paul, executive officer and secretary of the Minnesota Department of Health: This situation has seemed serious to the health officers for a long time. We have tried to warn the practicing profession and I am glad to see that organized medicine is now thoroughly aroused.

One thing we must all remember. The public will look at health and medical problems from a national rather than from a local point of view. When Minnesota people hear on the radio that one-third of the people of the United States lack adequate medical care, that only five per cent of those who need it receive pneumonia serum, they are going to apply those figures, based on the national W.P. health survey, to Minnesota. We must not be too irritated on that account.

Figures Do Not Apply

Actually we know that those figures do not apply to Minnesota at all. Incidentally, even a United States Public Health official who was organizing the "doorbell survey" was unable to answer all of the 62 questions that untrained numerators were required to ask in their house-to-house survey. That fact indicates that the figures so widely quoted may not always be accurate or reliable.

It is practically impossible to find out by a survey just how much disease there is and to estimate on that basis just how extensive the medical facilities must be to take care of it. It IS possible, however, to compare death rates and, even more significant, the rate of deaths at which no physician is in attendance.

Few Unattended Deaths

We have just discovered in a study made recently by one of our staff that only one-tenth of one per cent of deaths in Minnesota last year were unattended by a physician. That is an important finding, especially when it is compared with the record of Mississippi, where

15.5 of the death certificates were not signed by a physician last year.

In a situation of this sort the State Board of Health is between two camps. We have already done our best to work with the doctors in Minnesota. On the other hand, when large sums of money become available to the states, congressmen demand that the people in their districts get their share.

If our present plan for utilizing federal funds can be followed, we shall be doing the best that can be done, I believe, at the present time. It should be remembered that federal grants are not flat grants, they must be matched by state funds.

Surgeon General Parran is a very competent man but he is on the spot. In any case, he is bound to confer with the conference of state and provincial health officers before he recommends appropriations.

Lesson from Canada

It seems to me that we might take a lesson from Canada's system and experience. In Canada, the final decision on all extension of medical care still rests with the organized medical profession. In some instances legislation that was not approved by the physicians has been passed. But the doctors refused to work under the legislation and new regulations have had to be made. Undoubtedly we can do the same thing, if we wish, in the United States.

Every Precaution

Every precaution must be taken to avoid the appearance of a selfish motive before the public.

We have done our best to provide a good program along sound lines in Minnesota. If we have failed it is not because we have not tried or because we have lacked the close cooperation of the medical profession.

DR. W. A. COVENTRY, Duluth: In all this discussion, too little emphasis is placed upon preventive medicine, it seems to me.

Our programs of preventive medicine should be carried on vigorously and amplified if possible. For instance, better mental hygiene would do a good deal to prevent overcrowding of insane asylums and considerable research should be done on this line alone. There is no doubt that hospitals should make some arrangement

whereby they can give cheaper service, especially for the man in the low income group. The man on relief must, of course, receive care without cost.

DR. J. W. GAMBLE, Albert Lea: Doctors have been too close-mouthed. What we need now is some means of presenting our views to the public as impressively as the views of our critics have been presented. Newspapers, magazines, radio programs, have been full of criticism of the doctors. It is time for the doctors to take the public into their confidence.

DR. S. H. BOYER, SR., Duluth: We hear a great deal about "adequate medical service." But what is "adequate medical service"? Actually, we all know that service is a relative matter. What one person might consider adequate service another might regard as neglect. To one person four visits a day might be regarded as adequate service. To another one visit in two days might be ample. Adequate medical service is not an absolute but a relative matter and a matter which causes great difficulty whenever any group plan for medical service is contemplated.

DR. R. L. SCAMMON, Minneapolis, distinguished service professor of the graduate school of the University of Minnesota: We live in a mixed world. We use public water to bathe in a private bath with private soap. We go down to a breakfast which includes milk that is publicly inspected, in which, in fact, the only private thing is our spoons.

The real question is: where shall we draw the line between the things that are best as public functions and those that are best as private functions.

Medical Secrets

Medicine partakes conspicuously of both a public and a private function. It has always partaken of this dual function. In Rome there were codes for private functions of medicine. Even the barbarians set up their own codes. Such codes can be traced back to Greece and all over the civilized world.

Physicians, in fact, are often said to have medical secrets, to be in secret cliques. Now it seems to me, speaking not as a medical man —which I am not—but as a citizen, that these medical secrets are essential for the physician. In the same manner, a wife is permitted to have secrets and is not required to testify against her husband. A solicitor also has secrets and if he discloses confidential information given him by his client he may be called before the bar association. In the field of religious belief there are also inviolable secrets. We all have the right of confession, of pouring out our woes secure in the knowledge that our confessor or minister will not be obliged to disclose our confidences.

For Decent Reserves

The same thing is true for the doctor in his private practice. A great many people come to the doctor with all of their personal difficulties and it is necessary for him to preserve that confidence.

No doubt more criminals might be caught if the lawyer or the wife disclosed the information in their possession.

The point is—and a point which I wish to make at the start—there is a certain set of reticences that must be preserved no matter what the cost. These reserves are what make decent society possible.

The advance in the public field of medicine has been most remarkable. But there is another field, the field of private practice, and upon it rests the dignity of man. And while we recognize the field of public medicine we know there are diseases which cannot be cured.

None of us are going to live forever. Our population is changing. We are dealing more and more with degenerative diseases which we can't cure yet. The public as a whole does not understand that fact and it is purely misunderstanding that they do not keep the matter clearly in mind.

Plans Must Be Localized

Now as to insurance, about which I have been asked to speak to you today: I believe an insurance scheme could be worked out in this country but it would have to be a highly localized scheme because our people are so different in different localities. I believe also that it could be worked out so as to keep what I consider to be one of the decencies of civilization, the right of the individual to go to the physician of his choice.

In my opinion, however, we cannot expect to give an extremely high grade of medical care under such a system, any more than we could provide an extremely high grade of shoes or of housing.

Wealth Not Great

This country is the richest in the world and also the most populous of civilized countries. In population it is not to be compared with France or Germany; and, looked at from the point of view of the population, its wealth is not so great.

In the state of Minnesota the last figures we worked out for 1933 showed that the average family income was about $1,750 and that only six per cent of the people were earning $2,500 or more a year. If the total income were divided among the entire population, it would yield a mere $90 a year per person. Obviously, the difficulty in "soaking the rich" is that we should have to use bird shot to do it.

Under a system of voluntary insurance it is possible that the people who need the service most will not purchase it. Certainly life insurance under the voluntary system has not worked. Even in our most prosperous year, 1929, we could insure only enough people to protect us for thirteen months.

"Like a Dinosaur"

In any case there is only so much you can give, just as there are only so many shoes and so much food. Probably it is better to spread it. Certainly it is better to have a local rather than a national system. This is a large country and, like a dinosaur, its head is a long way from its feet.

The system of insurance in effect in England is extremely variable. It works well in the North and not in the South and the fault probably is neither with the system nor the physicians but rather with the English people. The system is largely affected, of course, by the caste system. Many men are eligible and won't accept it because they do not want to be identified with the working class. In any case, it is a grave mistake to think that the system worked out in one country can be lifted and applied as it is to another.

Essential Factors

We have some interesting samples of health insurance in this country but we cannot follow the plan of manufacturing people in any general form of insurance since the manufacturing companies select their people for insurance.

Perhaps the most important factors to be considered are these:

1. The plan would have to be localized.

2. It should not try to do too much, especially on the present income of the United States.

3. It would have to protect the confidential relationship between patient and physician.

In her recent report, Miss Roche gave 4½ per cent as the figure for medical expenditures in this country. That figure is probably wrong since it depends on a discredited study. But compare it with the German figure. In Germany about nine per cent of the worker's income is taken for health.

Everybody a Cousin

In the Scandinavian countries sickness insurance seems to work. I never could understand why, except that Sweden, for instance, is a small compact country and the age distribution is in the wealth-producing period. Also, Sweden did not get into the world war. Instead the Swedes devoted themselves to making money.

As in England, in Sweden everybody is cousin to everybody else. With that close relationship comes a sense of responsibility.

Professional Success

The difference between business and professional success is that success in business lies in making profits and success in a profession lies in the conduct of the job.

We should remember that there is all the difference in the world between maintaining standards which are occasionally violated and abandoning our standards altogether.

"BE ON GUARD"

(Monthly Editorial Prepared by the Medical Advisory Committee.)

Medicine is in the limelight. The public eye is focused on medical practice and medical men. Physicians and hospitals are being censured for the type of medical care which has been and is being given the people, especially those in the low income group.

716

Your Medical Advisory Committee finds that the great majority of the cases brought against members of our Association and reported to the committee come from the so-called indigent group.

It is easy for a lawyer to build up a case about this type of patient, sympathy is easily raised, and juries are readily swayed to give substantial verdicts.

Your committee warns you against any apparent neglect or indifference to them. Guard your words of advice carefully. Give the same careful consideration to their needs as you would to the man who can pay the highest fee, and keep records.

Remember, once having assumed the care of a case, you must continue attendance until discharged by the patient, until the patient has recovered, or another man has assumed the care with the consent of the patient or legal guardian.

MINNESOTA STATE BOARD OF MEDICAL EXAMINERS

Correspondence School Student Pleads Guilty to Unlawful Practice of Healing

Re: State of Minnesota vs. L. Leo O'Leary

L. Leo O'Leary, 23 years of age, entered a plea of guilty in the District Court, at Moorhead, Minnesota, on August 24, 1938, to an information charging him with practicing healing without a basic science certificate. O'Leary was arrested on August 16, 1938, following the filing of a complaint against him by Mr. Brist on behalf of the Minnesota State Board of Medical Examiners. O'Leary inserted a professional card in the Barnesville Record Review under date of July 7, 1938, reading as follows:

L. LEO O'LEARY
Drugless Therapy
Electro-Hydro, Therapy, Treatments
Dietetics and Baths
Office at Broadway Hotel
Hours 1-6 and by appointment
Phone 72

O'Leary also furnished the newspaper with a news item in which he referred to himself as a "drugless therapist" and that he had studied at the "National College of Drugless Physicians in Chicago." O'Leary was arraigned before E. U. Wade, Justice of the Peace at Moorhead, Minnesota, on August 17, 1938, at which time he waived his preliminary hearing and was held to the District Court under bond of $300.00, which he did not furnish. After eight days in the Clay County jail, O'Leary entered a plea of guilty before the Honorable Anton Thompson, Judge of the District Court. O'Leary stated that he started a three months correspondence course at the Swedish College of Massage in Chicago; that he was to pay approximately $30.00 for the course, but had only paid $3.00 and received a half dozen lessons. O'Leary maintained office hours only in the afternoon, devoting the mornings to the sale of aluminum ware. Judge Thompson,

OF GENERAL INTEREST

on being fully advised of the facts, sentenced O'Leary to a term of one year in the Clay County jail, suspending the sentence and placing the defendant on probation upon several conditions, the first one being that O'Leary is to refrain from practicing healing in any manner unless he is licensed. The Court, also, ordered O'Leary to pay his personal obligations at Barnesville, Minnesota, on or before March 1, 1939, and to pay the Court costs within 60 days. Judge Thompson, in no uncertain terms, told the defendant that the practice of healing, without being licensed, amounts to swindling and the obtaining of money under a false pretense.

The Minnesota State Board of Medical Examiners wishes to acknowledge the very fine cooperation extended by Mr. James A. Garrity, County Attorney at Moorhead, Minnesota, in the prosecution of this case.

OF GENERAL INTEREST

Dr. E. C. Hanson, formerly of Park Rapids, is now located at Austin, Minnesota.

* * *

Dr. R. H. La Bree of Minneapolis has joined the staff of the Fergus Falls State Hospital.

* * *

Dr. A. B. Rosenfield of Pequot, has been appointed school doctor for the pupils of the Hibbing schools.

* * *

Dr. Arnold Settlage, formerly of Stow, Ohio, has recently become affiliated with the Worthington Clinic.

* * *

Dr. Harry Palmer, formerly of Eveleth, has located at Blackduck, where he is taking over the practice of Dr. D. J. Jacobson.

* * *

Dr. D. W. Cummings, son of the late Dr. D. S. Cummings of Waseca, has returned to Waseca for the practice of medicine, after an absence of several years.

* * *

Dr. C. O. Erickson, formerly on the staff of the Fergus Falls State Hospital, has been appointed Assistant Superintendent of the Rochester State Hospital.

* * *

Dr. D. J. Jacobson, formerly of Blackduck, has located in Bemidji, where he will continue the practice of medicine.

* * *

Dr. James Chessen, of Duluth, has accepted a position at the Washington University postgraduate medical school, in the department of otolaryngology.

* * *

Dr. D. J. Jacobson, formerly of Blackduck, and Dr. W. M. Haller, who has been associated with the Civilian Conservation Corps at Pike Bay, Cass Lake, have opened a suite of offices in Bemidji.

* * *

Dr. Gordon R. Kamman, Saint Paul, opened new offices at 1044 Lowry Medical Arts Building, September 10. Dr. Kamman limits his practice to neurology and psychiatry. His office hours are from two until five.

* * *

Governor E. A. Benson has appointed Dr. John Esser of Perham to the State Board of Health to succeed

Dr. S. Z. Kerlan of Aitkin, who has left the state. Dr. A. G. Schulze of Saint Paul has also been appointed to the Board by the Governor to succeed Dr. N. G. Mortensen of Saint Paul.

* * *

Dr. V. E. Quanstrom has returned to Brainerd, where he will be associated with Dr. R. A. Beise. Dr. Quanstrom has recently completed several years of special work and study in surgery under Dr. Alton Achsner at the Tulane University, New Orleans.

After twenty-five years as chief of the Department of Obstetrics and Gynecology at the University of Minnesota, Dr. Jennings C. Litzenberg will complete his active service this month. An appreciation dinner will be held for him at the Minnekahda Club, Minneapolis, at 6 o'clock, Friday evening, October 14, the evening following the Homecoming Game with the University of Michigan. All former students and colleagues of Dr. Litzenberg are invited to attend. Application for tickets may be made to Dr. E. C. Maeder, 732 Eighth Avenue South, Minneapolis.

Silver Anniversary Dinner of the Glen Lake Sanatorium

The growth of Glen Lake Sanatorium, Hennepin County's tuberculosis hospital, from a three-cottage unit of fifty beds to a great, modern institution with facilities for the care of 750 patients, was reviewed at a silver anniversary dinner held at the sanatorium, September 9, honoring the twenty-five years of service of the Glen Lake Sanatorium Commission, its governing board.

E. C. Gale and J. R. Kingman, lay members of the commission, who have served continuously for the past twenty-five years, were guests of honor. Dr. F. H. Harrington, Minneapolis health commissioner, is the third member of the commission. Dr. S. Marx White and the late Dr. John W. Bell preceded him in that office.

The contribution which the sanatorium has made to the sum total of scientific knowledge on tuberculosis was emphasized by Dr. Donald Balfour, Director of the Mayo Foundation.

More than 350 representatives of local and state public health agencies, the medical profession, civic groups and church organizations attended the dinner.

NOTICE

Hereafter all communications to the Minnesota State Medical Association should be addressed to 493 Lowry Medical Arts Building, Saint Paul. Executive offices of the Association have been moved from 11 W. Summit Avenue, Saint Paul, to that address.

OCTOBER, 1938

717

REPORTS and ANNOUNCEMENTS

WOMAN'S AUXILIARY

Mrs. W. B. Roberts, President
2735 Irving Avenue South, Minneapolis.
Mrs. E. V. Goltz, Press and Publicity, St. Paul, Minn.

MEDICAL BROADCAST FOR OCTOBER

The Minnesota State Medical Association Morning Health Service.

The Minnesota State Medical Association broadcasts weekly at 9:45 o'clock every Saturday morning over Station WCCO, Minneapolis and Saint Paul (810 kilocycles or 370.2 meters).

Speaker: William A. O'Brien, M.D., Associate Professor of Pathology and Preventive Medicine, Medical School, University of Minnesota.

The program for the month will be as follows:

October 1—Pellagra.

October 8—Visual Errors.

October 15—Influenza.

October 22—How to Gain Weight.

October 29—Loss of Teeth.

THE MINNESOTA MEDICAL ALUMNI ASSOCIATION PROGRAM

From 8:30 to 12:00 on Friday morning, October 14, there will be a program of clinics to be held in Todd Amphitheatre of the University Hospitals, Dr. Harold G. Benjamin, chairman.

Clinics

DR. RALPH T. KNIGHT, Associate Professor and Director of the Division of Anesthesia.

DR. HORACE NEWHART, Professor of Otolaryngology.

DR. IRVINE McQUARRIE, Professor of Pediatrics.

DR. O. H. WANGENSTEEN, Professor of Surgery.

DR. J. L. McKELVEY, Professor of Obstetrics.

DR. CECIL J. WATSON, Associate Professor and Director of the Division of Internal Medicine.

DR. J. C. McKINLEY, Professor of Neurology and head of the Department of Medicine.

12:15 to 1:15—Luncheon in the Nurses' Hall at the weekly hospital staff meeting by courtesy of Mr. Ray Amberg, Superintendent of the Hospital.

1:15—Annual business meeting, Dr. Robert L. Wilder, President.

Additional Activities of the Homecoming Weekend

Appreciation dinner for Dr. J. C. Litzenberg, the retiring chief of the Department of Obstetrics, at the Minikahda Club at 6:00 p. m., Friday, October 14.

Following the homecoming game, Saturday, between Minnesota and Michigan, there will be a tea in the Nurses' Hall with dancing and refreshments. This event is sponsored by the nurses, who are inviting the attendance of student and graduate nurses, doctors, dentists, dental hygienists and medical technicians.

THE sixteenth annual convention of the Women's Auxiliary to the Minnesota State Medical Association was held in Duluth, June 29, 30, and July 1, with Mrs. J. F. Norman of Crookston, president, presiding. Registration at the Hotel Duluth, Wednesday, June 29, followed by the Executive Board meeting at 10:30 in the Royal Room of the Chamber of Commerce, opened the session. In the afternoon a delightful tea was given in honor of the visitors at the Woman's Club and the same evening a Public Health meeting was held in the Orpheum theater. Thursday morning at 10 o'clock the annual meeting of the Auxiliary was held at the Northland Country Club at which Mrs. M. G. Gillespie, president of the St. Louis County Auxiliary, gave the address of welcome with Mrs. C. L. Oppegaard of Crookston, responding. A memorial service was given by Mrs. W. W. Moir of Minneapolis. Reports from the various chairmen and county presidents were read and the meeting closed with the election of officers. A luncheon followed at the Northland Country Club, and members heard Dr. Howard W. Haggard, Associate Professor of Applied Physiology, Sheffield Scientific School, Yale University, speak on "The Social Side of Medical Progress." Newly elected officers were presented and the Auxiliary members were greeted by the newly elected president, Mrs. W. B. Roberts of Minneapolis. A post-convention Board meeting followed. The annual banquet was held at the Hotel Duluth at 6:30 that evening with Dr. J. M. Hayes, president of the Minnesota State Medical Association, as the toastmaster. Mrs. W. B. Roberts, the newly elected president of the Woman's Auxiliary, was presented and greetings were extended by Dr. Irvin Abell of Louisville, president of the American Medical Association, and an address by Dr. Howard W. Haggard. Dancing followed. Owing to the weather conditions the delightfully planned trip on Lake Superior had to be cancelled but a group of women enjoyed having luncheon on board the boat. The warm friendship and hospitality of the members of St. Louis County Auxiliary made up entirely for the lack of sunshine and pleasant weather conditions.

The following appointments have been made by the newly elected president, Mrs. W. B. Roberts. The medical advisory council will include Dr. J. M. Hayes and Dr. C. B. Wright of Minneapolis and Dr. W. A. Coventry, of Duluth. The advisory committee of the Auxiliary is composed of Mrs. Charles W. Mayo, Rochester; Mrs. A. A. Passer, Olivia; Mrs. Benjamin Davis, Duluth, and Mrs. Charles Bolsta, Ortonville. Mrs. W. W. Moir of Minneapolis has been appointed corresponding secretary and Mrs. M. S. Hirschfield of Duluth parliamentarian. Mrs. J. A. Thabes of Brainerd is historian. The committee chairmen chosen from various parts of the state are: Legislative, Mrs. E. A. Eberlin of Glenwood; Finance, Mrs. James Blake of Hopkins; Public Relations, Mrs. A. F. Branton, Willmar; Hygeia, Mrs. W. W. Will, Bertha; Health Education, Mrs. H. E. Wunder, Shakopee; Press and Publicity, Mrs. E. V. Goltz, St. Paul; Exhibits, Mrs. Harrold Wahlquist, Minneapolis; Archives, Mrs. S. S. Hesselgrave, St. Paul; Printing, Mrs. Frederick Erb, Minneapolis, and Revisions, Mrs. E. C. Eshelby, St. Paul.

Members of the Social Committee are: Mrs. Martin Nordland, Minneapolis; Mrs. E. M. Hammes, Saint Paul; Mrs. F. J. Elias, Duluth; Mrs. F. A. Figi, Rochester.

Elective members of the Executive Board include: Mrs. A. C. Baker, Fergus Falls, president elect; Mrs. John F. Norman, Crookston, past president; Mrs. Malcolm Gillespie, Duluth, first vice president; Mrs. J. J. Ryan, Saint Paul, second vice president; Mrs. G. E. Hertel, Austin, third vice president; Mrs. George Earl, Saint Paul, fourth vice president; Mrs. R. J. Josewski, Stillwater, recording secretary; Mrs. Russell Noice, Minneapolis, treasurer, and Mrs. T. M. Fleming, St. Cloud, auditor.

Mrs. Roberts asked the members to pursue definite health projects in the coming year and to fulfill the Auxiliary's dual purpose of assisting the State Medical Association and the county auxiliaries. She stated that the scope of the Auxiliary's service had widened from the original function of promoting fellowship and mutual understanding within the medical profession to include, now, an effort to create better understanding among lay groups of what the medical profession is trying to do for public welfare.

At the request of the Minnesota Medical Association, the Auxiliary will give special attention this year to the need for immunization against communicable diseases. The Auxiliary will continue its support of the campaign to control cancer and the fight against tuberculosis. Members are urged to undertake, in their everyday contacts, to spread the gospel of regular and thorough physical examinations by competent physicians as a preventative measure. Mrs. Roberts recommended popularizing legitimate and reliable health magazines, such as *Hygeia*, published by the American Medical Association, and *Everybody's Health*, issued by the Minnesota Public Health Association. As a special project, she suggested that the Auxiliary sponsor or stimulate interest in the showing of health motion pictures. "Any legitimate and ethical means at our command should not be overlooked to emphasize the unselfish and willing devotion of the honest medical practitioner to a suffering world."

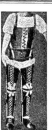
CLASSIFIED ADVERTISING

MINNESOTA STATE MEDICAL ASSOCIATION

Eighty-Fifth Annual Meeting
June 28, 29, 30 and July 1, 1938
Duluth, Minnesota

HOUSE OF DELEGATES

First Meeting
Tuesday Afternoon, June 28, 1938

THE first session was called to order by Dr. W. W. Will, Bertha, speaker of the house, at 3:30 p. m., Tuesday, June 28.

Following brief greetings from Dr. Irvin Abell of Louisville, Kentucky, president of the American Medical Association, and a report from Dr. F. J. Lexa, Lonsdale, chairman of the Committee on Credentials, showing a quorum of members to be present, Reference Committees were appointed and committee reports assigned to them as follows by the speaker:

Scientific Reference Committees

Medical Education Reports

A. E. Cardle...Minneapolis
(Appointed to act as Chairman in place of Dr. C. J. Ehrenberg, who was absent because of illness)
J. R. Aurelius...St. Paul
P. J. Hiniker...Le Sueur
H. A. Roust..Montevideo

Miscellaneous Scientific Reports

C. L. Roholt..Waverly
F. M. Gamble..Albert Lea
F. H. Magney..Duluth
C. O. Maland..Minneapolis
C. A. McKinlay..Minneapolis

Non-Scientific Reference Committees

Credentials Committee

F. J. Lexa...Lonsdale
B. A. McIver...Lowry
E. A. Thayer...Truman

Lay Education Reports

F. J. Elias..Duluth
(Appointed to act as Chairman in place of Dr. J. W. Helland, who was absent)
H. C. Cooney...Princeton
B. A. Smith..Crosby
E. J. Wohlrabe..Springfield

Medical Economics Reports

M. C. Piper...Rochester
G. I. Badeaux...Brainerd
H. W. Goehrs...St. Cloud
J. C. Jacobs...Willmar
A. G. Liedloff..Mankato

Officers and Council Reports

S. A. Slater..Worthington
E. S. Boleyn..Stillwater
W. F. Braasch..Rochester
A. J. Lewis..Henning
J. F. Norman..Crookston

State Health Relations Reports

A. H. Zachman..Melrose
O. W. Holcomb...St. Paul
R. H. Wilson..Winona

By motion duly seconded and carried, reading of the minutes of the last meeting of the House of Delegates was dispensed with and the meeting was recessed at 3:40 p. m. to permit the Reference Committees to con-

sider and prepare their reports on the committee reports submitted to them.

The meeting was re-convened at 7:55 p. m. by Speaker W. W. Will.

DR. WILL: I think we are all in full agreement that the House of Delegates wields a most far-reaching influence in our state. As I look over the group before me I see many who have been active in the affairs of our Association in the past and I am encouraged to believe that all have been elected because of a keen interest in the welfare of organized medicine. I hope that all of you will make detailed reports of the business that is transacted here at the first meeting of your respective societies. I hope, also, that all of you will feel free to take an active part in the discussions and to make any criticism or suggestion that may occur to you, both as to the business under discussion and as to the conduct of the meeting. One of our councilors remarked to me today that he was surprised at the valuable suggestions offered by delegates at a preliminary group meeting in his district. If it is timidity that prevents the delegates from offering suggestions here, may I ask you gentlemen not to be timid. This is your meeting; it will be your fault if our discussion tonight does not cover the things in which you as delegates are interested.

Following a report by Doctor Lexa, chairman of the Committee on Credentials, which was accepted by the House and which showed that a quorum of members was present, Speaker Will called upon Dr. George Earl of St. Paul, Chairman of the Council, for a report of the day's Council meetings.

Doctor Earl reported as follows and his report was accepted by the delegates:

REPORT OF THE COUNCIL

Three hospital or medical service plans on the prepayment basis were discussed and motions that we secure more information about them were duly passed. They included the American Benefit Association plan, a plan offered by a commercial insurance company; the Hawaii Medical Service Association, sponsored by a group of laymen and some doctors acting as individuals; the Toronto Medical Society plan sponsored, as indicated, by the medical society of Toronto.

An estimate was submitted by R. R. Rosell, executive secretary of the Association, showing that this Annual Meeting will undoubtedly pay for itself and that it will be unnecessary to draw upon the fund of $1,500 allotted in the budget to Annual Meeting expense. An increase of 95 members over last year was also reported by Mr. Rosell.

The Minnesota Social Hygiene Institute of Minneapolis, likewise reported upon by Mr. Rosell, was thoroughly investigated by Dr. A. J. Chesley, executive officer and secretary of the Minnesota Department of Health and found to be a lay organization without qualified medical advice or sponsorship, organized without consulting any of the constituted health authorities for the purpose of public health education on venereal disease. The Council directed that an article on the subject be prepared with the approval of Mr. F. Manley Brist, attorney for the Association, and printed in MINNESOTA MEDICINE.†

It was agreed that copies of the 1938 Roster should be sent as usual to judges of the district courts and of the probate courts of Minnesota for their information and assistance.

It was suggested that members of the Council keep in touch with members of the State Legislature and also with Minnesota members of the House and Senate in Washington. They were urged to express their feeling about current policies that concern medicine or public health, to keep legislators informed about the policy of organized medicine on all these matters and particularly to express their appreciation for the efforts of these legislators to safeguard American medicine and protect the public health.

It was agreed by the Council that the fiscal agency account as reported upon by the Finance Committee is in excellent shape and that the financial condition of the Association as reported upon by the treasurer has been also entirely satisfactory so far this year.

The Council approved the organization of a club to be called "The Fifty Club" and to be made up entirely of members who have been licensed to practice fifty years in Minnesota. These members will be honored as a group by the Association in general on appropriate occasions.

The Council also voted a letter of thanks to be sent to Dr. J. T. Christison and Dr. W. F. Wilson for their gift to the Association of old copies of MINNESOTA MEDICINE and of the *St. Paul Medical Journal* so that files of Association publications might be complete in our state headquarters.

It was decided unanimously that a distinguished service award should be presented on occasion to members of the Association whose contribution to the work of the Association merits such recognition. The following resolution accompanied this action:

"RESOLVED that the Minnesota State Medical Association should provide an appropriate token to be awarded on occasion to members of the Association who have rendered special, valuable and distinguished service to the Association; also, that selection of candidates for this award be left in the hands of the Council."

Other resolutions passed by the Council which are of special interest to the delegates are quoted herewith:

"WHEREAS, the Finance Committee of the Minnesota State Medical Association have carefully investigated the books and records of the Minnesota State Medical Association with the assistance and advice of their auditor, Mr. Byers, and found all entries on the books and records of said Association to be true, correct and proper, and

"WHEREAS, the 'inventories' submitted by the Chairman of the Council have been fully explained and discussed with Mr. Byers, auditor, and it is understood that the items of furniture on this list are in the possession of the Minnesota State Medical Association and that the equipment has been fully accounted for, and

"WHEREAS, all trade contracts have been individually investigated and have been found without exception to be to the financial advantage of the Association, therefore be it

"RESOLVED, that our secretary, E. A. Meyerding, M.D., be highly commended for the manner in which he has handled all Association affairs, and be it further

"RESOLVED, that an expression of appreciation be extended to Doctor Meyerding for the efficient and competent service he has given the Minnesota State Medical Association, and that he be asked to extend this appreciation of the Minnesota State

† The article appeared on page 584 of the August, 1938, issue.

Medical Association to his office staff and business associates for their assistance."

* * *

"WHEREAS, the Finance Committee of the Minnesota State Medical Association has thoroughly investigated the costs of the publication of MINNESOTA MEDICINE by the Bruce Publishing Company, and has also obtained independent estimates on printing and office editorial work, and

"WHEREAS, they have found that the present costs are in no way excessive, although certain suggestions for economies may be suggested by the Editing and Publishing Committee, be it

"RESOLVED, that the Council of the Minnesota State Medical Association extend to the Editing and Publishing Company and to the Bruce Publishing Company their sincere commendation and also their gratitude for the services rendered in such a faithful manner over these many years in developing and producing a journal of exceptional merit."

It was suggested that the earlier action of the House of Delegates, setting apart the Herman M. Johnson Memorial Fund in perpetuity for a lectureship which should appropriately commemorate the work of the late Doctor Johnson and directing that only the income from the fund be used for the purpose, be recalled and re-emphasized at this meeting.

The committee reports, designated under the general title "Medical Education Reports" and reviewed by the Scientific Reference Committee under the chairmanship of Dr. A. E. Cardle of Minneapolis follow:

COMMITTEE ON CANCER

The Committee on Cancer and the Council of the Minnesota State Medical Association have extended their coöperation to the Women's Field Army of the American Society for the Control of Cancer as a means of educating the public in the prevention and cure of cancer.

As part of this coöperation a specimen talk for use of physicians in addressing lay audiences on the subject of cancer was prepared by the committee and sent to every member of the Association with a letter from the committee setting forth its relationship and that of the Council to the Women's Field Army.

It was agreed that county and district medical societies should be requested to coöperate in the educational campaign of the Women's Field Army, also the Women's Auxiliary and that the Councilor in each district should be chief advisor as to plans and policies.

It was also decided that a Speakers' Bureau to be used by the Field Army should be on file at the State Office and that county medical societies in each instance should be consulted as to whether the speaker chosen is satisfactory to them.

It was determined by the Council, meeting with the Committee on Cancer, that the executive committee of the Women's Field Army should consist of the chairman of the Committee on Cancer, the State Commander of the Women's Field Army, the president-elect and secretary of the Minnesota State Medical Association, the state chairman of the American Society for the Control of Cancer, the state treasurer of the Women's Field Army, the chairman of the Committee on Public Health Education of the State Medical Association and representatives of the Field Army, which should be selected by the women's organization and approved by the Committee on Cancer and the Executive Committee as originally constituted. This committee held its first meeting in June, 1938.

Two state-wide cancer meetings under the auspices of the Women's Field Army were held during the year. One was held in Minneapolis, December 8, with Mrs. Marjorie B. Illig of New York, national commander of the women's organization and Dr. F. L. Rector of

Evanston, field representative of the American Society for the Control of Cancer, as guest speakers.

The other was held on the University of Minnesota campus with Dr. C. C. Little, managing director of the American Cancer Society, as principal speaker.

MARTIN NORDLAND, *Chairman*

The Reference Committee recommended acceptance of the report, recorded its appreciation of the interest and coöperation of the Women's Field Army and urged that all members of the Association make use of material available at the State Office to extend cancer education and coöperate with their local committees which are working on the cancer problem. The report was accepted.

COMMITTEE ON DIABETES

Revision of the booklet "Diabetes, How to Make It Harmless" was discussed at a meeting of the committee, June 4, and delayed by decision of the committee because treatment is in a state of flux at present. Members will study revision during the coming year. They propose, also, to draw up a series of short paragraphs for lay education on control and treatment of diabetes; to ask approval of the delegates for an effort to obtain a dietitian or nurse dietitian to be paid out of relief funds for the education of diabetic relief clients; to attempt to determine the attitude of industry toward diabetics and their employment.

H. B. SWEETSER, JR., *Chairman*

The Reference Committee recommended acceptance of the report, suggested that the problem of obtaining help for the education of relief clients is a local problem and should be handled locally, and agreed with the committee that the medical profession should stand ready to help both employer and employe to solve the diabetes problem as it relates to industry. It was further noted that the diabetes booklet in its present form is valuable and should be distributed continuously while the process of revision is carried on. The suggestion was made, however, that the term "harmless", be avoided in the title of the revised publication. The report and suggestions of the Reference Committee were accepted by the delegates.

COMMITTEE ON SYPHILIS AND SOCIAL DISEASES

The work of the Committee on Syphilis and Social Diseases is largely advisory at present since there seems to be no need, currently, to expand the venereal disease program of the State Board of Health in Minnesota; furthermore, no funds are available for any additional program.

The program of the State Board of Health has been well established for many years and has the approval of the Committee. At the suggestion of representatives of the American Social Hygiene Association, a special educational campaign has been carried on jointly in two or three localities of the state by the Junior Chamber of Commerce and the local medical society. The campaign carried on in Saint Paul by the Ramsey County Medical Society and the Junior Chamber of Saint Paul was notably successful.

Current public interest in the control of venereal disease has been utilized by fakers and commercial organizations, among the latter being the Minnesota Social Hygiene Institute, which proved, upon investigation, to have no qualified medical backing. Every effort should be made to eliminate unnecessary and unauthorized undertakings of this sort.

S. E. SWEITZER, *Chairman*

The Reference Committee approved the report, commending the committee for its work, and the delegates accepted it. The hope was expressed that the committee would continue the work of investigating non-medical organizations that might in the future attempt to exploit the program of venereal disease control.

Dr. T. H. Sweetser, chairman of the Committee on State Health Relations, said from the floor that the State Board of Health, from whose meeting he had just come, would consider the venereal disease program the next morning in the light of the new legislation on the matter just passed by Congress. The Board had expressed itself as anxious to have members of the Committee on Syphilis and Social Diseases present at the morning meeting so that they might have the opinion of the committee as well as of the Council, which had also been invited to attend. Members of the Board also suggested, according to Doctor Sweetser, that the House of Delegates might wish to make some official statement, concerning lay associations that are collecting money, ostensibly to further the venereal disease program but actually for commercial purposes.

The speaker recommended that the Committee on Syphilis and Social Diseases attend the State Board of Health meeting and make whatever recommendations to the House that they should see fit.

COMMITTEE ON DEAFNESS PREVENTION AND AMELIORATION

Activities of the Committee on Deafness Prevention and Amelioration during the past year have included exhibits at the state meeting of 1937 in Saint Paul and at the Minnesota State Fair in September of the same year. Also demonstration hearing surveys in several colleges and communities, in connection usually, with public health or parent-teacher meetings. The committee also worked for passage of a bill to provide means for a more adequate public health program including hearing testing in the schools. The bill failed of passage but much interest was created in the problem, particularly of hard-of-hearing children in the schools.

Increasing interest in acquirement of modern equipment for testing hearing on the part of schools has been demonstrated in the past year. In the opinion of the committee every community having a school population of 2,000 or more should own its own equipment for testing hearing. The need is especially urgent in rural districts.

The work of the committee should be continued and a reasonable grant made to carry out its activities.

HORACE NEWHART, *Chairman*

The Reference Committee approved the report, commending the committee for its work, recommended acceptance of the report and appropriation of the grant requested for continuance of the work. It was suggested that any information in the possession of the committee on mechanical devices for testing the hearing and also for the aid of the hard-of-hearing be placed at the disposal of the profession. The report was accepted.

Doctor Newhart emphasized in a supplemental discussion of his report the need for additional funds. He emphasized, also, the need to rouse local interest in each community in the work of the committee. It is the hope of the committee that a state-wide program can be established within the next few months; but it cannot be done without the active aid and leadership in each locality of members of the profession. The co-operation of the delegates was earnestly invited.

COMMITTEE ON MATERNAL AND CHILD WELFARE

With the collaboration of the Committee on Maternal Welfare and the Committee on Hospitals and Medical Education of the State Association, also of the University of Minnesota, the Minnesota Department of Health conducted the first series of postgraduate courses, so-called "refresher courses," in obstetrics and pediatrics in the state in May and June of 1937. These courses were sufficiently successful to warrant similar courses this year but with the difference that the 1938 courses were all given on one day instead of a weekly intervals. In 1937 the courses were given in Worthington, Brainerd, St. Cloud, Fergus Falls, Grand Rapids and Mankato. In 1938 they were given in Crookston, Winona, Hibbing, Willmar, Albert Lea, Fergus Falls, Worthington and Bemidji. The total attendance in 1937 was 1,005, a weekly average of 167½. Complete attendance reports have not been obtained as yet for this year's courses, but the indications are that the course was well received.

The newly organized State Society of Obstetrics and Gynecology held its last semi-annual meeting in St. Paul in April. Largely as a result of the efforts of this society the Central Association of Obstetricians and Gynecologists will hold its annual three-day meeting in Minneapolis next October, a further evidence of the growing interest in maternal welfare in Minnesota.

Maternal mortality rate for 1937 in Minnesota was 3.0 per 1,000 live births and the infant rate was 40.8. This is by far the lowest rate reported by any state in the United States.

R. D. MUSSEY, *Chairman*

The Reference Committee commended the work of the committee, endorsed the postgraduate lecture courses and recommended their continuance and the acceptance of the report by the delegates. The report was accepted.

The committee reports designated as "Miscellaneous Scientific Reports" and reviewed by the Scientific Reference Committee under the chairmanship of Dr. C. L. Roholt of Waverly, follow:

COMMITTEE ON HOSPITALS AND MEDICAL EDUCATION

The new experiment in postgraduate medical education, now in its second year at the Center for Continuation Study, University of Minnesota, under the direction of Dr. W. A. O'Brien, also, the postgraduate courses in obstetrics and pediatrics carried on in key communities throughout the state under the direction of the Division of Child Hygiene of the State Board of Health, are new centers of activity in this type of education.

This committee and the State Office have assisted in both programs. The committee also consulted with Dr. Hamilton H. Anderson of the Council on Medical Education and Hospitals, American Medical Association, concerning a survey of postgraduate education in Minnesota which later was made in coöperation with the State Office. A résumé of this survey was printed in the *Journal of the American Medical Association,* March 5, 1938, page 136B.

It seems obvious that the postgraduate courses sponsored and financed solely by the State Association are not now needed in Minnesota.

JAMES B. CAREY, *Chairman*

The Reference Committee recommended acceptance of the report with the following substitution for the final paragraph of the report:

"It appears to the committee to be too early to state that postgraduate courses sponsored and financed solely by the state association are not needed."

The delegates accepted the report with the change recommended.

SUB-COMMITTEE ON PUBLIC HEALTH NURSING

In conjunction with a representative of the Public Health Nursing Department, a set of Orders and Policies to guide nurses employed in boys' and girls' summer camps was formulated and copies sent to the members of this committee for their suggestions and approval. All committee members heard from approved, and mimeographed copies of the subject matter will be sent to nurses so employed.

H. F. BAYARD, *Chairman*

In compliance with the recommendation of the Reference Committee the delegates accepted the report.

COMMITTEE ON MILITARY AFFAIRS

The current status of Medical Reserves in Minnesota may be detailed as follows: For the Army—6 Colonels, 13 Lieutenant Colonels, 12 Majors, 48 Captains, 304 First Lieutenants. For the Navy—24 Lieutenant Commanders, 12 Lieutenants and 3 Lieutenants, Junior grade.

The profession is to be commended for careful examination of C. M. T. C. applicants. Medical Reserve Officers who are designated by the Chief of Staff of the First Reserve Area to serve on Boards for Appointment and Promotion are urged to adhere to regulations strictly so that personnel in the Reserve Corps may be of the type desired for service in the Army.

The ninth successive Medico-Military Inactive Duty Training Course of the Mayo Foundation was held this year at Rochester with 32 states represented and a total of 1,164 enrolled during the past nine years for the course. Several other medical centers throughout the country have also instituted courses recently. They are patterned after the original "Skinner Plan" employed since 1929 by the Mayo Foundation.

Funds allotted by War Department to the Surgeon General have been inadequate for training of medical reserve officers ordered to Flight Surgeon's School for practical training. Also, the War Department ruling grounding all but five of the 285 flight surgeons in the regular army, national guards and reserves, will handicap the aviation medical service, in the opinion of the committee, since pilots should be observed under flying conditions as well as on the ground. Every effort should be made to have this ruling annulled.

Reserve officers should avail themselves of all opportunities to participate in army maneuvers,· since much can be learned when serving with the troops in the way of organization, instruction, sanitation and many other details that cannot be learned from books. Medical officers participating in the Fourth Army Maneuvers at Fort Ripley last August acquitted themselves creditably. In the four concentrations of the army there were 1,803 reserves, of whom 16 per cent were in the medical department, ordered to active duty.

Twenty-six medical reserve officers are on CCC duty in Minnesota at the present time. A number of officers on CCC duty have successfully passed army examinations and have entered the regular establishment for their professional careers.

Re-establishment of the medical R. O. T. C. on a voluntary basis at the University has resulted in an enrollment that is far below the enrollment when the training was compulsory. Only 17 medical students enrolled for the training last fall, with 16 for the winter quarter and 13 for the spring quarter. This training should be established on a compulsory basis in order to qualify students for leadership in any branch of the service of the United States in time of emergency.

The bill for amending the National Defense Act to provide uniforms and other allowances to the officers of the Reserve Corps is noted by the committee. It provides for an allowance for each hour of credit earned in Army Extension Courses by members of the Officers' Reserve Corps who are eligible for active duty in excess of the annual minimum of 20 and not to exceed $75 in one year, as well as allowance for uniforms.

Attention of all Reserve Corps officers in the association is called to the Annual Convention of the Association of Military Surgeons to be held at Rochester, October 13, 14 and 15.

LT. COL. F. L. SMITH, *Chairman*

In compliance with the recommendation of the Reference Committee the report was accepted by the delegates.

HISTORICAL COMMITTEE

Two more county histories and several other manuscripts of historical interest have been received by the committee during the past year.

Installments of the "History of Medicine in Minnesota" have appeared regularly since January, 1938, in MINNESOTA MEDICINE, and sufficient material is on hand to continue the installments for at least two years.

Criticisms and correction of the published material are invited so that, should the history later be published in book form, they may be incorporated in an appendix.

The committee will continue to gather data and hopes to receive additional manuscripts from individual members of the Association. It also wishes to thank the Council for its coöperation and support, which have made possible publication of the material.

J. M. ARMSTRONG, *Chairman*

Complying with the recommendation of the Reference Committee, the report was accepted by the delegates.

COMMITTEE ON FRACTURES

A definite fracture program for Minnesota is suggested by the committee to include the following:

I. Creation of a permanent State Fracture Committee to consist of a chairman, appointed by the president and one member from each constituent society.

II. Formation in each constituent society of a fracture committee which should have its representative on the state committee for chairman and which should draw up a definite fracture program for the society, including an annual fracture symposium to be held at one of the regular society meetings.

III. Adoption of the following statewide program to be carried out by the state committee in coöperation with the constituent societies:

A. *First Aid and Transportation.*

1. Adoption throughout the state of the Keller-Blake hinged, half-ring splint for the lower extremity, and the Murray-Jones hinged ring splint for the upper extremity, these splints to be of the size and specifications used by the United States Army.

2. Education of profession and public in use of the splints.

3. Equipment of ambulances throughout the state with these splints; also industrial plants. Hospitals should be equipped likewise for the purpose of exchange with ambulances when patients are brought in with the splints on, since the splints cannot be removed

724

for some time and the ambulance must be on its way.

4. Coöperation with the Red Cross in its First Aid Station work throughout the state (splints are now available at these stations), with the Highway Department and the Boy and Girl Scouts in their First Aid educational program.

B. *Diagnosis.*

1. Adoption of standardized surgical directions to insure proper films and promotion of frequent x-rays to determine reduction and progress of healing.

C. *Hospital Equipment.*

1. For treatment of fractures of the long bones all hospitals should have overhead frames for suspension and traction, simple splints, Thomas arm and leg splints, equipment for skeletal traction; a portable x-ray apparatus.

D. *Treatment.*

1. Liberal constructive discussions should be allowed at society and hospital staff meetings.

It is further suggested by the committee that every annual meeting program should include a fracture symposium and that an exhibit showing first aid in transportation, x-ray diagnosis, hospital equipment, treatment, et cetera, should be arranged by the committee for each meeting.

O. W. YOERG, *Chairman*

The suggestion of a permanent state fracture committee was especially commended by the Reference Committee and, complying with its recommendation, the report was accepted by the delegates.

COMMITTEE ON ASPHYXIA AND ASPHYXIAL DEATH

The increasing use of automobiles and of gas in the home has increased both morbidity and mortality from asphyxia and the committee notes a growing need for the medical profession to give special thought to the subject.

Carbon monoxide is the chief source of poisoning. Most common causes are illuminating gas, exhaust gas from internal combustion motors and coal gas from defective furnaces or stoves.

One thousand asphyxia deaths are estimated to occur weekly in the United States, of which 50 per cent are due to carbon monoxide inhalation, either accidental, suicidal or homicidal. The interiors of about 5 per cent of automobiles on the highways have been found to contain a sufficiently high concentration of carbon monoxide to produce such symptoms as dizziness or collapse. The blood of about 49 per cent of 426 garage employes studied recently was found positive for carbon monoxide, the percentage in the blood of the positive reactors ranging from 5 to 30 per cent.

Recognition of chronic poisoning which develops insidiously due to repeated exposure to sublethal concentrations of gas over a long period of time is important, as well as recognition of acute poisoning. Much still remains to be learned about the subject, but it has entered today into the domain of everyday practice, and the committee hopes to make studies, formulate plans for public education on the subject which may in time serve to reduce the incidence of asphyxia and asphyxial death.

A. E. CARDLE, *Chairman*

Stressing the importance of further study in this field and the need for funds to carry out such work, the Reference Committee recommended acceptance of the report. The report was acceptd.

Committee reports designated "Lay Education Reports" and reviewed by the Non-Scientific Reference Committee under the chairmanship of Dr. F. J. Elias of Duluth acting for Dr. J. W. Helland of Spring Grove, follow:

COMMITTEE ON PUBLIC HEALTH EDUCATION

There is good reason to believe that public health education is the greatest problem that faces the doctor today. When the neglected illness is thoroughly investigated, it usually develops that ignorance or carelessness and not actual lack of medical facilities was the cause of the neglect. The conclusion is inescapable that public health education is fundamental to the solution of the medical problem of this country rather than subsidies to physicians, new laws or new taxes.

It becomes increasingly clear to members of this committee, furthermore, that it is the doctors and not the nurses, social workers or lay health agencies who must direct the educational work.

The Committee on Public Health Education carries on certain state-wide activities which can best be handled from state headquarters. These activities have expanded but will not be truly effective until every individual member is supplementing them by his own efforts in his own community—by initiative in bringing preventive measures to his people, by working intelligently with local health and welfare agencies, and by individual instruction which will bring the people in his community to the doctor promptly, whether or not they are able to pay full fees for his services.

If the patient's income is not sufficient to pay full private fees then the doctor himself must know all of the facilities of the community and state in order to utilize the aid of welfare and relief agencies efficiently for his patient.

Where improvements are needed the doctor must be the first to work intelligently and conscientiously with the responsible officials to improve the situation.

Certainly it is illogical and unjustifiable to embark upon radical and expensive legislative changes until our established agencies have had a chance to show their effectiveness for all the people.

Committee activities for 1937-1938 include the following:

1. The *News Service* prepared under the auspices of the editorial subcommittee which goes weekly to all newspapers in Minnesota, designed especially to provide health instruction and instruction on disease prevention.

2. *Speakers' Bureau* made up of a list of capable speakers from all parts of the state on file at the State Office and available for talks on health and preventive medicine before lay groups of all kinds.

3. *College Lecture Course* designed to reach young men and women in the colleges, who will be the teachers and professional men and women of the future. A series of four or five talks given annually in the majority of the colleges of the state, honorariums and traveling expenses of speakers paid by the Minnesota State Medical Association, arrangements and booking made by the Minnesota Public Health Association.

4. *Speakers' Library*, a file of material maintained at the State Office for use of speakers who are requested to make public health talks before lay audiences.

5. *Hygeia, Everybody's Health.* After a lapse of several years *Hygeia* is now being sent to the members of the State Legislature by order of the Council. Through a special arrangement with the Minnesota Public Health Association, *Everybody's Health* will go with it at a special rate secured for both publications.

6. *4-H Club.*—Annual physical examinations of county contestants for state honors among 4-H Club members in Minnesota. More than 200 boys and girls were examined in 1937 by a group of 11 specialists. Physicians' time is compensated out of the budget of this committee. Arrangements are made by the Minnesota Public Health Association, which also contributes use of its headquarters.

7. *Literature.*—A folder called "Your Child's Health," which was prepared under the supervision of the Editorial subcommittee, was distributed widely in the state this year in coöperation with the Minnesota Public Health Association.

Attention of the members is called especially to the large number of agencies and campaigns independent of Organized Medicine that are now directing their attention to public health education and promotions. In general, these agencies have enlisted the advice and assistance of the State Association. They have great potentialities for good but only if sponsored and directed by physicians. Chief among them are: The Women's Field Army of the American Society for the Control of Cancer; the Syphilis and Venereal Disease campaign sponsored nationally by the United States Public Health Service and the American Social Hygiene Association; the Pneumonia campaign, a campaign for universal typing of pneumonia cases and use of serum for appropriate cases sponsored by large insurance companies and health agencies everywhere and locally by the Minnesota State Department of Health; the Maternal and Child Health program sponsored nationally by the Committee on Maternity and Child Health and materially assisted by new programs financed by Social Security funds—the film "Birth of a Baby," departure in education by motion picture, marked the campaign this year; the Diabetes control campaign, sponsored by a special society in New York fostered in Minnesota by the State Association.

The practicing physician must be thoroughly informed on the objectives and accomplishments of all of these campaigns and programs. Beyond all this, he must be an apostle in his own community to extend information concerning all medical services and all accepted preventive measures. Much is demanded of him, but much will be lost, also, to himself and to the public he serves if he fails to assume this obligation.

L. R. CRITCHFIELD, *Chairman*

SUB-COMMITTEE ON RADIO

Considerable interest has been shown by county medical societies during the past year in the possibility of establishing radio programs in addition to the state association sponsored broadcasts of Dr. W. A. O'Brien from WCCO. In accordance with an action of the Council the committee has encouraged this interest and assisted in obtaining broadcasting material. Arrangements are now under way looking to the possibility of extending Doctor O'Brien's broadcasts by special wire to station KDAL in Duluth.

From May 8, 1937, to June 11, 1938, inclusive, this committee sponsored 42 radio talks by Doctor O'Brien over WCCO in Minneapolis. In addition, there were joint broadcasts on the last Saturday of each month with the Minnesota State Dental Association, amounting to 12 in all. The speaker was Dr. W. A. O'Brien, Associate Professor of Pathology, Preventive Medicine and Public Health of the University of Minnesota. As in the past, the radio station made no charge for the use of its facilities.

The subjects for the period included:

Child Health Day, Some Major Health Problems, Nervous Exhaustion, Avitaminosis, Water Cures, Diverticulitis, Fourth of July Injuries, Dysentery, Pre-School Examinations, Coronary Occlusion, Sore Throat, Diphtheria and Smallpox, Duodenal Ulcer, Insomnia, Heart Disease, Hand Infections, Dietary Dangers, Acute Abdominal Conditions, Diabetes Mellitus, Emotional Stability, Tuberculosis, Nasal Obstruction, Typhoid Fever, Public Health Objectives, Pneumonia Types, Measles Prevention, Early Tuberculosis, Infant Feeding, Scarlet Fever, Asthma in Children, Acute and Chronic Alcoholism, Geriatrics, Communicable Disease Control, Early Diagnosis Campaign, Glaucoma, Brain Tumors, Periodic Health Examinations, Air and Sun, Research and the Hospital, Chronic Illness, and Burns.

On April 2 the committee also sponsored a special broadcast commemorating the tenth anniversary of this radio health education series. Speakers at the regular broadcasting period in the morning were Dr. J. M. Hayes, president of the State Association, Mr. Max Karl, Director of Education of WCCO, and Dr. Robert Burns, chairman of the sub-committee on Radio, together with Doctor O'Brien. At noon representatives of the medical organization, civic organizations, the state dental association, the radio stations, the University of Minnesota and the press were invited to a luncheon to commemorate the event. The Minnesota State Medical Association enjoys the distinction of sponsoring the oldest local broadcast except the market report to be given from Station WCCO. More than 500 talks have been given by Doctor O'Brien, and the program continues to have excellent following. In spite of the fact that there is no attempt to solicit mail, there is a regular flow of questions from listeners. In addition, Doctor O'Brien receives numerous requests to speak in person before all manner of organizations, also to participate in broadcasts sponsored by other organizations and agencies.

The Committee desires to thank Station WCCO for its unfailing courtesy and coöperation and its sincere effort to maintain a definite place on the air for the program. The time, 9:45 a. m. Saturday, has been occupied continuously for many months.

R. M. BURNS, *Chairman*

SUB-COMMITTEE ON SPEAKERS' BUREAU

Speakers and materials have been supplied to all organizations that have requested the service. As far as possible speakers have been chosen from within the neighborhood from which the request came for obvious reasons of economy, though it is occasionally necessary to send speakers on special subjects from a distance.

Many more speakers could be utilized in this work and any person who can give a good talk himself or who knows of someone who is qualified is requested to communicate with the Sub-Committee on the Speakers' Bureau.

F. H. MAGNEY, *Chairman*

With regard to the report of the Committee on Public Health Education and the two sub-committee reports the Reference Committee declared as follows: That the report of the committee as a whole portrays evidence of an exhaustive and well-defined program and of outstanding accomplishments; that the college lecture courses described therein show that a series of well chosen subjects has been delivered by eminently well-qualified members of the profession; that the continuance of the excellent type of education carried on by the radio sub-committee and Doctor O'Brien is of vital importance to the Association and that extension of the program, particularly to the Duluth station, would be a valuable asset if it could be arranged; that, in connection with the work of the Speakers' Bureau, a speakers' bureau should be created within each component society with a view to extending health education by platform talks throughout the state. In accordance with the recommendation of the reference committee the report was approved.

At the invitation of the Speaker, Dr. F. J. Savage of Saint Paul gave the following supplementary report in the absence of Dr. L. R. Critchfield, chairman of the Committee on Public Health Education:

I wish to express the thanks of Doctor Critchfield to Doctor Meyerding and his staff and to Mr. Rosell and his staff for their help in the past year in making

726

our program a success. I wish also to give due credit to the affiliations with the Minnesota Public Health Association in putting over the work and to hope, also, that the association may continue.

—

The committee reports designated as "Medical Economic Reports" and reviewed by the Non-Scientific Reference Committee unnder the chairmanship of Dr. M. C. Piper follow:

COMMITTEE ON MEDICAL ECONOMICS

Members of the Medical Economics Committee and the sub-committees, as provided in the recently adopted constitution, held their first general meeting on Sunday, April 3, of this year in Saint Paul: This meeting was quite unique in the annals of medical organization since the work of the economic sub-committees which, though distinct, often overlaps and causes resultant confusion, could thus be coördinated and programs adjusted. Each sub-committee held its own round table discussions in the course of the morning, calling upon officers, councilors or representatives of other sub-committees for assistance as it might be needed. A general luncheon meeting for all followed, at which the Survey of Medical Facilities was outlined and discussed. Among the speakers were Dr. R. G. Leland, director of the Bureau of Medical Economics of the American Medical Association, Dr. C. B. Wright, trustee and Dr. R. L. Scammon, chairman of the Minnesota State Planning Board.

Details in the conduct of the survey were largely left in the hands of the Executive Secretary, Mr. R. R. Rosell, by the Committee on Medical Economics, which has general supervision of the work. Following is a brief summary of progress:

Information concerning scope and purpose was given initially in the *Journal of the American Medical Association.* The proposal was made first in Minnesota at the February County Officers' Conference, and since then it has been repeatedly publicized in MINNESOTA MEDICINE and in bulletins from the Executive Secretary's office.

Much credit goes to Secretary Rosell for his energetic conduct of the Survey, both from his office and in the field.

Council members have been asked to assume responsibility for the study in their own districts and several have held councilor district meetings to explain requirements to constituent county societies and to stimulate them to complete their portion of the work.

As a result, the Survey has made satisfactory progress in Minnesota. It is in advance here of many states, but much still remains to be accomplished, and this meeting should afford an opportunity for anyone who wishes it to get information and assistance. An exhibit on the survey and proper methods of filling out the Forms is on view in the exhibit hall.

The work of the editorial sub-committee has continued with the able supervision of Mrs. Fitzgerald, and we trust that the members are carefully reading the medical economics columns in which progress in medical economics is publicized each month. Members of the editorial sub-committee are Dr. W. F. Braasch, Dr. A. R. Barnes, Rochester; Dr. A. N. Collins, Duluth; Dr. Lennox Danielson, Litchfield; Dr. E. A. Meyerding, Saint Paul; and Dr. E. S. Platou, Minneapolis.

W. F. BRAASCH, *Chairman*

SUB-COMMITTEE ON PROFESSIONAL EDUCATION IN MEDICAL ETHICS AND SOCIAL AND ECONOMIC TRENDS

Education of undergraduates of the University of Minnesota Medical School in subjects related to medical ethics and to social and economic trends has been under discussion. Heretofore lectures on these subjects have been given periodically to sophomores. Dean H. S. Diehl of the University Medical School is now working on a schedule of similar lectures for seniors which shall include also, at the suggestion of the committee, consideration of medical jurisprudence. The committee recommends that sterilization by vasectomy, except for purely medical reasons, be considered unethical practice by the House of Delegates.

ERLING W. HANSEN, *Chairman*

MEDICAL ADVISORY SUB-COMMITTEE

The Medical Advisory Sub-Committee has had numerous meetings with various other groups interested in lessening of malpractice suits against members. Articles have appeared in MINNESOTA MEDICINE, papers have been given at various society meetings for the purpose of better coöperation among members. A detailed report is to be given verbally before the delegates at this meeting.

B. J. BRANTON, *Chairman*

SUB-COMMITTEE ON STATE HEALTH RELATIONS

The usual assortment of problems related to its work have been referred to this committee and the committee has handled them in coöperation with other committees and with officers of the State Society. We have kept in close touch, also, with the State Board of Health, a representative of the committee having been present at virtually every meeting of the Board.

A survey of medical care at the State Tuberculosis Sanitorium was made by this committee in response to a request of the State Board of Control made to the Council and referred to us. This survey consumed a great deal of time and effort and was, we trust, satisfactory to those concerned. Thanks are especially due to Doctors Tuohy and Geer, who worked with the committee in the undertaking.

The committee is now making a preliminary study of the possibility of developing a program of periodic health examinations for Legionnaires that will be satisfactory to the profession. The request for assistance came from the Rehabilitation Committee of the State Department of the Legion, and we are coöperating with this committee. Various officers of the state association have been kind enough to work with the committee in this preliminary study.

T. H. SWEETSER, *Chairman*

SUB-COMMITTEE ON LOW INCOME AND INDIGENT PROBLEMS

There are three classes to be considered in any discussion of the problem of ability to pay for medical services.

First: Those who are unable to pay any fee whatever. We believe it is the obligation of the federal, state and local governments to provide adequate medical care for this group. In Minnesota this problem has been well handled.

Second: Those who are able to pay moderate fees but are not able to assume unusual obligations incurred by sickness and its accompanying misfortunes; this is the largest group of all.

Third: Those who are able to pay for services rendered. They are omitted for obvious reasons from discussion at this time.

It is generally agreed that medical care of the second group, the "low-income group" is the real problem, and it varies in every part of the United States. Virtually every state in the Union has devised and tried out schemes for more adequate care of the low income group. Many of these schemes have failed. Some have helped in the solution of the difficulty in certain localities. The American Medical Association has

watched the progress of all these schemes and has carefully correlated them with their effects; but no national solution has been found or advised either by the federal government or by the association, though the American Medical Association has volunteered to coöperate with the government in an endeavor to find a solution to the problem.

Various plans for Hospital Insurance are now in operation, such insurance being handled by the hospital groups without outside aid. If some plan of sickness insurance should be devised that would apply in all parts of the United States, the medical profession would demand some part in management of the program. It is a well known fact that the political management of sickness insurance would be a disaster, as it has proved to be by experience with such "set-ups" in foreign countries.

That furtherance of preventive medicine is a function of the federal governmnt is generally agreed. America leads the world in this field today; but much still remains to be done. Why not a program directed toward less sickness as a means of reducing the costs of medical care to all? Is not our problem essentially one of disease prevention with good or better medical care to all, rather than one of medical fees?

Surveys on medical care have been conducted in many states and cities by lay people without the aid of the medical profession. It is well for us to have their side of the story, but as in all other stories, there is another side. And the American Medical Association, with its state affiliates, is making an intensive survey by questionnaires to physicians, hospitals, nurses, health departments, welfare agencies, public and parochial schools and through colleges and universities to discover as nearly accurate data as possible on the needs.

Perhaps from all this a real evaluation of needs and costs to the low income group may be elicited. Then, possibly, a scheme may be devised whereby sickness insurance may assist in providing care which is in the reach of all. There are two tenets that physicians will insist upon in any case. One is that the federal government shall not assume complete control of any plan that may be evolved; second, that the principle already held essential by the government, that the patient shall have free choice of physician, must be maintained.

Knowing well the burden placed upon those in the low-income group, the physicians of America are only too anxious to coöperate with the proper authorities to provide adequate and competent medical care to all.

The possibility of a program of rehabilitation of unemployable relief clients, similar to one now functioning successfully in West Virginia, has been discussed by this committee. The following recommendations were made:

1. That examinations made of all relief clients by the C.W.A. several years ago are now too remote to be of any value in laying plans for a rehabilitation program in Minnesota.

2. That the Minnesota State Medical Association will coöperate in such a program if the State Relief Administration believes the program worthwhile; but that it will be necessary to re-examine all relief clients as a first step toward formulating a program.

At the request of the Farm Security Administration, a plan for providing medical care for clients of the administration was drawn up by the committee and is now under discussion. In general, the plan provides for medical care for the clients at a 40 per cent reduction from prevailing fees in the locality to be paid within 90 days. The Administration, according to the plan, is to provide the doctors with names of the clients in their communities and to make it clear to them that medical care at such fees is only by special arrangement for the period of their association with the Farm Security Administration. Similar plans are in operation in other states.

W. A. COVENTRY, *Chairman*

SUB-COMMITTEE ON INDUSTRIAL RELATIONS

The following resolution is submitted by the Committee for action by Council and House of Delegates:

"WHEREAS in practice, the medical profession has always been in favor of the freedom of patients to choose their own medical advisers and

"WHEREAS only recently a law has been enacted in Minnesota giving the indigent the right to choose his own physician and

"WHEREAS there seems to exist an impression that the Minnesota State Medical Association is not fully in accord with this opinion.

"THEREFORE, Be It Resolved that the Minnesota State Medical Association declare itself in thorough accord and support of the principle that, in the interest of good public policy, the patient shall be permitted to choose his own physician, in cases involving liability and compensation insurance, as well as in private practice."

The Committee also recommends to the Council and the House of Delegates that insurance practice and compensation practice be subject to the code of ethics that governs private practice and offers for their consideration the "Interpretation of the Code of Ethics" which has been in force in the Hennepin County Medical Society since April, 1935, which is as follows:

"Physicians representing insurance carriers or employers in compensation cases or in cases involving public liability are expected to observe the rules laid down in Article IV, Section 3, Principles of Medical Ethics of the American Medical Association the same as physicians in private practice. A physician representing an employer or an insurance carrier may visit and examine as a consultant a patient in charge of another physician but should never take charge of or prescribe for the patient until after the other physician has relinquished the case or has been properly dismissed. This consultation should be arranged in the usual way by obtaining the consent of the attending physician. A request by an employer or an insurance carrier that a physician representing them take charge of the case shall not be considered a proper dismissal of the physician originally in charge. A physician representing an employer or an insurance carrier should never take charge of a patient who has been in charge of another physician unless the latter has been definitely discharged by the patient. In that case it shall be the duty of the physician representing the employer or the insurance carrier to explain to the patient that he has the privilege of choosing his own physician and to inquire whether he changed his physician by reason of duress, or intimidation, or misrepresentation. If the patient chooses to retain his own physician, it shall be unethical for the physician representing the employer or the insurance carrier to take charge of the case. Any case of doubt concerning professional judgment or management of the case or ethics as provided in Article 5, Principles of Medical Ethics of the American Medical Association should be referred to the Board of Censors of the Hennepin County Medical Society through the Ethics Committee for final decision."

A plan similar in general outlines to the Wisconsin plan for handling compensation insurance should be presented to the State Association for consideration. It is the opinion of the committee, however, that the problem differs from Wisconsin in Minnesota and it therefore suggests that a register be kept in every local medical society in the state showing the physicians who desire to engage in practice in which insurance companies are involved. Membership on this list would be optional with each physician; but any member in good standing in his local society should be eligible to enter his name. These names need not be posted or published but should be available for reference by employers, insurance companies or patients. Each local society should be privileged to decide whether it would adopt the plan and it should further have the privilege of adopting its own fee schedule.

M. S. HENDERSON, *Chairman*

SUB-COMMITTEE ON CONTRACT PRACTICE

Two years ago the chairman of the Committee on Contract Practice presented to the House of Delegates the standards relating to contract practice as simplified and revised by the Judicial Council of the American Medical Association for adoption all over the state. They were adopted at that time by the delegates and by a number of county and district societies in the state.

A report on the status of this action in all the counties of the state would be appreciated by the committee so that the matter can be presented again to societies that have not already acted.

The association of certain physicians with a fraternal organization which includes medical care in its benefits has been reported as a possible infringement during the past year. In some instances, physicians have been retained by the organization to take care of members and their families, thus introducing a third party into the relationship and also preventing free choice of physician to the patient. In both these particulars such a contract violates the official standard.

The matter has been under consideration by the Committee on Public Policy, however, with the result that the project has already been abandoned in several communities. Assurance has been given that it will be abandoned universally in the state by June 1 of this year.

The importance of the free choice of physician as a fundamental to the practice of good medical care cannot be brought too frequently to the attention of the physicians, in the opinion of the committee, or to the attention of others concerned in the delivery of medical care.

A so-called "hospital service contract" which includes medical services is being offered currently by certain insurance companies. The committee believes that the fee schedule for medical services should be eliminated from the contract and that the whole matter should be brought to the attention of the delegates.

F. A. OLSON, *Chairman*

EDITING AND PUBLISHING COMMITTEE

Although business conditions in 1937 were adverse with regard to the sale of advertising—this applies especially to the last half of the year—your Editing and Publishing Committee reports some increase in the total revenue from advertising and subscriptions.

MINNESOTA MEDICINE averaged almost 100 pages an issue for the year, the total number of pages printed being 1,168. This is an average of 97.3 pages for each issue. Of this number 826 pages were devoted to reading matter and 340 to advertising. The reading pages included 109 scientific articles in addition to several articles and abstracts of articles published in the Proceedings of the Minnesota Academy of Medicine and the Minneapolis Surgical Society, numbering twenty-six in all. Eight case reports were published. This does not include the case reports included in the body of numerous scientific papers. In addition, the usual sections features such as editorials, reports and announcements of societies, news items, book reviews and the Medical Economics section were given adequate space. The Medical Economics section this year totaled 79 pages, or an average of 6.6 pages each issue. Illustrations published with the various papers numbered 232, or an average of almost 20 an issue.

At the close of 1937, records showed the total number of paid membership subscriptions to be 2,147, with about 115 subscriptions carried the first part of the year as delinquent accounts. There were 180 non-member subscriptions. Miscellaneous distribution, including single copy sales, exchanges, complimentary copies, advertisers' checking copies, et cetera, numbered 303 copies, leaving a surplus of about 150 copies for possible distribution in filling orders for back copies and for sample copies to prospective subscribers and advertisers. The total average distribution was 2,891 copies. At this time the total has increased to a point where 3,100 copies of the journal are required each month, and it appears that to meet requirements, at least that many copies will be required of each monthly issue during 1938.

Herewith please find a financial statement showing the total income and expense. This shows a breakdown of all the expenses incurred in connection with the publication of the journal during 1937 in every detail.

Effective with January 1, an increase in advertising rates announced more than a year ago, became effective. This should have a good effect upon 1938 income, and it is reasonable to expect, your Committee believes, that the advertising volume for this year should show a substantial increase over that of 1937. Of course it is understood that no definite assurance can be given to this effect owing to the uncertainties of business conditions. Up to and including the June number of this year, we have a net increase in display advertising of $350.00 over the corresponding period for last year, so it seems only reasonable to estimate a $500 or $600 increase for the year in advertising receipts.

The journal is also carrying eight pages in each issue of the Minnesota Medical History. This material is being kept standing in page form for the possible publication of a book after the work has been completed and presented through MINNESOTA MEDICINE. It is felt that the sale of this book will enable the state association to recover all the costs incurred in the publication of the history in MINNESOTA MEDICINE with a reasonable probability of a net profit.

Some economies have been effected and plans approved for a possible increase in revenue from sources other than advertising and subscriptions which your committee is confident will show a larger net return for 1938 than has been earned during the past three or four years.

However, it is only fair, in considering costs and income of your journal, to bear in mind that MINNESOTA MEDICINE is produced in such a style as to reflect a great credit upon the medical profession of this state; that it is well printed on good quality of paper stock, with an attractive cover and good typography throughout. No state journal in organized medicine has a higher standing. It is much better illustrated than the general run of medical publications. Obviously the cost of these illustrations amounts to a considerable sum during the year, but we believe that the membership desires that a high standard be maintained.

STATEMENT OF CASH RECEIPTS AND DISBURSEMENTS

MINNESOTA MEDICINE
For the Period
January 1, 1937, through December 31, 1937

SOURCE OF CASH RECEIPTS -
Display Advertising	$ 8,562.20
Member Subscriptions	4,293.50
Non-member Subscriptions	425.20
Illustrations	49.55
Miscellaneous Income	7.83
Bad Accounts Recovered	83.05
(See Schedule A)	
Dividend	505.85
Gross Cash Receipts	$13,927.18

Less:
Discounts and Commissions
Advertising	$1,262.20	
Subscriptions	10.17	
		$ 1,272.37

Net Cash Receipts ... $12,654.81

CASH DISBURSEMENTS
Journal Expense	$12,031.38
(See Schedule B)	
Cash Surplus for Period	$ 623.43
Accounts Receivable January 1, 1937	$1,096.00
Accounts Receivable December 31, 1937	$1,278.79

SCHEDULE A
BAD ACCOUNTS RECOVERED
Palmer Company	$20.20
Minneapolis Sanitarium	47.00
Willows Sanitarium	15.85
	$83.05

BAD ACCOUNTS CHARGED OFF
Radioear Company	$76.00

SCHEDULE B
JOURNAL EXPENSE
Paper Stock	$ 1,328.38
Printing Expense	5,306.66
(Includes composition, make-up, lock-up, press-work, bindery work, addressing wrappers and inserting magazines in mailing envelopes)	
Editorial Salary—Dr. Drake	1,200.00
Bruce Publishing Co. Service Fee	1,680.00
(Covers business management, stenographic service, mechanical editing of all material, ordering all cuts, making of dummy, mailing all proofs, bookkeeping, billing and collections, keeping up mailing list, etc.)	
Bruce Publishing Co.	132.00
(Telephone, telegraph, addressograph plates, etc.)	
Advertising Commissions	1,123.14
(Including 5% received from advertising placed through CMAB)	
Illustrations	720.15
Mailing Envelopes	133.26
Second Class Postage	209.54
Stationery	18.55
2% Social Security Tax on labor costs	127.20
Bond—J. R. Bruce—Years 1937 and 1938	50.00
Enlargement of Cover for Exhibit	2.50
	$12,031.38

STATEMENT OF INCOME AND EXPENSE AND PROFIT AND LOSS

MINNESOTA MEDICINE
For the Period
January 1, 1937, through December 31, 1937

INCOME	ACCRUAL BASIS	
Display Advertising	$ 8,815.30	
Member Subscriptions	4,293.50	
Non-member Subscriptions	425.20	
Illustrations	49.55	
Miscellaneous Income	13.52	
Bad Accounts Recovered	83.05	
(See Schedule A)		
Dividend on Advertising from the American Medical Association	505.85	
		$14,185.97

EXPENSE		
JOURNAL Expense	$12,031.38	
(See Schedule B)		
Discounts and Commissions		
Advertising	1,262.20	
Subscriptions	10.17	
Bad Accounts Charged Off	76.00	
(See Schedule A)		
		13,379.75
Profit for Period		$ 806.22

J. T. CHRISTISON, Chairman

The Reference Committee made the following recommendations and comments concerning the reports of the Medical Economics Committee, its sub-committees and the Editing and Publishing Committee:

That the House of Delegates might wish to have more detail as to the progress of the Survey of the Need and Supply of Medical Care than is given in the rather generalized report of the Committee on Medical Economics though the committee realizes that the survey is still in its infancy. A definite stimulus to action seems to be needed since, in some instances, it is understood that the councilors have not yet met with the various local societies to explain objectives and methods.

—That the individual societies should appoint committees of review to analyze and consolidate reports as they come in. The Committee feels that Minnesota is fortunate in having within its ranks the national chairman of the Survey, that Doctor Braasch has undertaken a tremendous job and that the State Association should make every effort to complete its survey in the spirit in which it has been undertaken.

—That the Medical Economics feature of MINNESOTA MEDICINE is essential and should be continued.

—That the activities of the Sub-Committee on Professional Education in Medical Ethics and Social and Economic Trends should be extended in that members of county and district societies should meet with groups of internes for discussion of these problems while they are on their interne service. The Committee suggests further that county societies make it a part of their program to encourage new members in their communities, to call on them personally and to assist them in becoming acquainted with the relation of all these matters to the practice of medicine and to medical jurisprudence.

—That the Medical Advisory Committee is doing valuable work and the Committee hopes it will be continued.

—That the report of the Sub-Committee on State Health Relations be accepted as submitted.

—That a careful perusal of the report of the Sub-Committee on Low Income and Indigent Problems be recommended to all members. The Committee wishes to thank the Sub-Committee for its classification of indigency and suggests that the compilation of Survey Blanks will be simplified if this classification is followed. The Committee makes note of a new group of citizens forming itself into a position to request medical care at a 40 per cent discount of fees and asks an explanation of who may be included among the clients of the Farm Security Administration.

—That the resolution relative to choice of physicians proposed in the report of the Sub-Committee on Industrial Relations be adopted, also the code of ethics governing insurance and compensation practice and that the report as a whole be accepted.

—That the committee approves the principles proposed in the report of the Industrial Relations Committee and believes that the medical fee schedules presented in hospital service contracts of insurance companies should be considered by the House of Delegates and that such practices should be discouraged.

—That the report of the Editing and Publishing Committee be adopted and that the committee wishes to express its appreciation for the excellence of our state publication. The delegates accepted the reports with the recommendations of the Reference Committee.

Dr. W. F. Braasch, chairman of the Committee on Medical Economics, offered the following supplementary report on the Survey:

I can truthfully assure you, in the first place, that our progress with the Survey in Minnesota compares very favorably with other states in the Union. While the Medical Economics committee has general guidance, the work is largely centered in the office of the Executive Secretary, Mr. Rosell, and really he has done a very good job, proceeding systematically to coöperate to the fullest extent with committees, county societies and with allied agencies.

Only one of the nine survey forms prepared by the American Medical Association has been sent to each individual doctor in the local societies to fill out. The other forms have been sent through state organizations and agencies concerned with the activities in question. On the progress made by these coöperating agencies we can report with some degree of accuracy. The interest exhibited by these organizations and the promptness with which the forms have been filled out and returned is significant and encouraging.

Form No. 1, covering actual experience of individual doctors, has been answered fairly well. Some fail, however, to answer questions 7, 8 and 9, which call for their own solutions as to problems involved. These should not be left blank. There must be a solution to the problems involved in medical care for the indigent and we must have the help of the general practitioner in finding the solution.

Form No. 2 on hospital facilities and activities has been sent to all members of the Minnesota Hospital Association by Mr. A. M. Calvin, secretary. We understand a satisfactory return is coming in.

Form No. 3, concerned with nursing, has been sent for information on public health nursing to Miss Olivia Peterson, director of public health nursing of the State Board of Health, and to the Minnesota Registered Nurses Association for information on private duty nursing. Returns have been received from 35 counties this week by Miss Peterson and from four of the nine districts covered by the Registered Nurses Association.

Form No. 4 covering official health activities is in charge of Dr. A. J. Chesley, executive officer of the State Board of Health and member of the American Medical Association's advisory committee on the Survey, who has sent it to all community and county health officers of the state and received returns from 68 counties and seven communities.

Form No. 5 on public welfare activities is in charge of officials of the State Relief Agency, who has sent forms to relief workers in every county and received returns from 65.

Form No. 6 on health activities in the schools is in charge of the State Department of Education for the public schools. To date, 80 per cent of city and town schools and all county superintendents of the state have returned forms. One hundred and fifty of the 300 parochial schools who received forms direct from the state office have made returns.

Form No. 7 on health services in the colleges also went direct from the state office to the 25 colleges and universities of the state. Twenty-two have made returns.

Form No. 8 on medical service arranged for or provided by industrial, fraternal, mutual benefit, group hospitalization, community health or other similar organizations, or by county medical societies, is being handled direct by the state office.

Form No. 9 on activities and experience of wholesale and retail druggists was received at a later date than other forms, but is now in the hands of the State Pharmaceutical Association, and group meetings are being held in various parts of the state to stimulate interest and returns from the members.

As I have said before, to be accurate and to give a reliable picture of conditions all over the state on which to build improvements or readjustments, this Survey must be honest and it must represent all districts and classes. It was not planned as a statistical exercise but as an earnest and sincere effort to evaluate medical service in every county in the state and, as such, it is of importance to every member. Upon the accuracy and honesty with which the work is done will depend the future of medical practice in Minnesota.

Dr. B. J. Branton, chairman of the Medical Advisory Sub-Committee, presented the following supplementary report:

First, we wish to commend the spirit of coöperativeness that is becoming more and more evident among our members. This spirit will eventually eliminate virtually all unwarranted malpractice cases in the state.

Second, we call your attention to the lessening of the size of verdicts awarded in malpractice cases during the past year. Many cases, of course, have not been brought to trial at all, even after papers were served. Many others have been settled as nuisance cases for a very few dollars. When it came to settlement, many $15,000 to $20,000 cases have been settled for from $50 to $150.

Third, the committee selected by the Minnesota State Bar Association to work with our committee is doing everything in its power to curtail illegitimate cases. In this connection, I wish to urge all of our members to become better acquainted with members of the Bar Association. Interprofessional meetings should be encouraged and will do much to iron out difficulties encountered by both professions. There are 1,700 members of the Bar Association in the state, men of the same caliber and type as our members, and they welcome an opportunity to become better acquainted.

Contacts with insurance company representatives and this committee have been mutually advantageous, also. The insurance representatives have brought to my attention the following matters which should be considered by all of us.

One is that a great many suits are being brought in order to avoid having to pay medical and hospital bills. The patient is disgruntled and brings suit for malpractice, often as a counter action when he is sued for the bill. In the case of such patients trouble can be avoided by waiting until the 25th or 26th month has passed before putting the bill in the hands of a lawyer.

Another is that many suits are being brought by indigent patients who are looking for easy money. The doctor should be very careful in handling both disgruntled and indigent patients.

A third is that reports for industrial and compensation cases and insurance companies should be made in detail so that the doctor will not be obliged to testify from memory on the witness stand or before a referee. Be sure, also, that you are testifying only as to the facts of the case and that you are not favoring either side. There is always the possibility that the patient may not get as much money as he anticipated from the insurance company and then he may turn and sue for malpractice, especially if the doctor has elaborated too much on the condition of the patient.

The professional testifiers among doctors are becoming fewer in number. Some of them have seen the error of their ways when their insurance has been taken away from them.

Our committee has learned much from our many outside contacts during the past year and we hope to be of service to our members. Any member who is sued should notify the state office at once. He will then receive a questionnaire which should be made out and returned immediately. The committee will then be at your service and every means will be taken to assist you.

Dr. T. H. Sweetser, chairman of the Sub-Committee on State Health Relations, presented the following supplementary report:

I understand that the State Board of Health proposes to establish another public health district in the Southeastern part of the state to include Dakota,

Goodhue, Olmsted, Winona and, I think, Mower counties. They propose to establish an Arrowhead district in the Northern part of the state also.

We have discussed the matter of periodic health examinations for Legionnaires with the State Rehabilitation Committee of the Legion and have carefully examined the forms proposed by the Legion to see if they are complete and yet do not entail an excessive amount of work for the physician. We have advised, also, that the details be left for decision with the local medical society and that fees should be fixed in consultation with the local societies. It was agreed that Legionnaires who can afford to pay should be handled as private patients and that the legion would step in and help those who are unable to pay private fees; also that the physician-patient relationship should be preserved and that records should be kept by the physician who would be glad to furnish any information asked for by Legion officials or the Veterans' Administration upon request of the patient.

I am outlining all this so that you may have advance information in case the Legion post in your locality comes to you.

Doctor Piper requested from Doctor Coventry, chairman of the Sub-Committee on Low Income and Indigent Problems, an explanation of the status of Farm Security clients, also who would pay their loans.

DOCTOR COVENTRY: The government lends certain farmers certain amounts of money to maintain them on their farms until they shall be self-supporting. The money is not loaned for crop restriction or anything of that sort; it is merely done in preference to putting the farmer on direct relief.

DOCTOR PIPER: I was wondering if the special fee for examinations for Legionnaires—I understand two dollars was suggested—would apply to Farm Security clients, also. Or is it only for Legionnaires?

DOCTOR SWEETSER: Only for Legionnaires; but they all want a reduced rate. I don't know how the rest of you feel, but I don't believe that examination should be given for anything like two dollars. We are going to refer the fee question, however, to the local societies.

DOCTOR PIPER: The examination calls for blood test, urinalysis and physical examination, does it not? There are more organizations each year asking for special fees. Just now it is the Legion and Farm Security clients.

DOCTOR SWEETSER: I believe the fee for the examination for Legionnaires should be at least five dollars. If the fee is proper and our suggestions are followed I believe we could have no serious objections to the plan.

Doctor Piper also asked for an explanation of the "Wisconsin Plan" mentioned in the report of the Sub-Committee on Industrial Relations. The chairman was not present and the Speaker suggested that the committee make a supplemental report on the subject to be sent to the delegates.

Committee reports designated as "Officer and Council Reports" and reviewed by the Non-Scientific Reference Committee under the chairmanship of Dr. S. A. Slater of Worthington, follow:

731

REPORT OF THE CHAIRMAN OF THE COUNCIL

The most urgent business of the Council this year has undoubtedly been the reorganization of the state office made necessary by the leave of absence granted to Dr. E. A. Meyerding, who served us so long and so ably as secretary.

Office management was placed in the hands of Mr. R. R. Rosell, who previously served as assistant to Doctor Meyerding and who had established many close and valuable relationships with the official agencies whose activities involve medical care.

This action was taken on the recommendation of Doctor Meyerding at the meeting of July 25, 1937. As executive secretary, Mr. Rosell took over active direction of all organization activities on September 1 under instruction and advice from the Council and committee chairmen. On December 1, Mr. Rosell and Mrs. Sylvia Holliday were duly bonded for handling of funds and transfer of accounts was made.

Hand in hand with office reorganization, a cut in expenditures to keep within the income of our association was undertaken by the Finance Committee of the Council. A new budget drawn up on an annual instead of a biennial basis was recommended by the Finance Committee and adopted by the Council. This budget under which we are now operating provides for a saving over and above routine running expenses of the association of a sufficient amount to wipe out a deficit of recent years. We are living within the new budget and we hope the end of the fiscal year will see us in good financial condition. Thanks are due especially to the Finance Committee for its work in bringing about this essential adjustment.

It was the expressed wish of the Council that our Association should continue to work with the Minnesota Public Health Association just as we work with other health agencies to the end that all public health work in Minnesota should be effective and authoritative. This type of coöperation is a very important part of our function as a state medical association and is now being extended rapidly to include an intimate advisory participation, also, in the lay education program of the Women's Field Army of the American Society for the Control of Cancer.

Women's Field Army: At a joint meeting of the Council, the Committee on Cancer and representatives of the Women's Field Army, an executive committee was formed for the cancer organization to consist of certain designated officers of the State Medical Association, the American Society for the Control of Cancer and the Women's Field Army. The committee is in direct charge of the program of the field army and controls expenditure of funds (see Report of the Committee on Cancer for details).

In addition to routine work of the Council which includes, approval of applications for affiliate membership, ruling upon problems of ethics and organization brought by county societies, approval of expenditures, several notable special actions were taken as follows: The Herman M. Johnson Memorial Fund was set aside in perpetuity, only the income to be used for the annual memorial lectureship.

An investigation of medical service at Ah-Gwah-Ching, state sanatorium for the tuberculous, was requested by the State Board of Control and assigned to the Committee on State Health Relations of which Dr. T. H. Sweetser of Minneapolis is chairman. A thorough and impartial investigation was made and the present director endorsed with valuable suggestions as to improvements in personnel and equipment needed at the institution. The report was turned over with the approval of the Council to the State Board of Control.

The advice and coöperation of the Council on many other phases of its program was asked of the Council by the Board of Control, including approval of its program for crippled children and for rehabilitation of

tuberculous patients and appointment of a special committee to consult with the Department of Public Assistance of the Board on matters relating to standards of disability.

A special committee was appointed at the request of the Minnesota Hospital Service Association to study hospitalization problems in rural districts; inquiries concerning the advisability of approving commercial hospital insurance plans have come to the Council and the Council has been of the unanimous opinion that such approval should never be given, on principle, by members of the profession, noting further that lapses and loopholes have been discovered in some actual policies which might work hardship upon all parties concerned.

A joint committee of the state association and members of the Minnesota State Bar Association was suggested by the latter body and approved by the Council, which delegated the Medical Advisory Sub-Committee of the Medical Economics Committee to represent the medical body in this joint group.

The general plan proposed by the Committee on Diabetes for establishment of a Council on Diabetes of the Minnesota Public Health Association which should unite diabetics and function as an educational body received approval of the Council with the suggestion that, since Christmas Seal funds of the public health association may not be used for diabetes work, the Committee seek aid from other organizations such as the State Board of Health and also of philanthropically minded individuals for support.

Approval of the postgraduate courses now in their second year in obstetrics and pediatrics financed by Social Security funds and directed by Dr. E. C. Hartley, director of the Division of Child Hygiene of the State Board of Health.

The Council agreed to abide by the verdict of the Minnesota Society of Obstetrics and Gynecology on the suitability for public showing of the film "Birth of a Baby," and, as a result, the society having officially approved the film, it was shown to thousands of people at various points in the state this year.

A special committee was appointed to study the question of standards for physiotherapists looking to the possible licensure of this new professional group.

The Council directed all members, old and new, to fill out the new application blanks drawn up to obtain more extensive biographical information from our members, the blanks to be used as the basis for a new biographical file of members in the State Office.

The Council disapproved the suggestion which came from representatives of an out-of-state organization for a formal inter-professional organization in Minnesota, approving instead a letter sent to all county and district societies in Minnesota by Dr. F. J. Savage, chairman of the Inter-Professional Committee, suggesting frequent informal inter-professional gatherings in all localities for the purpose of better understanding and for the joint promotion of community welfare.

The plan for periodic examinations of all Legionnaires was approved in principle and referred to the Committee on State Health Relations for consideration of detail in conference with Legion officials (see Report of the Committee on State Health Relations).

The Council approved joint subscription to *Hygeia* and *Everybody's Health* on a special offer made by the Minnesota Public Health Association by which both magazines will be sent to members of the Legislature this year.

The term of office of the Chairman of the Council was set at three years, the incumbent being ineligible to immediate reëlection to office.

A total of ten all-day meetings were held by the Council during the year requiring a substantial sacrifice of time and money on the part of all. Other officers and committee chairmen also devoted large amounts of time and service to the work of the Association and the Council votes thanks to them for their contribution and also to the Executive Secretary and his staff for faithful and efficient service and splendid co-operation with the Council during the past year.

GEORGE EARL, *Chairman.*

The Reference Committee recommended adoption of the report with the following changes:

—That paragraph five of the report be eliminated and that the following paragraph be substituted (this substitution was submitted by Chairman Earl, himself):

"It was the expressed wish of the Council that our Association should continue to work with the Minnesota Public Health Association. The advantage of the past coöperation between the Minnesota Public Health Association and the Minnesota State Medical Association is fully recognized and it is desirable that the co-operation continue as far as possible."

—That the part of the paragraph on group hospital service referring to commercial hospital insurance plans be eliminated.

—That the following comment should be made on the paragraph on postgraduate courses:

"Although your committee appreciates the value of refresher courses of this type when controlled by the State. Association, nevertheless, we believe that other postgraduate courses sponsored by the State Association as in the past should not be neglected."

The delegates accepted the report with the changes and comments recommended by the committee.

REPORT OF THE COUNCILOR OF THE FIRST DISTRICT

Notable activity in the membership and in the component societies was noted during the year.

1. *Care of the indigent.*—County Commissioners have probably been as coöperative as necessities for economy would permit; an insufficient amount of money is available, however, for medical care of the indigent. In addition, relief clients have learned to demand the best and frequently ask for special tests, et cetera, that are not absolutely necessary, thus adding to expense in the individual case.

2. *Syphilis.*—Local health officers have complained of lack of coöperation financially in some instances, on the part of the local medical group, in the treatment of syphilis. County medical societies and local groups may have to make some more satisfactory financial arrangements with health officers if the campaign against syphilis is to be a success.

3. *American Medical Association Survey.*—Component societies in this district have been informed concerning details and some counties in the district have been active in carrying it on. Certain points that may be helpful have been brought out in discussion with physicians.

a. Local health officers may have difficulty in obtaining required information and should consult the State Board of Health on procedure.

b. Local town and village physicians should at some time review blanks filled in by schools, lodges and other local organizations in order to be sure that the local situation has been accurately covered and blanks gathered through state organizations should have approval of local physicians before tabulation is carried out.

c. Patients who are temporarily delinquent in accounts should not be reported as permanent medical indigents since many of these temporary delinquents have paid something on old bills and desire to be financially independent.

4. *Campaign of the Women's Field Army.*—Your councilor assisted in obtaining speakers throughout the district for the campaign of the Women's Field Army of the American Society for the Control of Cancer. The campaign in this district was successful.

Your councilor has been chiefly active during the past year in the study of finances of the Association as chairman of the Finance Committee of the Council. Report of the study is made by the Chairman of the Council.

H. Z. GIFFIN, *Councilor, Fifth District.*

REPORT OF THE COUNCILOR OF THE SECOND DISTRICT

All societies of the second district have been very active this year. All have held many meetings and several individual counties have organized medical clubs which meet six or seven times a year.

Dentists, lawyers and district judges of the locality were present at a well-attended and successful interprofessional meeting held by the Southwestern Minnesota Medical Society composed of medical men from six counties of the district this spring.

The Survey is under way in the district and I expect to be able to give a report of progress at the time of the state meeting.

L. L. SOGGE, *Councilor, Second District.*

REPORT OF THE COUNCILOR OF THE THIRD DISTRICT

Several important district meetings have been held during the past year, notably the meeting at Willmar at which all secretaries and presidents of the component societies met with Mr. Rosell and the Councilor to discuss phases of the economic situation as they affect medicine. Meetings of this type are of value, I believe, and should be held frequently.

The membership in the district has remained practically the same and a tendency to be closer in thought is notable among the members. Altogether, there is an unusually fine feeling, I believe, within the entire district.

B. J. BRANTON, *Councilor, Third District.*

REPORT OF THE COUNCILOR OF THE FOURTH DISTRICT

No complaints have been referred from this district for reference to the Council during the past year. Societies are active and membership somewhat higher than last year.

We have seen an improvement, also, in the handling of medical care for the indigent though conditions are not yet entirely satisfactory and we look to more satisfactory arrangements in all our counties.

J. S. HOLBROOK, *Councilor, Fourth District.*

REPORT OF THE COUNCILOR OF THE FIFTH DISTRICT

All societies of the Fifth Councilor District are active with the possible exception of Dakota County, where the situation is peculiar in that the county is relatively small in population and some of the physicians, being so close to the Twin Cities, are affiliated with the Ramsey and Hennepin County Medical Societies. The Dakota County society is primarily interested in problems related to care of the indigent and other such matters that must be handled on a county basis.

The problem of care of the indigent differs in status in the rural districts from the status in Ramsey County, where long established charitable institutions and agencies have had charge of the work for many years and have, with few exceptions, continued to carry the indigent load. In the country districts, progress has been made in improvement of relationships with official agencies.

The Survey has been presented to all of the societies in this councilor district and here, too, progress is being made, particularly in the East Central and the Washington County Societies.

GEORGE EARL, *Councilor, Fifth District.*

REPORT OF THE COUNCILOR OF THE SIXTH DISTRICT

Forms for the American Medical Association Survey have been placed in the hands of Wright county members by Doctor Catlin of Buffalo, and I am now beginning to receive returns. The entire membership of the Hennepin County Medical Society has received the forms but no returns are available as yet.

The Hennepin County Medical Association has appropriated $1,000 to defray cost of collecting and tabulating results of approximately 10,000 tuberculin tests applied by private physicians in their own offices. This action is, in effect, a tuberculosis survey in private practice for which aid has been requested by letter from both the state and the Hennepin County tuberculosis organizations. If the project is successful I may suggest that a similar survey for the state be carried on under the sponsorship of the state medical association with the aid of the state tuberculosis association and interested parties.

C. A. STEWART, *Councilor, Sixth District.*

REPORT OF THE COUNCILOR OF THE SEVENTH DISTRICT

Both membership and attendance in this district are at a higher level than before, due chiefly to the activities of the secretaries of the two constituent medical societies, Doctor Badeaux and Doctor Libert, and also to a growing interest in the problems of medical economics. Care of the indigent by county physicians obtained formerly in two counties, and in a third county physicians were not paid either by county or township for care of the poor. In one of the two counties, free choice of physician was restored a year ago and in the other it was restored following passage of the "choice of vendor" clause. Negotiations are under way in the first for a better percentage basis for physicians and elimination of certain objectionable features; in the second, the plan is operating much more satisfactorily than before. In the third, there is a prospect of payment for medical services as a result of conferences between township and county officials and committees of the medical society.

The feeling of comradeship among physicians in this district appears widespread and sincere.

E. J. SIMONS, *Councilor, Seventh District.*

REPORT OF THE COUNCILOR OF THE EIGHTH DISTRICT

Satisfactory relations exist between members in this district and between the profession and the public, and, on the whole, between the profession and the relief agencies. The swing seems to me to be towards the profession, generally, rather than away.

This condition can be ascribed to a considerable extent to the efficient work of the society, especially its Executive Secretary and special committees; also, fair treatment accorded the profession by the Governor and the State Relief Agencies, as well as the high standard of service rendered to the people by the profession.

W. L. BURNAP, *Councilor, Eighth District.*

REPORT OF THE COUNCILOR OF THE NINTH DISTRICT

Medical affairs have gone smoothly in the district. Meetings have been well attended, programs have been instructive and papers carefully prepared during the past year.

The Range Medical Society, an affiliate of the county society, has been active, also, holding well attended meetings with varied and interesting programs and conducting, all during the spring, postgraduate meetings with outside lecturers.

The relief situation has been handled as well as could be expected in the past although there are rumors of trouble which we hope will not materialize in the future.

BERTRAM S. ADAMS, *Councilor, Ninth District.*

In compliance with the recommendation of the Reference Committee the Councilors' reports were accepted by the delegates.

REPORT OF THE TREASURER

The officers and Council of the Minnesota State Medical Association have been troubled for a number of years over the increasing deficit in the finances of the Association at the end of each fiscal year. During this year they have undertaken to reorganize our expenditures and set up a budget which should keep our expenditures within our annual income.

You will note on the enclosed auditor's statement, dated December 31, 1937, that an apparent surplus of $2,144.72 appears. This surplus does not represent a true picture of the finances of the organization.

This figure occurs on the books of that date because $3,135.00 had been taken in in dues for 1938 but had already been used to defray expenses for 1937. In addition, the statement shows an item of $1,953.51 in the savings of the American National Bank. In reality, $1,927.42 of this amount represents the money contributed for the H. M. Johnson Memorial lectureship fund which has been set aside by resolution to be used only in promoting that lectureship and does not represent income for the general purpose of the organization. Further, the statement shows a note for $1,000 borrowed from the bank in October, 1937, as *cash receipts.* This loan was necessary to tide the Association over until the first of the 1938 dues should come in. Thus, at the end of 1937, the Minnesota State Medical Association had overdrawn close to $4,000.

The new budget drawn up for 1938 by the Finance Committee of the Council has so reduced expenditures that this deficit will be wiped out, the Association will be able to live within its income during 1938 and have a small surplus at the end of the year.

MINNESOTA STATE MEDICAL ASSOCIATION
STATEMENT OF CASH RECEIPTS AND DISBURSEMENTS
FOR THE YEAR ENDED DECEMBER 31, 1937

CURRENT FUNDS

Cash on Hand, December 31, 1936.......		$ 6,354.83
Cash Receipts, Year 1937:		
Dues collected, year 1936 and prior......$	216.25	
Dues collected, year 1937...............	31,134.50	
Dues collected year 1938...............	3,135.00	
Total dues collected \$34,485.75		
Contributions to Johnson Memorial Fund...	343.89	
Sale of diabetes books.................	84.44	
Bruce Publishing Company (Minn. Medicine)	774.36	
Transferred from Technical Exhibit Fund for credit of Annual Meeting expense	4,534.68	
Borrowed on notes payable.............	1,000.00	
Interest on savings accounts...........	54.43	
Dinner tickets (Annual Meeting)........	265.69	
Sundry items	20.77	
Total receipts		41,564.01
		$47,918.84

Cash Disbursements, Year 1937:
Special committees:

Educational Fund	$10,123.52
Historical	1.50
Hospital and medical education	58.82
Medical economics	1,487.82
Medico-legal advisory	290.81
Medical relief	272.96
Public Health education	4,634.21
Radio	386.22
State Health relations	159.62
Unbudgeted committees	1,018.18
Minnesota Medicine	4,293.50
Furniture and fixtures	209.30
Dues refunded	30.25
Advance to employee	200.00
Expenses, Johnson Memorial Fund	10.55
Diabetes books	16.90

Conferences and meetings:

Annual Meeting	5,873.83
Council Expense	412.35
A.M.A. delegates	235.05
County society meetings	72.47
Other conference expense	81.05
County officers' meeting	366.88
Special session, House of Delegates	8.03

Administrative expenses:

Secretary's salary	2,800.00
Secretary's travel expense	356.73
Field secretary's salary	3,600.00
Field secretary's travel expense	1,776.55
Field secretary, balance of 1936 salary	300.00
Treasurer's salary	100.00
Stenographic service	3,056.55
Rent	636.00
Office supplies and printing	838.74
Postage	531.51
Telephone and telegraph	729.20
Miscellaneous expense	805.02

Total disbursements	$45,774.12

Cash on Hand, December 31, 1937:

American National Bank, Checking account	$ 64.94
American National Bank, Savings account	1,953.51
Farmers and Mechanics Bank Savings account	99.45
First Nat'onal Bank Savings account	26.82

Total Cash on Hand	$ 2,144.72

W. H. CONDIT, Treasurer.

In compliance with the recommendation of the Reference Committee the Report of the Treasurer was accepted by the delegates with the following change. That the first paragraph should read as follows:

"The officers and Council of the Minnesota State Medical Association have been concerned for a number of years over the increasing cost of conducting the affairs of the State Association and balancing the budget. During this year they have undertaken to reorganize our expenditures and set up a budget which should keep expenditures within our annual income."

The Reference Committee also made note of the following: "In the opinion of your committee, if it should become necessary to secure funds to defray increasing expenses in order to balance the budget, the advisability of a small assessment might well be considered."

REPORT OF THE EXECUTIVE SECRETARY

On July 25, the Council granted the request of Dr. E. A. Meyerding for a year's leave of absence and instructed Mr. R. R. Rosell, assistant to the secretary, to take over the duties of executive secretary of the organization. Subsequently, in the interest of economy, the Finance Committee, with the approval of the Council, also ordered a complete separation of office management from the Minnesota Public Health Association, including a separation of bookkeeping. This separation was completed as rapidly as possible and the Executive Secretary's office, although still housed as a tenant in the building owned by the Minnesota Public Health Association, has been independently administered to conform to the budget adopted for 1938 by the Council and with the limited office force allowed by that budget.

Recognizing the need for retrenchment, the Executive Secretary's office has endeavored to cut expenses wherever possible without curtailing, in any way, essential activities of the Association. These activities have, in fact, expanded since last September to meet the growing demands made upon the State Medical Association for advice and coöperation by all federal and state agencies concerned in any way in the provision of medical care.

Among the new activities within the State Office itself is the inauguration of a new biographical file of members with the new application blanks duly filled in with requested biographical information as backbone of the file. Magazines and newspapers have been clipped for personal information about members to add to the file, which consists of a stout manila envelope for each member. It has been suggested that the Women's Auxiliary aid by providing a clipping service by members throughout the state.

Following logically upon institution of the new file, the State Office has also assembled a complete set of MINNESOTA MEDICINE since the date of its first appearance in 1918, early issues being the gift of Dr. W. F. Wilson; also a complete set of its precursor the St. Paul Medical Journal, gift of Dr. J. T. Christison. Both are now suitably bound. Thanks to these members, the State Office, which should be the repository of many historical records about medicine in Minnesota, is now equipped with a complete file of its publications and with the beginnings, at least, of a biographical file of its members.

Launching the Survey of the Need and Supply of Medical Care in Minnesota is also an important new activity of the last few months reported upon elsewhere in the committee reports.

Tabulation of replies and information secured still remains to be done. Special funds may need to be appropriated to complete the work uniformly without wasteful loss of time.

As a result of action taken by the Executive Secretary and our attorney, Mr. F. Manley Brist, a new ruling on state income tax exemptions has been made permitting Minnesota doctors to claim exemption in making out state income tax statements on expenses incurred in attendance at medical meetings and in postgraduate education.

One of the principal functions of the State Office other than its routine office functions in respect to collection of dues, issuance of membership certificates, maintenance of the roster, has become the maintenance of close contact and understanding between the State Association and the public and private agencies engaged in ministering to the welfare of the needy and the indigent.

In Minnesota, we have had the opportunity to present the enlightened medical point of view in advance of new programs and regulations. The result of this mutual confidence and understanding in the midst of changing conditions is that no hasty proposals for state supported sickness insurance or politically installed coöperatives have emanated from any of the leaders in political or welfare work. Such alternatives have been relinquished in favor of an honest attempt to deal with medical problems fairly and realistically and with the advice of physicians whose interests lie in the advancement of the public good and of medical science and not in the advancement of party machines and political jobs.

The appreciation of all physicians is due to the public officials who have worked so willingly and courteously with representatives of our Association. The situation with respect to our relations with these officials is in such marked contrast to the situation a few years ago that it would seem to deserve to be marked by the House of Delegates at this meeting.

As welfare work is now organized in Minnesota, virtually all official services with the exception of direct relief and WPA are under the direction of the State Board of Control. The special thanks of our organization should be extended to Mr. C. R. Carlgren, chairman, to Dr. H. E. Hilleboe, director of Services to Crippled Children, and to Mr. R. E. Youngdahl, director of the Division of Public Assistance, for the understanding and good will they have displayed in working with our organization.

Among marked gains made during the past year was the inclusion in the Extra Session Laws of 1937 on relief of the choice of vendor clause which reads that "all counties shall permit free choice of vendor to relief clients for relief orders, provided the vendors chosen conform to the regulations of the Executive Council and of the responsible relief agency."

Equally important was the ruling of the Attorney General on this clause by which the right of a person on relief to select his own physician is established.

Thanks to the firm stand of S.R.A. officials that state aid could and would be withheld from any county that failed to conform to this interpretation even prior to the ruling of the Attorney General, difficult situations have been cleared up in many Minnesota counties. Remaining sore spots are quite likely to be cleared up as a result of the unequivocal ruling of the Attorney General, which ruling was secured largely through the personal effort of Mr. Brist, who has worked in the closest coöperation with the State Office on all phases of our program during the past year.

The actual state of medical relief and public assistance in general, so far as medical service is concerned, is indicated with reasonable accuracy in the booklet called "Facts and Figures" and issued last February by the State Office. Not only case loads and money spent, county by county, are included, but a brief and complete explanation of the functions and source of funds of each of the more or less entangled agencies that make up the welfare picture in Minnesota.

Responsibility for a knowledge of these agencies and functions must be assumed by the individual practice physician.

The doctor's individual relationship to the community has changed in the last ten years and it is surely as much a part of his practice to know how to direct his patients who need help to the agency that will provide that help as it is to know how to treat the same patient medically. The State Office stands ready to answer inquiries but complete information on the part of the physician, himself, will contribute overwhelmingly to the successful working of the plan for medical care of relief and low income patients in Minnesota.

It is obvious, also, that physicians thus informed will be able to lay their fingers upon weak spots in the system and take the lead in correcting them.

One of the most effective approaches to the problem of medical care for the under-privileged is a vigorous, well-organized State Board of Health, and Minnesota has been exceedingly fortunate for many years in having such a board under the leadership of Dr. A. J. Chesley. Doctor Chesley works closely with the State Office and with the practicing physician.

The Executive Secretary has spent a considerable portion of his time in personal investigation of malpractice cases referred to the Medical Advisory Committee and also in attendance at meetings of county and district societies and at out-of-state conferences such as the Secretaries' Conference of the American Medical Association, conferences of insurance representatives and the Wisconsin State Medical Society at Madison. The State Office also arranged many committee meetings and conferences, the largest of which, outside of the state meeting, is, of course, the annual County Officers' Conference, at which attendance this year was nearly 100.

Membership of the organization is now 2,467 (2,363 active members plus 105 affiliate and associate members), representing an increase of 95 members over

last year. There are 3,884 physicians licensed to practice medicine in the state and of the 1,417 who are not members a percentage are not engaged in practice in Minnesota; others are ineligible to membership for various reasons. A special effort should be made to enroll the remaining eligibles this year so as to increase income and cement the strength of the Association in the state.

It is now possible to report that the income from the fine technical exhibit at this meeting will cover all expenses incident to the Duluth meeting. Thus, no funds will be needed from the budget of the Association to finance the meeting. The Committee on Scientific Assembly has arranged a distinguished program and the local arrangements committee under the chairmanship of Dr. Russell J. Moe of Duluth has worked actively and enthusiastically with the committee and the State Office to make the four-day stay in Duluth pleasant and profitable.

Credit is due also to the State Office staff for the efficiency with which they have assumed new responsibilities and carried on the above full program with a smaller personnel and a minimum of extra help. A considerable saving in expenditures for office help has been made as a result over a like period last year.

The current outlook for maintaining accepted standards for medical practice is good. The load of the needy in the state has reached very close to half a million, however, and the relief picture becomes increasingly complicated. Medicine cannot hope to steer a straight course in the confusion of politics and scarcity of funds to meet the needs unless physicians are clear and definite in their public policy and unless they present a united front.

What may happen in Washington or even in our neighbor state, Wisconsin, cannot be foretold now. Whatever may be in store for us in Minnesota depends very largely upon the public spirit with which we shape our policy and advance to meet the need.

R. R. Rosell, *Executive Secretary.*

The Reference Committee recommended that the report of the Executive Secretary be accepted with the following two notations:

With reference to the paragraph which reads: "The situation with respect to our relations with these officials is in such marked contrast to the situation a few years ago that it would seem to deserve to be marked by the House of Delegates," the Committee said.

"The Committee wishes to commend the progress that has been made and hopes it will continue."

At the conclusion of the report the Committee also added this comment:

"Without wishing to detract in any way from the excellent work of the Executive Secretary, your Committee believes that attention should be called to the fact that much of the efficiency of the Secretary's office is based on a continuation of the activities and system established by the retiring Secretary, Dr. E. A. Meyerding."

The delegates accepted the report and comments.

REPORT OF THE SECRETARY

As your Secretary has been on leave of absence since September 1, 1937, pending acceptance of his resignation, his report will cover briefly certain activities from January 1, 1937, to September 1, 1937. The customary detailed report of the activities of the Secretary's office and Council activities will come from the Executive Secretary's office.

Those who took part in the organization of your

Association in 1924 know how little we had with which to start. To compare the Association at that date with the present Association, the progress, growth, harmony, and united activity that exists, seems astounding. We truly have a great State Medical organization, a fact recognized throughout the United States and making the organization the envy of all of the other states.

This great development is not the work of any one man but of a large group of unselfish, self-sacrificing medical men, and we have many of these left in the organization—the type' of man who places the organization before any personal ambitions he may have.

This report would not be complete unless we mention some of this group of great workers who have made your present Association. Among them are: E. S. Boleyn, Charles Bolsta, S. H. Boyer, W. F. Braasch, W. L. Burnap, R. M. Burns, J. T. Christison, L. R. Critchfield, Carl B. Drake, George Earl, M. S. Henderson, H. M. Johnson, Starr Judd, O. E. Locken, the Mayos, J. A. Myers, N. O. Pearce, F. J. Savage, C. L. Scofield, L. L. Sogge, Theodore Sweetser. H. Longstreet Taylor, G. S. Wattam, W. W. Will, H. M. Workman, C. B. Wright, and others whose names will occur to you at this time.

Their hope and our hope is that their efforts will be appreciated and that the present group who are responsible will be as unselfish in promoting the best interests of our State Medical Association as were their predecessors.

Growth of Economic Problems.—With the increasing activity of Federal and State Welfare Agencies, our governmental administrators are becoming more intimately concerned with the health and medical care of the public, and medicine is consequently becoming deeply affected and influenced by these agencies.

We do not intend to go into detail but if you will consider the advances made in medical relief, the extension of the various state departments through federal aid in the care of the crippled and handicapped children, the many medical activities that have become part of the program of the State Board of Control, the increase in the activities of the State Board of Health, extending even to the education of the physician and allied groups, you can readily see that these proposed aids for medical care are only forerunners for more complete socialized medicine.

Therefore, it behooves the medical profession to become as compact a unit as possible so that its experience may be used to the best advantage for the public.

Contact Committees.—Your Secretary believes that the most important single accomplishment in his thirteen years' service in this office, was the organization of the County Contact Committees of three.

The necessity of the profession in each County organizing some kind of a group—may it be a medical club, a contact committee, or call it what you may—is of the utmost importance. This group must take upon itself the responsibility of looking after the interest of the profession and the health of the public within the boundaries of their County.

Public Health Education.—A few years ago, the public health education campaign which the Minnesota State Medical Association was able to put on with the Minnesota Health Association seemed to be a rather extensive program. Today, with the millions of dollars of federal funds being spent directly by the government for the work of the state and other official agencies, it is becoming more and more difficult for groups like organized medicine and the Christmas Seal organization to make their part of the public health education program noticed. Careful thought and planning are more essential now than ever before.

It is with extreme regret that your Secretary has noticed the growing separation of the Minnesota State

Medical Association and its committees from the Minnesota Public Health Association. I can assure you, however, that the Minnesota Public Health Association, its officers, Executive Committee and members, will at all times stand ready to coöperate to the fullest extent with the medical profession. I, personally, shall make every endeavor to maintain whatever contact I can with organized medicine.

The relationship between the Minnesota Public Health Association and the Minnesota State Medical Association is emphasized by the medical men in the personnel of its officers and executive committee.

Speakers' Bureau.—One of the outstanding accomplishments of the past thirteen years has been the development of speakers who can satisfactorily present medical subjects to lay groups. We now have a considerable number of medical men who are acceptable to the laity.

One of the principal factors in the development of these speakers has been the College Lecture Course. Another was the short courses in public speaking which were given several years ago in various parts of the state. Many of the profession have now taken up public speaking due to the interest developed.

As time progresses, it will become increasingly important to have more medical men who are qualified to present our problems before lay audiences.

The development of medical speakers for lay groups has, thus far, been confined to scientific lines. Unfortunately, the opportunity to develop speakers on economic problems has not as yet presented itself. This is an important problem which confronts the medical profession now. It should be given immediate attention.

College Lecture Course.—The Minnesota Public Health Association and the Minnesota State Medical Association for the fourth consecutive year have sponsored the Health Lecture Course in colleges throughout the state.

This course consists of four monthly health lectures extending from October through January. College officials have been most enthusiastic in their praise of this project and its effectiveness as a means of student health education.

The Minnesota State Medical Association pays the honorarium and traveling expenses of the physician lecturer. The cost of the 1937-1938 course will be approximately $1,150.00 with an average cost of $16.45 per lecture.

The Minnesota Public Health Association does all the administrative work, the organization, planning, booking of speakers and publicity. A conservative estimate of the value of these services is well over $1,500.00. This may seem expensive. We believe, however, that this course is one of our most valuable programs.

We sincerely hope that the College Lecture Course will be continued as long as the schools wish to receive it.

Annual Meeting.—Some eight years ago, members of the Council and a group of members of the Minnesota State Medical Association suggested that a large institute of some kind which should represent the entire Northwest might be possible and advisable. In accordance with the policy of the American Medical Association, it was suggested that this meeting should be held under the auspices of the State Association. The Secretary was urged to build up such a meeting and attempted to comply.

Records show that the enlarged meetings of the Association since that date have been more and more successful and that the cost has not exceeded that of previous small meetings.

Previous to the 1932 meeting in Saint Paul, much of the annual meeting was conducted under the supervision of the local arrangements committee. This included the handling of all exhibits, scientific, commercial, et cetera. Beginning in 1932, practically the complete supervision of the meeting was placed in the hands of your Secretary.

Audit—Oct. 4, 1924—Sept. 10, 1925—Local Supervision
Convention Expense—Minneapolis................$1,775.99
  (listed Convention Expense on this audit)
1926—Convention Expense—St. Paul................. 1,150.13
  (listed Convention Expense on this audit)
1927—Annual Meeting Expense—Duluth............. 1,420.38
1928—Annual Meeting Expense—Minneapolis......... 1,242.08
1929—Annual Meeting Expense—St. Paul............ 1,921.11
1930—Annual Meeting Expense—Duluth.............. 1,844.80
1931—Annual Meeting Expense—Minneapolis......... 1,459.13
1932—Annual Meeting Expense—St. Paul—State Supervision 1,513.13
1933—Annual Meeting Expense—Rochester—State Supervision 462.44
1934—Annual Meeting Expense—Duluth—State Supervision 1,544.00
1935—Annual Meeting Expense—Minneapolis—State Supervision 1,711.11
1936—Annual Meeting Expense—Rochester—State Supervision 393.83
1937—Annual Meeting Expense—St. Paul—State Supervision 867.60

Registration: The following comparison of registration is not only interesting but valuable:

Year	Registration	Place
1924	306	St. Cloud
1925	736	Minneapolis
1937	4256 (including physicians, Women's Auxiliary, exhibitors, members of allied professions attending the Congress of Allied Professions)	St. Paul

The 1937 meeting in Saint Paul will be memorable for many reasons. It gave unprecedented program representation to the scientific, social and economic problems of medicine. No other state medical association has been able to gather together at one time and for such a purpose so many organizations and groups who are today allied in the delivery of medical care to the people. Incidentally the participation in the meeting of so many organizations coming from many states made it possible to secure the St. Paul Auditorium for the meeting without charge—a saving of approximately $1,000 in the cost of the meeting.

Interprofessional Relationship Committee.—You are familiar with the report of the joint session of the Congress of Allied Professions held May 3, 1937, at the Lowry Hotel. Dr. Frank Savage, as chairman of the Interprofessional Relationship Committee, has done an outstanding piece of work. Other efforts are being made along this line that should be followed up. During the entire period of your Secretary's service, public health meetings and interprofessional meetings of various types, such as meetings between the dental profession, the legal profession, pharmacists, etc., have been held throughout the state. I would urge that such meetings be continued. Invitations should be given to the various county health officers and public workers to sit in with the medical profession so they can get better acquainted.

Committee on Medical Economics.—Minnesota was the first in developing the type of Committee on Medical Economics which has proved so successful. The co-ordination of the various sub-committees centralizes and makes possible a uniform and conservative program in our state.

We have been fortunate in having had as chairman, W. F. Braasch, M.D., whose long experience in medical economics, both state and national, and well known executive ability have been invaluable in keeping us in close touch with happenings in this field throughout the country.

Committee on State Health Relations.—Your chairman of the Committee on State Health Relations is not only very competent, but a very energetic and thorough chairman. Theodore Sweetser, M.D., of Minneapolis, has done a splendid job. He has devoted unlimited

time and effort to our Association. We owe a great deal to Doctor Sweetser.

New Constitution.—Your new constitution is not only one of the most advanced, but it has many unique features. The various graphs, showing the functions of the various committees, give at a glance the operation of our Association.

Every member should look over this constitution. It is a truly noteworthy document and is being copied by many other state organizations. In the main it was adapted from the constitution of the American Medical Association, especially in regard to the duties of the president and other high officers.

Housing Minnesota State Medical Association.—For almost fourteen years the Minnesota State Medical Association has been housed with the Minnesota Public Health Association. The administration of these two has been as one. We believe that this arrangement has been to the benefit of all.

Radio Broadcasting.—The Minnesota State Medical Association is unusually fortunate in having two members who are especially interested in radio broadcasting. R. M. Burns, M.D., chairman of your Radio Committee, is not only interested, but is well informed and has done much to put our radio program in the foreground. Doctor Burns is well able to meet any situation that may arise in the radio program.

Wm. A. O'Brien, M.D., is the foremost health commentator in the United States and we are very fortunate to have such a gifted speaker devoting himself to the dissemination of authentic health information.

Tribute to Dr. H. M. Workman.—Everyone who has been closely associated with the Minnesota State Medical Association during past years appreciates the great sacrifices and worth of that grand old man, Dr. H. M. Workman. Throughout his professional career he was intimately associated with guiding the policies, finances and management of this organization.

During that time his experiences taught him much regarding the medical profession, its members and the relationship with the public.

He was very fixed in certain of his policies, especially regarding the finances of your organization. As I grow older, I appreciate more and more that his attitude came from the wisdom of his many years of experience.

It was Doctor Workman who always believed that the medical profession should be organized as county units. Your county contact committees are an adaptation of his belief. He believed that the medical dues and funds were the most precious treasure that the medical man possessed and must be guarded in every possible manner.

All of us would do well at the present time to follow closely the policies of Doctor Workman. Personally, I am grateful to have had Doctor Workman as my medical economic preceptor.

Financial Obligations.—For more than 13 years your Secretary has had practically complete responsibility of the business and office details of your organization, the only exceptions being the Committee on Public Policy and Legislation, Chairman, Dr. H. M. Johnson and now Dr. L. L. Sogge, and the Publishing and Editing Committee of MINNESOTA MEDICINE. The Council usually met four times a year. Policies were formulated by the Council at its meeting and in the interval by your officers.

The Finance Committee of the Council has had direct supervision of the making of the Budget and has been directly responsible to the Council for the expenditures of the same. Other expenditures required a vote of the Council as a whole.

The only protection against political, legislative and governmental experimentation, including national, state and local, is that provided by your membership dues which amounts to some thirty thousand dollars—a very insignificant sum to pay for an insurance premium to protect the health of the public and the standing of our profession.

We used what we thought was the greatest economy and efficiency in handling your funds and affairs. I am proud of my record, and I am proud of the resolution passed by your Council as published in MINNESOTA MEDICINE in January, 1938.

It has been reported that some of you have said that the affairs of our State Association are a small business because only thirty thousand dollars is involved, but let me tell you that it is by far the most vital business in the state as far as the interests of the medical profession and the individual doctor are concerned. It is the only protection the doctor has against the inroads on his freedom and the attacks that are being made on him today in his relation to the public.

Insurance Premium.—The Minnesota State Medical Association has about 2,500 members from the total of more than three thousand medical men practicing in Minnesota. A conservative estimate of the cost of preparing a medical man to practice is at least fifteen thousand dollars; it is probably much more. The profession has an investment of some forty-five million dollars in the original preparation to practice medicine.

In addition, there are many hospitals, clinics, and other institutions that are dependent upon the medical profession. Your medical school, University Hospital, Mayo Clinic, State institutions, church institutions, hospitals, are all more or less dependent on the independence and successful future of the medical profession. Undoubtedly the total investment dependent upon the medical profession runs into hundreds of millions of dollars in Minnesota.

You will agree that every precaution, every effort and the best possible personnel should be sought to protect medical care of the people of Minnesota.

Finance and Reserve Fund.—During my term of office, the expenditures seldom exceeded our income. Most of the budget items, supervised by your Secretary, were underspent. At each Council meeting regular reports of the budget and finances were submitted. The Finance Committee of the Council received special reports in addition. It was necessary to borrow money only twice to tide over the year end. Your auditors, Shannon & Byers, in their annual audits, including 1936, stated: "The books and records of account are adequate for the needs of the Association and have been neatly and accurately maintained."

The Fiscal Agency account was increased some $20,000 odd. Special credit belongs to Dr. Frank Savage during his term as Chairman of the Finance Committee, and Dr. C. B. Wright as Councilman, for the growth of reserve fund. To Dr. H. Z. Giffin, Chairman of the Finance Committee since 1932, belongs the credit for his interest and study of the investments of this fund. We believe that the Fiscal Agency Fund should be several times the present amount.

Conclusion.—The finances, both current and reserve, should receive the most careful attention. Every effort should be made to increase both, to meet the many emergencies that will arise.

The strength of the medical profession lies in its unity. No other group has the training to care for the health of the public as ours has. Consequently, a solid front will permit our profession to guide its own destinies and protect the health of the public.

The medical student should have some training in medical ethics, economics and public relations.

Every medical unit, no matter how small, must appreciate its importance in the problems that confront the medical profession today. These problems may be local or national.

Small groups increase their strength by alliances. Every opportunity must be taken by our profession to

have the public appreciate our importance in the social and political organization.

Those responsible for the leadership should leave no stone unturned in protecting our interests both inside and outside the organization.

E. A. MEYERDING, *Secretary*

In compliance with the recommendation of the Reference Committee the report and also the resignation of the Secretary to take effect at once were accepted by the delegates.

Chairman S. A. Slater read the resignation of Doctor Meyerding as follows:

It is with deep regret that I tender my resignation, to become effective at once, as Secretary of the Minnesota State Medical Association. You are cognizant of the fact that I submitted my verbal resignation May 5, 1937, and that I have been on leave since September 1, 1937, and I now deem it wise in justice to myself to make this leave permanent. In justice to the organization, I ask the House of Delegates to accept my resignation this evening so that some one can be elected this week to fulfill the office.

In the summer of 1924, I unofficially assumed the duties as your Secretary. On the first of January, 1925, I officially became your Secretary, a period of practically fourteen years in which I served as executive officer of the Minnesota State Medical Association.

I look upon my work with the Medical Association during these years as the happiest and most interesting in my life. The friendships that have come about through close association in the work will mean much to me throughout my life. I wish to take this opportunity to extend thanks to the members of the Medical Association for the fine coöperation which made it possible for our organization to develop into one of the most progressive in the country. I wish especially to thank the officers and members of the Council and others who have given long hours and much energy in volunteer service.

I am proud of my association with the Minnesota State Medical Association and the American Medical Association and my profession. It is a satisfaction to have been of some assistance in solving our many problems, organizing, developing, and aiding in establishing before the Minnesota public the greatness of our profession.

While I am now stepping out of official service with the Medical Association, my interest and coöperation in the work will continue. Some of you will remember that in my earlier years I frequently paraphrased Decatur's memorial speech as follows:

"Our profession, in her intercourse with those outside, may she always be in the right; but right or wrong, our profession."

I shall always adhere to this precept.

At all times I shall be at your service, and shall be only too happy to assist in any way possible. In leaving, I urge close coöperation and harmony in order that our Association may continue to keep its place in leadership.

E. A. MEYERDING, *Secretary.*

The Non-Scientific Reference Committee on reports designated as "State Health Relations reports," of which Dr. A. H. Zachman of Melrose was chairman, reported as follows:

INTERPROFESSIONAL RELATIONSHIP COMMITTEE

Our major objective has been to foster establishment of local interprofessional relations committees in every county. In the past two or three years the state committee has met with groups of nurses, pharmacists, and hospital administrators for the discussion of common problems. Valuable as these meetings have been in the creation of better feeling and better understanding, it has been the feeling of the committee that the value would be greater if the same type of meeting could be extended to every county of the state. These local interprofessional meetings could render major service in the preservation of medical standards in times of legislative stress, in spreading sound doctrine to offset possible radical demands for state medicine, in backing the American Medical Association in their present study of medical care and, later, in their conclusions on the solution of the problem.

At a meeting of nurses in Minneapolis, attended by your chairman, government aid to tax-supported hospitals for the purpose of paying salaries of nursing instructors was advocated by the state director of education. This program was proposed on the basis of a report by his department on nursing education in Minnesota. The average nurse, according to this report, appears to be a downtrodden individual who sometimes works 84 hours a week, is poorly fed, badly housed, exploited and inadequately trained by the hospital and who graduates with health seriously impaired and without proper education. Not all hospital people or superintendents of nursing agreed with the report. One of the latter agreed that it might be true in isolated cases but that, in general, the report was incorrect. Mr. Amberg, superintendent of the University hospitals, showed that nursing education has been improved, hours reduced and curriculum revised, with students rotating on the various services. Cost of training has increased at the University hospital by $20,000.

At Nassau hospital in Mineola, Long Island, four graduate Minnesota nurses were found recently to be in charge of departments because, according to the chief of staff, "they seem to be the best trained women we can find."

A number of grievances from pharmacists were brought out in discussion following an address by the chairman before the Minnesota State Pharmaceutical Association, April 26. It was suggested that these grievances should be ironed out locally in interprofessional meetings between doctors and pharmacists; also that, although they had been informed two years ago that space would be allowed them to discuss these matters in MINNESOTA MEDICINE, no advantage had been taken of the offer.

F. J. SAVAGE, *Chairman.*

In compliance with the recommendation of the Reference Committee, the report was accepted by the delegates with following comments by the Reference Committee.

"We feel that the meetings sponsored by the Interprofessional Relationship Committee will work to the mutual satisfaction and benefit of all interested groups, namely, nurses, pharmacists, hospital administrators and dentists and also the legal profession, which happened to be left out, perhaps inadvertently, by the committee, but which we shall like to add to the group.

"We feel, also, that the report on nursing education in the state is decidedly biased and does not represent the true condition in the field of nursing education. We recommend that the delegates familiarize themselves with this nursing education report so that they can discuss it intelligently if the need should arise."

CHAIRMAN SAVAGE (supplementary report): One cannot read Doctor Earl's report or Mr. Rosell's report without being impressed with the fact that we can do much for the future of the medical man by these friendly get-togethers. The plan for these local interprofessional meetings met with the approval of the Council. The purpose is to create good feeling and an intelligent understanding of medical problems and the result should be the creation of a friendly body of people throughout every county in the state which should be of tremendous assistance in the shaping of our public policy. I know of two such meetings, one in Doctor Sogge's district and the other in Winona. There may have been more.

DOCTOR SOGGE (speaking at the request of the Speaker): Eighty-eight were present at our interprofessional meeting in Worthington, including the judge of the district. I agree with Doctor Branton that an intimate relation between the doctors and the attorneys in a community is a fine thing. The attorney who knows the doctor's problems is not going to be so quick to start a lawsuit in town, even though it may appear to be a chance to make some money. I am very enthusiastic about interprofessional meetings and so, I believe, was every doctor, druggist and attorney who attended our meeting. We are going to try to have one every year.

DOCTOR GIFFIN: I have a communication from Doctor Wilson of Lake City telling of a meeting held there by their interprofessional relations committee, attended by fifty people, including physicians, dentists, nurses, pharmacists, hospital executives and representatives of the various relief agencies. The problem of medical care for the indigent was discussed. Every profession and agency was represented by a speaker and a much better understanding was created on their joint difficulties.

DOCTOR WILSON (speaking on the subject at the request of the Speaker): We had a worthwhile meeting with the pharmacists at Winona this year. Two speakers from the state pharmaceutical association spoke, and we discussed each other's points of view and enjoyed the whole meeting very much. Six months later the pharmacists invited us to a meeting with them. The meeting was addressed by medical men and valuable discussion followed. I think these meetings should be promoted throughout every county in the state.

An oral report on the work of the Committee on Public Policy was given by Doctor Sogge, chairman, and Mr. F. Manley Brist, attorney for the Minnesota State Medical Association, and accepted by the delegates. No transcription was made of this report.

No report was presented by the Committee on University Relations.

The Necrology Report was presented as follows by Dr. Richard Bardon, representing the Historical Committee:

NECROLOGY REPORT

During the last year, the Association lost forty-four members by death. Thirty-six of these were active members and eight were formerly active members or members who had retired from the Association. The list of deceased members follows:

MEMBERS

Carl M. Anderson, Rochester; J. Fowler Avery, Minneapolis; John T. Bowers, Bemidji; Charles W. Bray, Biwabik; Edward J. Brown, Minneapolis; Charles P. Dolan, Worthington; Charles A. Donaldson, Mesa, Arizona; Frederick C Drenning, Duluth; Julian A. DuBois, Sauk Center; George Edward, Canton; Martin J. Fiala, Duluth; Herman W. Froehlich, Minneapolis; John J. Gelz, St. Cloud; Clarence W. Golden, Tyler; Frank B. Hicks, Grand Marais; Earl Jamieson Walnut Grove; DeWitt C. Jones, St. Paul; Raymond W Lagersen, Minneapolis; Hans M. Lichtenstein, Winona; Frederick W. Logan, Blue Earth; Elias P. Lyon, Minneapolis

Martin L. Mayland, Faribault; Patrick H. Mee, Osseo; Clarence R. Morss, Zumbrota; Henry T. Norrgard, Milaca; Homer F. Peirson, Austin; Donovan Penheiter, Bagley; Ralph St. J. Perry, Minneapolis; Clarence E. Persons, Marshall; William C. Portmann, Jackson; John T. Rogers, St. Paul; Philemon Roy, St. Paul; Roy A. Schnacke, McGregor; Oscar H. Ternstrom, Minneapolis; Henning F. B. Wiese, Minneapolis; Warren Wilson, Northfield.

FORMER MEMBERS

Frederick H. Aldrich, Belview; George S. Cabot, Jamestown, North Dakota; F. Emerson Daigneau, Austin; Joseph E. H. Garand, Dayton; Amos Leuty, Morris; Ira M. Roadman, Minneapolis; Jorgen G. Vigen, West Los Angeles; James D. Weir, Beardsley.

At the request of the Speaker, the delegates stood with bowed heads for a moment in tribute to the memory of these deceased members.

NATIONAL HEALTH CONFERENCE

Following announcements of the next day's committee meetings the Speaker introduced Doctor Abell, president of the American Medical Association, who spoke as follows:

Mr. Speaker, members of the House of Delegates: Perhaps you will be interested in the background of the National Health Conference which is meeting in Washington, July 18, 19 and 20.

As most of you know, we have been advocating a federal department of health headed by a cabinet minister since 1875. The request has been made to successive administrations and refused on the ground, I believe, that the money expended by federal health agencies did not justify creation of a separate department. The validity of this excuse may be doubted when we consider the various agencies of the federal government today whose functions involve health or medical care. Of the beds available for medical care in this country, approximately a million are controlled by government agencies, including state and municipal governments. In addition, of course, there are the public health functions in the charge of the Department of the Treasury; the food and drug administration of the Department of Agriculture; the maternal and child welfare agencies of the Department of Labor; the Coast Guard Service in the Department of Commerce; Indian welfare in the Department of the Interior; medical service for the Army and Navy under the War Department; medical service for veterans under the Veterans' Administration; and there are also medical functions involved in the work of other bureaus such as the Resettlement Administration and the WPA. The aggregate expenditure for all these must amount to a considerable sum.

The result is that an Inter-Departmental Committee has been appointed during the present administration in Washington to recommend ways and means of co-ordinating all of the health and welfare activities of the federal government. This committee consists of representatives of five departments; Agriculture, Labor, Commerce, the Treasury and the Social Security Board. The chairman is Miss Josephine Roche. A technical committee on medical care was appointed by the committee and it was under the auspices of this technical committee that the National Health Survey, carried on almost entirely by WPA workers, was made. This survey, designed to present a cross-section of the country, was carried on, I believe, in only nineteen states.

The report of the Inter-Departmental Committee presented to the President in February, and whether or not one agrees with all of the suggestions and data contained there it is one, I think, which should be considered carefully by everyone who is interested in the health movement in this country.

It starts by paying a tribute to the medical profession for its accomplishments in bringing about the decrease in mortality and the increase in longevity. It then takes up special problems in the control of various communicable diseases. Tuberculosis can be reduced 50 per cent below the present level, for instance, by correcting conditions in industrial life that tend to make people susceptible to it, according to the report. Syphilis, malaria and diseases of childhood are considered; also the degenerative diseases of advancing age—cancer, diabetes, arteriosclerosis, arthritis, nephritis—in relation to the income of the various groups of the population, pointing out what has long been patent to every thoughtful person, that the amount of disease is much higher among the lower income and indigent group than among those of higher incomes above $3,000 a year.

The fact that adequate fuel, food, clothing and shelter may in themselves be a factor in the health of people in the lower income brackets is not considered.

The number of physicians in the country is considered to be adequate by the report, though better distribution should be made. The number of dentists, now about 70,000, is believed to be only about half the number required, and hospital beds are inadequate. In the larger centers, of course, hospital beds are considered abundant for the needs, but the statement is made that in rural communities there are some 18,000,-000 people who live thirty miles or more from the nearest registered hospital. This last finding is not in harmony with findings of the bureau of medical economics of the American Medical Association, which show that there are only thirteen counties in which the population density is five to each square mile and the total population, some 68,700 in which the people live thirty miles or more from a registered hospital.

The report considers that public health nurses should be increased from 18,000 to 65,000; that hospitals and diagnostic services should be made within easy access of all communities.

The entire program of recommendations should be met by tax funds or Social Security funds, according to the committee.

Some further interesting observations by Miss Roche made in an address in New York before the American Public Health Association, indicate that the 40,000,000 people in the United States whose family incomes are less than $1,000 a year are considered indigent by the committee. The group of 50,000,000 with family incomes of less than $2,000 are considered medically indigent; in other words, they are able to buy food, clothing, shelter, but not medical care.

One may, perhaps, differ with Miss Roche in this matter. In New York City, $2,000 a year may well constitute medical indigency. In some communities, however, $2,000 constitutes independence and in others affluence. Thus, I am sure we cannot all subscribe to the statement that the 50,000,000 people with an annual income of $2,000 are medically indigent. Furthermore, one does hate to believe that 90,000,000 out of the 130,000,000 people in this country are worthy objects of federal bounty and medical service. I know of no way to reach an estimate of the cost of such service to 90,000,000 people, though possibly costs of medical service to government employes in the Canal Zone may provide an indication.

As you know, all of the inhabitants of the strip of land ten miles on either side of the Canal, together with Cristobal on the East and Balboa on the West, are government employes. There are no indigents and no one who has not adequate food, clothing and shelter. The government provides complete medical services at a cost, without including construction and equipment costs, of approximately $25 a year per person. To provide such care for 90,000,000 people would cost $252,000,000 a year without considering for a moment the funds needed for construction and maintenance of buildings and equipment.

Now the Inter-Departmental Committee has called a

conference to be held in Washington to present, according to the invitation, ways and means to prevent loss of efficiency in our people from illness and for reduction of economic burdens caused by illness. Also, proposals embodying such a program to be made to representatives of the government.

Of course, nobody knows what those proposals will be. I feel, however, that this conference will enable us to know what the attitude of the government toward the practice of medicine will be, and I sincerely hope that some proposal will be made for the improvement of the condition of the indigent, at least, upon which all of us may agree.

The following resolution proposed by Dr. B. A. Smith of Crosby was adopted by the delegates.

"The House of Delegates of the Minnesota State Medical Association wishes to express its appreciation to Mr. C. R. Carlgren, chairman, and through him to Mr. B. E. Youngdahl, Director of the Division of Public Assistance, and to Dr. H. E. Hilleboe, Director of Services for Crippled Children, as well as the entire State Board of Control for their sympathetic and intelligent understanding of medical problems of Minnesota, and for their fine coöperation with the Minnesota State Medical Association in the handling of all medical phases of their work."

The following resolution was proposed by Doctor Zachman and adopted by the delegates with the suggestion that the name of Dr. S. E. Gilkey, medical advisor of the State Relief Agency, be included in the resolution.

"The right to choose his own physician is recognized as fundamental to good medical care for all classes of patients, and the thanks and appreciation of all physicians are due especially to Mr. Aufderheide and his associates of the State Relief Agency for the vigorous manner in which they have interpreted and enforced the provision of the new relief law guaranteeing this right to relief patients in Minnesota. Appreciation is also due to these officials for the readiness and understanding with which they have assisted physicians wherever possible to improve the standards of medical care for the needy."

Following reports by the delegates to the American Medical Association, Dr. W. F. Braasch, Dr. J. T. Christison and Dr. W. A. Coventry, of the meeting of the American Medical Association in San Francisco, the meeting adjourned to be re-convened at 6 p. m., Wednesday, June 29, 1938.

HOUSE OF DELEGATES

Second Meeting
Wednesday, June 29, at 6 p. m.

By motion duly made and seconded it was unanimously agreed to dispense with reading of the minutes of the last meeting.

The Council having no further report for the House of Delegates, the Speaker called for announcements of the next day's events.

The following resolutions were proposed by delegates and adopted by the house:

"The interest and devoted effort displayed by every member of the St. Louis County Medical Society, and particularly by the committee on local arrangements, has added materially to the value of our program and to the comfort and convenience of all who are in attendance at this great meeting. The thanks and appreciation of this House and also of the Association are hereby extended to them for the splendid arrangements made by them for this meeting."

"In its generous contribution of space for our sessions and in its courteous attention to the comfort of our members, the Hotel Duluth has contributed greatly to the success of this meeting. The thanks of the House of Delegates is hereby extended for this service."

"Proper newspaper reports of the proceedings of a state

742

medical meeting add greatly to the interest of our members and they serve also as an important avenue of public education on public health. The House of Delegates extends its appreciation to the *Duluth Herald and Tribune*, especially, and to other Minnesota newspapers for their generous contribution of space to information about this meeting."

* * *

"An unprecedented amount of radio time has been put at the service of our Association at this meeting by stations WEBC and KDAL, not only for advance announcements, but to permit the public to listen to our distinguished guests on medical problems of interest to audiences. The thanks of this House is extended to both stations for their fine coöperation in this matter."

* * *

"The thanks of the House of Delegates should also be extended to the Duluth Chamber of Commerce for their excellent coöperation in all of the arrangements for this meeting and for the efficient help they have given us in registration of members."

* * *

"The thanks of the House of Delegates should be extended to the Minnesota Arrowhead Association for their courtesy in extending the facilities of their offices in the Hotel Duluth for this meeting and for their contribution to the pleasures and comfort of those who attended the meeting."

* * *

"The thanks of this House should be extended to the Kiwanis Club of Duluth for their courtesy and friendliness in presenting the beautiful basket of flowers for our platform."

ELECTION OF OFFICERS

The Speaker then called for nominations for the office of president-elect.

Dr. George Earl of Saint Paul was nominated for the position of *president-elect* by Dr. R. B. Hullsiek of Saint Paul in behalf of the delegates from the Ramsey County Medical Society.

There being no further nominations, it was moved, seconded and carried that the nominations should be closed and that the secretary should cast a unanimous ballot for Doctor Earl for the office of president-elect.

Dr. J. C. Jacobs of Willmar was similarly nominated for the position of *first vice president* and, there being no further nominations, it was moved, seconded and carried that the nominations be closed and that the secretary be instructed to cast a unanimous ballot for Doctor Jacobs for first vice president.

Dr. A. M. Hanson of Faribault was nominated for the position of *second vice president* and, there being no further nominations, it was moved, seconded and carried that the nominations be closed and that the secretary be instructed to cast a unanimous ballot for Doctor Hanson for second vice president.

Dr. B. B. Souster of Saint Paul was nominated by Doctor Hullsiek for the position of *secretary* to fill out the unexpired term of Doctor Meyerding, whose resignation had been accepted by the House, and also to serve for the year 1938-39. There being no further nominations, it was moved, seconded and carried that the nominations be closed and that the secretary be instructed to cast a unanimous ballot for Doctor Souster for secretary.

Dr. W. H. Condit of Minneapolis was nominated to succeed himself for the position of *treasurer* and, there being no further nominations, it was moved, seconded and carried that the nominations be closed and that the secretary be instructed to cast a unanimous ballot for Doctor Condit.

Dr. A. W. Adson of Rochester and *Doctor Will* were nominated for the position of *speaker of the House of Delegates*.

Dr. Joel Hultkräns, vice-speaker, was asked by Speaker Will to take the chair and, upon Doctor Adson's request that his name be withdrawn from the nomination, it was moved, seconded and carried that the nominations be closed and that the secretary be instructed to cast a unanimous ballot for *Doctor Will* to succeed himself as *speaker of the House of Delegates*. Doctor Will resumed the chair and *Dr. E. A. Meyerding* of Saint Paul was nominated for the position of *vice speaker*. It was moved, seconded and carried that the nominations be closed and that the secretary be instructed to cast a unanimous ballot for Doctor Meyerding for vice speaker.

Dr. H. Z. Giffin of Rochester, *councilor of the first district, Dr. L. L. Sogge* of Windom, *councilor of the second district,* and *Dr. B. S. Adams* of Hibbing, *councilor of the ninth district,* were nominated to succeed themselves as councilors of their respective districts. It was moved, seconded and carried in each case that nominations be closed and that the secretary cast unanimous ballots for each as councilors.

Dr. E. M. Jones of Saint Paul was nominated as *councilor of the fifth district* to succeed Dr. George Earl, previously elected to the position of the president-elect, and it was moved, seconded and carried that the nominations be closed and that the secretary be instructed to cast a unanimous vote for Doctor Jones as councilor of the fifth district.

Nominations were called for to fill the positions of two *delegates to the American Medical Association* with their *alternates* whose terms expired.

Dr. W. F. Braasch of Rochester and *Dr. W. A. Coventry* of Duluth, and *Dr. W. L. Burnap* of Fergus Falls, alternate to Doctor Braasch, were nominated to succeed themselves. It was moved, seconded and carried in each case that the nominations be closed and that the secretary be instructed to cast a unanimous ballot for each.

Dr. Joel Hultkrans of Minneapolis was nominated to succeed Dr. George Earl as *alternate* to Doctor Coventry and it was moved, seconded and carried that the nominations be closed and that the secretary be instructed to cast a unanimous ballot for Doctor Hultkrans for the position of alternate to Doctor Coventry.

PLACE OF MEETING

Invitations from the Hennepin County Medical Society from Dr. J. M. Hayes of Minneapolis, president of the Minnesota State Medical Association, and from the Minneapolis Civic and Commerce Association to the Minnesota State Medical Association to hold its 86th Annual Meeting in Minneapolis were presented by Dr. C. A. Stewart, councilor of the sixth district.

It was unanimously voted to hold the 86th Annual Meeting in Minneapolis.

* * *

In the absence of Dr. A. J. Chesley, secretary and executive officer of the State Board of Health, Doctor Adson was asked by the speaker to give a report of the morning meeting of the State Board of Health.

DOCTOR ADSON: I am sorry, Mr. Speaker, that Doctor Chesley is not here to give you the details of the meeting. The chief subject under discussion was the additional federal appropriation for control and treatment of syphilis which will be put at the disposal of the State Board of Health. I haven't the figures with me but I believe the amount is approximately $42,000. No great expansion in the work of the board can be carried on, as you know, until the present building program is completed. After that, it is the plan to add two assistants (clerks and technicians) with the intentions of using the money only to advance the present program.

Those of you who heard Doctor Irvine today fully appreciate the fine program carried on in Minnesota by the State Board of Health and also the fine interest and coöperation of the board with organized medicine. The fact that the State Board of Health is willing to coöperate with us and to listen to the problems that confront us in the practice of medicine is one of the finest compliments that can be paid them. It is our hope that the medical men in the rural communities particularly will likewise coöperate with the board in its work.

It has been proposed that the new funds be used in some instances to assist those who have no money so that the doctor can be compensated for his work in the treatment of syphilis. At the present time, it is not the intention, as I understand it, to set up any additional clinics anywhere in the state for treatment of syphilis. Instead, the facilities already in existence will be utilized and the general lines of the program that has been in existence here for some twenty years will be followed. Perhaps, Doctor Braasch has something to add on this subject.

DOCTOR BRAASCH: I don't know whether we all appreciate what a valuable man Doctor Chesley is in this community. He is president of the national association of health officers and undoubtedly the outstanding man in the departments of health of the country today. He has received many offers to go to other branches but has elected to remain here. And his work in maternal and child welfare and in child health, as shown by the statistics, is a record in itself. If you visit the State Board of Health exhibit in one of the booths at this meeting you will see what progress has been made in this state.

Furthermore, Doctor Chesley has coöperated fully with the medical profession here and has worked for our joint interests in Washington. I think it no more than right that this House of Delegates should extend a vote of confidence and thanks to him for his work in our behalf and on behalf of the public welfare.

DOCTOR SWEETSER: In seconding this motion, I would like to mention the fact, as chairman of the Committee on State Health Relations, that Doctor Chesley has invited a member of our committee to each Board of Health meeting since the formation of the committee. He has worked hand in hand with our committee all of the time.

The vote of thanks was unanimously carried by the House of Delegates and the meeting adjourned.

MINNESOTA MEDICINE

Journal of the Minnesota State Medical Association, Southern Minnesota Medical Association, Northern Minnesota Medical Association, Minnesota Academy of Medicine and Minneapolis Surgical Society

| Volume 21 | NOVEMBER, 1938 | No. 11 |

THE INFLUENCE OF AGE-DETERMINED FACTORS ON THE DEVELOPMENT OF TUBERCULOSIS*

ARNOLD RICE RICH, M.D.

Associate Professor of Pathology and Bacteriology, The Johns Hopkins Medical School

Baltimore, Maryland

IT IS now well known that at different periods of the life-span there are striking differences in the clinical manifestations, the prognosis, the character of the lesions, the mortality rate and the epidemiology of tuberculosis.

The recognition of the existence of these age-period differences has become essential for the proper interpretation of the disease, whether by the clinician, the pathologist or the epidemiologist. For the proper understanding, and for the most effective control of the disease it is of great importance that we learn precisely to what these age-period peculiarities are due. Unfortunately, our information about this matter is sadly deficient at present. The problem is a large one, with many ramifications; and each particular age-period is sufficiently complex to warrant an extended discussion of the factors peculiar to it. I cannot hope, therefore, to do justice to the consideration of all of the different age periods in a single lecture; but it may be worth while to attempt a review of the situation, even though no other end is achieved than that of defining and emphasizing the rather narrow limits of our present information regarding this important and arresting subject.

One of the most fundamental questions involved in the problem, and one that has aroused much interest and speculation, is that relating to the degree of native resistance to tuberculosis possessed by the human body at the different periods of life. By "native resistance" we mean,

of course, the inherent ability of the body to destroy or to prevent the progressive proliferation of the bacillus on first contact with it. Is this inherent ability different at different periods of life, independently of external circumstances? Throughout the following discussion we shall pay particular attention to this question.

The characteristic and consistent differences in the tuberculosis mortality rate at the different periods of life have been regarded by many as sufficient evidence that there are corresponding differences in native resistance at the various age periods. Simple mortality rates, however, do not in themselves throw any certain light upon differences in native resistance, for they are influenced too greatly by the complicating factor of resistance acquired through previous infection, by the external influences that are peculiar to each age period and which exert a potent effect upon resistance, and, most important, by the incidence of infection in the population at the different age periods. Resistance is the ability to restrain the progress of infection. In a consideration of resistance at a given age period, therefore, we are interested not in the number of deaths in relation to the total number of individuals of that age (i.e., the general mortality rate), but only in the number of deaths in relation to the *infected* portion of that age group. In other words, the only figures of any suggestive import in relation to resistance are those which tell us whether a larger or a smaller proportion of the *infected* population in a given age period die from the disease, as

*The John W. Bell Tuberculosis Lecture, delivered before the Hennepin County Medical Society, Minneapolis, Minn., April 4, 1938.

TABLE I. TWENTY RECENT TUBERCULIN SURVEYS

List restricted to surveys in which final test dose was not less than 1.0 mg. O.T. or equivalent amount PPD.

Place of Survey	Author	Date	Per Cent Positive Reactions in Each Age Group								
			0 to 4	5 to 9	10 to 14	15 to 19	20 to 24	25 to 29	30 to 34	35 to 39	40 and over
Rural Alabama*	Aronson	1933	27.3	36.4	44.4	76.2	84.2	53.8	81.8	80.0	81.0
Rural Florida*	Aronson	1933	17.7	20.6	22.3	62.1	61.7	81.4	72.4	65.7	83.3
Rural Michigan	Aronson	1935	6.1	9.6	17.8	26.4	41.0	52.4	54.4	72.1	76.4
Rural Tennessee*	Aronson	1933	–	36.8	60.8	67.4	–	–	–	–	–
Rural New York Schools	Korns	1931	–	7.0	10.8	16.0	–	–	–	–	–
Rural Minn. Schools	Leggett and Callahan	1931	–	–	–	31.5	–	–	–	–	–
Philadelphia Clinic*	Aronson and Nicholas	1933	14.1	20.0	42.8	–	–	–	–	–	–
Philadelphia Schools*	Hetherington, et al.	1934	–	60.2	76.0	83.0	–	–	–	–	–
Schools near Boston	Aronson et al.	1933	–	28.5	41.5	62.6	–	–	–	–	–
Waverly, Mass. Institution	Aronson et al.	1933	–	39.4	55.7	75.5	–	–	–	–	–
Minneapolis, Minn. Schools	Harrington et al.	1937	–	14.5	20.2	–	–	–	–	–	–
Pine City, Minn. Schools	Leggett and Callahan	1931	–	–	22.3	32.6	–	–	–	–	–
Univ. Wisconsin and High School	Stiehm	1935	–	–	19.4	23.3	36.8	50.1	–	–	–
New York City Schools	Barnard et al.	1931	–	–	67.3	–	–	–	–	–	–
Yale Univ. Students	Soper and Wilson	1932	–	–	–	53.5	58.1	–	–	–	–
Bellevue Hosp., N.Y. Entering nurses	Amberson	1936	–	–	–	57.9	–	–	–	–	–
St. Paul, Minn., Hosp. Entering nurses	Greer	1934	–	–	–	30.0	–	–	–	–	–
18,774 Students in 20 Colleges	Long and Seibert	1937	–	–	–	44.6	–	–	–	–	–
Univ. Pa. 1st year Medical Students	Hetherington et al.	1935	–	–	–	–	85.0	–	–	–	–
47,358 tests in 30 states	Whitney and McCaffery	1937	24.6	23.3	33.4	36.3	–	–	–	–	–
Average			17.9	28.6	38.9	48.6	61.1	–	–	–	–

*White subjects only.

compared with the mortality rate of the infected population in a different period of life. It is this relationship that we shall first proceed to examine.

At the very outset of this enquiry we encounter the first of our many difficulties and uncertainties, in the circumstance that no accurate information exists regarding the incidence of infection in the different age groups of the population at the present time. There are no recent representative autopsy studies of the matter, and no sufficient number of properly carried out and properly distributed tuberculin surveys made since 1930; and in the face of the rapidly declining tuberculosis mortality, figures for some years back cannot with propriety be mixed with the more recent ones.

In Table I, I have assembled the results of twenty representative tuberculin surveys reported in this country since 1930. The gaps in the available material are impressively evident. Particularly is there a dearth of representative material relating to adults, for the figures for college students can hardly be regarded as a fair average of the population. In the past, when it seemed established that the great majority of adults were infected, the position was adopted that nothing profitable could be learned from further tuberculin-testing of adults, and it became the practice to concentrate attention upon the incidence of infection in children. This attitude has persisted up to the present. In view of the markedly altered mortality rate of today however, it becomes highly desirable that both rural and urban surveys of the incidence of infection in adults of all ages be undertaken again and on a country-wide scale.

Studies of the incidence of infection in the first year of life are also urgently needed. At present there are only fragmentary figures of unrepresentative material, so that any estimate of the present day incidence of infection in the first year must represent only an individual guess.

In attempting to form an opinion regarding the incidence of infection from tuberculin surveys, there arises the important question as to the frequency with which a negative test may occur in persons who have been previously infected. It is commonly assumed that only in exceptional cases will the test be negative in healthy persons who have been previously infected, if 1.0 mg. of Old Tuberculin be used. Certainly, in the past, our information tended to support that view, but in the face of the markedly changed conditions it becomes possible that the results of the tuberculin test in present day surveys no longer mirror so well the actual incidence of infection. One disturbing element is that we do not know the average duration of tuberculin sensitiveness following a slight, well-resisted infection, and this clearly is a matter of importance in the interpretation of the results of tuberculin tests in terms of incidence of infection.—

That hypersensitivity, once established, by no means invariably remains at a level detectable by the routine tests has long been well known. This was plainly shown by Austrian[4] fifteen years ago, and all investigators who have studied the matter thoroughly are agreed on this, though there are differences of opinion as to the usual duration of manifest hypersensitivity, and the frequency with which it falls to a level too low to be detected by the routine tests. Evidence is rapidly accumulating, however, which leaves no doubt that hypersensitivity to tuberculin may be lost with a frequency which, under present conditions of infection, has to be seriously considered in any evaluation of the results of tuberculin surveys. To make this clear it will suffice to call attention to a number of recent studies, all carried out by experienced and able investigators. Barnard, Amberson and Loew[5] found that of 184 school children between twelve and fifteen years of age who had tuberculous lesions demonstrable by x-ray, 6 per cent failed to react to 1.0 mg. of Old Tuberculin. Wells and Smith[58] found demonstrable x-ray lesions in 5.5 per cent of 128 individuals negative to 1.0 mg. of tuberculin. The careful studies of Opie and his associates[25,38] on children between five and nineteen years showed that 15 per cent of 186 who were negative to 1.0 mg. of tuberculin had definite x-ray evidence of tuberculous infection. Crabtree, Hickerson and Hickerson[15] have recently

reported a study in persons over four years of age who were negative to 1.0 mg. of carefully standardized tuberculin. Seventeen per cent of those tuberculin-negative individuals were found to have calcified lesions on x-ray examination. Dr. Gauld, of the Department of Epidemiology in the Johns Hopkins School of Public Health, has recently shown me the results of an extensive study, soon to be published, in which an even higher percentage of definite calcified lesions in the lungs and bronchial nodes was found in healthy individuals completely negative to 1.0 mg. of carefully standardized Old Tuberculin; and Nelson, Mitchell and Brown[36] have recently reported similar results.

Since it is well known that the x-ray reveals the primary lesion in only a small percentage of all who do react to tuberculin and are therefore known to be infected, it is clear that the total number of infected persons among those who fail to react must be much larger that the number discovered by x-ray in the above-mentioned studies.

It can hardly be objected that the x-ray interpretation of all of these experienced students of tuberculosis were erroneous, and that the lesions observed in their tuberculin negative subjects were not really tuberculous. As a matter of fact, I know that in Dr. Gauld's study the figures for the presence of calcified tuberculous lesions in negative reactors were so high that he had the plates checked by four independent specialists in different cities in order to rule out errors of individual interpretation. But even such a possible objection is met by investigations in which the change from the hypersensitive to the tuberculin negative state has been directly observed. Thus, Lloyd and MacPherson[30] report from England that of 303 healthy London children who reacted to 1.0 mg. of Old Tuberculin in 1930, 2 per cent were negative to that dose two years later; and Aronson,[2] who has had so extensive an experience in tuberculin surveys in this country, has followed eighty-seven tuberculin-positive urban children for a period of five years, during which time 9 per cent became negative to 1.0 mg. of carefully standardized Old Tuberculin. In a private school that was free from cases of open tuberculosis, Horan,[27] tested 197 adolescent boys yearly for three successive years. During this time 14 per cent of those who were tuberculin-positive on the first test had lost their hypersensitivity to 1.0 mg. of tuberculin. In a recent study, Paretsky[41] reports that out of a group of tuberculin-positive children that were followed up to five years, 80 became negative to 1.0 mg. of Old Tuberculin. Sixty-four per cent of these were retested with 10.0 mg. and failed to react. In animals remaining in good health after having resisted a tuberculous infection, hypersensitivity may fall to so low a level after the lapse of one to two years following infection, that very large doses of tuberculin fail to produce any reaction; and it is very important to remember in relation to the human being that it has been demonstrated by Willis[54] that the animals that lose their sensitivity with the passing of time retain in high degree the resistance to reinfection that was conferred by the original infection. Sewall and his co-workers[47] and Boquet[7] have likewise shown that as hypersensitivity declines acquired resistance remains intact; and numerous studies from our own laboratory, confirmed by many subsequent investigations, have demonstrated that when hypersensitivity is deliberately abolished by proper desensitizing procedures, immunity to reinfection remains in high degree.[44] In the human being, therefore, not only is a negative tuberculin test no proof that the individual has never been infected, but it is also no proof that acquired resistance is lacking.

These considerations obviously have an important bearing upon the proper interpretation of the results of tuberculin surveys. In the first part of this century, when the mortality and morbidity from tuberculosis were very high, and open cases were far more numerous in the population than they are today, individuals who became infected once had a greater opportunity to become infected again and again throughout their lives, and so to have their hypersensitiveness frequently restimulated. Today, however, the spectacular decline in mortality and morbidity (and, therefore, in the number of open cases) has greatly decreased the opportunities for chance contact with the bacillus. The marked diminution in the number of open cases must influence not only the total number of individuals who will become infected at each age period, but also the number and frequency of repeated reinfections. Under these conditions it is reasonable to believe that a correspondingly larger number of individuals in the population today are escaping the hypersensitivity—reanimating influence of reinfections after having lost

the sensitivity conferred by a primary infection. It cannot be assumed, therefore, that the number who fail to react to tuberculin in a given survey in this country today approximates the number who have never been infected as closely as may have been the case in the early part of this century.

It is highly desirable to learn to what degree any present day diminution in the number of positive reactors reflects an actual decline in the number of primary infections, and to what degree it is due to a lessened opportunity for reinfections which maintain hypersensitivity at a level detectable by the routine tests. Large scale minute studies of the incidence of primary infections and reinfections in routine autopsies, such as those that were carried out some years ago during the period in which the opportunities for infection were much greater, are urgently needed in order that we may gain a better insight into the actual present-day incidence of infection in the different age groups.

In order to make clear how badly such studies are needed, I shall only remind you that for many years throughout the world it has been regarded as an established fact that the so-called adult type of pulmonary tuberculosis, characterized by apical or sub-apical localization, prominent fibrosis, the failure to involve regional lymph nodes appreciably, and by little tendency to generalization, develops only as a result of *reinfection* in persons who previously have had a partially immunizing, primary infection; and that if progressive disease develops directly as a result of *primary* infection, it will have the characteristics familiar in progressive childhood tuberculosis, namely, localization anywhere in the lung with the apex as the least frequent site prominent caseation and little fibrosis, marked involvement of regional lymph nodes, and marked tendency to generalization. Now there is much experimental, clinical and pathological evidence in support of this deep-rooted belief, and as long as practically all individuals in urban communities were known to have had a primary infection by the time adult life was reached there was little to disturb that view. At present, however, we are told, on the basis of tuberculin surveys, that only about half of all young adults carry a primary infection. If this be true, and if our long-held attitude toward the adult and childhood type of tuberculosis be correct, we should today be encountering on all sides, both

TABLE II.

U. S. Registration Area, 1932

Age	Total Deaths From Tuberculosis	Estimated Per Cent Infected*	Tbc. Deaths per 100,000 Persons of this Age			Tbc. Deaths per 100,000 Infected Persons of This Age
			Male	Female	Both Sexes	Both Sexes
0–1	834	1	43.0	38.1	40.6	4060
1–4	1718	10	19.9	20.5	20.1	201
5–9	989	25	8.2	7.8	8.0	32
10–14	1332	35	8.7	14.0	11.3	31
15–19	4912	45	31.2	55.2	43.3	96
20–24	8853	55	68.0	98.1	83.3	151
25–29	8672	65	83.2	97.1	90.3	135
30–34	7787	75	93.0	82.1	87.5	114
35–39	7566	85	99.4	68.2	84.0	100
40–44	6746	90	107.0	62.9	85.7	94
45–49	6014	90	113.2	58.8	87.0	96
50–54	5143	90	115.6	58.5	88.2	98
55–59	4304	90	124.3	61.9	94.3	104
60–64	3395	90	118.6	65.2	92.6	103
65–69	2756	90	119.1	83.6	101.9	113
70–74	2301	90	138.5	100.5	119.7	133
75 and over	2101	90	116.6	102.9	109.4	121

*Estimated from recent tuberculin surveys. The figures for some of the age periods are probably too low. See text for question of reliability of tuberculin surveys as indicators of the true incidence of infection.

clinically and pathologically, many instances of progressive tuberculosis of the childhood type developing in the great number of young adults who, according to the tuberculin surveys, have never had a previous, immunizing infection. This, however, is not the case. Young adult tuberculosis, both at the bedside and at the autopsy table, has today precisely the same characteristics as that during the period when primary infection in urban adults was almost universal. In this connection it is of particular interest to note that in the recent study carried out by Myers and his co-workers[33] on tuberculous infection developing in young adults who were regarded as never having been previously infected because they were negative to tuberculin shortly before the lesions appeared, in the overwhelming majority of those cases the lesions were apical or sub-apical and were typical of the adult type of the disease. Were these, then, really instances of primary infection, or were they instances of reinfection in individuals who had lost their hypersensitivity? This question has to be considered the more seriously since Arborelius[1] has described cases of apparently true primary infection occurring in tuberculin-negative young adults from rural districts in

Sweden, and in those cases the lesions were never apical but were typical of those characteristic of primary infection in childhood; and instances of typical, progressive childhood-type tuberculosis in young adults were observed at autopsy by Hart[24] in the German army during the World War.

These circumstances should make it clear that either our long-held concept of the pathogenesis of adult type tuberculosis requires a drastic revision, or else that many individuals who today are tuberculin negative have really been infected, and have retained their acquired resistance to the degree that determines the peculiarities of adult type tuberculosis, but have lost their hypersensitivity, and under present conditions of diminished opportunity for reinfection they remain tuberculin negative for longer periods than would have been the case formerly. Only a minute search for healed lesions with the aid of the x-ray in routine autopsies can settle this matter, and studies of this nature are at present being carried out in Baltimore. Needless to say, similar studies should be undertaken in widely different parts of the country, in order that a representative survey may be possible.

In order to determine the mortality in the infected portion of the population at each age period it is necessary to be able to compare the total deaths from tuberculosis in the entire population at a given age period with the number of infected persons in that age period. In view of the above circumstances it is obviously impossible to pretend to deal with any degree of accuracy with the question of the country's "average" incidence of infection at the different age periods. One can only form an individual impression of the matter from a study of the available urban and rural tuberculin surveys, making allowances for the circumstances discussed; and it is hardly to be expected that there will be any general agreement among the individual impressions so formed. It is such an impression, and no more than that, that is given in Table II. The estimate of the incidence of the infection for each age period has been made as conservative as has seemed compatible with present-day information, and it is probably too low in certain instances. In the older age groups we still have to do with individuals who have had to pass through the period of high exposure risk of the latter part of the last and the early part of the present century, and we cannot expect the incidence of infection in those individuals to reflect as well the more recent lowering of exposure risk.

While the figures in Table II relating to the proportion of infected persons in the population at each age period are admittedly based upon data that leave much to be desired, they nevertheless provide at least a relative view of the situation as it exists today, and it is important to make an attempt to view it from this particular standpoint. Certainly, any correction of the figures for the incidence of infection in any of the age periods within limits that, in either direction, are within range of probability, would not alter appreciably the general trend that the figures express. The figures showing the mortality rate of the infected portion of the population are markedly different from the ordinary mortality rates of the total population, and they bring out more clearly than do the latter figures the following facts which have been recognized by clinicians and students of the epidemiology of tuberculosis:

1. That tuberculosis is most fatal during the first year of life;

2. That it is much less dangerous, but still

markedly so during the succeeding several years;

3. That the period between five years and puberty is a strikingly "safe" period, during which the mortality from the disease decreases in spite of the fact that the incidence of infection increases. In this period of life the tuberculosis mortality rate reaches its lowest point.

4. That following the age of puberty there occurs a sharp increase in the death-hazard among those infected.

5. That the increase in the tuberculosis mortality-hazard continues steadily into adult life, reaching a peak in the middle twenties, after which it continues at an elevated level throughout the remainder of the life span, but with variations that depend upon sex, occupation and economic conditions.

6. That in old age there occurs a second peak of mortality-hazard.

From the above facts it is clear, then, that by far the most dangerous age period in which to be infected, from the standpoint of the chance of succumbing during that age period, is that of the first five years of life, and most particularly during the first year; and that by far the safest period is that between five years and puberty. From puberty onward the chance of dying if infected increases rapidly until it reaches a peak, the precise age period of which is inconstant in the total population and may be different for each sex at different periods of time. The mortality rate among the infected is always high in old age, but it may be lower than the first adult peak. How are these age peculiarities to be explained, and what relation if any, do they bear to age-determined differences in native resistance?

Factors Influencing the High Mortality in Infancy

Regarding the extraordinarily high mortality among those who become infected during the first year of life, it is altogether probable that this is due in part to the fact that since infants cannot move about to court infection they are ordinarily exposed either to heavy and continued infection (phthisical member of the household; contaminated milk, in localities which bovine tuberculosis is prevalent) or none at all. This explanation was suggested long ago by Römer,[46] and it is a reasonable one. In addition, it may be suggested that sin malnutrition affects resistance to tuberculosis adversely at all ages, the frequency of nutritional disturbances in infancy may play a rôle in favoring progressive infection in this period. In infancy, as is well known, malnutrition frequently results from conditions other than an insufficient supply of food in the home. High atmospheric temperature, artificial feeding, and acute infections of even slight degree, such as otitis media, are factors which often precipitate a diarrhea that prevents the proper assimilation of food, with consequent malnutrition not infrequently of severe degree. After the first year, debilitating diarrhea occurs less frequently as a complication of these conditions. It is not altogether improbable, therefore, that the greater frequency of malnutrition during the first year may influence to some degree the chance of development of progressive tuberculosis among those who become infected during this period of life.

But these factors of dosage of bacilli and liability to malnutrition do not dispose of the possibility that, in addition, the native resistance of the healthy infant may be lower than that of the older child or adult. Is there any reason to believe that this may be the case?

There is not at present any actual *proof* that the infant has a lower native resistance to tuberculosis than have older individuals. Obviously, it is practically impossible to obtain direct and controlled evidence regarding the degree of native resistance in the human being, for the only way in which the effectiveness of the mechanism of immunity can be accurately determined is by observing the result of a standardized test infection. Neither the clinical nor the pathological aspects of the accidentally acquired disease can help us here, for none of the variables, including the important one of dosage, are controlled.

If we turn to animal experiment for an answer to the question we find that while it has often been demonstrated clearly that young animals are more susceptible to many acute infections than are adult animals, the several experiments which have so far been carried out on tuberculosis have failed to show any convincing differences between the resistance of young and older animals. It may be fairly said, however, that none of the few recorded experiments on this subject are sufficiently satisfying to be regarded as at all conclusive.

Nevertheless, there is evidence from a different direction which, it has seemed to me,[45] can profitably be applied to the problem under consideration, and which renders it altogether likely that the native resistance of the infant to tuberculosis may be lower than that of the older individual. It is essential to bear clearly in mind the fact that any consideration of *native* immunity in a chronic disease involves, inescapably, a consideration of *acquired* immunity. In an acute infection which rapidly runs its course to a fatal termination, native immunity can be studied uncomplicated by acquired immunity, although even here this is true only when an infecting dose is chosen which will not permit survival for more than a day or two. Even in an acute infection, antibody-formation will be initiated as soon as the bacteria have multiplied to numbers sufficient to liberate an appreciable amount of antigen. It is well known, for example, that antibody-formation is often demonstrable a few days after the onset of lobar pneumonia in the human being. When protective antibody has begun to appear, acquired resistance has, of course, already entered the picture. In a chronic infection, in which the bacteria multiply in the body for weeks and months, it is clear that acquired resistance resulting from the infection itself will always have developed to some degree before the disease has run its course. This is strikingly true of tuberculosis. There is unassailable evidence that during the course of primary infection, in both the human being and the experimental animal, acquired resistance usually appears to a very definite degree, even in the case of infections that result fatally. The degree to which acquired resistance develops during infection; and the rapidity of its appearance, are important factors in the progress of the disease; and in many cases in the human being this factor of acquired resistance undoubtedly plays a dominant rôle in determining whether the infection will be restrained and arrested or whether it will progress to a fatal termination. In tuberculosis, therefore, it is essential to consider whether an observed degree of resistance to a primary infection is due chiefly to natively existing elements of immunity, or to circumstances that influence the degree to which acquired immunity develops following infection, and the rapidity with which it makes its appearance. Since this is the case, it is obvious that if the mechanism for developing acquired immunity were less efficient in infancy than in later life, the infant would unfailingly be less able to resist infection than the older child or the adult. Is there, then, any evidence that this situation actually exists?

Up to the present no satisfactorily controlled experiments dealing with the comparative ability of very young and older animals to develop acquired resistance to the tubercle bacillus have been carried out. There is, nevertheless, important evidence that the immunity response of human infants and very young animals to other bacteria and antigens is much less efficient than that of older individuals of the same species. Freund,[20] Kligler and Olitzki[29] and others have shown that very young animals cannot form antibodies to bacteria, bacterial toxins or foreign proteins nearly so effectively as older animals. This is true of birds as well as of mammals; and it is likewise true of the human being. It has been shown by Halber and his collaborators[23] and others that the human infant is deficient in the ability to form agglutinins in comparison with older children; and Ramon and his collaborators[35] and others have shown that the infant is distinctly less able to form diphtheria antitoxin than is the adult. Davies[17] found that infants in the first year of life failed to produce protective antibody in response to the injection of a pneumococcal antigen that was highly effective in stimulating the formation of protective antibody in older individuals, and Dr. Lloyd Felton, of our department, in a recently completed study, has had the same experience.

In connection with the evidence that infants cannot form antibody as effectively as older individuals, it may be stated that we have recently shown experimentally that the acute splenic tumor of bacterial infections represents a reaction to foreign antigens, and can be readily produced by introducing into the tissues foreign protein, whether of bacterial or non-bacterial origin.[43] It is of interest, therefore, that in infants acute splenic tumor rarely becomes so well developed during infection as it does in adults.

The fact that infants are relatively deficient in the ability to form protective antibodies as compared with adults has an important bearing upon the problem before us; for regardless of the lack of absolute parallelism between antibody titre in tuberculosis as measured by present *in vitro* tests, and resistance to infection as

measured by the body's ability to restrain the growth and spread of the bacilli, it is altogether likely that antibody-formation plays an important rôle in immunity to tuberculosis, as it does in immunity to other infections, even though the rôle that it plays in tuberculosis is not yet manifest in all of its relations. It must be remembered that there is no strict and constant parallelism between the serum antibody titre and resistance to infection even in the case of infections in which antibody is well known to play a highly important rôle in a defense. Time does not permit me to enter into a discussion of the function of antibody in resistance to tuberculosis. Here, I wish only to recall to you the fact that infants and young animals have been shown to be natively deficient in the ability to develop acquired immunity and to produce protective antibodies of every type so far investigated, and to point out the reasons for believing that a deficiency of this nature can play an important rôle in determining the well recognized greater susceptibility of the infant to primary tuberculous infection.

It is of interest in this connection that the deficiency in antibody-formation has been found to be particularly striking in infants under six months of age, and Brailey,[10] in the out-patient clinic of the Johns Hopkins Hospital, has found that the mortality from tuberculosis was more than twice as high in infants known to have been infected during the first six months of life as in those whose infection was first discovered between the ages of six months and two years.

Until more evidence is accumulated, we cannot speak with absolute certainty of the rôle that specific age susceptibility may play in the higher tuberculosis mortality rate of infected infants. It is, however, difficult to believe that the infant, with a deficient immunity-producing mechanism, can be natively as resistant to infection as the older child or adult with their more effective immunity mechanism; for in tuberculosis, the rapidity with which an effective degree of acquired resistance develops following infection plays a very important rôle in determining the outcome of a primary infection. Indeed, the well known fact that other infections (e.g., whooping cough, measles, chicken-pox, scarlet fever, diphtheria, pneumococcal, staphylococcal infections, et cetera) are much more fatal in young infants than in older children, is, in itself, evidence that the native ability of the infant to resist infections in general is deficient (Table III).

TABLE III
Figures for the Last U. S. Census Year (1930)

	Deaths Per 100,000	
Age	Combined Infections	Lobar Pneumonia
0-4	255	56
5-14	47	8
15-24	106	15
25-34	129	23
35-44	126	32
45-54	142	56
55-64	165	90
65-74	223	166

With no intent to disparage the investigation of the possibility of protective immunization by means of BCG or vaccines made of killed bacilli, which most assuredly should be studied until their potentialities and limitations are soundly established, it may nevertheless be pointed out that in administering these immunizing agents to new-born infants, as is ordinarily practiced, they are being applied to subjects who, in the light of all available evidence, have far less power of reacting to immunizing antigens than have individuals at any other period of life. This should be taken into consideration not only in regard to the dosage and the period of immunization, but also in drawing conclusions as to the immunizing power of these vaccines from the results obtained in newborn infants. Used at a later period their efficacy would, in all probability, be much greater.

One final point deserves comment in relation to the matter under discussion. For a long period of time the high mortality of infants with *clinical* tuberculosis led to the universal belief that infection in infancy was practically invariably fatal. More recent follow-up studies of tuberculin-positive infants have shown plainly that this is not the case, and this point has been stressed by Myers[32] and others. However, even in the literature of recent years one may still encounter the statement that the newly-born infant is completely devoid of resistance. Gottstein,[22] in his recent excellent monograph on the epidemiology of tuberculosis, states that at least 80 per cent of all infants infected in the first year of life die of the disease. There are

enough studies at present to make it clear that this is far from the case. In a recent follow-up study, Brailey,[10] in the Johns Hopkins Clinic, found that of sixty-six infants who became tuberculin-positive during the first year of life, two-thirds were alive and well at the end of the five years. Had it not been for a large admixture of negro infants in the series the survival rate would undoubtedly have been higher, for 82 per cent of the white infants survived the five-year period as contrasted with only 57 per cent of the negroes.

The Lübeck disaster of 1930 was, itself, highly instructive in this connection. In that unfortunate episode, as is well known, 251 newborn infants who were to have received prophylactic doses of the avirulent BCG bacillus, by mouth, were given by error cultures that were contaminated with virulent human type bacilli. Seventy-two of these children died with extensive tuberculosis within the first year, after which time there were no more deaths from tuberculosis. At the end of four years, when an extensive and minute official report was prepared,[18] it was found that 71 per cent of all of these children who had been infected with presumably large doses of virulent bacilli in the first few days of life were alive with no clinically active lesions, though the presence of arrested calcified lesions, often extraordinary in extent, was demonstrable in most of them. It is, therefore, obvious that it is by no means true that the infant is "completely devoid of resistance." On the contrary, in spite of the very high mortality among infected infants as compared with older individuals, and while there are very good reasons, given above, for believing that the native resistance of the infant is decidedly lower than that of the older child, a large majority of those infected in infancy are able to resist the infection.

Factors Influencing the Mortality Rate Between One and Five Years of Age

During the second year of life the external influences which act in infancy to favor a high death rate among those who become infected with the tubercle bacillus are still operative to some degree. The free excursion of the child into the outside world is still restricted and, as in the case of the infant, though to a lesser degree than during the first year, the most frequent source of infection will still be a phthisical member of the household or contaminated milk, with the opportunity for heavy and repeated infection inherent in these sources. However, the more independent locomotion of the child at this age increases somewhat its chances of acquiring slight first infections, particularly among the poorer classes. Nutritional disturbances due to diarrhea are less frequent than during the first year but are still fairly common and may serve to depress resistance in a portion of those who become infected with the tubercle bacillus. On the other hand, the ability to develop immune antibodies is distinctly higher in the second year than during the first six months of life, though not yet quite so well developed as in later childhood. These various factors all tend to bring it about that the mortality among those infected during the second year, though still high, is nevertheless much lower than that among those infected during the first year. In Brailey's study mentioned above,[10] the mortality of children who were first found to be tuberculin-positive in their second year was far lower than those in whom infection was discovered during the first six months of life.

After the second year of life the death rate of those who become infected falls markedly. It is reasonable to believe that this is due, in part at least, to the fact that the ability to move freely outside the home is accompanied by the opportunity for acquiring single, slight infections which can be well resisted, in contrast to the situation that obtains during the first two years. In addition, it is pertinent to point out that children between two and five years of age have a decidedly greater ability to form immune antibodies than have infants.[28]

Factors Contributing to the Low Mortality Rate Between Five Years and Puberty

The tuberculosis mortality rate among the infected population in the decade between five years and puberty is markedly lower than that in any other decade of the life span (Table II). The reasons for the low death rate in this period are certainly not all clearly understood at present, but there are at least several circumstances which may be regarded as playing a rôle in this direction.

In the first place, while there is ample evidence from tuberculin tests and autopsy studies that free movement in the outside world during this period is accompanied by a great increase in

primary infections, far fewer of these infections produce progressive, fatal disease than in infancy. We may assume, therefore, that a smaller percentage of the infections acquired during this decade are dependent upon heavy and continued exposure in the home, and that a much larger percentage represent the results of single, chance contacts in the outside world leading to slight infections which can be successfully resisted.

This decade is the one during which the individual, exposed freely to contact with the outside world, is most protected against the vicissitudes of life. These are years during which most children are protected in the home and in school, and during which they are, in general, spared from the cares, stresses, strains, debilitating influences and occupational hazards of later life. They have ample time for invigorating play out of doors, and have little to interfere with needed rest or regular and sufficient sleep. Many of the known factors which tend to depress resistance to tuberculosis are, therefore, in abeyance during this decade.

In addition, there is very good evidence that during this period of life the mechanism for developing acquired resistance (so-called "serological maturity") becomes fully established. It was pointed out above that infants and very young animals have a deficient immunity mechanism, and it is interesting to note that at the various periods of life there is a definite correlation between the titre of natural agglutinins, as exemplified by the blood groups, and the power to form antibodies against bacteria and their products. Thus, the new-born infant's deficient antibody-producing power is paralleled by the fact that the isoagglutinins that determine the blood groups are rarely present at birth. In general, the isoagglutinin titre is quite low and in some instances still zero between six month and one year of age; from one to two years parallel with the increase in antibody-producing power, the isoagglutinin titre rises; and i reaches its height precisely during the perio under present discussion, namely, between fiv and ten years of age.[51] There is no evidence tha after this period of life any further increas occurs either in isoagglutinin titre or in im mune antibody-forming power.

While there are probably other and as y undetermined factors, it is reasonable to belie that the above circumstances play a significa rôle in determining the lower tuberculosis mortality rate during this period of life, which is one of amazing safety as regards most infections, as can be readily seen in Table III. The careful study of the reasons for these marked differences in the mortality from various infections in the different age periods is clearly of the greatest importance for preventive medicine and public health.

Factors Influencing the Rise in Mortality Rate in Adolescence

The close relationship between the age at which the tuberculosis mortality curve begins to rise sharply and the period at which the puberty readjustments of the body take place, suggests at once that the state of pubescence may be accompanied by a depression in resistance to the infection, and that we are faced here with an age-period determined level of resistance. While no absolute proof of this exists at present there are circumstances which render it altogether probable.

In the first place, while the mortality rise at puberty and during adolescence can be accounted for partly by the fact that the freer excursion into the outside world at this period is accompanied by an increase in the opportunities for contact with open cases, it is perfectly clear that this factor alone is insufficient to account for the phenomenon. The increase in mortality far outstrips the increase in infection, and this is true regardless of what tuberculin surveys are used for the estimation of the incidence of infection. Furthermore, we have already seen that in the period between five years and puberty a great increase in incidence of infection is actually accompanied by a decrease in mortality—a fact which stresses the importance of factors other than mere infection incidence in the determination of the relative mortality rate of the different periods of life.

That a certain amount of active tuberculosis appearing at this period represents the evolution of infections acquired earlier in life cannot be questioned, but there is no reason for believing that this increment is great enough to account for the observed abrupt mortality rise unless we assume at the same time that resistance becomes depressed at this period, and so permits a greater number of infections to undergo progression than would have done so had resistance not flagged.

For a better understanding of the level of native resistance at the different periods of life after childhood, we need to know much more about the ultimate fate of those who become infected for the first time at each age period. Superficial studies of this matter, which ignore factors such as family contact, economic status, etc., can be very misleading. In time, the careful, long-period method of individual family study of the type now being carried out in various cities will provide invaluable information regarding the question. In relation to the matter before us, we may cite a study carried out by Opie and McPhedran[39] on persons living in contact with open tuberculosis and followed for a period of ten to fourteen years after the beginning of exposure. Of those first exposed between birth and nine years of age, 9.9 per cent developed clinical tuberculosis, of those first exposed between ten and fourteen years of age, 20 per cent developed the disease. In this particular study, exposure to familial infection in the unstable period immediately preceding and at the time of puberty was twice as dangerous as was exposure prior or subsequent to this period.

It may further be noted that while the tuberculosis mortality-rise following the low mortality period of childhood is marked in males, it occurs at a somewhat earlier age and is more pronounced in females. In females, the puberty alterations likewise occur earlier and are more profound than in males. Since there is no significant difference between the incidence of infection in males and females at this period of life these facts, in themselves, are highly suggestive that the state of pubescence plays a rôle in altering the resistance of the individual.

Suggestive evidence of the relation of pubescence to resistance is also provided by clinical and pathological experience. From the clinical side it has long been recognized that the period of pubescence is accompanied by a tendency to the exacerbation of latent lesions and the more rapid progression of active ones, and that this danger tends to be more pronounced in the female. On the pathological side it is familiar that progressive lesions of reinfection which develop at this period of life frequently have characteristics which are not encountered in typical white adult reinfections—features which indicate a higher degree of resistance than that seen in progressive first infections of childhood, but a lower degree of resistance than that in adult reinfections. It is not uncommon, for example, to find in this age-period progressive apical lesions quite like those that are characteristic of adult tuberculosis, though often with rather more prominent caseation and rather less prominent fibrosis; but associated with this type of pulmonary lesion there may be enlarged, caseous peribronchial lymph nodes—a finding that is foreign to typical adult tuberculosis, but is the rule in the progressive tuberculosis of the non-immunized child. In most instances the enlarged lymph nodes are not completely caseous, as they so frequently are in progressive tuberculosis of the young child, but show instead rather large areas of caseation embedded in non-necrotic node tissue. It may be recalled that the adult negro has a tendency to develop precisely this type of the disease on reinfection, and there is very good evidence, which I have assembled elsewhere[45] and which time prevents reviewing here, that the negro's level of native resistance is definitely lower than that of the white, and that dosage and living conditions are altogether inadequate to explain the differences in disease in the two races.

In precisely what manner pubescence acts to influence resistance to tuberculosis, as it apparently does, is at present obscure. The problem hardly lends itself to direct experimental investigation, for the period of pubescence in laboratory animals is of such brief duration. In the attempt to eliminate sexual factors, several investigators[9, 13, 16, 31] have studied the effects of tuberculous infection in castrated animals, but the results have been contradictory.

Approaching the problem from the opposite angle, Vercesi and Merenda[52] and Repetti[42] found that an excess of the female hormone had no effect upon native resistance to tuberculosis in experimental animals; and Dr. L. A. Gray and Dr. C. B. Brack, in our laboratory, have recently shown that acquired resistance is likewise unaffected in animals kept continually in a state of hyperoestrinism. Furthermore, Gray and Brack, in carefully controlled experiments, have so far been unable to confirm the recent report of Steinbach and Klein[49] that antuitrin increases resistance to the experimental disease.

These experiments, of course, demonstrate no more than the failure of an excess of these two particular hormones to affect resistance under the experimental conditions. They neither produce the state of pubescence, nor invalidat the view that resistance in the human being i altered at this period of bodily readjustment.

In summary, the sharp rise in mortality tha follows the childhood period of relative safet and continues into adult life is accompanied b clinical and pathological evidences of deficien resistance, and is associated with the followin circumstances: (1) a progressive increase i the incidence of infection; (2) apparently specific adverse effect of the state of pubescenc on resistance; (3) the beginning of exposure t the stresses and strains associated with th struggle for existance and with childbearing That other less evident factors may be opera tive cannot be denied. The most earnest stud should be devoted to an elucidation of th factors which influence the development of pr gressive tuberculosis at this time of life, fo the precise reasons for the disastrous effec observed during this period, and later in lit as a result of infection at this period, are sti for the most part obscure, and the problem i one not only of extraordinary theoretical ir terest, but of the utmost importance from th standpoint of human welfare.

The Relative Degree of Native Immunity in Adult Life

Following adolescence the tuberculosis mo tality rate continues to rise steadily into adu life. The age period at which the peak of tl rising curve is reached varies in different plac and at different times, but except in commur ties where economic conditions and industri hazards are particularly bad, the mortality pe is ordinarily reached in the middle twenties, a at a somewhat earlier age in the female than the male.

The high mortality rate in the middle twent is due in part to the rising incidence of inf tion, but the rate of increase in mortality d nitely outstrips the rate of increase in infectic incidence. Other factors, therefore, undoubte play a dominant rôle in determining the rise mortality rate at this period of life. The eff of general and specific occupational hazar childbearing and the care of a family, and pressure of the stresses and strains of the str gle for existence are now in full play. In ad tion, there is no doubt that many cases of tul culosis having their inception during the susce ible period of adolescence reach a fatal termination in young adult life and so add to the number of fatalities in this period.

Time does not permit me to enter into a discussion of the highly important problems involved in the effect of these various factors upon resistance to tuberculosis. Little is known of the manner in which most of them lower resistance. Even deleterious factors as familiar as malnutrition and physical exhaustion exert their adverse effects in a manner that is still almost completely obscure; and this is likewise true of those factors which at present can be expressed only in rather vague terms such as "over-stress and strain," and "the run-down state"; terms which, however unscientific, nevertheless express very real hazards in the body's struggle to hold a tuberculous infection in check.

. I believe that there can be little doubt that childbearing plays a definite rôle in influencing the female mortality rate in the general population. Without questioning the fact that the danger of childbearing may be reduced to a minimum for many tuberculous women *if adequate care is provided before and after labor*, as the studies of Jennings, Mariette and Litzenberg[28] and of others plainly show, it is nevertheless beyond question that childbearing may be attended by a variety of circumstances which can affect tuberculosis adversely if adequate rest and care are *not* assured—and certainly they are not assured in the case of most tuberculous women who become pregnant. Among these adverse conditions I need only mention the physical exertion of carrying the fetus about in the latter months of pregnancy in the performance of the usual household tasks; the exhausting strain of labor; the loss of nutritive materials to the fetus and to the nursing infant, particularly in undernourished women; and the effort and broken sleep involved in caring for the infant after it is born, while the mother is still below par physically. All of these conditions contain factors that are well known to affect tuberculosis adversely, and it may be pointed out that the curve of female tuberculosis mortality bears an interesting relation to the frequency of childbirths at the different ages. At the end of the active reproductive period the female tuberculosis mortality falls sharply below that of the male. I have recently made an analysis of the relation of the female tuberculosis mortality to the birth rate and to certain other factors in the individual states of

the Union, and, while other factors undoubtedly are highly important, it is at least interesting that there is a definite correlation between the birth rate among women past 30 and the length of the period during which the female tuberculosis mortality remains above that of the male in the individual states. When it is realized that each year in the United States approximately one out of every ten females between the ages of fifteen and thirty become pregnant, the opportunity for pregnancy to coincide with and to exert its deleterious effects upon tuberculosis in the female becomes impressively evident.

I cannot enter further into the various external factors that influence the development of tuberculsis in adult life but we must, for a moment, consider the question of the level of native resistance in young and middle aged adults, for this is a matter of considerable theoretical and practical import.

There are those who maintain that the previously uninfected adult is more susceptible to tuberculosis than is the child, and that it is dangerous, therefore, to adopt measures that will tend to postpone infection until adult life, particularly since an earlier resisted infection may confer some degree of acquired resistance upon the otherwise highly susceptible adult. Aschoff[3], for example, pleading this view, writes:

"We must, however, remember that with the prevention of the primary infection in childhood the adult is sent forth into life unprotected against this disease, which will then attack him with infinitely greater virulence than the usual familial infection, so to speak, in infancy."

This view that the adult has a lower native resistance than the child has many adherents. It has been based upon two facts: (1) that the tuberculosis mortality rate of young adults is much higher than that of young school children; and (2) that the adults of primitive African peoples in regions previously free from tuberculosis have developed a rapidly progressing type of disease with a very high mortality rate when tuberculosis was first introduced among them. The fear has therefore been entertained that if primary infection in childhood be prevented in our own communities, individuals who become infected in later life will fall victim to a similar devastating form of the dsease because they will lack the protection conferred by the acquired resistance that results from childhood primary infection.

In my opinion, there is no sound foundation for that view. In the first place, in transferring the observations on primitive races to civilized whites, no account is taken of the important evidence, to which I have already referred, that the native resistance of the negro is lower than that of the white race which has passed through centuries of contact with the tubercle bacillus. I have discussed our uncertainty regarding the significance of a negative tuberculin test, and it is a very real uncertainty; but, unless all present-day tuberculin surveys are completely misleading, there must now be a large number of individuals in the population who are being infected for the first time in adult life, and if white adults are really as susceptible as are the adults of primitive races we should at present be encountering on all sides cases of fulminant, primitive type tuberculosis in young white adults. In even the relatively small body of Senegalese troops brought into contact with tuberculosis apparently for the first time during the World War (only 5 per cent were tuberculin positive), devastating, rapidly progressing tuberculosis with caseation of regional lymph nodes and widespread generalization was soon impressively evident.[8] In the great group of tuberculin negative white adults at the present time, on the contrary, the development of this type of tuberculosis is extremely rare, and there is no evidence whatever to indicate that cases of this sort are any more frequent in adults than would be expected as a result of primary infection in a similar number of school children. Finally, it should be noted that there are no observations demonstrating that when tuberculosis is first introduced among natives living under primitive conditions the adults are any more severely affected than are the children.

In brief, the observations on tuberculosis in primitive peoples provides no justification whatever for assuming that the previously uninfected adult, whether white or negro, is any more susceptible, natively, than is the child of the same race.

Regarding the argument that the higher tuberculosis mortality among adults is evidence that adult *native* resistance is lower than that of children of school age, it is hardly necessary to point out that such a deduction is unwarranted, for it neglects entirely the important extraneous factors mentioned above which act to depress resistance in many adults, and from which the

child is spared. In the face of such complicating influences, simple mortality rates provide no trustworthy gauge of the comparative degree of native resistance in adult and child.

If there is no acceptable evidence that adults have less native resistance than have children of primary school age, there is, on the other hand, no valid evidence that they are natively *more* resistant to primary infection, as some have assumed. This view that children have less resistance than adults has arisen partly from the failure to separate the highly susceptible first several years of life from the much more resistant primary school age, and partly from the observed tendency of progressive primary infection in childhood to spread throughout the body, in contrast to the more effective localization of the disease in adults. It neglects, however, the influence of resistance in the adult acquired by previous infection.

At present we possess insufficient information to permit us to speak with certainty about the relative level of resistance in previously uninfected adults as compared with children of the same race, and we shall remain unable to speak with accuracy about this important matter until we have more certain information regarding the frequency of *arrested* primary infection in adults, and the clinical and pathological manifestations of *progressive* primary disease in adults. I tend to believe, however, that the information that we do possess indicates that there is no significant difference between the child of primary school age and the healthy adult in native ability to resist a primary infection. The higher mortality from tuberculosis in adult life appears to be referrable to circumstances which depress resistance rather than to an innate, age-determined deficiency in native resistance. The influence which these external conditions exert upon tuberculosis mortality becomes particularly apparent in the fourth decade for at this period the male tuberculosis mortality rate continues at a high level, whereas the female rate declines; and in parallel fashion, the industrial hazards to which males are exposed continue in full force, whereas the re productive activity of females declines. Fur thermore, the death rate of males at this pe riod tends to be decidedly higher in urban an industrial centers than in rural communities— tendency that is not shared by the females livin under the same economic conditions, but largel

758

spared from the laboring hazards of the male (Table IV).

TABLE IV. DEATHS FROM TUBERCULOSIS

Per 100,000 White Individuals 30-35 Years of Age. 1932.

	Males	Females
Predominantly Rural States	62.6	73
Predominantly Urban States	86.2	75

Now even though there is at present no reason for believing that the normal adult has a lower *native* resistance than the child, we must not be misled into believing that infection carries no more risk for young adults in general than for children, for there is very definite evidence that it does. I do not think that any of the studies so far made which purport to show that primary infection carries no more of a hazard for young adults than for school children are sufficiently representative or extensive enough to permit us to accept that view. This is one of the situations upon which the figures for the mortality rate of the *infected* portion of the population throw important light, for they show clearly that the death rate among infected young adults is much higher than that of infected children of primary school age. Since the death rate of infected young adults is much higher than that of infected children it is obvious that *on the average* it is more dangerous to be an infected young adult than to be infected in the safe period of childhood. This is doubtless due in large part to the fact that the adverse circumstances discussed above, from which the child is ordinarily spared, often conspire to thwart the protective action of native and acquired resistance in adults. Even though native resistance, when unhampered, may be quite as good in adults as in children, since many more young adults are exposed to the conditions that affect tuberculosis adversely than are children of primary school age, it is reasonable to expect that primary infection in adult life will develop into progressive disease more frequently than in childhood.

It cannot with propriety be argued that the lower mortality rate of children as contrasted with that of adults is due to an inherent benignity of primary infection as contrasted with the malignity of reinfection, as some would have us believe.[34] Those who claim that primary infection is harmless and reinfection disastrous apparently limit their gaze to the examples of well resisted primary infections and to devastating reinfections. Certainly, they appear to ignore the many devastating primary infections so familiar in childhood, and they likewise gloss over the tremendous number of perfectly benign reinfections encountered in adults—the familiar, completely arrested apical scars of reinfection found so commonly at autopsy in individuals bearing older, calcified primary lesions. The truth, of course, is that the overwhelming majority of all tuberculous infections, whether primary or secondary, pursue a perfectly benign course to healing and permanent arrest, and there is no acceptable evidence whatever that reinfection is any more dangerous than primary infection, providing the dosage and the bodily vigor of the individual are the same in both instances. On the contrary, the entirety of the experimental and pathological evidence that we possess teaches us that, other things remaining the same, reinfection is decidedly less dangerous than primary infection.

In regard to the effects of hypersensitivity, in spite of the many assertions about its protective rôle, no one has yet brought forth proof of any sort that hypersensitivity is necessary for any of the protective effects of immunity. Our own numerous experimental studies of the matter, which I have reviewed in another place[44] and into which I cannot enter here, together with the subsequent similar investigations of Siegl,[45] Birkhaug,[6] Clawson,[24] Branch and Enders,[11] Higginbotham[26] and others, have demonstrated plainly that hypersensitivity is not necessary for any of the manifestations of immunity; and it has been known since the time of Koch that the hypersensitive state is responsible for exaggerated tissue destruction at sites where many bacilli are present. It does not at all follow, however, that the hypersensitivity produced by a primary infection "sets the stage" for devastating disease of reinfection, as some maintain.[34] I think that it is important in these matters to keep the known facts strictly where they belong. Reinfection is always instituted by only a relatively few bacilli, and a few bacilli provoke only a negligible immediate tissue damage even in the hypersensitive body. Serious damage from hypersensitivity becomes evident in reinfection only after a sufficient time has elapsed to permit the bacilli to multiply to large numbers; and it must be remembered that after a similar lapse of time following the entry of the bacilli of even a primary infection, hypersensitivity will be just as highly developed. The amount of damage done by hypersensitivity, whether in primary or in reinfection, depends upon the degree to which the bacilli proliferate after reaching the tissues. If it is true that chronic phthisis occurs only in those who bear an earlier primary lesion, it is no less true that the acute, devastating, "childhood type" of progressive disease, with rapid local necrosis and caseation, and marked tendency to generalization occurs, in civilized races, only in those who have *not* had a previous primary infection.

The important and complex problem of the advantages and disadvantages conferred by a primary infection is bound up inextricably with the moot question whether adult tuberculosis results predominantly from exogenous or from endogenous reinfection. If phthisis is exogenous in origin, and rarely arises from activation of a primary lesion, as Opie[37] and many others believe, then it is obvious that a primary, arrested, immunizing infection could be no liability, and would be of great service in protecting against further infection from without, even though the protection were not always an effective one. If, on the other hand, adult tuberculosis is always the result of the lighting up of primary infections years after their establishment, as Fishberg[19] and others believe, then a primary infection would entail a large element of liability; though even in this case it would not necessarily be altogether disadvantageous, for if progressive tuberculosis can no longer be acquired from without, once a primary lesion has been established, then individuals with primary leisons would at least be protected against the danger of progressive infection acquired through contact.

The truth in all probability, lies in a midposition between these extreme views. There are probably many cases in which tuberculosis arises from the escape of bacilli from latent lesions of primary infection; many cases in which reinfection from without leads to progressive disease in individuals in whom the resistance conferred by a primary infection has become depressed by adverse conditions; and many cases in which the immunizing power of a permanently arrested primary lesion serves to protect the individual from further contact in-

fection. There is now a great body of unassailable experimental and pathological evidence that infection does confer a very decided degree of resistance to reinfection, and it is without question true that the overwhelming majority of individuals who develop a primary lesion arrest the infection successfully and never develop progressive disease thereafter throughout their lives. That the resistance conferred by an arrested infection fluctuates under various influences, and is not effective in all cases in preventing the later development of progressive disease is, of course, perfectly obvious; and until we learn, if ever we shall, whether or not primary infection occurring in adult life would progress to a fatal termination more frequently than adults now develop fatal reinfection, statements purporting to define the virtues or the vices of primary infection can be no more than individual guesses.

In expressing my own belief that a primary infection does exert an immunizing effect which may be very valuable in many individual cases, I should like to stress the fact that there is no incompatability whatever between this view and the belief that all individuals should avoid spontaneous and uncontrolled infection as far as is reasonably practicable; for although the immunizing effect of a primary infection is a fact which can be demonstrated experimentally with the greatest of ease, in spontaneous human infection we can neither regulate the size nor the time of the immunizing dose, nor can we preserve all infected individuals from the external influences that act to rob them of their resistance while they still carry bacilli in their arrested lesions. Those who regard a primary infection as only a liability often seek to imply that all who recognize that infection does confer some resistance to reinfection are in favor of rushing every child into exposure to infection in order that the protective primary complex may be obtained as soon as possible. Of course this is in no sense the case. There must be few, if any, experienced students of tuberculosis today, whatever their beliefs about the primary complex, who favor any other course than that of protecting all persons from infection as far as is reasonably practicable.

Resistance in Old Age

I must devote a few remaining moments to the peculiarities of tuberculosis in the final period of life. After sixty, the tuberculosis death rate tends to rise sharply, though in communities with an excessively high death rate in earlier adult life this tendency may be masked.

with less manifest symptoms than are usual in earlier years has led to the frequent statement that the disease is more benign at this period than in other periods of adult life. The high

TABLE V. FREQUENCY OF MILIARY TUBERCULOSIS IN THE AGED

Race	Age	Cases of Pulmonary Tuberculosis	Miliary Tuberculosis		Enlarged Caseous Nodes	
			No.	%	No.	%
White	25-50	71	3	4.0	1	1.4
White	60 and over	46	9	19.5	3	6.5
Negro	25-50	86	14	16.3	17	19.7

Certainly, there is no question here of increased exposure to infection as a cause of the rise in mortality rate. On the contrary, the aged tend to withdraw from active contact with the world. A rising mortality rate in the face of diminished exposure to infection is not, in itself, the presence of factors that depress resistance, but is there, in addition, any clinical or pathological evidence that resistance is depressed?

In the aged, tuberculosis often tends to progress with strikingly little in the way of symptoms aside from the cough which, in itself, is often not severe. The disease is therefore frequently unsuspected, even when well advanced and with abundant bacilli in the sputum. A tuberculous grandparent with "chronic bronchitis" to which no attention had been paid, has often been found on investigation to have been the source of fatal tuberculous infection for children living in the same house. This peculiarity of the disease in old age makes it of great importance to investigate carefully the reason for a persistent but otherwise symptomless cough in the aged, particularly if they are in intimate contact with children.

I think that it is probable that the rather symptomless course is due in no small measure to the circumstance that not only do the aged engage in less physical exertion than do younger adults, but even in their normal state they are much more easily fatigued, and the contrast between the degree of fatigability in health and that after the onset of tuberculosis is much less noticeable than in younger age periods.

The fact that, clinically, tuberculosis may run a chronic course in the aged and may be borne

mortality rate hardly substantiates that view, and there is, in addition to the high mortality rate, some evidence from the pathological side that the resistance of the aged often tends to be less effective than in earlier adult life. Since the better the resistance the greater is the ability to localize the process, it is of interest that there are indications that the aged more often fail to immobilize their bacilli and to localize their lesions than do younger adults. Thus, Taubert,[50] Oppenheim and LeCoz[40] and Braun[12] have commented upon the frequency of fatal miliary tuberculosis in old age. Dr. R. H. Follis, Jr., and I have recently studied a series of consecutive autopsies on cases of progressive pulmonary tuberculosis from this standpoint. The results are presented in Table V, where it will be seen that the frequency of miliary tuberculosis in the old age group was much higher than that at other periods of adult life in the white race, approximating that in the natively less resistant adult negro. The series here presented is a small one, and does not pretend to fix a mathematical percentage incidence for general application. Together with the observations of the above mentioned investigators, however, it does serve to indicate plainly that miliary tuberculosis tends to be a much more frequent complication of pulmonary tuberculosis in old age than at any other period of adult life. Enlargement and caseation of regional lymph nodes, another evidence of deficient resistance, was likewise somewhat more frequent in our old age group, but decidedly less frequent than in the negro adult. Both Braun[12] and Taubert[50] comment on the occurrence of caseation of lymph nodes in old age—an event of great rarity in earlier adult life in the white.

More extended studies of the pathology of tuberculosis in advanced years of age is highly desirable. The available evidence, however, together with the rising death rate in the absence of increased exposure, serves to indicate that the aged have a lower degree of resistance than have the middle-aged. Precisely what the factors are that may be responsible for a decline in resistance in old age is not definitely known, but there are a number of circumstances which might well be operative in this direction. Old persons ordinarily remain indoors much more than younger adults; loss of teeth and of appetite not so infrequently result in varying degrees of malnutrition; diabetes, which appears to exert an unfavorable effect upon resistance to tuberculosis, becomes much more prevalent in old age. In the last U. S. mortality reports there were twenty-five deaths from diabetes per hundred thousand individuals in the forty-five to fifty-five year age period; eighty-seven deaths in the fifty-five to sixty-five year age period; and 177 in the sixty-five to seventy-five year age period. While factors such as these may contribute to the lowering of resistance in old age, they are certainly not the only ones concerned. There are reasons for believing that, in addition, specific though imperfectly understood bodily alterations associated with senility itself may act to impair the body's defence against infection.

In the first place, the lowering of resistance at this period of life is not peculiar to tuberculosis, but is evident in the case of other infections, of so widely different a character as dysentery, erysipelas and pneumonia (Table III). The susceptibility of old persons to pneumonia is familiar even to the layman.

It is probable that physical and mechanical bodily alterations attendant upon senility, such as enfeebled circulation and senile tissue alterations (e.g., atrophy of the epidermis, senile emphysema), may be partly responsible for the more ready establishment of certain infections in certain tissues in old persons. In addition, and more important, a generalized lowered functional capacity of the organs and tissues characterizes senility, and there is no reason to doubt that the immunity mechanism shares in this general decline. In this connection it is important to point out that in very old age the isoagglutinin titre tends to decline to a level approximating in feebleness that present in infancy.[51] The parallelism between the isoagglu-

tinin titre and the ability to form protective antibodies against bacteria and their products was pointed out above, and it is not surprising there-fore that it has been established that persons of advanced age are decidedly deficient in the ability to form antibodies against bacterial products in comparison with younger adults.

In this connection, it may also be recalled that there is much evidence that the lymphoid tissue is concerned in some way in resistance to infection in tuberculosis and in other bacterial disease. The rôle of the lymphoid tissue in resistance cannot be discussed here, but I may recall as evidence of that rôle the fact that in animals raised from birth in a strictly sterile bacteria-free environment, the most striking deviation from the "normal" is an extraordinary incon-spicuousness of the lymphoid tissue of the entire body;[21] and, on the other hand, the fact that marked proliferation of the lymphoid tissue both the spleen (acute splenic tumor) and the regional lymph nodes occurs not only during in-fection, but also, as we have recently shown, during antibody formation induced by even non-bacterial antigens. It is pertinent, therefore, that in old age there occurs a marked atrophy of the spleen and other lymphoid tissue, and that lymph-oid proliferation during infections tends to be less conspicuous than at younger age periods.

The peculiarities of susceptibility and resist-ance at the various age periods, and the manner in which external factors act to alter resistance constitute perhaps the most important problem in tuberculosis today, not only from a theoretical but, indeed, from a highly practical standpoint, and they deserve the most serious and intense investigation. In this review of the general out-lines of the problem, I have sought chiefly to stress the narrow limits of our present informa-tion, rather than to attempt to provide a set of comfortable, theoretical explanations for the complex and incompletely understood phenom-ena.

References

1. Arborelius, M.: Klinische Studien über Tuberkuloselion bei Erwachsenen, besonders mit Hinsicht auf Vorkommen von Primärinfektionen. Acta. Soc.-Med. canae, 55:115, 1930.
2. Aronson, J. D., and Dannenberg, A. M.: Effect of vaccination with BCG on tuberculosis in infancy and child. Am. J. Dis. Child., 50:1117, 1935.
3. Aschoff, L.: Lectures on Pathology. New York: Paul Hoeber, Inc., 1924.
4. Austrian, C. R.: Observations on children admitted tuberculosis dispensary. Tubercle, 6:29, 1924.
5. Barnard, M. W., Amberson, J. B., Jr., and Loew, M.: Tuberculosis in adolescents. Am. Rev. Tuberc., 23, 1931.
6. Birkhaug, K.: Allergy and immunity in experimental tuberculosis. Acta Tuberk. Scand., 11:25, 199, 1937.

7. Boquet, A.: Surinfection tuberculeuse du cobaye par voie sous-cutanée. C. R. Soc. Biol., 109:363, 1932.
8. Borrel, A.: Pneumonie et tuberculose chez les troupes noires. Ann. Inst. Pasteur, 34:105, 1920.
9. Bourgeois, P., and Boquet, M.: Influence des hormones sexuelles et de la castration sur l' evolution de la tuberculose experimentelle du cobaye. C. R. Soc. Biol., 122:369, 1936.
10. Brailey, M.: Mortality in tuberculin-positive infants. Bull. Johns Hopkins Hosp., 59:1, 1936.
11. Branch, A., and Enders, J, F.: The immunization of guinea pigs with heat-killed and formol-killed tubercle bacilli. Am. Rev. Tuberc., 32:595, 1935.
12. Braun, E.: Die Haufigkeit der Miliärtuberkulose im Greisenalter. Corr.-Blatt f. Schweiz. Aerzte, 47:1121, 1917.
13. Bricker, F. M.: Die Tuberkulose und die Geschlechtsdrüsen. Zeit f. Tuberk., 40:198, 1924.
14. Clawson, B. J.: Relation of allergy to general resistance in streptococcic infection. Jour. Inf. Dis., 53:157, 1933; 33:1, 1937.
15. Crabtree, J. A., Hickerson, W. D., and Hickerson, V. P.: Tuberculosis studies in Tennessee. Am. Rev. Tuberc., Vol. 28, 1933, Supp. No. 6.
16. Cristofoletti, R., and Thaler, H.: Experimentelle und Klinische Beiträge zur Frage nach dem Beziehungen zwischen Tuberkulose und Schwangerschaft. Monat. f. Geb. u. Gyn., 34:513, 1911.
17. Davies, J. A. V.: The response of infants to inoculation with Type I Pneumococcus carbohydrate. Jour. Immunol., 33:1, 1937.
18. Die Säuglingstuberkulose in Lübeck: Arb. a. d. Reichsgesundheitsamte, Vol. 69, 1935.
19. Fishberg, M.: Pulmonary Tuberculosis. Philadelphia: Lea and Febiger, 1932.
20. Freund, J.: Influence of age upon antibody formation. Jour. Immunol., 18:315, 1930.
21. Glimstedt, G.: Bakterienfreie Meerschweinschen. Acta Path. et Microbiol. Scand., 1936, Supp. 30.
22. Gottstein, A.: Allgemeine Epidemiologie der Tuberkulose, Berlin: Julius Springer, 1931.
23. Halber, W., Hirzfeld, H., and Mayzner, M.: Untersuchungen über die Antikörperentstehung bei Kindern im Zusammenhang mit dem Alter. Zeit. f. Immunitätsforsch., 53:391, 1927.
24. Hart, C.: Pathologisch-anatomische Beobachtungen über die Tuberkulose am während des Krieges sezierten Soldatenmaterial. Zeit. f. Tuberk., 31:129, 1920.
25. Hetherington, H. W., McPhedran, F. M., Landis, H. R. M., and Opie, E. L.: A survey to determine the prevalence of tuberculosis infection in school children. Am. Rev. Tuberc., 20:421, 1929.
26. Higginbotham, M. W.: A study of the heteroallergic reactivity of tuberculin desensitized tuberculous guinea pigs in comparison with tuberculous and normal guinea pigs. Am. Jour. Hygiene, 26:197, 1937.
27. Horan, T. H.: The incidence of tuberculous infection and disease in a private school for boys. Am. Rev. Tuberc., 32:166, 1935.
28. Jennings, F, L., Mariette, E. S., and Litzenberg, J. C.: Pregnancy in the tuberculous. Am. Rev. Tuberc., 25:673, 1932.
29. Kligler, I. J., and Olitzki, L.: Antikörperbildung junger und erwachsener Tiere. Zeit. f. Hyg., 110:459, 1929.
30. Lloyd, W. E., and MacPherson, A. M.: A reinvestigation of children previously examined by tuberculin tests. Brit. Med. Jour., 1:818, 1933.
31. Mautner, H.: Über Beziehungen der Geschlechtsdrüsen zur Tuberkulose-Disposition. Monatschr. f. Kinderkeilk, 21:38, 1921.
32. Myers, J, A.: Panel discussion on resistance to tuberculosis during childhood. Jour. Pediatrics, 10:267, 1937.
33. Myers, J. A., Diehl, H. S., Boynton, R. E., and Trach B.: Development of tuberculosis in adult life. Arch. Int. Med., 59:1, 1937.
34. Myers, J. A., and Harrington, F. E.: The effect of initial tuberculous infection on subsequent tuberculous lesions. Jour. A.M.A., 103:1530, 1934.
35. Nattan-Larrier, L., Ramon, G., and Grasset, E.: L'anatox. ine tetanique et l' immunité antitetanique chez la mère et le nouveau-né. Ann. Inst. Past, 41:848, 1927.
36. Nelson, W. E., Mitchell, A. G., and Brown, E. W.: Intracutaneous tuberculin reaction associated with calcified inthrathoracic lesions. Am. Rev. Tuberc., 37:311, 1938.
37. Opie, E. L.: Present concepts of tuberculous infection and disease. Am. Rev. Tuberc., 32:617, 1935.
38. Opie, E. L., and McPhedran, M.: The contagion of tuberculosis. Am. Rev. Tuberc., 14:347, 1926.
39. Opie, E. L., McPhedran, F. M., and Putnam, P.: The fate of persons in contact with tuberculosis. Am. Jour. Hyg., 26:644, 1935.
40. Oppenheim, R., and LeCoz, C.: Frequence de la tuberculose pulmonaire des vieillards. Prog. Méd., 27:5, 1911.
41. Paretsky, M.: The disappearance of specific skin hypersensitiveness in tuberculosis. Am. Rev. Tuberc., 33:370, 1936.
42. Repetti, M.: Influenze della vitamina della fecondazione e degli ormoni sessuali sulla tubercolosi sperimentale. Ann. di. Ostet. e. Ginecol., 57:1489, 1935.
43. Rich, A. R.: Acute splenic tumor produced by non-bacterial antigens. Proc. Soc. Exp. Biol. and Med., 32:149, 1934.
44. Rich, A. R.: Studies on the dissociation of hypersensitivity from immunity. Rev. d' Immunol., 3:25, 1937; Inflammation in resistance to infection. Arch. Pathol., 22:228, 1936.
45. Rich, A. R.: Immunity in tuberculosis. Diseases of the Respiratory Tract. Philadelphia: W. B. Saunders Co., 1936, p. 215.
46. Römer, P. H.: Experimentelle Tuberkuloseinfektion des Säuglings. Beit. z Klin. d. Tuberc., 17:345, 1910.
47. Sewall, H., de Savitsch, E., and Butler, C. P.: The time-interval between primary infection and superinfection as a factor in immunity to tuberculosis. Am. Rev. Tuberc., 29:373, 1934.
48. Siegl, J.: Allergie und Immunität bei der Tuberkulose. Beit. z. Klin. d. Tuberk., 84:311, 1934.
49. Steinbach, M. M., and Klein, S. J.: The effects of gonadotropic hormones in the treatment of experimental tuberculosis. Jour. Exp. Med., 65:205, 1937.
50. Taubert, R.: Über Alterstuberkulose. Münch. Med. Wchnschr., 72:798, 1925.
51. Thomsen, O., and Kettel, K.: Die Starke der menschlichen Isoagglutinine und Antisprechenden Blutkorperchen-rezeptoren in verschiedenen Lebensaltern. Zeit. f. Immunitätsforsch., 63:67, 1929.
52. Veressi, R., and Merenda, P.: Sul comportamento della infezione tubercolare sperimentale delle cavie trattate con ormoni gravicidi. Riv. Med.-Soc. della Tuberc., 10:42, 1933.
53. Wells, C. W., and Smith, H. H.: The intensity of the tuberculin reaction and frequency of demonstrable tuberculous lesions. Am. Rev. Tuberc., 34:425, 1936.
54. Willis, H. S.: The waning of cutaneous sensitiveness to tuberculin and the relation of tuberculoimmunity to tuberculoallergy. Am. Rev. Tuberc., 17:240, 1928.

THE ROENTGENOGRAPHY OF PULMONARY TUBERCULOSIS*

With a New Method for Group Surveys

HOLLIS E. POTTER, M.D.

Chicago, Illinois

AS WE gather here today to discuss certain x-ray aspects of pulmonary tuberculosis let us pause for a moment in memory of our mutual and beloved friend, Dr. Russell D. Carman, in whose honor this hour has been set aside. I presume I knew Russell Carman rather intimately before most of you. I knew him best in the years before he came to Minnesota and in those years I can assure you he was quite as interested in the x-ray diagnosis of pulmonary disease as he later became in gastro-intestinal lesions. I may say quite truly that I gained quite a bit of inspiration from his early work on pleurisy and tuberculosis of the lungs and if he were here today I am sure he would heartily approve of spending this hour on the subject of tuberculosis.

*The Russell D. Carman Memorial Lecture presented before the annual meeting of the Minnesota State Medical Association, Duluth, Minnesota, June 29, 1938.

I am sure he would agree with me when I say with no reservations that in all the special fields of medicine where our poor attempts at x-ray diagnosis have gained foothold there is no disease in which we are able to render a more decisive and more valuable service than in the handling of adult pulmonary tuberculosis. Russell Carman and I were active in an era before 1910 during which the average clinician hooted the idea that significant tuberculous lesions could be fairly demonstrated by x-rays in a case where the more classical symptoms and signs were absent. This was the day of the so-called tuberculosis specialist whose very livelihood depended on a public recognition of his superhuman skill in physical diagnosis. He could not afford to recognize any method which would tend to amplify, replace, or debase his special attainments. Fortunately for the human race the specialists of this character are now either dead or very few in number. The most dependable tuberculosis workers of today are free to admit that most early pulmonary tuberculosis should be seen and not heard.

In fact it was not until some of our foremost clinical workers in the tuberculosis field incorporated the x-ray into their own routine practice, checked it carefully against other tangible factors in the diagnosis and followed up their results in an open minded manner that the x-ray method became widely accepted, so that it is now considered the one most important factor in the diagnosis. In this connection, I cannot too strongly express my gratitude for the work done and reported by Dr. Lawrason Brown and his associates at Saranac. It is true that the technic of the old days produced results that were far less convincing than are the brilliant sharp films of today, but the widespread acceptance of the x-ray method has been brought about quite as much by the study and educational work of clinicians and roentgenologists as by the outstanding technical improvements.

As we admit, therefore, that x-rays are rather widely used in general practice and most lavishly used in hospitals and sanatoria, what valuable message might I succeed in bringing you today? What great lesson has the medical world yet to learn about x-rays in relation to tuberculosis? My answer is that too few of the medical men yet understand the low percentage of early cases that are really diagnosed in general practice. One authority states that in a hundred consec-

utive chest cases where the diagnosis of tuberculosis is correct, less than 5 per cent are discovered in an early stage, less than 15 per cent are discovered at a moderately advanced stage and more than three-fourths are far advanced. Such a startling percentage of advanced cases at first discovery is most often to be explained by the lack of symptoms on the part of the patient sufficient to make him call on his doctor. The balance are either unrecognized by his doctor or sympathetically minimized until the pathologic process gives outspoken signs and symptoms. The insidious onset of so many of these cases demands that if 25 to 40 per cent are discovered early it must be done by some widespread survey in which the doctor goes to the people rather than waiting for the people to come to the doctor. Somewhere our system is wrong and medical practice and medical ethics must be modified to meet the facts. My message then is obviously to encourage some proper system of group surveys and to insist on a more widespread use of x-rays in private work. Personally, I cannot anticipate the discovery of an outstanding majority of these cases in a minimal stage because a real percentage of them are serious from the start and could never be classified as minimal or benign.

I will skip the old controversial question as to whether tuberculosis can be shown earlier by x-rays or by some other method except to express a firm belief that by x-rays the parenchymal lesions can be shown, if not identified, in more than 95 per cent of the cases. Roentgenologists are often criticized for venturing an opinion as to the identity of tuberculosis as shown on x-ray films and severely censured when trying to estimate its probable activity. Regarding the identity there may often be a reasonable doubt. When the lesions are simple and show characters more or less typical for tuberculosis I describe them as "tuberculoid" in type and leave it for the clinician and the future to determine whether actually "tuberculous." Regarding questions of activity, chronicity and healing would maintain that the competent roentgenologist can contribute most valuable information on these points. Frequently, when the state of activity is indeterminate from the study of a single set of films the true condition may be learned from films made after a short period of time. He who can see no difference in character between a frankly active and a near-heal lesion is not in a position to criticize another who in the light of considerable experience ventures a guarded opinion on one of the intermediate stages.

All things considered, I would mention about ten diagnostic aspects of work in adult pulmonary tuberculosis in which x-rays may be found most helpful.

1. In the negative findings, or determining the absence of a significant lesion.
2. In determining the presence and extent of involvement.
3. In recognizing the probable identity of the lesions in a majority of the cases.
4. In the differential diagnosis.
5. In recognizing the general pathologic form of the disease as an aid in its classification.
6. In recognizing evidences of activity, chronicity, and healing.
7. In the recognition of cavities.
8. As an aid in prognosis.
9. As a guide in determining and following up the surgical procedures.
10. In recognizing evidences of unfavorable advance, dissemination or complications.

Let us, now for the moment, turn back the chest wall and observe some of the basic facts regarding tuberculosis. We find that pathologically there are four main types of the disease, each having its own prognostic implications, but that in many advanced cases the lesions of various types are found together in the same person. At the onset the pathologic type is determined as a resultant between two opposing forces. On the one hand the invading force is measured by the number and virulence of the tubercle bacilli. Opposed to this is the resistance of the invaded host. We find that the architectural pattern of the lesions tends to conform to the mechanics of whatever portion of the lung is invaded, whether a whole lobe, a sub-lobar division, a single lobule or a single acinus.

In the simple or exudative type a minor focus of tuberculosis is completely surrounded and overshadowed by a diffuse homogeneous exudate, the so-called peri-focal reaction or collateral inflammation. On x-ray films it gives a diffuse homogeneous shadow like pneumonia. Only at a later period may further films disclose its tuberculous character by showing a small mottled and nodular residue after resorption of the reactive exudate.

The exudative-productive type is also relatively benign. Its scattered lesions for a time show a melted homogeneous appearance at periphery as from peri-focal exudate, but later, upon clearing, a more resistant nodular central zone appears which remains for some time before complete healing. These productive or proliferative features distinguish it from the exudative type. Upon complete healing it leaves but slight scar either linear or nodular. In these simple forms the intensity of the process does not reach the stage of real necrosis, and cavity formation.

Much more serious is the third type often called the caseous-pneumonic type. In this type more or less massive necrosis does occur and if the patient survives the first onslaught, caseation, liquefaction, evacuation and cavitation follow in due order. In fact, necrosis is its outstanding feature whether this be a necrosis of a whole lobe as in the form called acute pneumonic phthisis or a necrosis involving individual scattered lobules as in the form called acute bronchopneumonic phthisis. The caseation and cavity formation in these cases account for the condition which results in the prolonged or lifetime disability seen in those sub-types known as chronic ulcerative and chronic fibro-ulcerative tuberculosis. These cavity cases fill our clinics and sanatoria. These call for our mechanical and surgical handling.

In the first stages of caseous-pneumonic tuberculosis the density conditions are uniform throughout the involved area so that x-ray appearances may quite simulate the simple exudative type. In the course of a short time, however, when caseation, liquefaction, and evacuation have taken place, a central clear zone indicates the presence and general features of cavity. Gradually the peri-focal exudate may be resorbed and the external portion of the single or multiple cavities become well defined. Delayed absorption and atelectasis are not uncommon in the portions distal to the cavity.

The fourth general type is known as chronic proliferative tuberculosis. It is the result of a long series of super-infecting doses over a long period, seldom accompanied by any show of peri-focal exudate and mainly visible in the form of discrete linear or nodular scars. Starting often in the apex, the lowermost lesions may show diffuse borders testifying to their more recent activity.

No one who gets this bird's-eye view of the

pathology can fail to appreciate the seriousness of the caseous-pneumonic form and no one can fail to recognize the outstanding importance of the necrosis and cavitation sequence. The cavity is perhaps the key lesion upon which prognosis and therapy so largely depend. The early cavity is ragged at margin, irregular in form and tends to lie in the center of a- mass shadow of more or less homogeneous density. The early detection of cavity is difficult but important because collapse therapy may then be instituted before adhesions are formed and before a resistant cavity wall is developed. Cavities larger than a .cherry seldom heal spontaneously, since they lie in an area of negative pressure, and a valve-trap mechanism in the bronchus may even result in their distention and enlargement. It seems futile to attempt a classification of adult pulmonary tuberculosis without recognizing the cavity as the key lesion.

X-ray interpretation of tuberculous chest lesions is best conducted by one quite familiar with their various pathologic forms in the many and various stages of activity, chronicity and healing, but his ability will depend most particularly upon a vast experience in observing the x-ray findings alongside the clinical state of patients throughout that entire period of time required for their recovery or their death. This experience is greatly amplified by post-mortems on the fatal cases he has studied during life, but in the post-mortem he must not be confused by the pronounced terminal changes which were no part of the picture until the end. He learns to recognize consciously or unconsciously certain shadow structure criteria which are fairly characteristic though not pathognomonic of the disease. He observes the number, size and distribution of the lesions; their outline form and density; the character of their margin; their internal pattern of structure; and their relationship to other pulmonary structures. Certain combinations of these topographic, density and outline form characters are so often repeated in his experience that they come to have important meaning in respect to the kind as well as the degree of pathologic activity.

Topographically the novice who recognizes the single rule that primary adult reinfections are to be found above the hilum is much more often right than wrong. Our older conception that these changes were oftenest in the apex has been broadened to include the subclavicular region and particularly the shoulder periphery. Cavities which represent the climax of the invading process are far up, far back, and far out in more than 95 per cent of cases. Primary reinfections, whether exogenous or endogenous, are rare in the base of the white man's chest and probably less rare in the colored.

Dunham taught us to consider certain of these simple upper lung field lesions in terms of a fan whose handle lies at the hilum and which then spreads out toward the upper periphery as the invaded lobules enlarge. In many others, however, one fails to get the complete fan form but simply sees a large number of more or less discrete nodular deposits, commonly called apical or sub-clavicular infiltrations. In an especially allergic individual the field of involvement may for a time give the impression of a simple pneumonia of lobular or sub-lobar size because of the diffuse over-shadow cast by the exudate.

In a more severe case the involved area is homogeneous and denser until after evacuation of a liquefied area at the center, when our first sign of cavity is noted. Areas peripheral to the cavity may be largely resorbed or may remain in shadow. When patches of clearing occur on the side toward the hilum they must not be misinterpreted as cavities although they present somewhat similar appearance on a single film.

In the secondary reinfections and spread of the disease, new fan-like areas may be seen on the opposite side in apex, mid-lung field or base which often look quite similar to the first upper lesion. In the more advanced caseous-pneumonic cases with multiple cavities and lesions of every age intermingled or superimposed, the picture may become too complex for detailed analysis of each individual lesion.

The roentgenologist is justified in making inference of favorable resolution and healing when exudates become absorbed and the residual nodes shrink down over a period of time to a small nodular or linear form. Larger nodes that persist are eyed with suspicion because of the experience that caseous areas do not always evacuate but are sometimes encapsulated, and may undergo a breakdown at any favorable time. By the same token lesions which show discrete linear or small nodular characters over a longer time may be considered as "arrested," or, finally, as "apparently healed."

From the foregoing statements one can readily see that information obtained from films made at first discovery of tuberculosis is greatly amplified by any subsequent films which reveal a forward or backward trend in the disease. Made from time to time at intervals depending on the activity of the case they aid greatly in prognosis and in a way provide a graphic pathologic history of the disease.

My time is rather too short to point out the weak aspects of the x-ray in detecting tuberculosis but I wish to focus your attention on one peculiar paradoxical situation in which the tubercle bacilli are microscopically apparent in the sputum yet the x-rays show no pulmonary changes. I mean real radiographs and plenty of them on one day. Whether you are a conservative or a liberal you have to look this paradox in the face. It has been explained by pathologists in the last few years by the fact that occasionally a caseous lymph gland ulcerates directly into a bronchus and gives the positive sputum findings. The x-ray examination gives negative findings because on that day there was no pulmonary lesion, the bacilli coming from the gland.

Radiographs then made in a month may show a positive lesion of typical character at some point in the lung. We can only explain this as a dissemination from the gland through the bronchi into the lung similar to the dissemination from a cavity, and we may be thankful that such cases are so rare as to change our accuracy less than 1 per cent.

A very common mistake in the past has been to interpret incorrectly the ordinary prominent linear structures proceeding downward from the hilum as tuberculosis when the upper lung fields were clear. The term "peribronchial tuberculosis" was coined to designate this type of the disease and it was not until the pathologist declared there was no such type and clinicians found it did not progress or change with the years that the term was discarded and the finding discounted.

One outstanding weakness in the x-ray system is the absence of information we can get regarding the chain of lymph glands which lie about the trachea and bronchi, and so often harbor sizable areas of highly infected caseous material. While these encapsulated foci seldom break down and directly infect the adjacent lung areas, they nevertheless act as reservoirs of infection

which may be transferred elsewhere by the blood stream. It is probably only fair, when we emphasize so strongly the value of x-rays in detecting tiny lesions in the parenchymal portions of the lung, that we as freely admit our great limitations in detecting the inside structure and true nature of these all-important tracheo-bronchial lymph nodes.

In the next few moments, I wish to present for your consideration and criticism a series of experiments carried out in the laboratories of the General Electric X-ray Company at Chicago. I wish to emphasize that I did not personally conduct these experiments but acted in an advisory capacity. It is through the courtesy of their president that I am now able to make this first public mention of the work. When entirely completed an account of this work will undoubtedly find its way into the proper technical and medical prints.

The experiments consist of new attempts to photograph the fluoroscopic image directly from the screen. Almost since the discovery of x-rays men in various countries have attempted this with various poor degrees of success. Of late years they have tried to make moving pictures of the heart, lungs and stomach for teaching purposes or even for diagnosis. Our efforts were limited to obtaining the finest possible single miniatures of the chest hoping they would still be large enough and of such excellent quality that they could be used in place of the large, bulky and more expensive films now used. We think we have overcome many of the past difficulties in a very fair way.

Heretofore, the first great obstacle in obtaining brilliant and valuable miniatures from the fluorescent screen has been a limitation in speed. The capacity of generators and the capacity of tubes has been enormously increased but not enough to compensate for the limited brilliancy of the fluorescent screen, the speed of available lenses and the speed of such available photographic film as might be considered adaptable.

The first step was to obtain the most rapid screen possible. The ordinary green fluorescent screen was laid aside and a brilliant blue-violet fluorazure screen made of particularly large crystals of calcium fluoride was substituted. Without the usual blue covering material intended to reduce lag, this screen as developed by a competent manufacturer increased the speed seven-fold when used together with a film especially sensitive to blue and violet.

Using this screen, we then tested out all the very high speed films in the world's market. The tests were made with an f 1.5 lens which would cover one frame of a 35 mm. movie film. A rotating anode tube receiving 400 ma. at proper voltage was found to deliver through the average chest at four feet sufficient x-rays to fully expose certain of the films in a tenth of a second. It may sound peculiar, but the film which showed the greatest speed and best working qualities was no other than our common everyday x-ray film. Many of us do not know that this film is critically sensitive to the particular color values emitted from this fluorazure screen.

But the diminutive 35 mm. size was obviously too small for direct diagnostic reading and all attempts to enlarge these films to a three or four inch square size brought out so much obnoxious grain that they were considered of no practical value.

We next concentrated on the lens problem, trying to find a lens of sufficient speed that would cover a larger film without subsequent enlargement. Tests on an f 2.0 lens that would cover a two-inch square film showed that a chest exposure could be obtained in about two-tenths of a second but the films look a little starved and were too small for large film substitutes. Their enlargements, however, gave much less grain prominence.

Using the same power and distance factors, an f 3.5 lens which would cover a four-by-five film was then used. This gave rather good miniatures in half a second. They seemed quite large enough for direct reading and showed no appreciable grain. The films, however, often showed movement in the lower pulmonary structures just as half-second films do in the larger sizes and it was considered necessary to consult lens manufacturers about a lens of f 1.5 speed that would cover a three or four-inch square film.

At first, we were told that no lens of this character had ever been constructed but possibly could be. Shortly, it was learned that one lens of this speed which would cover a three and a quarter-inch square film had been constructed for rapid night photography from aeroplanes and we were extremely fortunate in obtaining a short time loan of this lens to continue the experiments. Naturally, it was a very large lens, having a diameter of about six inches and weighing no less than twenty-six pounds. Now, using the same rapid screen, a rotating anode tube and the same power and distance factors, a series of chest miniatures was then obtained which seem to answer all requirements. They are brilliant, fully exposed in a tenth of a second or less and quite free from grain. We are pleased to submit these films for your inspection and criticism. Although but three and a fourth inches square they show, with faithfulness, every detail present in standard sized films of the same chests.

A lens of this large size was then immediately ordered and has been recently delivered. It differs from the borrowed lens in that it has a higher light gathering power and is designed to focus the blue-violet light which altogether doubles its efficiency. The next experiment will be to place the equipment in a local tuberculosis sanitarium where a large series of films will be made from pathologic chests to be compared for readability with the standard sized films at hand. These may then be submitted to a group of experts for evaluation.

Should miniature films of this size and quality prove to be an adequate and practical substitute for our present standard sized films in the case-finding program of a tuberculosis survey you will quite agree that the filing and storage problem will be greatly simplified. The material expense for a single film is reduced to about five cents. This means that in a thousand cases the film cost alone will be lowered from about six hundred dollars to about fifty dollars.

THE FOOT AND ANKLE*

Their Discomforts, Deformities and Disabilities

PHILIP LEWIN, M.D.

Chicago, Illinois

I HAVE chosen a subject which is large both anatomically and geographically. I wish I could cover the subject from every practical point of view, including the orthopedic, industrial, surgical, roentgenologic, dermatologic, genitourinary, obstetric, gynecologic, neurologic, sociologic, economic and arthritic aspects, but that is obviously impossible. I have tried, however, to keep uppermost in my thoughts the function of the foot and ankle, which means their physiologic activity, their usefulness and comfort; in short, their "performance."

It is important to be able to arrive at a fair estimate of percentage of partial or total disability in order that both the patient and the employer be treated fairly.

A man who has had a fracture of the leg, thigh or foot, after weeks of treatment, may appear to have an excellent cosmetic and roentgenographic result, but he says his foot hurts and he can't walk; he doesn't walk and he won't work. I am interested in what can be done to give him a good functional result.

The relation of feet and their defects to other complaints such as backache, sciatic pain, knee pain and hip pain, is sometimes very close and occasionally brilliant results follow correction of foot imbalance. While I feel that the foot condition should not be underestimated, I do not lay too much stress upon this part of the examination, because the local complaint, such as backache and sciatic pain, must be thoroughly investigated, independently.

It would be impractical to consider foot lesions apart from the leg because the functions of the two members are closely associated. Every organ or tissue may react upon the general health, usually by the infectious, glandular or metabolic routes, but the feet, in addition, may react mechanically.

Foot abnormalities may be indicators of disturbances of the general health. Just as the eye specialist may, from an eye examination, suspect a serious lesion of the kidneys, so the

orthopedic surgeon may find evidence of disturbances of the general health, which, if thoroughly investigated, may reveal important facts. A doctor's wife consulted me because of a simple metatarsalgia. She had a spastic condition with disturbed skin sensation and some ataxia. I advised a neurological examination, which revealed evidence of a tumor of the spinal cord, which was proved by operation.

The foot cannot be treated as an isolated member, but must be considered a part of the human organism. This is especially true of mechanical disturbances of the feet and legs which are aggravated by constitutional abnormalities such as infections in the teeth, throat, sinuses, ears, glands, chest, stomach and intestines, genitourinary tract, and disturbances of the circulatory apparatus.

It is possible to judge some of the mental and physical characteristics of an individual by his gait.

An employer when engaging an individual will observe if that person has a springy gait or if he has a slouchy, dull, rigid gait. If one observes a large number of people walk into a room that has a runner of carpet, he will see some trip, proving that many people do not lift but drag their feet.

Shoe fitting is an art that requires years of experience, a proper determination of the type of shoe and a complete stock in order to fit the foot properly. Much progress has been made, through coöperation of shoe manufacturers with the orthopedic profession, in the manufacture of shoes for children and men, but women's shoes are still far from perfect. There is no one brand or type of shoe that is appropriate for every type of foot. Important advances were made in the solution of the static foot problem by the work of The American Posture League which divided feet into straight, inflare and outflare varieties. High heels tend to produce sway-back.

In many of our United States a license is required of every blacksmith who shoes horses, but I want you to show me one state in which

*Read at the annual meeting of the Minnesota State Medical Association, Duluth, Minnesota, June 30, 1938.

NOVEMBER, 1938

769

the human shoe fitter is required to have any special qualifications.

The chief foot defects are: Congenital defects, deformities and disabilities; acquired deformities and disabilities; diseases of bones, joints, muscles and nerves; traumatic conditions of bones, joints, muscles and nerves; paralytic conditions; circulatory disturbances, and tumors.

Congenital defects include absence of toes, constricting bands, supernumerary toes, syndactylism, congenital hypertrophy, congenital overgrowth of leg and foot, overlapping toes, and bipartite sesamoid bones.

Congenital deformities include various types of talipes.

Acquired deformities may be due to tuberculosis, syphilis, infantile paralysis, spastic paralysis, infections, flat-foot, metatarsal depression, bursitis, hallux valgus and exostoses.

The important traumatic conditions are fracture, dislocation, epiphyseal separation and epiphysitis. Warts, papillomas, corns of both the hard and the soft varieties and most circulatory disturbances are acquired.

Diseases of the foot are chiefly tuberculosis, syphilis, osteomyelitis, epiphysitis or osteochondritis such as Köhler's tarsal scaphoiditis. Freiberg's infraction of the metatarsal head, apophysitis of the os calcis, arthritis due to gonococcus, staphylococcus, streptococcus, metabolic and traumatic causes are common in the foot.

Tumors of the foot are chiefly lipomas, fibromas, osteomas, angiomas, sarcomas, melanomas, and melanoblastomas.

In 1781, Peter Camper, Professor of Medicine in Amsterdam, published a book entitled "A Dissertation on the Best Form of Shoes." According to Bick, it included a detailed anatomic study of the foot and its arches, and illustrated many of the distortions caused by pointed shoe toes, tight shoes, and other defects of the last. James Lowie, an Edinburgh shoemaker, quoted from an English translation as follows: "Shoes which are not adapted to the foot of each individual are defective; and a shoemaker who would excel in his art ought to have an exact knowledge of the diversity of form, more especially if he wishes to prevent corns upon the joints, and between the toes, inflammation of the roots of the nails, especially of the great toes, and painful callosities. . . .

He will prevent all these annoyances by giving a proper form to his shoes." Camper, who was a scientist, an anthropologist and an anatomist, virtually introduced the subject of static foot deformity. Following him, LaForest, a Frenchman, wrote a book, and from that period on, increasing studies on foot mechanics appeared.

The importance of foot disabilities other than those causing obvious gross deformity such as club-foot, was not appreciated until 1781, when Camper wrote his memorable Dissertation on the Best Form of Shoes.

The study of the mechanics of human gait offers the only physiological basis for an intelligent approach to the treatment of static foot disorders.

In 1836 the Weber brothers published a volume on the mechanics of locomotion, containing the first serious scientific study of human gait. They stressed the importance of the pendulum action of the lower extremities during locomotion, and described in great anatomic detail the muscular and articular structures involved.

Janssen suggested the study of gait by means of serial pictures, but the first successful application of the method was that of Carlot, in Paris. He made graphic records of the human gait by means of shoes built with rubber soles in which were placed air compression chambers, for the heel and forefoot. Carlot published his observations in 1872. Three years later Marey published another volume on locomotion in man and animals in which Carlot's air chambers were also used. Bradford was among the first of the American orthopedic surgeons to study the problem. Muybridge was said to have been the first to use an electric photographic method for recording gait (1925). This has been modified and improved from time to time. The most recent advance in the study of gait has been made by R. Plato Schwartz and his co-workers whose electrobasographic methods of recording gait, described in 1933, has offered refinements in study not previously possible.

Along with the development of methods for recording gait, the study of foot function from the anatomico-physiological viewpoint has proceeded with parallel progress. Duchenne, during his classic investigations on muscle function, was the first to note a specific relationship between muscular imbalance in the leg, and the everted foot. He felt that the most important factor in locomotion was well coördinated muscle control of the limb and its individual segments. Delpech, the master of French orthopedics, made a similar observation, so that the myogenic etiology of static foot deformity was early impressed upon French students. Toward the end of the nineteenth century, Royal Whitman distinguished between true flat-foot, and a pseudo flat-foot, in which the foot and leg become everted, painful, and, in advanced cases, more or less rigid.

The concept of the "weak foot," flaccid in its early stages and rigid in advanced cases, has almost entirely superseded the older concept of flat-foot.

Against the myogenic theory of static foot deformity has been brought the hypothesis of the stretched plantar or calcaneo-navicular ligaments. According to this hypothesis, the pain and disability of foot dysfunction is due to a gradual elongation of the tarsal ligaments, consequent upon faulty habits in walking and standing, or the use of improper shoes. Keith, however, emphasized what Duchenne had suggested, the fact that the interosseous ligaments are but secondary supports in weight bearing extremities, and are only called into play when the musculature of the part becomes ineffective. He referred to them as the "fatigue structures." As such, he maintained that their being stretched, or elongated by persistent passive strain, must of course presuppose inadequacy of the muscles concerned. The osseous theory of this deformity, which gave to it the popular name of "fallen arches," was based on the assumption, held especially in England, that the bony longitudinal arch of the foot was a true arch with the navicular or head of the astragalus as its keystone. This theory was refuted by the British orthopedists, Golding Bird, Adams, and Walsham, but it is constantly reiterated in the literature, especially in connection with operative methods of treatment. The literature of the nineteenth century contained a tremendous bibliography of books, monographs, theses and papers on the subject of foot deformity, a good proportion of which dealt with flat-foot. However, the work of Whitman and the advent of roentgenography invalidated many of the purely speculative concepts. In 1885, Shaffer described a painful static foot deformity of no specified etiology characterized by a high longitudinal arch, extended proximal phalanges, almost a mild pes cavus, the so-called

hollow foot. Although its etiology has never been determined, except for the hypothesis of short shoe-wear, Shaffer thought its pathogenesis to be a contracted tendo achillis. In 1876, T. G. Morton introduced into the literature the term metatarsalgia, a type of foot disability in which severe pain occurred in the region of the meta-tarsal arch. Morton believed the symptoms to be neuralgic in character, and described pain radiating into one or more toes due to pressure on the digital nerves as they passed between the heads of the metatarsal bones. Goldthwait, in 1894, and Robert Jones, in 1897, demonstrated that this was primarily due to a prolapse of the metatarsal arch. Another lesion giving similar symptoms had previously been described by Breithaupt (1885). This lesion, known variously as marchfoot or pied force, was fairly common among soldiers following long marches, and was treated as a strain or sprain until roentgenography disclosed its true pathologic change to be an infraction of a metatarsal bone, in which the fracture is not perceptible until some time after the appearance of symptoms. It resembles to some extent Kümmel's disease in the vertebræ.

To Hugh Owen Thomas, the great Liverpool surgeon, all static deformities of the foot were a problem of joints and ligaments rather than muscles. In the treatment of flat-foot, he introduced the raised and forwardly extended inner border of the heel of the shoe. During the middle of the last century the use of "arches" came into vogue. These "arches" or foot plates act as braces for the bones and ligaments of the longitudinal arch "which has broken down," or, as in the Whitman brace, serves to actively invert the foot, thereby bringing it into normal relationship and relieving the supporting musculo-tendon mechanism of undue strain. There has been a constant controversy between those who advocate rigid plates, and those who advocate non-rigid supports. The spring-arch first appeared rather generally in the literature during the nineties. Any reasonable support in an adult, adjusted with a proper appreciation of the mechanics of the deformity, can become suitable for the particular case. Foot supports have been made from steel, duraluminum and other metals, celluloid, leather, cork, wood and rubber. Thomas said: "It isn't the apparatus, it is the principle underlying its application that is important."

In children, adolescents and young adults, the tendency has been away from rigid supports, and in favor of exercises aimed at strengthening the involved muscles. Although foot plates are frequently used for temporary assistance, in younger patients many orthopedists feel that the raising of the inner border of the sole is sufficient to invert the calcaneus during the period of exercise or other physical therapy. These exercises are planned to strengthen specifically the anterior and posterior tibial muscles, and in some instances the intrinsic muscles of the foot. It is felt with increasing confidence that, at least in younger patients, such treatment affords an effective cure. Many surgeons vary their methods with the individual patient. Plates, manipulations, and exercises assisted frequently by physical therapy are used interchangeably. The painful foot represents a large proportion of private practice in probably every orthopedist's office. By the time these patients reach the orthopedist, the disability requires far more attention than the simple application of a rigid support.

The rigid or spastic flat-foot presents a difficult problem. To Royal Whitman is due credit for valuable study of this deformity, and the most effective methods of treatment. In such cases, correction by the simple use of foot plates or braces is impossible. Most cases, however can be improved by manipulation under anesthesia, followed by a plaster-of-Paris boot to maintain the over-corrected (inverted) position. After removal of the plaster the foot is stretched daily for a prolonged period of time, and the foot braces are worn as described by Whitman. For the very resistant cases, in which recurrence follows even the most painstaking treatment, operation becomes necessary.

Surgery of the Foot

Bone operations designed to correct deformities of the foot are, because of the highly specialized anatomy of the part, peculiar to themselves and represent a course of development in many instances quite distinct from the general rule of operations applied elsewhere upon the skeleton. Bick recalls that Fabricius Hildanus removed a fractured talus in 1608 to overcome the resulting disability. In 1741, Broglie repeated the procedure in a similar case of long standing with the intent of correcting the deformity. The operation was again performed by Marrigue in 1782, and Desault in 1788. Broca, in 1852, and Lund, in 1872, advocated the removal of the astragalus

for local destructive disease, and in 1857 Cock suggested the extirpation of the astragalus, scaphoid, cuneiform and cuboid for the same indication. In 1857, Solly removed the cuboid in an attempt to correct the deformity of club-foot. In 1878, Albert, a Viennese orthopedic surgeon, conceived the idea of employing a stabilizing operation for the relief of paralytic deformities of the foot. In order to accomplish this he adapted his method of arthrodesis to the bones of the tarsus, denuded the articular surfaces of their cartilages, and allowed fusion to occur during a period of immobilization. In the same year, and later in 1888, Golding Bird performed a similar operation, but applied it to severe flat-foot deformity. He removed the navicular, and in some cases also the head of the talus. The earlier case was probably the first occasion in which surgery was used for the correction of flat-foot. In 1884, Ogston performed a talo-navicular arthrodesis, also for flat-foot, by resecting the head of the astragalus, and denuding the articular surface of the navicular. He continued this procedure, but later, when necessary, he secured the two bones by an inserted ivory peg. He then sutured the surrounding soft parts, and immobilized the foot. Shortly after this, Stokes advised merely the removal of a wedge from the head and neck of the astragalus. In advanced cases of valgus deformity, Trendelenburg advocated fracturing the tibia and fibula above the ankle joint, permitting union with the foot adducted.

In 1901, Royal Whitman performed the first astragalectomy on a paralytic foot in a case of calcaneus deformity. In this operation he not only extirpated the astragalus, but, by displacing the foot backwards, gained the advantage of a direct line of support from the tibia through the mid-tarsus. It secures excellent stabilization without obliterating motion at any of the tarsal joints; and can be performed in children at any age. In 1908, Jones described a fusion operation for calcaneo-cavus, and later Dunn devised a similar procedure for several types of paralytic foot deformity. Goldthwait, also in 1908, tried the effect of fusing the ankle joint in cases of complete paralysis of the foot. In 1911, Lorthoir reported eight cases in which the astragalus was removed, denuded of cartilage on all sides, and replaced. The intent here was to effect a multiple arthrodesis. In 1913, G. G. Davis, of Philadelphia, described a type of fusion operation, or arthrodesis, which, unlike those of his contemporaries, involved only the subastragalar joint. Whitman's operation, and the arthrodesing types of operation, have formed the basis for many subsequent modifications since developed by Hoke of Atlanta, Ryerson of Chicago, and others. Hoke's arthrodesis is one of the most important contributions to this subject. According to his technic, the head of the talus is removed, and reshaped to accommodate itself to the deformity. It may be replaced or if advisable left out altogether. The articular surface of the navicular is denuded to allow for subsequent talo-navicular fusion. Secondly, the articular surfaces of the cuboid-calcaneal joint are fused, and lastly the subtalar joint is arthrodesed. Ryerson conceived the idea of constructing a bone ledge at the anterior border of the talus to check dorsiflexion in cases of paralytic pes calcaneus. In addition to these basic procedures, Jones, Garre- and Kuttner, Perthes, Schwarz, David, Gill, Putti, Ombredanne, Steindler, Campbel, Zadek, Lambrinudi, Mayer and others have advised numerous modifications and additions to the surgical correction of paralytic or severe static deformities of the foot. Among these operations are Jones' transverse osteotomy of the tarsus, Zadek's wedge osteotomy, Steindler's stripping of the plantar fascia for the correction of cavus, and Campbell's bone block for equinus. This latter has recently been simplified by Wagner. Mayer of New York formerly corrected such deformity entirely by tendon transplantation, but has recently added to his original procedure a modification of Hoke's operation. Gallie, Whitman, and others have likewise devised methods of relieving such deformities by means of muscle-tendon operations, but in general these have not met with the same acceptance as have procedures practiced upon the bones and articulations. In 1921, Soule proposed driving a bone pin through the navicular into the talus in cases of marked valgus deformity. Gleich sawed the calcaneus in an oblique direction and shifted the posterior fragment forward. The non-operative treatment of club-foot is not far different today from what it was during the Hippocratic era. As early as the sixteenth century, corrective braces were used, and these have been modified ever since. Paré, Glisson, Hunter, Venel, and Scarpa have all devised apparatus for this purpose. Theories of etiology have been numerous and variations of therapeutic measures

have, to some degree, depended on the contemporary theory in vogue. The possibility of intrauterine mechanical restraint was held by Hippocrates, Scarpa, and Paré. Bessel-Hagen, in 1899, restudied the subject in the human fetus, and came to the same conclusion. Arthur Keith believes that the phylogenetic evolution of the human foot adequately explains the condition of club-foot if one assumes a developmental rest of the fetal foot at an anthropoid stage.

Hugh Owen Thomas advocated the immediate forcible correction of the deformity, to be followed by a retention splint devised to maintain an over-corrected position. For this purpose, he constructed an osteoclast of special design, the "Thomas Wrench." Grattan, of Cork; Bradford, of Boston; and Lorenz, of Vienna, adopted the method in their extensive practices, and also designed similar, though modified, osteoclasts. Lorenz later made use of a padded pyramid over the apex of which he "broke" the deformity. According to Brockman, the French orthopedic surgeon, Guerin, in 1836, was the first to use a plaster bandage to splint the corrected club-foot. However, it was not until twenty years later that plaster-of-Paris was introduced and became popular in the treatment of these cases. A great step forward was made after overcoming considerable resistance, when the advisability of treatment at the earliest possible moment was realized. Until the end of the nineteenth century, treatment was deliberately delayed until early childhood. The practice of correction in early infancy has done more than anything else to solve the problem of club-foot. Zadek and Barnett, who studied a large series of end-results, found that the subcutaneous section of the tendo achillis and posterior capsule of the ankle joint was of additional advantage in certain cases. Failure to correct equinus is a cause of recurrences.

A notable advance was the introduction of operative methods for correction of cases seen in late stages with bone deformity. The use of achillo-tenotomy, as introduced by Stromeyer and others, will be discussed later. Many operations aimed at the correction of the malformation of the tarsus were popular during the nineteenth century. Augustoni and Morestin attempt to improve the position of the foot by removing the astragalus; Championniere removed several bones of the tarsus in addition to the astragalus; Gibney excised only the head of the astragalus, or in other instances the proximal end of the fifth metatarsal; Muller, Robert Jones, and many others practiced the removal of wedges, cut from almost every conceivable angle, to produce purely mechanical or cosmetic correction of the deformity. In addition, the intra-articular surfaces of almost every tarsal joint, and combination of joints, have been resected and arthrodesed.

In 1892, Bradford wrote: "The literature of the treatment of club-foot is, as a rule, that of unvarying success. It is often as brilliant as an advertising sheet, and yet in practice there is no lack of half-cured or relapsed cases, sufficient evidence that methods of cure are not universally understood. In all methods related to the treatment of club-foot, time and painstaking attention to the details of after-care are probably the most important factors in success.

An important stimulus has been introduced by Kite, of Decatur, Georgia. Severe operations necessarily entail considerable mutilation of the internal architecture of the foot. While such operations may give excellent cosmetic results, they almost invariably leave feet that are more or less permanently and recurrently painful. Kite proposed to first correct the deformity by slow conservative manipulations, without anesthesia. Each small correction is followed by a plaster to hold the new position. After repeated corrections over a period of time he found that the parts were susceptible to remarkable reformation. After maximum correction has been obtained, a period of observation is allowed. If a tendency to recurrence appears, the foot is surgically fused before the deformity appears. Under this method, a simple anthrodesing operation is sufficient to maintain correction, and more extensive surgery is no longer necessary.

The operative experience gained in the treatment of paralytic and congenital foot deformities has been applied to other foot disabilities. Numerous operations have been devised to overcome the malformation of rigid or exaggerated flat-foot, traumatic pes valgus, severe hallux valgus and other distortions. The present ingenuity applied to surgical procedures upon the bones of deformed feet is of temporary utility, since outstanding success follows only the proper early application of methods conceived for the prevention of bone deformity consequent to weight bearing.

Physiology

The physiology of the foot is concerned chiefly with the mechanics of weight-bearing and flexible locomotion. The structure of the foot furnishes spring to the step, which prevents jars to brain, spinal cord and abdominal and pelvic organs. Brown says the functions of the normal foot, which is certainly one of the most marvelous machines in Nature, are: weight-bearing during standing and locomotion, the provision of a spring to reduce jars and assist propulsion during movement, and action as a pivot to assist the turning of the body. There are few movements which do not combine all three of these. These functions do not depend entirely on the foot itself, but on the brain and spinal cord, so that an anatomically intact foot does not insure a perfectly functioning foot. The integrity of structure and function are not identical.

Disturbances of physiology involve mechanical stress and strain on muscles, ligaments and capsules of the bones and joints.

Two bones of great importance are the astragalus and os calcis; the former because it is the mortise bone between the leg and the foot. The astragalus articulates with the tibia, fibula and scaphoid. It articulates with the os calcis in three places. Although it cannot move itself, because it has no muscle attachments, it is subjected to the superincumbent weight of the entire body. The os calci is important because of its attachments for the achilles tendon and plantar fascia. It furnishes the initial bearing surface of the foot as it strikes the ground in walking. The scaphoid and first cuneiform bones owe their importance to the attachments of ligaments, and especially the tendons of the peroneus longus, and the anterior and posterior tibial muscles. The longitudinal arch is composed of the os calcis, astragalus, scaphoid, first and second cuneiforms, first metatarsal and proximal phalanx of the great toe. When a foot is in action it is supported chiefly by muscles, but when standing, chiefly by ligaments. Hoke emphasized the importance of three tendons: those of the anterior and posterior tibials and the flexor hallucis longus.

Terminology

The generic term for foot deformities is "talipes" derived from talus (astragalus) and pes (foot). If the toes are at a lower level than the heel, the term equinus is used; if the heel

774

is lower than the toes, the term calcaneus is used. In addition to either of these positions, if the foot is rotated on the long axis of the foot, the terms varus and valgus are used.

Inversion of the foot occurs when the inner border is elevated. Eversion occurs when the outer border is elevated. When a foot is inverted, there is a tendency for the fore part of the foot to approach the mid-line of the body, that is, adduction. This movement occurs chiefly at the tarso-metatarsal articulations. With eversion, there is a strong inclination to the opposite movement at these joints, namely abduction. When a foot is inverted and adducted, there is usually an upward and outward rotation of the medial bones of the mid-tarsal region, namely, the scaphoid, and the first and second cuneiform bones. This constitutes supination. If a foot is everted and abducted, the reverse occurs, that is, downward and inward rotation of the medial mid-tarsal bone, producing pronation. A foot that is inverted, adducted and supinated is in varus position, and a foot that is everted, abducted and pronated is in valgus position.

Shoes and Their Modifications

As a general proposition one may say that a shoe should be straight-lasted, round-toed, have a moderate height of heel and a rigid shank. It must be narrow in the heel and through the waist of the foot, but wide through the ball. There is comparatively little difficulty in obtaining proper shaped shoes for children and men; but for girls and women the matter is entirely different. Women are the victims of two things: one is style and the other is the shoe salesman. Women prefer to fit the eye rather than the foot and please the eye rather than their husbands. "There is no shoe too small for an ambitious foot."

Shoes are modified, for the most part, in the regions of the heels, soles, counters, and big toe. The chief modification of the heel is the Thomas heel, which is longer and higher on the inner than the outer border. This compels the individuals to walk over the proper walking angle so that a weight-bearing line dropped from the middle of the patella, bisects the tibia and the astragalus. The chief modification of the sole is the elevation of the outer border where the highest point of the wedge should be under the base of the fifth toe.

Modification of the counter includes the removal of the counter for irritation of the heel; and the prolongation of the counter on the inner border to protect and support the scaphoid, cuneiform I and base of the first metatarsal. Modification in the region of the big toe joint consists in a rigid sole to prevent motion in the big toe joint. This procedure may be beneficial in relieving the pain in cases of osteoarthritis of the big toe joint. The chief modification of the sole is what is known as a metatarsal bar or metatarsal cleat which consists of a strip of leather or rubber secured between the layers of the sole, at a point just behind the heads of the metatarsal bones. The so-called Denver bar is very effective.

Old Shoes

How much a man is like old shoes!
For instance, each a soul may lose.
Both have been tanned, both are made tight
By cobblers. Both get left and right.
Each needs a mate to be complete,
And both are made to go on feet.
They both need healing, they both get sold,
And both in time turn all to mould.
With shoes the last is first; with men
The first shall be the last; and when
The shoes wear out they're mended new;
When men wear out they're men dead, too.
They both are trod upon, and both
Will tread on others, nothing loth,
Both have their ties, and both incline,
When polished, in the world to shine;
And both peg out—Now, would you choose
To be a Man, or be his shoes?—M. C. Dodge.

* *

Note: Much of the historical material has been derived from Bick, Edgar M.: Source book on orthopædics, Baltimore, Williams and Wilkins, 1937. The author gratefully acknowledges permission to use this source in his paper.

AUTHENTIC BIOGRAPHIC DATA*

MONTE C. PIPER, M.D.

Rochester, Minnesota

THE constitution of the State Medical Association asserts that the purposes of the organization are the promotion of the science and art of medicine, the protection of public health, and the betterment of the medical profession.

The Council of the State Association adopted, last year, the new application blank for membership because sufficient record of the life histories of the members was not being maintained. Mr. Ralph K. Lindop remarks in "The Legal Aspects of Records" that, "it may be safely laid down as a general principle that whenever there is a duty to do, there is also a duty to record the things done." John G. Bowman, Director of the American College of Surgeons, says that, "record means Authentic Evidence" and, as refers to hospitals, "the record department is directly responsible for the reputation of the hospital." Fred G. Carter adds, "Records protect the physician in his practice." Likewise, the Council felt that records would be of value in protecting the reputation of the medical profession.

There is much evidence of record of achievement in the progress of science and teaching but there is no systematic uniformity in recording the progress of the members of the profession as a whole. While a doctor is attending school and applying for licenses, numerous records are made. His qualifications are recorded in an exacting manner but after he has graduated and has become elected to membership in the Medical Association, there is no further uniformity in system of recording his progress and activities. He is turned loose, as it were, to practice his profession with the assurance that he is qualified and, unless he is outstanding in some manner, his identity may be all but lost. True, he is protected by the licensing board of the state and the state journal is sent to his address; his colleagues know of his activities to some degree but authentic evidence or record is no longer maintained.

The old application blank for Association membership contained very little information

not included in the records of the licensing board and this new blank is only slightly more comprehensive than the old one, but it is a beginning, at least, for "the betterment of the profession." The new blank is designed to collect further historic and genealogic data and reveal something of the progress of each individual in medicine.

One is struck with wonder that, in the three thousand years of medical organization, there seems to be no evidence of concerted successful recording or compilation of the progress or failure of individual members. It is true that there is a vast amount of information about a few and much information regarding some physicians but there is certainly a paucity of information regarding many. Newspapers and magazine articles form the chief source of recorded data, but the doctor must "break into print" occasionally to be thus recorded. Large newspaper offices maintain very extensive reference libraries formerly called "morgues," some with as many as two million references. The American Medical Association has maintained a library of clippings and other information for thirty-two years. They have name cards with accumulated data concerning every doctor of whom they have ever had record and, now, there are accumulated about a million references. The library is admirably systematized, supervised, and kept alive, but its data come from printed or written reports.

The State Board of Medical Examiners is now keeping clippings and other data that their efficient office staff finds by searching publications. With the new application blank of the State Medical Association, each name is supplied with a large envelope in which all obtainable information will be filed. These, however, are only records of something remarkable enough to be printed or written about. There is no uniformity of purpose of these records except the accumulation of references.

Ramsey County Medical Society has compiled some biographic data and has a very fine album of photographs of many of its members. Hennepin County has photographs of all of its former presidents and attempted, for a time, to keep

---

*From the Section on Obstetrics and Gynecology, The Mayo Clinic, Rochester, Minnesota. Read before the annual meeting of the Officers of the County Medical Societies of the State, Saint Paul, Feb. 26, 1938.

776

MINNESOTA MEDICINE

a rather complete biographic record of all members but it has not been continued. The University of Minnesota Press has recently published "Physicians of The Mayo Clinic and The Mayo Foundation." This new volume contains the photograph and complete biographic and bibliographic data on all Members of the Staff of The Mayo Clinic and Fellows in the Foundation. No doubt, other groups have some system of keeping alive active records, but publications of these systems have not been found. The majority of members of the profession are unrecorded, perhaps throughout life, unless some event in their lives seems of sufficient importance to be "written up."

There is no uniform record of progress. Cities, villages, counties, and states do not attempt to maintain a measurement of the progress of professional men other than tabulations of qualifications. So far as has been ascertained, hospitals do not maintain a personal record of their staff except the professional qualifications and accomplishments of each member, if such pertain to the care of patients. The reputation and success of a hospital depends entirely on the quality of its staff members. One would suppose that hospital managements would be concerned about the health, the civil activities, the recreations and leisures and the families of so important a part of their organization.

The Medical School of the University is starting a five-year follow-up of its graduates to ascertain their successes and the shortcomings of their scholastic training. The General College of the University has made a critical survey of a group of graduates that preceded the depression and a similar group of students who have graduated since the depression to ascertain their attitudes toward the education obtained. This survey was made by use of a very comprehensive and painstakingly prepared questionnaire. It would seem that no better estimate of the usefulness of an education could be obtained than by those who have had an opportunity to apply that education to life.

Sir Richard Livingstone says there is a "threefold function of man: to make a livelihood, to be a citizen, to be a man . . . At present life is so arranged that most of us do our thinking in youth at an age when we are not best fitted for it, and having left the University think, systematically, no more. What wonder that middle life finds so many unaware of recent progress

in their own field, unapt for new experiments and ideas, deeply embedded in a rut, while progress waits impatiently for their death and the arrival of the next generation . . . In every point except the economic one adult education has the advantage . . . It is given to students who desire it, who have the mental development to receive it, and have the experience of life to value and interpret it."

There are many members of the doctors' guild who are doing valiant work, are of much influence for progress and good example in their communities, who have the love and respect of those who know them and have success. Of these, there is very little, if any, written record. Such lives should contribute a part historically, for history is the study of change in humanity, the development of human society in space and time.

The historical committee has made diligent effort to assemble facts of medical history in this state over the approximate period of 1850 to 1900, and they have succeeded to a remarkable degree. Those who have undertaken the task must have given freely of effort and time. The records they are able to obtain of the pioneers are written records in some form or other. But a knowledge of others, of whom there is so little written or recorded, has vanished with the passing of the friends and relatives who remembered them.

The new application blank will contain a uniformity of data which will be available as a starting point or a foundation on which may be added further information of the past as well as of the future. It is the desire of the Council that all members of the Association fill in these new blanks as completely as possible. Data other than what is requested in the questions will add much more to their value. Some seven county societies have already completed these blanks in large numbers. Others have voiced objections to filling out another blank and, probably, that objection is largely due to a misunderstanding as to the use that is to be made of these blanks. Previous members are asked to comply, so that uniform biographic data may be obtained of all. Records exist of your training period. Why should there be objection to keeping record of your progress?

This new movement has, as its object, uniformity in recording; it should be dedicated to all of the profession, quoting Dr. Henry E.

Sigerist, "To the unknown doctor, who, in unselfish and inconspicuous activities, fulfils the teaching of the Great Doctors."

The great teachers are conspicuous and there is much record of them but there are great physicians whose contribution to the welfare of their communities should not go unrecorded. Assuming that this foundation is established by collecting the data of the new information blank, why should not the medical association, of which we are members, continue to record a system of progress and build a structure showing advancement on that foundation? It would seem that such a procedure would be of present-day value as revealing cumulative authentic evidence in the future of progressiveness of the profession as a whole.

Such evidence might be obtained by various methods, but the one which suggests itself at present as being the most feasible would be a survey at stated intervals, perhaps once every five years. It would be feasible because all members would participate in personally supplying the desired information. Dr. R. G. Leland, Director of the Bureau of Medical Economics, says, "A knowledge of the competence of the members of the medical profession should be of value primarily to the public—but this knowledge should be compiled by the profession itself."

A committee consisting of the chairmen of several existing committees and including those of medical education and of history together with others interested in the subject could compile a suitable questionnaire or invoice sheet. This committee, probably, would wish to obtain assistance in compiling that form from the medical school and other departments of the University. Such a questionnaire of census could be filled out by individual members with the understanding that personal identity be treated confidentially. Conscientiousness and integrity would be assumed in compilation by each member. It would be a coöperative method and each member would be requested to contribute to its compilation. Such an attempt to keep a record of progress would be a new venture entirely, for there seems to be no published evidence of such an effort previously having been tried or, at least, carried on. Such an investigation might reveal professional achievements, courses of study taken, participation in

medical societies, honors attained, articles published, type of medical reading, value of certain journals, attitude toward preventative medicine, maternal and infant welfare, workmen's compensation and contract practices, hospital facilities, coöperation with other doctors, fitness for the chosen field or specialty, personal inspirations or inhibitions, civic activities and rewards, fluctuations in compensation, influence of relief problems, ancestors in the medical world or other geneologic factors influencing ambitions, progress of one's family, children studying or practicing medicine. Likewise, the investigation might reveal general achievements like recommendations of measures to advance the standards of medicine, improvements in medical school curricula by stressing some factors and curtailing others, postgraduate studies of practicing physicians, adult education, evaluation of fitness of some physicians in their field, health of doctors, occupational diseases, hobbies, recreations, trends, illness, and prevalence of hereditary influences on some diseases.

It is a sad commentary when cardiologists show that physicians succumb to hypertensive heart disease and coronary disease more frequently than those of any other vocation. The cumulative strenuousness and unremitting responsibility of the physician's life seem to be taking their toll of doctors. There are probably many other valuable factors which could be worked out. Supposing some such survey had been conducted over the past twenty-five years and included in its scope twenty-five to fifty thousand physicians. There could be evolved from statistical study of such records answers to many of the criticisms which have been aimed at the medical profession by some members of the medical profession and by the social reformers of recent years. The officers of the American Medical Association would, no doubt, welcome such information if it were available.

The success of such a survey or questionnaire would depend on the ease with which the questions could be answered. If they could be answered readily, without too much trouble, most men probably would be willing to fill out the blank. If questions were cumbersome and involved, many probably would defer answering them, and, finally, forget to answer them. But, if it is to be a record of progress, it would have a certain appeal.

Doctors should be qualified to keep records. It is important regarding the care of the patients and should be important to one's own life. When the American College of Surgeons, in 1913, required the records of 100 cases in order to qualify for membership, it afforded stimulus to hospitals and physicians to keep accurate records and these records have been an invaluable stimulus in the furthering of medical studies. The recording of the individual physician's activities will also be of great aid to future historical committees. Much information of this nature is disappearing as the older generation passes on and it should be collected while it is still available. The historical committee cannot reach it all.

There is an organization which could render very valuable assistance, if it could be prevailed on to undertake the task. Our wives are organized as Women's Auxiliary and, if they would undertake to collect this information, it would be a valuable assistance and, assumedly, an enjoyable project for their activities.

Perhaps some form could be supplied with an individual physician's name and address filled in and this could be allocated to the Auxiliary of the respective county unit. No doubt the historical committee would welcome such assistance.

References

1. Bowman, J. C.: Case records and their use. Bull. Am. Coll. Surg., 4:1-14, (Jan.) 1919.
2. Carter, F. C.: Why records? Hosp. Management, 43: 53-56, (June) 1937.
3. Leland, R. G.: Personal communication to the author.
4. Lindop, R. K: The legal aspect of records from a life insurance company's viewpoint. Hosp. Management, 42: 51-55; 61-62, (Sept.) 1936.
5. Livingstone, Sir Richard: The future in education. Nature, 138:601-602, (Oct. 10) 1936.
6. Sigerist, H. E.: Medical societies, past and present. Yale Jour. Biol. Med., 6:351-362, (Jan.) 1933-1934.
7. Sigerist, H. E.: The Great Doctors. A biographical history of medicine. New York: W. W. Horton and Co., Inc., 1933, 436 pp.

NUTRITION IN PREGNANCY*

RUSSELL J. MOE, M.D.

Duluth, Minnesota

IN spite of much valuable laboratory and clinical research on the problem of nutrition in pregnancy, it is only within recent years that we have begun to apply these findings to obstetrical practice. We, as practitioners, have failed to give proper attention to the dietary requirements during pregnancy. In view of the fact that an adequate protective diet is an important part of good prenatal care, it behooves us to give this problem the attention it rightly deserves.

It is an accepted fact that many of the complications and disabilities associated with pregnancy, labor and lactation are due directly or indirectly to improper or inadequate nutrition. This often begins in the early prenatal period, especially with multiparous, overworked women, and with women who are naturally substandard or chronically undernourished. There are still some misconceptions among medical men as to what constitutes the nutritional needs of the pregnant state. In general, this question may be answered by the statement that the mother should be supplied with the various foods necessary for her own metabolism, and in addition, those needed for the growth and development of the fetus.

Foods may be considered under two main types: (1) the "protective" foods, consisting chiefly of those containing "good" protein, minerals and vitamins; (2) the "energy-bearing" foods, such as carbohydrates and fats. The ideal diet includes sufficient "protective" foods to prevent the development of deficiency diseases, as well as the proper proportion of "energy-bearing" foods, to maintain the growth and activity of the body. Actual starvation from lack of sufficient calories is practically unheard of today. The real danger lies in the fact that individuals in the low income group are forced to substitute the lower priced carbohydrates for the higher priced foods containing protein, minerals and vitamins.

Protective Foods

The highly protective foods include milk, cheese, eggs, meat, butter, fresh green vegetables and raw ripe fruit. Sunlight may also be considered an adjunct to the above list, because it generates vitamin D in the organism. The value of milk as a food for pregnant and lactating moth-

*Read before the annual meeting of the Minnesota State Medical Association, Duluth, Minnesota, June 29, 1938.

DIETARY SCHEME FOR THE PREGNANT AND NURSING WOMAN

A. Protective Foods:

Food	Amount	Protein	Calcium	Phosphorus	Iron	Iodine	Vitamin A	Vitamin B_1	Vitamin B_2	Vitamin C	Vitamin D	Calories	Remarks
		Grammes			Milligrammes		International Units			International Units			
Milk	1,000	32	1.2	0.9	2.4	0.02–0.05	Rich (1,000-3,000)	Good (50-75)	Rich	Poor	Poor	660	(a) Calculations for lean meat.
Meat (or fish or poultry)	120(a)	22	—	0.3	5.0 / 2(a₁) 1.5	—	Poor	Poor(b)	Rich	Poor	None	240	(a₁) One-half calculated as available iron.
Eggs (one)	50	6	—	0.1	0.4	—	Rich (1,000-1,300)	Good (about 15)	Rich	None	25-40	70	(b) Except glands (liver and kidneys) and pork muscle.
Cheese (c)	30	8	0.3	0.2		—	Rich (800-1,000)	Poor	Good	Poor	Poor	125	(c) Calculated as cheddar cheese.
Green and Leafy Vegetables	100(d)	1	0.1	—	1.2	—	Rich (1,000-1,500)	Good	Good	Poor	None	30	(d) Estimated on basis of ⅓ cabbage, ⅓ lettuce, ⅓ spinach.
Potatoes	250	6	—	0.2	2.0	—	Poor	Good	Good	Good	None	250	(e) Calculated as beans.
Legumes, Dried	10(e)	2	—	—	0.2	—	Poor	Good	Good	None	None	35	
Cod Liver Oil	3.5	—	—	—	—	Richest source	Rich (1,800-3,500)	None	None	None	Rich (about 300)	30	
An available source of Vitamin C (from raw fruits and vegetables)										To yield 250-500			
TOTAL YIELD		77	1.6	1.7	10.2	Adequate	Over 5,000	Over 150	Adequate	Over 500	About 300	1,440	

B. Supplementary energy-yielding foods by means of which the individual's energy requirements can be met.

Food	Amount	Protein	Calcium	Phosphorus	Iron	Vitamin B_1	Calories	Remarks
Cereals as needed:								
Highly milled	250(f)	28	—	0.2	2.5	Rich (about 250)	1,000	(f) Calculated as white flour.
or Whole Grain	250(g)	—	0.1	0.9	9.0		1,000	(g) Calculated as whole wheat.

Fats as needed.
Sugar as needed.

The estimates are based on data in Sherman's "Chemistry of Food and Nutrition," 4th edition, 1933. The figures for milk are calculated for a content of 3.2% protein and 3.5% fat. The figures for vitamins, however, are converted to international units and must be regarded as rough approximation only.

TABLE I. NUTRITIVE VALUE OF FOODS[4]

Food	"Good" Protein	Minerals	A	B	C	D	
Milk	++	+++	+	+	+∅	+∅	
Cheese	++	+++	+	+	—	—	
E Eggs	++	++	+	++	—	++	
Liver	++	++	+	++	—	+	
E Fat fish (herring, etc.)	+		+	+	—	++	Highly protective foods
Green vegetables	+	+++	+	+	++	—	
Raw fruit	+	+++	+	+	++	—	
E Butter	—	—	+	—	—	+∅	
Cod liver oil	—	—	+++	—	—	+++	
Yeast	+	+	—	++	—	—	Less protective foods
Meat (muscle)	+	§	—	+	§	—	
Root vegetables, tubers			+*	+	+	—	
Legumes (dry peas)			—	+	—	—	
E Cereals (whole meal)	+	§	§	+	—	—	
E Cereals (white bread)			—	—	—	—	Non-protective foods
E Cereals (polished rice)			—	—	—	—	
E Nuts	§		—	++	—	—	
E Sugar, jam, honey			—	—	—	—	
E Margarine, olive oil and other vegetable oils			—	—	—	—	

E = foods of high energy value
+++ signifies very rich
++ signifies rich
+ signifies present

§ signifies present in traces
— signifies absent
∅ signifies in summer
* signifies if yellow in color

---

ers is well recognized. A committee report of the League of Nations on the relation of nutrition to health states that the use of the milk from cows or other mammals in the diet of the human race is as old as the history of mankind, and during the long ages in which it has been thus used its value has ever been highly esteemed. A land "flowing with milk" was the ideal of pastoral tribes in ancient times, and will still remain the ideal if the balancing of nutrition and health of the people receive due consideration. The report continues with the statement that modern scientific research has entirely confirmed the empirical conclusion drawn from human experience as to the dietary value of milk. Milk, which is designed to afford complete nutrition to the mamalian young, is known to contain all the factors needed for satisfactory nutrition, combined in a suitably proportioned mixture of protein of "good" quality, fat, carbohydrate, mineral salts and vitamins. In this respect, milk is the nearest approach we possess to a perfect and complete food. No other food that can be used as a substitute is known. The administration of calcium in any form or dosage cannot completely replace milk. The patient who will drink one quart of

cow's milk daily during pregnancy and lactation will satisfy her calcium and phosphorus requirements in a form which is especially easy of absorption and assimilation. In addition, she will obtain valuable protein food, in the form of lactalbumin and casein, both of which are not only present in large quantities but possess a highly nutritive value. We must also be mindful of the fact that in milk there is no loss of protein by cooking, such as occurs with the protein of muscle meats.

The vitamin content of cow's milk varies with the seasons of the year. However, the reduction of vitamin D in winter milk is easily overcome by the daily administration of two or three teaspoonfuls of cod liver oil or its equivalent. It is neither necessary nor desirable to give large doses of cod liver oil or its concentrates routinely to pregnant women. Vitamins are not a panacea for all the ills that beset women during pregnancy. Just as in all other conditions, judgment must be used in their administration. Naturally, associated fever or vomiting may call for special measures and larger dosages until equilibrium is attained. There is accumulating evidence to the effect that increased ossification of the fetal skull, leading to a higher incidence of dystocia, may be due to excessive calcium and vitamin therapy.

It should be understood, however, that certain women present more or less chronic deficiences of iron, protein and vitamins; and just as they need large doses of iron so a few may need, temporarily at least, large doses of vitamins. If we simply evaluate the condition of the tongue, the fingernails, in association with determining the presence or absence of free hydrochloric acid in the stomach and the hemoglobin level, we gain a valuable estimate of our patient's dietary efficiency.

Cheese, which may be considered as concentrated milk, contains the "good" protein, as well as the calcium salts and vitamins of milk. Small portions of cheese may well be included in the diet two or three times a week. Butter is a valuable food, because it is composed of the most easily digestible fat, and is an additional source of the fat soluble vitamins A and D.

Eggs are another important source of good protein, as well as valuable minerals and vitamin B. They are usually well tolerated, and may be prepared in a number of ways to entice the individual who will be benefited by them.

While ordinary muscle meat is inferior to milk or eggs in nutritional value, it does serve as an important source of protein and iron. We are all aware that many of our patients are instructed by their lay advisers to eat little or no meat during their pregnancy. The results of these curbstone consultations are undoubtedly reflected in some of the anemias seen during pregnancy. It is estimated that two grams of protein per kilo of body weight are needed by the maternal organism and the growing fetus. The daily requirement of protein for the patient of average weight would therefore be between one hundred and thirty and one hundred and fifty grams. Furthermore, all this should be absorbed. Liver, kidney and sweetbreads have a logical use, since they are rich in minerals and vitamins not found in muscle meats.

Green leafy vegetables and raw ripe fruits are highly acceptable, particularly because of their vitamin A and B content. They also contain the antiscorbutic vitamin C if taken in the uncooked form. The abundance of minerals adds greatly to the value of vegetables and fruits. Calcium is

present in oranges, while grapes and apricot: rich in iron.

In many parts of the world it is desirab complement the vitamin intake, especially ing the winter and spring months, by the ad istration of cod liver oil or other fish liver Some of the vitamins taken by the patient be lost, however, if she routinely uses mir oil to overcome constipation. The fat solubl tamins A and D are soluble in mineral oil.

While a patient may have an adequate ir of vitamins, the constant presence of miner: in the bowel may cause that patient to ha deficiency. As a result of the absorption of mins by the mineral oil the amount availabl· metabolism is utilized only in part.

In goitrous regions it is advisable to re mend either the use of iodized salt or tw three minims of Lugol's solution a week.

Energy-bearing Foods

The energy-bearing foods include cerea their various forms, sugar, potatoes and These foods should be added to the prote foods in a quantity sufficient to satisfy the er requirements during pregnancy. An analys the cereal foods reveals that many of their uable elements are lost in the process of mi White flour, for instance, is rich in carbohy but lacking in the B vitamins contained i husk and germ of the grain. There is also a nite reduction in the mineral content of the ly milled grains when the bran and gern cast off. The accompanying table shows c the relatively large amounts of minerals in bran and wheat germ as compared with th white flour. A finely textured white bre produced at the expense of these valuabl· stituents.

It is apparent that there is some variat the value of the different carbohydrate Sugar and milled cereals predispose to disease when introduced to people in 1 districts or countries where tooth decay w: viously unknown. Contrary to popular potatoes are of distinctly more value than or milled cereals, in that they do not pre(to dental caries. In addition, they are a v: source of iron, and, according to some a ties, retain a high proportion of their vit: content even after cooking. Certainly, tl ance of evidence indicates that we are n

TABLE II.. MINERAL COMPOSITION BY WEIGHT OF
WHEAT AND WHEAT PRODUCTS[7]

	Whole wheat	Wheat flour (white)	Wheat bran	Wheat germ
Potassium ...	0.473	0.115	1.217	0.296
Sodium	0.039	0.060	0.154	0.722
Calcium	0.045	0.020	0.120	0.071
Magnesium ..	0.133	0.018	0.511	0.342
Phosphorus ..	0.423	0.092	1.215	1.050
Chlorine	0.068	0.074	0.090	0.070
Sulphur	0.005	0.177	0.247	0.325
Iron		0.001	0.008	

ing the problem of dental caries by the administration of excessive amounts of calcium and vitamin D. Proper dental hygiene and eating of
foods that require more chewing seem to be the
factors which promote alveolar circulation and
dental metabolism.

Another factor in the dietary management of a
pregnant woman is the observation of the weight
curve. A woman of normal weight is expected
to gain from twenty-five to thirty pounds during
her pregnancy, while a woman who is overweight
to start with should be expected to gain less than
that amount. Conversely, a woman who is underweight may well gain more than thirty pounds.
By recording the average weight of the patient
before her pregnancy and the weight at each prenatal visit, the physician is readily made aware
of any abnormal weight gain, which will indicate
one of two conditions: either an abnormally
high carbohydrate intake, or an impending toxemia with its disturbed water metabolism.

The size of the fetus apparently is not affected
much by the weight gain of the mother. Our
present evidence indicates that the mother's metabolic rate may be a more important factor in
determining the weight of the baby.

Summary

1. The diet of the expectant mother should
include a quart of whole milk daily, to furnish
the necessary calcium and phosphorus as well as
"good" protein and vitamins.

2. A generous helping of meat is necessary
for an adequate protein intake. The lay and
medical advice to avoid meat has been very pernicious.

3. Eggs and cheese will furnish additional
protein and valuable minerals.

4. Fresh leafy vegetables and raw ripe fruit
are necessary for their vitamin and mineral con-

tent. The vitamin needs should be determined
for each individual.

5. The vitamin content of the diet should be
conserved by avoiding the routine use of mineral oil.

6. In goitrous regions small doses of iodine
are valuable adjuncts to the dietary.

7. The substitution of coarse cereals and potatoes is to be recommended to replace the highly
milled cereals and sugars.

8. Small doses of cod liver oil are of definite
value during the winter and spring months.

9. The routine use of large doses of calcium
and concentrated vitamins should be condemned.

10. Observation of the patient's weight during pregnancy will indicate excessive gains, as
well as give warning of impending complications.

Bibliography

1. Bell, Lennox G.: Protein requirements in normal nutrition. Can. Med. Assn. Jour., 38:387-389. (April) 1938.
2. Brehm, Wayne: Potential dangers of viosterol during pregnancy, with observations of calcification of placentæ. Ohio
State Med. Jour., 33:990-994, (Sept.) 1937.
3. League of Nations: Interim report of the mixed committee on the problem of nutrition. Geneva, (June) 1936. Official No. A. 12, 1936, II B.
4. League of Nations: Final report of the mixed committee
on the relation of nutrition to health, agriculture and economic policy. Geneva, 1937. Official No. A. 13, 1937, II A.
5. McCorrison, R.: Nutritional needs in pregnancy. Brit. Med.
Jour., 2:256-257, (Aug. 7) 1937.
6. McGonigle, G. C. M.: Dietary requirements of pregnancy.
Brit. Med. Jour., 2:259-260, (Aug. 7) 1937.
7. Sherman, H. C.: Chemistry of Food and Nutrition. Appendix B, Table 61 (4th ed. New York, 1933).
8. Sontag, L. W., Seegers, Walter H., and Hulstone, Lois:
Dietary habits during pregnancy. Am. Jour. Obst. and
Gynec., 35:614-621, (April) 1938.

Discussion

DR. E. C. HARTLEY, Saint Paul, (read in his absence
by Dr. V. O. Wilson): Doctor Moe has reviewed con-
cisely the important points to be considered in the
nutrition of the expectant mother.

In my discussion I wish to draw your attention to
two points which are significant.

First: The subject is one of more importance than
would appear to the casual observer. The studies of
the Mixed Committee of the League of Nations bear
witness to the far-flung bearing which nutrition has on
health, on agriculture and on the economic policy of
nations. Its more intimate relations to health are the
immediate concern of a growing number of publications devoted entirely, or in part, to the complex relationship between nutrition and health.

Second: The importance of nutrition reaches its
peak in the pregnant woman. Here the protective and
the growth factors in nutrition have their greatest significance. Our point of view here is both absolute and
relative. The absolute requirements of the pregnant
woman as compared to the non-pregnant woman are
summarized in a chart from the League of Nations
"Report on the Physiological Bases of Nutrition."

By relative requirements I mean those individual variations which the physician so frequently meets, and
which he should recognize so that he may guide the
patient in the necessary adjustments in her diet.

Dietary deficiencies in the pregnant woman may be
due not only to a failure to eat the proper foods in
adequate amounts. It is often due to a failure to utilize
such foods after they are eaten. In either case there
are usually clinical signs obvious enough to guide the

783

physician in correcting the deficiency. I agree with Doctor Moe that the indiscriminate use of calcium and vitamin D in pregnancy is neither desirable nor necessary. It is equally true, however, that the calcium requirements of every pregnant or nursing mother cannot be met by the classic dole of one quart of milk daily. The need for extra amounts of calcium is indicated by definite clinical signs. So, also, are the needs for extra amounts of iodine, or of iron.

The protein requirements of the pregnant, and

especially the nursing mother, are of great importance. Meat and eggs should be included on an equal plane with milk, and there is no great urgency in curtailing them too drastically at the first sign of toxemia.

The response of individuals to pregnancy, as we all know, is exceedingly variable. This variability extends to their nutritional needs, and we must be ready to recognize this variability and to adjust our patients to such a standard as will be optimum in individual cases.

INFLAMMATORY LESIONS OF THE CERVIX AND VAGINA*

LEE W. BARRY, M.D.

Saint Paul, Minnesota

TO the physician, the different inflammatory lesions of the cervix and vagina are oftentimes of minor importance. This is not the viewpoint of the patient. The resulting pelvic discomfort and especially the leukorrhea drive her from doctor to doctor in search of a cure. The constant vaginal discharge violates her ideals of cleanliness. She longs for the day when she can dispense with douches and the constant wearing of a sanitary napkin. The physician who affects a cure renders a worth-while service by restoring her health and happiness as well as her waning confidence in the medical profession.

The inflammatory lesions of the cervix, which will be considered, are cervicitis and endocervicitis (acute and chronic), the various erosions, cystic changes, lacerations, eversions, ulcerations, polypi and hypertrophy.

Injuries to the cervix during childbirth and gonorrhea are the two greatest causes of cervicitis and endocervicitis. Inflammation of the cervix may be classified as acute, sub-acute and chronic. In acute cervicitis, treatment should be restricted to a minimum, reliance being placed mainly upon cleanliness. Treatment with strong chemical solutions or with a thermal cautery should never be attempted. The cervical canal should not be invaded, because of danger of carrying infection into the uterine cavity with subsequent tubal, ovarian, or peritoneal involvement.

At the present writing, sulfanilamide is popular in the treatment of acute gonorrhea. Orr[18] treated thirty females with sulfanilamide, with cures in 26, or 86.6 per cent, of the cases. No local treatment of any kind was given. For the first four days, eighty grains of sulfanilamide were given in twenty grain doses, every four

hours, from 8 a. m. to 8 p. m.; forty grains daily were given for the next four days, and the doses were then reduced to twenty grains daily for the following seven days. The total dosage of sulfanilamide given to each patient was 620 grains during a period of fifteen days. In all the cured cases, smears became negative within two weeks. Many other writers have reported similar results, which would seem to indicate that sulfanilamide is a very valuable drug in the treatment of acute gonorrhea in the adult female.

The use of the Ferry-Corbus filtrate[3] is still an unsettled procedure. The hyperpyrexia of Bierman and Horowitz,[2] Desjardins,[6] Stuhler,[16] et al, has cured gonorrheal cervicitis, in 45 to 86 per cent of the cases, but the treatment is not without danger and requires a corps of well trained attendants to constantly watch the patient while a rectal temperature of 106 to 107 degrees is maintained for four to six hours. To obtain a cure the treatment must be repeated four or five times, at intervals of three to four days, at the end of which time the patient begins to wonder which is worse, the disease or cure.

Just what proportion of acute cervical infections become chronic is difficult of determination. However, it may be stated that practically a third of the women who visit the gynecologist do so because of a chronic endocervicitis.

Chronic cervicitis, endocervicitis, the chronic cervical erosions of whatever variety, and the cervical ectropions, may be treated with 50 per cent phenol, 5 to 30 per cent silver nitrate solution, zinc sulphate, either in a strong solution or by means of a zinc sulphate saturated porous pencil introduced into the cervix. All of the above treatments, result in a fair percentage of cure. Tincture of iodine, mercurochrome, argyrol and

---

*Read before the Annual Meeting of the Minnesota State Medical Association, Duluth, Minnesota, June 29, 1938.

ichthyol have been proved to be practically worthless.

In the last decade the treatment of the above conditions has been fairly well standardized in nearly all the large gynecological clinics. This standard treatment consists in linear cauterization of the cervix with a fine nasal tipped electro-thermal cautery. Incisions are made in the cervix with a cautery tip about one-fourth of an inch apart. The incision is begun in the cervical canal, one-half inch from the internal os, and is prolonged well over the outside of the cervical lip until it reaches the normal vaginal epithelium. If properly performed, one cauterization results in a cure in approximately 80 percent of the cases. Surgical diathermy with its more expensive equipment and more complicated technic gives about the same percentage of cures. After cauterization, the cervix should be observed at weekly intervals for about three months. Cervical stenosis may be prevented by keeping the cervix dilated up to 4 mm. at monthly intervals for one year after cauterization. The first one or two menstrual periods after cauterization may be very profuse, but this rarely ever results in any serious consequences. Cauterization of the cervix is contra-indicated: (1) where there is an acute infection of the cervix; (2) immediately before or immediately following a supra-vaginal hysterectomy; (3) in the presence of an acute or sub-acute salpingitis; (4) during pregnancy or within six weeks following delivery.

Nabothian cysts are best treated by puncturing the cyst with the cautery tip, pressure being exerted until the whole cyst cavity is thoroughly cauterized.

Lacerations of the cervix should not be repaired in the presence of an existing inflammation; too often, the diseased portion of the cervix is rendered inaccessible to treatment as a result of the surgical repair. Cure the cervicitis first and repair the cervix later.

Ulcerations of the cervix are simple, chancroidal, syphilitic, tuberculous, and malignant. Simple ulcers are rather obscure as to their origin and a cure is usually spontaneous without treatment. The chancroidal ulcer, due to Ducrey's bacillus, is usually multiple; the margins are ragged and undermined. Treatment with pure formalin is a specific.

Primary syphilitic ulceration of the cervix oc-

curs more frequently than is generally suspected. The ulcer is round, slightly depressed, and is surrounded by a white wheal-like area at the periphery. Leutic secondaries cause shallow ulcerations of the cervix which are very fleeting in character. They often disappear spontaneously in the course of a week or ten days. Tertiary syphilitic ulceration of the cervix may occur from five to forty years or more after the primary lesion, resulting frequently in a massive sloughing of the cervix and surrounding tissues. Diagnosis is best confirmed by finding the spirochetæ pallida in any of the above lesions. In the presence of the primary and tertiary ulcers the Wassermann reaction is usually negative. If the lesion is syphilitic, constitutional anti-leutic treatment should be instituted at once.

Tuberculosis of the cervix is rare and is usually secondary to tuberculosis elsewhere in the genital tract. The four forms of cervical tuberculosis are: the miliary, ulcerative, papillary, and interstitial. Diagnosis is confirmed by biopsy. Treatment by cautery or surgical removal of the lesion results in a cure in about two-thirds of the cases. Radium and x-ray have been used with considerable success. Many clinicians however, maintain that in tuberculosis of the cervix panhysterectomy is still the treatment of choice.

A biopsy is indicated in any cervical ulcer which fails to react to treatment. Many ulcers apparently inflammatory in character are proved by the microscope to be malignant. The microscope is many times more accurate than the most accomplished clinician.

Cervical polypi occur in the cervical canal at any age. They usually result from a chronic cervical discharge. Quite frequently they are multiple. When removed, their bases should be cauterized. All polypi should be examined microscopically, as a certain proportion are malignant. The incidence of malignancy increases with the age of the patient. To rule out malignancy, absolutely, it is a good policy to curette the uterus after the removal of a polypus, and have the curettings examined by a competent pathologist.

Hypertrophy of the cervix results from a chronic cystic and interstitial inflammation of the cervix. The cervix may reach enormous proportions, at times almost filling the vagina. Treatment is by electrical conization or surgical amputation. In conization, one may employ either Hyams'[11] or Crossen's[4] technic. In amputating, one may use the Sturmdorf or the Schroeder operation. Sloughing and alarming postoperative hemorrhage are not uncommon after the latter operation. These complications may be minimized by using non-absorbable sutures, cutting them long, and delaying their removal until the fifteenth to the twentieth postoperative day.

Inflammation of the vagina may occur in a localized, acute or chronic form, giving the mucosa a spotted or mottled appearance; or the process may be diffuse. Although containing no glands (excepting Bartholin's and Skene's glands), the vaginal mucosa, when inflamed, exudes an acid transudate varying in amount and consistency.

Considering the proximity of the vagina to the irritating discharges from the urethra and rectum, and also the trauma to which it is subjected in childbirth, coitus, surgical procedures, and discharge from the cervix and uterus, one wonders that vaginitis is not more frequent. This immunity to infection is largely dependent upon the nature of the lining epithelium and its acid secretion.

Vaginitis may be caused by the various pyogenic cocci and bacilli, the micrococcus catarrhalis, Vincent's bacillus, Ducrey's bacillus, the tubercle bacillus, the diphtheria bacillus, various saprophytes and yeasts, and at least one protozoan, the trichomonas vaginalis.

In adults, the vaginal mucosa is strongly resistant to gonorrheal infection. This is not true in young girls up to ten years of age, in whom the gonococcus is the most common cause of vaginitis. In schools and institutions, gonorrheal vaginitis frequently assumes epidemic proportions. Sporadic cases are also frequent.

Hess,[7] in 1916, Stein, Leventhal and Sered,[15] in 1929, and Reichert,[14] in 1937, found an involvement of the cervix in these young girls in as high as 98 per cent of the cases, and suggest that the condition be termed cervicovaginitis rather than the commonly used vulvovaginitis, but TeLinde,[17] in a recent paper, claims that involvement of the endocervix is comparatively rare clinically.

Local treatment with 1 per cent of silver nitrate in equal parts of vaseline and lanolin injected into the vagina affords a high percentage of cures; 1/1000 merthiolate cream has been used with a great deal of success. If the cervix is involved, metaphen 1/500, 2 per cent acriflavine, or 1 per cent silver nitrate solution may be applied through a Kelly cystoscope.

Estrogenic hormones in doses of 1,000 international units, hypodermically, tri-weekly, give good results. Vaginal estrin suppositories containing 1,000 I.U. of amniotin have been found superior to the hypodermic injections, according to TeLinde.[17] Some clinicians think the cure results from a thickening of the vaginal mucosa; others, to an increase in the acidity of the vagina. Excellent results have been obtained by Karnaky[12] with the use of Floraquin-Searle tablets. Daily introduction of two or three tablets into the child's vagina can be done by the mother at home. This necessitates only weekly visits on the part of the child to the doctor's office. Good results are attributed to the maintenance of the vaginal pH at 4, which acidity favors the growth of Döderlein's bacillus and inhibits the growth of the gonococcus.

Hoffman, et al,[10] at the Cook County General Hospital, treated a group of twenty-five children, suffering from acute vulvovaginitis with sulfanilamide in daily dosage of ¾ grain per pound of body weight, in four equally divided doses every six hours for two days, after which the dosage was gradually diminished. They report seven of the twenty-five cured in an average of 17.3 days, and nine in an average of 42.9 days. Only two of the nine remaining patients were cured by further administration of the drug. None of the children (aged three months to ten years) suffered any toxic reactions.

In the last fifteen years, the trichomonas vaginalis has assumed an important rôle as the cause of vaginitis. It has been variously estimated that from 15 to 40 per cent of the cases of vaginitis are caused by this protozoan. Considerable controversy exists as to the exact causative agent and its origin. Clinically, with a trichomonas vaginalis infection, the discharge is foamy, bubbling, and greenish yellow in color and has a sweet odor. There are small reddened punctate areas throughout the vagina, and the cervix is reddened to such an extent as to be designated as a strawberry cervix. Probably no other genital infection has been treated with such a multitude of remedies. Hesseltine[14] has recently studied the curative effect of three arsenical, one silver picrate, and two lactos preparations, and found that cures resulted from any of the preparations, in 85 to 90 per cent c the cases. He claims superior results in a series of his cases from the introduction of one tablespoon of a powder, consisting of 95 per cent lactose and 5 per cent citric acid into the vagina after it has been wiped dry. The patient is instructed to insert a 30 grain tablet of this mixture into the vagina each night upon retiring.

At the University of Minnesota Health Service the routine followed in the treatment of trichomonas vaginalis consists of 5 grams of silver picrate powder (Wyeth) insufflated into the vagina after a thorough cleansing with hydrogen peroxide solution. The patient is instructed to insert a 2 grain suppository of silver picrate into the vagina each night for six consecutive nights. The patient then returns for another insufflation, again followed by suppositories for six nights. Winther[18] reports a cure in all of the twenty cases studied, with no recurrence for six months following treatment.

To Hesseltine, Borts, and Plass[9] must be given credit for calling our attention to the frequency of mycotic infections of the vagina. Perhaps 10 per cent of the cases of vaginitis are due to the two yeast organisms: the oidium albicans and the monilia. Yeast infections are very common in diabetes and in pregnancy and may persist for some time after delivery. The discharge is scanty and there are areas of involvement of the vaginal wall which have the appearance of cottage cheese. Itching is intractable and is the predominant symptom. Painting the vagina with Lugol's iodine solution in 0.25 to 0.5 of 1 per cent solution is almost a specific; a 1 per cent solution of gentian or crystal violet also yields excellent results.

Senile vaginitis develops after the menopause. The cause is unknown. The vagina is chronically inflamed. The walls bleed easily, and ulceration with adhesions often exist. Davis[5] has treated this condition with hypodermic injections of 100 rat units of estrogenic hormone two to three times a week, together with an additional 75 units, introduced daily in the form of vaginal suppositories. A cure usually results in two to four months. Adair and Hesseltine[1] report similar results with 95 per cent lactose and 5 per cent citric acid powder treatments given in the office at intervals of one to three weeks, together with the daily introduction at home by the patient of 1 to 2 gram pills of the same preparation.

Conclusions

1. The two most common causes of cervicitis and endocervicitis are injuries during childbirth and gonorrhea.

2. Sulfanilamide in appropriate dosage apparently effects a cure in acute gonorrheal cervicitis and vulvovaginitis in a high percentage of cases.

3. Hyperpyrexia effects a cure in 45 to 86 per cent of the cases in acute gonorrhea. The objections to this form of treatment are the danger of collapse on the part of the patient, the expense of the apparatus used, and the number of attendants necessary.

4. About one-third of the patients who visit the gynecologist do so because of chronic cervicitis. Cure is best obtained by linear cauterization of the cervix. Tincture of iodine, mercurochrome, argyrol and ichthyol have been proved to be practically worthless.

5. Lacerations of the cervix should never be repaired in the presence of existing inflammation.

6. Hypertrophy of the cervix may be treated by conization or amputation.

7. Estrogenic hormones in doses of 1,000 I.U. in vaginal suppositories, introduced daily, have been found to be superior to hypodermic injections of the same substance in the treatment of vulvovaginitis. Maintaining the vagina acidity at a pH of 4 or less, with Floroquin-Searle, as recommended by Karnaky, also gives good results.

8. Trichomonas vaginitis responds to treatment with citric acid and lactose preparation, or to silver picrate.

9. Iodine in the form of Lugol's solution is a specific for the monilia and oidium albicans infections of the vagina.

10. Senile vaginitis, may be treated with estrogenic hormones or citric acid-lactose preparations.

References

1. Adair, Fred L., and Hesseltine, H. Close: Histopathology, and treatment of vaginitis. Am. Jour. Obst. and Gynec., 32:1-21, (July) 1936.
2. Bierman, W., and Horowitz, E. A.: Treatment of gonorrhea in the female by means of systemic and additional pelvic heating. Jour. A.M.A., 104:1797-1801, (May 18) 1935.
3. Corbus, B. C., and O'Conor, V. J.: Intradermal injections of gonococcal bouillon filtrate; experimental report. Jour. Urol., 24:333-342, (Aug.) 1930.
   Also Cummings, R. E., and Burhans, R. A.: Experiences with gonococcus filtrate (Corbus-Ferry) and other forms of intradermal therapy in the treatment of gonorrhea. Jour. A.M.A., 104:181-186, (Jan. 19) 1935.
4. Crossen, R. J.: New electrode for conization of cervix. Jour. Missouri Med. Assn., 32:125, 1935.
5. Davis, M. E.: Treatment of senile vaginitis with ovarian follicular hormone. Surg., Gynec. and Obst., 61:680-686, (Nov.) 1935.

6. Desjardins, A. W.: Fever therapy. Proc. Staff Meet., Mayo Clinic 10:196-199, (March 27) 1935.
7. Hess, Alfred: Vaginitis in infants. Am. Jour. Dis. Child., 12:466, (Nov.) 1916.
8. Hesseltine, H. Close: Evaluation by controlled series of vaginal trichomoniasis therapies. Jour. A.M.A., 109:768-771, (Sept. 4) 1937.
9. Hesseltine, H. C., Borts, J. C., and Plass, E. D.: Pathogenicity of Monilia (Castellani) vaginitis and oral thrush. Am. Jour. Obst. and Gynec., 27:112-116, (Jan.) 1934.
10. Hoffman, Samuel J., Schneider, Maurice, Blatt, Maurice L., and Herrold, Russell D.: Sulfanilamide in the treatment of gonorrheal vulvovaginitis. Jour. A.M.A., 110:1541-1543, (May 7) 1938.
11. Hyams, M. H.: New instrument for excision of diseased endocervix with surgical diathermy. (Preliminary report) N. Y. State Jour. Med., 28:646, 1928.
12. Karnaky, Karl J.: Gonorrheal vaginitis of children. Arch. Pediat., 54:34, (Jan.) 1937.
13. Orr, Harold: Sulfanilamide in the treatment of gonorrhea. Can. Med. Assn. Jour., 37:364-366, (Oct.) 1937.
14. Reichert, J. L., Epstein, I. M., Jung, Ruth, and Colwell, Charlotte A.: Infection of the lower part of the genital tract in girls. Am. Jour. Dis. Child., 54:459, (Sept.) 1937.
15. Stein, I. F., Leventhal, J. L., and Sered, Harry: Cervicovaginitis. Am. Jour. Dis. Child, 37:1203, (June) 1929.
16. Stuhler, L. G., and Popp, W. C. Fever therapy for gonococcic infections. Jour. A.M.A., 104:873-878, (March 16) 1935.
17. TeLinde, Richard W.: The treatment of gonococcic vaginitis with the estrogenic hormone. Jour. A.M.A., 110:1633-1638, (May 14) 1938.
18. Winther, Nora: The treatment of trichomonas vaginitis with silver picrate. Minn. Med., 19:731-735, (Nov.) 1936.

Discussion

Dr. W. F. Mercil, Crookston: On entering into the discussion of Dr. Barry's paper, one feels that his admonition to concern ourselves very definitely with the causation and proper treatment of leukorrhea is a timely one. The mere suggestion to the female to "take a douche for your discharge" is not satisfactory to the more exacting woman of this day. Certainly, a thorough investigation, the determination of the etiology, and the proper applications of the new and old principles of therapy are essential factors in maintaining the proper confidence of the laity in our profession.

Acute gonococcal cervicitis and endocervicitis is not commonly seen in the early stage. Most patients seek medical attention after a six weeks period, when smears are usually negative. The incidence of this acute disease in the female has been reduced markedly in the past ten years in our locality. The high doses of sulphanilimide seem to be the most effective. The use of local applications in chronic cervicitis, endocervicitis, and eversions of the cervix has been quite disappointing. Linear cauterization with the thin nasal cautery tip has been routinely employed with good results. One must bear in mind the possibility of lesions higher up in the female genital tract, and not treat too readily the more obvious cervical lesion. Crossen leans to

the idea that conization will be the accepted method of treatment in the more intensive cervical lesions.

In the diagnosis of various inflammations of the cervix and vagina, the appearance of the local lesions may be quite similar and our clinical impressions do not coincide with the laboratory findings. I believe this to be especially true in the cases of trichomonas vaginitis. One sees a patient with the symptoms of burning and itching and an irritating odorous discharge. On inspection, one may see the chafing of the inner thigh regions and vulva, and further, the typical, foamy, yellowish discharge, with redness of the vaginal wall, and fail to find the trichomona on repeated hanging drop preparations. Douches taken as early as twenty-four hours before examination will often be the cause of our failures in establishing a microscopic diagnosis. Repeated infections, or reinfections, may be due to poor hygiene. We instruct our patients to wipe the anus from front to back in an effort to prevent reinfection of the vagina from the anus. The growing number of reports in the literature of trichomonas in the male genital tract of interest, and reinfection from that source should not be overlooked. The urinary bladder is also to be considered as a possible source. Catheterized specimens of urine have been shown to contain the trichomonas in as high as 10 per cent of cases.

This brings us to the problem of curability of this disease. We can assure our patient of relief from symptoms temporarily, and in some cases get seemingly permanent benefits; but, in my experience, in the great majority of cases there is either a reinfection or a return of the previous infection. One hesitates to assure the patient of a permanent cure on the basis of the present methods of therapy. Insufflation with silver picrate, or Devegan powders, have been most effective. Care should be exercised to avoid too strenuous insufflations during pregnancy.

Yeast infestations are more common in pregnancy. The intense itching, if not due to the trichomonas, can usually be traced to the monilia infection. In our series, 1 per cent solution of gentian or crystal violet were applied locally with good results. In two cases, no definite benefit was obtained until local water-cooled ultra-violet applications were used, and with three treatments all symptoms and local inflammatory reactions subsided. This method of therapy would seem to be of benefit in certain highly resistant forms of yeast infections.

In the treatment of senile vaginitis, we prefer the local instillation of estrogenic suppositories, rather than its hypodermic use as this seems to be sufficient in most cases.

OBSTETRIC HEMORRHAGE[*]

ROY E. SWANSON, Ph.D., M.D.

Assistant Professor of Obstetrics and Gynecology, University of Minnesota

Minneapolis, Minnesota

IN the last few years, both the medical profession and the lay people have shown an ever increasing interest in maternal mortality. The recent excellent maternal mortality rates reported for Minnesota are to be taken, we hope, as a measure of better and more conservative obstetric practice in this state. It can be said, with-

out fear of contradiction, that much of the credit for this trend is due to the type of teaching given by our retiring chief, Jennings Crawford Litzenberg. For many years, he has taught a most conservative type of obstetrics; and nothing could be more fitting than to have his last year at the University marked by the lowest maternal mortality rate in the history of the state.

*Read before the annual meeting of the Minnesota State Medical Association, Duluth, Minnesota, June 29, 1938.

Among the outstanding causes of death in pregnancy, labor and the puerperium are sepsis, toxemia and hemorrhage. Hemorrhage and sepsis are very closely correlated in many cases, since the factors causing hemorrhage are many times factors in fatal sepsis. Sepsis which otherwise would not have resulted fatally may, if preceded by severe hemorrhage, lead to death. Sepsis so often results from meddlesome interference or major operative procedure with consequent abnormal blood loss and trauma, and so often follows toxemia, that it is difficult to evaluate the part each one plays in many deaths.

The recent and at times brilliant results that sulfanilamide has given in the treatment of puerperal sepsis will probably reduce the fatalities from this cause and will give hemorrhage a higher rate as a cause of death in labor.

The prevention and prompt treatment of hemorrhage should help to reduce maternal mortality. All procedures which are associated with the possibility of obstetric hemorrhage should be approached with the greatest caution even though methods for its treatment are immediately at hand.

Obstetric hemorrhage can most easily be discussed under the following headings: abortion, ectopic pregnancy, placenta previa, ablatio placentæ, and postpartum hemorrhage.

Abortion

Approximately 25 per cent of all maternal deaths are due to abortion. The criminal abortionist plays a large part in this with the introduction of infection and his refusal to take part in the treatment of subsequent hemorrhage. Sepsis, of course, plays a leading rôle. Death from hemorrhage following abortion should be rare, yet it causes about 10 per cent of deaths due to abortion. Prompt reporting of any bleeding in early pregnancy will save many lives. Facilities for curettage, packing the uterus and blood transfusions are essential. A firm stand on the part of the medical and legal professions in opposition to the professional abortionist would reduce maternal mortality in the United States by thousands yearly. Recent advances in the teaching of birth control will do much to avoid unwanted pregnancy. In time, it will cause a marked reduction in induced abortion. Spontaneous abortions are much better cared for since these patients are in most instances under adequate care. In the criminal abortion, however,

the patient is as a rule away from home and friends, and is in no position to get good medical care until she is in extremis.

Litzenberg's classification of abortions into the decidual stage of pregnancy; the attachment stage of the placenta; and third, the placental stage, offers help in the treatment of this condition. In the decidual stage, present during the first six weeks of pregnancy, an abortion is likely to be complete with little bleeding, and curettage is rarely indicated. During the second six weeks, good attachment has taken place and an abortion at this time often causes hemorrhage and pain, and placental remnants are apt to remain. In the third type, after the third month, the abortion is more like a normal labor and the placenta is usually expelled completely. There is not much danger of hemorrhage unless the placenta fails to separate completely.

Ectopic Pregnancy

Death from ectopic pregnancy is due chiefly to neglect on the part of the patient, and errors in diagnosis. Approximately 60 per cent of these deaths are due to hemorrhage. Any bleeding in pregnancy, at any stage, must be considered of sufficient importance to warrant prompt investigation and diagnosis. Where a diagnosis is doubtful, sharing of the responsibility can easily be had through consultation. With the history of a missed menstrual period, moderate vaginal bleeding and abdominal pain, ectopic pregnancy must be considered. The patient should preferably be sent to a hospital for careful observation. When the diagnosis is established, prompt operation is indicated and transfusion may be necessary. The replacement of blood loss by saline, glucose, acacia, or, better, blood transfusion is not to be neglected before, during, or after the control of internal bleeding. Since 60 per cent of deaths in this condition is due to hemorrhage, it is obvious that this procedure must have been neglected. It is not usual for a patient to die at the first rupture. This fact gives us, as a rule, adequate time to prepare for operation. Fewer deaths should occur from hemorrhage in ectopic pregnancy.

Placenta Previa

Any bleeding in the third trimester of pregnancy should be considered serious until a diagnosis is made. The diagnosis should be possible placenta previa until proven wrong. This attitude should necessitate immediate hospitalization except under unusual circumstances. No extensive examination should be made until this is done and all preliminary preparations for transfusion, bag or section are made. This diagnosis is not always easy. Usually the only symptom is painless bleeding which is frequently negligible at the onset. The presenting part is usually not engaged except in the marginal type. The rectal finger should feel a mass in front of the presenting part, and this examination usually should cause more blood loss. X-ray assistance may be had in vertex presentations by injecting silver iodide into the bladder. One may, by this means, especially in central attachment of the placenta, show the placenta between the bladder and the fetal head. This test is by no means pathognomonic and should only be used as an additional aid in the diagnosis.

The treatment of placenta previa has been more or less standardized. Williams taught that when such a diagnosis is made, the uterus should be emptied at once. At the University, Litzenberg allows time for observation and preparation of the patient, depending, of course, on the severity of the case. In central attachment, cesarean section is the procedure of choice. In partial or lateral attachment, this is also the most acceptable, especially in the primigravida. In marginal types, if the patient's condition permits, vaginal delivery may be the wisest choice where the head is engaged. Either the membranes may be ruptured or a bag inserted, and version performed later if necessary. Packing before delivery should be condemned except in rare instances. Braxton Hicks version is rarely resorted to in well trained communities. The uterus is best packed when delivery has been accomplished. In many instances the placenta must be manually removed in the presence of brisk post-partum hemorrhage. The mortality rate in the babies is high both because of blood loss and prematurity as well as from trauma. Since this is true, most of our efforts are expended in the interest of the mother. Prompt diagnosis, well planned treatment in a hospital, and blood transfusion will save many mothers in this serious condition. The prognosis is always serious. Even under good management the mortality varies between 3 and 10 per cent, and as high as 40 per cent in those poorly managed. The

mortality rate can be reduced by prompt recognition of the dangers of blood loss, hospitalization and courageous treatment.

Ablatio Placentæ

Ablatio placentæ or premature separation of the normally placed placenta is the accidental hemorrhage of our fathers. This term, accidental hemorrhage, was used to designate a condition in contradistinction to that seen in placenta previa. It represents hemorrhage from a normally placed placenta, the hemorrhage being either concealed or visible. It results in the frequent death of the baby and premature labor. The concealed type, characterized by a uterus of board-like consistency, is the most dangerous and usually requires cesarean section with hysterectomy if the uterus is apoplectic. In these severe cases the uterus fails to contract and the mother may die in spite of packs, pituitrin and blood transfusions. The milder types may be treated by bag and version if labor is not already in progress. Ablatio placentæ occurs late in pregnancy or during labor. There may be a great blood loss with acute anemia and shock, especially in the concealed type. When one finds a firm board-like enlarging uterus with signs of shock, the diagnosis is simple and the treatment is section. The prognosis for the mother is grave, the death rate running from 35 to 50 per cent in the severe type. The fetal mortality runs from 80 to 95 per cent. Here again hospitalization and prompt treatment are essential. Blood transfusions are extremely important in the severe concealed types.

Postpartum Hemorrhage

Postpartum or postnatal hemorrhage usually occurs during, or immediately after, the third stage of labor. It may be divided into primary hemorrhage occurring during the first twenty-four hours, secondary from twenty-four hours to two weeks, and puerperal from two to six weeks postpartum. Hemorrhage postnatally may be considered to exist when more than 500 c.c. of blood is lost. The normal blood loss should not exceed 300 c.c. The danger does not always lie in the amount of blood loss, but the condition of the patient before the blood loss. The predisposing causes are usually listed as due to blood diseases, anemias, cardiac disease, debility, malnutrition, multiple pregnancy, repeated pregnancies, atony, and certain types of women such as blonds and redheads.

The immediate and local causes are, in general, excess use of pituitrin, prolonged anesthesia or labor, atony, overdistension of the uterus, lacerations, operative delivery, improper conduct of the delivery of the placenta before its normal separation, and retained placenta.

The best treatment for postpartum hemorrhage is its prevention. Be on the lookout for it and treat it promptly. Give plenty of rest and fluid in long, fatiguing labors. Avoid the excessive use of oxytoxic drugs during labor. In operative deliveries, do not use too much haste, and avoid trauma. Do not attempt to deliver the placenta, if possible, until it is separated. Look the placenta over carefully to rule out retained portions. Use ergot and pituitrin by hypo immediately after the birth of the baby in difficult and fatiguing labors. Watch the uterus after delivery and hold it, if possible, for one hour after delivery. Have a speculum and big pack always available for packing the uterus. In patients who have had antepartum bleeding, always be prepared for postpartum hemorrhage. Hemorrhage in the presence of a well contracted uterus calls for inspection of the cervix and ligation of bleeding vessels. The essential treatment for the hemorrhage is blood transfusions, fluids, morphine, and good nursing.

Discussion

Dr. A. K. Stratte, Pine City: Dr. Swanson has covered the subject very completely, and there is very little to add. I wish to emphasize a few points he has mentioned, especially as they affect the general practitioner, namely, adequate prenatal care, conservative use of instruments and oxytoxics, and the proper diagnosis of emergencies when they arise. As he stated, there has been a marked improvement in maternal mortality rates, especially in this section; but fewer deaths should occur from obstetrical hemorrhages. During the past few years, perhaps more spectacular advancement has been made in other branches of medicine than in methods employed in the treatment of these conditions. Were all the available knowledge put into common usage, the mortality rate would be appreciably reduced. For example, in reference to placenta previa, Dr. Swanson states, "The mortality

rate varies between 3 and 10 per cent and as high as 40 per cent if poorly managed."

Wherein lies this great discrepancy and where can the blame be placed? First, failure to recognize or heed the warning of third trimester bleeding, which is usually not severe at the onset. Second, failure to place the patient in a hospital under the care of a man capable of handling the case. Some general practitioners who willingly refer cases to specialists in other branches of medicine, do not call in an obstetrician even though it is clearly indicated. How else can the large variance of 3 to 40 per cent mortality rates in placenta previa be explained? The average general practitioner cannot be expected to carry the equipment, nor have the training necessary to care properly for these emergencies in the home.

The final diagnosis of bleeding in the third trimester should never be attempted in the home, because of the increased hemorrhage which usually follows examination. However, certain signs might give you a fairly accurate opinion of the cause.

In placenta previa, hemorrhage is apparent, intermittent and painless. The uterus is normal in size, shape, and consistency. On the other hand, in premature separation of a normally implanted placenta, hemorrhage, though usually apparent, may be concealed, the pain is sudden in onset, severe and continuous in nature, and the uterus is often larger than normal, hard and sensitive.

The initial hemorrhage usually being slight, morphine may be administered and removal to a hospital can usually be safely accomplished. Packing should be avoided unless the hemorrhage is excessive. Prevention of obstetrical hemorrhages begins with thorough painstaking prenatal care. Harris states that premature separation of the placenta occurs four times as frequently in toxemic patients as in those in which toxic manifestations are absent. Bleeding, no matter how slight, during any of the three trimesters should not be regarded lightly.

Postpartum hemorrhages are chiefly of two types, traumatic and atonic. If the uterus is hard, the bleeding comes from laceration, which should be searched for with the aid of a speculum, and repaired.

In the absence of trauma, the bleeding is usually atonic. Normally, bleeding is controlled by three factors: (1) contraction of the uterine muscle fibers; (2) retraction of uterine muscle fibers; (3) clotting which occurs in the vessels.

The contraction and retraction of the muscle fibers of the uterus produce a compression and kinking of the arteries, and this controls the bleeding. Conditions which prevent these normal functions are toxemias, uterine exhaustion, and adherence of the placenta to the uterine wall with a partial separation. Prophylactic treatment consists in proper prenatal care, to avoid or detect toxemias which predispose to the atonicity of the uterus. Exhaustion during labor should be avoided by rest and intravenous glucose. Avoidance of haste in expressing the placenta, conservative use of instruments and oxytocis will reduce postpartum traumatic hemorrhages. More accurate clinical diagnosis would necessitate fewer retrospective diagnoses on the death certificate.

◆ CASE REPORT ◆

RUPTURE OF DUODENUM IN A THREE-YEAR-OLD CHILD

O. S. WYATT, M.D.

Assistant Professor of Surgery, University of Minnesota
Minneapolis, Minnesota

BEING unable to find a report in the literature of a rupture of the duodenum in a child so young, I felt that this case warranted reporting.

This three-year-old boy was first seen by Dr. Lane Arey of Excelsior, Minnesota, about 5 p. m., May 9, 1938. The history obtained was that the lad, while climbing up the side of a large flower urn, pulled it over on top of himself, so that it struck him across the upper abdomen and lower rib margin on the right side. He ran at once to his mother complaining of pain in the "tummy." He was seen by Dr. Arey within fifteen minutes and complained only of abdominal pain. His appearance, pulse, and blood pressure were normal. He was taken home and put to bed. At 8 p. m., three hours after the accident, he was again seen by his attending physician. He was complaining of severe abdominal pain, presented a picture of severe shock, and the right half of his abdomen was rigid. His blood pressure was 112 systolic and pulse rate 140 per minute. He was taken at once to Janney Children's Hospital, and I had the privilege of seeing him about 9:30 p. m., four and one-half hours after the accident. He was very apprehensive and alert. He presented a typical shock facies, abdominal pain was severe, B.P. 100 systolic, pulse 160. Examination of the chest was negative. Examination of the abdomen revealed a mild contusion across the lower rib margin on the right side. The abdomen, moderately distended in the epigastrium, was otherwise normal in appearance. Percussion revealed no fluid level and liver dullness was questionable.

Palpation revealed marked rigidity of the entire right abdomen, and moderate rigidity of the left. He was extremely tender in the right upper quadrant, moderately so in the right lower quadrant, and no tenderness was elicited in the left abdomen.

Flat plates were made of the abdomen but they revealed no gas beneath the diaphragm.

Our impressions were that this boy had a ruptured liver, with the possibility of a ruptured hollow viscus.

Operation.—After transfusion had been started, an upper right rectus incision was made under ether anesthesia.

Upon opening the peritoneal cavity no free blood was encountered, but a copious amount of dirty serous fluid. After aspiration of the free fluid, inspection of the liver revealed that it was normal. However, a great deal of plastic exudate was found in the region of the hepatic flexure, along the entire ascending colon, and down into the right lower quadrant. Even the appendix was covered with a plastic exudate.

Upon exploring in the region of the gallbladder, free bile was encountered and a large hematoma was noted on the anterior surface of the duodenum. There was also a large hematoma on the hepatic flexure of the colon, and in the retroperitoneal tissues. It was quite evident that the trauma was limited to this region.

Exploration of the duodenum for the possibility of a rupture revealed that bile was escaping into the peritoneal cavity. The duodenum was mobilized as much as possible and on the lateral surface of its second portion a longitudinal rent about 1.5 cm. in length was found through which bile was escaping. The mucosa was puckering through the opening. The tear was closed by whipping over Duloc sutures, and I was unable to express any more bile through it. Further examination of the duodenum revealed no more lacerations, and I could not express any bile from the lesser peritoneal cavity.

Inspection of the stomach, transverse colon, and terminal ileum revealed no other perforations. The omentum and mesentery were normal.

Soft rubber drains were placed in the region of the gallbladder and right lower quadrant. Closure of the abdominal wall was done in layers.

While the operation was going on the boy received between 350 and 400 c.c. of his father's blood. He left the table in good condition.

Naso-duodenal suction was employed on this boy for seventy-two hours, during which time he received intravenous feedings. His abdomen remained flat and at no time did he ever present any distention. On the fourth day the naso-duodenal tube was removed and feeding commenced by mouth. The convalescence was smooth with the exception of a slight wound infection, which healed by secondary intention in about eighteen days.

The patient was discharged on the twenty-fifth day. When seen three months after the accident he was in perfect health, and the mother states that she would never know that anything had ever happened to him.

Discussion.—This case is reported because of the interest it created, and likewise because the child in the case is probably the youngest on record.

Rupture of the duodenum is extremely rare following trauma to the abdomen. Rowlands reported only twenty-three cases of ruptured duodenum in 381 cases of ruptured intestines. Probably the reason that we see so few ruptures of the duodenum is that it is so well protected except where it crosses the vertebral column.

The symptoms in this case surely indicated an acute surgical abdomen, but because free gas was absent or undemonstrable in the peritoneal cavity, rupture of a hollow viscus could not definitely be diagnosed. The presence of free bile in the peritoneal cavity led us at once to suspect injury to the biliary apparatus or duodenum. We were fortunate in having a laceration which could easily be taken care of, and likewise fortunate that none were overlooked.

I consider it a privilege to be able to report this case and wish to express my sincere thanks to Dr. Lane Arey for his helpful assistance and suggestions.

HISTORY OF MEDICINE IN RAMSEY COUNTY

BY J. M. ARMSTRONG, M.D.

(Continued from October issue)

In the *Pioneer* for February 13, we note the following satirical squib:

"Dr. Charles M. Berg has slid off down the river. Berg was one of the large number of nice young men who flocked into Saint Paul last summer for office, but, like the majority, was disappointed. For several weeks past he has patronized the hotels, oyster shops, barbers, livery stables, and washwomen of Stillwater. It is said that he got into debt to about the amount of $1,000.00. Some ten days ago, the Doctor joined a trouting party to Rush river. Professing to have some business a short distance farther down the river, he left the party with somebody's horse and cutter and went down. The Doctor appears to have lost all command over the horse; for instead of returning to the fishing party next morning, a company of surveyors coming up the river reported that they met the Doctor near the foot of Lake Pepin, with his horse's head turned southward and under full speed. If the Doctor ever returns, he will probably sue the owner of the horse for the damage of running away with him."

It seems that the doctor, horse, cutter, and baggage went through an air hole in the river, but the doctor managed to extricate himself (*Pioneer*, March 13):

"The river below soon after opened and the ice commenced running. The Doctor acts like Croton oil and is bound to have a free passage through the world."

He sold his plunder at Prairie du Chien and when last heard of had reached Galena on his way to Philadelphia. Nothing further concerning Dr. Berg can be learned except that he was one of the organizers of the first Masonic lodge instituted in Saint Paul in 1849.

Both Dr. Potts and Dr. Day came to Saint Paul, as said before, in 1849, though Potts may possibly have been there previously, as he was married at Fort Snelling in 1847. In the *Pioneer*, under date of May 19, his professional card appears as follows:

Dr. T. R. Potts

Having made Saint Paul his permanent residence will attend to all calls in his profession in the town and county. He may be found at the store of Mrs. W. H. Forbes.*

Drs. Potts and Day apparently got an early hold on the community for we find them among the managers of a ball held July 4. Dr. Carli of Stillwater was also on the committee. This same year Dr. Day was appointed Register of Deeds for the newly organized county, and he recorded the first deed in Ramsey County. Dr. Potts was elected president of the Board of Trustees of the town. We may say he was Saint Paul's first mayor.

It is recorded also in the annals of Saint Paul that Dr. Day drew the plans for the first courthouse, for which he received the sum of ten dollars. This seems to be more of an exploit than the bare statement may indicate, as bids for plans

---

*Forbes represented the American Fur Company in Saint Paul and his store was known as the "Saint Paul Outfit." The store was on Bench Street (2nd Street) near Jackson.

were not advertised for till January 16, 1850, and had to be in the hands of the Commissioners by noon on the 20th. It is possible no others were able to compete on such short notice. Dr. Day was also one of the commission which built the court house, the construction of which was begun in 1885. His duties as Register of Deeds apparently were not strenuous. To correct the erroneous rumor that he had given up his practice, he published the following card:

"Dr. Day continues the practice of his profession at Saint Paul and will be found at his office on Third Street."

Dr. Dewey was not behind Drs. Day and Potts in social and political standing. In 1849, he was elected to represent Ramsey County in the first territorial legislature and served as a member of the executive committee of the Territorial Temperance Society, organized on October 30. At the same time that Governor Ramsey appointed Dr. Day Register of Deeds, he appointed Charles Bazille Coroner for the county. Judge Bazille, his son, stated that there were many offices to fill and few reliable men to fill them. When the appointment of coroner came up, someone remarked, "Give it to Bazille, he's the only white man left." There was some truth in the jest, as Bazille could not read or write. This same year the first dentist came to Saint Paul, though he did not become a permanent resident till 1851. His announcement under date of May 9, 1850, is curious. It reads as follows:

Dr. Jarvis

Dentist and Daguerrean

Will arrive in a few days and respectfully solicits from the citizens of Saint Paul, Stillwater, and The Falls of St. Anthony their patronage and support. He would particularly call their attention to the fact that he comes to stay and make Minnesota his home for life. His stock of materials, both in the Dentist and Daguerrean line, is most extensive and complete. Pictures taken in superior style in clear and cloudy weather.

5th Street near Jackson

This was Dr. William H. Jarvis, not only our first dentist but our first photographer. He was not the army surgeon of the same name stationed at Fort Snelling in 1836. In January, 1851, he opened a small drug store and advertised as a homeopathist; in August of the same year he opened a dental office in St. Anthony, intending to divide his time between the two places. In the spring of 1852 he closed out his daguerreotype business, and enlarged his drug store with capital furnished by Dr. J. H. Day, calling it "The Multum in Parvo Drug Store." After a number of years he gave up the drug business and opened a nursery on the west side of the river, raising vegetables and small fruit. He died in Saint Paul in the eighties. He is said to have been an Englishman and was born about 1828.

During the year 1849 a man whose name is still well known to the local medical profession located at St. Anthony and began the practice of medicine there. He received his diploma from Rush Medical College in 1850, and moved to Saint Paul in 1863. He is included here at this time because St. Anthony was then part of Ramsey County and his later activities were in Saint Paul. His name was John Henry Murphy.

John Henry Murphy was born January 2, 1826, at New Brunswick, N. J. He received part of his education at Quincy, Illinois, and boarded for a time with the parents of William W. Sweney while he and young Sweney studied medicine together under Dr. Abraham B. Hull of Marietta, Illinois. Following the custom of the day he established his practice before receiving his diploma, settling at St. Anthony. In 1850, he returned to Rush Medical College and completed his course. He practiced medicine at St. Anthony for ten years until the Civil War broke out and he went into the army. His family then moved to Saint Paul, and to the latter city he returned upon his discharge in 1863, to continue his practice until his death January 31, 1894. He was a member of the state constitutional convention and of the state legislature, and served for many years as Surgeon General of the state. He was also at one time president of the Association of Railway Surgeons, president of the Board of Pension Surgeons, and a member of the Saint Paul school board.

He was a large, uncouth man, uneducated, and possessed of a rather broad sense of humor. He had the reputation of being a great surgeon, and he firmly believed it himself. Although he did curious and bizarre things in surgery, his patients never seemed to hold it against him. He would do anything in a rough and ready way except eye surgery, and he firmly believed that all surgical patients in the community belonged to him by right, particularly fracture cases. It mattered not to him who their physician might be, or whether or not he was sent for. In many cases the ethics of practice as generally understood seemed to be absolutely incomprehensible to him. When a fellow doctor complained to him of a breach of etiquette such as stealing a surgical patient, he would make apologies, only to do the same thing again the next day, naively unaware that he had done anything wrong. In many ways he was a most lovable man, greatly liked and widely known. Probably there have been more curious stories told about Dr. Murphy than about any physician who ever lived in Saint Paul. Many young men, notably Edson Wait, James J. Dewey, Henry F. Hoyt, Ed. Whitcomb, James A. Quinn, and Clinton C. Miller, studied in his office. For many years in the early days he was the only physician in Minnesota who belonged to the American Medical Association. He served at different times as surgeon in the First, Fourth, and Eighth Minnesota Regiments and also was Division Surgeon. He was president of the Ramsey County Medical Society in 1874. At the time of his death he had perhaps a wider acquaintance than any man in the city.

Another physician came to Saint Paul with Governor Ramsey in 1849, Dr. Thomas Foster. He had practiced medicine in Pennsylvania but probably did not practice in Saint Paul. He came there as secretary to the governor, being at that time thirty-one years of age. In 1852 he was appointed physician to the Sioux Indians and later engaged in the drug business. As part owner and editor of the *Daily Minnesotian*, during the years 1857-61, he was one of the early newspaper men in the state. He served in the Civil War, attaining the rank of captain in the commissary department. In 1869 he established the Duluth *Minnesotian*, the first newspaper to be published in that city. He was born in Philadelphia, May 18, 1818, and died in San Francisco, March 31, 1903. He is said to have coined the phrase "The Zenith City of the Unsalted Seas" as descriptive of Duluth.

During this year cholera made its first appearance in Saint Paul. One of those who died was L. B. Larpenteur, the grandfather of the late A. L. Larpenteur. He was buried at the head of Jackson Street, about where the city market is now. Later his remains were removed first to a cemetery situated at the present location of St. Josph's Academy, and still later from there to Calvary Cemetery.

The year 1850 found a surgeon-dentist, Dr. A. G. Stiphers, announcing his skill in making artificial dentures:

"Scurvy and all other diseases of the gums, mouth and teeth cured, charges moderate, all work warranted."

Just how frequent scurvy was at that time is not known; but presumably it was not infrequent, as fresh vegetables were difficult to secure in the winter, and it was thought Minnesota was too cold for the raising of potatoes. Furs, cranberries, and pine lumber were the only products exported from the territory. In contrast to the difficulty of securing fresh provisions, whisky was cheap enough, twenty-five cents a gallon "and a better quality for twenty-eight cents." During this year also, Drs. Lee and Reynolds, both dentists of Dubuque, announced that one of them would spend a few weeks in Saint Paul and do dental work. A Dr. Todd who appears as a resident of Saint Paul and a member of a river excursion on July fourth was probably a clergyman, not a doctor of medicine. Although the town was but one year old, political squabbles and animosities were already rife, as is instanced by this note on the editorial page of the *Pioneer* for March 6:

"It is gratifying to learn that T. R. Potts, M.D., late of Galena, has been promoted to the office of Sioux doctor and Chief Surgeon to his Majesty Little Crow. It is a sphere for which he is better adapted than any other he has heretofore occupied."

What it was that excited this sarcastic tribute from the acid pen of James M. Goodhue, the paper does not state. Dr. Potts held this appointment till late in 1850, when Dr. Williamson was reappointed. Dr. David Day became the examining physician for the National Loan Fund Life Assurance Society of London and New York, the first life insurance company to establish an agency in Saint Paul. Late in December Dr. C. Rich opened an office in the building formerly occupied by Dr. Barbour's store on Third and Minnesota Streets. By 1850 Barbour had moved to another town, having sold his store to Wm. W. Hichcox. Sometime during the year Dr. William Wilson Sweney came to Saint Paul. He had been studying medicine under a preceptor for three years but had not as yet received a diploma. Dr. Sweney's activities are recorded in the section of this book relating to the medical history of Red Wing.

It may be of interest to insert here the deaths occurring in the "District of the County of Ramsey, Minnesota Territory," for the year ending June 1, 1850, as they appear in the census of 1850.*

Name	Age	Place of Birth	Days Ill	Cause of Death
Pierre Gervais	8	Minn. Territory	42	unknown
Magdeline Donna	60	Canada	15	fever
Atoine Bourais	80	Canada	30	pulmonary
Zoe Bivot	25	Canada	2	cholera
John Baptiste	2	Canada	30	pulmonary
Sophie Poncin	7	Minn. Territory	3	cholera
Alex. Ramsey, Jr.	4	Pennya	14	fever
W. A. Forbes	6/12	Minn. Territory	21	inflam brain
Phoebe Glass	8	Wisconsin	2	burned
Mary Jane Barber	5	Iowa	3	congestive
Albert Barber	2	Iowa	3	congestive
John Lurmley	23	Ohio	1	cholera
James Green	40	Pennya	1	cholera
Elijah Gladden	35	Ohio	5	cholera
Francis Robert	25	Missouri	90	consumption
James Goodhue, Jr.	2	Wisconsin	20	teething

In the manuscript division of the Minnesota Historical Society may be found the early account books of Dr. Potts. The first entry is dated May 20, 1849, the day after he arrived in Saint Paul. It seems worth while to give here some of the entries in his books. It should be noted that in all instances he gives the

---

*It is probable that the deaths from cholera occurred in the summer of 1849 rather than in 1850, at least John Lumley (not Lurmley) who worked for Larpenteur died in 1849. Barber should be spelled Barbour in the above.

names of his patients and the fee charged, but no case histories. His books are a veritable directory of Saint Paul at that time.

1849 June 11—Blister .50
    July 24—E. Rice—to obstet. 20.00
    Sept. 8—Visit to the Falls 9.00
    Sept. 27—Visit to Ft. Snelling 7.00
    Dec. 5—Visit & Med. 80.00 Sauk Rapids

1850 Jan. 29—Obstet & detention 35.00
    Feb. 28—to advice & med syphilis 25.00
    March 14—to visit and scarifying gums 1.00
    May 20—visit and consultation Dr. Day 5.00
    May 24—visit at night 2.00
    May 30—v. & opening abscess 3.00
    June 10—to visit & med (Falls) Smallpox 10.00
    July 20—obstet 10.00
    Aug. 6—obstet 5.00
    Aug. 6—extracting mote from eye 1.00
    Sept. 29—visit and Mendota 6.00
    Oct. 12—dressing wound 2.00
    Oct. 25—visit and blister 1.25
    Nov. 3—visit and consultation (Falls) 10.00
    Nov. 8—reducing luxation 10.00

1851 Jan. 15—J. M. Goodhue—to dressing wound 10.00
    April 25—D. A. Robertson—to visit and chloroform 1.00
    May 28—J. R. Brown—to extracting bone from throat 1.00
    Nov. 15—setting fracture 5.00

1852 Jan. 23—visit and cupping 1.00
    May 23—visit & setting arm 10.00
    July 25—E. Rice—consultation Dr. Day 5.00
    Oct. 29—Setting fracture 10.00

1853 Feb. 27—reducing hernia 5.00
    May 31—reducing fracture 10.00
    Sept 5—C. W. Borup—reducing fracture 20.00
    Oct. 28—reducing dislocation 5.00

1854 Jan. 4—Post Mortem of Philip Hull 20.00 (chg. County)
    June 26—to operation of trephining   10.00
    July 1—to consultation Dr. Day   5.00
                                     —————
                                    15.00
    Aug. 10—D. C. Dustin—to att'd & detent on self (cholera) 10.00

1855 Jan. 25—Consultation Dr. Goodrich 5.00
    March 15—Consultation Dr. Morton 5.00
    March 26—Consultation Dr. Wren 5.00
    April 3—tapping hydrocele 5.00
    April 4—to Morrison (Hospital) with Dr. Marsh 1.00
    May 16—Consultation Dr. Marsh 5.00
    July 12—Haskin (Winslow House) consultation Dr. Stewart 5.00
    Nov. 17—Seager
            To att. on wife 20.00
               By cash   10.00
             By copy of Shakespear   10.00
                              —————
    Nov. 20—Introducing catheter 5.00

His ordinary fee for a visit was $1.00. Sometimes a small amount, as 28 cents, was added for medicine; night visits were $2.00. The word "detention" means that he was detained for a long time. In the case of Dustin he spent the entire day with his patient. Mileage was charged for visits to St. Anthony, Fort Snelling, Mendota, and Sauk Rapids. This last visit evidently occupied three or four days as there are no entries on his books for one day before and two days after. It is interesting also to note that he never received his fee for this trip. ·The mention of chloroform in 1851 is rather early for this part of the country. The total of his charges for the year 1850 amounted to $1,224.53. He received during that period $69.80 in cash, a cupboard, one load of wood, and one dozen chickens. He seems to have made no particular effort to collect his accounts during the years 1849 and 1850, and his ledger was made up in 1851, probably by his wife. It is interesting to attempt to compare his book charges with those of today. The overhead charges in practicing medicine today are from 37 to 40 per cent, while his at that time could have been but a fraction of that. If one knew what percentage of his accounts he was able to collect and what was then the cost of living, one could arrive at a figure indicating the financial status of a physician in Saint Paul at that time. From the names on his books, only a few of which have been given, it appears that he had the best practice of any Saint Paul doctor during those years. During the months of June and July, 1850, are many charges for vaccination at one dollar each. It is also noted that on March 5, 1855, the writer's grandfather paid him $53.00 for attendance on his wife, who suffered from an attack of typhoid fever in the autumn of 1854.

1851

In April Dr. Barbour returned to Saint Paul and began again to solicit "a share of public patronage," announcing "he will practice upon the Eclectic Reform Principle, discarding mercury in all its forms." The name of the coroner for this year is not known, but a notice of an inquest to be held May 22 was signed Orlando Simons, Acting Coroner. Simons was not a physician. On May 29 Dr. Sweney returned to Saint Paul, after receiving his diploma from Rush Medical College. He opened his office on St. Anthony Street (West Kellogg Boulevard) next door below Mr. J. Irvine's (between Washington and Franklin Streets). Lee and Reynolds, the traveling dentists, again visited Saint Paul, and Dr. I. B. Branch, a Galena dentist, made a trip up the river and advertised he would be at the American House (N. E. corner Kellogg Boulevard and Exchange Streets) for a few days. Some time during the latter part of the autumn, Dr. Charles Rich moved from Saint Paul to Dubuque. He was evidently employed at some time during his stay in Saint Paul as county physician, for on one occasion he collected a bill from a patient, and also received $5.90 from the county for the same case. The *Pioneer* of September 4 makes the following comment regarding him:

"Dr. C. Rich and family left by the Nominee last week, being in debt to many people in St. Paul and especially to the printer. This reminds us of the old maxim 'Riches take to themselves wings and fly away' and we cannot help heartily and meekly responding 'Give us, Oh Lord, neither Poverty nor Riches.'"

The rapid growth of Saint Paul and the neighboring country is evidenced by the arrival of six more physicians later in the year. These men were Dr. James D. Goodrich (Sept. 25), Dr. John Harvey Day (Oct. 9), Dr. Albert G. Brisbine (Oct. 16), Dr. O. E. French (Oct.), Dr. R. Babbitt and Dr. Carlios (Nov.). Dr. Goodrich opened an office in the "Democrat Building, Wabashaw and Third Streets"; Dr. Day, "Office on Bench Street" (now 2nd Street) ; and Dr. Babbitt "in the rear of Levi Sloan's Store" (Kellogg Boulevard between Franklin and and Washington Sts.). Goodrich, Brisbine, Day, and Babbitt had simple cards in the paper announcing their arrival and where they might be found. Dr. French's announcement, however, is worth giving in full, as is also that inserted by Dr. Carlios. They are as follows:

HISTORY OF MEDICINE IN MINNESOTA

O. E. French, M.D.
Surgeon and Physician

Graduate of Harvard University, Cambridge, Mass. Dr. F. believes it is a duty, as a stranger, he owes himself and the community, as he intends to make Saint Paul his permanent residence, to state that he has had many years' experience in the hospitals and practice of the Eastern Cities, and also of the diseases of the Mississippi Valley,—is a graduate of the oldest and first University of the country, and was for a number of years the private pupil of the most eminent surgeons and physicians of New York, Boston and Philadelphia. Dr. French will give particular attention to diseases of women and children, and respectfully offers his services in the practice of Surgery, Medicine, and Midwifery to the citizens of Saint Paul and vicinity.

References

Drs. Crow, Ray, Robertson, Kittoe, etc., Galena; Messrs. Hollingshead, Rice, and Becker, Mr. Roberts, J. W. Simpson, S. H. Sargent, Gen. McBoal, St. Paul.

Dr. Carlios
Surgeon, Physician, and Accoucheur

A graduate of the Paris and Turin Universities has taken his residence in Saint Paul. He will take pleasure in exhibiting his diploma to anyone who desires to see it. Dr. C. will have his office at Mr. Turpin's on Fourth Street, Saint Paul; where he can be found and will promptly attend to every call.

N. B.—Dr. C. has instruments of the most approved kind for every surgical operation ever required.

It is interesting to compare these announcements with the modest professional cards of Goodrich, Babbitt, Brisbine, and Day. The claim of Dr. French that he was a Harvard graduate is verified by the catalogue of that university. He led a rather peripatetic existence, as shown by the attached biography. As to Carlios, Paris and Turin Universities are too far away to make the search for his name. In October, at the county election, P. T. Reid, a merchant, was elected coroner over W. Chapman, receiving 288 out of 534 votes.

One of the principal events of the year 1851 was the encounter between James M. Goodhue and Joseph Cooper, which occurred on January 15. Both men were wounded. The latter lived for a short time; the former died on August 27, 1852. Although his political friends asserted that his death was occasioned by the wounds he received, his survival for a year and a half makes such a statement ridiculous. Dr. Potts, who attended Goodhue, has left us the following statement of the case:

"You will see by the papers an account of a fight between Goodhue and young Cooper. The *Chronicle* today gives a long one sided account of the affair, and as old Jim is on his back and unable to write an account of the affray himself, some of his friends intend writing a short description of the affair and support it by a few affidavits. He shot Cooper above the bone of the pelvis and Cooper stabbed him in two places, one far back on the left side and the other about a half inch from the navel. Both wounds bled a great deal and gave people the impression that he was mortally wounded, and indeed he was under that conviction himself even after I had told him that neither of the wounds had penetrated any of the cavities. The morning after the affray he took a small dose of oil, and anxiously waited for the operation of it to find out whether the communication had been cut off. After it had operated he said, 'he was satisfied now that there was a communication between both ends yet' . . ."

(Dr. Potts to H. H. Sibley, then in Washington, Jan. 21, 1851.)

Reference may here be made to another misstatement concerning Goodhue. It is said in most accounts of him that he was buried somewhere on Dayton's Bluff. Actually, he was buried in Oak Hill Cemetery, which was organized the year of his death, and was situated between the present Mackubin and Western Avenues, on the west and east, and between Front and Maryland Streets on the north and south. This cemetery was soon abandoned and his remains were transferred in 1857 to Oakland Cemetery.

1852

There were now eleven physicians in Saint Paul. Dr. Sweney in January had associated with him a Dr. Abraham Hull, and the two men opened an office on St. Anthony Street over Sloan and Farrington's store (between Franklin and Washington). They advertised their services and also "an assortment of pure medicines for sale." Dr. Goodrich moved his office to the Saint Paul Drug Store (3rd and Cedar). Dr. Potts' announcement remained the same as it was in 1849. Either he was satisfied with Forbes' store for an office or he was careless in not changing his card in the paper. In the *Pioneer* under date of March 19 appears the following item:

"Hospital—In the rear of the American House, Mr. Rey, firm of Rey and Farmer, and Dr. Carlios, an eminent Medical and Surgical Practitioner from Paris, are laying the foundation of an extensive Hospital, upon ground given for the purpose by H. M. Rice, Esq."

This was the first promise of a hospital, but the plan seems not to have been executed. The records of the Abstract Office do not show that the land in question was ever transferred to the aforesaid gentlemen, and it is unlikely that the hospital was ever built, although Carlios rented Vital Guerin's house for his patients pending the completion of it. In May Drs. Hull and Sweney withdrew their card from the paper; presumably Hull left town. He may have been Dr. Abraham B. Hull, of Marietta, Ill., who was the preceptor of both Dr. Sweney and Dr. J. H. Murphy. There was no divorce law in Minnesota at this time. The legislature passed a bill granting A. Hull a divorce from his wife, Julia A. Hull. Governor Ramsey vetoed the bill on February 2, 1852. Presumably this was Dr. Hull. Late in the year Dr. Sweney went to Red Wing, where he remained till his death, August 12, 1882. In July Dr. Charles Ludwig Vicchers came to Saint Paul and opened an office on the corner of Fourth and Robert Streets, over Cathcart's and Tyson's store. In June Dr. French's advertisement was withdrawn. In May there were unclaimed letters in the post office for Dr. Hendee and Dr. Wm. Lewis. Probably they were connected with Owen's Geological Survey; at least there were unclaimed letters at Fort Snelling in 1849 for Dr. Lewis and Dr. B. E. Shumard, both of whom were connected with the survey. Shumard became a professor of obstetrics in a medical school in St. Louis, and in later years attained fame both as a geologist and as a physician.

Another dentist, G. W. Biddle, of Pittsburgh, located in Saint Paul in May, and Mrs. Biddle announced she would give instruction on the pianoforte. They established themselves at Hill and St. Anthony Streets. Biddle later bought some land above the present Seven Corners that had been preempted before the land was released by the government. Complications arose when someone staked out a claim on the property. This same predicament occurred to others; and they therefore organized for mutual protection to keep newcomers off. The organization was known as the Fort Snelling Claim Association. Biddle later located in Springfield, Illinois, and numbered among his patients Abraham Lincoln and his family. After several changes of residence and occupation he settled in Sparta, Illinois, where he was living in 1904, aged seventy-five years. In August, 1852, Dr. McLaren of Fort Snelling was ordered to Jefferson Barracks at St. Louis, and Dr. Ames, "a physician of excellent repute" of "All Saints" (Minneapolis), took his place as contract surgeon. In August, also, the Common Council of Saint Paul appointed a committee "for the purpose of investigating the facts connected with the appearance and progress of the smallpox in our city." The committee called in Drs. J. H. Day and Carlios, and made a canvass of all cases. They reported that the disease had made its appearance about two months previously, but that it was mild in form, and was not to be considered epidemic. There had been no new cases, they said, for two weeks. Of the twelve cases, eleven were now convalescing satisfactorily; one death was recorded, of "an infant previously afflicted with the measles." The Committee recommended care in the reporting of cases and stated that "a suitable place has been secured by the Board for the reception of patients." This place is said to have been a house at some place toward Fort Snelling from the present Seven Corners, but definite facts are not now available.

In August, or early September, Dr. Thomas Theodore Mann arrived from La Pointe, Wisconsin. He travelled by canoe through the Brule and St. Croix rivers to Stillwater, the immemorial route of the Indians from the Great Lakes to the Mississippi. An elaborate announcement of his intention to practice in Saint Paul appeared in the *Pioneer* for October 7, 1852:

Dr. Mann

Of Philadelphia offers his services, professionally to the citizens of Saint Paul. Residence at Mrs. Ford's, Fort Street, near the residence of the governor. Being a stranger in Saint Paul, Dr. M. bespeaks a share of their confidence, by presenting the following cards from men of eminence and distinction, furnished some years since in reference to a surgeoncy in the U. S. Army.

* * *

From Governor Shunk:

Hon. W. L. Marcy—Sir: Permit me to join his other friends in commending to your consideration the application of Dr. T. T. Mann for appointment of Surgeon. Dr. Mann's private worth and professional skill are amply sustained and show that his appointment will be a just recognition of his merits.

Yours very respectfully

Harrisburg, Nov. 23, 1846   (Signed) F. R. Shunk

* * *

From Col. James Page, Col. W. E. Patterson and others:

To the Hon. W. L. Marcy, Secretary of War: Dear Sir: We the undersigned being fully convinced that the professional standing of Dr. T. T. Mann, richly qualifies him for the commission of a Surgeoncy to one of the volunteer regiments, raised under Act of Congress passed at the last session, do most cordially unite in recommending him to your favorable notice as a gentleman of skill and experience, and who we believe would make an efficient medical officer. We shall be most happy to hear of his appointment.

(Signed) James Page	Richard Vaux	H. S. Patterson, M.D.
W. E. Patterson	Geo. McClellan, M.D.	Washington Atlee, M.D.
		W. R. Grant, M.D.

* * *

From Prof. Geo. McClellan, the most distinguished of American Surgeons:

From a long personal acquaintance I feel great pleasure in uniting with the above gentlemen in recommending Dr. Mann to the Commission he solicits.

(Signed) Geo. McClellan, M.D.

This announcement appeared again one week later (October 14). Anyone familiar with the history of Philadelphia will recognize the names of these men as very prominent either socially or professionally. Richard Vaux, known as "Dickie" Vaux, is said to have been the only American civilian who ever danced with Queen Victoria. In the late autumn Dr. Carlios' notice disappeared from the paper. In the same month Dr. Samuel Willey arrived in Saint Paul and almost immediately went into partnership with Dr. Brisbine; both were from Ohio. Their office was on St. Anthony Street, three doors below the American House.

Two physicians were married in Saint Paul during the year. Dr. Pugsley of Wisconsin, perhaps the first physician to be married in Saint Paul, took as his bride Miss Emeline Brewster. The service was held on June 10, 1852. On November 10 the Rev. Timothy Wilcoxson united in marriage Dr. C. L. Vicchers, a German physician, and Miss Anna Coulter.

(To be continued in the next issue)

EDITORIAL

MINNESOTA MEDICINE

OFFICIAL JOURNAL OF THE MINNESOTA STATE MEDICAL
ASSOCIATION

Published by the Association under the direction of its Editing
and Publishing Committee

EDITING AND PUBLISHING COMMITTEE
J. T. CHRISTISON, Saint Paul   C. B. WRIGHT, Minneapolis
E. M. HAMMES, Saint Paul   T. A. PEPPARD, Minneapolis
WALTMAN WALTERS, Rochester

EDITORIAL STAFF
CARL B. DRAKE, Saint Paul, Editor
W. F. BRAASCH, Rochester, Associate Editor
GILBERT COTTAM, Minneapolis, Associate Editor

Annual Subscription—$3.00   Single Copies—$0.40

Foreign Subscriptions—$3.50

Volume 21   NOVEMBER, 1938   Number 11

The Significance of the Apical Systolic Murmur

A SYSTOLIC murmur heard at the heart apex is not an uncommon finding in routine examination. Few physicians find them as frequently as Reid and Fahr, who have reported an incidence of 20 and 35 per cent in normal youthful patients.

At the turn of the century and even as late as the onset of the World War this finding was generally considered indicative of valvular heart disease and a student was frequently prohibited from strenuous athletics or a recruit was refused enlistment on this account alone.

Mackenzie was among the first to emphasize the importance of the functional capacity of the heart rather than the presence of murmurs and expressed the opinion that the presence of a systolic apical murmur in a normally functioning heart without enlargement or arrhythmia did not indicate organic valvular disease.

Cabot called attention to the rarity of uncomplicated mitral regurgitation in routine autopsies and does not believe that pure mitral insufficiency can be diagnosed during life. Personally we question the possibility of absolutely ruling out the presence of a slight leak in the mitral valve by autopsy examination.

Gradually the profession has come to accept Mackenzie's view of the significance of the apical systolic murmur. However, other factors than just the heart findings should be taken into consideration in evaluating a given case.

An analysis by Finberg and Steuer* of 100 youthful patients presenting a systolic apical murmur and observed over a period of years, is of interest. These were normal individuals except for the presence of the systolic murmur and except that 30 per cent of them showed a heart shadow over 50 per cent of the chest diameter on orthodiagraphic examination. Without going into details of the analysis, they concluded that the presence of the murmur in children under five years of age is not significant; that in youngsters with a systolic murmur and a history of rheumatic fever or chorea there is a 50 per cent chance of the development of mitral stenosis, aortic regurgitation or both; that in the 30 per cent showing heart enlargement some 40 per cent developed later serious valvular trouble; that a slight elevation of temperature (99 to 100) occurred in 70 per cent of the cases and proved of no prognostic value as to the later development of serious heart disease; that mitral stenosis or aortic regurgitation appeared on the average three or four years after first observation and that in only eight instances did the murmur disappear. Recently the same authors† reported the observation for over ten years of thirty-five of the original 100 patients without the discovery

---
*Finberg, M. H., and Steuer, L. G.: Apical Systolic Murmurs in Children. Am. Heart Jour., 7:553, (June) 1932.
†Steuer, L. G., and Finberg, M. H.: Further Observation on Apical Systolic Murmurs in Children. Am. Heart Jour 16:351, (Sept.) 1938.

of any new cases of mitral stenosis or aortic regurgitation.

The development of twenty-nine cases of mitral stenosis or aortic regurgitation or both in these 100 observed patients proves definitely that the group was not a normal one to begin with. Disregarding the twelve of the thirty patients with fluoroscopic evidence of heart enlargement who eventually developed mitral stenosis or aortic regurgitation or both, the number (17 per cent) that developed severe heart disease is still much too high for a normal group.

The conclusions drawn by the authors from this study are that as a group children with systolic apical murmurs are more likely to develop serious valvular disease. The statistical source of these authors might explain the apparent importance of a physical finding not commonly regarded as significant.

Biographic Data

PERUSAL of the files of most county medical societies would disclose a dearth of recorded information regarding present and past members. Attention is called to the situation in an article by Dr. Monte C. Piper entitled Authentic Biographical Data, which appears in this issue. Dr. Piper is the author of a new application for membership form which has been adopted by the Council of the State Association for use by all new members. This form is much more complete than the forms usually used by county societies, and its adoption gives uniformity to the information tabulated in all counties in the state. The form is made out in duplicate, one copy being filed by the local county and the other by the state office. Some counties have sent this form out to all county society members with the request that they be filled out for record purposes. Strange to say, many have neglected and some have even declined to fill out and return the forms. This is a thoughtless attitude when one considers the good reasons for the request.

We think Dr. Piper's suggestion that supplementary blanks be filled out periodically, is a good one. There is little space in the new application forms for information regarding a member's activities since graduation. If every five years a supplementary form were filled out giving information such as teaching positions, ar-

ticles published, society and staff membership, postgraduate studies, specialization, additions to the family, children studying or practicing medicine, there would be on file a gold mine of authentic information which would be available for various purposes.

One of the minor uses of such a file would be its use in the preparation of life sketches for publication on the death of a member. Too often the information available is a newspaper clipping or very scanty information supplied by a relative.

How scant is the available information about most of the pioneers. Such a store of reliable information would be of inestimable value to future medical historians.

One does not have to have any particular flare for medical history in order to derive considerable pleasure from looking over what meager biographical information is to be found in the files of the county societies.

It is to be hoped that a systematic effort is going to be made to obtain these supplementary reports and that members will coöperate by filling out the blanks already sent them, and any that may be sent them in the future.

The Saint Paul Profession and City Council

THE City of Saint Paul acts as its own insurance company in complying with the provisions of the Workman's Compensation Law regarding injuries sustained by its employes. On the grounds that certain members of the Ramsey County Society have rendered excessive bills for professional services to injured employes a threat was made a year ago by the Corporation Counsel to appoint one surgeon on a salary basis to care for all injured city employes. As a result, a committee of the Ramsey County Medical Society has been conferring with city authorities for several months in an effort to promote fair dealing and coöperation between the local profession and the city authorities. The committee offered to investigate any medical bills considered by the city to be excessive and attempt unofficially to adjust fees to the satisfaction of surgeons and city officials alike. Several bills were subsequently referred to the doctors' committee and the reductions recommended in certain cases after conference with the surgeons were as a rule agreed to.

Matters were apparently proceeding smoothly until October 4, when out of a clear sky the Council of the City of Saint Paul voted to appoint five Saint Paul surgeons to care for city accident cases on a fee basis—against the known wishes of the Saint Paul profession and also against the wishes of the city employes. Both these bodies wanted to maintain the free choice of surgeon for the individual employe.

At a special meeting of the Ramsey County Medical Society held October 12 to consider the action of the City Council a resolution was passed calling attention to the fact that this action of the City Council attempted to deprive 99 per cent of the physicians and surgeons in Saint Paul from rendering services to their patients who are city employes; that this action is not in accord with laws of the State of Minnesota, whereby an employe "should have the option or unquestioned right to choose his medical attendant or accept the one tendered him by the employer—" or as the State Supreme Court has held "the statute contains no language unconditionally requiring the latter (employe) to accept the physician tendered him or relinquish the right of reimbursement altogether. . . . The fact that the employer in this case is a municipal corporation and employs a physician for all such cases, paying him a fixed salary, cannot alter the construction given the statute." The resolution further calls attention to the fact that the Central Council of Public Service Employes has gone on record as being almost unanimously opposed to the action taken by the Council; that the members of the Ramsey County Medical Society are taxpayers and in addition furnish at no expense to the taxpayers the entire medical staff of the Ancker Hospital and the resolution declares the society opposed to such an un-American and undemocratic action that aims at the destruction of the principle of free choice of physician. It was further resolved that no member accept the appointment by the city; that the individual society members pledge themselves to continue to render services to city employes and use the services of the proper tribunals to collect fees if necessary; and that the society continue to coöperate with the city to eliminate abuses on the part of members and others in furnishing medical and surgical attention on the basis of free choice of physician by the employe.

Five surgeons were appointed by the Corporation Counsel and printed cards were distributed to employes with the names of the surgeons and instructions to patronize only the surgeons named if the employe expected his medical fees to be paid. Some, perhaps all, of the surgeons have declined the appointment and there the matter rests at the present time.

———

Charts prepared by the Children's Bureau at Washington showing the infant mortality in the various states for 1936, show Connecticut heading the list with 42 per 1,000 live births and Minnesota, Oregon, Nebraska and New Jersey tied for second place with 44. The rates are as a whole lower for the northern states, and Arizona, New Mexico and South Carolina had the highest mortality, 120, 122 and 81 respectively.

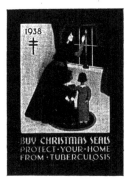

———

MEDICAL ECONOMICS

Edited by the Committee on Medical Economics
of the
Minnesota State Medical Association
W. F. Braasch, M.D., Chairman

LETTERS FROM NEEDY PATIENTS

SOME of the most illuminating and valuable information secured in the course of the Minnesota State Medical Association's Survey on Need and Supply of Medical Care has reached the State Office as a result of a newspaper appeal for information to all Minnesota newspapers, September 21.

This appeal was approved at the special meeting of county-officers and delegates held in Saint Paul September 10 and released to all Minnesota newspapers September 21.

To date 200 responses have reached the State Association and each mail brings additions.

Text of News Appeal

Following is the text of the appeal:

Have you ever been deprived of a doctor's care when you needed it? What was the reason?

The Minnesota State Medical Association is now engaged in a state-wide study of medical needs in Minnesota and, in a statement issued today, asked the co-operation of patients themselves in an effort to make the study useful and complete.

Anyone who has any complaint to make or who has had any difficulty in securing medical care is asked to take part in the study by answering the above questions in a letter addressed direct to the Minnesota State Medical Association.

Communications will be kept confidential if the writer wishes and the Association will investigate the complaint and give whatever assistance is possible to the writers.

In addition, the data thus gathered will be used to round out the most complete study ever made of this much discussed problem. Upon findings, the doctors plan, according to the statement, to base recommendations for changes and improvements wherever they may seem to be needed, to the end that nobody in Minnesota may be deprived of good medical care.

Replies should be sent to the Minnesota State Medical Association, Saint Paul.

Between Restrictions

It was to be expected, of course, that a certain number of these letters would come from the

NOVEMBER, 1938

chronic complainers and those who embrace all opportunities to describe their symptoms.

The great majority, however, give concrete instances of a condition suspected for some time by physicians but never before so impressively backed up by names, dates and details.

This is the condition: While people on the direct relief rolls are provided with the medical service they need — letters are conspicuously missing from recipients of direct relief—the people who are on WPA and those who are on the Old Age Assistance rolls are much too often caught between the restrictions.

In the case of Old Age Assistance, a definite provision is made in the regulations for budgeting an allowance for medical service for illnesses of a chronic or recurring nature. For emergencies the regulations definitely assign responsibility to the County Welfare Board. These regulations are clearly not recognized in a considerable number of Minnesota counties, nor are they understood by the recipients of aid.

Provided in the Law

There is, of course, no reason why these elderly people should lack medical aid in Minnesota. The law was carefully written to provide for it and the regulations adopted by the State Board of Control are explicit on the subject. It is clear, however, that missionary work is needed with county commissioners and other members of the welfare boards in a number of counties to show them their responsibility and explain to them the regulations.

The problem of medical care for WPA workers may be more difficult to solve under present regulations, but a determined effort on the part of doctors and local officials in each community should serve to create a definite understanding and a plan by which medical care can be supplied universally to these workers.

For Glasses, Dental Care

Need for glasses and dental care bulks very large in all these complaints. It is clearly very difficult for many County Welfare Boards to find funds for such non-emergent needs as these. This is a special problem for physicians, dentists, welfare boards and representatives of optical houses to work out together in each community.

In addition to the letters from those who are already recipients to some degree of some form of aid, there is a residum of letters from people who are not on the public rolls; who fear to run up doctors' bills and who are actually in serious need of medical attention. In several cases these people warmly praise their doctors, acknowledge readily that the doctor would give them the service they need if they were to apply to him regardless of their ability to pay. Nevertheless, they cannot bring themselves to ask more of that already overburdened friend.

These letters are in the minority, of course, but they should have the careful consideration of medical society representatives who investigate all these cases.

Procedure

The procedure to be followed in this investigation was outlined definitely at the special Council meeting held in Minneapolis, October 15.

Copies of the letters from each councilor district will be sent to the respective councilors and by the councilor to the officers or contact committees of the county or district society concerned.

These officers will be asked to investigate and report on each case to the councilor. Wherever advice as to official procedure would help, then the local physician will be asked to find a way to give that advice and assist the writer of the letter.

The importance of careful, sympathetic, well-considered action on each case cannot be over-estimated.

Reputation at Stake

The request for information was officially ordered at the special meeting of county officers and delegates in Saint Paul, September 10. As a result, many honest appeals for aid have been made. They must be carefully and honestly answered. The reputation and honor of the Minnesota State Medical Association and its members is at stake.

806

GROUP HOSPITALIZATION IN MINNESOTA

Group Hospital insurance was approved in principle at the special House of Delegates meeting in Chicago. It is, of course, already established and working successfully in a good many cities, notably in Minneapolis, St. Paul and Duluth.

Requests for extension of the service have been received by the Minnesota Hospital Service Association from a number of Minnesota communities.

The question of whether or not group hospitalization can be organized and operated with equal success in the rural districts was discussed at length at a joint meeting of the Council, the Council Committee to Study Group Hospitalization and a committee from the Minnesota Hospital Service Association in Minneapolis, October 15.

No definite action was taken by the assembled group, but the hospital service representatives indicated that they will make a further study of plans for extension into rural communities and report the results to the joint committees.

Any plan of organization that may be agreed upon will be submitted to the local county or district medical society concerned before action is taken.

REACHING THE STUDENTS

The Minnesota State Medical Association will continue the college lecture courses carried on in former years under the joint auspices of the medical association and the Minnesota Public Health Association.

The importance of reaching the college group prompted arrangement of the new courses by which, at the direction of the Council, two lectures will be offered to each college each year.

A carefully selected list of subjects has been prepared under the direction of the Committee on Public Health Education and four speakers have been chosen to present each subject. College authorities will thus have the opportunity of a wide range of subjects and speakers from which to make selections.

Reaching college students who will become the teachers, professional men and leaders of the next generation, is one of the most important parts of the health education program. Lectures to students are regarded by the Council as essential to this program.

SECOND CONGRESS

Dates for the 86th Annual Meeting of the Minnesota State Medical Association are May 31, June 1 and 2.

The place is the Minneapolis Auditorium and preliminary plans outlined by the Committee on Scientific Assembly provide for a program of unique proportions.

In addition to the usual fine scientific program there will be a Second Congress of Allied Professions occupying a full day of program time. All of the allied professions including dentistry, nursing, pharmacy, social welfare, hospital administration, will participate in this program which takes on a vital importance this year, in view of new programs now under discussion for medical care.

Specific Objective

The First Congress, held in Saint Paul three years ago, provided opportunity for expression of varying points of view toward the general problems of medical care. The 1939 Congress will have a more specific objective.

The theme of the meeting as outlined at a recent gathering of the Committee on Scientific Assembly is as follows: What has Minnesota accomplished to date in each of the fields of public health and medicine? Where does each program need improvement and what form should that improvement take?

Whatever enabling legislation Congress may pass at Washington this winter, the extent and character of the program in Minnesota will depend upon the legislative and health authorities in Minnesota. Official policies are certain to be greatly influenced by the discussions at this Congress.

Health Show

A second unique feature of the Minneapolis meeting will be an extensive health show. This show will occupy the entire basement of the Auditorium and will be open to the public for the entire three days of the meeting. During the daytime, groups of children from the Minneapolis schools will be escorted through the show by arrangement with the hygiene department of the schools and Minneapolis Board of Health.

The assistance of all of the health and welfare agencies in the state is being solicited to make the show complete.

STATISTICS OR SOUND JUDGMENT

(Monthly Editorial Prepared by the Medical Advisory Committee)

Happy is the medical man who never has trouble of any kind, who is always sure of his ground, who never makes a mistake in diagnosis, and whose patients always make a 100 per cent recovery. He has either to see his first day of practice or is in retirement. Every conscientious man in active work has periods of mental depression because of his failures.

Action recently brought against a surgeon in this state and reviewed by the Medical Advisory Committee brings out the following pertinent facts:

First.—A chronic lesion can become an acute one and conversely an acute one can become chronic.

Second.—In all conditions, acute or chronic, careful taking of a history of both past and present illnesses is essential before an operation.

Third.—Examination and confirmatory diagnosis should be made by the operating surgeon within the twenty-four hours preceding surgical treatment. Even though he has full confidence in the ability of the referring physician, the consulting surgeon should make his own diagnosis in order to plan his operative procedures.

If one remembers these three facts fewer operations will be performed without justification. Moreover, less censure will be meted out to the profession because of poor results following surgical intervention.

Statistics and numbers of cases should not be a substitute for sound judgment.

MINNESOTA STATE BOARD OF MEDICAL EXAMINERS

Sheriff Beihoffer, Strong Foe of Quacks, Dies Suddenly

Alfred T. Beihoffer, sheriff of McLeod county, Minnesota, for the past twelve years, died suddenly Sunday, October 17, 1938, while pheasant hunting near Wood Lake with a number of friends. Sheriff Beihoffer, while not enjoying the best of health, the past few months, was active in his office the day before his death. He suffered a heart attack while sitting in his car and died in a few moments.

Sheriff Beihoffer was known throughout his county as a sincere, hard-working and courageous law enforcement officer. He was best known to the medical profession for the splendid coöperation he gave the Minnesota State Board of Medical Examiners in the arrest and prosecution of quacks in his county. Two of his most notable cases were the cases of State of Minnesota vs. Robert McGraw and State of Minnesota vs. Herman Feenstra. McGraw was a well known Negro quack who was twice prosecuted at Glenwood and escaped conviction both times. McGraw was fined and sent to jail at Glencoe and left the state after serving his jail sentence. Feenstra was arrested by Sheriff Beihoffer in August, this year, after he had disappeared and forfeited a $2,500 cash bond at Brookings, South Dakota. He was sentenced to four years at Glencoe on a charge of criminal abortion.

Sheriff Beihoffer was born July 17, 1882, in Glencoe township, McLeod county. He spent his entire life in his home county. He is survived by his widow, Mrs. Alice Beihoffer, a son, Arnold, his 85-year-old father, one brother and four sisters, including Mrs. S. E. Allen, welfare worker for McLeod county.

In addition to the tragic loss suffered by his family, the people of McLeod county and the state of Minnesota have lost a faithful public servant, and the medical profession a loyal friend, in the death of Sheriff Beihoffer.

Minneapolis Woman Found Not Guilty of Obtaining Morphine from Physicians by Fraud and Deceit

Re: State of Minnesota vs. Helen Genevieve Rudd

After deliberating more than nineteen hours, a jury in the court of the Honorable Mathias Baldwin, Judge of the District Court, Minneapolis, found Helen Genevieve Rudd not guilty of obtaining morphine by fraud, deceit and misrepresentation under the new 1937 Minnesota Uniform Narcotic Drug Act.

The defendant was arrested July 7, 1938, following a joint investigation of the matter by the Federal Bureau of Narcotics and the State Board of Medical Examiners. The defendant has been in the Hennepin county jail since that time in default of bail. About a week before her trial began, she entered a plea of guilty to the charge before Judge Day, but upon being questioned by the Court prior to being sentenced stated she was unable to state the circumstances surrounding the obtaining of the two prescriptions that were the basis of the charge. Thereupon the Court ordered the plea of guilty stricken and the case set for trial.

The case was well tried for the state by Mr. Arthur Markve, assistant county attorney. The evidence offered by the State showed that the defendant had been attended by six Minneapolis physicians from the middle of April, 1938, and June 30, 1938, a period of six weeks. She was complaining of pain that indicated to each of the physicians called that she had a kidney stone. From five of these physicians she received morphine either in the form of hypos or by prescription. She received twelve prescriptions for morphine from four different physicians in thirteen days, May 6 to May 19, also one on June 30, a total of 78¾ gr. One physician testified that he wrote a prescription on May 6 and another on May 7 after the defendant had stated to him that she had lost the first one. This was denied by the defendant; she admitted getting the prescription but denied she stated she had lost the first one.

The defendant was convicted in Federal court in Minneapolis in December, 1934, on a charge of forging and altering narcotic prescriptions. She served fourteen months in the Federal Industrial Institution for Women at Alderson, West Virginia, on that charge. She is married and lives with her husband and one daughter at 2527 First Avenue South, Minneapolis. She is thirty-nine years of age, about 5 feet 2 inches in height and weighs about 155 pounds. She appears to be older than the age stated.

The State Board of Medical Examiners urges every physician to refrain from administering, furnishing or prescribing morphine for this woman. If a call is made for a physician, he should insist on a complete examination, including x-ray, and hospitalization, if necessary before any narcotic is given.

ALCOHOL IN RELATION TO TRAFFIC ACCIDENTS

RICHARD L. HOLCOMB, Evanston, Ill. (*Journal A. M. A.*, Sept. 17, 1938), reports the results of a study of the drinking of drivers involved in personal injury accidents and of the drinking of drivers in the general population. The second study served as a control of the first, allowing conclusions to be drawn as to the part alcohol plays in accidents. A total of 270 persons were tested in the first study. Drivers involved in personal injury accidents who accompanied the persons injured to a hospital or drivers who themselves were injured were tested by urinalysis for alcohol. A total of 1,750 persons were tested in the second study. Drivers were chosen at random from an area comparable to that of the first study. A complete testing laboratory, with the Harger "drunkometer," was set up in a trailer, allowing breath tests for alcohol to be made immediately. 1. The highest percentage of drinking drivers occurs in the early morning hours and over the week-end. 2. The largest number of drinking drivers occurs in the early evening and over the week-end. 3. The peak age for drinking drivers is from 25 to 30. 4. Women drink and drive as much as men when the number of women driving at various hours of the day is considered. 5. The percentage of drinking drivers in the general population varies as does the percentage of drinking drivers in the personal injury accident group but falls considerably lower at all times. 6. The percentage or number of drivers involved in personal injury accidents varies as does the percentage or number of drinking drivers. 7. As the blood alcohol content increases, the number of drivers appearing in the personal injury accident group increases out of all proportion over that in the general driving population. 8. As alcohol increases, accidents increase and at a rate somewhat proportionate to the increase in alcohol. 9. Equal percentages of drinking drivers are found in the accident group and in the general population group at a point near 0.5 part of alcohol per thousand parts of blood, indicating that alcohol in that amount is not necessarily a significant cause of accidents. 10. The data gathered in this study confirms a self-evident fact, that alcohol is a major cause of automobile accidents.

Dr. Roy A. Hoffman of Minneapolis was married on October 16 to Miss Lolita B. Wilkinson of Cloquet.

* * *

Dr. John C. Fueling of Bovey is taking a postgraduate course at Columbia University.

* * *

Dr. A. R. Ellingson of Detroit Lakes was recently elected a fellow of the American College of Surgeons.

* * *

Dr. O. F. Mellby of Thief River Falls has been amed chief of staff at Mercy Hospital.

* * *

Dr. Stanley Peters of Virginia has moved to Silver reek, N. Y.

* * *

Dr. O. H. Jones has opened offices in Madison Lake or the practice of medicine. He recently completed is internship at St. Mary's Hospital, Minneapolis.

* * *

Dr. Carl G. Wingquist has opened offices at Crosby. Ie formerly practiced at Carlton, Minnesota, and Los ingeles, California.

* * *

Dr. Harold Hullsiek of Saint Paul has resumed prac- ce following an absence of four months from his of- ce.

* * *

Dr. George Kaiser of Saint Paul has become asso- ated with Dr. W. E. Macklin of Litchfield. Dr. aiser is a recent graduate of the University of Min- :sota medical school.

* * *

Dr. E. H. Hansen, formerly of Minneapolis, has ened offices in Marshall. Dr. Hansen graduated from ulane University, and served his internship at the ity and County Hospital in San Francisco.

* * *

Dr. W. E. Richardson of Philip, South Dakota, has pened an office at Rushford, for the practice of medi- ne. Dr. Richardson practiced at Slayton and Pipe- one, before going to Philip, South Dakota.

* * *

Dr. L. F. Hawkinson, who has been associated with e Brainerd Clinic at Brainerd, Minnesota, will leave ovember 15 for Oakland, California, where he will tablish practice.

* * *

Dr. I. L. Oliver of Graceville was recently elected to e American College of Surgeons and attended the eeting in New York City, where he received his fel- wship.

* * *

Dr. John East has located in Northome for the prac- ce of medicine. He is a graduate of the school of edicine of the University of Oklahoma, and served s internship at Ancker Hospital, Saint Paul.

Dr. L. J. Hoyer, formerly of Howard Lake, has lo- cated at Windom. Dr. Hoyer recently completed a postgraduate course in surgery and bone fracture at the Cook County Graduate School of Medicine at the Mayo Clinic.

* * *

Dr. D. J. Jacobson, formerly of Blackduck, has lo- cated at Bemidji, where he will continue the practice of medicine. Before leaving Blackduck, Dr. Jacobson was the guest of honor at a dinner given by the Black- duck Community Club.

* * *

Dr. Harlow B. Thompson has opened offices at Ada for the practice of medicine. He is a graduate of the medical school of the University of Oregon, and served his internship at the Tacoma General Hospital and Pierce County Hospital at Tacoma, Washington.

* * *

Dr. Samuel T. Sandell has become associated with Dr. H. E. Binet of Grand Rapids. Dr. Sandell is a graduate of the medical school of the University of Minnesota and served internships at Ancker Hospital in Saint Paul, and the Glen Lake Sanatorium in Hen- nepin County.

* * *

The American Medical Association and the National Broadcasting Company are broadcasting at 1 p. m. each Wednesday, over the Blue Network, a radio pro- gram entitled "Your Health." The program is not one of health talks, but of dramatization written and produced by radio artists prepared from information furnished by the Bureau of Health Education of the American Medical Association.

* * *

Graduate Fellowships in Anesthesiology have been established by the Medical School and Graduate School of the University of Minnesota for physicians who de- sire to prepare themselves for the practice of this specialty. The fellowships offer an abundance of clin- ical training in all types of local, regional and general anesthesia and gas therapy, and also adequate related graduate work in chemistry, anatomy, physiology, pharmacology. Applicants must have served at least one year in a rotating internship.

* * *

The Squibb Institute for Medical Research, a new $750,000 modern building especially adapted for re- search, at New Brunswick, New Jersey, was dedicated with appropriate ceremonies October 11, 1938. Air conditioning and accurate control of temperature and humidity will make research possible the year around. The aim of the founders of the Institute is to create in the medical and biological fields an industry-support- ed research enterprise analogous to the Bell Telephone and General Electric laboratories in the sphere of physics.

Dr. Litzenberg Honored

An appreciation dinner was given in honor of Dr. Jennings C. Litzenberg on the evening of October 14, 1938, at the Minikahda Club, Minneapolis, by some 200 former pupils and friends in celebration of his completion of twenty-five years as chief of the Department of Obstetrics and Gynecology of the University of Minnesota.

Following his gradution from the University of Minnesota medical school in 1899, Dr. Litzenberg acted as assistant to Dr. L. J. Cooke, the medical director of athletics, before he specialized in obstetrics and gynecology. It was fitting that Dr. Cooke should act as Master of Ceremonies at the testimonial dinner, which he did with much display of wit and humor. After-dinner speeches were made by Dr. Lee W. Barry of Saint Paul, who outlined changes in obstetrical procedures which have taken place in the past twenty-five years; by Dr. William A. O'Brien, who wittily described a picture of Dr. Litzenberg. Dr. Litzenberg projected on a screen and purported to be the portrait of the honored guest to be presented to the University; by Dr. John L. McKelvey, who is Dr. Litzenberg's successor as chief of the department, in which he paid graceful tribute to his predecessor, giving him a large share of the credit for the low infant and maternal mortality in Minnesota. Although not appearing on the printed program, Mr. John Powell, a life-long friend, contributed a nice tribute to Dr. Litzenberg, and all those present were amused by the witty remarks of Dr. Litzenberg's son, Carl, a professor of English at the University of Wisconsin. In responding, Dr. Litzenberg disclaimed credit for the high standing of obstetrics in Minnesota, and gave credit to the ability of his departmental staff.

The dinner, sponsored by a committee of which Dr. S. B. Solhaug was chairman, was a great success and all who attended derived great satisfaction from being able to show their appreciation of "Litz."

* * *

Dedication of Mayo Foundation House

On September 23, at Fourth Street and Seventh Avenue Southwest in Rochester, in the stone house which had been their home since 1917, Dr. and Mrs. William J. Mayo received members of the staffs of The Mayo Clinic and The Mayo Foundation in order formally to dedicate the building and grounds as Mayo Foundation House.

On the occasion, short addresses were delivered by representatives of The Mayo Foundation, The Mayo Clinic and The Mayo Properties Association. Dr. Mayo responded in part as follows:

"When my brother and I built our homes, we built them not merely for the purpose of living in them ourselves, but with the idea that they should be of such character as would make them suitable gathering places where the staff of the Clinic and the fellowship men might meet men of science from this country and abroad and cultivate those social contacts which are so important a part of professional life.

"And so with this Foundation House, which we have given over to be used for continuation and extension of educational and related social functions which are in

(Continued on Page 812)

In Memoriam

Martin C. Bergheim
1886-1938

DR. Martin C. Bergheim, Hawley, Minnesota, died October 4, 1938, of bronchopneumonia, at the age of fifty-two.

Dr. Bergheim was born in Madison, South Dakota, January 23, 1886. He graduated from St. Olaf Colege in 1912. The following three years he acted as principal and athletic coach at Lamberton, Minnesota. In 1916 he entered the University of Minnesota medical school and graduated in 1919, serving as interne at the Providence Hospital at Detroit, Michigan. He was a member of the Phi Beta Pi medical fraternity.

Dr. Bergheim practiced medicine at Raymond, Minnesota, for a year before locating in 1921 at Hawley, where he had since practiced. In 1922 he contracted scarlet fever and his health was permanently impaired as a result although he carried on an active practice.

A member of the Lutheran Church, Dr. Bergheim also belonged to the Masonic and Eastern Star lodges. He was a member of the Clay-Becker County Society, the Minnesota State and American Medical Associations.

Dr. Bergheim is survived by his widow; two daughters, Gail Marie and Jeanne Marie; his father, C. N. Bergheim; two brothers, Richard and Nordahl of Madison, South Dakota; and six sisters.

Dr. Bergheim's kindness and patience in dealing with his many patients will long be remembered in the community in which he lived.

F. C. Bowman
1849-1938

DR. F. C. Bowman, of Duluth, passed away on October 4, 1938, at the age of eighty-nine.

Dr. Bowman was born on a farm at Hebron, Maine, and in 1857 came to Minnesota, attending high school in Litchfield, Minnesota. In 1875 he began the study of architecture at the University of Minnesota, earning his way by working as a janitor, carpenter, assistant chemist and contractor. In 1879 he began the study of medicine at the Hahnemann Medical School.

Dr. Bowman arrived in Duluth in March, 1881, having had to pawn his watch to finance the price of railway ticket to Minnesota. The first few months o practice in Duluth were difficult and it was onl through the assistance of Luther Mendenhall, a pionee Duluth banker, that he was able to continue practice

During the more than half century of practice i Duluth, Dr. Bowman was active in civic affairs. I the late 1880's he was a member of the Board of Edu cation of Duluth, and in the 1890's was a member o the State Board of Medical Examiners.

Dr. Bowman was a member of the First Methodi Church and of the Scottish Rite of Duluth, and als of the Golden Fleece lodge, A. F. and A. M. of Litchfield. For many years he was a member of the Saturday Lunch Club also. He is survived by his widow; a daughter, Mrs. L. H. Jones of Coral Gables, Florida; two sons, Lawrence and Leslie, of Duluth.

Henry Martyn Bracken

1854-1938

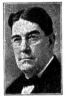

D R. Henry Martyn Bracken, former Secretary of the Minnesota State Board of Health and a resident of Minneapolis from 1885 until 1923, died at his home in Claremont, California, September 25, 1938, at the age of eighty-four.

Dr. Bracken was born February 27, 1854, the son of a physician and as a boy lived in Jersey, Ohio, where he received his preliminary education except for a year at Elders Ridge Academy. He taught in a summer school at the age of seventeen and then returned to the Academy, where he graduated in 1872, delivering a Greek oration. His father died the same year and he returned to teaching at Boonton, New Jersey, but in 1874 entered the medical department of the University of Michigan for a year. After teaching another year he entered the College of Physicians and Surgeons, New York, where he graduated in 1877.

Following graduation Dr. Bracken went to Venezuela as mine surgeon, but shortly left for Edinburgh for further medical study and in 1879 passed the examination of the Royal College of Surgeons. After spending the summer as physician in a boys' boarding school at Uppingham-by-the-Sea, he sailed as ship surgeon on the "Moselle" to Central and South America and the West Indies. During the three years as ship surgeon he contracted both yellow fever and malaria.

In the fall of 1882, Dr. Bracken returned to practice in a New England town, but being dissatisfied went to Sonora, Mexico, in 1884, as camp surgeon in a mining camp. Owing to the activities of the Apaches under Geronimo, the mines closed in 1885 and Dr. Bracken returned to New York for more postgraduate study. In December, 1885, he came to Minneapolis with his wife whom he had married in 1884 before going to Mexico.

Upon organization of the Medical School of the University of Minnesota in 1887, Dr. Bracken was appointed Professor of Materia Medica and Therapeutics and lectured also on Public Health and Preventive Medicine. He remained on the faculty until 1907 when he resigned to devote his time to the State Board of Health. He was elected to this board in 1895 and became its Secretary and Executive Officer in 1897, succeeding Dr. Charles N. Hewitt. During his incumbency, which lasted until 1919, the present divisions of the board, with the exception of the Division of Child

Hygiene, were created. The mortality from typhoid, diphtheria, and the other contagious diseases of childhood and also from tuberculosis were unbelievably high at the turn of the century and proved a serious problem in State Board activities. Dr. Bracken was particularly concerned with the care of lepers in Minnesota and was instrumental in the establishment of a national leprosarium. He took a leading part in national health affairs and in 1912 was president of the Conference of State and Provincial Health Authorities of North America.

In 1916, Dr. Bracken volunteered his services to the medical corps of the British Navy but was not accepted on account of his age. Again in 1917, he volunteered his services to the Medical Corps of the United States Army, but was considered of much greater value in his official position. On September, 1919, he retired as State Health Officer and was commissioned as surgeon in the Reserve Corps of the United States Public Health Service and was assigned to the Veterans' Bureau. In 1923, he resigned and moved to Claremont, California, where he maintained his interest in Public Health, lecturing at Pomona College, and making a thorough review of the official records of the Minnesota State Board of Health from 1872 through 1936.

Dr. Bracken took an active part in the American Medical Association's public health program, was a member of the first Board of Directors of the National Tuberculosis Association, and in 1906 organized the Minnesota's Association for the Prevention and Relief of Tuberculosis, now the Minnesota Public Health Association. He also organized the Minnesota State Sanitary Conference and was its secretary.

A few years ago Dr. Bracken returned for a visit with his nephew, Dr. William Henry Condit of Minneapolis. At this time he appeared hale and hearty, attended with Dr. Chesley, present secretary of the State Board of Health, several county society meetings, and enjoyed meeting many of his old friends. Besides his nephew, Dr. Condit, Dr. Bracken is survived by his widow.

John Folta

1901-1938

D R. John Folta of Ceylon, Minnesota, died suddenly from coronary thrombosis at the home of his brother, Andrew Folta, in Minneapolis, on October 14, 1938.

Dr. Folta was born in Morrison County, Minnesota, in 1901, the son of Adam and Anna Folta, his parents being natives of Austria. At the age of sixteen he entered Baldwin-Wallace College near Cleveland, Ohio, and later Berea College, where he received his B.A. degree in 1923. He received his M.D. degree at the University of Minnesota Medical School in 1929, and after serving one year as interne in St. Luke's Hospital, Duluth, he became associated with Dr. Arnt G. Anderson, Minneapolis, for a year.

Dr. Folta began practice at Ceylon in 1930 and the

following year purchased the practice and hospital of Dr. Bailey when the latter moved to Fairmont. Since July, 1937, Dr. I. Fisher had been associated with him in practice.

In 1930 Dr. Folta married Dorothy Thompson of Duluth. He is survived by his widow; two sons, Russell, aged 6, and Richard, aged 3; his father, three brothers and a sister.

Dr. Folta was keenly interested in athletics, having played football in his student days, and had gone to Minneapolis chiefly to attend the Minnesota-Michigan game. He was a member of the Masonic Lodge of Sherburn, the Blue Earth Valley Medical Society, Minnesota State and American Medical Associations.

Albert Henry Parks

1880-1938

DR. Albert Henry Parks was born in Battle Creek, Michigan, April 15, 1880, the son of Reuben B. and Celia Burr Parks. He was graduated from the Battle Creek High School in 1898 and after two years at Albion College he entered the University of Michigan, where he graduated June 25, 1904, receiving a Bachelor of Arts degree. He received his M.A. and M.D. degrees from Northwestern University in 1906. After serving his internship in St. Luke's Hospital, Chicago, he was licensed to practice in the State of Minnesota on April 12, 1907 and in California, February 23, 1922.

Dr. Parks was a member of the Hennepin County Medical Society, Minnesota State Medical Association, American Medical Association, Sigma Chi Fraternity, and the Phi Beta Pi Fraternity.

During the period from 1908 to 1915 when Dr. Parks was assistant city physician, Hopewell Hospital for tuberculous patients was opened and he was put in charge of the medical treatment of these patients, also acting as superintendent of the institution.

He was a founder and first president of the Lake Harriet Commercial Club, a founder and first president of the Lake Harriet Lodge A. F. and A. M. 277; and from 1910 to 1911 was national president of the Phi Beta Pi medical fraternity.

In 1913 and 1914 he served as alderman of the 13th Ward, resigning in 1915 to give his attention to practice.

In June 1917 he was appointed a member of the local draft board of the 13th Ward of Minneapolis. In June 1918 he resigned and on August 1 was commissioned captain in the Medical Section of the Officers' Reserve Corps, receiving his honorable discharge on April 15, 1919.

Dr. Parks was appointed chief of the Surgical Service, Division "B" of the General Hospital Staff, Minneapolis, January 14, 1918. He was a member of the Staff of St. Barnabas Hospital for five years and was a member of the Surgical Staff of Asbury Hospital from the beginning of his practice until his retirement, serving as Chief of Staff during the year 1932. The last years of his surgical practice were spent here, where he endeared himself to the hospital personnel

and to the staff of doctors. He was appointed ber of the Board of Public Welfare during t 1923.

The following articles were written by him Among his written contributions may be liste Medico Legal Expert, written for the Medic Journal; Brotherhood, written for the Phi I Quarterly; and Economic Therapeutics, read the Asbury Hospital Staff and the Hennepin Medical Society and published in Minnesota M in 1932.

Dr. Parks was married to Katherine Ba graduate nurse from Abbott Hospital, Minr on September 1, 1909. Their only child is a d: Mrs. Jean Parks Forrest of Minneapolis.

Dr. Parks used unusual foresight in preparir self for his profession, obtaining his B.A., M. M.D. degrees and serving his internship in one leading hospitals. When he began to practice City of Minneapolis he continued to reëducate by his association with the General Hospita carried out a program for the young physici was ideal. In his private practice from the v ginning there was ample evidence of his good p tion and that he was applying the highest ethic: ciples of medical practice.

Dr. Parks felt, also, a civic duty which was by his willingness to serve the public hospita public welfare board, and the city council.

He was devoted to his family and knowing t condition of his health might separate them warning, he, as long ago as 1929, wrote and s farewell message to his wife and daughter, beautiful and well deserved tribute to them bof died August 30, 1938, after an illness of five y

One of Dr. Parks' outstanding characteristi his praise of others and his personal modest; other virtue was his great generosity. He remembered for his gracious manner, his tho ness of others, and his pleasant companion; well as for his painstaking care of his patie his scientific attainments.

Dr. Parks was a colorful figure in his pro a clever surgeon, an astute diagnostician, and consultant. My association with him in sur Asbury Hospital during his last active years inspiration.

CLAUDE C. KEN

OF GENERAL INTEREST

Mayo Foundation House

(Continued from Page 810)

the best interest of the purposes of the Fou This house was built with the intention of such use: fireproof, of large size, suitable for the ment of the opportunities which we hope realized."

The donors have provided a sufficient endow maintenance of the house and garden and ha up their residence in a new and smaller Their former home, now Mayo Foundation H ready is in daily use as a meeting place for and for other groups engaged in educational :

MEDICAL BROADCAST FOR NOVEMBER

The Minnesota State Medical Association Morning ealth Service.

The Minnesota State Medical Association broadcasts eekly at 11:00 o'clock every Saturday morning over :ation WCCO, Minneapolis (810 kilocycles or 370.2 eters) and Station WLB, University of Minnesota 760 kilocycles or .395 meters).

Speaker: William A. O'Brien, M.D., Associate Pro:ssor of Pathology and Preventive Medicine, Medical :hool, University of Minnesota. The program for the onth will be as follows:

November 5 Good Posture.
November 12 Gall Bladder Disease.
November 19 Sinusitis
November 26 Development of Teeth.

CIENTIFIC EXHIBIT
MERICAN MEDICAL ASSOCIATION

Application blanks are now available for space in the cientific Exhibit at the St. Louis Session of the Amer:an Medical Association, May 15-19, 1939. Attention ; called to the fact that the meeting is a month earlier :an usual, and applications close January 5, 1939. lanks will be sent on request to the Director, Scienific Exhibit, American Medical Association, 535 North)earborn St., Chicago, Ill.

PAN-PACIFIC SURGICAL ASSOCIATION

The third Congress of the Association will be held in Honolulu, September 15 to 28, 1939. An invitation is :xtended to all surgeons in the State Association to :ake part in this meeting, which will be attended by)utstanding surgeons from Australia, New Zealand, China, Japan, Java, Canada and the United States. There will be sections on fractures and orthopedics, ;eneral surgery, gynecology, neurosurgery, ophthalmol)gy, otolaryngology, plastic surgery, thoracic surgery and roentgenology. A visit to the "Paradise of the Pacific" is an additional attraction. Dr. Forrest J. Pinkerton, Young Building, Honolulu, is secretary of: :he Association.

NORTH DAKOTA SOCIETY OF OBSTETRICIANS AND GYNECOLOGISTS

The biannual meeting of the North Dakota Society of Obstetricians and Gynecologists was held Friday, October 28, at the Fargo Country Club, Fargo, North Dakota.

Dr. W. F. Mengert, of the University of Iowa Medi:al School, spoke on "Toxemias of Pregnancy" and Dr. J. C. Litzenberg, Emeritus Professor of the Department of Obstetrics and Gynecology of the University of Minnesota, addressed the meeting. Case reports

were presented by Drs. J. F. Hanna, G. W. Hunter, B. M. Urenn and J. R. Dillard.

Officers for the ensuing year are: Dr. J. F. Hannar, Fargo, president; Dr. John H. Moore, Grand Forks, vice pesident; and Dr. A. C. Orr, Bismarck, secretaryteasurer.

SCOTT-CARVER SOCIETY

At the Scott-Carver Medical Society meeting held in Montgomery, October 11, Dr. George Eitel, Minneapolis, spoke on "Traumatic Surgical Emergencies," and Dr. Ernest Meland, Minneapolis, talked on "Urological Emergencies."

WABASHA COUNTY SOCIETY

The seventieth annual meeting of the Wabasha County Medical Society was held at Wabasha, Thursday afternoon and evening, October 6, 1938.

At the-business session, the following officers were elected for the coming year:

President—Dr. B. J. Bouquet, Wabasha
Vice President—Dr. E. W. Ellis, Elgin
Secretary-Treasurer—Dr. W. F. Wilson, Lake City
Delegate to State Association—Dr. E. C. Bayley, Lake City
Alternate—Dr. R. H. Frost, Wabasha
Censor for three years—Dr. G. W. Holt, Wabasha
Censors continuing in office—Dr. J. R. Slocumb, Plainview, and Dr. B. A. Flesche, Lake City.

One new member was received into the society, Dr. Robert A. Glabe of Plainview.

Dinner was served at Hotel Anderson through the courtesy of the Wabasha members. Among the guests were Dr. A. J. Chesley and Dr. R. N. Barr of the Minnesota Department of Health, and Dr. Roy Flannagan, of Richmond, Virginia, liaison officer of the relief forces of that state. Upon invitation, each of these guests made a few appropriate remarks.

At the scientific session in the evening, the following program was presented:

President's Address—"Coöperation Within the Society"—Dr. H. T. SHERMAN, Plainview.

"Epidemic Encephalitis"—Dr. GORDON R. KAMMAN, Saint Paul.

"Granulocytopenia, With Case Reports"—Dr. B. A. FLESCHE, Lake City.

"Practical Points in Pediatric Practice"—Dr. EDWARD DYER ANDERSON, Minneapolis.

"Roentgen Therapy in Malignant Disease"—Dr. W. C. POPP, Mayo Clinic, Rochester.

The Women's Auxiliary held their sessions in connection with this meeting. Entertainment for the ladies was provided at the home of Dr. and Mrs. Ochsner.

In all, there were thirty-two in attendance, including nineteen physicians, three dentists and ten doctors' wives.

WASHINGTON COUNTY

The regular meeting of the Society was held September 13. A report was given by Dr. E. V. Strand,

Bayport, and by the secretary of the State House of Delegates meeting held in Saint Paul, September 11. The scientific program was given by Dr. Gordon R. Kamman, Saint Paul, who devoted most of his time to a consideration of vitamins and then discussed some recent experiences with acute encephalitis.

Dr. Leo James Conlin, Lake Elmo, was elected to society membership.

* * *

The guest speaker at the meeting held on October 11 was Dr. Raymond N. Bieter of the Medical School, who spoke on "The Chemistry and Therapeutic Use of Sulfanilamide."

The booklet on Maternal Care and Complications edited by Dr. Fred Adair and distributed by the Minnesota State Department of Health through Dr. Chesley, was given to the society members.

Mr. Manley Brist of Saint Paul was a welcome guest.

WOMAN'S AUXILIARY

Mrs. W. B. Roberts, President
2735 Irving Avenue South, Minneapolis.
Mrs. E. V. Goltz, Press and Publicity, St. Paul, Minn.

Mrs. William B. Roberts, State President of the Women's Auxiliary of the Minnesota State Medical Association, was the guest delegate of the Auxiliary to the northern Minnesota district August 29 and 30, which was held in Crookston. The Northern Minnesota District Medical Society met at that time and members of the Auxiliary were entertained delightfully by the members of the Auxiliary of the Red River Valley Medical Association. Women from various parts of the northern territory of Minnesota attended and special guests besides Mrs. Roberts were Mrs. E. M. Hammes and Mrs. George Earl of Saint Paul. Mrs. Roberts was the house guest of Mrs. J. F. Norman, past president of the State Auxiliary. An attractive luncheon was held at the Hotel Crookston for the visitors, and Mrs. Roberts addressed the group. Following the luncheon a tour was arranged for the visitors, taking in the interesting points of the city and community. Later in the afternoon a bridge-tea was held at the home of Mrs. O. E. Locken. Honors in bridge were won by Mrs. Clarence Jacobson, Mrs. H. H. Hodgson and Mrs. Roberts. Presiding at the tea table, which was attractively arranged with zinnias, were Mrs. C. L. Oppegaard and Mrs. B. Borreson of Thief River Falls. Mrs. C. L. Oppegaard was the social chairman and was assisted by Mrs. G. A. Morley and Mrs. C. G. Uhley (registration); Mrs. O. L. Bertelson and Mrs. M. O. Oppegaard (transportation); Mesdames Hodgson, L. L. Brown, O. K. Behr, R. O. Sather and B. Borreson of Thief River Falls (luncheon); and Mesdames J. F. Norman, W. G. Paradis, W. F. Mercil, S. H. Stuurmanns of Erskine and Mrs. O. E. Locken of Crookston (bridge-tea). In the evening the doctors and their wives enjoyed a dinner together. The Red River Valley Auxil-

iary is noted for its hospitality and sociability, and Mrs. Roberts reports a most interesting and enjoyable meeting.

―――――

The members of the Woman's Auxiliary to the Clay-Becker Medical Society had their regular summer meeting, August 15, when the Clay-Becker Medical Society convened. A joint dinner was held at the Pelican bone Lodge, which was followed by a talk by Dr. J. T. Hayes, who spoke of the work done by the organization, and also on the technical subject "Gallbladder Diseases." The business session of the Auxiliary was devoted mainly to philanthropic plans for the coming winter. Attending from Detroit Lakes were Mrs. L. J. Flancher, Mrs. Arnold Larson, Mrs. O. O. Larsen and Mrs. A. R. Ellingson; from Hawley, Mrs. C. W. Simson, Mrs. V. D. Thysell and Mrs. M. C. Berghei. After the business session cards were enjoyed by the members.

―――――

Mrs. Roy Andrews, a member of the Blue Earth County Auxiliary, attended the annual American Medical Association meeting in San Francisco.

―――――

On September 26 the Woman's Auxiliary of the Minnesota State Medical Association held its first Executive Board meeting at the Minikahda Club, Minneapolis, at 10:30 a. m. Mrs. William Roberts, the president presided. Reports of the county presidents were read and the activities for the year discussed. Following the meeting a luncheon was served at the club with Mrs. Charles C. Tomlinson of Omaha, Nebraska, president of the Women's Auxiliary of the American Medical Association, the honored guest. Dr. J. M. Hayes, president of the Minnesota Medical Association, spoke. Following the luncheon Mrs. J. M. Hayes was hostess a beautifully arranged tea for the visitor, at her home 2821 Benton Boulevard. Mrs. Martin Nordland of Minneapolis was the social chairman.

―――――

The Woman's Auxiliary of the Mower County Medical Society held its fall meeting October 3 at Austin Country Club. Thirteen members and f guests were present and luncheon was served at o'clock followed by a business meeting. Mrs. F. Robertson, president, presided and gave a report of state board meeting held in Minneapolis September 25. Bridge followed and prizes were won by Mrs. Leck and Mrs. G. E. Hertel. Out-of-town guests were Mrs. A. E. Henslin of LeRoy and Mrs. J. Thomson of Brownsdale The next meeting will October 31.

―――――

A tea held at the home of Mrs. Edward Sch Saint Paul, September 26 honored the national president of the Woman's Auxiliary, Mrs. Charles C. Tomlinson of Omaha. The tea was given by the members of the Ramsey County Women's Auxiliary.

ALLERGIC DISEASES: THEIR DIAGNOSIS AND TREATMENT. , By Ray M. Balyeat, assisted by Ralph Bowen. Illustrated with 132 engravings, including 8 in colors. 4th ed., rev. and enl. $6.00. Philadelphia: F. A. Davis Co., 1936.

In writing this book the author seems to have had in mind a manual for allergic patients. However, much of the text seems to be more scientific and more specialized than most laymen would be able to understand. For the professional man the book contains a large fund of information, but there is much of it that is simpler than a physician needs. There is a wealth of information in this book, but it is not as available as it should be either for the doctor or for the patient. Many of the points are illustrated with case histories, which is not good for laymen, as it serves as a patent medicine advertisement. There is advice given in this book which does not seem in agreement with the feeling of the profession as a whole; i.e., birth control is recommended for people with migraine as a means of preventing it in the offspring. This seems to a reviewer as radical treatment for a condition that is an inconvenience rather than a disease. On the whole this volume is not particularly recommended either for the patient or for the professional man.

DIABETES; A MODERN MANUAL. Anthony M. Sindoni, Jr., M.D. 240 p. charts, $2.00. New York: Whittlesey House, 1937.

This book is put out primarily to teach the diabetic patient how to take care of himself while under a physician's care. The material is well written and in simple language so that the intelligent diabetic individual can understand it. The section containing answers to typical questions asked of physicians should be a great help to the patient in having a better understanding of the disease and what is required of him to remain in good health. The section on diet including menus and recipes is very complete and well written. The book is one that is not only valuable for the patient, but is also of value to the physician who needs all the assistance he can get in handling the problem of diabetes.

JOHN R. MEADE, M.D.

A MANUAL OF OPERATING ROOM PROCEDURES. Alvina W. Hoppe, Science Instructor, Jewish Hospital, St. Louis, and Lucile M. Halverson, Supervisor of Operating Rooms, University of Minnesota Hospitals, Minneapolis. The University of Minnesota Press (Humphrey Milford, Oxford University Press, London), 1937. Price $2.00.

As the title indicates, this volume is intended for the surgical nurse in the operating room. The supervision of a modern operating room requires much attention to detail if an operation is to proceed smoothly. The duties of the operating room personnel are outlined in detail, the care of materials, the preparation of patients, tray set-ups and, under separate headings, instructions for practically all operations are given in minute detail. Representing, as it does, the technic used in two outstanding hospitals, its pages reflect the careful thought given by the authoresses. The volume should be of great value to surgical nurses, particularly those in charge of operating rooms.

C. B. D.

MATERIA MEDICA AND PHARMACOLOGY. H. A. McGuigan and E. P. Brodie. 580 p. Illus. $2.75. St. Louis, Mosby, 1936.

This book is an outgrowth of Brodie's Materia Medica for Nurses, but is much more complete. It has left out many of the older drugs which were used without any basis, but which have been handed down as being of value. The book is well written and the subject matter well classified. The sections on the action of drugs on the nervous system and on the vascular system are very complete. The illustrations make it easier for the students to understand the actions of drugs. The book should make a very good textbook for both medical students and nurses.

JOHN R. MEADE, M.D.

ENDOCRINE THERAPY IN GENERAL PRACTICE. 192 p. illus., $2.75. E. L. Sevringhaus, M.D., F.A.C.P. Chicago: Year Book Publ. Co., 1938.

This small book does not attempt to cover the entire field of endocrine literature but manages, in an easy-to-read form, to simplify and correlate the most important fundamental facts to serve as a background for intelligent endocrine therapy by the general practitioner. The author fully understands that any book written about glandular therapy is quickly outdated.

One of the most likely criticisms of this volume will undoubtedly be that the handling of the material is too elementary. This criticism is valid; but nevertheless the same criticism will recommend the book to those practitioners who on looking up references in the field of endocrine therapy are likely to become perplexed by the confusion that exists in terms, nomenclature, indications, and dosages. A careful reading may well result in a better understanding of indications and avoid the dangers of enthusiastic overtreatment as a result of commercial exploitation of endocrine products.—M. L. STRAUS, M.D.

A PEDIATRICIAN IN SEARCH OF MENTAL HYGIENE. Bronson Crothers, M.D., New York, $2.00. The Commonwealth Fund, Oxford University Press, 1937.

The fascinating title of this small volume recommends it at once. Anyone—pediatrician or other—whose resurgent hopes send him forth on so commendable a search deserves company.

The author "starts with a general survey of the situation as it relates to the practice of medicine and then goes on in a rather casual way to discuss the medical school and the teaching hospital." He closes with a description of a scheme for coöperation between psychologist and pediatrician as worked out at the Children's Hospital in Boston. That the author has achieved a sympathy with the psychologist may be surmised

from his comment on the enterprise: "With full expectation of harmony on both sides, friction became evident almost from the start. Since this friction has, we both now believe, led us to an adequate and effective measure of coöperation, it is I think worth considering."—E. C. HARTLEY, M.D.

CLASSIFIED ADVERTISING

MINNESOTA MEDICINE

Journal of the Minnesota State Medical Association, Southern Minnesota Medical Association, Northern Minnesota Medical Association, Minnesota Academy of Medicine and Minneapolis Surgical Society

| Volume 21 | DECEMBER, 1938 | No. 12 |

THE ROLE OF INSECTS AND ALLIED FORMS IN THE TRANSMISSION OF DISEASES DUE TO FILTERABLE VIRUSES*

WM. A. RILEY, Ph.D.

Chief of the Division of Entomology, University of Minnesota

Saint Paul, Minnesota

THE fact that there exists among horses in Minnesota an epizoötic disease known technically as equine encephalomyelitis and that during the five summers preceding 1938 it affected approximately 50,000 of these animals and killed 10,000 of them on farms in this state is a matter of very serious concern for our farmers and through them it affects all of us as an economic problem.

Repeatedly during the course of the epizoötic in Minnesota and elsewhere the question has been raised as to whether this disease was transmissible to man. There have been a number of instances in which this seemed clearly indicated and Eklund and Blumstein (1938) report on six cases of "an unusual encephalitis occurring among farmers in Minnesota localities where equine encephalomyelitis was prevalent." The blood serum of one of three patients was shown by Dr. Ten Broeck, of the Rockefeller Institute, to neutralize the western strain of equine encephalomyelitis. Within the last few weeks there have been additional clear-cut demonstrations of this relationship. First, Fothergill, Dingle, Farber and Connerley reported that they had recovered the virus of the equine disease from the brain of a Massachusetts child who had succumbed to a case of encephalitis, during a period when there was an unprecedented outbreak of the horse disease. This finding was promptly confirmed by Webster and Wright, who described positive findings in four additional cases. They report that the virus from the brain tissue

of human cases is highly infectious for mice by the nasal route and by injection. And now, Schoening, Giltner and Shahan, using virus originally obtained by Fothergill from the brain of a child, have infected two horses, and through failure to infect one which was immune to the so-called eastern virus, have shown that the Massachusetts cases in man are of the eastern type. Incidentally, they report that all five strains recovered by the Bureau of Animal Industry from Massachusetts horses during the outbreak of 1938 were definitely of this same eastern type.

This brings again to the foreground the question as to the method, or methods, of transfer of this and related diseases. There is general agreement today that these infections are due to filterable viruses and there are many workers who are convinced that they are transmitted in nature primarily or even solely by insects and allied forms. To what extent has this arthropod transmission been demonstrated and what species may be regarded as clearly under suspicion in this region?

It must be recognized at the outset that the problem is not a simple one. The fact that an insect is a blood sucker does no more than place it in a list of forms to be considered. The abundance of the species, its seasonal distribution in relation to the outbreaks of the disease, its ready access to diseased and healthy animals, frequency of blood meals and longevity, the ability of the virus to exist in the insect, and its particular host specificity are among the points which must be considered.

Laboratory experiments, important as they

*A paper presented before the Minnesota State Sanitary Conference, November 4, 1938.

may be, are by no means sufficient to demonstrate that a given disease is commonly transmitted by an insect in nature. Indeed, the results obtained may be sufficient to blind workers to the possibility of other, and more important methods of spread of the disease. The type of so-called experiment which consists merely of grinding up insects which have fed on diseased animals and injecting a suspension into healthy animals, *unless supported by other conclusive evidence*, proves no more than that the minute quantity of blood which the insect may have sucked up is infective. One ten thousandths of a c.c. of blood from an animal with South African horse sickness was shown by Theiler to be sufficient to infect a healthy horse. A fully fed mosquito may contain twenty times that amount.

The studies on the method of spread of yellow fever will long remain the outstanding illustration of the development of our knowledge regarding the insect transmission of a virus disease. As far back as 1853 the French physician, Louis Daniel Beauperthuy, though believing in the telluric origin of the disease, argued in the most explicit manner that it was transmitted by mosquitoes. Thirty-eight years later, Carlos Finlay postulated the existence of "something tangible, which requires to be conveyed from the sick to the healthy before the disease can be propagated" and reached the conclusion that the carrier of yellow fever was the mosquito known today as *Ædes ægypti*. We all know how brilliantly this work was supported and placed on a firm foundation by the American Army Commission. For more than a quarter of a century following, it was a dogma of preventive medicine that only through the agency of mosquitoes of this species could yellow fever be transmitted. Today we know that eighteen different species of mosquitoes are efficient transmitters of the virus under experimental conditions and that some of these, or others as yet unidentified, are responsible for transmitting in nature the yellow fever which lurks in the jungles. They are not only the close relatives of *Ædes ægypti* but include anopheline and culicine, as well as ædine mosquitoes. The latest reported addition to the group is *Ædes triseriatus*, a species occurring in this state and through the northeastern United States.

It must not be overlooked that Bauer (1928) demonstrated that the virus was able to penetrate the unbroken skin of a macacus monkey.

In several instances in recent years investigators have contracted the disease in the course of autopsies or of laboratory work with the virus, in the absence of infective mosquitoes.

Following quickly after the work of the Army Commission came Graham's conclusive demonstration that dengue, or "break-bone" fever, is mosquito borne. Later investigations showed that, as in the case of yellow fever, the patient was infective to the insect only during the first three or four days of the disease and that there must be an incubation period of at least eight days before the mosquito could transmit it. Graham thought that it was carried by *Culex quinquefasciatus* but later workers have considered that he was using, at least in part, the *Ædes ægypti*. In all of the subsequent work this species or its very near relative in Asia, *Ædes albopictus*, have been shown to be primarily implicated in the spread of the disease. The trend of the present-day investigations of yellow fever should warn us not to make dogmatic statements regarding other suggested vectors.

In the meantime, Theiler and various other workers turned their attention to the possibility of the dreaded South African horse sickness being transmitted by insects. Pitchford (1903), claimed that he had transmitted it by allowing Anopheles and *Ædes ægypti* to feed on healthy horses forty-eight hours after feeding on diseased animals. Rickmann (1911), and subsequent workers have not been able to confirm this, although it has been widely credited by field workers. Other investigators have reported direct transfer by the bites of stableflies (*Stomoxys calcitrans*), horseflies (Tabanus spp.), "punkies" (Culicoides spp.), and hornflies (Hæmatobia). The question has not yet been settled definitely despite thirty-five years of intensive study.

In view of the successes which had rewarded the search for insect vectors of various diseases, virus and others, it was inevitable that attention should be directed towards such a transmitter of poliomyelitis. C. W. Howard and Clark (1912) early presented the results of studies on this phase of the problem. They dealt especially with the housefly, bedbug, head and body lice, and mosquitoes. Lice and mosquitoes were found not to take up or maintain the virus but the bedbug took it from infected monkeys and could maintain it in a living state within the body, up to seven days. The housefly was shown

tained in experimental studies of equine encephalomyelitis.

All attempts to implicate mosquitoes, stableflies, houseflies, fleas or other blood-sucking insects were negative.* It cannot be claimed that
the conclusions were final but there is little reason to suppose that arthropod transmission plays
a significant, if any, rôle in the spread of men-
ingo-encephalitis in man.

When it comes to the problem of equine encephalomyelitis there is tangible evidence that
mosquitoes and, possibly, other arthropods, must
be considered as incubators and potential carriers
of the infection. This evidence we shall review
briefly and then consider more particularly the
local situation as regards possible vectors and
their control.

Haring, Howarth and Meyer (1931), the first
to definitely describe the disease, mention the
possibility of its being spread by insects, and
Meyer (1932), noting that the virus circulates in
the blood, says: "Hence the rôle of biting insects
deserves consideration." He also, at this early
date, mentions three suspected cases in men handling infected horses but did not have available
brain tissues for testing for the virus.

In connection with this pioneer work, Herms,
Wheeler and Herms undertook studies of possible arthropod vectors. In a very carefully
planned series of experiments they tested the
hornfly, *Hæmatobia serrata* (= *Lyperosia irri-
tans*), a horsefly, *Tabanus punctifer*, the stablefly,
Stomoxys calcitrans, and two species of common
mosquitoes, *Ædes dorsalis* and *Anopheles ma-
culipennis*. Only negative results were obtained.

Except for the work with mosquitoes, the tests
by Herms, Wheeler and Herms were conducted
in 1932, though not published before October,
1934. In the meantime Kelser, in 1933, had announced that he had succeeded in transmitting
the virus of equine encephalomyelitis from an
inoculated guinea pig to a horse by the bites of
Ædes ægypti. Mosquitoes fed on the horse during the period of high temperature and subsequently fed on a normal animal likewise produced the disease. The mosquitoes were infectious as early as the sixth day after feeding on
the diseased animal.

An important contribution by Giltner and Shahan (1933) showed that there were two strains

*The epidemiological study of St. Louis encephalitis by Casey
and Broun (*Science*, November 11, 1938) concludes that "Every
known feature of its epidemiology is common to mosquito borne
diseases." Experimental evidence is not educed.

of the virus, a western and an eastern one, which were serologically and immunologically distinct. The eastern type is much the more virulent and is rather narrowly limited, but the western type has spread eastward.

In 1934 Merrill, Lacaillade and Ten Broeck reported that both strains were transmissible by the salt marsh mosquito, *Ædes sollicitans,* and the western strain by *Ædes cantator.* Ten Broeck and his associates followed this with a series of papers in which they presented critical data relative to the period of infectivity of the horse and the multiplication and persistence of the virus within the insect host, and Madsen and Knowlton (1935), working in Utah, demonstrated that two species of native mosquitoes, *Ædes nigromaculis* and *Ædes dorsalis* were capable of transmitting the western type of virus from infected to healthy mosquitoes.

Of special interest to residents of Minnesota is the fact that Kelser, in 1935, was able to infect one of three guinea pigs by bites of *Ædes vexans.* Unfortunately, this work was interrupted by removal to Panama, where experiments were continued with another species, *Ædes tæniorhynchus,* which proved capable of transmitting the western, but probably not the eastern, strain of the virus. A single mosquito biting a normal guinea pig but once, produced encephalomyelitis and death of the pig in five days.

In the meantime Simmons, Reynolds and Cornell (1936) reported successful transmission to guinea pigs of the western type virus by *Ædes albopictus,* an Asiatic species closely related to *Ædes ægypti.*

To date, then, we have proof that at least eight species of Ædine mosquitoes are able to take up, incubate, and convey, under laboratory conditions, the virus of equine encephalomyelitis. These are *Ædes ægypti* ("Stegomyia"), *A. albopictus, A. cantator, A. dorsalis, A. nigromaculis, A. sollicitans, A. tæniorhynchus* and *Ædes vexans.* That several of these play an important rôle in nature cannot be doubted, although it is far from established that mosquito transmission is the only, or even the most important method of spread of encephalomyelitis to animals or to man.

Of the eight species listed, *Ædes vexans, Ædes dorsalis* and *Ædes nigromaculis* occur commonly in Minnesota. Overwhelmingly dominant in most parts of the state is *Ædes vexans,* a marsh-breeding species, which is noted for its

migratory habits. In the course of studies aided by WPA on the pest mosquito problem of the Minneapolis-Metropolitan Area this past spring and summer, we found 98.28 per cent of the 337,960 mosquitoes trapped and identified were of this species. *Ædes dorsalis* was represented only to the extent of 0.26 of one per cent and *Ædes nigromaculis* by 0.01 of one per cent. These figures would vary, dependent on local conditions, but the great dominance of *vexans* remains as great in the regions where the three species are common.

Ædes vexans is known to deposit its eggs in low-lying ground where they may lie dormant not only for the remainder of the year but even for several years, until heavy rains create temporary pools which persist until the developmental cycle is completed. In warm weather this period may be as brief as four or five days. On emergence, the adults readily migrate for a distance of fifteen miles or more.

The vast areas of low-lying ground suitable for breeding places but not readily identifiable as such until there come periods of excessive rains, the value of the marsh hay and other crops of such areas, the expense of extensive drainage operations and the conflicting interests of various groups, make the problem of control of this and related species a difficult one which cannot be considered in detail at this time. In our urban areas a considerable reduction of pest mosquitoes will result from normal growth and from careful consideration of the problem in connection with planning for parks, lakes and streams, reservoirs and similar developments.

To the present no mention has been made of other possible vectors of the disease, though many insects have been submitted to us with the inquiry as to whether they are of importance in this respect. Some of them such as plant feeding leaf-hoppers, or spittle insects, could be immediately dismissed because of their habits and their distribution. Horseflies cannot be regarded as unworthy of consideration. They have been shown definitely to be direct carriers of anthrax and of several protozoal infections, but there is no experimental evidence incriminating them in the case of encephalomyelitis.

Some species of Simulium flies, commonly known as buffalo gnats, turkey gnats, or black-flies, are vicious blood suckers and there are notable instances of their attacks resulting in the death of large numbers of horses, mules, cattle and hogs in the Mississippi Valley. Whenever they are abundant, many young chickens and turkeys succumb to their attacks. In spite of numerous suggestions that the deaths of these various animals are due to a virus transmitted by the Simulium, the whole picture is such as to support the view that the fatalities are due to the poisonous saliva injected by enormous hordes of attacking insects. The distribution of the species attacking horses does not in anywise correspond with the geographic distribution or observed characteristics of the spread of equine encephalomyelitis.

In view of the ease with which the infection is transferred experimentally by nasal secretions, one cannot entirely rule out the possibility of mechanical carriage by houseflies, stableflies and similar insects, but if it occurs, it must be exceptional.

Syverton and Berry (1936) report the transmission of the western strain of the virus to Richardson's ground squirrel by ticks which had engorged as nymphs for forty-eight hours on infected guinea pigs. The evidence is altogether too scant to justify drawing conclusions from these results but they raise anew the question as to whether there is a reservoir host which maintains the virus in nature. Certainly this transmission cannot account for the spread of the disease in a more direct manner.

By way of summary, it may be said:

1. That the epidemiological evidence indicates that arthropod vectors play a rôle in the spread of encephalomyelitis to animals and to man.

2. Mosquitoes of the genus Ædes most nearly meet the requirements for this transmission and there is conclusive experimental evidence that they are capable of taking up, incubating and increasing the virus, and then transmitting it to healthy laboratory animals and to horses.

3. There is no satisfactory evidence that other arthropods are implicated, unless under very exceptional conditions.

Difficulties in the way of accepting the theory that ædine mosquitoes are the most important carriers are:

1. In spite of numerous attempts, infective mosquitoes have never been found under natural conditions.

2. Our native ædine mosquitoes, and specifically, those shown to be potential carriers, do not winter as adults. Since diseased horses are infective to mosquitoes only in the first few days, there must be some explanation for the survival of the infection over winter.

3. The possibility of ticks being effective transmitters under natural conditions is very remote.

4. The readiness with which the virus is transmitted by the nasal route suggests that in the case of encephalomyelitis as in that of poliomyelitis, there are important methods of spread, other than by arthropods, even though mosquito transfer is clearly possible.

INFLUENZA, RABIES, AND ENCEPHALITIS*

CARL M. EKLUND, M.D.

Epidemiologist, Division of Preventable Diseases, Minnesota Department of Health
Minneapolis, Minnesota

DURING the past decade great advances have been made in the study of virus diseases. Quantitative methods of studying immunity and physical methods such as the use of the ultra centrifuge and ultra filtration have been introduced.

Growth of virus in tissue cultures and on the chorio-allantoic membranes of the developing chick is receiving much study and is used both for isolation and preparation of virus for vaccine. This latter point is of great interest. Vaccine used for immunization against virus diseases at present contains much foreign material, and growth of virus in tissue culture cuts this to a minimum.

During the past year the State Board of Health has been especially interested in three of the virus diseases: influenza, rabies and encephalitis.

*Read at the Minnesota State Sanitary Conference, November 4, 1938, Minneapolis, Minnesota.

Influenza

About a year ago an influenza research laboratory was established in the State Department of Health.

The history of influenza virus research is very recent.

In 1931, Shope reported isolation of a virus which, in conjunction with H. influenzæ, suis, has caused influenza in swine in the middle west each fall since 1918.

In 1933, Laidlaw, Smith, and Andrewes reported isolation of a virus from human cases of influenza by means of intranasal inoculation of ferrets. They showed it to be closely related to the swine influenza virus.

In 1934, Francis reported isolation of the same virus from human influenza patients in Philadelphia and Puerto Rico.

In 1936, human influenza virus was transmitted to man accidentally from a ferret and produced clinical influenza. Russian human volunteers were infected by the human influenza virus. Influenza virus has been isolated in Russia, Germany, Australia, Alaska, and various parts of the U. S. A.

Strains of virus, while very closely related, do show a difference. Many problems need study:

1. There is the question of the existence of different strains which is of great importance in the production of vaccines.

2. Not all influenza-like diseases yield, on study, an influenza virus, yet some resemble influenza so closely in every respect that it seems certain they must be due to a virus, which, however, may be different from the influenza virus now known.

3. Clinically, it would be desirable, if possible, to differentiate the members of the influenza group from which it is possible to isolate a virus, from the rest of the group. Careful clinical studies are needed in association with influenza virus studies.

4. The whole group of respiratory diseases, included under the term "cold" and upper respiratory infection, need study from virus standpoint.

Present studies here are limited to those carried on in institutions since it is possible to study the clinical side better in such surroundings.

Rabies

We have been free from rabies since 1931 with the exception of one case in 1933 in a dog imported from Texas. This year, since May 4, positive diagnosis of rabies has been made in 105 dogs and 2 cattle. One hundred and sixty-nine people who have been in contact with the animals have taken rabies vaccine, and of these, thirty-one are said to have been bitten or scratched. In the lay mind, rabies causes greater apprehension than any other disease, and because of this, treatment is often demanded where degree of exposure does not justify treatment. Before giving antirabic treatment, the physician should question the patient carefully as to the type of exposure and type of lesion and examine the patient for lesions through which saliva may have entered. Risk of serious reactions from rabies vaccine, while not great, should be borne in mind when considering the use of antirabic vaccine in cases where exposure is slight.

Although rabies is a disease long studied problems in connection with the disease still require study:

1. The evidence of various strains and the question of various clinical forms of rabies in different outbreaks in dogs.

2. Incidence in various wild animals, and question of reservoir in wild animals.

3. Use of mice makes possible a study of immunity following the use of various type of vaccine, both in men and animals. Over 200 people have had rabies vaccine. Opportunity exists for study of immunity in them. A better vaccine is still desired, on which gives higher immunity and less reactions. It is hoped that it will be possible to study some of these problems here.

Encephalitis

During the past five years, great advance have been made in the study of encephalitis. Up to 1933 the diagnosis of encephalitis of the non-suppurative type was clinical and pathological. The history of encephalitis is quite recent.

In 1917, Economo reported clinical and pathological findings in cases of encephalitis occurring in Austria. The disease has been often named after him although epidemic or lethargic encephalitis is the usual name now used. 1918 and 1919 and the early '20's, there was great deal of this type of encephalitis reported. The disease has tended to occur sporadically since this time. This type of encephalitis has its greatest incidence in winter and spring and affects the younger age groups, fifteen to forty-five years of age. The disease is of slow onset, with low fever. It has a protracted course and numerous sequelæ. Eye muscle paralyses are common. Mortality is uncertain because of the existence of mild or questionable cases but is probably about 20 per cent. At the time the disease first appeared there were reports of transmission to animals and that it was due to a filterable virus. No further work was done.

In Japan, epidemics of another type of encephalitis have been occurring since 1871. The greatest epidemic occurred in 1924. It has been called summer encephalitis, because it occurred when the hot months were drawing to a close. It is acute in onset and short in course. The cranial nerve paralyses, so common in the Economo type, are rare in this type. Mortality has been, however, 60 to 90 per cent in various epidemics. The incidence and mortality increased directly with age. Sequelæ were few. The Japanese suggested that Economo encephalitis be called Type A, and that this be called Type B.

In 1933, an outbreak of encephalitis occurred in Missouri in St. Louis County and City. Over one thousand cases were reported. It started in July and the peak of incidence of disease occurred in late August. It resembled the Japanese type closely in time of appearance, age incidence and clinical course. There was sudden onset with headache, nausea or vomiting, and a temperature of 104-105°. Then there was drowsiness which might proceed to coma, or instead there might be delirium or restlessness. There was usually a short course, and the mortality was about 20 per cent. The sequelæ were few. Neurological findings outside of stiff neck and positive Kernig were not striking. There may have been absent abdominal reflexes, positive Babinski, or changed tendon reflexes. Paralysis of cranial nerves was uncommon.

A virus was soon isolated by Muckenfuss, Armstrong, and McCordock, and shortly after by Webster at the Rockefeller Institute. Monkeys and mice were found susceptible. It was shown that protective antibodies were present against the virus in blood obtained from convalescents.

In 1937 a similar epidemic occurred in St. Louis, and the same virus was again isolated.

In 1934 and 1935 other epidemics occurred in Japan and a virus was isolated that was shown to be distinct from the St. Louis type.

Equine Encephalomyelitis

Western Strain.—In 1931, Meyer, Haring, and Howitt reported the discovery of a virus as the cause of an epizoötic of encephalomyelitis among horses and mules in the San Joaquin Valley of California during the summer of 1930.

In 1933 the disease appeared along the eastern seaboard. In this year, TenBroeck and Merrill, and Biltner and Shahan reported the isolation of an eastern strain of equine encephalomyelitis virus which, though similar to the western strain, differed serologically. The disease in horses was more acute and fatal and the virus appeared to be more virulent for laboratory animals than the human strain.

The viruses of equine encephalomyelitis differ immunologically from the viruses of lymphocytic chorio-meningitis, the St. Louis type of encephalitis, Borna disease, vesicular stomatitis and poliomyelitis.

Present epidemiological and experimental evidence points to spread by an insect vector and not by contact. Experimentally, mosquitoes can be infected and transmit the virus to laboratory animals and horses. A. ægypti, A. sollicitans, A. nigromaculis, A. d o r s a l i s, A. albopictus Skuze, A. vexans, and A. tæniorhynchus, can transmit the western strain; A. cantator and A. sollicitans, the eastern strain. To date no one has found infected mosquitoes in localities where equine encephalomyelitis is prevalent.

Meyer, in 1932, suggested the possibility of human infection from the equine strain. He briefly reported three cases of encephalitis occurring in men closely associated with horses having encephalomyelitis. No virus was isolated or protective antibodies demonstrated.

Equine encephalomyelitis was very prevalent in Minnesota during the summer of 1937. During the last week of August and the first two weeks of September 1937, six cases of human encephalitis, all farmers, were reported from a county in Northwestern Minnesota. Five had had contact with sick horses. The sixth had had no contact with sick horses at the time of onset of his illness. He drove a tractor on a farm in North Dakota not far from the Minnesota border. There was much equine encephalomyelitis in this locality.

Blood was collected from three of the recovered patients during January 1938. Dr. C. TenBroeck of the Rockefeller Institute demonstrated neutralization of the Western strain of equine encephalomyelitis virus by one of the sera. Blood was collected again in May 1938 from this patient and neutralization again demonstrated by Dr. TenBroeck. This was the patient who had had no contact with sick horses and had been sick about three weeks.

Four mosquitoes shown to transmit the western strain occur in Minnesota: A. vexans, A. nigromaculis, A. dorsalis, and A. tæniorhynchus. Of these only A. vexans is a common mosquito.

Eastern Strain.—In late August and early September 1938, equine encephalomyelitis invaded southwestern Massachusetts for the first time. At the same time a highly fatal encephalitis among children appeared. Only meager clinical reports have been made to date. Drs. Fothergill, Dingle, Farber, and Connerly at Harvard isolated the eastern type of equine encephalomyelitis virus from the brain of a patient.

Drs. Webster and Wright at the Rockefeller Institute confirmed this, and in addition isolated the virus from the brains of four other patients. In addition, virus was sent to the Division of Animal Husbandry at Washington, D. C., and the above work was confirmed, using horses as experimental animals.

Summary

In summary, under the infectious non-suppurative type of encephalitis, the following known types of virus may be listed:

1. Economo or lethargic encephalitis, probably caused by virus.
2. Japanese type, virus isolated, protective bodies present against it in the serum of recovered patients.
3. St. Louis type, virus isolated, protective bodies present against it in the serum of recovered patients.
4. Encephalitis caused by eastern and western strains of equine encephalomyelitis virus, protective bodies present against them in the serum of recovered patients.

NOTE: After presentation of the above paper, isolation of the Western strain of virus from the brain of a twenty months old child was reported by Dr. B. F. Howitt of California.

EMERGENCY TREATMENT OF INJURIES*

H. M. LEE, M.D.

Minneapolis, Minnesota

THE susceptibility to injury is universal; there is no immunity. The treatment of the injured is chiefly the concern of the medical profession but not of the surgeon alone. This is especially true in smaller towns and rural communities. In the larger cities and industrial centers the major portion of the care of the injured has fallen to the general surgeon. In the last decade or two the industrial injuries at least have passed largely into the hands of the industrial surgeon. Even the laity must assume some responsibility in emergency treatment of injuries. It is not only frequent but almost the rule that some immediate care is rendered by laymen before skilled medical service is available. Many industrial plants and commercial institutions employ a lay person with some instruction in first aid. A nurse is frequently employed for

*Read at the annual meeting of the Minnesota State Medical Association, Duluth, Minnesota, June 30, 1938.

this purpose. I am certain that the morbidity in accidental injuries has thereby been reduced. The public generally has been enlightened along many medical lines, but I believe that with such general and only superficial information as we can broadcast, the importance and necessity of skilled medical care for every type of injury should be stressed. It is often the apparently insignificant but neglected puncture wound which leads to disaster. In my short discussion, I shall make no attempt to describe detailed surgical procedures applicable to the endless number of specific injuries which we encounter. I shall attempt rather to review and discuss certain principles of treatment applicable to types of injury, surgical principles most of which are neither new nor original but which, like a prayer, may bear repetition. For the purpose of this paper, injuries may be classified roughly according to anatomic location such as:

1. Head injuries
2. Injuries to chest and abdomen.
3. Injuries to the back.
4. Injuries to the extremities.

Injuries to the extremities are by far the most common and therefore of great importance, both from this and an economic standpoint. The symptoms and signs of injury requiring our immediate attention are: pain, hemorrhage, and shock.

Pain naturally varies in degree depending upon the severity and location of the injury, and the susceptibility of the individual to painful stimuli. There are certain portions of the body surface such as the lips, fingers, external genitalia, and the perianal region which are more richly innervated with pain fibers than are others. Likewise, there are some organs more sensitive to pain than others. For instance, bones give rise to pain more readily than do muscles. The sensitivity of the testis and blood vessels forms a tremendous contrast to the relative insensitivity of the fascia, cerebral cortex, and cartilage. The difference in susceptibility to pain in individuals is well recognized. Paralleling this phenomenon there is also the well known fact that there is a marked difference in susceptibility to drugs among individuals.[3]

Hemorrhage may be from the gaping margins of an open wound, into deep structures, or into closed cavities such as the cranial, thoracic, and abdominal. The natural processes which some into play to control and to arrest hemorrhage often do not suffice and then the surgeon must resort to artificial methods of controlling hemorrhage. Intravenous injections of calcium chloride or repeated small transfusions of whole blood may be indicated. At times, there may be troublesome bleeding from arteries which do not permit clamping or transfixing. In such a case a piece of fresh muscle rubbed on a piece of gauze and quickly applied will often promote clotting. Recognition of internal hemorrhage is often difficult. Here, the careful observation of blood pressure is of help. An increasing pulse rate should lead one to suspect bleeding. Pallor, anxiety, restlessness, and thirst are signs of continuing hemorrhage. Obviously, its control is urgent.

Shock is not always easy to differentiate from severe hemorrhage. In shock, however, the onset is usually abrupt. The patient is apathetic, but

not unconscious. There is no restlessness or anxiety, but rather, indifference. The temperature is subnormal, and there, too, the blood pressure is low. The treatment is external heat, judicious use of morphine (except in head injuries), elevation of the foot of bed, and blood transfusions.

The emergency treatment of injuries then, generally speaking, resolves itself into: (1) the management of symptoms as they present themselves; and (2) to the more deliberate and planned treatment of the injury itself. This planned treatment must consist of careful examination of the injury by inspection, frequently palpation, demonstration of function or loss thereof, and x-ray examination. The importance of this step is obvious. Many wounds have been sutured leaving severed tendons or nerve trunks unrecognized beneath the sutured skin. Foreign bodies in the depth of the wound are frequently over-looked. Fractured bones may be left unreduced and unsplinted. The next logical step is directed toward the prevention of infection in the clean wound and to combat infection in the contaminated wound. The former is accomplished by strict attention to asepsis, such as the proper preparation of the surgeon's hands, the wearing of a mask covering nose and mouth, a surgeon's cap, and aseptic care of patient's skin surrounding wound. This last is accomplished by careful cleansing of the skin with soap and water,[8] great care being taken not to wash dirt into the open wound. This can be done by carefully covering the wound with sterile dressings, and when an extremity is involved it should be raised as the skin proximal to the wound is cleansed and lowered for the washing of the region distal to the wound. The clean wound is then swabbed with an antiseptic which will not damage the tissue cells by precipitating protein. For this purpose I prefer one of the newer organic mercurial germicides. The wound is then closed not too tightly, loose dressings applied, unless temporary pressure is required to control bleeding.

The contaminated or potentially infected wound must receive the best care the surgeon's skill and experience can muster. How frequently we have seen extensive crushing lacerated wounds tightly sutured and snugly bandaged without proper preparation, and consequent disaster. The proper treatment of such a wound, after adequate examination, should consist in not only proper preparation of the surgeon as for a major operation but meticulous cleansing of the wound itself as well as the surrounding skin. This is accomplished again by thoroughly cleansing of the wound with neutral white soap and water or normal salt solution,[10] débridement of the devitalized skin and muscles, insertion of Carrel-Dakin tubes, and leaving the wound open or only partially closed, with loose dressings, immobilization, elevation, and irrigation every two hours with Dakin's solution.

Severed tendons and nerves should be sutured as early as possible. For this purpose, fine silk is recommended.[8] This applies at least to reasonably clean wounds or where there is a reasonable likelihood that the wound will heal without any severe infection. In contaminated wounds a secondary suture is advisable. A period of at least three weeks must elapse after the original wound is completely clean and healed. Suture of the extensor tendons on the dorsum of the hand to about the proximal phalanges offer the best prognosis.[11] Here, if the gap is not too great, union may occur even without suture. These tendons are free, isolated, and accessible. In the case of the middle phalanx of the fingers division of the tripartition of the extensor aponeurosis with its different insertion for each partition, causes a quite characteristic and prognostically very unfavorable injury. Injury to the flexor tendons of the hand and fingers offers a worse prognosis due to their ensheathed condition. In addition, the palm of the hand shows a structure very appropriate for the protection of sensitive structures, but very inappropriate surgically. Tendons should be sutured within six hours from time of injury if primary suture is done. The part should be immobilized for ten or twelve days in position to relieve tension, and splinted for three weeks. Essentially, the same rule applies to both severed tendons and nerves.

The treatment of localized infections and frankly infected wounds is not ordinarily considered emergency treatment, but frequently patients with such conditions do not seek any medical care until infection is well established. The treatment may depend somewhat on the location of the infection. In general, a spreading infection should be allowed to localize before any incision is made.[6] Infections about the face, mouth, and neck should be treated very conservatively. Blair has stated that he has never seen a fatality in such a case treated conservatively, that is, where the infection has not been pinched, punctured, or incised or otherwise traumatized. The treatment should consist of application of heat, ultra-violet rays, rest, and fluids. Sulfanilamide may be indicated. Infected wounds and spreading infections in other locations are also best treated by hot packs consisting of light moist dressings kept warm with a heat cradle or lamp, and elevation. The matter of hot packs is of some importance in its application. These are best applied as light moist dressings kept warm with a heat cradle, frequently moistening the dressings with sterile water, normal saline, or boric acid solution. Frequently, hot packs are applied in great bulk. These gradually cool and before long the wound is enveloped in a cold pack. The purpose of the hot pack is to produce active hyperemia and this is facilitated by elevation of the extremity to relieve the passive hyperemia.

Ochsner's solution, properly applied, is of definite therapeutic value in spreading infections with lymphangitis and induration.

X-ray treatment of infections is apparently of real benefit.[4] Koch[6] gives a half erythema dose and has found this to be of definite value.

Localized infections and tendon sheath infections require immediate incision and drainage. Hot packs, as described above, and elevation is indicated.

Recently, Wangensteen at the University of Minnesota, has described treatment of acute infections by rigid immobilization of the extremity in plaster-of-Paris casts holding the extremity in elevation. He has shown that this type of treatment is of definite value.

Burns, especially if at all extensive, are best treated by the so-called tannic acid treatment. This was introduced by Davison about twelve years ago. Bettman has recently modified this treatment to the extent of applying silver nitrate after the application of tannic acid.[5] The technic of this treatment consists, first of opening all blebs, removing all burned and necrotic tissue, cleansing the burned area of grease and dirt, then spraying the burned area with a freshly prepared 5 per cent aqueous solution of tannic acid and following this with application of 10 per cent silver nitrate with cotton pledgets. The patient is then placed on a sterile sheet and a heat cradle applied over the body. For small burns, I personally prefer nupercainal ointment. This relieves pain promptly, dressings do not stick to the wound, no heavy crusts form, and the wound is easily kept clean.

The emergency treatment of chest and abdominal injuries is an extensive subject in itself and will be discussed only briefly. (A recent article by Karl Meyer is made free use of.) Practically all penetrating wounds of the abdomen should be explored as soon as possible, taking into consideration, of course, the patient's general condition. Hemorrhage and shock must be treated first unless it is apparent that there is rapid and extensive internal hemorrhage which only immediate operation can control. Perforations of the bowel and stomach produced by stab or bullet wounds are closed. The most rapid method of accomplishing this is to make a long paramedian incision and at once eviscerate the intestines into warm wet towels. Small to moderate sized wounds of the liver are best sutured with catgut through pieces of muscle excised from the abdominal wall. Muscle may also be inserted into the wound cleft.

Both surfaces of the liver must be repaired. Large wounds of the liver must be tamponed with gauze, left as a drain, and a snug bandage applied about the abdomen for pressure.[7] Such abdominal wounds are not drained; only the abdominal wall. Wounds of the spleen of any degree are best treated by splenectomy. Wounds of the pancreas are sutured or tamponed and drained. In suspected rupture of the urinary bladder Butler recommends, if the urine contains blood or if no urine is obtained by catheter, the injection of 500 c.c. of 5 per cent sodium iodide solution and x-ray to make a positive diagnosis.[1] Wounds of the urinary bladder are closed with catgut in two layers and the bladder kept empty by means of a retained catheter for six or seven days.

In injuries of the chest it should be kept in mind that half of the ribs cover the abdomen so that penetrating wounds below the fifth rib must lead one to suspect injury to abdominal viscera. The usual policy in penetrating wounds of the lungs is conservative management.

Head injuries may vary from minor lacerations of the scalp to extensive skull fractures with varying degrees of brain injury. Severe head injuries must be treated by bed rest, ex-

ternal heat, intravenous administration of 50 to 150 c.c. of dextrose solution, probably lumbar puncture and drainage reducing the pressure 50 per cent and limitation of fluids.[2]

Craig advises against the use of morphine in severe head injuries.[2] He recommends the use of barbiturates. Sodium amytal intravenously may be given for quieting. The closest observation is indicated. I am omitting from my paper any discussion of back injuries and fractures.

Summary

1. Some general knowledge of first aid treatment of injuries on the part of the public is important.

2. All injuries should receive the most careful care in regard to general cleanliness and asepsis.

3. Skilled surgical care is indicated in all types of injuries.

4. Experience and judgment are important qualifications in determining the type of treatment indicated in infected wounds.

5. Immobilization, elevation, and heat are important therapeutic measures in treating injuries and infections.

Bibliography

1. Butler, Edmund: Injuries of chest and abdomen. Surg. Gyn. and Obst., 66:448-453, (Feb.) 1938.
2. Craig, Winchell M.: Adequate and inadequate treatment of injuries of the head. Minn. Med., 20:712-716, (Nov.) 1937.
3. Firor, Warfield M.: Lewis' Practice of Surgery, Vol. 1, Chap. 8.
4. Hanson, M. B.: X-ray treatment of acute infections. Minn. Med., 21:146, (Feb.) 1938.
5. Hedin, Raymond F.: The immediate and subsequent treatment of burns. Minn. Med., 21:229-236, (Apr.) 1938.
6. Koch, Summer L.: Care of infected wounds. Surg. Gyn. and Obst., 66:105, (Feb.) 1938.
7. Meyer, Karl, and Shapiro, Philip F.: Treatment of abdominal injuries. Surg., Gyn. and Obst., 66:245-256, (Mar.) 1936.
8. O'Shay, Maurice Culmer: Severed tendons and nerves of the hand and forearm. Ann. Surg., 105:228-242, (Feb.) 1937.
9. Power, D'Arcy: Short History of Surgery. London, 1933.
10. Reid, Mont. R., and Stevenson, John: Treatment of fresh wounds. Surg. Gyn. and Obst., 66:313, (Apr.) 1938.
11. Stahel. W.: Ueber Schnenverletzungen der Hand. Schweiz. med. Wchnschr., 67:51-54, (Jan. 16) 1937.

Discussion

DR. BENJAMIN F. DAVIS, Duluth: Amidst the avalanche of advice as to what to do, especially in certain classes of industrial emergencies, basic principles of surgery are frequently lost sight of. The demand to do something is so great that many times a something is done just because it is the fad of the moment, or worked out well in a previous case, regardless of the indications which a proper analysis of the particular case to be treated would show.

Consider the matter of wound infections. The arguments as to the type of disinfectant, if any, to be used, the type of drainage to be employed, how to apply hot moist dressings and so on are beside the point of minor importance. The question is, how long an interval has elapsed since this wound was inflicted, what is the character of the wound and what is the degree of contamination? Wounds seen within twelve to twenty-four hours of their infliction are in the stage of contamination. The bacteria are on the surface and careful mechanical cleansing of the wound with removal of devitalized tissue very frequently will permit of primary closure and primary union. Wounds seen in the next twelve to twenty-four hours will be in the stage of invasion. Bacteria may have penetrated beneath the surface cells and have been carried into the deepest recesses, and mechanical cleansing, other than complete debridement, may not suffice to remove all such organisms but probably will greatly minimize the degree of subsequent wound infection. Wounds seen after forty-eight to seventy-two hours, will almost certainly be in the stage of established infection. Mechanical cleansing will accomplish little, but adequate drainage, if infection is established, is essential.

The immobilization of infected wounds either by splints or casts is of prime importance and the essayist is to be commended for emphasizing a point which is too often forgotten.

Consider, now, the matter of head injuries, particularly when associated with loss of consciousness. Here, more than in any other field of industrial surgery, the temptation to fit the patient into some special form of treatment rather than to make the treatment fit the patient seems to be well nigh irresistible. Each case of head injury, with loss of consciousness, must be individualized. Frequent observations on the condition of the pulse, the respiration, the rectal temperature and the state of consciousness should be made. In the majority of instances, it will be possible, by this means alone, to estimate the danger of mounting intracranial pressure fairly accurately and to determine when surgical decompression becomes necessary and when less radical measures may suffice. I can best illustrate this idea by the means of two case histories:

Case 1.—This patient fell while in an alcoholic state, and struck his head against a curbstone. He was unconscious for five minutes, but on admission to the hospital his state of consciousness was good, his respiration normal, his temperature by mouth 99.6° F.,

and his pulse 60. He was discharged on the eighth day after his accident, "feeling fine except for slight headache," with his state of consciousness good, his respiration and temperature normal and his pulse 56. The following morning, however, this patient returned to the hospital, complaining of severe headache and vomiting. His state of consciousness, respiration and temperature were as before, and his pulse rate was 60. After thirty-six hours of rest in bed, the pulse rose to the seventies and the headache and vomiting ceased. This was a case of head injury with concussion, a moderate increase of intracranial pressure, well compensated (note the moderate bradycardia), and required no complicated or radical treatment.

Case 2.—This patient had had a mild headache for one week. Immediately after making a sudden effort, she clasped her hands to her head and complained of a sudden, severe headache. This was immediately followed by a clonic convulsion and unconsciousness. On admission to the hospital, the patient had regained consciousness; her temperature was 97.4° F., her respiration 29, her pulse 64. The spinal fluid was bloody. The patient became drowsy and gradually stuporous, as the pulse dropped to 48 and the respiration to 10. Breathing became of the Cheyne-Stokes type. This condition persisted for approximately 24 hours, when, without other change, the temperature rose to 100, the pulse to 140 and the patient died. Autopsy disclosed hemorrhage from a ruptured aneurysm of the right middle meningeal artery. This was a case in increasing intracranial pressure finally extending beyond the limits of physiologic compensation; the physiologic signs demanded radical treatment, but were disregarded.

I believe that each of these cases is typical of a certain group of head injuries and that in each the clinical story is clearly told by the obvious physiologic changes, which also clearly indicate the treatment demanded.

I am not taking issue with the essayist on any of the points which he has raised in his excellent paper. It is my purpose to stress the necessity for properly analyzing and diagnosing the conditions to be met and making the treatment fit the patient rather than to rely on stereotyped formulæ.

ABDOMINAL INJURIES*

E. MENDELSSOHN JONES, M.D.

Saint Paul, Minnesota

ABDOMINAL injuries caused by penetrating wounds or by contusion of the abdomen with resulting visceral damage are accompanied by a high mortality. In 1890 the mortality rate was about 90 per cent. This figure has gradually dropped until at present the rate for this type of injury throughout the United States is approximately 50 per cent. These patients are most frequently seen in industrial hospitals and in the large city hospitals. A group of seventy-one cases treated at Ancker Hospital in St. Paul were reviewed. This hospital has a large and very active emergency service. Despite the fact that

these patients are given immediate treatment and kept under constant observation it is startling to learn the high mortality encountered. What is the reason for this high mortality in an institution adequately equipped to care for such cases?

This group includes thirty-two patients who had received penetrating abdominal wounds, and thirty-nine patients who had abdominal contusions accompanied by visceral injury.

Twenty-eight of the patients with penetrating wounds were operated upon, four having been so badly injured that there was no possibility of giving any surgical relief. Fifteen of this group recovered and seventeen died, a mortality of about

*Read before the annual meeting of the Minnesota State Medical Association, Duluth, Minnesota, June 30, 1938.

TABLE I. ABDOMINAL INJURIES

Total number of cases	71
A. Penetrating wounds with visceral injury	32
Cases operated upon	28
Recovered	15
Died	17
Mortality	53.2%
B. Contused wounds with visceral injury	39
Cases operated upon	14
Recovered	7
Died after operation	7
Died without operation	25
Mortality	82.1%

TABLE II. PENETRATING WOUNDS

Gun shot wounds	27
Stab wounds	5
Cases operated upon	28
Not operated upon	4

Cases not operated upon, all gun shot wounds:
1. Died three hours after admission. Perforation of mesentery and kidney. Severe hemorrhage.
2. Died two hours after admission. Perforation of colon and jejunum. Severe hemorrhage.
3. Died seven hours after admission. Severe wounds of abdomen, chest and head.
4. Died four days after admission. Injury to lung, spleen, stomach, colon and small intestine.

TABLE III. PENETRATING WOUNDS OPERATION DEATHS

Died within six hours	4
Died within twelve hours	3
Died within twenty-four hours	3
Died after forty-eight hours	7
Died following operation	13

This group of patients had the following injuries:

Liver and duodenum	1
Small intestine	1
Small intestine and colon	3
Pancreas, duodenum and liver	1
Small intestine, iliac vein, severe hemorrhage	2
Stomach and small intestine	1
Colon	1
Small intestine and kidney	1
Liver and stomach	1
Colon and spleen	

TABLE IV. PENETRATING WOUNDS. OPERATION RECOVERIES

Cases operated with recovery	
Injuries to liver	3
Small intestine, spleen—spleenectomy	1
Small intestine	6
Colon and small intestine	1
Spleen and kidney—splenectomy	2
Stomach and duodenum	1
Stomach and transverse colon	1

53.2 per cent. A brief analysis of this group is shown in Tables I to IV.

It is interesting to note that the highest number of recoveries occurred in the patients in this group in whom the small intestine was the only abdominal viscus injured, and that only one of these died. Furthermore, all but two who died

TABLE V. CONTUSED WOUNDS OF THE ABDOMEN WITH VISCERAL INJURY

Seven patients recovered. All operated upon. This group had the following injuries:

Rupture of liver	1
Rupture of bladder	2
Rupture of small intestine	3
Rupture of spleen, splenectomy	1

Seven patients died following operation:

Died within six hours	3
Died within twelve hours	1
Died within twenty-four hours	1
Died after forty-eight hours	2

TABLE VI. CONTUSED WOUNDS. INJURIES FOUND IN PATIENTS WHO DIED AFTER OPERATION

Rupture of liver	2
Rupture of spleen, splenectomy	3
Stomach, small intestine and colon	1
Ruptured bladder	1
Died without operation	25
Died within six hours	15
Died within twelve hours	2
Died within twenty-four hours	3
Died within forty-eight hours	5

TABLE VII. CONTUSED WOUNDS. INJURIES FOUND IN NON-OPERATION DEATHS

Ruptured liver	11
Ruptured liver and spleen	3
Ruptured spleen	2
Rupture of small intestine and colon	1
Rupture of small intestine	2
Ruptured bladder	2
Rupture of kidney, spleen and liver	1
Rupture of kidney and liver	1
Retroperitoneal hemorrhage	1

Fourteen patients in this group had one or more complicating fractures.

had two or more structures injured, increasing the gravity of the problem and partially explaining the high mortality rate.

There were thirty-nine cases of contusion of the abdomen with visceral injury (Tables V to VII). Fourteen of these patients were operated upon with seven recoveries. Twenty-five died without operation and of this group fifteen died within six hours after admission. There were severe liver injuries in eleven instances in the non-operated group. Fourteen of these patients sustained one or more fractures in addition to the abdominal injury, again contributing to the appalling mortality rate. There is no question that many of the injuries we are called upon to treat today are more complicated and severe than those encountered before the advent of the high-speed motor car and the speed mania that has spread over the country. Many of the automobile injuries are of the crushing type and there is often injury to the liver or spleen with or without injury to any other abdominal viscus. In this group of thirty-nine cases there was either a liver or a spleen injury alone or combined in twenty-six instances. This fact in itself explains a great deal of the high mortality rate in this group.

There are no cases included in this series of simple contusion or concussion of the abdomen. In this type of injury the patient is "knocked out" for a few minutes and recovery is prompt. However, in the more severe cases the picture is more complicated, presenting marked pallor, anxious expression, severe pain in the abdomen, labored, shallow respiration, thin, rapid pulse, low blood pressure, subnormal temperature, and frequently nausea and vomiting. Usually patients with simple contusion recover in a few hours from the state of shock. The picture of shock in these cases is similar to that found when visceral injury is present and it frequently is three or four hours before a positive diagnosis can be made. The shock is likely to be less profound and the recovery is usually more rapid. Because of the difficulty in differentiation, an occasional unnecessary abdominal exploration is carried out.

When there is contusion of the abdomen with visceral injury, the primary shock above described is present and with proper shock treatment, recovery occurs in three to four hours. At this point it is necessary to determine, if possible, the extent of the visceral injury. Very close observation of the patient is absolutely essential and every clinical sign must be carefully observed. In this way the early warning signs following the initial improvement can be detected. An increase in the pulse rate with a decrease in its volume is found in cases of marked hemorrhage. Muscular rigidity is frequently present and tenderness over the injured area may often be found. In injuries to the spleen a severe pain in the left shoulder, with painful respiration and restricted diaphragmatic movement on the left confirmed by x-ray, is of valuable diagnostic importance. If, after careful analysis of all the findings, it is determined that there is severe intra-abdominal bleeding, immediate exploration should be done. However, should the symptoms not indicate a severe hemorrhage there is no immediate operative emergency to deal with and expectant treatment may be followed.

One must, however, bear in mind that in spleen injuries there may be a delayed hemorrhage necessitating surgical treatment. A recent example of this was a young man who was playing basketball and was struck in the abdomen by the head of an opponent. He was able to finish the game but did not feel right. He consulted his physician and was allowed to return to work the next day. About ten days after the injury he was admitted to the Ancker Hospital. He presented the picture of severe, intra-abdominal bleeding. His abdomen was explored and a spleen that weighed 760 grams was found fractured. The abdomen contained a great quantity of blood. A splenectomy was done. He developed post-operative pneumonia and after this subsided he was apparently making a good recovery. However, he again began running a high fever and a cause for the temperature was not found. He died about thirty days after admission. On autopsy many ulcerations were found in the intestines and eventually a diagnosis of typhoid fever was made. During the search for the cause of his temperature, a Widal test was made and reported negative.

It is very important to obtain an accurate history to determine if possible the degree of force and the direction of its application. When there is evidence of rupture of a hollow viscus, exploration must be performed as soon as the condition of the patient will permit. It has been shown that under these circumstances the mortality mounts greatly if this is not done within six hours after the injury.

The x-ray is a great aid in making a diagnosis of bowel or stomach perforation as free gas can often be observed under the diaphragm. Examination should be made with the patient in an erect position if possible, but if the patient is too ill he should lie on the right side, as a small amount of gas is more easily detected on the left side. Each case presents a different clinical problem and calls for the keenest clinical analysis by the surgeon. It is conceded that various clinical and laboratory methods are important but they do not replace keen clinical sense and interpretation. A recent experience was that of a man working with a motor-driven circular saw. A small piece of wood about four inches long and an inch wide flew from the saw and struck him in the abdomen. He had severe abdominal pain and was taken to a physician. The incident was treated lightly and he was sent home. His employer was not satisfied and wished further investigation. The patient, when admitted to the hospital, was having severe abdominal pain and had slight tenderness over the mid-abdomen. X-ray examination showed no free gas in the abdomen. In spite of this an exploration was done immediately and a laceration was found in the jejunum. This was sutured and the patient made a prompt recovery.

Injuries to the urinary bladder are frequently encountered, especially so in association with a fracture of the pelvis, and the repair should be done as soon as possible. Crushing injuries to the kidney are also common but do not often call for an emergency procedure as the injury is retroperitoneal and the compactness of the structure in this area aids in controlling the hemorrhage. An x-ray picture will sometimes show gas around the kidney and thus indicate rupture of the retroperitoneal portion of the duodenum or retroperitoneal portion of the colon.

Injuries to the gallbladder and bile ducts are not frequently encountered, but when present they must be cared for surgically. In pancreatic injury there may be a complete tear which sets free the pancreatic secretions, and pancreatic digestion and necrosis follow. Unless this damage is repaired and drainage established, the injury is usually fatal. There may be a less severe injury to the pancreas, resulting in the formation of a pancreatic cyst. Not infrequently mesenteric tears occur, resulting in severe hemorrhage demanding early surgical relief. Diaphragmatic hernia is another condition that must be considered in connection with contusion injuries to the abdomen. In a person receiving a severe blow to the abdomen a hernia through one of the diaphragmatic openings, usually the esophageal, may develop. When the abdominal injury is accompanied by a chest injury, there may be a rupture of the right or left hemi-diaphragm.

Bullet wounds or stab wounds of the abdomen may not injure any of the viscera, but if there is a perforating injury to a solid viscus, hemorrhage results, and peritonitis develops if there is perforation of a hollow viscus. Gunshot wounds are prone to give rise to tetanus, gas bacillus and other infections not only of the peritoneal cavity but of the abdominal wall. Unless one is positive that the wound has just grazed the abdominal wall without entering the peritoneal cavity, the abdomen should be explored immediately. Bullet

wounds may cause many perforations of the intestines and all the perforations must be closed. It has often been pointed out that in this type of injury there is an even number of perforations, and this is a valuable point to keep in mind. These openings are often very difficult to find. In discussing this point with Dr. John Noble, Pathologist at the Ancker Hospital, he commented on the number of cases that he has seen come to the autopsy table that have died of peritonitis because one intestinal perforation had been overlooked.

I realize the mortality rate of 53.2 per cent in the cases with penetrating abdominal injuries seems high, but it corresponds to other reports for similar cases. As pointed out previously, the highest number of recoveries occurred in the cases receiving only small bowel injury. The high mortality rate of 82.1 per cent in the group of contusions with visceral injury is explained by the severity of the abdominal injuries and also by the other severe injuries frequently sustained.

Summary

1. Abdominal injury complicated by visceral damage is accompanied by a high mortality.

2. Constant observation of these cases is necessary until the extent of the injury is determined.

3. The treatment of shock is the first consideration in cases of abdominal injury.

4. Abdominal exploration should be carried out as soon as possible in cases of severe intra-abdominal hemorrhage and in penetrating wounds of the abdomen.

Bibliography

1. Metz, Arthur R.; Householder, Raymond; and DePree, James F.: Treatment of abdominal trauma. Surg. Gynec. and Obst., 64:373-375, 1937.
2. Hanchett, McMicken: Abdominal trauma and its diagnosis. Industrial Med., 6:14-17, (Jan.) 1937.
3. Bisgard, J. Dewey: The traumatic abdomen. Nebraska State Med. Jour., 22:294-300, (Aug.) 1937.
4. Wangensteen, O. H.: Abdominal injuries. Internat. Surg. Dig., 21:323-335, (June) 1936.
5. Farley, J. B.: Diagnosis and treatment of traumatic injuries of intra-abdominal viscera. Colorado Med., 33:543-546, 1936.
6. Donald, D. C.: Traumatic injury of abdomen with extensive damage to colon and small bowel. Am. Jour. Surg., 36:514-519, 1937.
7. Thomson, John: Non-penetrating injuries to the abdominal viscera. Indiana Med. Jour., 29:229-232, 1936.

Discussion

Dr. Wm. C. Bernstein: It has been a pleasure for me to listen to Dr. Jones' very clear and frank discussion of abdominal injuries. Drawing on my limited experience, compared to his, it would be difficult for me to add much of consequence to his paper. However, I would like to discuss several points.

Practicing as I do in rural Southern Minnesota, I am often impressed with the large number of these major abdominal injuries which occur outside the industrial centers. Farm implements and farm animals account for a large number of these accidents but the ever increasing automobile hazard on the highways where strict traffic regulations are not enforced as they are in the cities furnish a great many cases of abdominal injuries. Gun-shot wounds of the abdomen during the hunting season are also becoming quite common. For this reason most small hospitals in rural Minnesota have become equipped to handle these cases as well as they are handled in any larger center. I say this without fear of contradiction.

Dr. Jones has stressed the point that close and undivided attention must be given to these patients during the first hours to determine whether the shock is due to the so-called "abdominal concussion" or to actual visceral damage. This brings up the question of blood transfusion in these cases. So often, we hear of large amounts of blood or other fluids being given to a patient for his hemorrhage where, in fact, the fluid is running out of his torn vessel as fast as it is being introduced into the vein. Many patients would be better benefited if the abdomen were opened, the bleeding vessels tied off, and the introduction of blood or other fluids then started. We must not forget that raising the blood pressure can easily start a vessel bleeding once more.

Finally, I would like to emphasize the point that many a patient's life has been saved by the good judgment of the surgeon in deferring operation. This is especially true in cases of retroperitoneal injury, including rupture of the kidney. Dr. Jones has mentioned the fact that due to the compactness of the structures, hemorrhage here often takes care of itself. I recall one case in point where a man had a ruptured kidney and was brought in in extreme shock. There is no question but what he would have died if we had operated on him. We treated him expectantly and when he was in good shape for operation he refused and has now worked hard for five years without an operation.

INTRACTABLE LOW BACK AND SCIATIC PAIN DUE TO PROTRUDED INTERVERTEBRAL DISKS: DIAGNOSIS AND TREATMENT*

J. GRAFTON LOVE, M.D.

Rochester, Minnesota

THE intervertebral disks act as shock absorbers; they probably were the first hydraulic shock absorbers invented. When one of these disks becomes injured and a portion of it protrudes, the patient may complain of backache or sciatic pain. For years, such patients have received the most varied treatment. The treatment in many cases has run the gamut of pharmacologic, orthopedic and physical therapeutic measures. Manipulations and adjustments by irregular practitioners likewise have been given credit for the relief and, in some cases, even for semimiraculous cures of some of these partially or wholly disabled individuals.

The more or less general use of roentgenography in studying the vertebral columns and sacro-iliac synchondroses of individuals whose chief complaints were backache and sciatica did much to clarify thinking concerning painful conditions of the spinal column. The condition known in the earlier literature as "railway spine" practically disappeared. Physicians and even laymen began to feel that if roentgenograms of the vertebral column gave evidence of a normal condition and no evidence of fracture, there could be no gross change in the skeleton to ac-

count for the pains in the back and legs. During the past few years tremendous progress has been made in diagnosis and treatment of many heretofore obscure painful conditions.

It is not my desire to increase the number of already alarmingly high industrial hazards nor to cause men and women to seek compensation that is not their just dessert. It is my desire only to call attention once again to a very common cause of partial or complete chronic invalidism. This cause is notorious for the paucity of objective findings in the course of the usual physical examination. Ordinary roentgenography, likewise, fails in the vast majority of cases to give a clue to the real pathologic condition which underlies the patient's disability.

Although lesions of the intervertebral disks as a cause of intractable sciatic pain have been recognized for many years and Adson, at the Mayo Clinic, in 1922, cured a dentist of intractable sciatica by removing a protrusion of a lumbar disk, it has only been within the last few years that a more general appreciation of the rôle of the intervertebral disks in the causation of compression of the spinal cord and nerve roots, with subsequent development of painful syndromes, has come about.[5]

Prior to the realization of the frequency with which intervertebral disks may be protruded and

*From the Section on Neurologic Surgery, The Mayo Clinic, Rochester, Minnesota. Read before the meeting of the Minnesota State Medical Association, Duluth, Minnesota, June 29 to July 1, 1938.

be the cause of low back and sciatic pain, laminectomy for removal of such cartilaginous protrusions was infrequent. Today, laminectomy for removal of protruded disks is one of the commonest of neurosurgical operations performed at The Mayo Clinic.

A clear understanding of the nature of the normal intervertebral disk and of its relationship to the two adjoining vertebral bodies, to the posterior longitudinal ligament, to the intervertebral foramina and to the spinal cord and nerve roots is essential to full appreciation of the rôle which the cartilaginous intervertebral disk plays in the production of chronic continuous or of intermittent and recurring low back and sciatic pain.

The intervertebral disk is composed of two parts: (1) the annulus fibrosus, a rather dense, elastic fibrocartilage, which is intimately attached to the margins of the adjoining vertebral bodies; (2) the nucleus pulposus, a very soft resilient tissue which is enclosed, and in the normal state is maintained by the annulus fibrosus. Normally, the posterior longitudinal ligament, which extends from the second cervical vertebra to the sacrum, and thus forms a part of the anterior wall of the spinal canal, aids in the maintenance of the intervertebral disk within its position. The spinal cord, surrounded by its meninges, lies directly posterior to the posterior longitudinal ligament and the paired spinal nerves emerge from the dural sac and leave the spinal canal at the intervertebral foramina. A more detailed study of the spinal nerves and their relationship[1] to the intervertebral spaces is necessary for a clear understanding of the way in which a particular protruded disk may involve a given nerve root. The fact that the spinal nerves do not come off at right angles and do not immediately leave the spinal canal opens the possibility of considerable variation occurring in the impingement of some of the disks on the nerve roots.

Intervertebral disks occur throughout the spinal column from the space between the second and third cervical vertebræ to the coccyx. Those present in the fixed vertebral segments (sacrum and coccyx) are rudimentary, however, and rarely, if ever, are protruded with the resultant production of low back and sciatic pain.

As far as is known, any of the others may be protruded, although there are certain disks which seem particularly vulnerable.[6] At the clinic we

have encountered several protrusions in the cervical and thoracic regions of the spinal column, but by far the largest number of protrusions encountered have been in the lumbar region.

Etiology and Pathology of Protruded Intervertebral Disk

The nucleus pulposus consists of a semisolid substance and when stress or strain is applied to the back the nucleus pulposus may be forced against the elastic annulus fibrosus and cause considerable stretching of this latter structure. When the stress is ended, normally the disk returns to its usual position. When unusual stress or strain is applied to the back the annulus fibrosus may be injured and then a portion of the disk escapes from its normal position between the vertebræ. The portion of the disk which escapes or protrudes may consist of a pea-sized fragment of fibrocartilage, or it may be several centimeters in length and breadth (Fig. 1). The majority of the protrusions, however, are small and their ability to produce symptoms depends on their relationship to nerve roots.

It is my feeling that true protrusions of intervertebral disks are a result of undue stress or strain placed on the fibrocartilaginous annulus fibrosus. The stress may be secondary to the lifting of a heavy object,[2] the cranking of a tractor, forceful unexpected sitting (such as on a slippery pavement) or to a blow on the back. Whether there is one or more than one predisposing cause which makes one individual more susceptible to this lesion than another I am unprepared to say. It is true that many of our patients at the clinic have had congenital anomalies of the spinal column, particularly in the region of the lumbosacral joint. These anomalies have consisted of the presence of four or six lumbar vertebræ instead of the usual five; partial or complete sacralization of the last lumbar vertebra; partial or complete lumbarization of the first sacral vertebra; incomplete fusion of the laminæ posteriorly, with the occurrence of spina bifida occulta and of anomalies of position of the articular facets, particularly of those of the fifth lumbar and first sacral vertebræ. About 25 per cent of our patients have been unable to recall an injury to the back even after a protruded disk has been removed.[7]

The cartilage which protrudes into the spinal canal and encroaches on the spinal cord or on one

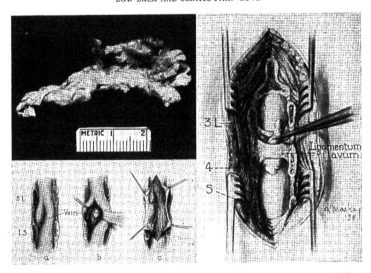

Fig. 1 (*upper left*). Protruded portion of lumbosacral disk removed at operation in a case in which backache and sciatica had endured for one year. Complete relief was obtained following removal of the protruded portion.

Fig. 2 (*right*). In this case a portion of a protruded disk had perforated an hypertrophied ligamentum flavum.

Fig. 3 (*lower left*). The findings at operation in a case in which backache and left sciatic pain had endured for twelve years. *a*, the characteristic enlargement of the nerve root; *b*, the thinned out posterior longitudinal ligament has been incised and the protruded portion of the disk is escaping; *c*, enlargement of the intradural portion of the fifth lumbar and first sacral nerve roots on the left. The remainder of the cauda equina is normal.

or more nerve roots may be small or relatively large, as large as a section of the cord itself. So far as I know, however, the entire disk never protrudes and since surgical treatment of this condition consists in removal of the protruded portion of the disk, the entire disk is never removed. Some of the protruded portions are so small that they may be overlooked on superficial examination of the intervertebral space. Some, however, are so large that they obstruct the spinal canal and appear and feel as if they were large, intraspinal neoplasms. At times the disk is so completely fragmented that loose fragments of cartilage may be found lying on the dorsal aspect of the dural sac. In one case, a piece of disk tissue was found, having perforated a ligamentum flavum (Fig. 2). In the majority of cases, however, the findings are similar and characteristic. The majority of the protrusions occur laterally (the central part of the posterior longitudinal ligament is strongest and there are deficiencies laterally) and thus the unilaterality of symptoms and signs is explained. The nerve root compressed by the protruded disk is always enlarged owing to injection and edema secondary to the compression (Fig. 3). The enlarged nerve root is usually elevated and appears more posterior than does its fellow of the opposite side. At times the enlarged nerve root is displaced mesially or laterally by the protruded disk. The variations of the relationship of the protrusion to the nerve root cause minor variations in the technic of removal of the protruded portion. Ordinarily the protrusion appears as a smooth, rounded or dome-shaped tumefaction, the resilience of which is easily tested when slight pressure is applied to it with an instrument. Occasionally, when the involved nerve root is retracted, one or more loose fragments of cartilage will pop out free into the canal and they are lifted from the wound with forceps. The usual condition, however, requires incision of the "cap-

834

sule" which allows the bulging cartilaginous fragments to escape. The capsule is a thinned portion of the posterior longitudinal ligament. The fragments unwind, as it were (Fig. 3b), as they

cord by an intraspinal neoplasm. If the protrusion into the spinal canal occurs laterally, as it most often does, then the early symptoms are those of irritation of a nerve root and, later,

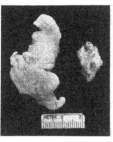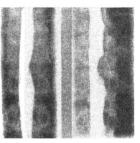

Fig. 4 (*left*). Protruded portion of fourth lumbar disk which had produced paraplegia and complete subarachnoid block. The smaller specimen represents the hypertrophied overlying ligamentum flavum.

Fig. 5 (*right*). Postero-anterior and antero-posterior roentgenograms which demonstrate a defect in the column of lipiodol opposite the eleventh thoracic intervertebral space. The patient had had backache without sciatica for ten years. At operation an hypertrophied ligamentum flavum was resected and a protruded portion of the eleventh thoracic intervertebral disk was removed. The patient has been relieved of his backache.

escape through the incision in the ligament, and they appear much like ragged pieces of tendon which have been matted together in a small ball. The protrusions vary in consistency from that of soft mucoid material to the bony hardness of complete ossification.

Microscopically, various degrees of degeneration are noted. There may be simple edema or there may be various stages of hyaline degeneration, calcification or ossification. The tissue contains both nuclear and annular material[1] and it is for that reason that we prefer to designate the lesion by the term "protruded disk" rather than "herniated nucleus pulposus," "rupture of the intervertebral disk," or any of the other terms used in connection with injury and extrusion of intervertebral fibrocartilage. True neoplasms of the disks occur, but that is another subject and is not to be considered in this paper.

Symptoms and Diagnosis

The symptoms produced by protrusion of an intervertebral disk vary according to the disk involved and the site at which the protrusion occurs in relation to the particular disk. If the protrusion occurs in the midline in the cervical or thoracic region of the spinal canal the symptoms are likely to be those of compression of the spinal

those of interruption of the impulses that travel along that nerve, owing to severe compression. Large protrusions in the lumbar region may give all the symptoms and signs of an intraspinal neoplasm and produce paraplegia by compressing the cauda equina and interrupting all nerve function below the level of the lesion (Fig. 4).

Of all the protrusions of disks for which we have performed laminectomy (more than 200) about 90 per cent have occurred in the lumbar region and the most common symptom has been sciatic pain.[3] The pain in the course of the sciatic nerve, on one side or, more rarely, both sides, may be and usually is associated with more or less pain in the lower part of the back. The low back pain is situated in the lumbar region, lumbosacral region, over the sacro-iliac synchondroses, or it may exist chiefly in the buttocks. A small percentage of patients have had low back pain without projection of the pain along sciatic nerves. When low back pain exists for a considerable period without projection along one or both sciatic nerves, the protrusion is more likely to be in the lower thoracic region than in the lumbar region (Fig. 5).

The patient who has a protruded intervertebral disk usually gives a history of trauma to the spinal column. However, about a fourth of the patients are unable to recall any distinct injury.

The pain of which these patients complain partakes. of the usual characteristics of root pain. That is, the pain follows the anatomic distribution of the peripheral nerve which has its origin in the nerve root involved. The pain is usually aggravated by coughing, sneezing and straining, or by anything that increases the pressure of the spinal fluid. Some of the patients state that they are unable to sleep at night because of exacerbation of their symptoms in the small hours. Others state that they are comfortable while recumbent.

If the lesion has been present for a long time, is large, or there have been repeated exacerbations of symptoms, weakness and numbness of the involved member may constitute a major complaint.

One of the most important points in the history of a patient who has a protruded disk is the fact that, in spite of treatment by the long accepted methods, the symptoms have persisted. When low back or sciatic pain fails to respond to the usual conservative orthopedic measures a protruded disk as the causative factor should be considered.

On examination, the patients frequently exhibit scoliosis and they move about cautiously in order to prevent jarring and thus exaggeration of their pain. When sitting down or rising from a sitting position they guard their motions. When a considerable number of these patients have been seen the diagnosis in a given case can be surmised after observing the patient rise from a sitting position and walk across a room. The posture and gait are often characteristic.

When the patient is disrobed and examined one notes, in addition to the scoliosis, spasm of the erector spinæ muscles. Raising of the straight leg produces severe pain, and motion of the involved lower extremity, as well as of the spinal column, is limited.

The neurologic findings vary considerably. In the presence of larger lesions definite paralysis exists. There may be more or less complete paralysis of both lower extremities. The vesical and anal sphincters likewise may be paralyzed. The majority of the patients, however, display few objective neurologic findings. The most constant finding is diminution or absence of the Achilles tendon reflex on the involved side. There may be or may not be sensory loss and tenderness along the course of the involved nerve.

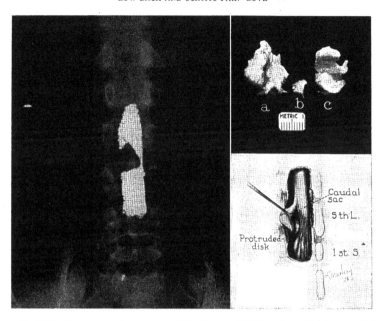

Fig. 6 (left). Postero-anterior roentgenogram showing defect in the column of lipiodol opposite the third lumbar intervertebral space on the left. This defect is characteristic of protruded intervertebral disks. The patient had sustained an injury of his back a year and a half previously and had suffered backache and left sciatic pain since.

Fig. 7 (upper right). Specimens, removal of which relieved a man of chronic backache and sciatica of one year's duration. a, protruded portion of fifth lumbar disk; b, corresponding portion of the ligamentum flavum between the sixth lumbar and first sacral vertebræ. This ligament was not abnormal. There were, in this case, six lumbar vertebræ; c, the ligamentum flavum between the fifth and sixth lumbar vertebræ. The ligament was markedly thickened.

Fig. 8 (lower right). Exposure, by means of hemilaminectomy, of a protruded lumbosacral disk. The patient had had backache and left sciatic pain for fifteen years. The study with lipiodol was negative because the caudal sac ended above the level of the protrusion.

extradurally. The defect produced in the column of lipiodol by a protruded intervertebral disk usually is characteristic (Fig. 6). The defect usually is anterolateral in position and is situated opposite the intervertebral space. In addition to the defect produced by the disk itself, often a defect owing to the enlarged, edematous, involved nerve root can be detected in the shadow of the lipiodol. Recently we have come to recognize defects attributable to hypertrophy of the ligamentum flavum. This abnormality of the overlying ligament is, I feel, a more or less constant accompaniment of protrusion of an intervertebral disk (Fig. 7). There are, however, cases in which hypertrophy of the ligamentum flavum causes low back and sciatic pain without associated protrusion of a disk. This condition, occurring as a single lesion, however, in our experience, is much less common than is hypertrophy of the ligament associated with true protrusion of the underlying disk. In every case careful search should be made to exclude an associated lesion of a disk.

As our experience has increased, on a few occasions we have advised laminectomy for protruded disk in the face of negative examination with lipiodol. Whenever this is done the patient should be advised of the possibilities and the operation should not be performed until every other condition which might account for the patient's symptoms is excluded.

Occasionally a patient will be encountered in

examination of whom a positive test is impossible for anatomic reasons. The caudal sac may end above the lumbosacral space and thus the lipiodol cannot reach the level of protrusion (Fig. 8).

Treatment

There is only one treatment for protrusion of an intervertebral disk that is producing compression of the spinal cord or of a nerve root. When a definite protrusion is demonstrated and a lesion at the level of the protrusion will explain the patient's symptoms and signs, laminectomy for the express purpose of removing the protruded portion of the disk should be performed. Anyone who has witnessed the operative removal of a protruded disk and seen the relationship of the abnormal cartilaginous mass to the spinal cord or nerve root, the edema, the enlargement and displacement of the nerve root and the complete relief of pressure following removal of the protruded portion will agree, I feel sure, that there is a definite anatomic and pathologic basis for the condition under discussion (Fig. 3). If there still should be any doubt, to see the patient when he leaves the hospital two weeks later, free of pain, free of scoliosis and smiling is sufficient to convince even the most skeptical.

In performing laminectomy for protruded intervertebral disk, removal of two spinous processes and of two pairs of laminæ is, in the majority of cases, sufficient to obtain adequate exposure. The articular facets should be preserved. Resection of the ligamentum flavum, which is found to be hypertrophied in most, if not in all cases, aids materially in obtaining satisfactory exposure of the involved nerve root and the underlying protruded part. Since most of the protrusions are lateral to the common dural sac, most of them can be removed extradurally before the dural sac is opened. Leaving the dural sac intact serves three distinct purposes: there is less bleeding from the extradural vessels while the hydrostatic effect of the cerebrospinal fluid is active; the cerebrospinal fluid acts as a buffer to protect the cauda equina while the dura mater is being retracted, and finally if one should be unfortunate enough to encounter a previously unrecognized extradural inflammatory lesion, the subarachnoid space and its contents would be protected from contamination.

After the protruded portion of the disk has been removed the dural sac is opened and the

interior inspected. Edema of the intradural portion of the involved nerve root is noted (Fig. 3c). The canal is carefully inspected to be sure that all pressure has been removed. The lipiodol is sucked out before the dura mater is closed. Bone graft or fusion is not necessary.

Following operation the patients are kept in bed for twelve days. They are allowed to leave the hospital on the fourteenth day and to return to their homes three weeks after operation. They are advised to refrain from heavy lifting or from placing stress or strain on their backs for three months. After this time they are encouraged to return gradually to their former activities. The period of hospitalization and period of convalescence is much shorter than it would be if bone grafting were performed. This is, of course, a tremendous saving in expense to the patient and he is enabled to return to work much sooner. The hypertrophied ligamentum flavum is resected in the course of exposing the protrusion.

Results

Our results justify continuation of our present treatment, namely, laminectomy and removal of the protruded portion of the disk. Most of the patients are completely relieved of their symptoms and are able to return to their former occupations. There has been one postoperative death in more than 200 laminectomies for protruded intervertebral disk. There has been one recurrence. This patient was completely relieved following a second operation.[4]

References

1. Kernohan, J. W.: Personal communications to the author.
2. Love, J. G.: Protrusion of the intervertebral disk (fibrocartilage) into the spinal canal. Proc. Staff Meet. Mayo Clinic, 11:529,535, (Aug. 19) 1936.
3. Love, J. G.: The rôle of intervertebral disks in the production of chronic low back and sciatic pain. Proc. Staff Meet. Mayo Clinic, 12:369-372, (June 16) 1937.
4. Love, J. G.: Unpublished data.
5. Love, J. G., and Camp, J. D.: Root pain resulting from intraspinal protrusion of intervertebral disks; diagnosis and surgical treatment. Jour. Bone and Joint Surg., 19:776-804, (July) 1937.
6. Love, J. G., and Walsh, M. N.: Protruded intervertebral disks: report of 100 cases in which operation was performed. Jour. Am. Med. Assn., 111:396-400, (July 30) 1938.
7. Walsh, M. N., and Love, J. G.: Protruded intervertebral disk as a cause of intractable pain. Proc. Staff Meet. Mayo Clinic, 13:203-205, (March 30) 1938.

Discussion

Dr. Harold O. Peterson, Minneapolis: I am sure that Dr. Love and his associates have had more experience with posterior protrusion of the intervertebral disc than any other person or group, and I heartily agree with everything he has said. Since my experience has been limited largely to the roentgen diagnosis of this condition I shall confine my remarks to this phase of the subject.

I was gratified to hear that Dr. Love is still as enthusiastic about the diagnosis and treatment of this condition as he was when the original reports were made. Although it is several years now since the first papers were published and even though the condition is known to exist by many it is still difficult in some places to obtain a satisfactory examination in order to establish the diagnosis. By a satisfactory examination is meant the injection of lipiodol into the spinal canal in sufficient quantities (5 c.c.) to permit a thorough radiographic examination.

This is due entirely to the fear of injecting a foreign substance such as lipiodol into the subarachnoid space. In a review of the literature one year ago I was able to find only a few isolated instances in which it was probable that permanent damage had followed its use. Those who had used lipiodol the most reported no serious consequences, although many patients had temporary ill effects which disappeared after the second or third day. Therefore, although there may be an occasional case which shows undesirable cord and nerve root damage subsequent to lipiodol injection, the information which can be obtained only by this method outweighs the danger of any possible ill effects.

The indiscriminate intraspinal injection of lipiodol into every patient with a backache is, however, not justified and it is for this reason that a thorough orthopedic and neurologic examination is necessary in every case to exclude all other possible explanations of the pain. Dr. Love has adequately outlined the indications for lipiodol study, and I merely wish to emphasize a few points. Lipiodol study of the spine should be reserved for those cases of chronic back pain which have failed to respond to conservative treatment and is contra-indicated in those patients with acute back pain of short duration. Ordinary roentgenograms must be taken of the spine before lipiodol injection is considered. I recall one case in which a diagnosis of metastatic malignancy was readily made on the films taken after lipiodol injection, there having been no previous films made. It should be understood, however, that a positive diagnosis of herniated disc cannot be made from the plain roentgenograms alone. Suggestive findings may be present in at least half of the cases consisting of narrowing of the intervertebral disc, straightening of the normal lumbar lordosis, and scoliosis.

The lesion which Dr. Love has described explains on a sound anatomic and pathologic basis many of the cases which have been heretofore loosely and incorrectly diagnosed as sciatica or sacro-iliac disease. It is difficult to understand how sacro-iliac disease, per se, can ever produce sciatic pain. It must be remembered, however, that all cases of low back pain, even if sciatic radiation is present, are not due to herniated discs. Since these cases are clinically indistinguishable in many instances from what is usually called sacro-iliac disease, sciatica and low back strain, it is essential that a lipiodol study be made. By this method of examination 90 to 95% of the cases can be correctly diagnosed and localized.

In closing I should like to emphasize the necessity of thinking of this condition in those patients who have intractable low back pain and especially where there is sciatic radiation. If the usual methods of treatment fail, lipiodol injection is indicated.

THE VALUE OF THE X-RAY IN GENERAL PRACTICE*

CHARLES G. SUTHERLAND, M.D.

Rochester, Minnesota

EARLY in the eighteenth century, a French physicist of peasant birth spent many hours on research concerning the passage of an electric current through a tube from which the air had been evacuated. A curious void contrivance which he constructed at that time and which not inappropriately was called the "electric egg" undoubtedly represented the earliest and humblest ancestor of the modern vacuum tube.

Nearly eighty years passed before further activities in this field of scientific research were initiated. The new light which Wilhelm Conrad Roentgen discovered, in 1895, was actually produced in 1785 and many times after that, but it was not recognized until the discovery by Roentgen. Roentgen gave the new light the name of "x-ray"; in his honor it was later called the "roentgen ray" and the new science which developed from his discovery was given the name of roentgenology.

*From the Section on Roentgenology, The Mayo Clinic, Rochester, Minnesota. Read before the annual meeting of the Minnesota State Medical Association, Duluth, Minnesota, June 29, 1938.

The possibilities of the x-rays as a diagnostic agent in medicine were discussed before the Berlin Medical Society the day previous to, and before the Society of Internal Medicine in Berlin the day of the announcement of the discovery. By the end of February, 1896, the method was in comparatively general use as a new diagnostic procedure in many countries.

The epochal feature of the roentgen rays was that they supplemented conjecture in medicine with visual and graphic factual evidence. Because of technical difficulties, it was many years before the application of the method became practical in routine investigation. The World War was probably a real factor in stimulating interest in this new field of investigation. The demand for machinery and accessories necessary to the production of roentgenograms and the visualization of various anatomic parts fired the imagination of the industrialist and encouraged the expenditure of time and money in research which resulted in the production of the paraphernalia required.

Concomitant with this industrial research went the correlation of roentgenologic findings and the already known facts of clinical and pathologic investigation. The pioneers in this work established new foundations in the appearance .of normal structures and the normal limit of their variations. They proved that the roentgenographic image was a reproduction in relief of the various components of the body, normal and abnormal. They found that the idiosyncrasies of individual disease entities, expressed in predilection for certain types of tissue and definite situation in particular structures, long known to the pathologist, could be graphically recorded. In short, they discovered that roentgenology afforded the opportunity to study pathologic changes in the living patient. Experience with the new method revealed a new and unique advantage: by serial roentgenography it was possible to study the changes resulting from the progression or regression of the individual morbid process and thereby evaluate specific forms of therapy and at the same time more accurately establish the prognosis.

Radiotherapy has become a definite factor in the establishment, or in the corroboration, of a diagnosis. For example, the changes produced by radiotherapy in Ewing's tumor are characteristic enough to be diagnostic.

With the aid of substances ingested or injected or autogenously produced after the injection or ingestion of chemical compounds, most of the viscera of the body were rendered visible in roentgenoscopic observation or in the roentgenogram. Other viscera were made visible by the introduction of air or gases. The anatomist, the physiologist, and the pathologist, working with the aid of roentgenography and roentgenoscopy, have added materially to the sum of knowledge of their special subjects.

The value of the roentgen rays in general practice is familiar to most of you; time will only permit discussion of a single phase of the subject, the use of the method in the diagnosis of lesions involving bone.

Let me sound a note of warning. The interpretation of roentgenologic findings is not to be undertaken lightly. It involves a serious responsibility. An error in conclusion may influence subsequent therapy to an extent that might be embarrassing and even disastrous to the interests of the patient and to professional reputation.

To avoid such disaster, one must have some knowledge of the fundamental changes in the architecture of bone peculiar to certain diseases. This point can best be illustrated by considering the salient features of the benign and malignant neoplasm of bone. The decision of paramount importance that one may be called on to make is whether a given lesion involving bone is inflammatory or neoplastic, and, more important still, if neoplastic, is it benign or malignant in nature. Of lesser importance, but still very helpful in later consideration, is whether the lesion is a primary neoplastic one or whether it is a secondary (metastatic) implant in bone from a malignant tumor in some remote part.

The importance of this statement lies in the fact that not infrequently in a case in which the lesion has been considered comparatively innocuous the roentgenogram reveals a primary malignant tumor or metastatic involvement. The metastatic involvement may be the first indication of a malignant lesion in the body and may institute a search for the primary neoplasm.

To lessen the confusion resulting from any elaborate attempts at classification, this discussion will be limited to the main groups of lesions recognized by the committee of the Clinical Pathological Association and their simulants. To enable consideration in sequence I have rearranged this classification as follows: (1) benign osteogenic tumors, (2) periosteal fibrosarcoma (extraperiosteal sarcoma), (3) noninflammatory conditions simulating benign lesions of bone, (4) giant cell tumor, (5) benign angioma, (6) myeloma, (7) malignant osteogenic tumors, (8) inflammatory conditions simulating malignant lesions of bone, (9) Ewing's tumor (Ewing's sarcoma), (10) malignant angioma, and (11) metastatic involvement.

Benign Osteogenic Tumors

The word "osteogenic" is used here, not in the sense of bone forming, but simply to designate a tumor arising from bone cells or bone-forming cells in contradistinction to tumors that originate in bone marrow cells or in the vessels of bone or bone marrow. The outstanding roentgenographic feature of a benign tumor of bone is the retention of the cortical contour. The cortex may be expanded or otherwise deformed but there is never any dissolution of its continuity. On the other hand, the almost pathognomonic

840

characteristic of the maligant osteogenic tumor is the definite break in the continuity of the cortical outline. This, with but few exceptions, which will be mentioned, is the prominent feature of malignant tumors of bone.

Turning to the pathology of these lesions, one finds that these features have been described. In 1925 Broders said: "The chief difference between the average benign neoplasm and the average malignant one is that the benign exerts more control over itself than the malignant. It cannot be said that any neoplasm has complete control of itself at all times, because the very fact that it grows shows that its control is not absolute, but, fortunately for the human race, the majority of neoplasms do reach a point of absolute self control, or, in other words, obey the law of limitation of growth. . . . Benign neoplasms produce a structure in which the cells are practically indistinguishable from the cells of normal tissues, although the arrangement is somewhat different, and unquestionably a number of benign neoplasms function to some extent like the tissues they so closely imitate . . . All benign neoplasms, like the tissues which they imitate, produce regenerative cells as well as differentiated cells; otherwise they could not grow, because the differentiated cells do not reproduce. It is also reasonable to believe that the regenerative cells of benign neoplasms are more active than the regenerative cells of normal tissues, and that the regenerative cells of certain benign neoplasms are more active than the regenerative cells of others, because they grow faster than others. It may be that the regenerative cells of benign neoplasms are more numerous than those of others.

"When benign neoplasms reach the point of complete self control, their cells either cease to regenerate or they differentiate beyond the point of regeneration. If all the cells of a benign neoplasm have differentiated beyond the point of regeneration, there is only one thing for the neoplasm to do, and that is to degenerate, and this probably often takes place, especially in myomas of the uterus. Degeneration seems to be one of Nature's methods of getting rid of neoplasms . . . In passing from benign to malignant neoplasia, the fact should not be lost sight of that the power of self control still exists, although to a gradually diminishing degree. A wart that has been slowly growing for a number

of years may show evidence of increased rate of growth, and after it has been excised and examined under the microscope, cells are observed at its base that differ from those found at the base of the ordinary benign wart . . . The regenerative cells at the base of this wart have undergone . . . anaplasia (undifferentiation), or a process of dedifferentiation . . . These anaplastic or dedifferentiated cells appear to represent a new type, and are observed in all forms of malignant neoplasia, although they vary in shape and size in different types of malignant neoplasms . . . These anaplastic or dedifferentiated cells have various potentialities . . . I wish to emphasize here a good potentiality, or the power to produce cells that differentiate or reach a state of maturity beyond their ability to reproduce. This differentiating or controlling quality ranges from practically nothing to almost 100 per cent. The cells of a neoplasm that show practically no tendency to control themselves rapidly infiltrate the adjacent structures and, by utilizing the vascular system as a means of metastasis, set up colonies in various parts of the body, which in turn keep on producing their own kind of cells, finally with a fatal result. On the other hand, if the cells of a neoplasm show a marked tendency to control themselves by differentiation the neoplasm will grow slowly, and show very little tendency to metastasize; or if some of the cells do metastasize, they will in turn set aside the large majority to differentiate and build a structure similar to that found in a normal organ, which functions to some extent. . . .

"Malignant neoplasms need not necessarily be preceded by benign neoplasms; the large majority are not. Many are preceded by destruction of tissue, but others spring up without the slightest injury, so far as we know . . . It would seem that this type can only be explained by heredity. These should be called true spontaneous neoplasms."

When one studies the so-called benign tumors of bone it immediately becomes apparent that the majority of them at least, if not all of them, occur in early life and at about the age of puberty. Most of them are situated at the growing ends of bone and in many cases there is a distinct tendency toward cessation of growth and even regression at about the period when the development of the skeleton is complete. All of these facts point to a disturbance in development of the cartilaginous elements in the formation of bone and joints. It may be difficult in some cases to draw the line between the abnormal and the normal state. For example, limited outgrowths of preëxisting cartilage occurring in the ribs and about the joints are distinguished as ecchondroses. True progressive neoplasms which are composed of cartilage appear in the same situations and also in tissues which normally do not contain cartilage; these neoplasms are called enchondromas or chondromas. Chondromas are familiar to most of us as single or multiple tumors of the hands and feet. In some chondromas the formation of cartilaginous matrix is imperfect and a simple hyaline material results. Roentgenographically such a tumor is transparent to the roentgen rays; it will only cast a shadow by virtue of its bulk. In cases of smaller tumors the only evidence in the roentgenogram may be a filling defect in the bone, which has a smooth margin; this is the result of erosion of the tumor by pressure. Calcification with the deposit of phosphate and carbonate of lime may cause incrustation of both the matrix and the cells and may produce a characteristic roentgenographic image. The tumor may be partly fibrillated and be recognizable as a fibroma. Mucinous material may take the place of the matrix; in such cases the prefix myxo is used in the pathologic nomenclature. Ossification of chondromas occurs; depending on the preponderance of bone or cartilage, the tumor is known as an osteoma or osteochondroma. These subdivisions of this group of tumors can all be recognized by their roentgenographic images.

The exostosis occurs in two forms: (1) the single outgrowth of bone which is capped by a cauliflower shaped excrescence of cartilage, and (2) the multiple symmetrically distributed lesions of the same type, which are familiar to most of us as multiple congenital exostoses or hereditary deforming chondrodysplasia. If one accepts Keith's explanation of the occurrence of the latter type, that is, a congenital defect in the periosteum which normally acts as a ferrule in the control of the architecture of bone, and if one accepts the opinion that benign tumors of bone are due to a disturbance in development of the cartilaginous elements in the formation of bone, then all the lesions which have been mentioned are in the same category. Their roentgenographic images confirm this opinion. The con-

trol stressed by Broders is perfectly apparent in the roentgenogram. In the benign osteogenic tumor the contiguous soft tissue structures are only invaded by the expansion of the cortex of the bone.

In the malignant osteogenic tumor, the tumor breaks through the cortex and "promiscuously" invades the surrounding soft tissue structures. The latter exemplifies the loss of control which Broders pointed out as the characteristic of the malignant neoplasm.

These two facts, the retention throughout or the dissolution at some point of the cortical contour, and the sharply demarcated or the promiscuous invasion of the adjacent soft tissue structures are the keynote of the roentgenologic differentiation of benign and malignant tumors.

The greatest value of the roentgen rays is, of course, in the decision of the nature of the morbid process. This establishes the prognosis. If the benign tumor is of the osteogenic type, the treatment will be conservative. Obviously, surgical intervention is contraindicated at least until mature growth is attained. Unless demanded because of mechanical interference with function or some other complicating factor, surgical removal of these tumors should not be attempted. Unless every last cartilage cell can be removed or destroyed, these tumors will recur. In recurrence, there not infrequently is a mutation of the cell and a chondrosarcoma or an osteochondrosarcoma results. These tumors grow slowly; a sudden acceleration of growth and occurrence of new symptoms call for roentgenographic examination and careful search for evidence of dissolution of the cortical contour and promiscuous invasion of the contiguous soft tissues, which indicate sarcomatous change.

Of the nonosteogenic tumors involving bone the benign hemangioma is comparatively rare. This neoplasm involves the shafts of long bones, the skull and the vertebral bodies. In the shafts of the bones it occurs in the region of the metaphysis; it expands the cortex but does not extend deeply into the medullary or cancellous spaces; the roentgenographic image is that of a "soap-bubble" and is somewhat similar to that of a giant cell tumor. In the vertebral body the image is characterized by vertical striæ on a background of decreased density. Pathologic fracture is commonly a complicating factor.

The two most important simulants of benign

epiphysis at the expense of the cancellous bone. Primarily it is traversed by trabeculæ which divide the tumor into several loculi. Later these trabeculæ may disappear and may be replaced by a homogeneous flat shadow in the roentgenogram, owing to a lysis in the central portion of the bone; this lysis may extend into the cortex and leave only a thin shell of bone. This thin shell of bone may be expanded until it becomes invisible in the roentgenogram and the tumor may extend beyond the cortex and push the soft tissues ahead of it. At this stage it may be very difficult to differentiate roentgenographically a giant cell tumor and a malignant neoplasm. In a case of giant cell tumor careful study of the outline of the soft tissue shadow will reveal that it has a smooth margin and is intact. A remnant of the cortical shell persists as a wavy outline of bone which passes over the soft tissue shadow at the proximal end of the bone. Occasionally, the shaft of the bone may be telescoped for some distance into the soft tissue shadow. In some cases the evidence of a benign tumor may all be masked and the roentgenographic interpretation may be extremely difficult, but a careful study of the soft tissue invasive shadow will usually reveal some evidence of the continuity of the outline of the shadow.

Periosteal fibrosarcoma (extraperiosteal sarcoma) occasionally presents a roentegenographic image that simulates very closely that of a benign osteogenic tumor or more often that of a giant cell tumor. Periosteal fibrosarcoma invades the bone from without and the destructive lesion in bone, when the bone is involved, is frequently the result of pressure erosion. In such cases the filling defect in the bone has a smooth margin and the continuity of the contour shadow is maintained.

Myeloma is the other malignant lesion that involves bone and simulates a benign tumor roentgenographically. In fact, myeloma violates every principle suggested for the differentiation of benign and malignant tumors. In the shafts of long bones and in the skull this lesion is characterized by multiple, small, discrete filling defects in the bone shadow and the margins are as clear-cut as if they had been made with a steel punch. In the ribs and the shafts of long bones a wide expansion of the shaft may occur and although the cortex may be markedly thinned the contour is always maintained just as it is in the benign osteogenic or giant cell tumor. The shaft of the bone may even be telescoped into the soft tissue shadow as it is in giant cell tumor. In the spinal column complete destruction of one or more vertebral bodies is suggestive of myeloma. In the shaft of long bones pathologic fracture may occur and this may be the first evidence of the morbid process. In the greater number of cases there is general involvement of most of the skeletal structures and there may be difficulty in distinguishing myeloma from the osteoclastic form of metastatic carcinoma. The roentgenogram of the skull offers the most conclusive evidence of the nature of the lesion.

The characteristics of malignant tumors of bone are best exemplified by osteogenic sarcoma. The gradually diminishing degree of the power of self control is apparent in the perforation of the periosteum and the promiscuous invasion of the contiguous soft tissue structures by the tumor mass. Roentgenographically these changes are demonstrable in the roentgenogram as a dissolution of the contour of the cortex and an inability to trace the outline of the soft tissue shadow. The elevation of the periosteum at the proximal end of the lesion is the remaining evidence of the defensive protective measure of the involved bone set up by the periosteum against the continuous aggression of the tumor elements. Sarcoma predominantly involves the metaphyseal portion of the shaft of long bones and extends into the diaphysis. It may involve the diaphysis. When it involves a large flat bone, such as the os innominatum, the filling defect in the bone has an irregular or serrated margin or fades imperceptibly into the surrounding bone, in contradistinction to the smooth margins and well demarcated outline of the filling defect in cases of benign tumors.

Several subdivisions of sarcoma are recognizable in the roentgenograms: (1) subperiosteal and medullary sarcoma; (2) periosteal sarcoma; (3) sclerosing sarcoma; (4) telangiectatic sarcoma (aneurysm of bone); (5) chondosarcoma, and the sarcomas involving the diaphysis.

Careful technic often is required to demonstrate a subperiosteal or medullary sarcoma. In one projection the evidence of the lesion may be so slight as to be missed; in another projection the break in the continuity of the cortex and the "promiscuous" invasion of the soft tissue structures will be easily recognized. The periosteal sarcoma exhibits a "sun-ray" of fine linear bony shadows radiating more or less at a right angle

to the axis of the shaft of the bone. In one projection it may be difficult to detect any break in the cortical contour, while in another characteristic features of the lesion are easily apparent.

The sclerosing sarcoma shows, as the name suggests, an intense eburnation of the involved portion of the bone. Particularly in the upper end of the tibia this tumor may be difficult to distinguish from syphilitic osteitis; only careful study in one of perhaps several projections will reveal the break in the continuity of the cortex. The invasion of soft tissues also tends to be much limited in comparison with other types of sarcoma; it may be so limited as to be difficult of recognition.

The telangiectatic sarcoma (aneurysm of bone) is characterized by a rather extensive bony proliferation in the soft tissues, which in the femur, for example, may very closely simulate a suppurative or other inflammatory lesion of the synovial membrane.

Chondrosarcoma, because of its preponderant cartilaginous content, occasionally offers difficulty in detection of the break in the cortical contour and the soft tissue invasion lacks the extent and the definitely promiscuous features of other types of sarcoma.

The sarcomas involving the mid-diaphyseal portions of the long bones have some of the characteristics of Ewing's tumor, a nonosteogenic tumor which was described as an endothelial myeloma or hemangio-endothelioma by Ewing in 1920.

Ewing's tumor tends to involve the mid-diaphyseal portion of the shaft of long bones, but it may involve any portion; not infrequently, it involves the metaphysis (the growing portion of bone at the junction of the epiphysis and the diaphysis). It rarely affects persons who ar more than twenty-one years of age. The bulk o the tumor lies beneath the periosteum; the tumo infiltrates the bone and the bone reacts vigorous ly with ossification. This reaction is attende with intermittent attacks of fever. The lesion i most often mistaken for osteomyelitis. Roentgen ographically, the medullary portion of the bon is not involved. This observation may be o value in the differential diagnosis. In a cas recently observed, in which the roentgenographi findings were typical of osteomyelitis of the mid shaft of the tibia and in which the pathologi reported that the changes were inflammator;

the patient returned within seven months with all evidences of a periosteal sarcoma.

Subperiosteal formations may be observed; these may be parallel to the bone (onion-skin laminations) or may be at right angles to the axis of the shaft, as are the miniature sun-ray spicules of bone in Ewing's tumor. The onion-skin laminations and the miniature sun-ray bony spicules have occurred synchronously in the same case. In some of the diaphyseal tumors atypical radiations of bony spicules are seen projecting at or nearly at right angles to the axis of the shaft of the bone; in my experience those have proved on pathologic investigation to be osteogenic sarcomas and this diagnosis has been corroborated by the reactions of the tumor to radiotherapy. A helpful point in differential diagnosis has been the soft tissue invasion shadow. In osteogenic sarcoma this is promiscuous in character; in Ewing's tumor it tends to be indefinitely demarcated. In Ewing's tumor the margin of the invasive shadow is not as sharply demarcated as that of a benign tumor and yet it is more distinct than the line of demarcation that marks the osteogenic sarcoma.

Ewing's tumor should not be confused with traumatic sclerosing osteitis or with infectious nonsuppurating osteomyelitis of Garre; these inflammatory lesions do not show any tendency to lamination of the expanded cortical shadow but exhibit a homogeneous flat density throughout. An intact subperiosteal hematoma is usually more closely confined in area and more frequently projects from only one aspect of the bone than is the case in Ewing's tumor. A ruptured subperiosteal hematoma presents lines of ossification that run parallel to the axis of the shaft, and are much coarser and more widely divided than the onion-skin laminations of Ewing's tumor. Green-stick fracture, with the formation of callus, may be difficult to distinguish from this malignant tumor.

The defensive mechanism of the bone against the advance of Ewing's tumor is very similar to that against the advance of a pyogenic infection; it consists of the creation of a bony shell which is called an "involucrum." An interesting fact is that Ewing's tumor, in contradistinction to osteogenic sarcoma, reacts favorably for a time to radiotherapy. Efficient treatment by this method apparently stimulates the defensive mechanism and results in marked accentuation of the density of the involucrum in

the roentgenogram. In all cases of doubt, therefore, a safe procedure is to institute radiotherapy in moderate dosage, as it will be beneficial if the condition is an osteomeylitis. One then should await the results as evidenced in serial roentgenography.

Under such a procedure, some tumors which roentgenographically appeared to be most typical of Ewing's tumor of the shaft were proved ultimately to be osteogenic sarcomas. If careful inspection of the roentgenographic image reveals involvement of the medullary portion of the bone, one should at least suspect osteomyelitis or osteogenic sarcoma.

The malignant angiomas have some of the characteristics of the telangiectatic sarcoma and of Ewing's tumor roentgenographically. Malignant angiomas exhibit an intense subperiosteal proliferation of bony tissue with a subsequent wide invasion of the soft tissues. Under treatment with radiotherapy these tumors show some response, but they do not respond as favorably as does Ewing's tumor.

Metastatic malignant tumors are the result of implants from malignant tumors in parts remote from bone. They have the histologic characteristics of the parent growth. Practically, only carcinoma metastasizes; occasionally one sees sarcomatous lesions in bone that have all the roentgenographic features of metastasis, but the consensus seems to be that these are multicentric growths. The malignant lymphomas (Hodgkin's disease, lymphosarcoma and leukemia) show involvement of bone in a small proportion of cases. Ewing's tumor also tends to involve the skull in the late stages of the disease.

Two distinct forms of metastatic carcinoma are seen. The osteoclastic (melting or melted ice) form is most frequently seen secondary to carcinoma of the breast; it is the usual form seen secondary to carcinoma of the kidney and genito-urinary tract, suprarenal gland, thyroid gland, bronchus and lung, uterus or adnexa, pancreas and biliary tract. Metastasis from carcinoma of the stomach is rare; when seen it has a distinctive roentgenographic image and shows some tendency to assume the features of the osteoplastic form. Occasionally, a slowly growing carcinoma of the breast will produce an image with some osteoplastic features. The lesions of the osteoclastic forms may be localized or there may be a general involvement of the skeletal structures. One portion of a bone may be completely destroyed, presenting a perfect picture of a malignant lesion that has produced complete dissolution of the cortical contour. There is seldom evidence of any reaction; the roentgenographic image is that of a complete melting away of the shadow of bone over a limited area. Metastasis is seldom seen in the bones of the extremities below the elbows and the knees; when it does occur there is often almost complete obliteration of the shadow of one or a portion of one of the bones, more frequently of the radius in the forearm and the tibia in the leg. Not infrequently, a faint shadow of the cortex will remain. Lesions in the proximal ends of the femur and humerus are the site of pathologic fracture; not infrequently the pathologic fracture may serve to call attention to the metastatic process and occasionally even to the presence elsewhere in the body of a primary malignancy.

In the spinal column the metastatic process may be confined to a single vertebral body or it may involve several isolated vertebræ. Compression of a vertebral body is noted in some cases in which there is evidence of extensive involvement of other vertebræ but no alteration in their architecture. This suggests that pathologic fracture must be a factor in some of the deformities noted. At necropsy, vertebræ have been examined and proved to be so friable that one could force the finger into the substance of the body but visualization of the lesion in the roentgenogram called for the closest scrutiny. Knowing this, one is justified in upholding a clinical diagnosis of metastasis in the spinal column even when it is impossible to visualize the lesion in the roentgenogram.

Localized lesions in the os innominatum, in the pubis, and in the ischium vary from extensive destruction of bone with irregular, serrated or indistinguishable margins to multiple punctate areas of varying size, or "melted ice" areas of varying dimension.

Localized lesions may occur in the ribs; these are usually multiple lesions scattered throughout several different ribs. Not infrequently, in cases in which patients are of advanced age and there is evidence of some general osteoporosis of bone and a diffuse fibrosis of the lung as a result of chronic bronchitis or other cause, the superimposition of the pulmonary markings on the more translucent bone will give the impression of metastasis in the ribs. In such cases, reëxami-

nation with heavier exposure and the int tion of the Bucky-Potter diaphragm wil reveal normal bone and obviate an er diagnosis.

In general involvement of most of the s structures, the bone usually will have a combed appearance; the dimension of th vidual defects varies widely; punctate are be noted in some parts, and there may filling defect of varying size in other par

The osteoplastic form of metastatic car is almost always secondary to carcinoma prostate gland. The roentgenographic im this form is that of a background of bc struction with a concomitant hyperplasia o The one process usually keeps pace w other, but not infrequently there are var in the degree of one or the other, with a ant diversity of the image. In early ca involvement is in the inner margin of th on one or both sides, under the overlyin of the sacrum. This may easily be misint ed as hypertrophic changes in the sac joints. The lesion may involve one pelv ment before spreading to other parts skeleton. In other cases splotches of hypr of bone which are scattered over the sha the ilium on one or both sides may be t evidence of metastasis. These splotcl increase in size and number simultaneou increasing evidence of destruction of bo the entire bony structure of the pelvis ai the upper portion of the femurs are i The destruction and the proliferation m cide to the extent that there may be geneous eburnation, often extending thr the skeletal structure. In the spinal colu vertebral body or several separate bodies involved; rarely this may be the only of metastatic involvement.

The recognition of the metastatic inv by roentgenographic examination may first intimation of carcinoma of the gland. Occasionally, carcinoma may demonstrable by physical examination, e metastasis in bone has been discovered

The noninflammatory condition whi lates osteoplastic metastasis is osteitis d (Paget's disease). In some cases this considerable difficulty in differential Both diseases affect men who are in period of life, and both are frequently i findings in routine examinations.

Osteitis deformans may, similarly to carcinomatous osteitis, involve a single pelvic bone before involving the whole skeletal structure; a coincidental secondary anemia is present alike in cases of benign osteitis and carcinomatous osteitis.

In benign osteitis, or osteitis deformans, the evidence of the trabecular elements of the bone is maintained or exaggerated; in carcinomatous osteitis it is always obliterated in cases in which the differential diagnosis is difficult. In osteitis deformans there is an enlargement of the shadow of the bone owing to subperiosteal deposition of osteoid tissue; in carcinomatous osteitis there is no enlargement of the bony shadow. In cases in which the femurs are involved, there is a widening of the cortex and a bowing of the shaft; this feature is absent in carcinomatous osteitis.

Roentgenographic examination of the cranium and the tibia will reveal pathognomonic roentgenographic images if the lesion is osteitis deformans.

Summary

In this necessarily brief review an attempt has been made to point out the salient roentgenographic characteristics of lesions involving bone. In competent hands the roentgenologic method is a rapid and accurate method of determining the etiologic factor in the majority of lesions involving bones and joints. Careful subsequent correlation of the roentgenographic, the clinical and all other findings should be carried out in every case before the ultimate diagnosis is arrived at, and before the therapeutic measures are instituted. Surgical intervention should always be preceded by biopsy under control of a tourniquet, and the decision as to the procedure should always await the results of microscopic examination of the excised tissue. Under such circumstances the roentgenogram is of inestimable value; in fact, one can truly say roentgenology has become one of the indispensable methods in general diagnosis.

References

1. Broders, A. C.: Cancer's self-control. Med. Jour. and Rec., 121:133-135, 1925.
2. Ewing, James: Neoplastic diseases: a treatise on tumors. Ed. 2. Philadelphia: W. B. Saunders Company, 1922, 1054 pp.
3. Geschickter, C. F., and Copeland, M. M.: Tumors of bone. New York: American Journal of Cancer, 1936, 877 pp.
4. Keith, A.: The true nature of the condition known as multiple exostoses. Tr. Med. Soc., London, 43:67-73, 1920.

THE ROENTGEN TREATMENT OF INFLAMMATORY DISEASES*

GAGE CLEMENT, M.D.

Duluth, Minnesota

IN considering the use of the roentgen ray in the treatment of inflammatory conditions, it must be borne in mind that a whole group of circumstances and developments must be evaluated. One of the first of these is that, until comparatively recently, roentgen rays were used more or less empirically. The instability of the old gas tube, the variation in the quantity and quality of the radiation it produced, the absence of the auto-transformer, the lack of knowledge of filtration as it affects wave-length and depth dose and the entire lack of scientific instruments for measuring roentgen dosage made x-ray therapy, in its early days, more or less unreliable.

Gradually x-ray equipment has been improved. The auto-transformer, the mechanical and valve-tube rectifier, the hot cathode tube, the spectroscope, the electroscope and the r-meter were developed gradually and today are accepted equipment in constant use. These have enabled the radiologist to duplicate, from day to day, the potentials and currents that are needed, and uniform settings and equivalent energies are obtainable at will. Contemporaneously have come methods of studying biological effects and the responses of various types of tissues to ionizing influences. Consequently roentgen therapy has been put upon a sound foundation and must be considered a scientific procedure.

During the development of these various steps in the physical progress of x-ray therapy, radiologists were more and more inclined to concentrate their efforts on the treatment of malignancies and more or less neglect the milder lesions. However, inflammatory lesions have

*Read before the annual meeting of the Minnesota State Medical Association, Duluth, Minnesota, June 29, 1938.

been treated since 1900 and the beneficial effects of the x-ray in acne, furunculosis and erysipelas are well known. Even the recently much-advertised therapy for sinusitis has been used by the radiologist for fifteen years. About eight years ago, Desjardins[2] summarized the results of several years of experience in treating inflammatory conditions and his explanation of the action of the roentgen rays is still authoritative. During this time, also, biophysicists, biochemists and pathologists have been studing the effects of roentgen irradiation on healthy and inflamed tissue. Their observations and recorded findings have brought roentgen therapy into the field of accepted therapeutic agencies.

In applying roentgen irradiation to inflammatory areas the method of application has much to do with the successful outcome of the therapy. It is not sufficient merely to subject the patient to more or less haphazard exposure under an x-ray tube, without giving thought to the invading organisms, the tissues involved or the lymph drainage system of the locality. The nature of the infection, its methods of spreading and the toxic manifestations it produces are important considerations. The depth of the infection in the tissues modifies, to a certain extent, the potential at which the machine is set; the acuteness or chronicity of the lesion indicates the interval of time between treatments; and the probable duration of the disease determines the number of r to be administered at each treatment. As a rule, smaller doses at rather frequent intervals produce better results than larger doses at greater intervals. This has been clearly shown by extensive experimental work carried out in Leningrad. It was noted that the dose-time interval is important. Small doses given every other day had much better effect than larger doses given every fourth day, although the total amount of radiation was the same. This is readily understood when it is realized that only a short time is required to break down the phagocytic cells of the blood, liberating the antibodies or other substances therein contained. These antibodies act as antitoxins and have definite phagocytic properties after liberation. It must be remembered that the metabolism and function of parenchymal and connective tissues are increased by inflammation; therefore, physically equal roentgen doses have much greater effect on inflammatory tissue than on normal tissue.

An editorial in the *Journal of the American Medical Association*[3] reads, in part, as follows: "Roentgen irradiation appears to be capable of aborting many of the early infections and of promoting the breaking down and localization of the more advanced lesions. The roentgen rays are not in themselves bactericidal. The favorable action is believed to be due to the breaking down of certain radio-sensitive cells and the consequent liberation of powerful antitoxic substances."

The amount of irradiation required in the treatment of infections is small as compared with the larger doses ordinarily considered in the treatment of malignant tumors. Surrounding normal tissue is included in the field of application and the lymph drainage areas must certainly be reached. It is advantageous to begin therapy in the lymph drainage areas if possible and then cover the focus of infection. This plan should be followed in such a manner that one area is treated daily, and no time interval of any magnitude intervenes. Kaplan[6] states that "while x-rays are not bactericidal, they possess the power to stimulate within tissues certain responses, as hyperemia and destruction of leukocytes and lymphocytes with the liberation of endotoxins which possess the power of phagocytosis. The employment of x-rays for the treatment of inflammatory conditions is rational procedure."

Time is an important factor in the treatment of infections. Roentgen therapy, in addition to all other kinds or types of therapy selected, should be started early. The most prompt effects and the best results are obtained by early application. It is a well known fact that x-rays increase both the local and general resistance to infection and the tendency toward secondary infection is lessened. This local increase of tissue resistance continues for three or four weeks, after which it gradually declines to normal. It exists only in the area treated and does not extend to adjacent tissues. There is no cumulative action which might lower tissue resistance. Healing takes place normally and neither the diseased tissue nor the healthy tissue surrounding it is injured by the treatment.

It must not be believed that roentgen therapy should be used to the exclusion of any other therapy, neither should it be used as a last resort; it should be considered an adjuvant and be thought of in every infection. Kelley and

848

Dowell,[7] in an analysis of fifty-six cases of gas bacillus infection, recommend that the patient be treated with x-ray as soon as the presence of the infection is suspected. They believe that such treatment, combined with serum treatment, tetanus antitoxin, local surgical procedures and antiseptics, removes the necessity of amputation. They report a mortality of less than 10 per cent.

In the treatment of lobar pneumonia, Powell[9] gives the results of the treatment of two groups of patients. In both groups the treatment by all other means of therapy remained the same, but one group received the serum and the other group roentgen therapy. In the group which received serum the mortality was 15 per cent, while in the group which received x-ray the mortality was 5 per cent. These statistics agree with those published elsewhere, particularly in Europe, where the mortality rate for all types of pneumonia without serum or x-ray treatment is given as 30 per cent, with serum 15 per cent and with x-ray 5 per cent. These results are due to an early crisis brought about by the x-ray therapy and it is explained by the statement that a certain lysin is liberated from the infiltrating leukocytes which causes rapid solution of the coagulum which is the principal component of the consolidation.

Recent experimental work by Fried[4] on guinea pigs with artificial pneumonia produced by emulsified cultures of hemolytic staphylococcus aureus showed marked consolidations in the control animals while the irradiated animals showed only scattered small areas of consolidation. The irradiated lungs showed less congestion, less edema, less infiltration of tissue and fewer abscess formations.

In substantiation of these findings and results I quote from Boyd[1]: "Acute inflammatory lesions * * * are amenable to radiation. Exposure at an early stage causes rapid resolution. It seems strange that an agent which destroys the inflammatory cells should benefit the lesion. The probable explanation is that protective substances are liberated by the disintegrating polymorphoneuclears and lymphocytes."

The infectious involvements of the nasal accessory sinuses, the mastoids and the middle ear are quite aggravating. After all other medical and surgical procedures have been used and have been found insufficient to relieve the symptoms, a majority of the patients can be benefited by roentgen therapy, provided care in its adminis-

tration is used. Many exorbitant claims have been made of the results obtained in the treatment of this class of infections and, as a result, some discredit has been reflected on roentgen therapy in all infections. The fact remains, however, that the method of application and not the therapeutic agent itself was at fault. Lucinian[8] reports favorably on the treatment of otitis media and catarrhal deafness, and the works of Woolley[10] and Hodges[5] on sinus infection are well known.

All types of infection have been successfully treated with roentgen rays. These include such conditions as arthritis, parotitis, bursitis, peritonsilar abscess, pyorrhea, endocarditis, bronchiectasis, puerperal mastitis, peritonitis, localized cellulitis, adenitis, endometritis and many others. There is a possibility that any infection may be treated by x-ray if the treatment is administered with caution and the general principles of small doses, repeated frequently, followed. Let me quote from the paper of Desjardins,[2] published seven years ago, whose description of the accepted physiological action of roentgen therapy in inflammation cannot be surpassed. He says: "The infiltrating cells contain or elaborate within themselves the protective substances or other means which enable them to destroy or neutralize the bacterial or other toxic products which give rise to the defensive inflammation. If these assumptions are well founded, it seems not unreasonable to deduce that irradiation, by destroying the infiltrating leukocytes, causes the protective substances contained by such cells to be liberated and to be made even more readily available for defensive purposes than they were in the intact cell."

Founded on such a reasonable premise, the clinical application of the roentgen rays in inflammatory reactions is practicable, efficient and scientific practice.

References

1. Boyd, Wm.: Text Book of Pathology. Lea and Febiger, 1934, p. 357.
2. Desjardins, A. U.: Radiotherapy for inflammatory conditions. Jour. A.M.A., 96:401-408, (Feb. 7) 1931.
3. Editorial: Furuncle of the face. Jour. A.M.A., 109:278-279, (July 24) 1937.
4. Fried, Carl: Treatment of experimental pneumonia by irradiation. Strahlentherapie, 58:430-448, (Mar. 20) 1937.
5. Hodges, Fred M.: Unpublished paper read before the International Congress of Radiology, 1937.
6. Kaplan, Ira I.: Radiation Therapy. Oxford University press, 1937, p. 451.
7. Kelley, J. F., and Dowell, D. A.: X-rays in gas gangrene. Jour. A.M.A., 107:1114-1117, (Oct. 3) 1936.
8. Lucinian, J. H.: The treatment of otitis media and mastoiditis by roentgen rays. Am. Jour. Roent. and Radium Therapy, 36:946-953, (Dec.) 1936.
9. Powell, Eugene V.: Unpublished paper read before the International Congress of Radiology, 1937.
10. Woolley, Ivan M.: Unpublished paper read before the International Congress of Radiology, 1937.

HISTORY OF MEDICINE IN RAMSEY COUNTY

BY J. M. ARMSTRONG, M.D.

(Continued from November issue)

1853

At the beginning of 1853 there were ten physicians practicing medicine in Saint Paul: Drs. J. H. Day, Goodrich, Barbour, Dewey, Vicchers, Potts, Mann, Brisbine, Babbitt and Willey. David Day was at this time at Long Prairie, and Borup was not practicing.

On March 17, Babbitt's card disappeared from the papers and Dr. Barbour's was discontinued a month later. Whoever was Coroner this year was apparently not filling his office, for on the 20th of April Dr. Mann was appointed by Truman M. Smith, Justice of the Peace, to hold an "inquisition" on the body of a man who met his death by the shifting of a cargo of lumber on one of the river boats. Two more physicians came to Saint Paul: Dr. Wm. H. Morton, of Patterson, N. J., on May 30, and Dr. L. C. Kinney in July. Dr. Kinney stated in his professional announcement that he had been in practice ten years, one of which he spent with the army in Mexico. He took an office in Holland Place, in a two-story frame building that stood on St. Anthony Street opposite the site now occupied by the West Publishing Co.

Dr. Morton seems to have been in no hurry to start in business, for his professional card did not appear in the paper till December 8, when he associated himself with Dr. Potts. They took an office over H. C. Sanford's store situated on Third Street just below Wabasha. Previous to this time Dr. Potts' professional card remained the same as it was in 1849.

This year marks the beginning of medical societies in Minnesota. At this point we must digress a little to settle a point in history which may as well be cleared up now as later.

Our present Minnesota State Medical Association was organized as the Minnesota State Medical Society on February 1, 1869. Its first volume of transactions was published in 1870. This first volume of transactions contains the minutes of the preliminary meeting held for the purpose of organization, a list of those signing the constitution, and the statement that Dr. Thomas R. Potts, president of the old Society organized in 1855, now defunct, presided at the formation of the present Society. In 1925, the Council of our present State Association, finding that the archives of the Association did not have a copy of the first volume, had it reprinted from the only copy available which was and is now in the Library of the Ramsey County Medical Society. As regards the date, 1855, the statement is erroneous, the date should be 1853. The *Pioneer* for July 28, 1853, states:

"In pursuance of a call publically given by the papers of the Territory, physicians representing different counties and towns met in St. Paul on Saturday 23, inst., at the Court House and made a temporary organization, by calling Dr. Potts to the chair and Dr. Anderson Secretary. The Convention then organized, soon admitted the propriety of forming a Medical Society, and went into a committee of the whole, Dr. Murphy in the chair, to deliberate upon forming a constitution. At half past twelve the committee rose, to meet at two o'clock at Dr. Mann's office.

"Afternoon Session—The attendance being punctual, the convention resolved itself at once into a committee of the whole, Dr. Murphy in the chair, when a plan of Constitution and By-laws was reported, accepted and the committee discharged, Dr. Potts in the chair. A Constitution made up mainly from those in force in Pennsylvania and Illinois, was now taken up and considered by sections, and with various additions and amendments adopted, together with a set of By-Laws and the American Association's Code of Ethics. Drs. Ames, Murphy, and Mann were now appointed a committee to select permanent officers and committees for the ensuing year: who reported—

"President—Dr. Potts, St. Paul
"Vice Presidents—Drs. Ames, All Saints, and Murphy, St. Anthony
"Corresponding Secretary—Dr. T. T. Mann, St. Paul
"Recording Secretary—Dr. Anderson, St. Anthony."

An abbreviated statement of the proceedings may also be found in the *Northwestern Medical and Surgical Journal* (Chicago) for August, 1853. Corroborating these we find the following from the pen of Dr. Wm. W. Finch, of Saint Paul, in "Physicians, the Climate and Diseases of Minnesota" (*Boston Medical and Surgical Journal*, Oct. 12, 1853):

"On the 23rd of July, 1853, the first Medical Society was organized in this territory and christened 'The Minnesota Medical Society.' Considering that there are scarcely twenty regular physicians in the territory, the meeting was well attended, matters were discussed in a friendly manner and the following officers chosen: Dr. Potts of St. Paul, President; Dr. Ames of Minneapolis, and Dr. Murphy of St. Anthony, Vice Presidents; Dr. Anderson of St. Anthony, Recording Secretary; Dr. Goodrich, Treasurer; Dr. Mann, Corresponding Secretary; and Drs. Day, Dewey, and Finch, Censors. The last five officers are residents of St. Paul. Though few in numbers, we mean to do what we can to sustain and advance medical science in this new territory, and we hope to receive the good wishes at least of the older societies in the states."

If these two citations are not sufficiently convincing that the society was founded in 1853, we find in the Transactions of the American Medical Association of the St. Louis meeting of 1854, that John H. Murphy, Falls of St. Anthony, attended the meeting as a delegate with credentials from the Minnesota Medical Society. Murphy was the first Minnesota physician to belong to the American Medical Association, but while this is true we must state for the benefit of those not informed that Minnesota Territory did not exist until 1849, and just previous to that date the eastern part of our state was part of Wisconsin Territory, and that Dr. A. E. Ames, of Wisconsin, was a member of the American Medical Association in 1848. Ames, however, at that time was not a resident within the present limits of Minnesota. From the *St. Anthony Express*, which contains the best account of this meeting, we learn that Dr. A. E. Johnson of St. Anthony also personally attended the meeting and that Dr. A. W. Daniels of St. Peter and Dr. O. P. Marsh of St. Paul signified their desire to belong and were marked present by request; and that Drs. J. H. Day, A. G. Brisbine and Samuel Willey of St. Paul, together with Dr. Carli of Stillwater and Dr. Chas. McDougall of Fort Snelling, were made charter members, though not actually present. Dr. McDougall had recently arrived at Fort Snelling, relieving Dr. Ames who was Contract Civilian Surgeon there till McDougall arrived. Dr. McDougall, a native of Indiana, entered the army in 1832 and retired in 1869. He was made a Brevet Brigadier General in 1865 for gallant conduct in the field. A meeting of the Society was scheduled for January 1854, but apparently was not held, though it is possible that some data regarding it may yet be found. Mrs. Abbott, widow of the late Dr. Everton J. Abbott and daughter of Dr. John Steele, says she remembers having a minute book of a medical society and using it for a scrapbook when she was a girl. The book was not destroyed till after Dr. Abbott's death when the family moved to another residence. Possibly, it was the minute book of this Society.

As regards the further activities of this Society, the St. Paul City Directory for 1856-1857 states:

Medical Society of Minnesota—organized December, 1855.
Officers for 1856-7:
    Dr. Thomas Potts, President
    Dr. J. H. Murphy, Vice President
    Dr. J. V. Wren, Recording Secretary
    Dr. James D. Goodrich, Corresponding Secretary
    Dr. David Day, Treasurer
    Dr. W. H. Morton, Dr. F. R. Smith, Dr. J. H. Stewart, Dr. A. E. Johnson, Dr. A. E. Ames—Censors
    Dr. R. W. Wing, Dr. O. P. Marsh, Dr. C. L. Anderson—Standing Committee.

Note that the date "1855" appears again. The word "organized" should be "reorganized" at a meeting held in December, 1855. However, the paper for January 5, 1856, says the meeting was held in Dr. Wren's office January 3, 1856, and gives the additional information that Dr. LeBoutillier was chosen essayist. Evidently, this is where the date 1855 came from in the 1869 transactions of our present Association, and also because of no meeting in 1854 a reorganization was effected in 1855. It is known that the Constitution and By-laws of this Society were printed in 1856, but no copy of it has yet been found. The last meeting of the Society was held at St. Anthony in 1857, the officers being the same as given in 1856 with the exception of the censors, who were Drs. W. H. Morton, F. R. Smith, J. H. Stewart, A. E. Johnson, and A. E. Ames. No account of this meeting can be found, the files of St. Anthony and Minneapolis papers being incomplete for that year.

There is evidence then that the Society was active during the years 1853-55-56 and 1857. Our information as to this Society ends here unless further research discloses more data. It will be noted that Dr. Potts was its first and last recorded president. It is probable that the reason Potts was elected president is that he was a much older man than any of the others. In fact, Minnesota at that time was populated chiefly by comparatively young men, and Potts, in 1853, was forty-three years of age and one of the oldest men here. It is further probable that the panic of 1857 killed the Society as it nearly killed all business activities in the Territory. The preceding remarks as to Doctor Potts and the demise of this Society are not founded alone on my own surmises, but Dr. C. E. Smith, Sr., and Dr. Alfred Wharton were of the same opinion. Both of these physicians knew of this Society but had no further recollection of it. St. Paul, in 1850, had a population of 1,294, Ramsey County (then including St. Anthony), 2,197, and the entire territory, excluding soldiers, but 4,780, while in 1860 St. Paul had 10,279 inhabitants and the county 12,150. So the proportion of physicians to the number of inhabitants was excessive, which accounts for the many changes. Every steamboat, however, during this period brought in a cargo of immigrants, speculators, and adventurers.

This same year (1853) Bishop Cretin laid the cornerstone of St. Joseph's Hospital on the same site as the present building, though it was not open to patients till the following year. This was the first hospital in the state other than the military hospitals. It served not only as a hospital but as a home for orphans and the aged and housed the sisters. For some years after 1859 it was occupied by St. Joseph's Academy. Until our city and county hospital (now the Ancker Hospital) was established in 1882, the city and county patients also were cared for at St. Joseph's.

In July, Dr. Babbitt moved his office from St. Anthony Street to Main Street (West Fourth), between St. Peter and Market Streets. It would seem that ten physicians were not enough for St. Paul, for in July, Dr. O. P. Marsh arrived and took an office on Third Street next to the Post Office (below Wabasha). In October the election returns showed that J. E. Fullerton, Whig nominee for coroner, was victorious over Patric Carey, the Democratic nominee. On November 17, the *Pioneer* published on its editorial page a "Business Directory" of St. Paul and gave the names of fourteen physicians. In addition to those already mentioned the names of Drs. Alfred Berthier, Wm. W. Finch, and David Day were listed. The latter had been physician to the Winnebago Indians at Long Prairie since the spring of 1852. He was still there in 1853, but it was stated in parentheses after his name that "he will take up his residence in St. Paul in the spring." Dr. Day was succeeded at Long Prairie by Dr. Frederick Andros, of Iowa, who had also preceded him in the same position. This same business directory also stated that the druggists in St. Paul were Bond and Kellogg, Wm. W. Hichcox, Wm. H. Jarvis, and John J. Dewey, and that the capital invested in the drug business in our city was $31,000. Kellogg soon went out of business and the firm became Bond and Axtell. At this time there were five physicians in St. Anthony: Drs. J. H. Murphy, A. E. Johnson, Charles L. Anderson, Kingsbury, and Z. Jodon. St. Paul consisted of 700 buildings and 4,700 inhabitants. Although Dr. Finch was in St. Paul before November 17, his professional announcement in the *Pioneer* did not appear till January 5, 1854. It is interesting in its reference to the use of ether.

"Being familiar with the use of ether, operations in surgery will be performed under its influence without pain, if desired."

The "if desired" seems incomprehensible to us now. Doctor Finch gave as reference Professor McClintock, of the Philadelphia College of Medicine, and Professor Perkins, of Vermont Medical College. Dr. Mann, late in the year, was appointed physician to the Sioux Indians, but retained his residence in St. Paul, since the Sioux were still living at Kaposia (Little Crow's Village). On November 10, Oakland Cemetery was ready for use. Governor Ramsey was president of the Association and Dr. Borup one of the Board of Trustees.

Harry Birmingham, who had been Assistant Surgeon at Fort Snelling for four years, located in St. Paul during the year. He never practiced there, however, but was in the drug business for a time. Dr. Thomas W. Foster, a resident of Hastings, was later a druggist in St. Paul. A son of Dr. Birmingham became a surgeon in the army and died in 1932. Dr. Henry Birmingham died in St. Paul, September 25, 1891. St. Paul, at the end of 1853, had thirty physicians. Three of them never practiced, and Wm. H. Jarvis, as a homeopath, probably did little except counter prescribing at his drug store. A homeopath at that time simply meant that a man bought a book on homeopathy and announced himself as a physician of that cult.

It was during this year that some Chippewa Indians hid under the wooden steps of the Pioneer Building all night in order to waylay any Sioux that might come into town the next morning from Kaposia. Early in the morning of April 27, a canoe containing Old Bets, her sister, and Wooden-legged Jim, her brother, landed at the foot of Jackson Street and the three walked up to the store of the Minnesota Outfit.

It was the intention of the Chippewas to ambush them at the landing, but the marsh between Fifth Street and Third Street prevented them, and the unsuspecting Sioux, circling the flooded area, reached the store before the Chippewas opened fire. Old Bets' sister was mortally wounded, and wooden-legged Jim had a splinter knocked off his wooden leg by a ball as he rushed out of the store to discharge his old pepper-box pistol. Dr. Goodrich dressed the woman's wounds, and at her own request she was taken back to Kaposià, where she died.

Two new life insurance companies entered St. Paul this year: the Mutual Life of New York, for whom Dr. Potts served as medical examiner; and the New England Mutual Life, who employed as examiner Dr. G. S. Sperry. Sometime during the year, Dr. Ebenezer Miller came to St. Paul from Vermont. He was the father of the late Dr. Clinton C. Miller. He never practiced medicine in St. Paul, however, and died in Louisiana, July 21, 1865. Among the distinguished visitors to St. Paul in 1853 was Dr. Marshall Hall of London, famous for his studies of the physiology of the nervous system.

1854

Although most of the physicians who were in St. Paul at the end of 1853 remained there during the following year, the practice of inserting cards in the papers went out of fashion, and the historian is forced to rely upon other sources of information. In February, Dr. Marsh's card disappeared, and a few weeks later advertisements inserted by Dr. Goodrich and Dr. Dewey were discontinued. By the end of the year only three physicians' cards were published in the *Pioneer*; those of Drs. Sperry, Kinney, and J. H. Day. Of these, the last mentioned had left town.

In February, smallpox became epidemic among the Chippewa Indians, and their condition became so bad that the governor appointed Dr. Mann to render medical aid to them. Mann, however, found it inconvenient to leave town and deputed Dr. J. H. Day to act in his place. Day left St. Paul on March 25, and returned sometime in April. He and his guide and interpreter first went to St. Croix Falls and then westward. It was a very arduous trip. The *Pioneer* for May 2 contained a long report made by Dr. Mann to Governor Gorman on the subject. The condition of the Indians was deplorable. Not only were they afflicted with the smallpox; they were destitute as well. In one village, Dr. Day found but seven out of a band of fifty-four alive.

A business directory published in the *Daily Times* for May 16 gave the names of fourteen physicians as follows: Brisbine and Willey, A. Berthier, J. H. Day, J. D. Goodrich, John J. Dewey, C. L. Vicchers, W. W. Finch, David Day, O. P. Marsh, T. T. Mann—Sioux physician, Potts and Morton, and Barbour. In June, Dr. Finch's card was withdrawn from the papers, though he was apparently still in St. Paul as late as October, when he went to Clinton Falls. Early in May the citizens of St. Paul began to be worried by the development of cholera along the river, and a health officer and city physician was appointed. The history of cholera in St. Paul will be discussed in another place.

On June 20, William W. Hichcox, the druggist, who was a man of violent temper, had a dispute with a drayman named Peltier over some drayage charges. As Peltier drove away from the drug store, Hichcox caught up an axe and followed him, running up alongside the cart. Peltier, sitting in the dray, caught up an iron dray pin and swinging it out to ward off the axe, struck Hichcox on the head, fracturing his skull. Hichcox's skull was trephined to raise the depressed bone, but he died on July 3. Charles Bazille, who was coroner at the time, impaneled a jury, and at his order a post-mortem examination was made by Dr.

Morton assisted by Drs. Goodrich, J. H. Day, and Marsh. Peltier was later tried for homicide but was acquitted on the plea of self-defense. Peltier left St. Paul after his acquittal and went to Canada, where he became a monk, a very learned man and teacher. Dr. William G. LeDuc of Hastings witnessed the encounter of the two men. The story of Peltier's later life is recorded from his testimony. It may be of interest to note here that while General LeDuc was attending Harvard Law School in 1849 he was engaged by the *New York Tribune* to report the trial in Boston of Professor Webster, who was charged with the murder of Dr. Parkman.

After Hichcox's death, Dr. David Day, who was appointed administrator of his estate, took over his drug business on the southwest corner of Third and Cedar Streets, and continued it until 1866. In August, a new physician came to town, a Dr. George Hadfield, homeopath. He took an office on Third Street, one door above Buell's store (presumably just below Wabasha). During August, also, Dr. Sperry, who already had been in St. Paul for some time, inserted his professional card in the paper as a "Homeopath, office on Third Street opposite C. E. Mayo and Co.; Residence at Winslow House." Later in the year he changed his announcement, inserting "M.D." after his name, and moved his residence to the Central House (Third and Minnesota Streets). Sperry got into some trouble and left town suddenly about 1859.

Dr. J. H. Day concluded that Kansas and Nebraska territories offered advantages over Minnesota, and in August he left St. Paul and settled at Leavenworth. Dr. L. C. Kinney bought out the World's Fair Drug Store at Third and Robert Streets from William H. Jarvis, and also opened a branch store in upper town at the Winslow Block. At the Democratic primaries in the autumn several candidates sought the nomination for the legislature, among them Drs. Willey and Goodrich. Neither man received the nomination or polled many votes, and both disclaimed any desire for the office—after the election. By a peculiar vote William H. Jarvis was chosen coroner. There were four candidates, H. A. Schlick, Lott Moffet, S. C. Cave, and William H. Jarvis. Jarvis received 342 votes and the other three one vote each. The year 1854 was a banner year for new physicians to locate at St. Paul, more so even than 1851. Among the men to arrive were the following: Thomas J. Vaiden (September 2 or 3), George W. Huntington (October 17), A. E. Boyd, and Louis Francis Tavernier. Dr. Thomas W. Foster, who had been living in Hastings, returned to St. Paul during the year and became actuary and executive for the Oakland Cemetery Association. He and Dr. David Day were also active in the organization of the Board of Trade on November 29. Dr. N. Barbour remained in town and became one of the officials of the Sons of Temperance.

As to Dr. Huntington little further is known. His card was discontinued in November, and he seems to have remained in St. Paul only a short time. Vaiden probably never practiced but interested himself in real estate. He was an elderly man with long dark hair, a gentleman, very reticent as to his affairs, and almost a recluse. More will be said of him later. Boyd remained in town a few years, practicing homeopathy, then moved to a farm in New Canada Township. Later, he came back to St. Paul, where he died June 4, 1888. It is said he knew Dr. Hadfield before coming to St. Paul. Neither he nor Tavernier, however, played any part in the medical history of St. Paul or Ramsey County. Tavernier left to practice at Fort Atkinson, Iowa, for a short time, but returned and died in St. Paul, January 26, 1870, aged fifty-three years. He was a French Canadian. Both Boyd and Tavernier left families in St. Paul.

(To be continued in January, 1939, issue)

EDITORIAL

MINNESOTA MEDICINE

OFFICIAL JOURNAL OF THE MINNESOTA STATE MEDICAL
ASSOCIATION

Published by the Association under the direction of its Editing
and Publishing Committee

EDITING AND PUBLISHING COMMITTEE

J. T. CHRISTISON, Saint Paul   C. B. WRIGHT, Minneapolis
E. M. HAMMES, Saint Paul   T. A. PEPPARD, Minneapolis
WALTMAN WALTERS, Rochester

EDITORIAL STAFF

CARL B. DRAKE, Saint Paul, Editor
W. F. BRAASCH, Rochester, Associate Editor
GILBERT COTTAM, Minneapolis, Associate Editor

Annual Subscription—$3.00   Single Copies—$0.40

Foreign Subscriptions—$3.50

The right is reserved to reject material submitted for editorial
or advertising columns. The Editing and Publishing Committee
does not hold itself responsible for views expressed either in
editorials or other articles when signed by the author.

Classified advertising—five cents a word; minimum charge,
$1.00. Remittance should accompany order.

Display advertising rates on request.

Address all communications to Minnesota Medicine, 2642 University Avenue, Saint Paul, or Suite 604, National Bldg., Minneapolis. Telephone: Nestor 2641.

BUSINESS MANAGER
J. R. BRUCE

Volume 21   DECEMBER, 1938   Number 12

The Oral Use of Neoprontosil in the Treatment
of Chronic Ulcerative Colitis

THE possible efficiency of certain sulfamido
compounds in the treatment of chronic ulcerative colitis was foreseen soon after clinical use
of these drugs was instituted. This interest in
the therapeutic possibilities of these drugs probably was aroused by the fact that these compounds were effective in the treatment of diseases resulting from infection with hemolytic
streptococci. It followed, therefore, that some of
the sulfamido compounds might be of value in
the treatment of chronic ulcerative colitis since
this disease may be due to a related organism.

The early experience of Bannick, Brown and

Foster, which has been confirmed by Collins and
others, seemed to indicate that sulfanilamide was
of definite benefit in ulcerative colitis. However,
as was pointed out later by Brown, Herrell and
Bargen, the occasional appearance of rather severe toxic manifestations subsequent to use of
this drug makes the use of sulfanilamide somewhat undesirable. In fact, the general experience
of most of those interested in this form of treatment leads, now, to the conclusion that sulfanilamide is not the drug of choice in treatment of
this disease. Especially is this true if patients
are acutely ill and if there is a rather extensive
ulceration of the colon.

In the search for a similar preparation which
might possess the therapeutic efficiency of sulfanilamide, without the severe toxic manifestations which prohibit its administration to severely ill patients, neoprontosil was suggested by
Bannick and Brown. At that time, however,
neoprontosil was available only in a 2.5 per cent
solution to be administered parenterally. The
inherent chronicity of chronic ulcerative colitis
and the necessity of long continued use of any
therapeutic agent were somewhat against any
parenteral medication. Then too, as was shown
by Rosenthal, 85 to 95 per cent of this drug,
when given parenterally to experimental animals,
was excreted in the urine within five hours.
This fact meant that the concentration of the
drug could not be held at a high level without
repeated injections at short intervals. The experimental work of Raizess and Rosenthal, working
independently, indicated that if the drug could
be given orally it would be more slowly absorbed
and thus would be retained in the body for a
longer time. Such retention would allow for
greater concentration and, therefore, for greater
therapeutic efficiency. Therefore, the material
was obtained in powdered (capsule) form and
was first administered clinically by Brown, Bannick and Herrell. In a representative group of
unselected cases of ulcerative colitis, the results
following oral administration of this material
were better than the most optimistic expectations.

The dosage employed was similar to that used
in the previous oral administration of sulfanilamide. To the average adult, amounts of between

856

4 and 5 gm. of this drug, divided into five equal parts, were given in each twenty-four hours. In other words, 15 grains (1 gm.) were usually given an hour before each meal, at bedtime, and at 2 a. m. Such a course was administered usually for ten to fourteen days. It seems apparent that if the drug is given an hour before the intake of food, most of the gastro-intestinal symptoms usually associated with sulfamido compounds will be eliminated. Subsequent to a course of this dosage, experience has indicated that a smaller dosage, of approximately 2.5 gm., given daily for another ten to fourteen days, is advisable. Following this again a larger dosage may be employed for at least the first three months of treatment.

In addition to the marked clinical improvement, the lack of toxic manifestations following the use of this drug is apparent. For example, Brown and Herrell reported, following administration of neoprontosil orally to nearly 500 patients, that depression of the leukocyte count was seen only once or twice. It is further interesting that among those individuals with chronic ulcerative colitis, whose stools are rather markedly hemorrhagic and number from four to fifteen per day, both quantity of blood and number of stools are markedly decreased by the third or fourth day of treatment. In other words, blood disappears from the stools of these individuals long before healing of a rather severely denuded bowel would seem possible. It is also interesting that the proctoscopic appearance of the mucous membrane in cases of rather severe ulcerative colitis has been reported to be normal often as early as two or three weeks following administration of neoprontosil. It is proper, however, at this point to emphasize a pertinent observation made by those individuals originally responsible for the administration of this drug in ulcerative colitis; namely, that it is impossible for any chemotherapeutic agent to restore to normal the physiologic function of a bowel which has become contracted and deformed by chronic ulcerative colitis of long standing. If, however, neoprontosil is used early in the course of chronic ulcerative colitis, rather remarkable results may be expected. It is further worthy of emphasis that those who are responsible for the use of neoprontosil have stated repeatedly that they do not pretend to have discovered the cause or the absolute cure of chronic ulcerative colitis; they do feel, however,

that continuous use of the drug is amply justified on the basis of clinical experience in the past year.

At present only impressions exist concerning the mode of action of neoprontosil in the treatment of chronic ulcerative colitis. Some general beliefs, however, are justifiable in view of what has been observed clinically and following use of the drug in experiments on animals. Certainly, the therapeutic response cannot be explained on the basis of the sulfanilamide which is made available in the systemic circulation by the breakdown of neoprontosil. In other words, it appears that neoprontosil has an action wholly independent of the available sulfanilamide. Neoprontosil often appears in the stools of human subjects as soon as twelve hours following its oral administration. The clinical results would seem to indicate that at least part of the drug is absorbed through the lower part of the intestinal tract and thereby exerts its efficiency to encourage healing of the mucous membranes. The experimental work of Marshall, however, would tend to indicate that absorption does not take place in the large bowel of experimental animals. This observation, of course, does not necessarily mean that absorption is not possible in the lower part of the intestinal tract of man. It is further possible that the mere presence of the drug in direct contact with the lower part of the bowel may exert a local action independent of that made possible by absorption into mucous membranes or into the systemic circulation.

Certainly, the marked clinical response reported following oral administration of neoprontosil in the treatment of chronic ulcerative colitis is stimulating and it is safe to say that this drug deserves clinical application in an effort to evaluate its efficacy.

WALLACE E. HERRELL.

Medicine and Music

GREAT musicians have seldom come out of medicine. Fritz Kreisler was a medical student but never graduated. His whole career has been centered in his violin; his medicine was merely a passing incident in his youth, wholly obliterated by his genius in his music.

Theodor Billroth (1829-1884) was a great surgeon and unusually well qualified as a musician. He was a close friend of Brahms and wrote a classic on the physiology and psychology of music entitled "Wer ist musikalisch?" which was published after his death. While his standing in the musical world did not compare with his fame in surgery he believed that the two were complementary and that the study of music greatly aided his inventive genius as a surgeon. That he had the inherent quality of a real musician is shown in the words he wrote a few hours before his death:

"It is night and everything has been quiet for a long time and now I am very calm. My mind begins to wander. An ethereal blue sky envelops me. My soul soars upwards. The most beautiful harmonies of invisible choirs are audible—in soft undulations like the breath of eternity! I also recognize voices and the gentle whisperings: 'Come, tired man, we will make you happy. In the charm of these spheres we will free you of the thoughts which have been of the greatest joy or deepest sorrow. You have felt yourself as a part of the universe, now be distributed through the universe and comprehend the whole.'"

He died, world-renowned in surgery, but with only local repute as a talented performer and music lover.

Alexander Borodin (1834-87) began his career as a general practitioner but soon dropped it to take up chemistry, in which he became quite eminent, contributing numerous articles to the literature and being credited with being the co-discoverer of aldol, with Wurtz. As a child he had shown marked talent for music and had been given instruction in the piano and cello, in both of which he became proficient. At thirteen he wrote a concerto for the flute. Later he joined the circle of Balakireff, enjoying the companionship of the youthful group which included César Cui, Moussorgsky, Rimsky-Korsakoff and Glazounoff, who laid the foundation of the modern Russian school. Borodin wrote his greatest compositions as recreation in the busiest period of his professional career and two of the best known of these, his third symphony and his opera *Prince Igor*, were unfinished at the time of his death. Both were capably completed by Glazounoff and Rimsky-Korsakoff and are often heard on the programs of the great symphony orchestras. Mr. Ormandy was especially fond of the Polévetzian Dances from *Prince Igor*.

So far as we have been able to discover, Borodin is the only physician in history who attained the highest rank in musical composition.

The one remaining example, and a very remarkable one, is that of Albert Schweitzer, who is still living. Educated originally for the ministry he had also studied organ music under competent teachers and later graduated in medicine. He became the world's foremost exponent of the organ music of J. S. Bach and prepared for publication the most comprehensive and scholarly edition of Bach's preludes and fugues extant. Some years ago he betook himself to the west coast of French Equatorial Africa and established a medical mission at Lambaréne, about seventy miles inland, incidentally building and setting up there a large, modern organ. Wanderers in the dense, almost impassable, forests around there have reported their amazement at hearing the air suddenly filled with the tremendous majesty of a Bach fugue played by a master.

At intervals Schweitzer emerges from his voluntary exile to give organ recitals in London or on the continent. Always he is greeted by large and appreciative crowds of educated musicians who grasp eagerly the opportunity to hear him. He does this to raise money for his mission and he never returns empty-handed.

When one considers the exactions of the musical profession in order to reach the upper strata of perfection it is not surprising that so few have been able to accomplish its highest attainment while at the same time carrying on the work of any kind of medical practice or professional research. Borodin and Schweitzer, one the composer, the other the performer, stand alone in this distinction.   G. C.

Typhoid Mary

THE death last month of Typhoid Mary on North Brother Island in the East River, New York, recalls the incident of her detection as a typhoid carrier in 1907.

An outbreak of typhoid fever had occurred in a household at Oyster Bay in the late summer of 1906. In early 1907 Dr. George A. Soper was delegated to trace the source of the infection which involved six of the eleven persons in one household. All six cases had developed in one week's time with no other cases in the neighborhood. After excluding the usual sources of infection, the evidence developed that three weeks before the first case developed a new cook, Mary Mallon, had been employed and had departed three weeks after the typhoid had appeared. When finally located in 1907, she was employed as a cook for a family in New York City and two cases of typhoid fever occurred in this family. One of the patients, the daughter of the employer, died of the disease. The cook refused to give information as to her past history, but the investigation disclosed that in seven of eight locations where she had been employed in the previous six years typhoid fever had developed a few weeks following her arrival and that she had left in each case a few weeks after the appearance of the disease. She had not contracted the disease at any of the discovered locations. She had been responsible for twenty-six cases with one death and doubtless many more which were not discovered.

Upon her refusal to be examined Typhoid Mary was forcibly taken into custody by the New York Department of Health, not however without a severe struggle. She was taken to the Detention Hospital where repeated examination of the feces proved her to be a typhoid carrier. It had been shown that the gallbladder is the most frequent harborer of typhoid bacilli in carriers, but Typhoid Mary refused operation. After several years she was released upon promising never to cook again. When this promise was broken she was again placed in detention for life.

It is reported that some two per cent of typhoid patients become carriers with the persistence of the infection in the gallbladder for months or even years following the acute fever. In 1908 Dean reported the case of an English doctor who twenty-nine years before had contracted typhoid fever in America and had had persisting gallbladder symptoms. Although the patient had carried on an active practice, he had not known of a case of typhoid fever for which he might have been responsible.

That a carrier of intestinal infection, especially one of low intelligence, little education and with no sense of responsibility, can be a menace to society was well illustrated in the case of Typhoid Mary. Her refusal to cooperate with authorities indicated a suspicion, at least, on her part that in some way she was responsible for the appearance of typhoid fever wherever she went. Her refusal to part with her gallbladder indicated an unusually long resisting stubbornness.

The American Journal of Medical Jurisprudence

A NOTHER medical journal, the *American Journal of Medical Jurisprudence*, was launched on its career with the appearance of its

first number in September, 1938. The tremendous increase in incidents in recent years that result in lawsuits involving medical practice is one of the reasons that such a journal is needed according to the first editorial by the editor, Dr. F. C. Warnshuis. It is believed that such a publication should be invaluable to the medical and dental professions, hospitals, druggist employers, employes, as well as attorneys! Subscription involves joining the American Medico-Legal Association with headquarters in Boston with a five dollar fee for registration and ten dollars annual dues which entitles the member to receive the journal monthly.

A perusal of the first issues of this new journalistic enterprise discloses an interesting array of articles involving various phases of medicolegal matters and the infant journal has our best wishes for a successful future. With the growth of the new journal's advertising section and a reduction in the subscription price we would predict a wider distribution.

A Coördinated Medical and Public Health Program

A T THE meeting of the House of Delegates of the American Medical Association in San Francisco last June a resolution embodying the so-called "Indiana Plan" was submitted.*

The purpose of the plan is the extension of preventive medicine through an active campaign of education not only of the laity but of the medical profession itself. A topic is chosen each month and all agencies of state and county medical societies concentrate on that topic. If, for instance, pneumonia is the subject chosen for January, this subject would be stressed by the Public Health committees of state and county societies before parent teachers or similar associations, or over the radio or in syndicated newspaper articles, and the subject would also be stressed to the profession at county society meetings and in the current issue of the journal.

The plan is being submitted to the county societies by the office of the State Medical Association. If the plan receives a favorable response on the part of the membership, it is safe to say the various committees of the State Medical Association will coöperate wholeheartedly.

---

*Plan in detail Journal of American Medical Association, 111:49, (July 2) 1938.

A Motivating Force

"Consumption is a very fatal disease as it is at present managed. . . . The nineteenth century is drawing rapidly to a close. It has the honor of having discovered the cause and also of having defined the methods which are capable of exterminating this form of human suffering, and it should not be left to the next century to see them put into execution. From numerous small beginnings this reform will rapidly gain in volume and momentum, and it is destined to sweep with irresistible force over all obstacles, until in every civilized portion of the globe tuberculosis has bowed down to the majesty of preventive medicine."

THUS wrote the late Dr. H. Longstreet Taylor of Minnesota, pioneer leader in the fight against tuberculosis, in the late nineties. However, it did remain for the next century to start the campaign of applying available knowledge to saving lives.

Strangely enough the motivating force was nothing more than a small scrap of paper, the tuberculosis Christmas Seal. This stamp, making every citizen a partner in the crusade, breaks through the wall of public indifference and brings the fight against tuberculosis close to the hearts of the people. It makes possible one of the most far-reaching health educational campaigns of all times. The fatalistic do-nothing attitude toward the great White Plague has given way to hope and action. Participation of citizens makes possible great victories.

Physicians have the aid of an aroused public in their efforts to set up machinery to fight tuberculosis. Sanatoria have made possible the isolation of spreaders of the disease. Intensive educational campaigns using all resources continue to create citizen interest and to disseminate information. The tuberculosis death rate has been halved and almost halved again. Definite programs of prevention and early discovery are in progress.

Of this program, Dr. Irvin Abell, Louisville, Kentucky, president of the American Medical Association, says:

"The splendid results achieved so far in the field of tuberculosis are gratifying, not alone to the profession, but to everyone interested in human welfare. The worthiness of the objective of the Christmas Seal Campaign is such as to appeal to the spirit of human kindness, which should be inherent in every individual, and consequently should have widespread endorsement. The National Tuberculosis Association, judged by its aim and accomplishments, is an institution deserving any and all possible assistance."

The importance of continuing the program is indicated in the following statistics:

Tuberculosis is still the first cause of death during the age period from fifteen to forty-five, although it has been reduced to seventh in importance as a cause of death in the entire population.

There are estimated to be more than 500,000 active cases of tuberculosis in the United States.

It is responsible for the death of 200 people every day, of one individual every seven and one-third minutes. Thirty years ago deaths occurred at the rate of one every three and one-half minutes.

Two-thirds of all the deaths from tuberculosis occur before the age of forty-five.

Considerably more than half of all the deaths from tuberculosis occur during the important productive years of life—between the ages of fifteen and forty-five.

Each year, tuberculosis claims the lives of forty thousand young people between the ages of fifteen and forty-five. In this state, the Minnesota Public Health Association, the affiliated unit of the National Tuberculosis Association, directs the state-wide sale of Christmas Seals.

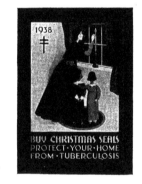

MEDICAL ECONOMICS

Edited by the Committee on Medical Economics
of the
Minnesota State Medical Association
W. F. Braasch, M.D., Chairman

THE A.M.A. IS INVESTIGATED

A N ARTICLE which was asserted to have been based on a thorough investigation of the American Medical Association appeared in the November issue of *Fortune*. The first portion includes a concise, if superficial, survey of some of the many activities of the American Medical Association. Unfortunately, the writer did not confine his observation to a thorough, impartial survey of the Association's numerous activities but went on to criticize the recent policies adopted by the Association and wound up with a plea for compulsory health insurance and medical reform. He used the stock arguments long employed by social reformers and included many of the statistical data which appeared in the National Health Report. He repeated the erroneous statement made by many lay observers that the policies of the American Medical Association are dictated by its officers. After all his investigation he failed to find out that the House of Delegates and constituent state societies are the predominant forces in the American Medical Association and not the officers.

Misconceptions

Included among many misconceptions is the appraisal of Doctor Fishbein and his influence on American medicine. Doctor Fishbein is given credit for being the dictator of the policies and opinions of the Association. He is described as a promotor who has "promoted the Association from a mild academic body to a powerful trade association." To those of us who are familiar with conditions existing at the headquarters of the American Medical Association, such statements are ridiculous. According to the author, Doctor Fishbein is guilty of influencing the opinions of the members of the American Medical Association, and of leading their opposition to governmental control of medicine. The author apparently is ignorant of the

basic principles of the medical profession when he refers to the practice of medicine as a "Business Government Problem."

The writer states that the policies adopted by the officials of the American Medical Association are generally regarded as being unprogressive and antagonistic to reform. That the officers have been severely criticized by members of the Association and that their future leadership is now seriously threatened. While there may be many who believe this to be true, the great majority of the members of the A.M.A. are largely in agreement with its policies. It must be admitted that the officers of the Association and the Board of Trustees have been conservative in their attitude toward the many radical solutions of the economic problems of medicine which have been proposed in the last few years. If they had not been so, American medicine would be in a thoroughly demoralized state today. The officers have always faithfully carried out the policies adopted by the majority of the members of the House of Delegates and when a reform was suggested which proved to be sound, none were quicker to adopt it and to promote it.

Survey Belittled

The article goes on to belittle the National Survey of Supply of Medical Service, which is being conducted by the physicians themselves. The absurd statement that the physicians cannot estimate the number of patients who have inadequate medical care as accurately as the doorbell surveys conducted by W.P.A. laymen sounds like a direct quotation from one of the medical proponents of medical socialization. References made to the advantages of a panel system of medical care are largely quotations from other superficial surveys made by American observers. The author apparently fails to realize the differences between the social conditions in Europe and in America; the political control of our governmental activities and its lack of an adequate civil service; the greater demands and the better standards of living among those with low incomes in America—all of which would make a panel system of medical care impossible in this country.

While investigating the American Medical Association the writer apparently had one eye on the activities going on there and the other on the theories of a host of medical social reformers. Instead of a survey of the American Medical Association, the article is just another bit of lay propaganda by another social reformer. Although the writer's arguments for socialization contain nothing new, the veneer of authenticity given by a so-called investigator might well deceive the uninformed.

W. F. BRAASCH.

TIME TO PUSH FORWARD

Election results and an altered Congress will undoubtedly combine to retard somewhat new welfare programs that require huge expenditures of money.

Legislation to provide for vast new health services will probably be introduced into Congress; but experienced observers are of the opinion that appropriations to finance them will not be so easily secured as formerly.

It is unlikely that any state will seriously consider health legislation before Congress has had time to act.

If, in the meantime, organized medicine pushes forward in its program for local adjustment and improvement where it may be needed, for close and sympathetic coöperation with official agencies and for extension of those services to the needy wherever reliable studies have shown that they are needed, it is unlikely that any radical and unnecessary legislative program will gain support either in Washington or in the state legislatures.

Survey Essential

In any discussions on this issue the first essential will be reliable figures. Failing these, WPA collected figures of the United States Public Health Service's "Doorbell Survey," are sure to be quoted—and believed.

The Survey of Medical Needs and Supply initiated by the American Medical Association and carried on in Minnesota by the Minnesota State Medical Association is designed to supply these figures.

Much information has already been gathered for this study but returns are still far from complete from the physicians themselves.

The importance of complete testimony from the doctors, themselves, has been repeatedly emphasized in these columns. Tabulations of all findings will be made in December. Members who have still not filled in Form No. 1 are urged to do so immediately and send them to the secretaries of their county societies.

ORGANIZED LABOR CONDEMNS SAINT PAUL CITY COUNCIL FIVE DOCTOR PLAN IN ACCIDENT CASES

The Saint Paul Trades and Labor Assembly has emphatically stated that it does not want any part of the plan concocted by Corporation Counsel John W. McConnelough and sponsored by Mayor William H. Fallon to deprive injured St. Paul city employes of their right under the laws of the State of Minnesota to choose their own physician, when injured in line of duty. Without a dissenting vote the Labor Assembly went on record as being opposed to the plan.

The resolution adopted by the Labor Assembly was presented by delegates of the Saint Paul Fire-Fighters' union. It called attention to the fact that the Ramsey County Medical Society had condemned the plan and that "city employes engaged in hazardous occupations are entitled to every protection of medical science." It also pointed out a well known truth "that personal confidence in one's physician is an important element in the treatment of any illness or injury." The resolution concluded by calling "upon the Labor members of the city council to demand a reconsideration of their action and to oppose adoption of any resolution calculated to destroy the right of any city employe to call his family physician for professional care in the event of any illness or injury suffered while in the performance of his official duties."

The Ramsey County Medical Society can well be proud that it took the initiative in condemning the plan and that it has the solid support of the Central Council of Public Service Employes and the Saint Paul Trades and Labor Assembly.

DENTISTS OPPOSE COMPULSORY CARE

The dentists of the United States joined the doctors in opposition to compulsory health insurance at their 80th annual meeting in St. Louis recently.

The following interesting recommendations by their special committee were adopted by the dental delegates at that meeting:

"We approve of the general expansion of public health services and, in addition, recommend the establishment of a Federal Department of Health with a secretary who shall be a graduate in medicine and a member of the President's Cabinet; and a first secretary who shall be a graduate in dentistry.

"In an expanded public health program which involves a consideration of the expenditure of millions of dollars for public health purposes, your Committee recommends that the problem of dental caries and other dental diseases be included.

"Your committee approves the proposed expansion of maternal and child health services provided that dental care of mothers and children be included.

"In any plan for extension of hospital facilities, your committee recommends that due consideration be given to inclusion of adequate facilities for dental services."

"Satisfactory Care Cannot Be Rendered"

With reference to the proposals for provision of medical care for the medically needy and a general program of medical care the committee made the following recommendations:

"Your committee is convinced that satisfactory dental service cannot be rendered under a compulsory health insurance system. *We therefore do not favor such a plan but do approve voluntary budget plans under professional control which will enable patients to apportion costs and timing of payments so as to reduce the burdens of dental costs and remove the economic barriers which now militate against the receipt of adequate dental care.*

Most Prevalent Disease

"The committee approves the recommendation that such a program should provide for continuing and increased incentives to the development and maintenance of high standards of professional preparation and professional service.

"In view of the fact that dental caries is the most prevalent disease of mankind, the American Dental Association strongly recommends that the Federal Government augment with a comprehensive research program the efforts of the organized dental profession to determine the cause of this disease."

863

EXPERT MEDICAL TESTIMONY

Malpractice by a physician is predicated on the fact that there has been negligence on the part of such physician, and the size of the verdict awarded the plaintiff must be contingent on the evident results from such negligence. Negligence must be based again on what is proper treatment in the locality in which the injury was alleged to have been sustained and what the average, ordinary and reasonably prudent man would have done in a like situation.

Results in given cases must be sustained or denied by expert testimony. The question is often asked, "What is expert testimony in a malpractice case?"

Expert testimony may or may not be the testimony of a specialist or so-called "expert." It is the opinion of any person qualified by training and education to give such opinion on the facts of the case. This opinion should preferably be given by a qualified practitioner of medicine whose practice is in the same community as the defendant. He is certainly better able to testify as to the usual proceedings in that community than one whose place of business is much removed or who is in a different type of practice.

It has never been the opinion of the Medical Advisory Committee that one practitioner should conceal the facts concerning malpractice by another where negligence is evident. Members of our association should at all times protect each other, however, against the unscrupulous bringing of malpractice suits for the profit to be obtained either from the alleged negligent doctor or his insurance carrier.

In Minnesota the high quality of medical work performed and the evident interest in postgraduate training has given and will give to the people of this state less cause for litigation as time goes on. The year 1938 has shown this to your committee. We have high hopes for the coming year.

WHY DO THEY DELAY?

A significant study of ten years' experience in the Massachusetts Cancer Clinics published recently in the *Journal of the American Medical Association* showed that a large percentage of persons who do not employ a physician fail to do so because they lack proper education rather than because they lack the funds.

uated from Syracuse University College of Medicine in 1898. He was licensed in Minnesota by examination in 1898. He resided in Saint Paul before returning to New York. His New York license was revoked in March, 1938.

Hopkins Physician's License Revoked

In the Matter of the Revocation of the License of George W. Moore, M.D.

The license to practice medicine and surgery held by George W. Moore, M.D., Hopkins, Minnesota, was revoked by the Minnesota State Board of Medical Examiners on November 4, 1938. Dr. Moore was found guilty by the Board of "immoral, dishonorable and unprofessional conduct," and specifically with "procuring, aiding and abetting a criminal abortion."

Dr. Moore was before the Medical Board in 1936 on a similar charge and after being reprimanded was placed on probation. The facts show, however, that Dr. Moore continued in this type of criminal practice. Dr. Moore offered no defense at the hearing except to state that he did not "care to discuss the matter."

Dr. Moore was born in Indiana in 1870 and graduated in Medicine from the University of Minnesota in 1892.

Physicians Licensed on November 4, 1938

October Examination

Anderson, John Adolph, U. of Minn., M.B. 1933; M.D. 1934, St. Paul, Minn.

Baker, Theodore, Jr., Jefferson Med. Col., M.D. 1933, Rochester, Minn.

Basom, William Compere, Baylor U., M.D. 1936, Rochester, Minn.

Becker, Arnetta Marie, U. of Minn., M.B. 1937; M.D. 1938, Minneapolis Minn.

Birge, Richard Fuller, U. of Neb., M.D. 1935, Rochester, Minn.

Bodaski, Albert Alexander, U. of Minn., M.B. 1937; M.D. 1938, Minneapolis, Minn.

Bond, John H., U. of Pa., M.D. 1936, Minneapolis, Minn.

Church, John Mark, U. of Chicago, M.D. 1938, St. Paul, Minn.

Cook, Paul Thomas, Northwestern U., M.B. 1937; M.D. 1938, St. Paul, Minn.

Daniel, Ruby Kathryn, Baylor U., M.D. 1928, Rochester, Minn.

Erskine, Gordon McClure, U. of Minn., M.B. 1937; M.D. 1938, Grand Rapids, Minn.

Field, Anthony Hugh, Marquette U., M.D. 1938, Minneapolis, Minn.

Fisk, Charlotte, U. of Iowa, M.D. 1932, Minneapolis, Minn.

Gardner, John Williams, U. of Ore., M.D. 1936, Rochester, Minn.

Grinley, Andrew Victor, Rush Med. Col., M.D. 1937, St. Paul, Minn.

Hammerel, John Joseph, Loyola U., M.D. 1938, St. Paul, Minn.

Henderson, John Warren, U. of Neb., M.D. 1937, Rochester, Minn.

Hertz, Myron Jacob, U. of Minn., M.B. 1938, St. Paul, Minn.

Ide, Lucien Waterman, U. of Iowa, M.D. 1937, St. Paul, Minn.

Karn, Jacob Francis, U. of Minn., M.B. 1938, Minneapolis, Minn.

Kaufmann, Mark Irving Herbert, McGill U., M.D. 1936, Oak Terrace, Minn.

Keating, Francis Raymond, Jr., Cornell U., M.D. 1936, Rochester, Minn.

King, William Lyon Mackenzie, U. of Toronto, M.D. 1937, Rochester, Minn.

Lander, Howard Hayes, Northwestern U., M.D. 1937, Rochester, Minn.

McKelvey, John L., Queen's U., M.D., C.M. 1926, Minneapolis, Minn.

McManamy, Eugene Patrick, McGill U., M.D. 1936, Rochester, Minn.

Morissette, Leopold, U. of Montreal, M.D. 1936, Rochester, Minn.

Mountain, George Elmer, Northwestern U., M.D. 1938, Rochester, Minn.

Nelson, Edward Norman, U. of Cincinnati, M.B. 1938, Minneapolis, Minn.

Novak, Milan Vaclav, U. of Minn., M.B. 1938; M.D. 1938, Minneapolis, Minn.

Peterson, Lowell John, U. of Minn., M.B. 1937, Minneapolis, Minn.

Pugh, David Graham, U. of Ind., M.D. 1932, Rochester, Minn.

Ramsay, Robert Matthews, U. of Manitoba, M.D. 1937, St. Paul, Minn.

Sather, Richard Norman, Rush Med. Col., M.D., 1937, St. Paul, Minn.

Seebach, Leslie G., U. of Minn., M.B. 1938, Minneapolis, Minn.

Sherman, Lloyd Frederick, U. of Minn., M.B. 1938, Minneapolis, Minn.

Sims, John LeRoy, U. of Texas, M.D. 1937, St. Paul, Minn.

Smith, Graham Gable, U. of Minn., M.B. 1938, Minneapolis, Minn.

Smith, Robert Lee, Jr., Stanford U., M.D. 1937, Rochester, Minn.

Stafford, Donald Edward, Harvard U., M.D., 1935, Rochester, Minn.

Stewart, Donald Edward, U. of Minn., M.B. 1937; M.D. 1938, Minneapolis, Minn.

Street, Bernard, U. of Minn., M.B. 1937, Minneapolis, Minn.

Utendorfer, Robert William, Northwestern, M.D. 1937; M.D. 1938, St. Paul, Minn.

Vadheim, James Lowell, U. of Minn., M.B. 1937, Minneapolis, Minn.

Vickers, Evelyn Smith, U. of Minn., M.B. 1936; U. 1937, St. Paul, Minn.

Walsh, William Vincent, U. of Minn., M.B. 1937; M.D. 1938, Minneapolis, Minn.

Westra, Jacob John, Rush Med. Col., M.D. 1937; Rochester, Minn.

Word, Harlan Lamar, U. of Okla., M.D. 1936, St. Paul, Minn.

Wulf, Robert Fischer, U. of Pa., M.D., 1936, Rochester, Minn.

By Reciprocity

Baumeister, Carl Frederick, U. of Iowa, M.D. 1933, Council Bluffs, Ia.

Frost, John Bert, U. of Wis., M.D., 1937, Minneapolis, Minn.

Gore, Herbert Robert, Long Island Medical Col., M.D. 1933, Rochester, Minn.

Settlage, Arnold Frederick Ernest, Harvard U., M.D. 1933, Worthington, Minn.

Walske, Benedict Raymond, Marquette U., M.D. 1937, Galesville, Wis.

National Board Credentials

Kenyon, Thomas Jackson, U. of Minn., M.D. 1938, St. Paul, Minn.

Reeser, Richard, Jr., Cornell U., M.D. 1935, Rochester, Minn.

Sundet, Nere Joseph, U. of Minn., M.B. 1936; M.D. 1937, Gary (Norman Co.), Minn.

Vinje, Ralph, Northwestern U., M.D. 1936, Bismarck, N. Dak.

866

OF GENERAL INTEREST

Dr. Owen W. Parker of Ely was elected president of the Minnesota State Sanitary Conference at its last meeting.

* * *

Dr. H. T. Sherman, formerly of Plainview, has moved to Spring Valley, where he will continue the practice of medicine.

* * *

Dr. Gordon Erskine has become associated with Dr. H. E. Binet, Grand Rapids. Dr. Erskine was formerly located in Minneapolis.

Dr. James R. Deagen, formerly of Cold Spring, has established an office in Freeport, where he will continue the practice of medicine.

÷

The engagement has been announced of Eleanor Mary Smith, St. Paul, to Dr. Clarence Dennis, St. Paul, son of Mrs. Warren A. Dennis and the late Dr. Dennis.

* * *

Dr. F. W. Engdahl, formerly associated with Dr. H. E. Binet at Grand Rapids, has moved to Ortonville, where he will continue the practice of medicine.

* * *

Dr. S. Sandell, formerly of Grand Rapids, is taking over the practice of Dr. A. M. Boe of Deer River, who is leaving Deer River because of ill health.

* * *

The Minnesota-Dakota Orthopedic Club met in Rochester on October 22. Several interesting papers were presented in the morning, followed by a luncheon.

* * *

Dr. Traugott Bloedell of Thief River Falls was married to Miss Marion Bernice Long of Minneapolis, on November 9. Dr. Bloedell is on the staff of the Bratrud Clinic.

Dr. Ralph Vinje of Bismarck, North Dakota, formerly a member of the Roan and Strauss Medical Clinic of Bismarck, has located at Ada for the general practice of medicine. He is a son of Dr. and Mrs. Syver Vinje of Hillsboro, North Dakota.

* * *

Dr. Charles B. Cunningham, obstetrician and gynecologist, has become associated with the Lenon-Peter-of the Sunnyside Sanatorium. Dr. Jennings was associated with Glen Lake Sanatorium for more than twenty years, and has been a member of the Board of Directors of the Hennepin County Tuberculosis Association, where he has taken an active part in the program for tuberculosis control in Hennepin County.

† †

Dr. Gilbert J. Thomas has returned from Houston, Texas, where he was a guest speaker at the Seventh Annual Postgraduate Medical Assembly of South Texas, held November 1, 2 and 3. Dr. Thomas spoke on the following subjects: "Non-Specific Renal Infection"; "Chronic Infection of the Prostate Glands; Their Relation to Other Foci of Infection"; "Sterility in the Male and the Responsibility of the General Practitioner in the Diagnosis and Treatment"; "Tuberculosis of the Genital Tract."

Dr. Thomas also spoke to the students at Baylor University by special request, on the subject of "Tuberculosis of the Kidney."

* * *

The detailed plans for the emergency care of visitors to the New York World's Fair include an automobile x-ray unit available to the eight first aid stations to be established on the grounds. X-rays will be taken and developed at once, not only in cases of severe injury, but where fracture is only suspected. It is estimated that such procedure will minimize the fake claims against the Fair itself or exhibitors. First aid in the form of oxygen for resuscitation will also be available in cases of asphyxiation from whatever cause, and inhalation anesthesia for emergency operations. According to estimates, some eighteen to twenty deliveries are likely to take place during the course of the fair.

The increasing demand for graduate training in the various fields of medicine is evidenced by the following tabulation of the graduate students in the Medical School of the University of Minnesota. This is exclusive of those who are registered under the Mayo Foundation division of the Graduate School.

The total number of candidates for graduate degrees in the fall of 1938 was 166. These are divided as follows:

I. Candidates for Doctor of Philosophy degrees: anatomy, 4; bacteriology, 12; internal medicine, 2; neuropsychiatry, 1; obstetrics and gynecology, 7; ophthalmology and otolaryngology, 1; pediatrics, 6; pharmacology, 3; general physiology, 9; physiological chemistry, 5; general preventive medicine and public health, 1; biostatistics, 1; surgery, 7; and radiology, 5.

II. Candidates for Master's degrees: anatomy, 14; bacteriology, 16; internal medicine, 5; neuropsychiatry, 2; dermatology, 2; ophthalmology and otolaryngology, 12; pathology, 8; pediatrics, 1; pharmacology, 1; general physiology, 12; physiological chemistry, 7; general preventive medicine and public health, 11; biostatistics, 2; surgery, 6; and radiology, 3.

In Memoriam

Leo Melville Crafts

1863-1938

D R. LEO MELVILLE CRAFTS was born in the City of Minneapolis in 1863, the son of Major Amasa and Mary J. Crafts. Some of his ancestors were among the founders of Boston and his parents early pioneers of Minneapolis.

Dr. Crafts was educated in the public schools of Minneapolis and graduated from the law department of the University of Minnesota in 1886 and from Harvard Medical School in 1890. He interned at the Boston City Hospital and also served there for one year as house physician.

He began the practice of his specialty in Minneapolis in the early nineties, serving as professor of Nervous and Mental Diseases in the Medical Department of Hamline University from 1893 to 1908, being Dean of the faculty from 1893 to 1903.

Dr. Crafts was a member of the staffs of most of the leading hospitals in Minneapolis and enjoyed a very large consulting practice. He was treasurer of the Hennepin County Medical Society for two years.

Dr. Crafts belonged to the Hennepin County Medical society, the Minnesota State and American Medical associations, the Massachusetts Medical society, the Harvard Medical and Boston Alumni associations.

He was a member of the First Congregational Church of Minneapolis for fifty-five years, being active in the Minnesota State Sunday School Association, serving as its president for three years. He was a member of the board of directors of the Minnesota National Park and Forestry Association, the old Minneapolis Commercial Club, the Auto Club, the American Legion and the Bloomington Golf Club. He also belonged to the Republican Party, the Sons of the American Revolution, Phi Rho Sigma, and Native Sons of Minnesota.

Dr. Crafts served during the war at Camp Funston and later with the United States Veterans' Bureau at Minneapolis.

On September 4, 1901 he married Amelia I. Burgess, who survives him.

Dr. Crafts practiced neurology in Minneapolis for almost half a century, and was at work in his office when he died on September 22, 1938, at the age of seventy-five.

Dr. Crafts came into the practice of his specialty well prepared. Few men of his time had his educational background. He was a gifted teacher who was able to impart enthusiasm as well as instruction to his students. He personified the highest ideals of medical ethics. As Dean of the medical department of Hamline University he gave a great leadership to his students and to his fellow faculty members as well. Dr. Crafts enjoyed a long and useful practice, being one of the most helpful consultants in his special field.

Dr. Crafts' kindly manner, courteous treatment of

others, his ample knowledge and his unlimited charity endeared him to his patients and his fellow doctors.

Following is a list of Dr. Crafts' contributions to medical literature:

1. Relation of Spinal Concussion to Chronic Diseases of the Spinal Cord, 1892.
2. The Sensory Manifestations of Hysteria, 1893.
3. Medical Education, 1898.
4. The Physician in Practice, 1898.
5. A Fifth Case of Family Periodic Paralysis, 1900.
6. Incipient Amyotrophic Lateral Sclerosis with Recovery, 1902.
7. Wear and Care of the Nervous System, 1906.
8. Nerve Stress and Longevity, 1906.
9. The Influence of Ductless Glands Over Metabolism, 1908.
10. Expert Testimony and The Medical Witness, 1909.
11. Mechanism and the Significance of the Reflexes, 1910.
12. The Problem of the Insane and the Defective, 1910.
13. Symptomatology of Traumatic Organic Lesions Affecting Sensorimotor Areas, 1912.
14. Possibilities in the Treatment of Epilepsy, 1915.
15. Myasthenia Gravis, with Report of Three Cases, 1917.
16. The Early Recognition of Multiple Sclerosis, 1917.
17. An Original Test for the Pathologic Great Toe Sign, 1919.
18. Mixed Cell Sarcoma of the Brain, 1922.
19. Epidemic Encephalitis: Some of the More Unusual of Its Widely Variant Syndromes, 1923.
20. Text Book on Epidemic Encephalitis, 1927.
21. Reflections on Sexology, 1936.

CLAUDE C. KENNEDY.

Raymond W. Lagerson

1896-1938

D R. RAYMOND W. LAGERSON, a practicing physician in Minneapolis for the past fifteen years, died at the University Hospital, March 13, 1938, following a cerebral hemorrhage.

Dr. Lagerson was born November 19, 1896, at Burns, Minnesota. He graduated from the high school at Anoka in 1915 and received his medical degree from the University of Minnesota Medical School.

A member of the staff of St. Barnabas Hospital for a number of years, he was also a member of the Hennepin County Medical Society, state and national medical associations.

Dr. Lagerson is survived by a daughter, Diane, a brother Leif Lagerson of Milwaukee, and five sisters, Mrs. Joseph Peterson, Mrs. Phil Peterson and Mrs. Earl Hunter of Anoka, Mrs. Frank Addington of Saint Paul, and Mrs. L. H. Nolte of Seattle.

Peter Lorentz Vistaunet

1871-1938

D R. P. L. VISTAUNET, one of the most prominent physicians of Thief River Falls, died on September 22, 1938, from pneumonia.

Dr. Vistaunet was born February 7, 1871, at Inneroi, near Trondhjem, Norway. At the age of seventeen he came to America and received his M.D. degree from the University of Minnesota Medical School in 1902.

On June 27, 1903' Dr. Vistaunet was married to Anna C. Hauglum. His wife and one son, Alv, and daughter, Liv, survive him.

Dr. Vistaunet was city health commissioner for several years. He was a member of the I.O.O.F., W.O.W. and Sons of Norway lodges. An able musician, he served as assistant leader of the Red River Scandinavian Singers' Association and directed the local Brage Chorus for many years. He was choir director in the Trinity Lutheran Church for about twenty years.

EDICAL BROADCAST
OR DECEMBER

The Minnesota State Medical Association Morning Health Service.

The Minnesota State Medical Association broadcasts eekly at 11:00 o'clock every Saturday morning over tation WCCO, Minneapolis (810 kilocycles or 370.2 eters) and Station WLB, University of Minnesota 760 kilocycles or 395 meters).

Speaker: William A. O'Brien, M.D., Associate Pro-essor of Pathology and Preventive Medicine, Med-al School, University of Minnesota. The program or the month will be as follows:

ecember 3—Occupational Skin Disease.
ecember 10—Tuberculosis.
ecember 17—Irritable Colon.
ecember 24—Medical Accomplishments.
ecember 31—New Year Resolutions.

. STARR JUDD LECTURE

Dr. Dallas B. Phemister of Chicago, Illinois, Pro-essor and Chairman of the Department of Surgery at he University of Chicago, will give the sixth E. Starr udd Lecture at the University of Minnesota in the edical Science Amphitheater on Wednesday, February , at 8:15 P. M. The subject of Dr. Phemister's lec-ure is "Pathogenesis of Gallstones." The late E. 5tarr Judd, an alumnus of the Medical School of the Jniversity of Minnesota, established this annual lec-ureship in surgery a few years before his death.

MINNESOTA PUBLIC HEALTH ASSOCIATION

In observance of the twentieth anniversary of the :ompletion of Minnesota's chain of public tuberculosis sanatoria, the Minnesota Public Health Association ledicated its annual meeting, held November 18, in the Twin Cities, to the surviving original board members)f each institution. Principal speakers were Dr. W. W. Bauer, Director of the Bureau of Health and Public Instruction of the American Medical Association, Chi-:ago, and Dr. H. E. Hilleboe, Director, Divisions of Tuberculosis and Services for Crippled Children, Min-iesota State Board of Control.

Dr. S. A. Slater, Worthington, President of the Association, presented the following pioneer sanatorium)oard members with life certificates in the organiza-:ion: Dr. E. L. Tuohy, Duluth, of Nopeming Sana-.orium, St. Louis County, the first county institution in .he state, established in 1912; Mrs. W. J. O'Toole, Mrs. .. P. Wolff, Mrs. Claude S. Brown and Mr. James :. Otis, all of St. Paul, Ramsey County Preventorium :stablished in 1915; Mr. L. E. Johnson, Wanamingo, ind Mr. M. W. Smith of Red Wing, Mineral Springs 5anatorium established in 1915; Mr. Edward C. Gale

and Mr. Joseph R. Kingman, Minneapolis, of Glen Lake Sanatorium, established in 1916; Mr. J. L. Wold, Thief River Falls, of Sunnyrest Sanatorium, established in 1916; Dr. E. W. Johnson, Mr. A. P. Ritchie and Mr. A. A. Tone, all of Bemidji, Lake Julia Sanatorium, established in 1916; Dr. C. L. Sherman, Luverne, Dr. A. L. Vadheim, Tyler, L. F. Johnson, Mankato, Dr. Thomas Lowe, Pipestone, G. S. Redmond, Pipestone, N. P. Minion, Bingham Lake, H. M. Burnham, Jack-son, S. S. Smith, Worthington, of Southwestern Min-nésota Sanatorium, established in 1917; Mr. E. W. Davis, Detroit Lakes, Dr. O. J. Hagen, Moorhead, Mr. John Nelson, Lake Park, of Sand Beach Sana-torium, established in 1917; Mr. L. Engstrom, Roseau, Donald Robertson, Argyle, and Dr. O. F. Mellby, Thief River Falls, of Oakland Park Sanatorium, established in 1918; Dr. W. W. Will, Bertha, of Fair Oaks Lodge Sanatorium, established in 1918; Dr. J. A. Thabes, Brainerd, Charles P. Delaittre, Aitkin, and Mr. Peter Larson, Aitkin, of Deerwood Sanatorium, established in 1918.

Dr. Hilleboe summarized the progress made in Min-nesota during its sanatorium and anti-tuberculosis cam-paign and the problem ahead in the following words:
"Since the establishment of Pokegama Sanatorium at Pokegama, Minnesota, in 1905, and the Minnesota State Sanatorium at Ah-Gwah-Ching, Minnesota, in 1907, with the capacity of sixty beds, farsighted county and state officials, public spirited citizens, and physi-cians have continued to develop the sanatorium pro-gram with the result that at the present time there are fourteen county sanatoria, one county preventorium, and one state sanatorium, with the total capacity of 2,254 beds available for the care of the tuberculous. In 1937 there were 912 deaths from tuberculosis. This means that there are more than two sanatorium beds available for each death from tuberculosis in any one year in Minnesota at the present time.

"With the establishment of adequate. sanatoria beds for care of tuberculous patients in need of hospitaliza-tion, our program is being directed in two other fields of endeavor. First, it is essential for control of the disease to diagnose early cases of tuberculosis so that the best possible chance of arrest of the disease may be obtained. After an adequate period of sanatorium care, another important factor in the control of tuber-culosis is being developed in after-care and rehabilita-tion of tuberculous patients. It is necessary to provide the necessities of life, medical supervision, and relief from mental anxiety for tuberculous patients dis-charged from sanatoria, particularly during the first five years after discharge, if best results are to be ob-tained. The needs of the tuberculous in Minnesota can be met only if a strong battle is waged against this dread disease along these three fronts."

CAMP RELEASE DISTRICT

At the meeting of the Camp Release District Medical Society, held on October 20, 1938, the following officers were elected for the coming year: H. A. Roust, Montevideo, president; George Tangen, Canby, vice president; Magnus Westby, Madison, secretary-treas-urer.

The following members were elected to the Advisory Committee: M. Hauge, Clarkfield; George Boody, Jr., Dawson; F. M. Burns, Milan; H. L. Herbert, Granite Falls; N. Westby, Madison; L. G. Smith, Montevideo.

The society held a meeting at Montevideo on November 3. Dr. Frederick H. K. Schaaf of Minneapolis spoke on "Cardiac Disorders."

EAST CENTRAL MINNESOTA

The East Central Minnesota Medical Society held a dinner and inter-professional meeting at the Episcopal Parish House in Anoka, Minnesota, on October 11, 1938. Problems common to the allied professions of medicine, law, dentistry, and pharmacy were discussed by guest speakers.

Guests of the Society were Dr. Wm. Dickson of Minneapolis, Vice-Chairman of the Legislative Committee of the State Dental Association; Dr. B. J. Branton, Willmar; Mr. H. H. Gregg, Minneapolis; Dr. F. J. Savage, St. Paul; and Mr. R. R. Rosell, Executive Secretary of the State Medical Association.

MOWER COUNTY

Newly elected officers of the Mower County Medical Society are: R. S. Hegge, Austin, president; J. M. Thomson, Brownsdale, vice president; Paul A. Robertson, Austin, secretary; A. E. Henslin, Le Roy, treasurer.

RICE COUNTY

At the meeting of the Rice County Medical Society, held in Faribault, November 3, Dr. Gordon R. Kamman of Saint Paul was the guest speaker. His subject was "Endemic Encephalitis."

SOUTHWESTERN MINNESOTA

The annual meeting of the Southwestern Minnesota Medical Society was held in Worthington on October 31. Doctors from six counties gathered for dinner and heard Dr. William A. O'Brien speak on "Socialized Medicine." Dr. J. D. Waller of Wilmont was elected president; Dr. B. M. Stephenson of Fulda, vice president; Dr. J. De Boer of Edgerton, secretary-treasurer; Dr. E. W. Arnold of Adrian, censor from Nobles County.

The members of the Woman's Auxiliary of the Society were present at the dinner, and were entertained afterward by Mrs. C. R. Stanley.

STEARNS-BENTON COUNTIES

The Stearns-Benton Medical Society held its monthly meeting in St. Cloud on November 17. Dr. W. W. Bill of Bertha, and Dr. E. J. Simons of Swanville, were the principal speakers.

WOMAN'S AUXILIARY

Mrs. W. B. Roberts, President
2735 Irving Avenue South, Minneapolis.
Mrs. E. V. Goltz, Press and Publicity, St. Paul, Minn.

The members of the Women's Auxiliary of the Hennepin County Medical Society, held their regular meeting Friday, November 4, in the Hennepin County Medical Library. On November 18 and 19 they sponsored the annual sale of articles made by the patients of Glen Lake Sanatorium, the proceeds going to the makers of the articles. The sale was under the leadership of Mrs. J. C. Davis, chairman, and Mmes. N. F. Lufkin, L. F. Richdorf, J. C. Miller, L. M. Larson, F. L. Jennings and Donald McCarthy.

* * *

The members of the Women's Auxiliary of the Scott Carver Medical Society held their first meeting of the season on October 11 at Montgomery, Minnesota. After having dinner with their husbands they met at the home of Mrs. Alvin Westerman and discussed plans for the year. The new officers are: Mrs. B. F. Pearson, Shakopee, president; Mrs. H. P. Fischer, Shakopee, vice president; Mrs. H. M. Juergins, Belle Plaine, secretary and treasurer.

* * *

The members of the Ramsey County Auxiliary held their first meeting of the fall in the Medical Society rooms in the Lowry Building, Monday, October 24. Mrs. A. E. Nichols, president, presided. During the afternoon a reading was given by Mrs. Roy Jones of Minneapolis. Members of the board for the coming year are: Mrs. A. E. Nichols, President; Mrs. Harry Ghent, president-elect; Mrs. Hugh Beals, vice president; Mrs. Charles Waas, recording secretary; Mrs. Mark Ryan, treasurer; Mrs. E. H. Boland, auditor; Mrs. E. C. Eshelby, parliamentarian; Mrs. Albert Schulze, historian; Mrs. B. J. Mears, magazine; Mrs. Herman Kesting, information; Mrs. Richard Aurelius, Christmas seals; Mrs. C. Neumann McCloud, hospitality; Mrs. Karl Wold, philanthropic; Mrs. Lloyd G. Dack, program; Mrs. Douglas Brand, year book; Mrs. Gordon R. Kamman, publicity; and Mrs. James Benepe, ways and means.

* * *

Mrs. Wm. B. Roberts, president of the Women's Auxiliary of the Minnesota State Medical Association, returned November 13 from an extensive trip in th East.

Oddities Called for in Drug Stores

Sterilized Ink for Stearate of Zinc.
Hyena Nursing Bottle for Hygeia Bottle.
Paralyzed Gauze for Sterilized Gauze.
Aspiration Tablets for Aspirin Tablets.
Polluted Water for Pluto Water.
Scott's Emotion for Scott's Emulsion.
Rooster Foam for Hennafoam.
Runaway Seeds for Caraway Seeds.
Cynical for Clinical Thermometer.
Exorbitant for Absorbent Cotton.

PROCEEDINGS OF THE MINNESOTA ACADEMY OF MEDICINE

Meeting of October 12, 1938.

The regular monthly meeting of the Minnesota Academy of Medicine was held at the Town and Country Club on Wednesday evening, October 12, 1938. Dinner was served at 7 o'clock and the meeting was called to order at 8 o'clock by the President, Dr. R. T. LaVake.

There were fifty-six members and one guest present. Minutes of the May meeting were read and approved as read.

The Secretary read a letter of resignation from Dr. George E. Senkler, with the recommendation from the Executive Committee that his name be placed on the Honorary Membership list. A motion was seconded and unanimously carried that this be done.

The Secretary introduced a proposed amendment to Article III, Section I of the Constitution to read as follows: "There may also be *ten* active members from the University faculty who are teachers of medicine not engaged in private practice." This had been approved by the Executive Committee and will be printed on the November programs. The Executive Committee also suggested the election of new members at the December meeting.

The Secretary was instructed to write a letter of appreciation to Dr. Archa Wilcox for the party held at Dr. Wilcox's summer home in July.

The scientific program followed.

PRIMARY CARCINOMA OF THE PANCREAS
JUSTUS OHAGE, M.D.

Dr. Ohage, of St. Paul, read his Inaugural Thesis on the above subject. (To appear in MINNESOTA MEDICINE at a later date.)

Abstract

A series of thirty-nine cases of primary carcinoma of the pancreas, proved by autopsy or operation, were reviewed.

Primary carcinoma of the pancreas is most common in the fifth and sixth decades; the average age of incidence in this series was sixty-one years. It is more common in males than in females; the ratio in this series was 2.5 to 1. The head of the pancreas is most commonly involved; only the head was involved in almost 60 per cent of the cases in this series.

The diagnosis of primary carcinoma of the pancreas is largely by exclusion. Most commonly it must be differentiated from stone in the common duct. For this purpose, the Watson test is very useful.

· Negative x-ray findings in the stomach and duodenum are also of great value as diagnostic aids.

Jaundice should not be considered as a cardinal symptom. At least four, and possibly seven, cases in this series had no jaundice and no involvement of the common duct.

The prognosis is grave but by no means hopeless. Surgical intervention is the best palliative means. Cho-
lecystoduodenostomy and cholecystojejunostomy are the operations of choice.

Discussion

DR. IRVINE MCQUARRIE (U. of M.): Do these malignant tumors ever originate from the Islands of Langerhans?

DR. OHAGE: Very rarely. Malignant tumors of the pancreas nearly always originate from the ducts of the gland or the parenchyma.

DR. MAX HOFFMAN (St. Paul): Dr. Ohage stated that five of the cases presented showed positive blood findings in the stool. I am impressed with the fact that in carcinoma of the head of the pancreas blood is frequently found in the stool, and it is a valuable diagnostic finding. I would like to ask Dr. Ohage if stools were examined in the entire series? Contrary to the textbook description of carcinoma of the head of the pancreas, intermittent jaundice is not rare, especially in the early states, and the presence of intermittent jaundice should not lead one away from the true diagnosis.

DR. OHAGE: Unfortunately, all of our cases did not have stool analysis and consequently I was unable to determine the exact percentage of cases which showed blood in the stool. In our series, five cases showed blood and absence of bile.

DR. MOSES BARRON (Minneapolis): Dr. Ohage stated that jaundice is not a constant finding in his series of cases. However, it is obvious that the jaundice is important in diagnosing carcinoma of the pancreas only when the tumor is in the region of the head of the organ. In a number of his cases the involvement was in the body and tail, and of course jaundice is of little importance when in these regions. Dr. Hoffman brought out the fact that occasionally there is an intermittency in the jaundice. That is true. Occasionally there develops collateral inflammatory edema as a result of the growth of these tumors. When the edema is present the bile ducts may be compressed, with jaundice resulting. When the edema subsides the ducts may reopen, and the jaundice may disappear. One cannot say dogmatically that because there is intermittency the jaundice is not the result of a tumor in the head of the pancreas.

DR. HENRY L. ULRICH (Minneapolis): I recall a case of carcinoma of the tail of the pancreas. All the symptoms were pleural. There were repeated effusions in the left chest which, as they progressed, became more and more mucoid in character. Not until the postmortem did we realize what we were dealing with. A primary carcinoma of the tail had walked up through the spleen and then the diaphragm and had involved the left pleura.

DR. OHAGE: In answer to Dr. Barron's discussion,

jaundice is practically always present in carcinoma of the head of the pancreas except in anomalous conditions, as in one case where the common duct passed completely over the head of the pancreas. If there is no involvement of the common duct by compression or extension of the malignant process, jaundice does not take place. Dr. Ulrich cited a case of carcinoma of the tail of the pancreas in which case the malignancy extended through the diaphragm into the lung. The patient showed no jaundice.

NAILING OF HIP FRACTURES
WALLACE COLE, M.D.

Dr. Cole, of St. Paul, reported on this method of operation in hip fractures, and showed lantern slides.

Discussion

DR. E. A. REGNIER (Minneapolis) : I wish to compliment Dr. Cole on this report of his method of nailing intracapsular hip fractures. Those of us who have taken an interest in this type of work have been bewildered by the numerous gadgets which have been devised. I have had the opportunity of seeing Dr. Cole's instrument used by his colleagues and I am frank to state that it is the best that I have seen.

While the conservative method of treatment recommended by Whitman is still usable and good in well-trained hands, I believe that the day is not far away when all these intracapsular fractures will be treated immediately by internal fixation. We now have evidence that the treatment by internal fixation will be attended by a high percentage of excellent results.

There are three or four factors, as Dr. Cole has stated, which recommend internal fixation. The first and most important of these is the immediate relief of pain, doing away with long periods of bed rest and sedation by the use of opiates. The second factor is the great economic saving to the patient both in money and period of disability. The third factor is that it obviates a prolonged period of rehabilitation of the patient due to prolonged incarceration in plaster. All these factors, assuming that an accurate reduction was obtained and the fixation was maintained, insure a bony union.

I have had a limited experience in nailing hip fractures by the direct exposure method. I have, in most instances, chosen to nail them by driving a nail over a previously inserted Kirschner wire. This method is just as satisfactory as the former, provided that ample radiographic studies are made to assure the operator of a careful reduction and an optimum position for the insertion of the nail. I think that Dr. Cole will agree that an accurate reduction of these fractures even by the open method is often very difficult. Again I wish to state that this instrument devised by Dr. Cole is unique in the versatility of its application and, if used according to instructions, is practically fool-proof.

The meeting adjourned.

A. G. SCHULZE, M.D.
Secretary.

BOOK REVIEWS

Books listed here become the property of the Ramsey and Hennepin County Medical libraries when reviewed. Members, however, are urged to write reviews of any or every recent book which may be of interest to physicians.

OUR COMMON AILMENT. Constipation and Its Cause and Cure. Harold Aaron, M.D., Medical Consultant to Consumers Union of United States. 192 pages. Price, cloth, $1.50. New York: Dodge Publishing Co., 1938.

THE 1938 YEAR BOOK OF GENERAL MEDICINE. Edited by George F. Dick, M.D., et al. 840 pages. Illus. Price, cloth, $3.00. Chicago: Year Book Publishers, 1938.

DOCTOR BRADLEY REMEMBERS. A Novel. Francis Brett Young. 522 pages. Price, cloth, $2.75. New York: Reynal & Hitchcock, 1938.

HOW TO CONQUER CONSTIPATION. J. F. Montague, M.D., Editor-in-Chief of Health Digest. Medical Director New York Intestinal Sanitarium, etc. 244 pages. Price, cloth, $1.50. Philadelphia: J. B. Lippincott Co., 1938.

CRIPPLED CHILDREN: THEIR TREATMENT AND ORTHOPEDIC NURSING. Earl D. McBride and Winifred R. Sink. 379 Pages. Illus. Cloth, $3.50. 2d edition. St. Louis: Mosby, 1937.

This book deals with the various phases of the handling of crippled children. It is intended for the training of nurses but contains more inaccuracies and dogmatic statements than one would expect in a text used for instruction purposes. The language has been simplified to such an extreme extent that the value of the work as a reference is lost. The illustrations for the most part are fairly good but do not, in all cases, adequately picture the condition under discussion.

The advisability of using such a book as this for distribution to social workers and the laity is questioned.

THE HORSE AND BUGGY DOCTOR by Arthur E. Hertzler, M.D. New York. Harper Bros. 1938.

The story of the early experiences of a small town doctor in the horse and buggy days, his difficulties in transportation and the establishment of a hospital, is written in a most entertaining style and so saturated with humor and horse sense that the book is being enjoyed not only by doctors but by the general public. A book of this sort, which should prove to be one of the best sellers, will do much to emphasize the importance of the personal relationship between patient and doctor, so essential to the best medical care.

C. B. D.

A PRELIMINARY REPORT ON THE INFLU-ENCE OF FOOD AND FUNCTION ON THE INCIDENCE OF MAMMARY GLAND TUMOR IN "A" STOCK ALBINO MICE*

IVAR SIVERTSEN, M.D.

AND

WALDON H. HASTINGS, M.S.

Minneapolis

SEVENTEEN years ago[4] a preliminary report was compiled on the relationship of muscular activity to carcinoma in man. In this paper it was suggested that the lack of muscular activity may be a definite factor in the causation of or susceptibility to cancer. When the adult males in Minnesota who died during the years 1918, 1919 and 1920 were divided into six groups according to the degree of muscular activity demanded by their occupations, it was found that the ratio of cancer incidence between the most physically active and the least physically active group was one to twelve.

During the ensuing years the exigencies of private practice have delayed a scientific study of this interesting disclosure. January 1, 1937, marked a new era and studies were resumed, this time with experimental animals. Because of the present difficulty in using controlled human subjects it was decided to secure pure strain mice having a high incidence of carcinoma for experimental work. The studies on these animals which I should like to discuss this evening resulted from the following observations: (1) the cancer death rate in males actively engaged in a gainful occupation is less than the death rate of those not actively engaged in a gainful occupation and is inversely proportional to the degree of muscular activity necessary for that occupation; (2) there appears to be a recent increase in cancer accompanying the advent of the age of machinery; (3) cancer has been recognized as a degenerative disease, and, knowing that degeneration takes place in all tissue that does not function, it is thought that food and function must be factors in maintaining a normal physiological condition of the human body.

History.—It is a general clinical observation that neoplastic tissue can proliferate in spite of unfavorable dietary and metabolic conditions. However, when these factors are carefully controlled their influence is seen on tumor growth.

Ball and Samuels[3] report a profound depression in the rate of growth of the Walker rat carcinoma 265 and a decrease in the number of positive growths on implantation, following the removal of the pituitary. Voegtlin and Thompson,[9] using the Marsh strain of

mice, found that tumorous animals fed a diet deficient in the essential amino-acid lysine showed striking inhibition of tumor growth. Maison and Pourbaix[4] found that feeding organs and extracts of organs had in some cases an acceleratory effect and in others an inhibiting effect on the growth of tar cancers in mice.

Sugiura and Benedict[8] have studied the influence of insufficient diets on tumor recurrence and growth in rats and mice. They found that transplants of the Flexner-Jobling rat carcinoma in rats fed a complete basic diet but limited in quantity to one-third that of the normal food requirement, survived less frequently and grew much more slowly than those in full-fed controls; that under-feeding, after engrafted tumors had well established themselves in the hosts, had no marked inhibitory effect on the subsequent rate of tumor growth; and that prolonged post-operative insufficient feeding had a distinct influence on the frequency of recurrences of spontaneous tumors in mice. Using 65 mice carrying spontaneous tumor they found that 73% of those under-fed were completely cured of the tumors, while on the other hand 18% of the normally-fed controls were free from tumor at the time of death. The average post-operative longevity in the under-fed mice was 142 days against 96 days for the full-fed controls. The gain of 46 days in the experimental animals corresponds to about 3.8 years of a man's life. In addition, the number of metastases found at autopsy was much less in the under-fed animals than in the full-fed controls.

Some studies have been made by Strong and Bittner on the "A" strain albino mice, inbred since 1912 and originally secured from H. G. Bagg. Strong[7] found that 90% of the breeding females of this stock had spontaneous mammary gland cancer. The average age of the tumorous mice varied significantly when different diets were fed. He also found that "A" strain mice kept on the same diet in New Haven, Connecticut, Bar Barbor, Maine, and Ann Arbor, Michigan, give the same age distribution of spontaneous tumor of the mammary gland. Bittner reports on 292 "A" strain mice, of which 88% of those living after four months developed mammary gland carcinoma at an average age of 11.5 months or 350 days. These mice were fed Purina Chow food ad libitum. About 68 per cent of 421 mice were cancerous at an average age of nine months when fed rolled oats, milk and salt. The increase in the percentage of tumors and the increase in the average age at the onset of the tumor in the mice on the Fox Chow diet was attributed to the better health of the animals, allowing more to live into the cancerous age.

Bittner concludes in this paper that, "Given the cancer susceptibility constitution and the subsequent irritating factors, the average age at the appearance of mammary gland tumors may possibly be influenced by the physical condition of the individual."

Experiments.—In view of the promising effects of these simple dietary experiments, twenty-six "A" stock

*From the Sivertsen Clinic (Sivertsen) and the Department of Physiology, University of Minnesota Medical School (Hastings).

mice were secured from Dr. Bittner, Jackson Memorial Laboratory, for a preliminary study on dietary and metabolic factors influencing tumor incidence. These mice normally have an incidence of 88 per cent spontaneous mammary gland tumors at an average age of 11.5 months.

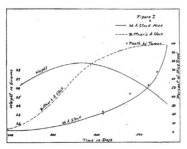

Fig. 1. Percentage of mice dead in the two "A" strain colonies and the average weight of the mice used in this experiment.

The animals were housed in wooden boxes, fed Purina Fox Chow food, and in every way possible were kept under the same conditions as other "A" stock mice reported in the literature. They were mated and produced one to three litters of young each. As Murray[2] and Bittner[3] have found no correlation between the average tumor age for animals and their breeding records, the males were removed from the colony after nine months. The only variables between this colony and Bittner's were the amount of a complete basic diet given per day and the amount of exercise.

To find the amount of food which the mice needed to maintain their weight equal to controls fed ad libitum, fourteen contemporary mice were chosen for a feeding experiment. At the beginning of the experiment Group I, consisting of seven mice, weighed an average of 27.13 grams. Group II, also seven mice, weighed an average of 27.81 grams. Group II mice fed ad libitum for eighteen days consumed 3.76 grams per day and weighed 27.83 grams at the end of that period. Group I mice were fed only enough to maintain their weight constant with those of Group II and consumed 1.94 grams per day. These mice weighed 27.16 grams at the end of the eighteen day period. Thus it was shown that mice fed ad libitum eat twice as much as is necessary to keep their weight constant. From time to time as the mice grew older this experiment was repeated and the diet of the "A" stock experimental animals was varied to meet the requirements of weight equal to mice fed ad libitum.

In addition to the restricted diet a large circular cage was constructed in which the mice were exercised daily

TABLE I.—NUMBER OF MICE DYING CANCEROUS AND NON-CANCEROUS, AVERAGE WEIGHT AND FOOD CONSUMED PER DAY BY EACH, IN MONTHLY PERIODS.

Age in months	No. dying non-cancerous	No. dying cancerous	Weight in grams (Average)	Food consumed grams per day
6.5	1		24.5	2
8.5	1		26.0	
10.5	1		28.0	2.5
12.5	2		28.0	3
13.5	2		28.0	3
14.5	2	2	26.5	
15.5	1		28.5	
16.5	1	1	27.0	
17.5		1	26.0	3
18.5	2	1	26.0	
19.5	9		25.0	3

for two hours. This exercising period was strictly supervised by a technician.

Results.—The results of our experiment are presented in Table I and Figure 1. Dr. Bittner's 292 mice fed Fox Chow ad libitum lived 358±8.1 days. Our mice lived 482±6.4 days. Two hundred and fifty-seven of Bittner's mice developed mammary gland cancer at an average of 351±3.6 days. Four of our twenty-six mice died of mammary gland cancer at an average age of 463±2.3 days. One of our mice died of primary lung tumor when 550 days old.

As our group of four mammary gland cancerous mice is quite small for significant comparison with Bittner's group we will take his group as standard and see what the chance is that four mice drawn at random from his group dying cancerous will live for an average age of 463 days. This probability is 0.00007, which means that the chances are seven in 100,000 that our four mice dying of cancer could be taken from Bittner's group. It is thus significant that the age at which our cancerous mice died was probably greatly increased by the conditions under which they existed.

In Bittner's group, twenty-four cancerous mice lived beyond 463 days. Of these, twenty-one died of cancer. In our experiment fifteen mice lived beyond 463 days, two developed mammary gland cancer and one lung cancer. This shows that the incidence of cancer has been decreased in mice living into the fatal cancerous age.

Conclusions

The incidence of mammary gland carcinoma in "A" strain albino mice has been decreased from 88 per cent to 16 per cent in the animals studied in this experiment. The average age at which these 16 per cent develop cancer has been significantly increased beyond the average age of Bittner's colony.

874

by Warren and Gates published in 1932, a total of 1259 cases have been reported. The survey by these authors was based largely on autopsy records as were Billroth's cases and many others. We feel fortunate therefore in being able to present the following report of a live patient.

A white woman, the wife of a physician, age sixty-four, para III, presented herself for examination August 7, 1929, complaining of a blood-tinged, watery vaginal discharge of two years duration. The discharge had not been offensive nor irritating. The past history is otherwise unimportant.

Physical examination revealed the following:

The external genitalia and vaginal walls were atrophic. On the posterior lip of the small cervix there was a flat nodule about one centimeter in diameter which was raised about two millimeters above the surrounding cervical tissue. The corpus was not enlarged and was regular in outline. The cervix and corpus were freely movable and there were no masses and no induration of the pelvic tissues. The entire cervical nodule was removed, and a diagnostic curettage was done on August 9, 1929. A large amount of necrotic tissue was obtained from the uterus. Frozen sections of the tissues were made and examined immediately by Dr. Floyd Grave, who made a diagnosis of adenocarcinoma of the uterus with a cervical metastasis. Radium cartridges prepared by Dr. Charles Drake were placed in the uterine cavity and in the cervical canal. A total dose of 1500 milligram hours was given. The radium was screened with 0.5 millimeter of silver and 1 millimeter of bronze encased in 1 millimeter of rubber tubing.

The patient was placed under the care of Dr. T. A. Peppard for treatment of a mild diabetes mellitus.

On November 12, 1929, a panhysterectomy was done. The uterus was slightly enlarged and boggy. There was a pedunculated tumor 3 centimeters in diameter, attached near the left uterine cornu. The tumor and endometrium were degenerating. A diagnosis of adenocarcinoma of the uterus was made after microscopic examination of sections. The patient made a good recovery from her operation and has had no evidence of any recurrence of this tumor.

In February 1935 at the age of sixty-nine she returned with a small epithelioma of the face. No pathologic sections were made of this growth. The patient was treated with roentgen rays by Dr. R. G. Allison, with recovery.

In April 1935 at the age of sixty-nine years she returned complaining of belching of gas, vague pain in the lower abdomen, considerable rumbling, vomiting on one occasion, weakness and constipation. The physical examination was essentially negative. Hemoglobin was 73 per cent; red blood cells—4,070,000; white blood cells—9,500 and differential count normal. The urine was normal.

X-ray examination revealed a carcinoma involving the pyloric end of the stomach and extending back on the greater and lesser curvatures about four or five inches. There was 80 per cent gastric retention at three hours.

At operation on April 25, 1935 the pelvic region was palpated and there was no evidence of recurrence of the carcinoma removed six years previously. The appendix was examined and did not appear abnormal. The gallbladder contained stones. The stomach contained a mass which began at the pylorus and extended upward about one and one-half inches on the lesser curvature and about five inches on the greater curvature. The lower half of the stomach was resected and an anterior Polya type gastroenterostomy with enteroanastomosis was made. The pathologic report by Dr. Margaret Smith was carcinoma of the stomach. Recovery was uneventful.

The fourth carcinoma appeared on the right leg about two inches below the knee as a small wart-like growth which continued to grow until it was about the size of an almond. There were no other symptoms. The patient came to the hospital because of an attack of pain in the right lower quadrant of the abdomen. She had had abdominal discomfort for two or three weeks. The distress shifted about, sometimes on the left side, sometimes on the right side and sometimes beneath the costal margin on the right side. During the past forty-eight hours it had increased in intensity, and on the evening of March 29, 1938 she had been nauseated. There was slight fever, slightly increased pulse rate and slight tenderness in the lower abdomen particularly on the right side. The leucocyte count was 20,000 with 88 per cent p. m. ns. The history of carcinoma of the uterus, carcinoma of the stomach and the existence of gallstones complicated the diagnosis. The age of the patient being seventy-two years and the previous record of examination of the appendix with normal appearance caused the consultants to be very conservative. Finally, however, on March 31, 1938, we opened her abdomen for the third time and removed an appendix which was one-half inch in diameter and completely filled with pus. The appendix was not ruptured, and it was possible to explore the abdomen. Although there were a moderate number of adhesions present, a fairly satisfactory exploration was made and neither the upper abdomen nor the lower abdomen showed evidence of metastatic growths. The appendix was removed in the usual manner. On April 14, 1938 the stomach was examined with the x-ray and it was felt that there was no evidence of carcinoma.

The tumor of the right leg was removed, and microscopic examination showed it to be squamous celled carcinoma. The patient left the hospital on April 17, 1938 and is still in good health at the time of this report.

Multiple primary malignancies occur in 2 to 4 per cent of persons suffering from cancer according to Warren and Gates. These authors made a survey of the literature and added forty cases from their study of a series of 1,078 post-mortem examinations on malignant disease cases. Among the 1,259 reported cases there were 242 cases of double carcinomata of different systems and sixteen of these were primary carcinomata of the stomach and uterus (including the cervix), and three were of the stomach and bladder. In 111 cases, three or more malignant tumors were found.

Warren and Gates conclude that multiple malignant tumors occur more frequently than can be explained on the basis of chance and that this may be explained by a predisposition or susceptibility to cancer in certain persons, or the action of some factor favoring the development of malignancy.

Our patient still has gallstones. Gallstones have been credited as a factor favoring the development of malignancy. The question naturally arises in view of her demonstrated ability to survive major operations as to whether or not we should advise removal of the gallbladder or let the gallstones prove their ability to produce carcinoma in the patient with a special previous disposition or susceptibility to carcinoma.

Discussion

DR. T. H. SWEETSER: I think that you may be interested in the case of a fairly young man, just turned forty, who has survived six major operations for three entirely different malignant tumors. In 1920 our fellow member, Dr. J. F. Corbett, performed the second and third operations for glioma of the brain and there has been no recurrence of that trouble in the intervening

eighteen years. In May of this year he referred the patient to me because of gross hematuria. Cystoscopy disclosed a papillary carcinoma of the bladder, and biopsy demonstrated it to be of Grade IV malignancy. I resected the bladder wall by open suprapubic cystotomy; he has had no signs or symptoms of recurrence thus far. Later he noticed blood in his stools, and proctoscopic examination by Dr. Corbett demonstrated an annular carcinoma at the lower end of the sigmoid colon. He has survived a two-stage removal of sigmoid and rectum, the growth microscopically having been of Grade IV malignancy. Of course, it is too early to say anything as to the final outcome. Such cases raise the question of the presence in certain people of some factor of susceptibility to malignancy in general. Incidentally, I understand that this man has also survived a serious automobile accident and an attack of acute pancreatitis.

DR. MARTIN NORDLAND: I would like to know how long this patient had any symptoms of appendicitis. I noticed in examining the specimen that the appendix was not sectioned and I wondered if she might not also have a carcinoma of this organ.

DR. R. C. WEBB: I wish to thank the members for the discussion, and I believe that if you were to check your records, more cases of multiple carcinoma could be reported from this society. We have seen four other cases of multiple carcinoma.

One patient, a woman of fifty-three years, was first seen in July, 1926 and a radical operation of the left breast was performed on July 3, 1926. She returned in January, 1928, one and one-half years later, with a small carcinoma in the lower outer quadrant of the right breast. This breast was likewise removed with a radical amputation. This patient is still living, ten and one-half years after the second operation. The fact that she is still living lends some weight to the argument that the second growth was a primary one rather than a metastatic growth.

An unmarried woman, aged forty-eight, was seen in March, 1933, with a large carcinoma of the right breast. A radical operation was done. No carcinoma was found in the axillary glands. This patient was examined at intervals of three months and in March, 1934, one year later, a small lump was felt in the upper outer quadrant of the left breast which was not adherent to the chest wall or to the skin. Radical breast amputation was done and in the left axilla several large hard glands which lay high up behind the vein and artery were removed. The patient died within six months. She was treated with x-ray following both the first and second operation.

Another patient, a woman sixty-six years of age, was seen in 1923. A skin tumor of the left forearm and skin tumor of the right side of the neck were excised with a margin of normal skin. Specimens were examined by Dr. E. T. Bell whose reports show that each was a basal cell carcinoma. This patient died ten years later of pneumonia. A postmortem examination showed no evidence of carcinoma of the internal organs.

Wynne reported a case* of primary carcinomata of the bladder and stomach before the Minneapolis Clinical Club in 1933. This case was discussed by Dr. J. C. Mc Cartney, Jr., who had made the pathological examination of the tissue removed at the operation and performed the autopsy five years later.

As to the appendicitis, this patient was admitted to the hospital March 29, 1938, but the appendix was not removed until March 31, 1938, about forty-eight hours after admission. She had had symptoms from her gall stones off and on, but on March 28 she had had pain in the lower right abdomen without nausea. The presence of the gallstones and the two previous operation

*Wynne, H. M. N.: A case of carcinoma of the bladder removed by operation with death from carcinoma of the stomach five years after operation. Journal-Lancet, 53:168, (March 15) 1933.

for carcinoma, together with out knowledge that her appendix was normal in appearance three years previously at the age of sixty-nine, rendered the diagnosis more difficult and confusing and accounted for the delay.

INCREASED BILE FLOW AND PRESSURE AS AN AID IN THE SURGICAL AND NON-SURGICAL MANAGEMENT OF BILIARY TRACT DISEASE

R. Russell Best, M.D. (by invitation)

Omaha, Nebraska

Summary of Presentation

Frequent opening of the common duct and cholangiography have proved that common-duct stones are more common than was formerly supposed, and that stones, mucous plugs, collections of inspissated bile and blood clots which remain post-operatively not infrequently produce symptoms simulating gallbladder disease. Cholangiograms have not only done much to prove this but have aided considerably in reaching a better understanding of the physiology and mechanism of the extrahepatic biliary tract. Spasticity of the sphincter of 'Oddi, or spastic biliary dyssynergia, may exist to the degree of completely blocking the lower end of the common duct, and increase in common duct pressure associated with this spasm may well be the cause of symptoms in the post-cholecystectomy syndrome. Various antispasmodic drugs have been used to relax the sphincter area, nitroglycerin and atropine being most commonly employed. Then by stimulating bile flow along the bile highways, namely the intrahepatic, hepatic and common ducts, a biliary flush has been obtained. This increased bile flow is accomplished by administering dehydrocholic acid (decholin and procholon). Studies have been made and curves plotted to show the increase of bile flow and bile pressure (Figs. 1 and 2). After three or four days administration of dehydrocholic acid, the pressure tends to return to normal, but after withdrawing it for a few days, the pressure may again be increased by its administration. Cases were presented in which delayed cholangiograms revealed single stones, multiple stones, or other debris in the common duct and which demonstrated the flushing out of these foreign bodies by increasing the bile flow and relaxing the sphincter area. In several instances where the stones were too large to pass through the relaxed sphincter area, the method was not successful.

Immediate cholangiograms are not taken as often since the introduction of this biliary flush, for the smaller foreign bodies which in the past probably remained in the common duct without being properly appreciated or suspected, may now be removed quite easily by this method without proving their existence. In every case with a common duct T-tube or catheter, a cholangiogram should be made before the tube or catheter is withdrawn. A 48 per cent hippuran solution has proved to be the most advantageous contrast medium, 15 to 40 c.c. usually being necessary. An immediate radiograph is taken, after which the con-

trast medium is permitted to escape from the tube for five minutes, and then the cholangiogram is repeated.

The following three-day regime is instituted some ten days after every cholecystectomy; it is also used in all patients who have previously had their gallbladders removed and that have residual symptoms, and in the routine medical management of gallbladder disease. It may be necessary to repeat the treatment a number of times or at intervals in some cases because latent infection of the ductal system may result in secondary formation of common duct stones and debris. This method may also prove to be the means of dislodging stones from the liver into the common duct.

1. Dehydrocmolic acid tablets, 3½ grain, are given t.i.d. after meals and at bedtime for three days.
2. One-half ounce of magnesium sulphate is given each morning.
3. One ounce of pure cream or olive oil is given before the noon and evening meals and at bedtime.
4. On the first day, 1/100 grain nitroglycerin is dissolved under the tongue t.i.d. before meals.
5. On the second day, 1/100 grain atropine is given in a little water before meals.
6. On the third day, the nitroglycerin is repeated.
7. If a T-tube or catheter is present in the common duct, or if a fistula exists, inject warm saline solution each day and follow with warm olive oil. Warm lipoiodine is beneficial at times.

Jaundice with complete obstruction of the common duct contraindicates this method of treatment.

Discussion

Dr. A. A. Zierold.—This evening I have heard a great deal that is interesting and stimulating. I cannot help but have a feeling of admiration for someone who can so boldly enter a field that is hedged about with so much controversy as is the biliary system.

Until about 1900 most surgeons felt that the treatment of fractures was reasonably good. They were quite satisfied with the results on the whole until the x-ray appeared. Immediately they became dissatisfied with their results. Widespread use of the cholangiogram may bring about a similar state of affairs. Either my experience has been too small or I have not been sufficiently accurate in my observations, but for the most part, I have been satisfied that people who had stones in their gallbladders and had them removed, had a reasonably good convalescence and subsequent course. After seeing Dr. Best's studies and hearing him talk, I am not at all so sure that this is the case. It may be that patients whom I assumed were symptom-free were going to someone else and detailing their symptoms to them.

Undoubtedly there must be a much greater number of cases with residual symptoms due to the original condition for which they were operated upon or treated than we appreciate. It seems also not unreasonable to suppose that of this number a great many must obtain relief spontaneously without any particular treatment. Undoubtedly a number of them must pass stones from time to time without any special treatment.

I am impressed with what Dr. Best said with regard to dysfunction of the sphincter of Oddi, which most satisfactorily explains for me the symptoms of the patient who presents for surgery with an apparently normal gallbladder without stones. It is much easier to reconcile their symptoms upon this assumption and I believe that in the absence of satisfactory x-ray findings and persistence of symptoms simulating colic a most exhaustive study should be conducted to determine whether or not this may not be a case of dysfunction of the sphincter.

With regard to the digestive symptoms of gallbladder disease, I cannot help but feel that these symptoms are of dysfunction of the common duct rather than symptoms of gallbladder disease itself. It is hard for me to believe or to consider the gallbladder disease

One thing I was interested in observing in Dr. Best's cholangiograms was the appearance of the pancreatic duct and I rather expected him to say something with regard to pancreatic reflux. It seems quite reasonable

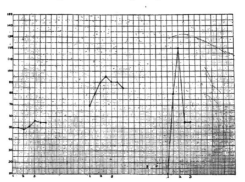

Fig. 1. Following administration of dehydrocholic acid, the general level of the intraductal pressure is increased as compared with the control level. The intravenous injection of sodium dehydrocholate results in a sudden but not prolonged rise.

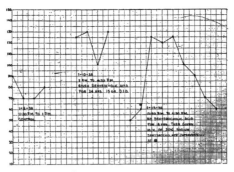

Fig. 2. Plotted curve of another patient, giving similar result. During the period of increased pressure and aided by a relaxed sphincter area a flushing out effect is provided.

which we characterize by stone formation, and fibrosis of the gallbladder wall, as an inflammatory or bacterial phenomenon. To my mind it is more the evidence of foreign body or chemical reaction. The treatment of it as an infectious process is rather difficult for me to accept. I am impressed more and more, particularly from what Dr. Best said, that many of the symptoms which we consider as chronic inflammatory disease of the gallbladder are disturbances of function or sphincter control of the emptying of the common duct.

to me that many changes in the duct as well as the gallbladder may be a result of a pancreatic reflux. The frequency with which pancreatic secretion may be obtained from the gallbladder bile is sufficient to make it a matter of importance and a matter worthy of further investigation.

I did not quite understand whether Dr. Best implied that the relaxation of the sphincter obtained by diet and nitroglycerin, atrophine, etc., was intended to overcome the spasticity of the sphincter only temporarily or permanently and whether it could be first

of us will solve our problems without the help of the other. As an illustration of this point I would like to mention not only Dr. Best's contributions but also Dr. Leven's recent studies in the University Hospital. When some of us were working out the development of the sphincter of Oddi in the human fetus we came to the conclusion that the principal muscle in the duodenal portion of the bile passage lies around the common bile duct just before it joins the ampulla of Vater, and that this is the sphincter which causes the filling of the gallbladder. We also observed in these fetuses some muscle around the ampulla. But it was clear that the important muscle, physiologically, is the sphincter choledochus. Meanwhile Dr. Leven was finding that in 20 per cent of his cholangiograms there was indication of a reflux of contrast media into the pancreatic duct. This implied the existence of a strong sphincter ampullæ. With these new observations in mind Mr. Kreilkamp and I began examining macerated adult sphincters of Oddi, and found that one of every six autospy specimens exhibited a prominent sphincter ampullæ in addition to a well developed sphincter choledochus. It is quite possible, therefore, that the patients that show refluxes of this sort are those in whom there is an atypical development of muscle around the ampulla of Vater. What is physiologically important, therefore, is not always the most important clinically.

In conclusion, I would like to join Dr. Zierold in thanking Dr. Best for a most interesting and instructive evening.

DR. N. LOGAN LEVEN (by invitation).—I was very much interested in this excellent paper. This matter of evacuating stones from the common bile duct brings to mind a case reported by Neuwirt in 1930. In a case of persistent biliary fistula he demonstrated three stones in the common bile duct by injecting iodized oil into the fistula. He planned to operate on this case the next day but on the following morning he found a pea-sized gallstone at the external opening of the fistula. A second somewhat larger stone was found in the stool the following day. The fistula promptly closed and the patient remained well. He ascribed the passage of stones to the cholangiography. The viscid oily solution remained on the surface of the stone and the mucous membrane lining of the bile duct. It is natural that a stone which has become slippery passes more easily through a slippery passage than a rough surface stone, especially if through the injection of a large amount of fluid the pressure in the bile passages becomes raised. In this case a small stone plugged the fistula, allowing an increased intraductal pressure to occur.

A similar procedure has long been used in the removal of ureteral stones where in cases of smaller stones spontaneous passage of the stone may occur following injection of oil into the ureter.

I would like to ask Dr. Best whether he has ever seen a case following cholangiography of the syndrome simulating the acute pancreatic edema described by Zoepfel.

Mallet-Guy, Beaupere and Armanet, Walzel, Sturm and others have reported such cases. I had one case in a series of 200 cholangiograms where following reflux into the pancreatic duct the patient on the following day developed abdominal pain, nausea, vomiting and a temperature of 103.8 degrees. By the second day the symptoms had subsided.

DR. GEORGE S. BERGH.—The administration of a choleretic together with a drug intended to produce relaxation of the sphincter of Oddi, as Dr. Best has suggested as a means of favoring the passage of stones from the common bile duct into the duodenum, appears to be based upon physiologically sound principles. The objection that I would have concerns his selection of atropine as a drug to produce sphincter relaxation.

Although it appears to be fairly well established that atropine will produce relaxation of the sphincter in some laboratory animals, our experience, based upon direct observations in patients with choledochostomy tubes, indicates that this drug has no significant effect upon the sphincter in man. Amyl nitrite and nitroglycerin, on the other hand, will produce relaxation.

We have found that Dr. Boyden's fatty meal of egg yolks and cream sometimes will cause relaxation of a spastic sphincter when drugs such as amyl nitrite and nitroglycerin have failed. This suggests the possibility that such a meal might prove useful as a means of producing sphincter relaxation in cases similar to those presented by Dr. Best, but we have had no clinical experience with it along that line.

DR. R. RUSSELL BEST (closing).—Dr. Zierold mentioned a very practical point which was also brought out by Dr. Boyden—that probably stones and debris are often passed from the common duct with very little pain. I believe this is true, and it has no doubt been the saving point about gallbladder surgery. The purpose of this form of treatment is to flush out the ductal system, whether a spastic or atonic sphinc-

ter exists. Nitroglycerin and atropine, with or with out a biliary flush, are indicated in spastic dyssyn ergia. Those with an atonic spincter probably shoul have a biliary flush periodically in order to guar against an ascending infection.

In regard to the instrumentation advocated by sev eral authors, I might say that we use the smalle Bake dilators but never the large dilators, for I thin they tear the muscle. The cutting instrument show by Dr. Doubilet of New York might also prove harm ful.

We do not believe nitroglycerin relaxes the sphinc ter in all cases, and our investigation has shown th same to be true of atropine. Therefore, in our three day regime we have combined the two.

We have had quite a number of cases where th pancreatic duct was visible, as shown in the cholangic gram, but we believe there is no danger attached t the reflux of the opaque material into the pancreati duct.

* * *

The meeting adjourned.

HARVEY NELSON, M.D., *Secretary.*

● CLASSIFIED ADVERTISING ●

INDEX TO VOLUME 21

In Memoriam

N

O

P